THORACIC ONCOLOGY

Second Edition

Jack A. Roth, M.D.

Chairman and Professor
Department of Thoracic and Cardiovascular Surgery
University of Texas
M.D. Anderson Cancer Center
Houston, Texas

John C. Ruckdeschel, M.D.

Professor of Medicine
Director, H. Lee Moffitt Cancer
  Center and Research Institute
University of South Florida
Tampa, Florida

Thomas H. Weisenburger, M.D.

Clinical Professor
Department of Radiation Oncology
University of California
Los Angeles, California
Director of Radiation Oncology
Cancer Foundation of Santa Barbara
Santa Barbara, California

W.B. SAUNDERS COMPANY
A Division of Harcourt Brace & Company
Philadelphia London Toronto Montreal Sydney Tokyo

W.B. SAUNDERS COMPANY
A Division of
Harcourt Brace & Company

The Curtis Center
Independence Square West
Philadelphia, Pennsylvania 19106

Library of Congress Cataloging-in-Publication Data

Thoracic oncology / [edited by] Jack A. Roth, John C.
Ruckdeschel, Thomas H. Weisenburger.—2nd ed.

p. cm.

Includes bibliographical references and index.

ISBN 0–7216–4769–3

1. Chest—Cancer.   I. Roth, Jack A.   II. Ruckdeschel, John C.
III. Weisenburger, Thomas H.   [DNLM: 1. Thoracic
Neoplasms.   WF 970 T4875 1995]
RC280.C5T48 1995   616.99′494—dc20

DNLM/DLC   94–26869

THORACIC ONCOLOGY   ISBN 0–7216–4769–3

Last digit is the print number: 9   8   7   6   5   4   3   2   1

Contributors

Joseph Aisner, M.D.

Professor of Medicine, Oncology, Pharmacology, and Epidemiology and Preventive Medicine, University of Maryland at Baltimore School of Medicine; Professor, University of Maryland Cancer Center, University of Maryland Hospital, Baltimore, Maryland

Clinical Presentation of Lung Cancer; Multimodality Therapy of Malignant Mesothelioma

Jaffer A. Ajani, M.D.

Professor of Medicine, Chairman (ad interim), Department of Gastrointestinal Oncology and Digestive Diseases, University of Texas M. D. Anderson Cancer Center, Houston, Texas

Chemotherapy and Combined Modality Therapy for Squamous Cell Carcinoma and Adenocarcinoma of the Esophagus and Gastroesophageal Junction

Karen Antman, M.D.

Professor of Medicine and Pharmacology, Columbia University; Attending Physician, Presbyterian Hospital, New York, New York

Multimodality Therapy of Malignant Mesothelioma

Louis R. Bégin, M.D., F.R.C.P.(C.)

Associate Professor of Pathology and Surgery, Associate Member, Department of Oncology, McGill University Faculty of Medicine; Head, Divisions of Surgical Pathology and Diagnostic Electron Microscopy, The Sir Mortimer B. Davis—Jewish General Hospital, Montreal, Quebec, Canada

The Pathobiology of Esophageal Cancer

William J Blot, Ph.D.

Chief Executive Officer, International Epidemiology Institute, Ltd., Rockville, Maryland

Epidemiology and Genesis of Esophageal Cancer

Philip Bonomi, M.D.

Associate Professor of Medicine; Director, Section of Medical Oncology, Rush University Medical Center, Chicago, Illinois

Preoperative and Postoperative Therapy of Non–Small Cell Lung Cancer

Marvin H. Chasen, M.D.

Professor, Department of Diagnostic Radiology, University of Texas M. D. Anderson Cancer Center, Houston, Texas

Diagnostic Imaging of Esophageal Cancer

Robert A. Clark, M.D.

Professor of Radiology, University of South Florida Health Sciences Center; Professor and Chief of Diagnostic Radiology, H. Lee Moffitt Cancer Center and Research Institute, Tampa, Florida

Fundamentals of Diagnostic Imaging

Tom DeMeester, M.D.

Professor and Chairman, Department of Surgery, University of Southern California School of Medicine, Los Angeles, California

Preoperative Assessment of Patients Undergoing Lung Resection for Cancer

Gerald D. Dodd, M.D.

Professor of Radiology, Department of Diagnostic Imaging, University of Texas M. D. Anderson Cancer Center, Houston, Texas

Diagnostic Imaging of Esophageal Cancer

Per Dombernowsky, M.D., Ph.D.

Associate Professor, Copenhagen University; Physician in Chief, Department of Oncology, Rigshospitalet, Copenhagen, Denmark

Clinical Presentation and Natural History of Small Cell Lung Cancer

L. Austin Doyle, M.D.

Associate Professor of Medicine and Oncology, University of Maryland School of Medicine, Baltimore, Maryland

Clinical Presentation of Lung Cancer

Meade C. Edmunds, M.D.

Fellow, Gastroenterology, University of Virginia Medical School, Charlottesville, Virginia

Premalignant Lesions of the Esophagus

Donald R. Eisert, M.D.

Professor, Radiation Oncology; Chairman, Center for Radiation Oncology, Vanderbilt University Medical Center, Nashville, Tennessee
Treatment of Small Cell Lung Cancer

Robert J. Ginsberg, M.D.

Professor of Surgery, Cornell University Medical College; Chief, Thoracic Service, Department of Surgery, Memorial Sloan-Kettering Cancer Center, New York, New York
Surgery for Non–Small Cell Lung Cancer

Eli Glatstein, M.D.

Chairman and Professor, Department of Radiation Oncology, Harold C. Simmons Cancer Center, University of Texas Southwestern Medical Center at Dallas, Dallas, Texas
Malignancies of the Thymus

Melvyn Goldberg, M.D.

Professor of Surgery, Temple University School of Medicine; Chief, Thoracic Surgical Oncology, Fox Chase Cancer Center, Philadelphia, Pennsylvania
Surgery for Non–Small Cell Lung Cancer

Victor E. Gould, M.D.

Professor of Pathology, Rush Medical College; Senior Attending Pathologist, Rush–Presbyterian–St. Luke's Medical Center, Chicago, Illinois
Epithelial Neoplasms of the Lung

Geoffrey M. Graeber, M.D.

Professor of Surgery, Director of Surgical Research, Division of Surgery, West Virginia University School of Medicine, Morgantown, West Virginia
Malignant Tumors Involving the Heart and Pericardium

F. Anthony Greco, M.D.

Director, Sarah Cannon Cancer Center, Nashville, Tennessee
Mediastinal Germ Cell Neoplasms

Marc S. Greenblatt, M.D.

Biotechnology Fellow, Laboratory of Human Carcinogenesis, National Cancer Institute, Bethesda, Maryland
Carcinogenesis, and Cellular and Molecular Biology of Lung Cancer

Frederick L. Grover, M.D.

Chief of Surgery, VA Medical Center, Denver, Colorado
Superior Sulcus Tumors

John D. Hainsworth, M.D.

Associate Director, Sarah Cannon Cancer Center, Nashville, Tennessee
Mediastinal Germ Cell Neoplasms

Heine H. Hansen

Professor, Copenhagen University; Physician in Chief, Department of Oncology, Rigshospitalet, Copenhagen, Denmark
Clinical Presentation and Natural History of Small Cell Lung Cancer

Curtis C. Harris, M.D.

Chief, Laboratory of Human Carcinogenesis, National Cancer Institute, Bethesda, Maryland
Carcinogenesis, and Cellular and Molecular Biology of Lung Cancer

Waun K. Hong, M.D.

Professor of Medicine, Chairman, Department of Thoracic/Head & Neck, Medical Oncology, University of Texas M. D. Anderson Cancer Center, Houston, Texas
Chemoprevention of Lung Cancer

Michael T. Jaklitsch, M.D.

Fellow in Thoracic Oncology, Harvard Medical School; Fellow in Thoracic Oncology, Brigham and Women's Hospital, Boston, Massachusetts
Multimodality Therapy of Malignant Mesothelioma

David H. Johnson, M.D.

Professor of Medicine, Director, Medical Oncology, Vanderbilt University Medical School, Division of Medical Oncology, Nashville, Tennessee
Treatment of Small Cell Lung Cancer

David P. Kelsen, M.D.

Professor of Medicine, Chief, Gastrointestinal Oncology Service, Memorial Sloan-Kettering Cancer Center, New York, New York
Chemotherapy and Combined Modality Therapy for Squamous Cell Carcinoma and Adenocarcinoma of the Esophagus and Gastroesophageal Junction

Timothy J. Kinsella, M.D.

Professor, University of Wisconsin; Attending Physician, University Hospital, Madison, Wisconsin
Superior Vena Cava Syndrome

Ritsuko Komaki, M.D.

Professor, Division of Radiotherapy, University of Texas M. D. Anderson Cancer Center, Houston, Texas
Superior Sulcus Tumors

Louis A. Lanza, M.D.

Assistant Professor of Cardiothoracic Surgery, University of Iowa, Iowa City, Iowa
Resection of Pulmonary Metastases

Jin S. Lee, M.D.

Associate Professor of Medicine, Chief, Section of Thoracic Medical Oncology, University of Texas, M. D. Anderson Cancer Center, Houston, Texas
Chemoprevention of Lung Cancer

Barry S. Levinson, M.D.

Assistant Professor of Internal Medicine, Harold C. Simmons Cancer Center, University of Texas Southwestern Medical School at Dallas, Dallas, Texas
Malignancies of the Thymus

Scott M. Lippman, M.D.

Associate Professor of Medicine, Chief, Section of Head and Neck Medical Oncology, University of Texas M. D. Anderson Cancer Center, Houston, Texas
Chemoprevention of Lung Cancer

Richard W. McCallum, M.D.

Faculty, Program Director, University of Virginia, University of Virginia Medical Center, Charlottesville, Virginia
Premalignant Lesions of the Esophagus

Minesh P. Mehta, M.D.

Associate Professor, University of Wisconsin; Attending Physician, University Hospital, Madison, Wisconsin
Superior Vena Cava Syndrome

Stephen A. Mills, M.D.

Cardiothoracic Surgeon, Private Practice, High Point, North Carolina
Malignant Tumors Involving the Heart and Pericardium

Bruce Minsky, M.D.

Associate Professor of Radiation Oncology, Cornell University Medical College; Associate Attending Physician, Memorial Sloan-Kettering Cancer Center, New York, New York
Definitive Radiation Therapy and Combined Modality Therapy for Cancer of the Esophagus

Darroch W. O. Moores, M.D.

Clinical Associate Professor of Surgery, Albany Medical College, Albany, New York
Staging of Lung Cancer; Pleural Effusions in Patients with Malignancy

Mark G. Nelson, M.D.

Chief Cardiothoracic Resident, Division of Surgery, West Virginia University School of Medicine, Morgantown, West Virginia
Malignant Tumors Involving the Heart and Pericardium

Jonathan C. Nesbitt, M.D.

Assistant Professor, Department of Thoracic and Cardiovascular Surgery, University of Texas M. D. Anderson Cancer Center, Houston, Texas
Staging of Lung Cancer

Harvey I. Pass, M.D.

Head, Thoracic Oncology Section, Senior Investigator, Surgery Branch, National Cancer Institute, Bethesda, Maryland
Primary and Metastatic Chest Wall Tumors

Theodore L. Phillips, M.D.

Professor and Chairman, Department of Radiation Oncology, University of California at San Francisco, San Francisco, California
Definitive Radiation Therapy and Combined Modality Therapy for Cancer of the Esophagus

Joe B. Putnam, Jr., M.D.

Associate Professor, Department of Thoracic and Cardiovascular Surgery, University of Texas M. D. Anderson Cancer Center, Houston, Texas
Surgery for Carcinoma of the Esophagus; Resection of Pulmonary Metastases

Roger R. Reddel, M.D.

Laboratory of Human Carcinogenesis, Division of Cancer Etiology, National Cancer Institute, Bethesda, Maryland
Carcinogenesis, and Cellular and Molecular Biology of Lung Cancer

Carolyn E. Reed, M.D.

Associate Professor of Surgery, Medical University of South Carolina, Charleston, South Carolina
Cancer of the Esophagus: Clinical Presentation and Stricture Management

Thomas W. Rice, M.D.

Head of the Section of General Thoracic Surgery, The Cleveland Clinic Foundation, Cleveland, Ohio
Diagnosis and Staging of Esophageal Carcinoma

Tyvin A. Rich, M.D.

Professor of Radiotherapy, M. D. Anderson Cancer Center, Houston, Texas
Chemotherapy and Combined Modality Therapy for Squamous Cell Carcinoma and Adenocarcinoma of the Esophagus and Gastroesophageal Junction

Jack A. Roth, M.D.

Chairman and Professor, Department of Thoracic and Cardiovascular Surgery, University of Texas M. D. Anderson Cancer Center, Houston, Texas
Esophageal Cancer—Overview; Surgery for Carcinoma of the Esophagus; Chemotherapy and Combined Modality Therapy for Squamous Cell Carcinoma and Adenocarcinoma of the Esophagus and Gastroesophageal Junction

John C. Ruckdeschel, M.D.

Professor of Medicine, University of South Florida, College of Medicine; Chief Executive Officer, H. Lee Moffitt Cancer Center and Research Institute, Tampa, Florida
Lung Cancer: An Overview; Management of Disseminated Non–Small Cell Lung Cancer; Pleural Effusions in Patients with Malignancy

Alexander D. Soutter, M.D.

Attending Physician, Department of Surgery, Brigham and Women's Hospital, Boston, Massachusetts
Multimodality Therapy of Malignant Mesothelioma

David J. Sugarbaker, M.D.
Associate Professor of Surgery, Harvard Medical School; Chief, Thoracic Surgery, Brigham and Women's Hospital, Boston, Massachusetts
Multimodality Therapy of Malignant Mesothelioma

Henry Wagner, Jr., M.D.
Associate Professor, Radiology, University of South Florida; Program Leader, Thoracic Oncology Program, H. Lee Moffitt Cancer Center and Research Institute, Tampa, Florida
Preoperative and Postoperative Therapy for Non–Small Cell Lung Cancer

Garrett L. Walsh, M.D.
Assistant Professor, Department of Thoracic and Cardiovascular Surgery, University of Texas M. D. Anderson Cancer Center, Houston Texas
General Principles and Surgical Considerations in the Management of Mediastinal Masses

William H. Warren, M.D.
Rush Medical College; Associate Attending Surgeon, Rush–Presbyterian–St. Luke's Medical Center, Chicago, Illinois
Epithelial Neoplasms of the Lung

Paul F. Waters, M.D., F.R.C.S.(C.), F.A.C.S.
Professor of Surgery, University of California at Los Angeles School of Medicine; Director of Thoracic Surgery and Lung Transplantation, University of California at Los Angeles, Los Angeles, California
Surgery for Non–Small Cell Lung Cancer

Thomas H. Weisenburger, M.D.
Clinical Professor, Department of Radiation Oncology, University of California at Los Angeles School of Medicine, Los Angeles; Director of Radiation Oncology, Cancer Foundation of Santa Barbara, Santa Barbara, California
Definitive Radiotherapy and Combined Modality Therapy for Inoperable Non–Small Cell Lung Cancer; Overview of Malignancies of the Chest Wall and Pleura

Jorge A. Wernly, M.D.
Professor of Surgery and Pediatrics, University of New Mexico School of Medicine; Chief, Thoracic and Cardiovascular Division, Attending Surgeon, University Hospital, Lovelace Medical Center, Veterans Administration Medical Center, Albuquerque, New Mexico
Preoperative Assessment of Patients Undergoing Lung Resection for Cancer

Charles C. Williams, Jr., M.D.
Associate Professor of Medicine, Department of Internal Medicine, University of South Florida College of Medicine; Director, Hospice Care, H. Lee Moffitt Cancer Center, Tampa, Florida
Management of Disseminated Non–Small Cell Lung Cancer

Preface

The 6 years that have elapsed since the first edition of *Thoracic Oncology* have witnessed important developments in carcinogenesis prevention, and therapy of thoracic cancers. These developments persuaded the editors that a second edition was warranted. The underlying concept of the first edition was to develop a text emphasizing multimodality therapy and a multidisciplinary approach to patient care. This concept is now beginning to translate into improvements in patient survival. This is most apparent in lung cancer, in which preoperative chemotherapy regimens have resulted in significantly prolonged survival in nonrandomized and randomized clinical trials, and in esophageal cancer, in which induction chemotherapy has improved survival in patients receiving curative radiation therapy. Studies of the molecular basis of lung and esophageal carcinogenesis continue to advance. It is likely that these studies will contribute to improvements in the areas of diagnosis, prevention, and treatment. The identification and characterization of premalignant lesions and advances in chemoprevention research also have made important contributions.

We have retained the basic organization of the first edition. However, increased emphasis has been given to the practical aspects of patient care. Chapters on prevention and premalignant lesions of the esophagus have been added, while other chapters have been extensively rewritten. This edition is intended to provide a summary of the state-of-the-art care of thoracic oncology patients, and it is hoped that it will provide a stimulus for continued basic and clinical research that will result in the next generation of improved treatment modalities.

Contents

Part I

CANCER OF THE LUNG

1 LUNG CANCER: AN OVERVIEW

John C. Ruckdeschel, M.D.

In the first edition of *Thoracic Oncology* we attempted to bring together the discordant elements of lung cancer into a unified, multidisciplinary approach. We focused on the roles of the various clinical and basic scientists involved in lung cancer and, in so doing, discovered several leitmotifs that have continued to develop into recognizable themes. The same genetic changes that permit a mutational response to environmental carcinogens are now used as diagnostic tools, leading us toward enhanced early detection and prevention. We are not yet ready to stage the final performance for lung cancer but, with the advent of the first gene transfection trials, we are beginning rehearsals.

SECTION 1—BIOLOGY OF LUNG CANCER

In the late 1980s, our understanding of the biology of lung cancer had been enormously enhanced by the development of well-characterized lung cancer cell lines in the laboratories headed by John Minna and his colleagues. The emerging concepts of neuroendocrine differentiation and oncogene expression appeared to point the way to therapeutically useful interventions. Not all the approaches taken have been successful, however. Immunohistochemical determination of neuroendocrine differentiation has not proved useful yet as a prognostic marker nor as a reliable predictor of response to therapy. The first trials attempting to modulate malignant growth by interfering with specific growth factors have shown some tantalizing responses, but these methods are not yet capable of inducing sustained remissions. The growth in our understanding of lung cancer biology has increased exponentially from these initial discoveries, however, as demonstrated by Greenblatt, Reddell, and Harris in Chapter 2.

It now seems clear that the process of carcinogenesis is multifactorial and occurs in a series of sequential steps. The traditional concepts of initiation, promotion, and malignant conversion have been enhanced by an understanding that the changes that predispose a person to develop cancer may occur before initiation and that the malignant cell continues to mutate toward an ever more malignant phenotype. The sequence of these changes is now well described for colon cancer and is increasingly being elucidated for lung cancer. The development of reliable culture methods for normal human bronchial epithelial cells should further clarify this "domino effect" of genetic and phenotype changes.

Our understanding of the process of normal differentiation and how it is both perturbed and sustained during malignant transformation has also allowed the demonstration of several so-called intermediate markers of malignant conversion that can be used to assess the impact of a new generation of more specific chemopreventive agents. Although an increased risk of familial lung cancer can be demonstrated, the actual marker gene has not been found, nor is a good linkage gene yet available.

Smoking remains the major source of lung cancer, and it would now appear beyond doubt that passive or environmental tobacco smoke plays a significant role in the development of lung cancer as well. Although restrictions exist on smoking in public places, the practice is still widespread. The character Joe Camel is only one of many disreputable techniques employed to induce smoking in a new generation. There still exists no political will to stop the production of tobacco and, in deed, we continue to force other nations to accept our so-called "legal agricultural products" (i.e., cigarettes) as a requirement of trade agreements.

SECTION 2—DIAGNOSIS AND STAGING

In Chapter 3, Doyle and Aisner have updated their extraordinarily complete review of the signs and symptoms of lung cancer, and in Chapter 4, Gould and Warren have demonstrated how the multidirectional and unstable differentiation pathways for epithelial cancers of the lung might lead to differing clinical as well as histologic expressions. Their finding that epithelial cancers can apparently arise de novo from extrafollicular reticulum cells in mediastinal lymph nodes may explain some of the unusual presentations of lung cancer.

In Chapter 5, Clark reviews the technologic advances in computed tomography (CT) imaging (helical or spiral volumetric CT) that will lead to a reduction in respiratory artifacts and volume averaging. It is now clear that MRI is not superior to CT for routine assessment and may only play a role in resolving issues of chest wall, apical, and mediastinal invasion. The increasing usage of preoperative therapy may force a re-evaluation of these studies, however, because magnetic resonance imaging (MRI) can better distinguish tumor and fibrosis. Nesbitt and Moores update the now well-studied International Staging System and in Chapter 6, point out the remaining glitches.

SECTION 3—THERAPY

The first indications that combined modality therapies might enhance the outcome for patients with lung cancer were apparent when the first edition of *Thoracic Oncology* was being published. Those indications have now coalesced into a series of definitive reports. In Chapter 8, Ginsberg has updated his work on the surgical approach to lung cancer and the chapter is accompanied by a section by Wernly and DeMeester on preoperative evaluation. They point out that although the approach to the routine case of resectable lung cancer is now well standardized, the increasing use of preoperative therapy has required increasingly sophisticated preoperative and intraoperative assessment and techniques. At the earliest stages of lung cancer (T1N0), it appears that less extensive resections (e.g., segmentectomy and wedge resections) are indeed less, with increased rates of local recurrence and diminished survival. These results may temper the now headlong rush to employ video-assisted thoracoscopic (VAT) approaches to resection.

In Chapter 9, Wagner and Bonomi have carefully reviewed the literature on preoperative and postoperative adjunctive therapy. There is increasing evidence that preoperative therapy is superior to surgery alone in locally advanced cases. The data for postoperative therapy remain less clear. Weisenburger has reviewed the data for therapy of unresectable lung cancer and demonstrates the superiority of combined modality therapy to radiation alone in Chapter 10. Even in the area of chemotherapy for disseminated disease there has been progress, as outlined by Williams and Ruckdeschel in Chapter 11. When compared with palliative care only, survival is longer, symptoms are reduced, and in one analysis, the costs are less. The arrival of several new agents, including the taxanes, camptothecins, navelbine, and gemcitabine, are leading to potentially significant enhancements in outcome.

SECTION 4—SMALL CELL LUNG CANCER

In Chapter 12, Hansen and Dombernowsky clarify the innumerable clinical presentations of small cell lung cancer and how they influence patient evaluation. In Chapter 13, Johnson and Eisert review therapy of small cell lung cancer. Here, too, combined modality therapy (chemoradiation) appears superior to single modality therapy (chemotherapy alone) for limited disease. Surgery would now appear to play no role as an adjunct to combined-modality therapy, even though its use for very early lesions appears to be reasonable.

SECTION 5—SPECIAL CONSIDERATIONS

Grover and Komaki discuss both the traditional and newer surgical approaches to superior sulcus tumors as well as the use of combined-modality therapy in Chapter 14. In Chapter 15, Kinsella and Melita describe the therapy of superior vena cava syndrome, but their most important point is diagnostic; there is almost always time to make the histologic diagnosis before initiating treatment.

The final chapter in this section, which is written by Lee, Lippman, and Hong, is the introduction to the next edition. They demonstrate that it is in the arena of early detection and prevention that the biology and therapy of this disease will come together. They describe our current understanding of the efficacy of screening and how this understanding may be enhanced. They also describe the initial studies of chemopreventive agents and how their specificity will be enhanced as we better understand the biology of lung cancer.

All of this could, however, come crashing down if overzealous attempts to reduce the cost of health care are implemented. Bringing the fruits of bench research to the bedside requires research and access to patients with all stages of cancer, including those with premalignant lesions and those at high risk of developing cancer. We are too close to a solution to allow ourselves to ratchet down our research efforts for short-term, and ultimately false, savings. Quality and low cost may be able to coexist for routine care, but they cannot do so if advances in care are to be made through research.

BIOLOGY OF LUNG CANCER

2 CARCINOGENESIS, AND CELLULAR AND MOLECULAR BIOLOGY OF LUNG CANCER

Marc S. Greenblatt, Roger R. Reddel, and Curtis C. Harris

The study of bronchial carcinogenesis has expanded from the initial epidemiologic and toxicologic reports identifying tobacco smoke as the major cause of human lung cancer to include contributions from many branches of biomedical research, including epidemiologic and toxicologic evaluation of other chemical and physical carcinogens, clinical and pathologic observations, and in vitro and in vivo studies in cellular and molecular biology. Current models of cell function and carcinogenesis have integrated these data and provide coherent explanations for many of the early controversies of cancer research. A comprehensive approach to bronchial carcinogenesis incorporates the features of normal cellular behavior, general theories of carcinogenesis, and the properties of bronchial cells and lung carcinogens.

CARCINOGENESIS—GENERAL CONCEPTS

Cell and Molecular Biology—Relevant Principles

Normal cells are well regulated, responding to internal and external signals by activating or repressing genes that code for proteins that control cellular proliferation, differentiation, function, and death. Carcinogenesis is a multistep process by which a somatic cell becomes altered by changes in genes vital for growth control (known as oncogenes and tumor-suppressor genes) and no longer responds normally to regulation. An affected cell acquires a growth advantage over other cells; the clone of progeny derived from this abnormal cell expands and, through further damage, develops malignant characteristics—immortality, invasion, and metastasis (Fig. 2–1).[1]

Proto-oncogenes are the normal cellular genes that stimulate proliferation. When abnormally activated (e.g., by gene amplification or by mutations that enhance their functions), they are called oncogenes and lead to unregulated growth and malignancy. Tumor-suppressor genes are the normal cellular genes that inhibit proliferation; unregulated growth results from their inactivation. Abnormalities in these genes are the critical molecular events in carcinogenesis.[2] These genes control such cellular functions as recognition of external stimuli (e.g., erb-B/neu), transduction of these stimuli from the cell membrane to the cytoplasm and nucleus (e.g., ras), and control of gene transcription (e.g., p53) (Table 2–1, Fig. 2–2).[3] Confirmation of the hypothesis that alterations in oncogenes and tumor-suppressor genes are responsible for malignant transformation has come from studies of cultured cells, animal models, and human tumors. For example, multiple studies of in vitro and in vivo exposure to chemical carcinogens in a variety of rodent tissues have correlated malignant transformation with induction of activating ras point mutations.[4]

Cell Proliferation, Differentiation, and Death

Many epithelial tissues and other organs such as bone marrow contain stem cells (progenitor cells), which retain the potential for self-renewal, indefinite division, and differentiation into the cell types present in that organ. As normal cells differentiate, they acquire specialized functions and markers characteristic of

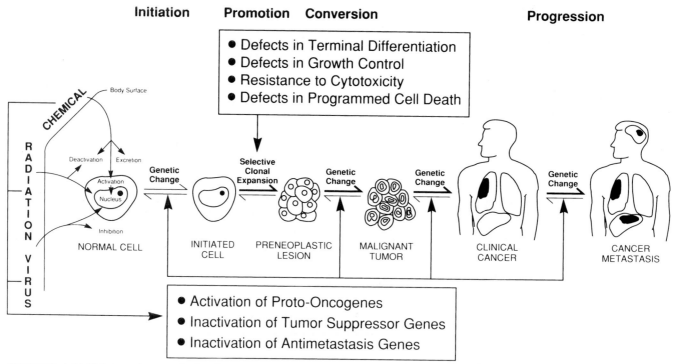

FIGURE 2–1. Multistep carcinogenesis. Carcinogenesis is a multistage process characterized by the accumulation of alterations to cellular proto-oncogenes and tumor-suppressor genes. The current model describes four conceptual steps: (1) tumor initiation, (2) tumor progression, (3) malignant conversion, and (4) tumor progression.

their tissue and lose the capacity of the stem cell for self-renewal and cell division; cells that can no longer divide are called terminally differentiated. Epithelial tissues can have a high fraction of dividing cells, because they must continuously replace discarded cells. Although stem cells are usually dormant and are not always easily discernible by morphologic criteria, they have a high proliferative potential and are thought to be susceptible to neoplastic transformation. In bronchial epithelium, it is not clear which cells are the targets for transformation to malignancy (see Bronchial Cell Biology later in the chapter).[5, 6]

Equilibrium within a tissue requires that some cells

die when they are no longer needed, and programmed cell death (apoptosis) is an integral part of the maintenance of homeostasis in all multicellular organisms. Apoptosis is an orderly cellular process that differs from toxic cell death, is controlled by spe-

TABLE 2–1. Classes of Oncogenes and Tumor Suppressor Genes, with Examples*

GROWTH FACTORS
sis
SIGNAL TRANSDUCTION PROTEINS
Growth factor receptor tyrosine kinases: *erb-B2 (neu), fms*
Non–receptor membrane–associated kinases: *src, fes*
Cytoplasmic kinases: *raf*
G proteins: *ras*
NUCLEAR PROTEINS
Transcription factors, DNA-binding proteins: p53, *myc*
Cell cycle regulators: p53, Rb
APOPTOSIS REGULATORS
p53, *bcl-2*
GENOMIC STABILITY REGULATORS
p53

*Over 100 oncogenes and approximately ten tumor suppressor genes are currently known; each category includes other genes. Only genes mentioned in the text are noted here.

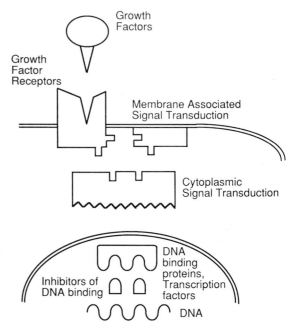

FIGURE 2–2. Functions of proto-oncogenes and tumor-suppressor genes. Examples of each class of genes can be found in Table 2–1.

cific genes, and is characterized by RNA and protein synthesis, specific morphologic features, and DNA fragmentation. It is a crucial process for proper organogenesis and function, and improperly regulated apoptosis appears to be an important feature of carcinogenesis in some systems.[7]

Cell Cycle

Cell division proceeds through discrete stages known as the cell cycle. These stages have been defined for decades, but the mechanisms involved in cell cycle control are still poorly understood. Recent research has identified numerous genes and proteins responsible for cell cycle regulation, including the retinoblastoma and p53 tumor-suppressor genes and the family of cyclins, proteins that accumulate during the cell cycle and are physically destroyed during mitosis.[8, 9] The study of the links between these genes, proteins, and processes and carcinogenesis is an area of intense interest at present.[10, 11] The phases of the cell cycle are shown in Figure 2–3 and include

1. G_0 phase—cells are dormant and perform specialized functions; they are not actively cycling but may be recruited to do so if necessary.
2. G_1 phase—the gap between mitosis and DNA synthesis, when proteins and RNA, most notably the enzymes required for DNA synthesis, are manufactured. The G_1 phase is of variable duration, and procession through the remainder of the cell cycle is controlled by a G_1 checkpoint, when the cell awaits the unknown signal that triggers entry into S phase.
3. S phase—DNA synthesis, lasting 10 to 12 hours, when the DNA content doubles from 2N (diploidy) to 4N (tetraploidy) in preparation for cell division.
4. G_2 phase—the period of 2 to 4 hours or longer following DNA synthesis, when the mitotic spindle is organized, protein and RNA synthesis continue, and cell volume increases. A second checkpoint occurs at the boundary between G_2 and M phases.
5. M phase—mitosis, the separation of DNA and cellular organelles into two daughter cells, lasting about 1 hour.

The growth rate of a tissue or tumor depends on the fraction of the cell population that is actively cycling, the duration of the cell cycle, and the cell death rate, all factors that vary among cell types and are frequently abnormal in malignant cells. Histopathologic evaluation of tumors often demonstrates increased numbers of cells in mitosis, and labeling of the DNA of intact cells with fluorescent dye can quantify their DNA content and demonstrate an elevated fraction of cells in S, G_2, and M phases.[5]

Cell Communication

Intercellular communication often involves two classes of cellular proteins: (1) cytokines, including positive and negative growth factors, which are secreted into the blood or pericellular regions; and (2) receptors (to cytokines and other effector molecules), which reside either on the cell surface or intracellularly and specifically bind with their ligands to receive these messages. Growth factors secreted into the pericellular region that stimulate nearby cells are called paracrine agents, whereas those that interact with receptors to stimulate the same cells that produce them are called autocrine agents.[12] A sophisticated network of proteins converts these molecular stimuli into specific cellular responses (e.g., DNA synthesis, replication, and production of growth factors and other proteins) by a series of processes known as signal transduction, which often involves changes in protein conformation, phosphorylation, and enzymatic or binding activity.[13] Mutations and altered expression of signal transduction genes such as the *ras* genes are often important steps in carcinogenesis.

Cell Immortalization and Neoplastic Transformation

Many lines of evidence indicate that carcinogenesis proceeds through a number of stages (see the discussion of multistep carcinogenesis later in the chapter). Clinicopathologic evaluation of phenotypic changes in many tissues may demonstrate premalignant changes (metaplasia, hyperplasia, and dysplasia), early noninvasive malignant features (carcinoma in situ), localized invasive carcinoma, and metastatic carcinoma.

When cultured in vitro, normal mammalian cells retain normal phenotypic properties, remain diploid, and have a limited life span, dividing a finite number

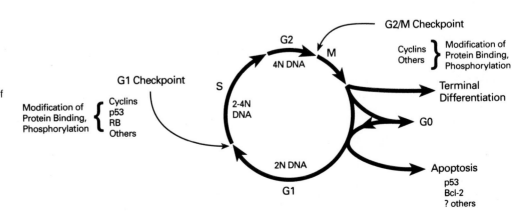

FIGURE 2–3. The cell cycle. Stages in the cell cycle are G_0, G_1, S, G_2, and M. 2N refers to diploid DNA, 2–4N to amounts of DNA between diploid and tetraploid, and 4N to tetraploid DNA. Cell cycle control genes whose products have been demonstrated to play a role in carcinogenesis are indicated (cyclins, p53, *RB*, *bcl-2*).

of times before undergoing senescence.[14] Experimental evidence of conversion to a malignant phenotype involves (1) loss of some normal cellular properties, analogous to metaplasia or dysplasia (e.g., altered responses to growth stimuli and changes in protein or antigen expression); (2) indefinitely increased in vitro life span with loss of senescence, or immortalization; (3) ability to form tumors in animals, or tumorigenicity; and (4) ability to metastasize.[15]

Spontaneous immortalization rarely occurs in human cells.[16] Immortalization was first accomplished experimentally by infection with a papovavirus, simian virus 40 (SV40), in human fibroblasts; the SV40 protein responsible for transformation was identified and named large T antigen (TAg).[17] Immortalized cells do not necessarily form tumors, however; tumorigenicity involves further genetic changes. In experimental models, tumorigenicity often correlates with the development of other abnormal growth characteristics, such as the capacity for in vitro anchorage-independent growth in soft agar.[15]

Tumorigenic cells continue to accumulate genetic abnormalities, probably owing to intrinsic genomic instability, that is often present in malignant cells and accounts for their frequent aneuploidy and clonal evolution.[18] Phenotypically this results in increasingly malignant behavior, such as invasion, metastasis, and drug resistance. These observations complement the animal studies of chemical carcinogens that led to the concept of multistep carcinogenesis.

Somatic Mutation Theory, Clonality, and Tumor Heterogeneity

A central concept of neoplasia is that tumors are monoclonal expansions[18]; that is, they arise from abnormal proliferation and transformation following mutations in a single somatic cell. Data from laboratory animals and humans strongly support this theory. Studies of mice that are heterozygous for two alleles of an isoenzyme demonstrate that tumors that develop in response to carcinogens express only one of those alleles.[4] Human hematopoietic malignancies have been extensively studied for clonality by examining isoenzymes of the glucose-6-phosphate dehydrogenase (G6PD) gene; in almost all cases, only one isoenzyme is found in the neoplastic cells of heterozygous individuals.[19] However, as tumor growth progresses, subclones develop as mutations occur in individual cells within the original population, resulting in heterogeneity of phenotypes and genotypes in the progeny of the original clone.[17] Studies of the heterogeneity of mutations or deletions within and between tumor populations can provide evidence for the clonality of the tumor, timing of critical genetic events, and the importance of specific genes and chromosomes in the various stages of each tumor's development. Finding the same mutation in all nodules of multifocal carcinomas suggests that they are part of the same malignant clone, whereas different mutations imply multiple clones and separate mutational events during some stage of carcinogenesis.[20]

Multistep Carcinogenesis

Carcinogenesis is a multistep process characterized by the accumulation of genetic and epigenetic damage in susceptible cells, which develop a selective growth advantage leading to clonal expansion and malignant transformation. The critical changes are alterations in the genes that control cellular proliferation and differentiation—the proto-oncogenes and tumor-suppressor genes (see Fig. 2–1).[1] This concept emerged from studies of chemical and viral carcinogenesis on animal models,[16] and it has been strengthened by more recent research on cultured cells and the molecular biology of oncogenes and tumor-suppressor genes.[21]

By the early years of this century, clinicians and laboratory investigators had observed long latency periods between exposure to chemical carcinogens and tumor development.[22, 23] The basis of the concept that carcinogenesis is a multistep process is found in Rous's study of chemical and viral carcinogenesis in rabbits in the 1930s. Rous noted that some chemical carcinogens caused either initiation, the first latent changes in cells, or promotion, the stimulation that induced growth of initiated cells, and that sequence and duration of carcinogen administration were important variables.[23–25] Subsequent studies of the initiators (such as polycyclic aromatic hydrocarbons [PAHs]) and promoters (such as croton oil) that were used in these early experiments have provided critical information on molecular mechanisms of carcinogenesis.[4] The current model describes four steps in carcinogenesis: (1) tumor initiation; (2) tumor promotion; (3) malignant conversion; and (4) tumor progression.[26] Models of age-dependent cancer incidence and molecular genetic studies suggest that six or more independent events may be necessary.[21, 27]

In most model systems, administration of initiators and promoters results in benign tumors, only a small fraction of which progress to malignancy.[4, 22] These models permit study of the characteristics and mechanisms of the stages of carcinogenesis. The most extensively investigated systems have been the induction of mouse skin papillomas and rat liver adenomas by chemical carcinogens. Bronchial carcinogenesis has been studied in mice, rats, hamsters, and dogs using cigarette smoke and purified chemical carcinogens.[4, 28–30]

Tumor Initiation

Tumor initiation is the first step in carcinogenesis, arising from irreversible genetic damage caused by chemical, physical, or microbial carcinogens. It is not yet possible to detect the individual cells that have been initiated. Early clonal expansions of altered cells can be identified by the change in phenotype caused by the mutation (e.g., altered differentiation, response to growth factors, or enzyme expression).[4, 22, 31, 32] Evidence for spontaneous initiation exists; promoters can induce a neoplastic clone in cells in vitro that have not been exposed to initiating agents.[33, 34]

Genotoxic agents produce initiated cells in a dose-dependent manner. They are most effective when administered immediately before or during S phase,[35] and cell division in the presence of the carcinogen is necessary to fix the genetic damage in the genome.[36] Most chemical carcinogens require metabolic activation by cells into their ultimate carcinogen form, and tissue specificity of these carcinogens is affected by intercellular differences in metabolism. Agents known as cocarcinogens are not carcinogens in themselves, but they enhance the formation of initiated cells when administered with an initiator, frequently by increasing the metabolic activation.[4, 22] Mechanisms by which carcinogens cause DNA alterations are discussed in DNA Damage and Repair.

Tumor Promotion

Tumor promotion is the selective, reversible clonal expansion of initiated cells due to a proliferative or survival advantage resulting from the initiating change. Promoting agents disproportionately increase the proliferative rate of initiated cells, resulting in a relatively larger subpopulation of cells with a genetic defect. Tissue specificity of promoting agents is often related to intercellular differences in mitogenic response, and promoters include a wide variety of chemical agents, hormones, and physical processes that increase target cell proliferation.[4] In the lungs and other organs, promoters may induce differentiation or cytostasis in normal cells whereas initiated cells are resistant.[32, 37, 38] In rat liver, promoters induce programmed cell death in normal but not in initiated cells.[39] These processes are reversible on withdrawal of the promoter.[4, 22, 40]

Pure promoting agents are not genotoxic, require frequent administration but generally not metabolic activation, and are not carcinogenic when administered alone.[4, 41] In a dose-dependent manner, they reduce the latency or increase the number of tumors formed following exposure to an initiator, and they induce tumor formation when administered with doses of initiators that are too low to be carcinogenic alone. Agents with both initiating and promoting actions exist and are called complete carcinogens.[22]

Some of the molecular mechanisms of tumor promotion have been studied extensively, but much remains unknown. The best studied promoters are the phorbol esters, a class of plant products which includes 12-O-tetradecanoylphorbol-13-acetate, or TPA, the promoter present in croton oil.[4] Phorbol esters bind to receptors present in cells of all vertebrates and activate an intracellular signal transduction system that normally responds to certain cytokines. The cellular receptor for TPA is protein kinase C, a family of kinases that phosphorylates a variety of substrates.[42] The resulting cascade of epigenetic changes, including altered prostaglandin synthesis, ion flux, and cell-cell communication, leads to cell growth and often altered differentiation.[4]

Malignant Conversion

Malignant conversion is the transformation by further genetic changes of a preneoplastic, initiated cell into one that expresses a malignant phenotype. Benign tumors induced by initiators and promoters in mouse skin and rat liver convert to malignancies with high frequency when they are re-exposed to an initiator. Prolonged administration of promoters also increases conversion frequency, although factors intrinsic to the early neoplasms may be even more important.[43-46] These data are consistent with epidemiologic data of cessation of cigarette smoking and the reduced, but not eliminated, incidence of lung cancer.[47] The withdrawal of the initiators and promoters present in cigarette smoke reduces the risk of conversion of initiated cells, but it cannot eliminate the risk because the converting mutations may have already occurred.

Tumor Progression

Tumor progression occurs through genetic events such as overexpression or activating mutations of oncogenes, and deletion or inactivating mutations of tumor-suppressor genes. These events are facilitated by genomic instability, an intrinsic feature of many malignant cells that results in increased chromosomal deletion, mutation, amplification, and nondisjunction.[10, 18] The p53 tumor-suppressor gene is one important regulator of this process, and p53 mutations can result in genomic instability and gene amplification in vitro.[48, 49]

Tumor invasion has been postulated to occur in three steps: (1) tumor cell attachment to extracellular matrix; (2) digestion of the matrix and adhesion molecules by tumor or induced host enzymes; and (3) movement of tumor cells into the modified matrix.[50] For metastasis to occur, tumor cells must additionally invade, survive, and then escape from the lymphatic or blood circulation, attach via cell surface adhesion molecules to a target tissue, and create a distant colony by producing, or inducing local production of, angiogenesis agents and growth factors.[51] Again, specific genes participate at all stages in this cascade, such as the multiple drug resistance (MDR) gene, which codes for a protein that acts as an efflux pump for macromolecules, including some antineoplastic agents.[52]

DNA Damage and Repair

Carcinogens may be chemical, physical, or biologic agents that, as discussed earlier, mutate cellular DNA, resulting in abnormal protein expression or function that increases the probability of the affected cells undergoing malignant transformation. Current research is examining the mechanisms by which carcinogens damage DNA, the roles of exogenous versus endogenous carcinogens, and the protective processes by which cells repair DNA abnormalities. These characteristics not only are important for understanding carcinogenesis and developing a comprehensive paradigm of cancer biology but also are relevant to theories and trials of chemoprevention, to the assessment of risk and recommendations for individual patients, and to societal policies regarding carcinogen expo-

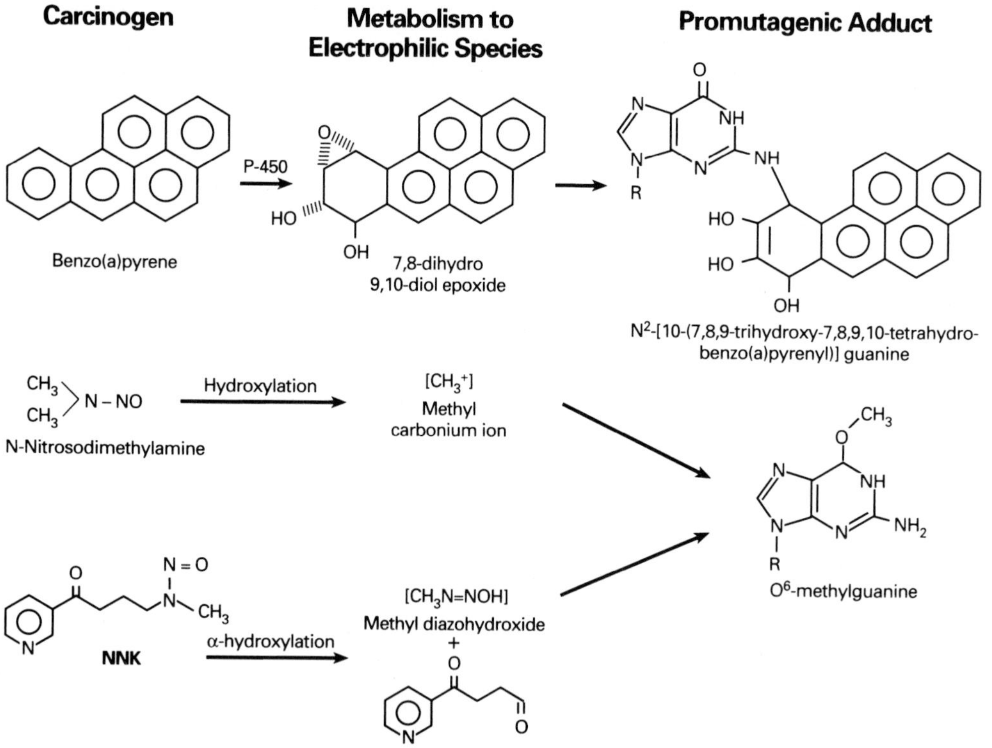

Carcinogen **Metabolism to Electrophilic Species** **Promutagenic Adduct**

Benzo(a)pyrene

7,8-dihydro 9,10-diol epoxide

N^2-[10-(7,8,9-trihydroxy-7,8,9,10-tetrahydro-benzo(a)pyrenyl)] guanine

N-Nitrosodimethylamine

Hydroxylation

[CH_3^+] Methyl carbonium ion

NNK

α-hydroxylation

[$CH_3N=NOH$] Methyl diazohydroxide

O^6-methylguanine

FIGURE 2–4. Examples of carcinogens and their metabolic activation to promutagenic DNA adducts. NNK = 4-(methylnitros-amino)-1-(3-pyridyl)-1-butanone.

sure. Strategies for measuring the damage caused by a carcinogen include tests for mutations in bacteria and eukaryotic cells, evaluation of chromosome damage, and direct assays of the breaks and cross-links formed by carcinogens.[1]

Types of DNA damage include deletion, insertion, and base substitution, either transition (change of a pyrimidine to another pyrimidine or of a purine to another purine) or transversion (change of a pyrimidine to a purine or vice versa).[53] Some carcinogens produce characteristic mutations, and the study of mutation patterns may offer clues to the etiology or mechanism of damage.[1] Chemical carcinogens usually form complexes with bases in DNA (and other macromolecules) known as adducts, which lead to base substitutions. Ionizing radiation and some chemicals result in oxygen-free radicals, which cause DNA strand breakage, nucleotide base changes, and deletions.[26] Ultraviolet radiation causes pyrimidine dimers, which often result in tandem CC to TT mutations.[54] Endogenous mutagenic processes include the generation of oxygen radicals and the spontaneous deamination of methylated cytosine residues (see Endogenous Mutagens). Thus, even in the absence of exogenous carcinogen exposure, there is a need for DNA repair to ensure the integrity of the genome. Most of these mechanisms of DNA damage have been demonstrated in bronchial carcinogenesis (see Endogenous Mutagens).

Metabolism of Chemical Carcinogens

Almost all chemical carcinogens are metabolized, both activated from an inactive procarcinogen to a mutagenic form (the ultimate carcinogen) and detoxified to inactive metabolites.[22] Differences in enzyme expres-

sion and activity among species, individuals, and tissues are thought to be responsible for the organ specificities of many carcinogens and for some of the differences in individual susceptibility to cancer.[1]

Research on early carcinogens that are not highly chemically reactive revealed the creation of high-energy electrophilic groups that proved to be responsible for the mutagenic properties of chemical carcinogens (Fig. 2–4).[55–57] For the PAHs and other agents, metabolic activation is accomplished by cytochrome P450 enzymes, which produce highly reactive diol-epoxides[4]; other compounds, such as aromatic amines, are activated by P450 and other enzymes, resulting in hydroxylation, esterification, and acetylation.[22] Carcinogen metabolism in most laboratory animals is similar to that in humans, so extrapolation of animal data is generally valid.[14] Interindividual variations in activity of these enzymes may be important determinants of cancer risk (see Metabolic Variations).

Adduct Formation

The most common mechanism by which chemical carcinogens and their metabolites cause mutations is by forming adducts with the bases in DNA, interfering with DNA synthesis and eventually inducing coding errors during DNA replication. Examples of carcinogen-DNA adducts are shown in Figure 2–4. Certain base sites are more susceptible to electrophile attack and adduct formation by specific agents, producing a specific spectrum of mutations. For example, the ultimate carcinogen of benzo[a]pyrene (BP), anti-benzo[a]pyrene-7,8-diol-9,10-epoxide, reacts almost exclusively with the 2-amino position of deoxyguanine, and N-nitrosamines preferentially attack the N^7 and O^6 position of guanine, the N^1, N^3, and N^7 positions of adenine, the O^4 position of thymidine, and the N^3 position of cytosine.[4, 58] In general, the level of adduct formation in model systems correlates with a compound's carcinogenicity. Specific adducts such as O^6-methylguanine persist and are associated with mutagenicity and carcinogenicity, whereas others are more readily repaired and are not mutagenic.[4, 59–61]

Some of the mechanisms by which DNA adducts interfere with DNA replication and cause mutations are known (Fig. 2–5). If they are not removed, adducts create physical changes that result in improper reading of the DNA sequence by DNA polymerase. For small adducts induced by alkylating agents, the polymerase may simply misread the base pairing owing to the altered hydrogen-bonding properties of a base containing an additional methyl or ethyl group. In this way, for example, methylguanine may be mispaired with thymine rather than cytosine, and if this pairing is not corrected, the next round of DNA synthesis will substitute an adenine for the original guanine. Experimental evidence has confirmed such G to A transitions as the most common mutations induced by alkylating agents.[60]

A different model exists for mutagenesis from larger compounds, whose bulk prevents the polymerase from reading the code at all (a noninstructive site). DNA polymerase appears to fill noninstructive sites preferentially with adenine (the so-called A rule), which pairs with thymine in the next round of DNA synthesis, resulting in a transversion of guanine to thymine.[62]

Measurement of carcinogen-DNA adducts allows correlation of specific DNA damage, dosimetry, and carcinogenicity. Adduct formation is a necessary but not sufficient criterion for initiation, and dose-response studies have shown that adduct formation reflects exposure for several important carcinogens.[63, 64] In experimental systems, there is general correlation between the formation and persistence of adducts in tissues and the number of tumors formed. Adduct measurements in populations exposed to carcinogens, such as cigarette smokers or persons with occupational exposure,[65–68] may allow more specific assessment of the risk of an individual within an exposed population.

Oxygen Species, Free Radicals

Ionizing radiation and some chemical carcinogens cause mutations by reduction of molecular oxygen via single electron transfer to highly reactive oxygen radicals that attack DNA. Active oxygen species cause DNA strand breakage and at least three base modification products, 5-hydroxymethyluracil, thymine glycol, and 8-hydroxydeoxyguanine. Transition metals, such as iron, copper, and manganese, act as single electron donors and facilitate the generation of the most reactive of these species, the hydroxyl radical OH·. Two important lung carcinogens that act through these species are cigarette smoke, which contains large quantities of active oxygen species, and ionizing radiation from radon gas.[26]

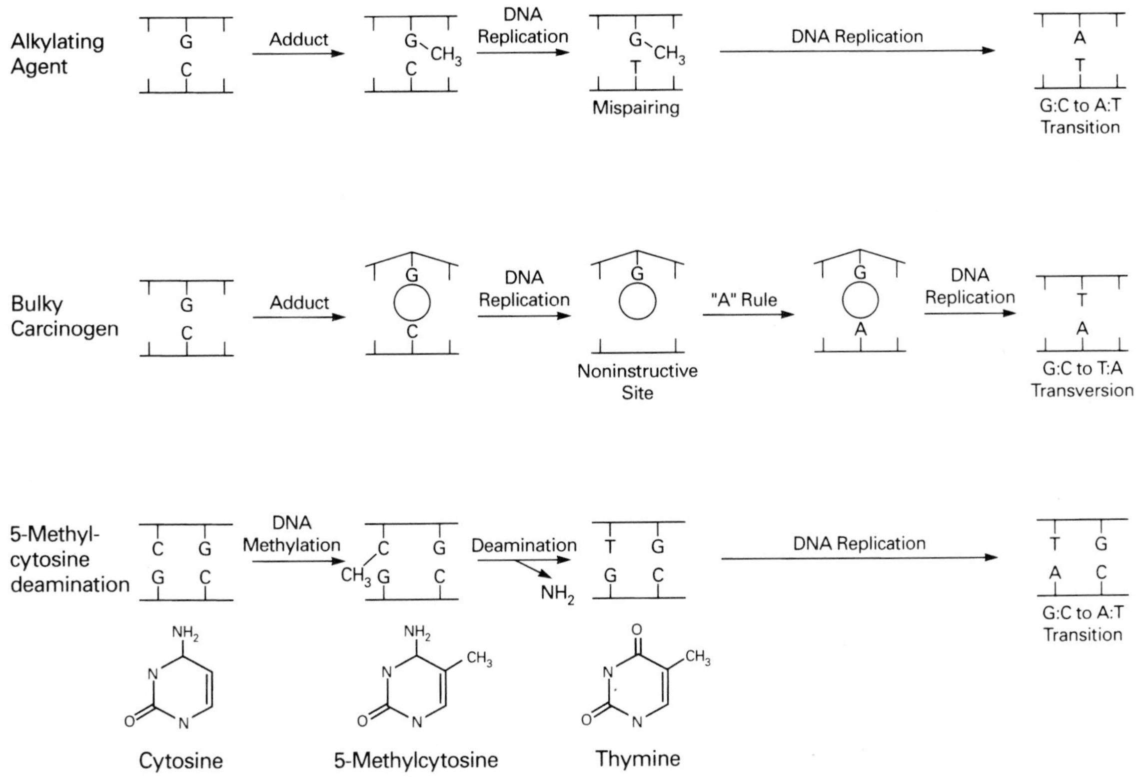

FIGURE 2–5. Mechanisms of base substitution mutations. The mechanisms are described in the text. Note that the methylation of guanine by alkylating agents represents formation of a promutagenic adduct, whereas the methylation of cytosine is a normal process by which cells regulate gene expression. The process is only mutagenic if deamination occurs and is not repaired. All mutations must be fixed in the daughter cells by DNA replication.

Most oxygen species are efficiently eliminated by the enzymes superoxide dismutase and catalase, which catalyze reactions in which the oxygen molecules react with themselves. Hydroxyl radicals, however, must be eliminated by nonenzymatic quenching systems, particularly glutathione. Glutathione is a small molecule with a sulfhydryl side group that donates an electron to free radical groups, quenching them while becoming oxidized. Reduced glutathione must be replenished by enzymes such as glutathione-S-transferase.[26] Low levels of glutathione correlate with elevated levels of DNA damage in cells exposed in vitro to oxidative stressors such as cigarette smoke condensate,[26, 69] and the presence of inactivating mutations in glutathione-S-transferase may be important in lung carcinogenesis (see Metabolic Variations).[70, 71]

Pyrimidine Dimers

Ultraviolet irradiation causes dimerization of adjacent pyrimidine bases into cyclobutane dimers, which are converted, via unknown mechanisms, into C to T or CC to TT transition mutations.[54, 72] Several recent studies have presented evidence that activated oxygen species also can induce tandem mutations by an unknown mechanism.[72, 73]

Endogenous Mutagens—Deamination, Oxygen Species, and Nitric Oxide

Not all mutations are caused by exogenous carcinogens; some normal cellular processes can be mutagenic. The most studied mutation at this time is the phenomenon of deamination of 5-methylcytosine (see Fig. 2–5). Methylation of DNA is one epigenetic mechanism that controls gene expression. Methylated cytosine residues, especially those at CpG dinucleotides (a cytosine followed by a guanine), can spontaneously deaminate to thymine, which, if it is not repaired, will result in a G:C to A:T transition.[74] This process is induced in vitro by nitric oxide, a ubiquitous, although short-lived, product of nitric oxide synthase with important homeostatic regulatory functions.[75] Although chemical carcinogens may affect 5-methylcytosine deamination,[76] the rate of these transitions at CpG dinucleotides is thought to reflect the background rate of deamination. Characteristics of the local DNA sequence or other factors produce so-called hot spots with a high frequency of CpG transitions. In some human tumors, these mutations may be significant; for example, G:C to A:T transitions at CpG sites compose half of all p53 mutations in colon cancer.[77, 78]

Other cellular processes generate mutations or mutagenic agents. DNA polymerase infidelity and depurination may cause spontaneous point mutations.[79, 80] Macrophages and gastrointestinal enzymes produce N-nitrosamines; inflammatory processes and lysosomal digestion release oxygen radicals; and membrane metabolism creates peroxyl radicals.[26, 81] Studies of constitutive cellular genes suggest a baseline mutation rate of approximately 10^{-5}.[53] This background level of mutations implies that populations will always exhibit a baseline rate of cancer, even in the absence of carcinogen exposure.

DNA Repair

DNA repair may be defined as the cellular responses that restore the normal nucleotide sequence and stereochemistry of DNA following damage.[82] Three different types of repair are known: (1) base or nucleotide excision repair, (2) mismatch repair, and (3) postreplication repair. The most common mechanism, excision repair, was first described in 1964 for ultraviolet-induced dimers, and it is also responsible for the repair of many carcinogen-DNA adducts. In postreplication repair, the DNA polymerase skips a region of damage and leaves a gap on the new DNA strand. This site may then undergo genetic recombination, or single base gaps may be filled in by an adenine nucleotide; both events can lead to genetic changes.[83]

DNA repair is closely linked to other cellular pathways that control gene expression. DNA of actively transcribed genes is preferentially repaired, as is the transcribed DNA strand.[82, 84] Several recently described genes code for enzymes exhibiting both DNA repair and gene transcription activities, suggesting a potential molecular mechanism for control of cellular proliferation until repair is accomplished.[85, 86] DNA repair involves at least 30 genes in yeast, and probably more are required in the repair of mammalian cells.[82] Differences in DNA repair activity are another potential source of individual cancer susceptibility, and inherited abnormalities in DNA repair confer an increased risk of cancer.[26]

HOST FACTORS AND CANCER RISK

Individual differences clearly exist among the population in susceptibility to cancer, because the same level of carcinogen exposure (e.g., tobacco smoking) produces malignancies in some persons but not in others. Traditional epidemiologic studies of cancer incidence, which identify risk in populations, are now supplemented by research in molecular epidemiology, which attempts to identify individuals at elevated risk and the molecular basis for cancer susceptibility.

Inheritance and Lung Cancer

Patterns of inheritance have long been observed in many human cancers, including carcinoma of the lung. The first case-control study, performed in 1963, found an increased relative risk of mortality from lung cancer in relatives of both smokers and non-smokers.[87] Other epidemiologic studies have confirmed this association in both men and women, and have estimated the relative risk of a positive family history at 2 to 3.[88–92] Statistical modeling of epidemiologic data from these families suggested the existence of a rare major autosomal codominant allele that produces earlier age at onset of lung cancer in affected families.[93] Hypotheses to explain these data include the possible inheritance of mutated oncogenes or tumor-suppressor genes, variations in carcinogen metabolism, abnormalities of DNA replication or repair, or other differences in pulmonary physiology that might predispose an individual to the effects of carcinogens.

Germline Mutations and Polymorphisms in Oncogenes and Tumor-Suppressor Genes

Inheritance of germline mutations that alter the function of tumor-suppressor genes is responsible for several types of human malignancies, such as retinoblastoma (RB gene)[94] and the Li-Fraumeni syndrome (p53 gene),[95] in which affected individuals develop an assortment of cancers, most commonly sarcomas and breast carcinoma. No such direct relationship has yet been demonstrated for lung carcinoma.

Gene polymorphisms represent a source of genetic variation that can be studied for clues to an individual's risk of disease. Polymorphisms in several specific oncogenes and a variety of other genetic markers have been examined to determine whether or not certain alleles are associated with an increased lung cancer risk. Three groups of investigators have found an association between the inheritance of rare (not activated) polymorphic alleles of the H-ras oncogene and increased risk.[96–99] This relationship was not noted for tested alleles of L-myc and p53.[96, 100, 101] Data in animals support the notion that a particular oncogene allele may be more vulnerable to activation. Some mice that are susceptible to developing lung cancer contain a specific K-ras allele, and the majority of tumors contain ras mutations in the susceptible allele.[102, 103] Studies of variations in alleles of other molecules such as cell surface antigens have produced conflicting results. No causal relationship can be ascribed to these genes, because they may merely represent linkage with the critical, unidentified gene.[92]

Pre-existing Lung Disease

Several studies demonstrate increased lung cancer risk in patients with chronic obstructive pulmonary disease, controlling for age, sex, and smoking habits.[90, 104–107] One possible explanation for this association is that chronic obstructive pulmonary disease results in poor clearance of the particulates present in tobacco smoke, and thus an increased exposure to carcinogens. Alternatively, it may reflect inheritance of a gene (or linked inheritance of two genes) responsible for increased risk of each disease.[92, 108] An elevated risk of lung carcinoma has also been reported in patients with diffuse pulmonary fibrosis, both isolated and that associated with systemic sclerosis.[92, 109]

Until the 1980s, pre-existing scars, most commonly from infarcts or tuberculosis, were thought to give rise to up to 7% of lung carcinomas.[110] Recent studies of matrix collagen indicate that frequently the connective tissue is produced by, or in response to, the cancer, and most cases of so-called scar carcinomas are now believed to be de novo cancers with secondary scarring.[111–114]

Metabolic Variations

Exposure of populations to specific carcinogens such as PAHs, N-nitrosamines, and aromatic amines is clearly related to cancer risk.[115] Determination of an individual's exposure is more difficult, because it requires sensitive and specific assays to detect the biologically relevant damage or a reliable surrogate marker. Ongoing studies are attempting to correlate biochemical markers of carcinogen exposure, such as DNA adducts, with an individual's cancer risk.[63, 116, 117]

Epidemiologic evidence exists linking lung cancer with certain biochemical or physiologic phenotypes that suggest mechanisms of enhanced carcinogenesis. Because most chemical carcinogens undergo metabolic activation and detoxification, individual variations in enzymes responsible for these reactions may contribute to cancer susceptibility through differential carcinogen metabolism. These variations have been measured by both biochemical detection of metabolites and molecular studies defining an individual's genotype.[115] One example is the N-acetyltransferase gene, which has alleles responsible for fast versus slow acetylation. Slow acetylators have a higher risk of bladder carcinoma, and fast acetylators have an elevated risk of colon cancer, which is thought to be due to differential metabolism of aromatic amines.[115] No association has been found for lung cancer.[118, 119]

Clear association of carcinogen metabolism with risk of lung carcinoma has been difficult. Polymorphisms of two enzymes have been linked to elevated lung cancer risk in multiple studies. The cytochrome P450 enzyme debrisoquin 4-hydroxylase (CYP2D6) is responsible for the metabolism of debrisoquin, an antihypertensive, and numerous other drugs, possibly including N-nitrosamines present in tobacco smoke. Debrisoquin hydroxylation varies widely among individuals, and several case-control studies have associated the phenotype of extensive metabolism of debrisoquin with an increased risk of lung and other cancers, although not all studies have confirmed this finding.[120–124] The specific genotypes associated with increased risk have not been identified,[125] and it is not clear whether this risk is related to carcinogen metabolism by CYP2D6 or to linkage with a different susceptibility gene. Low phenotypic activity of glutathione-S-transferase, and a genotype coding for an inactive enzyme, also have been correlated with mutagenicity, increased DNA adducts in lung tissue, and increased lung cancer risk in some but not all studies.[70, 71, 126, 127]

Several enzymes are involved in carcinogen metabolism and also occur in polymorphic forms that alter biochemical phenotypes, but their relationship to cancer risk is uncertain.[128–131] These include the P450 enzyme aryl hydrocarbon hydroxylase (AHH, a product of the CYP1A1 gene). Several inherited syndromes of deficient DNA repair are associated with an elevated risk of cancer.[26] The role of DNA repair enzyme activity in cancers unrelated to these syndromes is unknown.

Finally, studies have reported elevated levels of bombesin-like peptides, neuropeptides that are growth factors for small cell lung cancer, in the lungs and urine of smokers compared with nonsmokers. Some individuals exhibit marked elevations and may represent a subgroup of smokers at increased risk for lung cancer, perhaps as a result of tobacco-induced endogenous tumor promotion by these peptides.[131, 132]

Immune Factors and Cancer

Cancer incidence is increased in inherited and acquired immunodeficiency syndromes, suggesting a role for immune surveillance in cancer suppression, but the details of this process are unclear.[133–134] Animal studies suggest that individual differences in immune function can determine susceptibility to chemical carcinogens.[135]

Studies of immune function in patients are inconclusive regarding its importance in the pathogenesis of lung cancer. Infiltration of all immune effector cells has been seen in non–small cell lung carcinomas, but is rare in small cell carcinomas, which express class I major histocompatibility antigens in low levels in vitro.[136, 137] Bronchoalveolar lavage shows changes in T-lymphocyte subsets and cytokines in lung cancer patients, and the cytotoxicity of pulmonary alveolar macrophages and natural killer cells is often abnormal in cancer patients.[133, 138–140] It is unknown whether these changes represent impaired immune surveillance predisposing to the development of lung cancer or tumor-induced functional changes.[133]

BRONCHIAL CARCINOGENESIS

Carcinogens Involved in Bronchial Carcinogenesis

Tobacco Smoke

Epidemiologic and experimental data have unequivocally established tobacco smoking as the primary cause of lung carcinoma, a fact widely recognized since the national reports were generated in Great Britain and the United States in the 1960s.[141, 142] Tobacco smoking is now thought to be responsible for 90% of lung carcinomas in males and 78% in females.[143]

Experimental Studies. Cigarette smoke is a complex mixture with thousands of constituents. Dozens are known to be carcinogenic, but the contributions of the majority to bronchial carcinogenesis are not known (Table 2–2). For experimental purposes, cigarette smoke is divided into two fractions: (1) the volatile fraction, or vapor phase, compounds of which more than 50% passes through a Cambridge glass fiber filter; and (2) the particulate phase, or cigarette smoke condensate (CSC), which is retained by the

TABLE 2–2. Carcinogenic Compounds in Tobacco and Tobacco Smoke

POLYCYCLIC AROMATIC HYDROCARBONS	
Benz[a]anthracene	Dibenz[a,h]anthracene
Benzo[b]fluoranthene	Dibenzo[a,i]pyrene
Benzo[j]fluoranthene	Dibenzo[a,l]pyrene
Benzo[k]fluoranthene	Indeno[1,2,3-cd]pyrene
Benzo[a]pyrene	5-Methylchrysene
Chrysene	
AZA-ARENES	
Quinoline	Dibenz[a,j]acridine
Dibenz[a,h]acridine	7H-Dibenzo[c,g]carbazole
N-NITROSAMINES	
N-Nitrosodimethylamine	N'-Nitrosonornicotine
N-Nitrosoethylmethylamine	4-(Methylnitrosamino)-1-
N-Nitrosodiethanolamine	(3-pyridyl)-1-butanone
N-Nitrosodiethylamine	N'-Nitrosoanabasine
N-Nitrosopyrrolidine	N-Nitrosomorpholine
AROMATIC AMINES	
2-Toluidine	4-Aminobiphenyl
2-Naphthylamine	
ALDEHYDES	
Formaldehyde	Crotonaldehyde
Acetaldehyde	
MISCELLANEOUS ORGANIC COMPOUNDS	
Benzene	2-Nitropropane
Acetonitrile	Ethylcarbamate
1,1-Dimethylhydrazine	Vinyl chloride
INORGANIC COMPOUNDS	
Hydrazine	Cadmium
Arsenic	Lead
Nickel	Polonium-210
Chromium	

Data compiled from references 26 and 259.

filter.[26] These fractions have been tested for transforming activity, mutagenesis, adduct formation, and effects on DNA strand breakage and on lung cells in vitro and in vivo.[26, 144]

Cigarette smoke contains tumor initiators, promoters, and cocarcinogens.[144] The particulate phase retains initiating and promoting ability, while the volatile phase contains initiators but is unable to promote tumors in cells pretreated with initiating agents.[145] Chromosomal damage resulting from CSC was first demonstrated in the root tips of onions, and mutagenicity has since been noted in Salmonella, yeast, and many other eukaryotic cells.[144, 146] CSC causes squamous differentiation and malignant transformation in rodent and human lung cells in culture.[144, 147, 148] In addition to mutagenicity and tumor promotion, cigarette smoke causes defects in DNA repair in human lymphocytes and hamster lungs.[144] DNA adduct levels are higher in the lungs of smokers than in nonsmokers, although it is not known which adducts are important in human lung carcinogenesis.[65, 68]

Some of the carcinogens found in tobacco smoke (Table 2–2), most notably nitrosamines and PAHs, have been purified and tested in model systems. Nitrosamines are derived from organic nitrogenous bases (such as nicotine) known as alkaloids. They include 4-(methylnitrosamino)-1-(3-pyridyl)-1-butanone (NNK), a potent carcinogen present in high doses in tobacco smoke.[26, 149] NNK exhibits specificity for lung carcinogenicity in rodent models, and causes malignant transformation in rodent and immortalized human bronchial cells.[26, 148, 149] Another N-nitroso compound, N-nitroso-N-methylurea (NMU), also causes bronchial carcinoma in hamsters, alone and in synergy with BP.[150] Many PAHs are found in tobacco smoke, including BP, which is a complete carcinogen in bronchi of hamsters. Several other PAHs are initiators that induce benign bronchial tumors but whose metabolism and promoter activity in bronchial cells are unclear.[151] Catechols are a cocarcinogen in tobacco smoke that block the detoxification of BP.[152] Aldehydes (acrolein, benzoyl peroxide, formaldehyde, and hydrogen peroxide) are present in both CSC and the volatile phase. Aldehydes cause DNA strand breaks and the formation of alkyl-DNA adducts in human bronchial cells, and inhibit their colony formation.[153, 154] Formaldehyde and NMU exhibit synergy in their mutagenicity, perhaps because formaldehyde inhibits adduct repair.[155] Other mutagenic agents present in the volatile phase include active oxygen species and polonium-210, whose decay emits ionizing radiation that is a carcinogen in hamsters.[156, 157]

Environmental tobacco smoke contains the same constituents as inhaled mainstream smoke, although absolute concentrations are lower and relative concentrations differ; the quantities inhaled passively are estimated to be 1% to 10% (lower for some constituents, higher for others) of those inhaled by the smoker.[158, 159] Passive smokers have elevated biomarkers of tobacco exposure, including urinary cotinine, serum carcinogen, and carcinogen-protein adducts.[92, 160, 161] Particle size in environmental tobacco smoke is smaller, and inhaled particles may travel to peripheral lung regions more readily than with mainstream smoke.[158] This has been suggested as an explanation for the excess of peripheral adenocarcinomas seen in passive smokers.

Radon

Radon-222 is a colorless, odorless, inert gas that is a naturally occurring decay product (daughter) of uranium-238. Radon is present in most soils and rocks, and is released into indoor and outdoor air in amounts that are dependent on features of local geology and building construction. Decay of radon and two of its daughters results in the emission of alpha particle radiation, a potent physical carcinogen. If radon has been inhaled, this radiation may damage bronchial epithelial cells but rarely other cells, because radon is poorly absorbed. Quantitative radon exposure is expressed in working level months (WLM), a unit obtained by multiplying concentration of potential energy of alpha particles by duration of exposure.[162]

Conclusive epidemiologic evidence implicates occupational exposure to radon by uranium miners as a cause of lung cancer, an association first noted in miners of radioactive ores in Europe in 1879.[163] Multiple case-control studies have established a dose-response relationship, with an excess relative risk attributable to radon estimated at 0.5 to 3.0/100 WLM, and radon exposure and cigarette smoking increase risk synergistically.[162, 164] Radon concentrations in homes vary widely and fluctuate within a building, but they can reach levels as high as those detected in occupational settings.[162] Epidemiologic studies of domestic radon exposure and lung cancer risk have been inconclusive owing to methodologic inconsistencies, but early results suggest that domestic exposure also elevates lung cancer risk.[165] More studies are in progress.[166]

Few laboratory studies of radon-induced lung cancer have been performed, but existing information does raise some questions about the mechanisms of carcinogenesis. Exposure of rats to radon can induce lung cancer, and dose intensity per time appears to be important.[167, 168] Analysis of human tumors may reflect interactions between radon and tobacco carcinogens, because smoking is prevalent among miners.[162] Early studies of radon miners reported a large excess of small cell carcinomas (in smokers and nonsmokers) and no increase in adenocarcinomas, but newer analyses note a decline in the incidence of small cell cancer and an increase in squamous cell cancer.[169–171] The first molecular analyses of radon-induced lung cancer confirm the lack of *ras* mutations in small cell and squamous cell cancers and the importance of p53 mutations.[172] The frequency of p53 mutations in small cell cancers was lower than previously reported, however, suggesting possible differences in radon- versus tobacco-induced tumors. In miners from the Colorado Plateau who were exposed to high amounts of radon, one specific p53 mutation was observed frequently. Because these miners were heavily exposed to other carcinogens found in the mines, it cannot yet be concluded that radon was responsible for these mutations.[173]

Asbestos

Asbestos is a silicate fiber used widely in industry as an insulating agent. Through unknown mechanisms related to fiber length and structure, asbestos is a physical carcinogen for lung and mesothelial tissues, exhibiting a long latency period often in excess of 20 years.[174] The first conclusive report linking occupational exposure to asbestos with lung carcinoma appeared in 1955.[175] Subsequent studies have established that risk from occupational exposure to asbestos is synergistic with the risk from smoking.[176] Asbestos also appears to be a bronchial carcinogen in nonsmokers, although data are less conclusive owing to lower numbers of subjects. The role of low-level, nonindustrial exposure is likewise unclear. Mesothelioma is a well-recognized consequence of asbestos exposure in smokers and nonsmokers.[92, 177]

Experiments on the mechanisms of asbestos carcinogenicity have established that asbestos is a tumor promoter and mitogen for hamster tracheal epithelial cells and that it induces hyperplasia and dysplasia in cultured human bronchial cells.[178] Bronchial epithelial cells phagocytize asbestos fibers, which may serve as a conduit for carcinogen absorption. Free radicals released by macrophages after phagocytosis of asbestos fibers have been implicated as a possible mechanism of carcinogenesis.[154] In mesothelial cells, evidence exists for mutagenicity and promoting activity.[154, 178, 179]

Other Environmental Agents

Additional environmental agents proposed as etiologic factors in lung carcinogenesis include metals, diesel exhaust, and miscellaneous other sources (Table 2–3). Metals can cause DNA damage (including mutations in the p53 gene[180]) by direct DNA binding, generation of free radicals, or interaction with DNA-binding proteins, and several metals are known to be carcinogens from epidemiologic and experimental data.[181, 182] Among these metals, occupational exposure to nickel, arsenic, chromium, and cadmium has been associated with elevated lung cancer risk.[177]

Increased risk from other occupational exposures has been reported but not confirmed.[177] Air pollution results in exposure to known carcinogens such as PAHs, asbestos, and metals, and has been associated with increased lung cancer risk, but case-control studies attempting to link pollution with lung cancer suffer from the inevitable presence of uncontrolled variables.[183–185] No associations have been found between specific pollutants and histologic type.[183] Epidemiologic studies in China implicate indoor air pollution, resulting from burning smoky coal to heat homes and cooking with rapeseed oil (both processes which release PAHs), as an etiologic agent.[186–188]

There is no epidemiologic evidence linking viruses with lung cancer, although reports describe the presence in lung cancer cells of DNA from human papillomavirus, which is strongly linked with other cancers.[189]

Dietary Factors and Cancer Risk

Epidemiologic evidence exists that dietary factors may either increase or decrease lung cancer risk, and experimental data suggest possible mechanisms. In the most powerful association, over 20 epidemiologic studies have demonstrated a statistically significant protective effect for fruit and vegetable intake, with a relative risk of about 0.5 for high- versus low-intake groups.[190, 191] A possible biologic rationale for this phenomenon is the effect of retinoids, particularly beta-carotene. Retinoids have long been known to inhibit tumor formation and regulate differentiation, including reversal of squamous metaplasia of bronchial cells in smokers.[192, 193] Many studies have failed to demonstrate conclusively any benefit of dietary retinoids or elevated serum retinol (vitamin A) levels, but high intake and serum levels of beta-carotene, a dietary vitamin A precursor that is also a powerful scavenger of free radicals, are clearly associated with a decreased incidence of lung carcinoma.[190, 194–196] Chemoprevention trials of beta-carotene, retinoic acid, and other agents are under way. One study of smokers in Finland reported no benefit from vitamin E and an increased lung cancer risk from beta-carotene.[197] Several studies suggest a protective effect for dietary vitamin C, an antioxidant.[190] Elevated fat and cholesterol intake has been associated with an elevated risk of lung carcinoma in several studies, but these data are inconclusive.[198]

Bronchial Cell Biology

Cell of Origin of Bronchogenic Carcinoma

The approach to the identification of the cell of origin of bronchogenic carcinoma began with histologic analyses of lung cancer and preneoplastic changes. These studies included examination of morphologic responses to growth factors, differentiating agents, and carcinogens in animal models; in vitro kinetic studies to determine which bronchial cells proliferate and their growth properties; and molecular studies of human tumors and model systems.[199, 200] Early models postulated that different stem cells transformed into the various histologic types of lung cancer. However, observations of tumors and individual cells with mixed features, and the evolution of cell types within individual cancers suggested the possibility of one pluripotent stem cell that could transform into all histologic types of lung cancer. To date, the identity of the lung stem cell remains unclear; more than one type of bronchial cell may indeed undergo malignant transformation, beginning with squamous metaplasia and progressing through dysplasia to carcinoma (Fig. 2–6).[201, 202]

Animal Models

Animal models for human lung cancer include the mouse, the rat, the hamster, and the dog. Although these systems allow in vivo evaluation of carcinogens and biologic parameters (such as preneoplastic lesions) not possible in humans or in vitro studies, direct extrapolation of animal data to human disease must be tempered by recognition of interspecies differences. For example, mouse cells have a higher susceptibility to mutation in general and lung cancer in particular, although hamster susceptibility to lung cancer is similar to that of humans.[28, 29]

TABLE 2–3. Environmental Agents Linked to Lung Carcinogenesis

ESTABLISHED RISK FACTORS	POSSIBLE RISK FACTORS
Arsenic	Acrylonitrile
Asbestos	Beryllium
BCME and CMME	Cadmium
Environmental tobacco smoke	Coal combustion products
Mustard gas	Cooking oil vapors
Nickel	Diesel exhaust
PAHs	Dietary cholesterol
Radon	Dietary fat
Tobacco smoke	Urban air pollution
Vinyl chloride	**POSSIBLE PROTECTIVE AGENTS**
ESTABLISHED PROTECTIVE AGENTS	Dietary beta-carotene
	Dietary vitamin C
Dietary fruits and vegetables	

BCME = bis(chloromethyl) ether; CMME = chloromethyl methyl ether; PAHs = polycyclic aromatic hydrocarbons.
Data compiled from references 177, 184, 185, 194, 195, 198, 260, and 261.

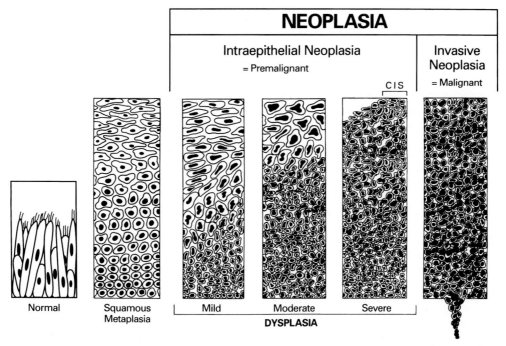

FIGURE 2–6. Bronchial histology—progression of neoplasia. Normal pseudostratified bronchial mucosa (left) responds to a variety of injurious stimuli with hyperplasia, stratification, and squamous metaplasia. Early benign neoplastic changes, called dysplasia, are characterized by nuclei that are enlarged, irregular, and darkened on hematoxylin/eosin staining. Dysplasia is divided into three stages: mild, involving one-third of the mucosal thickness; moderate, involving two-thirds of the mucosal thickness; and severe, extending through the full thickness of the mucosa. Mild dysplasia frequently regresses, whereas severe dysplasia generally progresses to malignancy. When the mucosa no longer shows evidence of maturation from basal to superficial surfaces, it is called carcinoma in situ (CIS). When CIS invades the basement membrane, it is called invasive carcinoma. (Adapted from Boone CW, Kelloff GJ, Steele VE: Natural history of intraepithelial neoplasia in humans with implications for cancer chemoprevention strategy. Cancer Res 52:1651, 1659, 1992.)

Normal Human Bronchial Epithelial, Lung Cancer, and Other Cell Lines in vitro

Despite the failure to identify the bronchial carcinoma progenitor cell in vivo, recent advances in the culture of human tracheobronchial cells permit the study of specific biochemical and molecular events associated with proliferation, differentiation, and transformation under more controlled conditions than animal models. Normal human bronchial epithelial (NHBE) cells grown in serum-free medium divide 20 to 30 times, and before terminal differentiation and senescence, their characteristics can be studied and compared with those of transformed cell lines and others derived from carcinomas.[26]

Effects of Differentiating Agents, Cytokines, and Carcinogens on NHBE Cells. Serum inhibits proliferation and induces terminal squamous differentiation of NHBE cells; the primary compound in serum responsible for these effects is transforming growth factor-β (TGF-β), a cytokine produced by a variety of normal and malignant cells.[32] TGF-β receptors are present on lung and many other cells, but its signal transduction pathways are unclear. TGF-β alters phosphorylation of the retinoblastoma protein, which may account for its growth-arresting activity.[200] Conditions that inhibit squamous differentiation include high cell density, high retinoid levels, and agents that elevate cyclic adenosine monophosphate levels.[32, 200]

Other cytokines also affect growth and maturation of NHBE cells. Epidermal growth factor (EGF) and TGF-α stimulate proliferation and may be important autocrine and paracrine agents in lung regulation because they are produced by a variety of lung cells.[200] Other evidence suggesting the importance of these growth factors is the frequent overexpression and amplification of the oncogenes coding for the EGF and related receptors (*erb-B1, erb-B2*).[203] Insulin and insulin-like growth factors also stimulate bronchial epithelial cells in vitro; production of insulin-like growth factors by pulmonary macrophages may play a role in lung neoplasia in vivo.[200] Gastrin-releasing peptide (GRP, bombesin), an important autocrine growth factor for small cell lung cancer (SCLC), also stimulates NHBE cell growth.[204] Retinoic acid inhibits NHBE cell growth in vitro while inhibiting squamous differentiation in tissue explants.[32, 200]

Cigarette smoke, specific tobacco-related carcinogens, and other tumor promoters and bronchial carcinogens have been tested on NHBE cells. Aldehydes, CSC, and the tumor promoter TPA induce squamous differentiation.[147, 205] Tobacco-related aldehydes are cytotoxic to NHBE cells, causing DNA strand breaks and impairing DNA repair ability.[153, 154] Nickel sulfate treatment is also cytotoxic to NHBE cells but produces some transformed cells that are aneuploid, not dependent on EGF for growth, not responsive to TGF-β–induced differentiation, and nontumorigenic.[32]

Transformation of NHBE Cells. Although human bronchial cells are relatively resistant to transformation in vitro, introduction of several genes has produced immortalized lines with epithelial features. Transformation of NHBE cells was first accomplished by transfection with the H-ras oncogene.[206] These cells became tumorigenic, providing strong evidence for a crucial role for ras in bronchial carcinogenesis; the additional genetic events that may have contributed to tumorigenicity in these cells are unknown. Transfection of c-myc altered the phenotype of NHBE cells but did not immortalize them.[32] Nontumorigenic transformed bronchial cell lines have been obtained by transfection of NHBE cells with human papillomavirus[207] and SV40 TAg (BEAS-2B cells).[208] Because TAg and human papillomavirus proteins E6 and E7 bind to the p53 and retinoblastoma proteins, disruption of these pathways may contribute to bronchial cell transformation.[209]

BEAS-2B cells provide a model to study the features of the different stages of bronchial carcinogenesis. In contrast to NHBE cells, some BEAS-2B clones are unresponsive to the differentiating effects of serum, TGF-β, CSC, and TPA; this supports the concepts of selective expansion of initiated clones by tumor promoters and coupling of impaired differentiation with abnormal proliferation.[32, 147, 205] A second genetic event can confer tumorigenicity to BEAS-2B cells. This has been accomplished by transfecting an activated H-ras, K-ras, or c-erb-B2 oncogene, the combination of myc and raf oncogenes (but neither gene alone), or a mutant of the p53 tumor-suppressor gene.[210–213] The resulting tumors exhibit features of multiple differentiation pathways.[214] A subline of BEAS-2B has spontaneously become weakly tumorigenic, and these cells have lost chromosome 3p loci.[215] Because efficiency of tumorigenic conversion of immortalized cells is much greater than immortalization of NHBE cells, the immortalization step may be rate limiting in lung carcinogenesis.[212]

Tumor Cell Lines. In vitro cell lines have been established from SCLC, non–SCLC, and transformed NHBE cells, and they have been examined for morphology, growth factor production and responsiveness, and oncogene expression and activation.

Under defined culture conditions, cell lines can be established from the majority of clinical specimens of SCLC. At least three types have been characterized by biochemical and molecular features. So-called classic SCLC lines (SCLC-C) have the morphology of clinical SCLC. They express the neuroendocrine peptides GRP and dopa decarboxylase, and they do not overexpress c-myc. So-called variant SCLC lines (SCLC-V) comprise 30% of the lines, do not express GRP and dopa decarboxylase (although they do express other neuroendocrine markers), overexpress c-myc, and grow much more rapidly. Some SCLC-V lines also vary in

morphology, resembling large cell undifferentiated carcinomas.[216, 217] SCLC-C lines transfected with c-myc acquire some phenotypes of SCLC-V lines,[218] but c-myc amplification is rare in clinical SCLC, suggesting that it is an in vitro event related to tumor progression in cultured cells.[219]

Fewer lines have been established from non–SCLC. Morphologic features of all non–SCLC types have been noted, and biochemical studies have sometimes correlated morphology with expression of characteristic enzymes, such as markers of peripheral airway cells in adenocarcinoma lines or keratin production in squamous cell lines.[201, 202] Other lines are less differentiated or express mixed phenotypes. No specific markers for non–SCLC cells are known, although they may be distinguished from SCLC by expression of HLA-I antigens, which are absent in SCLC.[220] Tumors resulting from transformed NHBE cell lines are less well studied but are known to express phenotypes of all bronchial lineages, confirming the pluripotent differentiating ability of the lung cancer stem cell.[214]

Over 20 cytokine growth factors have been identified in lung cancer lines, and cells often produce both a cytokine and its receptor, suggesting that autocrine loops are an important mechanism of lung carcinogenesis.[203, 221] This may explain why serum often stimulates the growth of cell lines, which are also resistant to the differentiating effects of TGF-β.[32] The most studied of these factors is GRP, produced by clinical SCLC tumors, SCLC-C lines, some non–SCLC lines, and normal bronchial neuroendocrine cells. GRP is a potent mitogen for SCLC and NHBE cells, both of which express the GRP receptor.[204, 221] The GRP receptor is a G protein involved in the ras signal transduction pathway, accounting for participation of this pathway in SCLC biology despite the absence of ras activation.[221] GRP is likely an important autocrine agent for SCLC, may play a role in early lung carcinogenesis, and is being studied as a potential tumor marker.[131]

Retinoids, suppressors of squamous differentiation in normal bronchi,[200] have the same effect on some SCLC-C lines. When treated with retinoic acid, some SCLC-V lines adopt an SCLC-C phenotype.[222] Some cell lines express retinoic acid receptor,[223] and transfection of the receptor into a nonexpressing non–SCLC line inhibited its growth.[224] The recent identification of these receptors as transcription factors[200] promises further progress in understanding retinoid actions.

The relative roles of oncogenes and tumor-suppressor genes in cell lines, and the comparability of cell line oncogene data to human cancer data, are unclear. For example, ras activation is rare in squamous cell tumors but is common in squamous cell lines.[225, 226] When present, ras activation is probably critical to tumorigenesis, because inhibition of activated ras transcription restored normal growth characteristics to a non–SCLC line[227] and inhibited tumorigenicity of human tumor explants.[228] Several oncogenes have been found to be selectively expressed in SCLC or non–SCLC lines: in SCLC lines, c-myc, N-myc, L-myc, and c-myb; and in non–SCLC lines, *fur*, *sis*, *src*, and *erb-B1*. The *raf* oncogene is probably involved in both cell types.[220, 229] Tumor-suppressor genes have been implicated in lung carcinogenesis by cell fusion experiments creating NHBE and BEAS-2B/cancer cell hybrids.[230] Two tumor-suppressor genes, p53 and K-*rev*, have been transfected into lung cancer line, which suppressed their growth and tumorigenicity.[231–233]

Cytogenetics, Oncogenes, and Tumor-Suppressor Genes and Bronchial Carcinogenesis

A goal of molecular genetic research is identification of the precise molecular events responsible for malignant transformation and differentiation into various cell types, which might allow assignment of the risks associated with specific mutagens, identification of premalignant molecular abnormalities, and therapeutic strategies with molecular targets. Cytogenetic analysis has associated specific chromosomal aberrations with lung cancer, helping focus the search for specific cancer-related genes. Chromosomal translocations may either activate oncogenes or inactivate tumor-suppressor genes, and deletion or loss of heterozygosity of a gene locus often heralds the site of a tumor-suppressor gene.[203] Common sites of loss of heterozygosity and deletions in lung cancers frequently correspond to known tumor-suppressor genes, such as 13q (RB) and 17p (p53 and probably others).[234, 235]

Oncogenes: *ras*, *myc*, and Others. The most thoroughly studied oncogenes in lung cancer are the *ras* genes, of which K-*ras* is the most relevant. K-*ras* mutations are thought to be an early event in lung carcinogenesis, with important consequences for growth deregulation. Activating K-*ras* mutations are found in 25% to 30% of adenocarcinomas and in 15% of large cell carcinomas, but rarely in squamous cell carcinoma and never in SCLC.[226, 236–238] N- and H-*ras* are rarely altered. Other data implicate *ras* in the differentiation pathway of adenocarcinomas, as suggested by clinicopathologic and molecular epidemiologic studies. Transfection of activated K-*ras* into a SCLC line induces features of non–SCLC differentiation.[239, 240] *Ras* mutations are rare in nonsmokers, and 66% of *ras* mutations are G to T transversions, which are consistent with damage caused by bulky carcinogens in tobacco smoke.[225] Finally, two retrospective studies have correlated *ras* activation with poor prognosis.[241, 242]

Activation of other oncogenes has been demonstrated in many lung cancer cell lines and some primary tumors (Table 2–4). Overexpression of *myc* genes is present in 10% to 15% of primary lung cancers, and activated c-*myc* may correlate with prognosis.[203, 219] Expression of *erb-B2/neu* is common in non–SCLC and may be associated with shortened survival in adenocarcinomas.[26, 238] Other oncogenes observed to be activated in lung cancers and cell lines include *fur*, *fes*, and *sis* in non–SCLC; *myb* and *fms* in

TABLE 2–4. Examples of Oncogenes and Tumor Suppressor Genes Found to be Altered in Lung Cancer

	SCLC	NSCLC
Oncogenes		
	c-*myc**	K-*ras**
	L-*myc*	N-*ras*
	N-*myc*	H-*ras*
	c-*raf*	c-*myc*
	c-*myb*	c-*raf*
	c-*erb-B1* (EGF-R)	c-*fur**
	c-*fms*	c-*fes*
	c-*rlf*	c-*erb-B1* (EGF-R)*
		c-*erb-B2* (Her2, neu)
		c-*sis*
		bcl-1
Tumor-Suppressor Genes		
	p53*	p53*
	RB*	RB

*Most frequently altered genes in tumors or cell lines evaluated.
Data compiled from references 203, 219, 220, 238, and 253.

SCLC; and *erb-B1 (EGF-R)*, *raf*, and *rlf* (Table 2–4).[203, 219, 229, 243, 244] The biologic and clinical significance of most of these alterations remains to be determined.

p53. The p53 protein appears to have multiple critical regulatory functions, including transcription activation, control of progression through the cell cycle, and regulation of programmed cell death (apoptosis). It contains functional domains that are highly conserved in evolution. Nonmutated, wild type p53 protein is constitutively present in low quantities, forms multimers with itself, complexes with other cellular proteins, binds to specific DNA sequences, and activates the transcription of some genes while inhibiting others.[209, 245] It appears to function at the G_1-S checkpoint to prevent progression through S phase.[245] Mutations in the conserved regions change the conformation of p53 and alter its half-life and its DNA-binding, multimerization, protein-binding, and transcriptional regulation properties.[246, 247] Different mutations alter function differently, and some mutations of p53 cause it to behave as an oncogene, stimulating cell proliferation.

p53 mutations are found in 72% of cases of SCLC and 47% of cases of non–SCLC, including 35% of adenocarcinomas and 60% of squamous and large cell carcinomas.[78] Mutations, loss of heterozygosity, and abnormalities in p53 expression suggesting mutation are frequently found in bronchial dysplasia,[172, 248–250] implying that this gene is an early target for mutations in lung carcinogenesis and that study of its mutational spectrum might provide direct clues toward bronchial carcinogens. Such analysis indicates that the p53 gene is a frequent target for external carcinogens and suggests a distinct pattern of mutagens for different cell types. For example, in most cell types, the predominant mutations are the G to T transversions anticipated from bulky tobacco carcinogens, but in adenocarcinomas, G to A transitions are more common.

Other Tumor-Suppressor Genes: RB, 3P, 9P, MCC, APC. Several other known tumor-suppressor genes have been shown to be mutated or deleted in lung cancers. The best characterized is Rb, which is abnormal in over 90% of SCLC tumors and a minority of non–SCLC tumors and lines.[251–253] Studies demonstrating consistent chromosomal deletions or loss of heterozygosity suggest the participation of other tumor-suppressor genes in lung carcinogenesis. Strong evidence exists that an unidentified tumor-suppressor gene critical in SCLC and often non–SCLC development resides on chromosome 3p21.[253–255] Candidate genes in this region include a retinoic acid receptor and protein-tyrosine phosphatase-γ.[224, 256] Two tumor-suppressor genes on chromosome 5 that are important in colon carcinogenesis, MCC and APC, also show frequent loss of heterozygosity in SCLC.[257] Cytogenetic analyses frequently demonstrate losses of chromosome 9p in non–SCLC; a tumor-suppressor gene may reside in the interferon gene cluster in this region.[258] Other chromosomes frequently deleted in lung cancers (e.g., chromosome 11) may also contain tumor-suppressor genes.[203, 234]

The synthesis of clinicopathologic, epidemiologic, and laboratory data in lung cancer research promises insights into basic mechanisms of cell behavior, and opportunities for interventions including prevention, early diagnosis, and therapy. Specific issues being addressed include the identification of mechanisms of tobacco carcinogenesis and possible preventive strategies, the roles of diet and other environmental agents, identification of individual risk, the molecular pathways controlling proliferation and differentiation, and how these processes are affected by carcinogens and may be altered by therapies.

Acknowledgments

The authors would like to thank William Bennett, M.D., Stephane Minvielle, M.D., Steven Krasnow, M.D., and other colleagues for their helpful comments, and Dorothea Dudek for excellent editorial assistance.

SELECTED REFERENCES

Cell Biology, Oncogenes, and Tumor-Suppressor Genes

Aaronson SA: Growth factors and cancer. Science 254:1146, 1991.
Bishop JM: Molecular themes in oncogenesis. Cell 64:235, 1991.
Weinberg RA: Tumor suppressor genes. Science 254:1138, 1991.

General Carcinogenesis

Harris CC: Chemical and physical carcinogenesis: Advances and perspectives. Cancer Res 51:5023s, 1991.
Yuspa SH and Poirier MC: Chemical carcinogenesis: From animal models to molecular models in one decade. Adv Cancer Res 50:25, 1988.

Bronchial Cell Biology

Jetten AM: Growth and differentiation factors in tracheobronchial epithelium. Am J Physiol 260:L361, 1991.

REFERENCES

1. Harris CC: Chemical and physical carcinogenesis: Advances and perspectives. Cancer Res 51:5023s, 1991.
2. Bishop JM: Molecular themes in oncogenesis. Cell 64:235, 1991.
3. Park M, Vande Woude GF: Principles of molecular cell biology of cancer: Oncogenes. *In* DeVita VT, Jr, Hellman S, Rosenberg SA (eds): Cancer: Principles and Practice of Oncology. 3rd Ed. Philadelphia, J. B. Lippincott, 1989, p 45.
4. Yuspa SH, Poirier MC: Chemical carcinogenesis: from animal models to molecular models in one decade. Adv Cancer Res 50:25, 1988.
5. Baserga R: Principles of molecular cell biology of cancer: The cell cycle. *In* DeVita VT Jr, Hellman S, Rosenberg SA (eds): Cancer: Principles and Practice of Oncology. Philadelphia, J. B. Lippincott, 1993, p 60.
6. Jetten AM, Nervi C, Vollberg TM: Control of squamous differentiation in tracheobronchial and epidermal epithelial cells: Role of retinoids. Monogr Natl Cancer Inst 93, 1992.
7. Williams GT: Programmed cell death: Apoptosis and oncogenesis. Cell 65:1097, 1991.
8. Lewin B: Driving the cell cycle: M phase kinase, its partners, and substrates. Cell 61:743, 1990.
9. Sager R: Tumor suppressor genes in the cell cycle. Curr Opin Cell Biol 4:155, 1992.
10. Hartwell L: Defects in a cell cycle checkpoint may be responsible for the genomic instability of cancer cells. Cell 71:543, 1992.
11. Hunter T, Pines J: Cyclins and cancer. Cell 66:1071, 1991.
12. Mendelsohn J, Lippman ME: Principles of molecular cell biology of cancer: Growth factors. *In* DeVita VT Jr, Hellman S, Rosenberg SA (eds): Cancer: Principles and Practice of Oncology. Philadelphia, J. B. Lippincott, 1983, p 114.
13. Cantley LC, Auger KR, Carpenter C, et al.: Oncogenes and signal transduction [published erratum appears in Cell 1991 May 31;65(5):following 914]. Cell 64:281, 1991.
14. Hayflick L, Moorhead PS: The serial cultivation of human diploid cell strains. Exp Cell Res 25:585, 1961.
15. Harris CC: Human tissues and cells in carcinogenesis research. Cancer Res 47:1, 1987.
16. Reddel RR, Hsu IC, Mass MJ, et al.: A human bronchial epithelial cell strain with unusual in vitro growth potential which undergoes neoplastic transformation after SV40 T antigen gene transfection. Int J Cancer 48:764, 1991.
17. Defendi V, Naimski P, Steinberg ML: Human cells transformed by SV40 revisited: the epithelial cells. J Cell Physiol Suppl 2:131, 1982.
18. Nowell PC: The clonal evolution of tumor cell populations. Science 194:23, 1976.
19. Jandl JH: Blood. *In* Textbook of Hematology. Boston, Little, Brown & Co., 1987, p 335.
20. Oda T, Tsuda H, Scarpa A, et al: Mutation pattern of the p53 gene as a diagnostic marker for multiple hepatocellular carcinoma. Cancer Res 52:3674, 1992.
21. Fearon ER, Vogelstein B: A genetic model for colorectal tumorigenesis. Cell 61:759, 1990.
22. Pitot HC: Principles of carcinogenesis: Chemical. *In* DeVita VT Jr, Hellman S, Rosenberg SA (eds): Cancer: Principles and Practice of Oncology. Philadelphia, J. B. Lippincott, 1990, p 116.
23. Foulds L: The experimental study of tumor progression: A review. Cancer Res 14:317, 1954.
24. Rous P, Kidd JG: Conditional neoplasms and subthreshold neoplastic states. J Exp Med 73:365, 1941.
25. Rous P, Friedwald WF: The effect of chemical carcinogens on virus induced rabbit carcinomas. J Exp Med 79:511, 1944.
26. Willey JC, Harris CC: Cellular and molecular biological aspects of human bronchogenic carcinogenesis. Crit Rev Oncol Hematol 10:181, 1990.
27. Armitage P, Doll R: The age distribution of cancer and a multistage theory of carcinogenesis. Br J Cancer 8:1, 1954.
28. Malkinson AM: Primary lung tumors in mice: An experimentally manipulable model of human adenocarcinoma. Cancer Res 52:2670s, 1992.
29. Benfield JR, Hammond WG: Bronchial and pulmonary carci-

nogenesis at focal sites in dogs and hamsters. Cancer Res 52:2687s, 1992.

30. Steele VE, Nettesheim P: Tumor promotion in respiratory tract carcinogenesis. *In* Slaga TJ (ed): Mechanisms of Tumor Promotion. Boca Raton, Florida, CRC Press, 1983, p 91.

31. Yuspa SH, Harris CC: Molecular and cellular basis of chemical carcinogenesis. *In* Schottenfeld D, Fraumeni JF (eds): Cancer Epidemiology and Prevention. Philadelphia, W. B. Saunders, 1982, p 23.

32. Pfeifer A, Lechner JF, Masui T, et al: Control of growth and squamous differentiation in normal human bronchial epithelial cells by chemical and biological modifiers and transferred genes. Environ Health Perspect 80:209, 1989.

33. Schulte-Hermann R, Timmermann-Trosiener I, Schuppler J: Promotion of spontaneous preneoplastic cells in rat liver as a possible explanation of tumor production by nonmutagenic compounds. Cancer Res 43:839, 1983.

34. Popp JA, Scortichini BH, Garvey LK: Quantitative evaluation of hepatic foci of cellular alteration occurring spontaneously in Fischer-344 rats. Fundam Appl Toxicol 5:314, 1985.

35. Grisham JW, Greenberg DS, Kaufman DG, Smith GJ: Cycle-related toxicity and transformation in 10T1/2 cells treated with N-methyl-N'-nitro-N-nitrosoguanidine. Proc Natl Acad Sci U S A 77:4813, 1980.

36. Kakunaga T: The role of cell division in the malignant transformation of mouse cells treated with 3-methylcholanthrene. Cancer Res 35:1637, 1975.

37. Yuspa SH, Ben T, Hennings H, Lichti U: Divergent responses in epidermal basal cells exposed to the tumor promoter 12-O-tetradecanoylphorbol-13-acetate. Cancer Res 42:2344, 1982.

38. Willey JC, Moser CE, Jr, Lechner JF, Harris CC: Differential effects of 12-O-tetradecanoylphorbol-13-acetate on cultured normal and neoplastic human bronchial epithelial cells. Cancer Res 44:5124, 1984.

39. Bursch W, Lauer B, Timmermann-Trosiener I, et al: Controlled death (apoptosis) of normal and putative preneoplastic cells in rat liver following withdrawal of tumor promoters. Carcinogenesis 5:453, 1984.

40. Pitot HC, Glauert HP, Hanigan M: The significance of selected biochemical markers in the characterization of putative initiated cell populations in rodent liver. Cancer Lett 29:1, 1985.

41. Diamond L, O'Brien TG, Baird WM: Tumor promoters and the mechanism of tumor promotion. Adv Cancer Res 32:1, 1980.

42. Ashendel CL: The phorbol ester receptor: A phospholipid-regulated protein kinase. Biochim Biophys Acta 822:219, 1985.

43. Hennings H, Shores R, Balaschak M, Yuspa SH: Sensitivity of subpopulations of mouse skin papillomas to malignant conversion by urethane or 4-nitroquinoline N-oxide. Cancer Res 50:653, 1990.

44. Hennings H, Shores R, Wenk ML, et al: Malignant conversion of mouse skin tumours is increased by tumour initiators and unaffected by tumour promoters. Nature 304:67, 1983.

45. O'Connell JF, Klein-Szanto AJ, Digiovanni DM, et al: Malignant progression of mouse skin papillomas treated with ethylnitrosourea, N-methyl-N'-nitro-N-nitrosoguanidine, or 12-O-tetradecanoylphorbol-13-acetate. Cancer Lett 30:269, 1986.

46. Hennings H, Shores R, Mitchell P, et al: Induction of papillomas with a high probability of conversion to malignancy. Carcinogenesis 6:1607, 1985.

47. U.S. Dept. of Health and Human Services: The health benefits of smoking cessation. *In* DHHS, PHS, Centers for Disease Control, Office on Smoking and Health (eds): A Report of the Surgeon General. Bethesda, Maryland, DHHS Publication (CDC)90-8416, 1990.

48. Yin Y, Tainsky MA, Bischoff FZ, et al: Wild-type p53 restores cell cycle control and inhibits gene amplification in cells with mutant p53 alleles. Cell 70:937, 1992.

49. Livingstone LR, White A, Sprouse J, et al: Altered cell cycle arrest and gene amplification potential accompany loss of wild-type p53. Cell 70:923, 1992.

50. Liotta LA: Tumor invasion and metastases—role of the extracellular matrix: Rhoads Memorial Award lecture. Cancer Res 46:1, 1986.

51. Liotta LA, Steeg PS, Stetler-Stevenson WG: Cancer metastasis and angiogenesis: An imbalance of positive and negative regulation. Cell 64:327, 1991.

52. Deuchars KL, Ling V: P-glycoprotein and multidrug resistance in cancer chemotherapy. Semin Oncol 16:156, 1989.

53. Strauss B: The origin of point mutations in human tumor cells. Cancer Res 52:249, 1992.

54. Hall EJ: Principles of carcinogenesis: Physical. *In* DeVita VT Jr, Hellman S, Rosenberg SA (eds): Cancer: Principles and Practice of Oncology. Philadelphia, J. B. Lippincott, 1993, p 213.

55. Kennaway EL, Hieger I: Carcinogenic substances and their fluorescence spectra. Br Med J 1:1044, 1930.

56. Miller EC: Some current perspectives on chemical carcinogenesis in humans and experimental animals: Presidential address. Cancer Res 38:1479, 1978.

57. Miller EC: Studies on the formation of protein-bound derivatives of 3,4-benzpyrene in the epidermal fraction of mouse skin. Cancer Res 11:100, 1951.

58. Hecht SS, Foiles PG, Carmella SG, et al: Recent studies on the metabolic activation of tobacco-specific nitrosamines: prospects for dosimetry in humans. *In* Hoffmann D, Harris CC (eds): Banbury Report 23: Mechanisms in Tobacco Carcinogenesis. New York, Cold Spring Harbor Laboratory, 1986, p 245.

59. Hruszkewycz AM, Canella KA, Peltonen K, et al: DNA polymerase action on benzo[a]pyrene-DNA adducts. Carcinogenesis 13:2347, 1992.

60. Horsfall MJ, Gordon AJ, Burns PA, et al: Mutational specificity of alkylating agents and the influence of DNA repair. Environ Mol Mutagen 15:107, 1990.

61. Poirier MC, Beland FA: DNA adduct measurements and tumor incidence during chronic carcinogen exposure in animal models: Implications for DNA adduct-based human cancer risk assessment [see comments]. Chem Res Toxicol 5:749, 1992.

62. Strauss BS: The "A rule" of mutagen specificity: A consequence of DNA polymerase bypass of non-instructional lesions? Bioessays 13:79, 1991.

63. Wogan GN, Gorelick NJ: Chemical and biochemical dosimetry of exposure to genotoxic chemicals. Environ Health Perspect 62:5, 1985.

64. Beland FA, Poirier MC: DNA adducts and carcinogenesis. *In* Sirica AE (ed): The Pathobiology of Neoplasia. New York, Plenum Publishing Corp., 1989, p 57.

65. Phillips DH, Hewer A, Martin CN, et al: Correlation of DNA adduct levels in human lung with cigarette smoking. Nature 336:790, 1988.

66. Harris CC: Future directions in the use of DNA adducts as internal dosimeters for monitoring human exposure to environmental mutagens and carcinogens. Environ Health Perspect 62:185, 1985.

67. Perera FP, Hemminki K, Young TL, et al: Detection of polycyclic aromatic hydrocarbon-DNA adducts in white blood cells of foundry workers. Cancer Res 48:2288, 1988.

68. Mustonen R, Schoket B, Hemminki K: Smoking-related DNA adducts: ^{32}P-postlabeling analysis of 7-methylguanine in human bronchial and lymphocyte DNA. Carcinogenesis 14:151, 1993.

69. Moldeus P, Berggren M, Grafstrom RC: N-acetylcysteine protection against the toxicity of cigarette smoke and cigarette smoke condensates in various tissues and cells in vitro. Eur J Respir Dis 139(suppl):123, 1985.

70. Shields PG, Bowman ED, Harrington AM, et al.: Polycyclic aromatic hydrocarbon DNA adducts in human lung and cancer susceptibility genes. Cancer Res 53:3486, 1993.

71. Brockmöller J, Kerb R, Drakoulis N, et al: Genotype and phenotype of glutathione S-transferase class mu isoenzymes mu and psi in lung cancer patients and controls. Cancer Res 53:1004, 1993.

72. Reid TM, Loeb LA: Tandem double CC → TT mutations are produced by reactive oxygen species. Proc Natl Acad Sci U S A 90:3904, 1993.

73. Reid TM, Loeb LA: Mutagenic specificity of oxygen radicals produced by human leukemia cells. Cancer Res 52:1082, 1992.

74. Ehrlich M, Zhang XY, Inamdar NM: Spontaneous deamination of cytosine and 5-methylcytosine residues in DNA and replacement of 5-methylcytosine residues with cytosine residues. Mutat Res 238:277, 1990.

75. Wink DA, Kasprzak KS, Maragos CM, et al: DNA deaminating ability and genotoxicity of nitric oxide and its progenitors. Science 254:1001, 1991.

76. Wilson VL, Smith RA, Longoria J, et al: Chemical carcinogen-induced decreases in genomic 5-methyldeoxycytidine content of normal human bronchial epithelial cells. Proc Natl Acad Sci U S A 84:3298, 1987.

77. Hollstein M, Sidransky D, Vogelstein B, Harris CC: p53 mutations in human cancers. Science 253:49, 1991.

78. Greenblatt MS, Bennett WP, Hollstein M, Harris CC: Mutations in the p53 tumor suppressor gene: Clues to cancer etiology and molecular pathogenesis. Cancer Res 55:4855, 1994.

79. Loeb LA, Cheng KC: Errors in DNA synthesis: A source of spontaneous mutations. Mutat Res 238:297, 1990.

80. Loeb LA, Preston BD: Mutagenesis by apurinic/apyrimidinic sites. Annu Rev Genet 20:201, 1986.

81. Marnett LJ: Peroxyl free radicals: Potential mediators of tumor initiation and promotion. Carcinogenesis 8:1365, 1987.

82. Bohr VA, Phillips DH, Hanawalt PC: Heterogeneous DNA damage and repair in the mammalian genome Cancer Res 47:6426, 1987. (Published erratum appears in Cancer Res 48[5]:1377, 1988.)

83. Burt RK, Poirier MC, Link CJ Jr, Bohr VA: Antineoplastic drug resistance and DNA repair. Ann Oncol 2:325, 1991.

84. Hanawalt PC: Preferential DNA repair in expressed genes. Environ Health Perspect 76:9, 1987.

85. Xanthoudakis S, Miao G, Wang F, et al: Redox activation of Fos-Jun DNA binding activity is mediated by a DNA repair enzyme. EMBO J 11:3323, 1992.

86. Schaeffer L, Roy R, Humbert S, et al: DNA repair helicase: A component of BTF2 (TFIIH) basic transcription factor. Science 260:58, 1993.

87. Tokuhata GK, Lilienfeld AM: Familial aggregation of lung cancers in humans. J Natl Cancer Inst 30:289, 1963.

88. Ooi WL, Elston RC, Chen VW, et al: Increased familial risk for lung cancer. J Natl Cancer Inst 76:217, 1986.

89. Lynch HT, Kimberling WJ, Markvicka SE, et al: Genetics and smoking-associated cancers: A study of 485 families. Cancer 57:1640, 1986.

90. Samet JM, Humble CG, Pathak DR: Personal and family history of respiratory disease and lung cancer risk. Am Rev Respir Dis 134:466, 1986.

91. Horwitz RI, Smaldone LF, Viscoli CM: An ecogenetic hypothesis for lung cancer in women [see comments]. Arch Intern Med 148:2609, 1988.

92. Davila DG, Williams DE: The etiology of lung cancer. Mayo Clin Proc 68:170, 1993.

93. Sellers TA, Bailey-Wilson JE, Elston RC, et al: Evidence for mendelian inheritance in the pathogenesis of lung cancer. J Natl Cancer Inst 82:1272, 1990.

94. Friend SH, Bernards R, Rogelj S, et al: A human DNA segment with properties of the gene that predisposes to retinoblastoma and osteosarcoma. Nature 323:643:1986.

95. Malkin D, Li FP, Strong LC, et al: Germ line p53 mutations in a familial syndrome of breast cancer, sarcomas, and other neoplasms. Science 250:1233, 1990.

96. Weston A, Caporaso NE, Perrin LS, et al: Relationship of H-ras-1, L-myc, and p53 polymorphisms with lung cancer risk and prognosis. Environ Health Perspect 98:61, 1992.

97. Heighway J, Thatcher N, Cerny T, Hasleton PS: Genetic predisposition to human lung cancer. Br J Cancer 53:453, 1986.

98. Sugimura H, Caporaso NE, Hoover RN, et al: Association of rare alleles of the Harvey *ras* protooncogene locus with lung cancer. Cancer Res 50:1857, 1990.

99. Ryberg D, Tefre T, Skaug V, et al: Allele diversity of the H-ras-1: Variable number of tandem repeats in Norwegian lung cancer patients. Environ Health Perspect 98:187, 1992.

100. Weston A, Perrin LS, Forrester K, et al: Allelic frequency of a p53 polymorphism in human lung cancer. Cancer Epidemiology, Biomarkers, and Prevention 1:481, 1992.

101. Tamai S, Sugimura H, Caporaso NE, et al: Restriction fragment length polymorphism analysis of the L-*myc* gene locus in a case-control study of lung cancer. Int J Cancer 46:411, 1990.

102. You M, Wang Y, Stoner G, et al: Parental bias of Ki-ras oncogenes detected in lung tumors from mouse hybrids. Proc Natl Acad Sci U S A 89:5804, 1992.

103. Ryan J, Barker PE, Nesbitt MN, Ruddle FH: KRAS2 as a genetic marker for lung tumor susceptibility in inbred mice. J Natl Cancer Inst 79:1351, 1987.

104. Skillrud DM, Offord KP, Miller RD: Higher risk of lung cancer in chronic obstructive pulmonary disease. A prospective, matched, controlled study. Ann Intern Med 105:503, 1986.

104. Tockman MS, Anthonisen NR, Wright EC, Donithan MG: Airways obstruction and the risk for lung cancer. Ann Intern Med 106:512, 1987.

106. Kuller LH, Ockene J, Meilahn E, Svendsen KH: Relation of forced expiratory volume in one second (FEV_1) to lung cancer mortality in the Multiple Risk Factor Intervention Trial (MRFIT). Am J Epidemiol 132:265, 1990.

107. Nomura A, Stemmermann GN, Chyou PH, et al: Prospective study of pulmonary function and lung cancer. Am Rev Respir Dis 144:307, 1991.

108. Harris CC: Tobacco smoke and lung disease: Who is susceptible? Ann Intern Med 105:607, 1986.

109. Peters-Golden M, Wise RA, Hochberg M, et al.: Incidence of lung cancer in systemic sclerosis. J Rheumatol 12:1136, 1985.

110. Auerbach O, Garfinkel L, Parks VR: Scar cancer of the lung: Increase over a 21 year period. Cancer 43:636, 1979.

111. Shimosato Y, Suzuki A, Hashimoto T, et al: Prognostic implications of fibrotic focus (scar) in small peripheral lung cancers. Am J Surg Pathol 4:365, 1980.

112. Madri JA, Carter D: Scar cancers of the lung: origin and significance. Hum Pathol 15:625, 1984.

113. Barsky SH, Huang SJ, Bhuta S: The extracellular matrix of pulmonary scar carcinomas is suggestive of a desmoplastic origin. Am J Pathol 124:412, 1986.

114. Yoneda K: Scar carcinomas of the lung in a histoplasmosis endemic area. Cancer 65:164, 1990.

115. Shields PG, Harris CC: Molecular epidemiology and the genetics of environmental cancer. JAMA 266:681, 1991.

116. Carmella SG, Kagan SS, Kagan M, et al: Mass spectrometric analysis of tobacco-specific nitrosamine hemoglobin adducts in snuff dippers, smokers, and nonsmokers. Cancer Res 50:5438, 1990.

117. Foiles PG, Murphy SE, Peterson LA, et al: DNA and hemoglobin adducts as markers of metabolic activation of tobacco-specific carcinogens. Cancer Res 52:2698s, 1992.

118. Weston A, Caporaso NE, Taghizadeh K, et al: Measurement of 4-aminobiphenyl-hemoglobin adducts in lung cancer cases and controls. Cancer Res 51:5219, 1991.

119. Philip PA, Fitzgerald DL, Cartwright RA, et al: Polymorphic N-acetylation capacity in lung cancer. Carcinogenesis 9:491, 1988.

120. Horsmans Y, Desager JP, Harvengt C: Is there a link between debrisoquine oxidation phenotype and lung cancer susceptibility? Biomed Pharmacother 45:359, 1991.

121. Amos CI, Caporaso NE, Weston A: Host factors in lung cancer risk: a review of interdisciplinary studies. Cancer Epidemiology, Biomarkers and Prevention 1:505, 1992.

122. Ayesh R, Idle JR, Ritchie JC, et al: Metabolic oxidation phenotypes as markers for susceptibility to lung cancer. Nature 312:169, 1984.

123. Caporaso NE, Tucker MA, Hoover R, et al: Lung cancer and the debrisoquine metabolic phenotype. J Natl Cancer Inst 85:1264, 1990.

124. Wolf CR, Smith CA, Gough AC, et al: Relationship between the debrisoquine hydroxylase polymorphism and cancer susceptibility. Carcinogenesis 13:1035, 1992.

125. Sugimura H, Caporaso NE, Shaw GL, et al: Human debrisoquine hydroxylase gene polymorphisms in cancer patients and controls. Carcinogenesis 11:1527, 1990.

126. Heckbert SR, Weiss NS, Hornung SK, et al: Glutathione S-transferase and epoxide hydrolase activity in human leukocytes in relation to risk of lung cancer and other smoking-related cancers. J Natl Cancer Inst 84:414, 1992.

127. Zhong S, Howie AF, Ketterer B, et al: Glutathione S-transferase mu locus: Use of genotyping and phenotyping assays to assess association with lung cancer susceptibility. Carcinogenesis 12:1533, 1991.

128. Kawajiri K, Nakachi K, Imai K, et al: Identification of genetically high risk individuals to lung cancer by DNA polymorphisms of the cytochrome P450IA1 gene. FEBS Lett 263:131, 1990.

129. Uematsu F, Kikuchi H, Motomiya M, et al: Association between restriction fragment length polymorphism of the human

cytochrome P450IIE1 gene and susceptibility to lung cancer. Jpn J Cancer Res 82:254, 1991.

130. Kato S, Shields PG, Caporaso NE, et al: Cytochrome P450IIE1 genetic polymorphisms, racial variation, and lung cancer risk. Cancer Res 52:6712, 1992.

131. Aguayo SM, King TE Jr, Kane MA, et al: Urinary levels of bombesin-like peptides in asymptomatic cigarette smokers: A potential risk marker for smoking-related diseases. Cancer Res 52:2727s, 1992.

132. Aguayo SM, Kane MA, King TE Jr, et al: Increased levels of bombesin-like peptides in the lower respiratory tract of asymptomatic cigarette smokers. J Clin Invest 84:1105, 1989.

133. Pisani RJ: Bronchogenic carcinoma: Immunologic aspects. Mayo Clin Proc 68:386, 1993.

134. Groopman JD, Broder S: Cancer in AIDS and other immuno-deficiency states. In DeVita VT Jr, Hellman S, Rosenberg SA (eds): Cancer: Principles and Practice of Oncology. Philadelphia, J. B. Lippincott, 1989, p 1953.

135. Prehn RT: Immunological basis for differences in susceptibility to hydrocarbon oncogenesis among mice of a single genotype. Int J Cancer 24:789, 1979.

136. Ioachim HL, Dorsett BH, Paluch E: The immune response at the tumor site in lung carcinoma. Cancer 38:2296, 1976.

137. Doyle A, Martin WJ, Funa K, et al: Markedly decreased expression of class I histocompatibility antigens, protein, and mRNA in human small-cell lung cancer. J Exp Med 161:1135, 1985.

138. Okubo A, Sone S, Singh SM, Ogura T: Production of tumor necrosis factor-alpha by alveolar macrophages of lung cancer patients. Jpn J Cancer Res 81:403, 1990.

139. Hosker HS, Corris PA: Alveolar macrophage and blood monocyte function in lung cancer. Cancer Detect Prev 15:103, 1991.

140. Piazza G, Marchi E, Scaglione F, et al: Lymphocyte subsets in bronchoalveolar lavage fluid and in circulating blood in epidermoid bronchogenic carcinoma. Respiration 57:28, 1990.

141. U.S. Dept. HEW: Smoking and health: report of the advisory committee to the Surgeon General. In CDC (ed): PHS Publication No. 1103. Washington, DC, US Govt. Printing Office, 1964.

142. Royal College of Physicians: Smoking and Health Summary and Report of the Royal College of Physicians of London of smoking in Relation to Cancer of the Lung and Other Diseases. New York, Pitman, 1962.

143. Shopland DR, Eyre HJ, Pechacek TF: Smoking-attributable cancer mortality in 1991: Is lung cancer now the leading cause of death among smokers in the United States? J Natl Cancer Inst 83:1142, 1991.

144. DeMarini DM: Genotoxicity of tobacco smoke and tobacco smoke condensate. Mutat Res 114:59, 1983.

145. Hoffmann D, Wynder EL, Rivenson A, et al: Skin bioassays in tobacco carcinogenesis. Prog Exp Tumor Res 26:43, 1983.

146. Matsukura N, Willey J, Miyashita M, et al: Detection of direct mutagenicity of cigarette smoke condensate in mammalian cells. Carcinogenesis 12:685, 1991.

147. Miyashita M, Willey JC, Sasajima K, et al: Differential effects of cigarette smoke condensate and its fractions on cultured normal and malignant human bronchial epithelial cells. Exp Pathol 38:19, 1990.

148. Klein-Szanto AJP, Iizasa T, Momiki S, et al: A tobacco-specific N-nitrosamine or cigarette smoke condensate causes neoplastic transformation of xenotransplanted human bronchial epithelial cells. Proc Natl Acad Sci U S A 89:6693, 1992.

149. Hecht SS, Hoffmann D: Tobacco-specific nitrosamines, an important group of carcinogens in tobacco and tobacco smoke. Carcinogenesis 9:875, 1988.

150. Harris CC, Kaufman DG, Sporn MB, et al: Ultrastructural effects of N-methyl-N-nitrosourea on the tracheobronchial epithelium of the Syrian golden hamster. Int J Cancer 12:259, 1973.

151. Hoffmann D, Hecht SS, Wynder EL: Tumor promoters and cocarcinogens in tobacco carcinogenesis. Environ Health Perspect 50:247, 1983.

152. Hoffmann D, Melikian A, Adams JD Jr, et al: New aspects of tobacco carcinogenesis. Carcinog Compr Surv 8:239, 1985.

153. Saladino AJ, Willey JC, Lechner JF, et al: Effects of formaldehyde, acetaldehyde, benzoyl peroxide, and hydrogen peroxide on cultured normal human bronchial epithelial cells. Cancer Res 45:2522, 1985.

154. Harris CC, Willey JC, Matsukura N, et al: Pathobiological effects of fibers and tobacco-related chemicals in human lung cells in vitro. In Mohr U, Dungworth D, Kimmerle G, et al(eds): Assessment of Inhalation Hazards: Integration and Extrapolation Using Diverse Data. New York, Springer-Verlag, 1989, p 103.

155. Grafstrom RC, Curren RD, Yang LL, Harris CC: Genotoxicity of formaldehyde in cultured human bronchial fibroblasts. Science 228:89, 1985.

156. Little JB, O'Toole WF: Respiratory tract tumors in hamsters induced by benzo[a]pyrene and 21P alpha radiation. Cancer Res 34:3026, 1974.

157. Shami SG, Thibodeau LA, Kennedy AR, Little JB: Proliferative and morphological changes in the pulmonary epithelium of the Syrian golden hamster during carcinogenesis initiated by 210Po alpha alpha-radiation. Cancer Res 42:1405, 1982.

158. Byrd JC: Environmental tobacco smoke: Medical and legal issues. Med Clin North Am 76:377, 1992.

159. U.S. Department of Health, Education and Welfare: Smoking and health. In A Report of the Surgeon General. DHEW Publication No. (PHS) 79-50066, 1988, p 5.

160. Hammond SK, Coghlin J, Gann PH, et al: Relationship between environmental tobacco smoke exposure and carcinogen-hemoglobin adduct levels in nonsmokers. J Natl Cancer Inst 85:474, 1993.

161. Maclure M, Katz RB, Bryant MS, et al: Elevated blood levels of carcinogens in passive smokers. Am J Public Health 79:1381, 1989.

162. Samet JM: Radon and lung cancer. J Natl Cancer Inst 81:745, 1989.

163. Harting FH, Hesse W: Der lungenkrebs, die bergkrankheit in den schneeberger gruben. Vrtljschr Gerlichtl Med 30:296, 1879.

164. Moolgavkar SH, Luebeck EG, Krewski D, Zielinski JM: Radon, cigarette smoke, and lung cancer: A re-analysis of the Colorado plateau uranium miners' data. Epidemiology 4:204, 1993.

165. Pershagen G, Akerblom G, Axelson O, et al: Residential radon exposure and lung cancer in Sweden. N Engl J Med 330:159, 1994.

166. Neuberger JS: Residential radon exposure and lung cancer: an overview of ongoing studies. Health Phys 63:503, 1992. (Published erratum appears in Health Phys Mar; 64[3]:333, 1993.)

167. Morlier JP, Morin M, Chameaud J, et al: [Importance of the role of dose rate on tumor induction in rats after radon inhalation]. C R Acad Sci III 315:463, 1992.

168. Moolgavkar SH, Cross FT, Luebeck G, Dagle GE: A two-mutation model for radon-induced lung tumors in rats. Radiat Res 121:28, 1990.

169. Saccomanno G, Huth GC, Auerbach O, Kuschner M: Relationship of radioactive radon daughters and cigarette smoking in the genesis of lung cancer in uranium miners. Cancer 62:1402, 1988.

170. Butler C, Samet JM, Black WC, et al: Histopathologic findings of lung cancer in Navajo men: Relationship to U mining. Health Phys 51:365, 1986.

171. Saccomanno G: The contribution of uranium miners to lung cancer histogenesis. Recent Results Cancer Res 82:43, 1982.

172. Vahakangas KH, Samet JM, Metcalf RA, et al: Mutations of p53 and ras genes in radon-associated lung cancer from uranium miners. Lancet 339:576, 1992.

173. Taylor JA, Watson MA, Devereux TR, et al: Mutational hotspot in the p53 gene in radon-associated lung tumors from uranium miners. Lancet 343:86, 1993.

174. Craighead JE, Mossman BT: The pathogenesis of asbestos-associated diseases. N Engl J Med 306:1446, 1982.

175. Doll R: Mortality from lung cancer in asbestos workers. Br J Ind Med 12:81, 1955.

176. Berry G, Newhouse ML, Antonis P: Combined effect of asbestos and smoking on mortality from lung cancer and mesothelioma in factory workers. Br J Ind Med 42:12, 1985.

177. Whitesell PL, Drage CW: Occupational lung cancer. Mayo Clin Proc 68:183, 1993.

178. Gabrielson EW, Van der Meeren A, Reddel RR, et al: Human mesothelioma cells and asbestos-exposed mesothelial cells are selectively resistant to amosite toxicity: A possible mechanism for tumor promotion by asbestos. Carcinogenesis 13:1359, 1992.

179. Lechner JF, Tokiwa T, LaVeck MA, et al: Asbestos-associated

chromosomal changes in human mesothelial cells. Proc Natl Acad Sci U S A 82:3884, 1985.

180. Maehle L, Metcalf RA, Ryberg D, et al: Altered p53 gene structure and expression in human epithelial cells after exposure to nickel. Cancer Res 52:218, 1992.

181. Sunderman FW Jr: Carcinogenic effects of metals. Fed Proc 37:40, 1978.

182. Waalkes MP, Coogan TP, Barter RA: Toxicological principles of metal carcinogenesis with special emphasis on cadmium. Crit Rev Toxicol 22:175, 1992.

183. Becher H, Jedrychowski W, Wahrendorf J, et al: Effect of occupational air pollutants on various histological types of lung cancer: A population based case-control study. Br J Ind Med 50:136, 1993.

184. Jedrychowski W, Becher H, Wahrendorf J, Basa-Cierpialek Z: A case-control study of lung cancer with special reference to the effect of air pollution in Poland. J Epidemiol Community Health 44:114, 1990.

185. Pershagen G, Simonato L: Epidemiological evidence on air pollution and cancer. In Tomatis L (ed): Air Pollution and Human Cancer. Berlin, Springer-Verlag, 1990, p 63.

186. Qu YH, Xu GX, Zhou JZ, et al: Genotoxicity of heated cooking oil vapors. Mutat Res 298:105, 1992.

187. Xu ZY, Blot WJ, Xiao HP, et al: Smoking, air pollution, and the high rates of lung cancer in Shenyang, China. J Natl Cancer Inst 81:1800, 1989.

188. Mumford JL, He XZ, Chapman RS: Human lung cancer risks due to complex organic mixtures of combustion emissions. Recent Results Cancer Res 120:181, 1990.

189. Syrjanen KJ, Syrjanen SM: Human papillomavirus DNA in bronchial squamous cell carcinomas. Lancet 1:168, 1987.

190. Block G, Patterson B, Subar A: Fruit, vegetables, and cancer prevention: A review of the epidemiological evidence. Nutr Cancer 18:1, 1992.

191. Steinmetz KA, Potter JD, Folsom AR: Vegetables, fruit, and lung cancer in the Iowa Women's Health Study. Cancer Res 53:536, 1993.

192. Mathe G, Gouveia J, Hercend T, et al: Correlation between precancerous bronchial metaplasia and cigarette consumption, and preliminary results of retinoid treatment. Cancer Detect Prev 5:461, 1982.

193. Gouveia J, Mathë G, Hercend T, et al: Degree of bronchial metaplasia in heavy smokers and its regression after treatment with a retinoid. Lancet 1:710, 1982.

194. Le Marchand L, Hankin JH, Kolonel LN, et al: Intake of specific carotenoids and lung cancer risk. Cancer Epidemiology, Biomarkers, and Prevention 2:183, 1993.

195. Willett WC: Vitamin A and lung cancer. Nutr Rev 48:201, 1990.

196. Ziegler RG: Vegetables, fruits, and carotenoids and the risk of cancer. Am J Clin Nutr 53:251S, 1991.

197. The Alpha Tocopherol, Beta Carotene Cancer Prevention Study Group: The effect of vitamin E and beta carotene on the incidence of lung cancer and other cancers in male smokers. N Engl J Med 330:1029, 1994.

198. Goodman MT, Hankin JH, Wilkens LR, Kolonel LN: High-fat foods and the risk of lung cancer. Epidemiology 3:288, 1992.

199. Basbaum C, Jany B: Plasticity in the airway epithelium. Am J Physiol 259:L38, 1990.

200. Jetten AM: Growth and differentiation factors in tracheobronchial epithelium. Am J Physiol 260:L361, 1991.

201. McDowell EM, Trump BF: Histogenesis of preneoplastic and neoplastic lesions in tracheobronchial epithelium. Surv Synth Path Res 2:235, 1983.

202. Gazdar AF, Linnoila RI, Kurita Y, et al: Peripheral airway cell differentiation in human lung cancer cell lines. Cancer Res 50:5481, 1990.

203. Buchhagen DL: Molecular mechanisms in lung pathogenesis. Biochim Biophys Acta 1072:159, 1991.

204. Willey JC, Lechner JF, Harris CC: Bombesin and the C-terminal tetradecapeptide of gastrin-releasing peptide are growth factors for normal human bronchial epithelial cells. Exp Cell Res 153:245, 1984.

205. Miyashita M, Smith MW, Willey JC, et al: Effects of serum, transforming growth factor type beta, or 12-O-tetradecanoyl-phorbol-13-acetate on ionized cytosolic calcium concentration in normal and transformed human bronchial epithelial cells. Cancer Res 49:63, 1989.

206. Yoakum GH, Lechner JF, Gabrielson EW, et al: Transformation of human bronchial epithelial cells transfected by Harvey ras oncogene. Science 227:1174, 1985.

207. Willey JC, Broussoud A, Sleemi A, et al: Immortalization of normal human bronchial epithelial cells by human papillomaviruses 16 or 18. Cancer Res 51:5370, 1991.

208. Reddel RR, Ke Y, Gerwin BI, et al: Transformation of human bronchial epithelial cells by infection with SV40 or adenovirus-12 SV40 hybrid virus, or transfection via strontium phosphate coprecipitation with a plasmid containing SV40 early region genes. Cancer Res 48:1904, 1988.

209. Levine AJ, Momand J, Finlay CA: The p53 tumour suppressor gene. Nature 351:453, 1991.

210. Gerwin BI, Spillare E, Forrester K, et al: Mutant p53 can induce tumorigenic conversion of human bronchial epithelial cells and reduce their responsiveness to a negative growth factor, transforming growth factor type B1. Proc Natl Acad Sci U S A 89:2759, 1992.

211. Noguchi M, Murakami M, Bennett WP, et al: Biological consequences of overexpression of a transfected c-erbB-2 gene in "immortalized" human bronchial epithelial cells. Cancer Res 53:2035, 1993.

212. Amstad P, Reddel RR, Pfeifer A, et al: Neoplastic transformation of a human bronchial epithelial cell line by a recombinant retrovirus encoding viral Harvey ras. Mol Carcinog 1:151, 1988.

213. Pfeifer A, Mark GE, Malan-Shibley L, et al.: Cooperation of c-raf-1 and c-myc protooncogenes in the neoplastic transformation of SV40 T-antigen immortalized human bronchial epithelial cells. Proc Natl Acad Sci U S A 86:10075, 1989.

214. Pfeifer AMA, Jones RT, Bowden PE, et al: Human bronhcial epithelial cells transformed by the c-raf-1 and c-myc protooncogenes induce multi-differentiated carcinomas in nude mice: A model for lung carcinogenesis. Cancer Res 51:3793, 1991.

215. Reddel RR, Salghetti SE, Willey JC, et al: Development of tumorigenicity in SV40-immortalized human bronchial epithelial cell lines. Cancer Res 53:985, 1993.

216. Carney DN, Gazdar AF, Bepler G, et al: Establishment and identification of small cell lung cancer cell lines having classic and variant features. Cancer Res 45:2913, 1985.

217. Gazdar AF, Carney DN, Nau MM, Minna JD: Characterization of variant subclasses of cell lines derived from small cell lung cancer having distinctive biochemical, morphological, and growth properties. Cancer Res 45:2924, 1985.

218. Johnson BE, Battey JF, Linnoila I, et al: Changes in the phenotype of human small cell lung cancer cell lines after transfection and expression of the c-myc proto-oncogene. J Clin Invest 78:525, 1986.

219. Bergh JC: Gene amplification in human lung cancer: The myc family genes and other proto-oncogenes and growth factor genes. Am Rev Respir Dis 142:S20, 1990.

220. Makela TP, Mattson K, Alitalo K: Tumour markers and oncogenes in lung cancer. Eur J Cancer 27:1323, 1991.

221. Viallet J, Minna JD: Gastrin-releasing peptide (GRP, mammalian bombesin) in the pathogenesis of lung cancer. Prog Growth Factor Res 1:89, 1989.

222. Doyle LA, Giangiulo D, Hussain A, et al: Differentiation of human variant small cell lung cancer cell lines to a classic morphology by retinoic acid. Cancer Res 49:6745, 1989.

223. Nervi C, Vollberg TM, George MD, et al: Expression of nuclear retinoic acid receptors in normal tracheobronchial cells and in lung carcinoma cells. Exp Cell Res 195:163, 1991.

224. Houle B, Rochette-Egly C, Bradley WE: Tumor-suppressive effect of the retinoic acid receptor beta in human epidermoid lung cancer cells. Proc Natl Acad Sci U S A 90:985, 1993.

225. Rodenhuis S, Slebos RJ: Clinical significance of ras oncogene activation in human lung cancer. Cancer Res 52:2665s, 1992.

226. Mitsudomi T, Steinberg SM, Nau MM, et al: p53 gene mutations in non-small-cell lung cancer cell lines and their correlation with the presence of ras mutations and clinical features. Oncogene 7:171, 1992.

227. Mukhopadhyay T, Tainsky M, Cavender AC, Roth JA: Specific inhibition of K-ras expression and tumorigenicity of lung cancer cells by antisense RNA. Cancer Res 51:1744, 1991.

228. Georges RN, Mukhopadhyay T, Zhang Y, et al: Prevention of orthotopic human lung cancer growth by intratracheal instil-

lation of a retroviral antisense K-ras construct. Cancer Res 53:1743, 1993.

229. Kiefer PE, Wegmann B, Bacher M, et al: Different pattern of expression of cellular oncogenes in human non-small-cell lung cancer cell lines. J Cancer Res Clin Oncol 116:29, 1990.

230. Kaighn ME, Gabrielson EW, Iman DS, et al: Suppression of tumorigenicity of a human lung carcinoma line by nontumorigenic bronchial epithelial cells in somatic cell hybrids. Cancer Res 50:1890, 1990.

231. Takahashi T, Carbone D, Nau MM, et al: Wild-type but not mutant p53 suppresses the growth of human lung cancer cells bearing multiple genetic lesions. Cancer Res 52:2340, 1992.

232. Caamano J, DiRado M, Iizasa T, et al: Partial suppression of tumorigenicity in a human lung cancer cell line transfected with Krev-1. Mol Carcinog 6:252, 1992.

233. Cajot JF, Anderson MJ, Lehman TA, et al: Growth suppression mediated by transfection of p53 in Hut292DM human lung cancer cells expressing endogenous wild-type p53 protein. Cancer Res 52:6956, 1992.

234. Weston A, Willey JC, Modali R, et al: Differential DNA sequence deletions from chromosomes 3, 11, 13 and 17 in squamous cell carcinoma, large cell carcinoma and adenocarcinoma of the human lung. Proc Natl Acad Sci U S A 86:5099, 1989.

235. Biegel JA, Burk CD, Barr FG, Emanuel BS: Evidence for a 17p tumor related locus distinct from p53 in pediatric primitive neuroectodermal tumors. Cancer Res 52:3391, 1992.

236. Rodenhuis S, Slebos RJ, Boot AJ, et al: Incidence and possible clinical significance of K-ras oncogene activation in adenocarcinoma of the human lung. Cancer Res 48:5738, 1988.

237. Suzuki Y, Orita M, Shiraishi M, et al: Detection of *ras* gene mutations in human lung cancers by single-strand conformation polymorphism analysis of polymerase chain reaction products. Oncogene 5:1037, 1990.

238. Carbone DP, Minna JD: The molecular genetics of lung cancer. Adv Intern Med 37:153, 1992.

239. Mabry M, Nakagawa T, Baylin S, et al: Insertion of the v-Ha-ras oncogene induces differentiation of calcitonin-producing human small cell lung cancer. J Clin Invest 84:194, 1989.

240. Mabry M, Nakagawa T, Nelkin BD, et al: v-Ha-ras oncogene insertion: a model for tumor progression of human small cell lung cancer. Proc Natl Acad Sci U S A 85:6523, 1988.

241. Slebos RJ, Kibbelaar RE, Dalesio O, et al: K-*ras* oncogene activation as a prognostic marker in adenocarcinoma of the lung. N Engl J Med 323:561, 1990.

242. Mitsudomi T, Steinberg SM, Oie HK, et al: ras gene mutations in non-small cell lung cancers are associated with shortened survival irrespective of treatment intent. Cancer Res 51:4999, 1991.

243. Kern JA, Schwartz D, Nordberg JA, et al: p185neu expression in human lung adenocarcinomas predicts shortened survival. Cancer Res 50:5184, 1990.

244. Makela TP, Shiraishi M, Borrello MG, et al: Rearrangement and co-amplification of L-myc and rlf in primary lung cancer. Oncogene 7:405, 1992.

245. Montenarh M: Functional implications of the growth-suppressor/oncoprotein p53 (Review). Int J Oncol 1:37, 1992.

246. Vogelstein B, Kinzler KW: p53 function and dysfunction. Cell 70:523, 1992.

247. Lane DP, Benchimol S: p53: oncogene or anti-oncogene? Genes Dev 4:1, 1990.

248. Sundaresan V, Ganly P, Hasleton P, et al: p53 and chromosome 3 abnormalities, characteristic of malignant lung tumours, are detectable in preinvasive lesions of the bronchus. Oncogene 7:1989, 1992.

249. Nuorva K, Soini Y, Kamel D, et al: Concurrent p53 expression in bronchial dysplasias and squamous cell lung carcinomas. Am J Pathol 142:745, 1992.

250. Sozzi G, Miozzo M, Donghi R, et al: Deletions of 17p and p53 mutations in preneoplastic lesions of the lung. Cancer Res 52:6079, 1992.

251. Minna JD, Takahashi T, Nau MM, et al: The molecular pathogenesis of lung cancer involves the accumulation of a large number of mutations in dominant oncogenes and multiple tumor suppressor genes (recessive oncogenes)[Abstract]. J Cell Biochem 14C:I, 1990.

252. Harbour JW, Lai SL, Whang-Peng J, et al: Abnormalities in structure and expression of the human retinoblastoma gene in SCLC. Science 241:353, 1988.

253. Iman DS, Harris CC: Oncogenes and tumor suppressor genes in human lung carcinogenesis. Crit Rev Oncog 2:161, 1991.

254. Whang-Peng J, Kao-Shan CS, Lee EC, et al: Specific chromosome defect associated with human small-cell lung cancer; deletion 3p(14-23). Science 215:181, 1982.

255. Rabbitts P, Douglas J, Daly M, et al: Frequency and extent of allelic loss in the short arm of chromosome 3 in nonsmall-cell lung cancer. Genes Chromosom Cancer 1:95, 1989.

256. LaForgia S, Morse B, Levy J, et al: Receptor-linked protein-tyrosine-phosphatase, PTPγ, is a candidate tumor suppressor at human chromosome region 3p21. Proc Natl Acad Sci U S A 88:5036, 1991.

257. D'Amico D, Carbone DP, Johnson BE, et al: Polymorphic sites within the MCC and APC loci reveal very frequent loss of heterozygosity in human small cell lung cancer. Cancer Res 52:1996, 1992.

258. Olopade OI, Buchhagen DL, Malik K, et al: Homozygous loss of the interferon genes defines the critical region on 9p that is deleted in lung cancers. Cancer Res 53:2410, 1993.

259. International Agency on the Research of Cancer: IARC monographs on the evaluation of the carcinogenic risk of chemicals to humans. Tobacco smoking. IARC Monogr 38, 1989.

260. Emmelin A, Nystrom L, Wall S: Diesel exhaust exposure and smoking: A case-referent study of lung cancer among Swedish dock workers. Epidemiology 4:237, 1993.

261. International Agency for Research on Cancer: IARC monographs on the evaluation of carcinogenic risks to humans. Diesel and gasoline engine exhausts. IARC Monogr 46:132, 1989.

DIAGNOSIS AND STAGING

3 CLINICAL PRESENTATION OF LUNG CANCER

L. Austin Doyle and Joseph Aisner

With the exception of patients found to have lung cancer in screening programs for asymptomatic smokers, the vast majority of patients with lung cancer present with symptomatic disease. In 678 patients from Yale–New Haven Hospital and New Haven Veterans Administration (VA) Hospital who had bronchogenic carcinoma, Carbone and colleagues found only 7% of patients to be asymptomatic, whereas 27% had symptoms related to their primary tumor, 32% had symptoms related to metastatic disease, and 34% had systemic symptoms that suggested cancer, such as anorexia, weight loss, and fatigue.[1] The presence of symptoms was associated with significant differences in survival that were independent of anatomic stage among the subgroups. A subgroup of patients who had symptoms related to the primary tumor that lasted more than 6 months had the best chance of survival. In this group, 16% survived 5 years, compared with 8% who survived 5 years among patients with less than a 6-month history of symptoms related to the primary tumor at diagnosis. These findings indicate that a long duration of symptoms may correlate with a biologically more indolent or slower growing lung cancer, although an analysis of prognostic factors from the Eastern Cooperative Oncology Group (ECOG) trials did not corroborate this finding.

The symptoms of lung cancer develop gradually in most cases and are often attributed by the patient to a smoker's cough or a cold and, by the patient's physician, to tracheobronchitis, pneumonia, influenza, pulmonary infarct, or lung abscess. Thus, it is common for a patient to delay seeking medical attention for several months from the first recognizable onset of symptoms. Several additional months of symptomatic treatment and antibiotics frequently pass before the physician establishes the correct diagnosis. Although there are no pathognomonic signs or symptoms of lung cancer, some signs or symptoms are seen more frequently than others (Table 3–1). One study of 702 lung cancer patients in Charleston, South Carolina, found nine common symptom complexes at presentation.[2]

DIFFERENT PRESENTATIONS OF PRIMARY LUNG CANCERS BY HISTOLOGIC TYPES

Understanding the common radiographic appearance of the four major histologic types of lung cancer will

TABLE 3–1. Presenting Signs and Symptoms of Patients with Lung Cancer

FINDING	PERCENTAGE
Cough	74
Weight loss	68
Dyspnea	58
Chest pain	49
Sputum production	45
Hemoptysis	29
Malaise	26
Bone pain	25
Lymphadenopathy	23
Hepatomegaly	21
Fever	21
Clubbing	20
Neuromyopathy	10
Superior vena cava syndrome	4
Dizziness	4
Hoarseness	3
Asymptomatic	12

Modified from Hyde L, Hyde CI: Clinical manifestations of lung cancer. Chest 65:299–306, 1974; and Cromartie RS, Parker EF, May JE, et al: Carcinoma of the lung: A clinical review. Ann Thorac Surg 30:30–35, 1980. Reprinted with permission from the Society of Thoracic Surgeons.

help the physician to remember their primary signs and symptoms. Squamous cell cancers, in addition to having a central location, associated atelectasis, and hilar adenopathy, may occasionally cavitate. Adenocarcinomas tend to appear as well-defined peripheral nodules, with pleural and chest wall involvement if they are large. Large cell anaplastic carcinoma is usually seen as a large peripheral mass with pneumonitis and hilar adenopathy; because of the tendency to admix with other histologic types, however, large cell carcinoma may also be seen with more central presentations. Small cell lung cancer tends to present as a central lesion with atelectasis, pneumonitis, and mediastinal lymphadenopathy. Peripheral presentation of small cell carcinoma is uncommon. However, the various forms of lung cancer all can appear as either peripheral or central lesions, and using x-ray studies alone to categorize one form or the other is inappropriate.[1-3]

Although the majority of all lung cancers arise in peripheral bronchi,[4, 5] by the time a clinical diagnosis has been made, squamous cell and small cell lung cancer have generally extended centrally and appear as paramediastinal masses on chest radiographs. In contrast, adenocarcinoma and large cell anaplastic carcinoma remain peripherally located in most patients.[6, 7] Because of its peripheral location, adenocarcinoma is the form of lung cancer most likely to be asymptomatic at diagnosis. The difference between the primary site of squamous and small cell tumors in one group and that of adenocarcinoma and large cell carcinomas in the other leads to different patterns of presenting signs and symptoms (Table 3–2). The former group tends to present with cough, hemoptysis, wheezing, pneumonia, and dyspnea owing to atelectasis with loss of lung volume or chest pain.[8, 9] The pain may be related to involvement of mediastinal structures or perivascular or peribronchial nerves and tends to be vague, intermittent, and poorly localized. Bronchoscopy in these patients frequently shows fungating, friable masses that partially or completely occlude a lobar or main-stem bronchus. The bulky intrabronchial tumor involvement leads to hemoptysis, atelectasis, and postobstructive pneumonia. Tumors in the peripheral bronchi may grow large by the time of diagnosis and present with direct involvement of the pleura or chest wall. Dyspnea, when present in pe-

ripheral adenocarcinomas or large cell carcinomas of the lung, is most likely due to pleural effusions or pain-induced restriction of chest wall movement. An exception is bronchioalveolar carcinoma, which may present with cough, hemoptysis, and dyspnea resulting from an infiltrative process.[10] The nodular variant of bronchoalveolar carcinoma is less prone to such interalveolar dissemination, is more amenable to surgical resection, and is clinically indistinguishable from typical lung adenocarcinomas.[11] In the acinar filling variety of bronchioalveolar carcinoma, oxygen transfer across capillary membranes may be impaired by tumor cells growing along the alveolar surfaces, leading to arteriovenous shunting; cyanosis, dyspnea, and hypoxemia therefore may be prominent. The large quantities of foamy sputum (bronchorrhea) can exacerbate the hypoxemia and can lead to hypovolemia and electrolyte abnormalities. Confusion of this syndrome with pneumonia is common. In contrast to lung adenocarcinoma, pleural and chest wall involvement is not prominent with bronchioalveolar carcinoma. Some asymptomatic patients may have evidence of extensive pulmonary disease on a chest roentgenogram, which may show a solitary noncavitating nodule, multiple nodules, a persistent infiltrate, lobar consolidation, or a cavitary lesion.[12] Because the malignant cells are in the alveoli, an air bronchogram effect is commonly seen. One of the diseases that may be confused with adenocarcinoma of the lung is the epithelial form of mesothelioma.[13, 14] Mesothelioma grows in the pleura, and small tissue biopsy specimens may lead to confusion.

SPECIFIC SYMPTOMS FROM PRIMARY BRONCHOGENIC CARCINOMAS

Cough

Cough resulting from bronchial irritation is the most common early symptom of lung cancer; it was initially present in 73% of 2000 patients studied in one large cohort.[15] The cough may be productive or nonproductive and frequently is disregarded by the patients as being a so-called cigarette cough. The cough frequently goes away after a few days and returns intermittently. Sputum, when present, may be clear or may be mucopurulent if there is an associated infection. One effect of cigarette smoking is to paralyze the bronchial cilia, preventing effective cleansing of the tracheobronchial tree. Cigarette smoking also causes the production of excess mucus.

Mechanistically, coughing involves both afferent and efferent pathways. The afferent limb includes cough receptors within the sensory distribution of the glossopharyngeal, superior laryngeal, and vagus nerves.[16] The efferent limb includes the recurrent laryngeal nerve, which causes glottic closure, and the spinal nerves, which cause contraction of the thoracic and abdominal musculature. In lung cancer, cough is produced in part by inflammatory or mechanical stimulation of the cough receptors. Cough may be

TABLE 3–2. Signs and Symptoms Due to Primary Tumor

SYMPTOMS FROM ENDOBRONCHIAL AND CENTRAL TUMOR GROWTH	SYMPTOMS FROM PERIPHERAL TUMOR GROWTH
Cough	Sharp pain (pleura, chest wall)
Obstruction dyspnea	Restrictive dyspnea
Segmental atelectasis	Effusion: serous or bloody fluid
Segmental emphysema	Cough
Pneumonic (fever, productive cough)	Lung abscess from tumor cavitation
Dull chest pain	
Wheeze or stridor	

produced by a small tumor acting as a foreign body, or by ulceration of the bronchial mucosa. In some cases, nonproductive cough may be associated with invasion of the carina by the tumor.[16] Peripheral tumors, arising from small bronchi and bronchioles, usually become large without producing cough.

Severe paroxysms of coughing may lead to cough fractures, rupture of an emphysematous bleb, or cough syncope.[9] Rib fractures occur in the lateral portion of the rib at the point of maximal mechanical stress. Predisposition to the fractures results from coexistent osteoporosis or lytic metastases. Cough syncope is due to cerebral ischemia that occurs when coughing leads to diminished venous return to the heart and a resultant fall in cardiac output. These complications or any significant change in a smoker's cough demand evaluation for bronchial carcinoma.

Hemoptysis

Hemoptysis occurred as a presenting complaint in 29% of the lung cancer patients in the VA Lung Cancer Study Group series.[15] Different series report hemoptysis occurring in between 25% and 40% of lung cancer patients at the time of presentation.[2,17] Hemoptysis in a lung cancer patient may also result from coexistent nonmalignant processes such as tuberculosis, bronchitis, left ventricular failure, mitral stenosis, pulmonary infarct, bronchiectasis, lung abscess, pneumonia, bronchial adenoma, or benign bronchial erosion. In most large medical series, lung cancer is responsible for about 20% of all cases of hemoptysis.[18] Thus hemoptysis, even in patients who have another likely etiology, should be considered to be possibly due to lung cancer until radiographic and bronchoscopic evaluation proves otherwise. Hemoptysis is rare in patients with metastases to the lung.

Dyspnea

Dyspnea was found as an early symptom in 58% of lung cancer patients in a large series.[15] Some patients may have dyspnea due to underlying pulmonary disorders such as pulmonary fibrosis or chronic obstructive pulmonary disease. Others may decrease their physical activities gradually and thus avoid sensing dyspnea because they do not induce stress in themselves. Dyspnea in patients with lung cancer may also be due to congestive heart failure, coincidental pneumonia, atelectasis, or pulmonary emboli.

Central lung cancers cause dyspnea by means of obstruction with or without postobstructive pneumonitis. Peripheral tumors usually cause dyspnea on a restrictive basis with pain fixation or pleural effusions. Some patterns of dyspnea are not directly related to physical exertion and may be positional in nature. Occasional lung cancer patients are reported to have trepopnea, which is dyspnea and hypoxemia when the patient lies on the unaffected side, or platypnea and oxygen desaturation, which occurs when the patient sits up or stands.[18,19] It has been speculated that a shunt might be increased in the involved lung

field for cases of positional increase in obstruction by an endobronchial tumor or increased pressure on a pulmonary artery.[20]

Wheezing

Wheezing, stridor, or a sudden increase in dyspnea is highly suggestive of a partial bronchial obstruction. Wheezing is seen in only 2% of lung cancer patients at diagnosis and is most significant when it is unilateral or of recent origin.[15] Wheezing occurs when hilar tumors produce narrowing of a large bronchus or the trachea. Occasionally, segmental emphysema may develop distal to an endobronchial obstruction.

Fever

Lung abscesses can cause patients with bronchogenic carcinoma to develop febrile and toxic signs often associated with hemoptysis or purulent sputum. Abscesses associated with lung cancer typically develop within necrotic tumor cavities rather than distal to an obstructing tumor mass. Lung abscesses are most often associated with squamous or large cell anaplastic subtypes of lung cancer.[9] Lung abscess or significant cavitation within a tumor mass is found in 20% of tumors at necropsy, but in only about 8% of tumors radiographically.[21]

Fever in lung cancer patients may occur with other pulmonary conditions such as bronchitis, atelectasis, and postobstructive pneumonia. Fever may also be associated with the development of liver metastases, but other etiologies should be rigorously excluded before ascribing a fever to metastatic disease.

The findings of fever, pulmonary symptoms, and radiographic infiltrate usually prompt a trial of antibiotics. Resolution of signs and symptoms depends on the causative organism, the degree of bronchiolar patency, and the degree of compromise of bronchial peristalsis. A delay of over 1 month in the resolution of signs and symptoms of pneumonia, particularly in an at-risk individual such as a smoker over age 40, should be considered as suggestive of lung cancer and should lead to a careful evaluation.

SYMPTOMS FROM REGIONAL SPREAD IN THE THORAX

Many of the major presentations of all forms of lung cancer are related to the spread along interbronchial lymphatics to the mediastinal lymph nodes and the subsequent invasion of mediastinal structures (Table 3–3). The continuity of lymphatic channels along the tracheobronchial tree thus has great bearing on the spread of lung cancer. These include groups of lymph nodes that communicate via lymphatics accompanying the large pulmonary vessels, those in the mediastinal fat pads, and those that drain via folds of pleura, notably the inferior pulmonary ligament.[22] The last group puts pulmonary lymph in continuity with para-

TABLE 3–3. Signs and Symptoms from Regional Spread of Lung Cancer

NERVE ENTRAPMENT
Horner's syndrome (enophthalmos, meiosis, ptosis) due to involvement of the cervical sympathetic nerves
Ulnar pain and vasomotor signs with eighth cervical and first thoracic nerve invasion
Dyspnea, cough, and diaphragmatic paralysis from phrenic nerve involvement
Hoarseness and dysphagia due to left recurrent laryngeal nerve damage

CARDIOVASCULAR INVOLVEMENT
Venous distention and edema in face, neck, and chest due to superior vena cava obstruction
Tamponade, heart failure, arrhythmia with pericardial or myocardial extension

MEDIASTINAL INVOLVEMENT
Dysphagia due to esophageal compression or involvement
Hypoxemia and dyspnea from lymphangitic spread through the lungs
Wheezing, stridor from tracheal obstruction
Effusion: serous due to lymphatic obstruction, chylous due to thoracic duct involvement
Aspiration from bronchoesophageal fistula

esophageal lymph and with that related to the pericardium.

Lymphangitic carcinomatosis involving the lung parenchyma is associated with cough, dyspnea, and fever. Lymphangitic carcinomatosis has characteristic features on high-resolution computed tomography, with uneven nodular thickening of interlobular septa and bronchovascular bundles.

Metastases to the hilar lymph nodes were found to occur in about 90% of patients with lung cancer in an autopsy series.[23] Bronchial nodes, on the other hand, are found to be involved in 40% to 60% of cases at necropsy.[23] The scalene nodes are much less frequently involved but are sometimes positive in upper lobe lesions. When palpable, scalene nodes are positive in about 85% of cases.[24, 25] However, routine study of the prescalene nodes has been so unrewarding that the procedure generally is best avoided except in rare situations such as patients with roentgenographic findings of advanced lung cancer or those at poor risk for major surgical procedures, when a histologic diagnosis cannot be established by other means.[26]

The most common sites of visible or palpable lymph nodes are in the supraclavicular fossae, which may be involved in about 15% to 20% of patients with lung cancer during the course of their disease.[9] The drainage of the right lung, left lower lobe, and left lingula is to the paratracheal and mediastinal lymph nodes and then most frequently to the right supraclavicular lymph nodes.[27]

Pleura and Diaphragm

Pleural effusions are seen in about 12% of lung cancer patients at the time of presentation.[28] The effusion is most commonly secondary to involvement of the visceral pleura by tumor, but it may sometimes be associated with mediastinal lymphatic obstruction or obstructive atelectasis with pneumonitis. Pleural effusions may also be due to coexistent congestive heart failure, tuberculosis, or pulmonary infarction. Pleural effusions cause a restriction of lung expansion with decreased gas exchange, alter ventilation/perfusion relationships, and produce atelectasis. Although a small number of tumors with cytologically negative effusions are still resectable, in non–small cell lung carcinomas (adenocarcinoma and squamous and large cell carcinoma) any pleural effusion confers a poor prognosis.[28] In small cell lung cancer, an ipsilateral pleural effusion, regardless of whether or not it is cytologically positive, in a patient with disease confined to the chest does not negatively affect the prognosis.[29] Such an effusion, however, usually precludes thoracic irradiation.

Sharp pleuritic chest pain seen early in the natural history of pleural invasion may cease with the onset of pleural effusion. The pleural fluid in lung cancer is frequently bloody, and a hemorrhagic effusion in a patient over the age of 40 is most frequently due to pulmonary neoplasm or infarct. Complete evaluation of an effusion lacking an obvious etiology requires pleural biopsies as well as cytologic examination of the fluid and a careful evaluation of the pulmonary parenchyma.

Invasion of the diaphragm usually precludes curative resection, not because the diaphragm cannot be spared or reconstructed but because diaphragmatic extension usually signals wider spread of disease. The extensive venous and lymphatic drainage from the diaphragm almost invariably results in disease outside the scope of surgery. There are both subpleural and extrapleural lymphatic plexuses on either side of the diaphragmatic muscle. Once cancer cells have crossed both the visceral and parietal layers of pleura into diaphragmatic muscle, there is almost always invasion of the liver or metastases to the retroperitoneal lymph nodes or both.

Lung cancer may occasionally be associated with an ipsilateral spontaneous pneumothorax, which may be asymptomatic.[30, 31] Erosion of the visceral pleura by a peripheral lung cancer with the creation of a bronchopleural fistula is the most likely etiology, but postobstructive emphysema or severe coughing with rupture of emphysematous blebs may also be implicated.

Chest Wall

Chest pain is a common presenting feature in lung cancer. Chest pain was reported as an initial problem in 43% to 67% of patients.[15, 32] The pain is usually a dull intermittent ache lasting from minutes to hours on the same side as the tumor and is not related to cough or respiration. Although the pulmonary parenchyma is insensitive to pain, the peribronchial nerves associated with bronchi may give rise to painful sensations probably via the vagus nerves. When chest pain is severe, persistent, and well localized, it is usually related to invasion of parietal pleura or chest wall by tumor. Shoulder pain may be caused by Pancoast's tumor involving the apex of the lung or by tumor invading the diaphragm and irritating the central portion innervated by the phrenic nerve. Pain radiating from the shoulder down the arm is very characteristic of brachial plexus involvement. Chest pain in a patient with bronchogenic cancer may also be due to compression of a pulmonary artery by tumor, with or without resultant pulmonary infarction.[33]

Direct extension of lung cancer to the chest wall is generally a poor prognostic sign, although patients with T3N0 disease may have prolonged survival. Chest wall involvement, although sometimes resectable, is associated with a high recurrence rate.[34] Even though sections of chest wall may be technically resectable, intercostal venous drainage from chest wall lesions can infuse malignant cells into the systemic venous circulation via the azygos vein on the right or the hemiazygos veins on the left as well as anteriorly through the internal mammary veins.[35] Lymphatic spread from the chest wall can parallel the vessels just mentioned or follow other pathways. There is no single or localized pathway of lymphatic drainage from any given point on the chest wall.

Pericardial and Myocardial Metastases

Pericardial and myocardial metastases are a relatively unusual initial presentation of lung cancer, although they are found in 15% to 35% of lung cancer patients at necropsy, especially in patients with anaplastic histologic findings, left lower lobe primary cancers, or widely disseminated disease.[36] Pericardial involvement is more common than myocardial invasion. At necropsy, the pericardium is involved in 88% of heart metastases, whereas the myocardium is involved in 45%, usually by direct extension through the pericardium for all cell types.[36] Intracardiac metastases from lung cancer have occasionally been misdiagnosed as atrial myxoma.[37] Although cardiac metastases usually are not diagnosed antemortem, a retrospective review showed that only 4% of patients pathologically proved to have cardiac metastases have both absence of clinical signs or symptoms related to the heart and a normal electrocardiogram.[36] Therefore, any new cardiac finding in a lung cancer patient should prompt consideration of cardiac involvement by tumor.

The two most common presentations of pericardial involvement in lung cancer are the sudden onset of an arrhythmia (usually sinus tachycardia or atrial fibrillation) or the recognition of increased cardiac diameter on a chest roentgenogram, with or without symptoms of right-sided congestive heart failure and tamponade. These conditions may be associated with signs of pericarditis such as paradoxical pulse, distant heart sounds, pericardial friction rub, cardiac percussion dullness lateral to the apex impulse, Kussmaul's sign (distention of cervical veins during inspiration) from obstruction of venous return to the right side of the heart, and Ewart's sign (dullness to percussion and bronchial breathing beneath the angle of the left scapula). The effusion is readily confirmed by echocardiography, and if pericardial tamponade is impending, a definitive diagnosis and therapy may be obtained with pericardiocentesis and decompression plus cytologic analysis of the pericardial fluid. Rarely, lung cancers also can perforate through the pericardium to form a bronchopericardial fistula and cause pneumopericardium.[38]

Superior Vena Cava Syndrome

The pathologic and physiologic description of superior vena cava (SVC) syndrome is covered in depth in Chapter 15. Almost half of all patients with SVC obstruction have small cell lung cancer; squamous cell cancer is the next most common histologic finding. SVC syndrome is a presenting sign in about 4% of all lung cancer patients.[15]

The SVC is joined by the azygos vein just before entering the pericardial sac, and the clinical picture of SVC obstruction depends on whether the obstruction is proximal or distal to this junction.[39, 40] Obstruction above the junction causes distention of the arm and neck veins; a dusky suffusion and edema of the face, neck, and arms; and dilated tortuous collateral vessels on the upper chest and back. Obstruction proximal to the venous junction is a more serious clinical picture, involving more extensive collateral circulation along the anterior and posterior abdominal walls to reach the systemic circulation via collaterals to the inferior vena cava.

The diagnosis of SVC obstruction is strongly suggested by the demonstration on physical examination of elevated venous pressure with delay of venous return in the arm and normal venous pressure in the leg. Associated symptoms include headache, dizziness, drowsiness, vertigo, blurred vision, dyspnea, chest pain, cough, or dysphagia.[41] The patient may have edema of the eyelids, conjunctival suffusion, proptosis, or papilledema. Associated upper airway obstruction or signs of cerebral edema are very poor prognostic signs.[39] SVC syndrome by itself does not confer a poor prognosis and can in some cases call attention to a small tumor.[42] Patients may have long-term survival with SVC syndrome in both small cell and non–small cell histologic types. Even with a rapid onset of the SVC syndrome, histologic or cytologic confirmation of the tumor is important and can usually be accomplished before the initiation of definitive treatment.

Tumor compression or invasion of the SVC may lead to venous stasis and secondary thrombus. Caval thrombus is found in greater than one-third of such patients at necropsy.[40] The presence of thrombus makes it difficult to evaluate the extent of tumor involvement by angiographic studies, which are already technically difficult to perform in the SVC syndrome. SVC syndrome is also associated with spinal cord compression and pericardial metastases in lung cancer patients who therefore require careful neurologic and cardiac evaluations.[43]

Isolated axillary and subclavian venous occlusions without SVC syndrome can occur, but usually these develop only in the context of recurrent lung cancer.[44] Most of the patients had upper lobe or superior sulcus non–small cell lung cancers. Embolism in this circumstance is rarely detected clinically.

Pancoast's Tumors

Pancoast's tumors are discussed in depth in Chapter 16. Tumor in the apex of the lung may involve the first thoracic and eighth cervical nerves by local extension, causing pain in the shoulder and the portion of the arm innervated by the ulnar nerve.[45, 46] There may be erosion of the first and second ribs. Paravertebral tumor extension with sympathetic nerve involvement may lead to Horner's syndrome. In addition, there may be muscular atrophy and decreased range of motion in the arm and shoulder; the patient may walk supporting the elbow of the affected arm. A reflex sympathetic dystrophy or "shoulder-hand syndrome" may be apparent with paresthesias, cool, mottled skin, flexion contractures, palmar fasciitis and other vasomotor features.[47, 48] A classic presentation of this syndrome in a patient with radiographic abnormalities consistent with lung cancer requires little further diagnostic evaluation.[49] Superior sulcus syndrome is seen initially in only 4% of lung cancer patients.[15]

Horner's Syndrome

Superior sulcus tumors, by means of paravertebral extension, may compromise the sixth cervical and first thoracic segments of the sympathetic nerve trunks and plexus, resulting in Horner's syndrome. Patients have unilateral enophthalmos, ptosis, meiosis, and ipsilateral anhidrosis.[15] With early involvement, mydriasis (pupillary dilatation on the affected side) may result. Similarly, mild sympathetic nerve irritation may stimulate localized sympathetic overactivity with ipsilateral hyperhidrosis of the face, thorax, or arm associated with thoracic scoliosis concave to the affected side.[50] Eventually, the tumor causes outright destruction of the sympathetic fibers with anhidrosis. Rarely, a provocative sweat test shows anhidrosis on the ipsilateral side and hyperhidrosis on the contralateral side as a reflex compensatory mechanism.[51] Horner's syndrome is often associated with radiographic evidence of destruction of the first and second ribs.

Recurrent Laryngeal Nerve Involvement

Hoarseness is another common presentation and disease complication for lung cancer. Hoarseness, usually due to recurrent laryngeal nerve involvement, is more common with lung cancers arising on the left side, because the left recurrent laryngeal nerve has a greater intrathoracic course than the right; the left recurrent laryngeal nerve passes around the aortic arch at the level of the carina, whereas the right recurrent laryngeal nerve loops around the subclavian artery in the base of the neck. One large series of lung cancer patients reported huskiness of the voice in 19% of patients, but only 3% had true hoarseness.[15] Because most lung cancer patients are heavy smokers,

examination of the vocal cords for a separate laryngeal primary cancer and for mobility is required.

Phrenic Nerve Involvement

Occasionally, lung cancer produces diaphragmatic paralysis or paroxysmal contractions (hiccups). Involvement of the phrenic nerve by bronchogenic carcinoma can lead to paralysis of either the right or left hemidiaphragm. The diagnosis is made by physical and radiographic findings of an elevated hemidiaphragm and paradoxical motion on respiration or sniffing.[52] The paradoxical motion can be clearly shown by the use of fluoroscopy. The absent or paradoxical diaphragmatic excursion leads to a decreased vital capacity and a sensation of dyspnea. Phrenic nerve paralysis is seen in approximately 1% of all lung cancer patients at the time of their first examination.[15]

Vagus Nerve Involvement

The vagus nerve, which contains visceral as well as somatic afferents, may be involved by compression and infiltrations, and is thought to be involved in some cases of referred lung cancer pain. A series of 16 lung cancer patients with facial pain unrelated to local metastases has been described.[53] These patients complained of aching pain in the ear and temporal regions. The facial pain was predominantly on the right side, which might be explained by the close anatomic relationship of the right vagus nerve to the trachea and mediastinal lymph nodes. The left vagus nerve is separated from these structures by the large blood vessels. The facial pain in most cases was relieved by thoracic irradiation or surgery.

Esophageal Involvement

Regional spread of lung cancer to the posterior mediastinal lymph nodes can produce displacement or extrinsic compression of the esophagus, leading to dysphagia. In a series of 615 consecutive patients hospitalized for bronchogenic carcinoma, dysphagia was noted in 2.2% and was found to correlate well with advanced disease and inoperability.[15] Dysphagia may also be a manifestation of paralysis of the recurrent laryngeal nerve, which partly innervates the cricoid muscles and proximal esophagus. In this case, dysphagia occurs for both solids and liquids, and aspiration is common. A pharyngoesophageal myotomy may effectively palliate symptoms in many cases.[54] An unusual complication of lung cancer is the formation of a bronchoesophageal fistula, which may lead to recurrent aspiration pneumonitis.

SYMPTOMS FROM EXTRATHORACIC METASTASES

The rates of hematogenous metastases to common sites such as brain, bone, liver, adrenal gland, and kidney roughly parallel the distribution of the cardiac output at rest. Necropsy studies find lung cancer metastases in nearly every organ of the body (Table 3–4). The frequency of extrathoracic metastases varies according to the histologic findings and the degree of differentiation of the cancer. In squamous cell lung cancers, poorly differentiated tumors have a much greater risk of extrathoracic metastasis than do the well-differentiated ones. Small cell lung carcinomas have a much greater propensity to metastasize to some organs such as the pancreas, testis, thyroid, and breast than do non–small cell lung cancers.

Symptoms arising from metastases often dominate the clinical picture, complicate the diagnosis, and make therapy futile. The size of the primary tumor often does not correlate with the extent of spread: large tumors may not be attended by metastases and, conversely, small asymptomatic primary lung cancers may have widespread metastases.

Central Nervous System Metastasis

Ten per cent of all lung cancer patients are found to have central nervous system (CNS) metastases at the time of diagnosis, and another 15% to 20% are discovered to have such metastases during the course of their disease.[55] CNS metastases are seen most commonly in small cell lung cancer, less commonly in large cell anaplastic carcinoma and adenocarcinoma, and least commonly in well-differentiated squamous cell lung cancer. The presenting symptoms from brain

metastases are most commonly those of increased intracranial pressure and include headaches, diplopia, blurred vision, nausea, vomiting, changes in mentation and level of consciousness, weakness, and malaise. Patients with brain metastases less commonly present with focal neurologic findings such as seizures, cranial nerve abnormalities, hemiparesis, cerebellar abnormalities, or aphasia. The symptoms from brain metastases in peripheral lesions may significantly predate the onset of chest symptoms. Tumors of the lung usually metastasize to the frontal lobes of the cerebrum and far less frequently to the cerebellum. In 30% of cases, the metastases are seen as solitary by a computed tomographic (CT) scan. Although a scan of the head is not routinely indicated in non–small cell lung cancer in the absence of neurologic symptoms or deficits, one study of 50 asymptomatic patients with non–small cell lung cancer revealed that three (6%) had occult brain metastases shown by a CT scan.[56]

Brain metastases are clinically detected in about 15% of patients with small cell lung cancer at the time of diagnosis and develop clinically in an additional 20% of patients during the course of the disease.[57] In addition, as modern treatment regimens have led to improved survival for small cell lung cancer patients, the frequency of brain metastases has increased with the duration of survival.[58] Multiple cerebral metastases are noted in most cases, and at necropsy, cerebellar and pituitary metastases are noted in 44% and

TABLE 3–4. Metastatic Patterns Found at Autopsy in Patients with Lung Cancer

SITE OF METASTASIS	PERCENTAGE OF PATIENTS WITH METASTASIS			
	Squamous Cell Carcinoma	Adenocarcinoma	Large Cell Carcinoma	Small Cell Carcinoma
Number of patients studied	(N = 126)	(N = 100)	(N = 80)	(N = 102)
Hilar, mediastinal lymph nodes	77	80	84	96
Pleura	34	60	67	34
Chest wall	20	20	20	13
Diaphragm	9	11	15	14
Alternate lung	21	60	34	34
Cardiovascular system (total)	21	26	33	21
Pericardium	20	25	25	18
Myocardium	8	11	20	14
Limited to thorax	46	18	14	4
Liver	25	41	48	74
Adrenal	23	50	59	55
Bone	20	36	30	37
Kidney	21	23	28	22
Central nervous system	18	37	25	29
Meninges	0	10	9	3
Dura	0	5	9	1
Gastrointestinal tract	12	5	20	14
Esophagus	13	8	3	14
Pancreas	4	12	22	41
Thyroid	4	2	6	18
Spleen	3	6	13	10
Parathyroid	1	0	0	1
Pituitary	1.6	4.5	3	15
Abdominal lymph nodes	10	24	30	52
Testes	0	0	0	7
Skin	0	0	6	0

Modified from Matthews MJ: Problems in morphology and behavior of bronchopulmonary malignant disease. *In* Israel L., Chahanian P (eds): Lung Cancer: Natural History, Prognosis, and Therapy. New York, Academic Press, 1976, pp 23–62.

16% of patients, respectively.[59] Necropsy series involving treated patients have suggested a CNS metastasis rate as high as 80%.[58]

Additional major presentations and complications of CNS metastases are those that involve the spinal cord along its axis. Spinal cord involvement generally takes two forms: epidural metastases causing cord compression and leptomeningeal involvement. Two additional rare complications occasionally are seen: compression of an anterior spinal artery causing a transverse myelitis (Brown-Séquard syndrome) and intramedullary metastases.

Epidural metastases are manifested initially by the presence of back pain in over 95% of patients. Weakness, autonomic dysfunction, and sensory loss, including ataxia, are late findings. Older, unselected series suggest that up to one-half of patients may present with these findings.[59] In most instances, the deficits are caused by direct extension of tumor from the vertebral body into the extradural space. However, in selected instances, particularly small cell lung cancer, tumor can encroach on the extradural space via the neural foramen and be associated with spinal cord compression and a paraspinal mass in the absence of vertebral destruction. It has been clearly demonstrated that patients with back pain and vertebral destruction on plain roentgenogram have an incidence of extradural spinal cord compression greater than 50%, even in the presence of a normal neurologic examination.[60] Patients with radicular pain have a greater than 60% incidence of epidural metastases. When these patients are treated with radiation therapy before the development of myelopathic signs, virtually all of them remain ambulatory until death from their systemic disease.[61] Therefore, physicians caring for lung cancer patients with back pain should not wait for the appearance of weakness or autonomic dysfunction but should proceed immediately to a diagnostic evaluation that includes, at a minimum, a plain x-ray study of the spine.

Radicular back pain is relatively more common in cervical and lumbosacral regions than in the thoracic spine. In the thoracic area, radicular pain is almost always bilateral and is sharply localized. The pain of an epidural tumor frequently is worse in the recumbent position and often awakens the patient or requires the individual to sleep sitting up.

Leptomeningeal carcinomatosis is frequently seen in small call lung cancer. Although the condition is uncommon at presentation, it develops later with progressive or relapsing disease.[62] Changes in mental status, limb weakness, sensory loss, bowel or bladder dysfunction, back pain and paresthesia, and headache are common findings.[62] An isolated case of cranial nerve palsy is rare. In another series, 137 patients with small cell lung cancer had a 9% incidence of leptomeningeal disease, with most diagnoses made by means of cerebrospinal fluid (CSF) cytology.[63] A mass lesion in the brain must be excluded before performing a lumbar puncture in a lung cancer patient with neurologic findings, particularly if there is evidence of elevated intracranial pressure on funduscopic examination.

Bone Metastases

Bone is a common site of metastases in lung cancer. In a large VA Lung Cancer Study Group series, necropsy results showed a 25% incidence of bone metastases.[15] The most common sites of bone metastases are the spine (70%), pelvic bones (40%), and femur (25%), whereas other long bones of the extremities, the scapulae, the sternum, and the small bones of the wrists and feet are less commonly involved. Peripheral bone metastases distal to the elbow and knee are uncommon, but osteolytic metastases to the fingers and toes with progressive destruction of the distal phalanges occasionally are seen.[64] Although most bone metastases of lung cancer are osteolytic, some, especially those of adenocarcinoma and small cell lung cancer, can be osteoblastic.[65] Metastatic lung cancer may rarely present as monarticular arthritis with cancerous deposits in the juxta-articular bone or synovial tissue.[66, 67] Physical examination of the affected joint reveals inflammation and effusion. The knee and hip are the two most commonly involved joints. In the majority of cases, malignant cells are demonstrable in the effusion. Therefore, patients with lung cancer who develop an effusion in the joint should have cytologic evaluation of the fluid before anti-inflammatory therapy is initiated.

Some patients with back pain secondary to vertebral metastases have false-negative skeletal roentgenograms and bone scans[68] because plain films cannot detect bone metastases unless 50% or more of the bony cortex is destroyed. For patients with documented lesions in the vertebrae and back pain, myelography should be obtained. One series showed that more than 80% of such patients had early evidence of epidural or leptomeningeal involvement.[69] Magnetic resonance imaging is also highly sensitive in defining bone involvement by metastatic lung cancer.

Liver Metastases

Hepatic metastases are frequent in lung cancers of all histologic types, although they are more evident clinically late in the disease than early as a presenting manifestation. At necropsy, liver metastases are seen in 35% or more of lung cancer patients.[15] The characteristic symptoms of liver metastases are liver enlargement, pain, hardness, and palpable nodularity. Mild elevation of the transaminases aspartate aminotransferase and alanine aminotransferase can be seen, but elevation of the alkaline phosphatase is most common. Carcinoembryonic antigen is also likely to be elevated. Hectic fevers can also occur as part of liver metastases, but this must be a diagnosis of exclusion. Jaundice and ascites are relatively uncommon occurrences, and jaundice, which may be due to extrahepatic biliary obstruction from periportal lymph nodes, usually is accompanied by other signs of liver failure. Some signs and symptoms of liver involvement are ambiguous. Anorexia may be a sign of liver metastases or may be secondary to the metabolic effects of the tumor. Similarly, hepatomegaly may be related to cirrhosis, fatty liver, or congestive heart failure, and fever may be due to any number of other causes.

Liver metastases from lung cancer rarely have been associated with lactic acidosis, presenting with hyperpnea, circulatory collapse, and death.[70] In lung cancer, lactic acidosis appears as a result of the failure of a liver, damaged by extensive metastatic disease, to clear and reuse the quantity of lactate normally generated by anaerobic glycolysis rather than from extensive lactate production by the tumor itself.

Adrenal Metastases

Adrenal hypofunction is seen more frequently in association with lung cancer than with any other metastatic tumor but is still an uncommon finding clinically, because patients are asymptomatic unless more than 90% of the gland has been replaced. With modern CT scanning techniques, adrenal metastases are being seen more commonly and are noted in up to 15% in some series.[71] Up to 27% of lung cancer patients have adrenal metastases at necropsy, the majority of these with bilateral disease.[2] Percutaneous biopsy of the adrenal gland has been advocated when preoperative CT evaluation for non–small cell lung cancer reveals unilateral adrenal enlargement in the absence of other metastatic disease.[71] The tumor metastases are usually situated in the adrenal medulla and consequently may relatively spare cortical functions. Symptoms of organ failure (Addison's disease) include weakness, fatigue, anorexia, nausea and vomiting, abdominal pain, hypotension, and pigment changes in the skin and mucous membranes. Associated laboratory findings include hyponatremia, hyperkalemia, moderate metabolic acidosis with a normal anion gap, and high urine sodium and low potassium levels with evidence of extracellular fluid volume depletion.

Gastrointestinal Metastases

Metastases to the gastrointestinal tract and abdominal lymph nodes are common, but they are usually clinically silent or cause nonspecific symptoms that do not lead to antemortem diagnosis. Twelve per cent of lung cancer patients have gastrointestinal metastases, with 33% of those with large cell anaplastic carcinomas manifesting this finding.[72] The proximal portion of the large intestine is involved more frequently than are the rectum and sigmoid colon. Intestinal obstruction or perforation is rare: The latter occurrence is associated with an ominous prognosis.[73] The stomach is involved in 2% to 4% of cases at necropsy, and such involvement often is associated with epigastric pain, nausea, and vomiting.[74] The spleen is involved in 5% to 7% of cases, but most of the metastases are very small. Splenic ruptures are very rare, but occasionally they are seen with small cell lung cancer.[75] Small cell lung cancer also has a predilection for metastasis to the pancreas and constitutes 70% of all lung cancer metastases to that organ. Most pancreatic metastases are small, and obstructive jaundice is uncommon.

Three cases of clinical acute pancreatitis occurred in a series of 40 patients with small cell lung cancer.[76] The two patients in whom necropsy was granted had small cell involvement of the pancreas. Lung cancers, particularly adenocarcinomas, may uncommonly produce amylase, which can cause concern about pancreatitis but can be distinguished immunologically as the salivary isoform of amylase.

Skin and Soft Tissue Metastases

Skin metastases were seen in 1% of patients in one large lung cancer series and are seen in about 3% in necropsy series.[32] In a series of 36 necropsied patients with cutaneous metastases, the lung was the primary site in 47%.[77] Therefore, lung cancer should be strongly considered in the evaluation of cutaneous metastases, particularly those appearing on the chest, head, or neck. Skeletal muscle metastases may also occur, but they are particularly rare. Lung cancer is the most common primary tumor to metastasize to the soft tissues of the oral cavity, particularly the gingiva and tongue.[78] The scalp is another area of soft tissue involvement and thus should be palpated for subcutaneous nodules, which should be biopsied for histologic confirmation.

Other Metastases

Small cell lung cancer has a propensity to metastasize to endocrine organs, and a careful examination of the thyroid is important in all patients with small cell cancer.[75] Usually, thyroid metastases will not be clinically evident or associated with disturbances of thyroid functions.

Choroidal metastases occur in 0.5% of all lung cancer patients, although special studies may reveal a higher incidence. The chief complaint is of blurred vision or spots before the eyes. Lung cancer is the most common tumor that metastasizes to the choroid in men and is second, after breast cancer, in women. Choroidal metastases are usually found in connection with widespread disease and thus tend to occur late in the clinical course, but occasionally they may be seen at initial diagnosis of the disease.

Kidney metastases are found in 15% to 20% of patients in necropsy series of lung cancer. The tumors are small and usually asymptomatic. Lung cancer may also metastasize to the ovaries and uterus in 1% to 2% of cases each; metastases to the uterus rarely are associated with uterine bleeding. Small cell lung cancer can metastasize to the testes, but the tumors are usually under 1 cm in size and asymptomatic. Rarely, lung cancer will metastasize to the penis, where it can cause ulceration and difficulty in urination.

PARANEOPLASTIC SYNDROMES

Paraneoplastic syndromes are the distant effects of a neoplasm unrelated to the actual dissemination of tu-

TABLE 3–5. Paraneoplastic Syndromes in Lung Cancer Patients

ENDOCRINE
Hypercalcemia (ectopic parathyroid hormone)
Cushing's syndrome
SIADH
Carcinoid syndrome
Gynecomastia
Hypercalcitonemia
Elevated growth hormone
Elevated prolactin, follicle-stimulating hormone, luteinizing hormone
Hypoglycemia
Hyperthyroidism

NEUROLOGIC
Encephalopathy
Subacute cerebellar degeneration
Progressive multifocal leukoencephalopathy
Peripheral neuropathy
Polymyositis
Autonomic neuropathy
Eaton-Lambert syndrome
Optic neuritis

SKELETAL
Clubbing
Pulmonary hypertrophic osteoarthropathy

HEMATOLOGIC
Anemia
Leukemoid reactions
Thrombocytosis
Thrombocytopenia
Eosinophilia
Pure red cell aplasia
Leukoerythroblastosis
Disseminated intravascular coagulation

CUTANEOUS
Hyperkeratosis
Dermatomyositis
Acanthosis nigricans
Hyperpigmentation
Erythema gyratum repens
Hypertrichosis lanuginosa acquisita

OTHER
Nephrotic syndrome
Hypouricemia
Secretion of vasoactive intestinal peptide with diarrhea
Hyperamylasemia
Anorexia-cachexia

SIADH, syndrome of inappropriate antidiuretic hormone.

mor cells (Table 3–5). They are clinically important in at least 10% of patients with lung cancer. Small cell lung cancer is more closely associated with paraneoplastic syndromes than is any other human cancer. Occult metastatic involvement by tumor, complications of therapy, vascular abnormalities, fluid and electrolyte disturbances, and infections can all mimic paraneoplastic syndromes. Paraneoplastic syndromes may be due to the production of biologically active substances by tumor cells or in response to tumor cells, but in many cases, the mechanism is unknown.

Some tumors may produce more than one hormone and have multiple paraneoplastic syndromes with overlapping effects (Table 3–6). The biologic correlate to this is the discovery that some small cell lung cancer cell lines have been found to secrete 10 or more biologically active peptides in cell culture.[79]

Some paraneoplastic syndromes are strongly linked to particular histologic types of lung cancer.[80] Squamous cell cancers are associated with ectopic parathyroid hormone–like secretion and hypercalcemia, whereas lung adenocarcinomas are particularly associated with hypertrophic pulmonary osteoarthropathy and periostitis. Small cell lung cancers are associated with ectopic adrenocorticotropic hormone (ACTH) secretion producing Cushing's syndrome; ectopic arginine vasopressin, causing a syndrome of inappropriate antidiuretic hormone and hyponatremia; and the Eaton-Lambert myasthenic syndrome (see Chapter 12). Paraneoplastic syndromes are often the first indication of the presence of tumor and may antedate the demonstrable tumor by a period ranging from months to years. Consequently, their presence may lead to the discovery of treatable lung cancers. Paraneoplastic syndromes can be confused with the signs or symptoms of metastatic disease, preventing appropriate curative therapy from being undertaken. For example, neurologic paraneoplastic syndromes, such as cerebellar or cortical degeneration or arterial emboli from marantic endocarditis, can be mistaken for brain metastases. Hypertrophic pulmonary osteoarthropathy can cause pain, tenderness, and swelling over affected bone along with a positive bone scan and may be mistaken for bone metastases.

Anorexia and Cachexia

Lung cancer patients often are weak and cachectic with a decrease in muscle mass, a marked decrease in body fat by skinfold thickness, and reduced levels of nutritional cofactors such as folic acid and vitamin C.[81-83] These findings correlate with the general systemic signs of the disease: unexplained malaise, fati-

TABLE 3–6. Frequency of Peptide Hormone Elevation in the Blood of Lung Cancer Patients

HORMONE	PERCENTAGE OF PATIENTS WITH SIGNIFICANTLY ELEVATED LEVELS			
	Small Cell Carcinoma	Squamous Cell Carcinoma	Adenocarcinoma	Large Cell Carcinoma
ACTH	30–69	0–80	17–75	26
ADH	32	—	—	—
Beta-human chorionic gonadotropin (β-hCG)	1–32	19	17	26
Calcitonin	48–64	9	0	11
Growth hormone	0	3	0	0
GRP	74	17	20	7
IGF	27	11	Not done	Not done
Lipotropin	54	33	20	Not done
Neurophysins	65	14	29	20
NSE	69	Not done	Not done	Not done
PTH	27	32	0	17

GRP, Gastrin-releasing peptide; IGF, insulin-like growth factor; NSE, neuron specific enolase; PTH, parathyroid hormone.
Modified from Bunn PA, Minna JD: Paraneoplastic syndromes. *In* DeVita VT, Hellman S, Rosenberg SA (eds): Cancer: Principles and Practice of Oncology, 4th Ed. Philadelphia, J.B. Lippincott, 1993.

gability, reduced ability to work, and often a low-grade fever. Tumor cachexia has been associated with expression of tumor necrosis factor, interleukin-1, and various prostaglandins. Some lung cancer patients also appear to have a hypermetabolic state similar to that of hyperthyroidism, and 1.4% of lung cancer patients reportedly are hyperthyroid.[84]

Ectopic Parathyroid Hormone Secretion

Hypercalcemia in patients with lung cancer is most often due to bone metastases; however, squamous cell lung cancer is known to secrete a parathyroid hormone–like polypeptide (Table 3–7). Of the 10% of lung cancer patients who develop hypercalcemia, approximately 15% may develop this disorder because of tumor production of parathyroid hormone or other humoral substances, including prostaglandin E_2.[85] A gene encoding a parathyroid hormone–related peptide has recently been identified and cloned from lung cancer cells.[86] Although hypercalcemia is occasionally seen with small cell lung cancer, it is almost always in association with bone or bone marrow metastases.[87]

In the hypercalcemia of lung cancer, neurologic symptoms, nausea, anorexia, constipation, and dehydration generally dominate the clinical picture. Some symptoms associated with chronic hypercalcemia (e.g., hyperparathyroidism) such as pruritus, hypertension, or nephrolithiasis are only rarely seen in the hypercalcemia of malignancy.[88] The signs and symptoms of the more acute hypercalcemia of malignancy include irritability, confusion, lethargy or coma, anorexia, constipation, nausea, and cardiac arrhythmias. Polyuria, polydipsia, decreased tendon reflexes, and disorders of speech and vision are also noted. Accompanying hypophosphatemia is seen with ectopic parathyroid hormone secretion. Although the prognosis for patients with lung cancer and hypercalcemia is usually dismal, cases have been reported in which hypercalcemia remitted completely with lung resection.[89]

Hypocalcemia may also occur with osteoblastic metastases in lung cancer but only rarely causes tetany. Although up to two-thirds of small cell lung cancer patients have elevated levels of an immunologically detectable calcitonin-like hormone, it is noteworthy that there is only a single report of a patient who had small cell lung cancer with coexistent hypocalcemia and hypercalcitonemia.[90]

Syndrome of Inappropriate Antidiuretic Hormone Secretion and Cushing's Syndrome

Elevated levels of antidiuretic hormone (e.g., arginine vasopressin) are noted in up to 70% of patients with lung cancer, but clinical manifestations of hyponatremia, which are predominantly of the small cell subtype, are seen in only 1% to 5% of lung cancer patients (see Chapter 12).[91–94] Many lung carcinomas contain pro-opiomelanocortin, or so-called big ACTH polypeptide, a precursor for corticotropin. This prohormone contains four repetitive sequences based on the ACTH-MSH core. The importance of the promolecule is that it can be split into many biologically active fragments, including ACTH, melanocyte-stimulating hormone (MSH), β-lipotropin hormone (β-LPH), β-endorphin, and met-enkephalin. Corticotropin has been demonstrated in the tumor tissue and sera of up to 50% of patients with lung cancer.[95] Although over 70% of patients with lung cancer have elevated corticotropin on sensitive radioimmunoassays, less than 2% have clinical symptoms of hypercortisolism.[96–100]

Carcinoid Syndrome

Carcinoid syndrome, resulting from the ectopic secretion of vasoactive peptides, is most commonly associated with bronchial carcinoid but has also been reported in small cell lung cancer.[101] Recent literature suggests that some of these cases may fit into the spectrum of atypical carcinoid or neuroendocrine carcinoma. The symptoms include prominent facial and upper body flushing, episodic tachycardia and wheezing, hyperperistalsis and diarrhea, facial edema, weight loss, and anorexia. Patients may have associated left-sided cardiac lesions, including mitral and aortic stenosis. Osteoblastic bony metastases are often seen in these patients. The biochemical basis of this disorder appears to be the release of serotonin (5-hydroxytryptamine), 5-hydroxytryptophan, bradyki-

TABLE 3–7. Endocrine Paraneoplastic Syndromes in Lung Cancer

SYNDROME	HORMONE	HISTOLOGIC TYPE(S)	INCIDENCE (PERCENT)
Cushing's syndrome	ACTH	Lung cancer—all types	0–2.0
		Small cell lung cancer	(6.0)
Gynecomastia	β-hCG	Lung cancer—all types	0.5–0.9
		Small cell lung cancer	(2.0)
Hyperthyroidism		Lung cancer	0–1.4
Syndrome of inappropriate antidiuretic hormone secretion	AVP	Lung cancer—all types	0.9–2.0
		Small cell lung cancer	(9.0)
Nonmetastatic hypercalcemia	PTH	Lung cancer—all types	1.0–7.5
		Squamous cell lung cancer	(15.0)

ACTH, adrenocorticotropic hormone; β-hCG, beta-human chorionic gonadotropin; AVP, arginine vasopressin; PTH, parathyroid hormone.
Modified from Rees LH: The biosynthesis of hormones by nonendocrine tumours—a review. J Endocrinol 67:143–175, 1975. Reproduced by permission of the Journal of Endocrinology Ltd; and Richardson RL, Greco FA, Oldhan RK, Liddle GW: Tumor products and potential markers in small cell lung cancer. Semin Oncol 5:253–262, 1978.

TABLE 3–8. Differential Diagnosis of Neurologic Syndromes in Lung Cancer Patients

Syndromes due to effects of primary or metastatic tumor
Syndromes due to endocrine or metabolic tumor products (antidiuretic hormone, calcium, glucose, electrolytes)
Syndromes due to embolic infarction (septic emboli, marantic endocarditis)
Syndromes due to thrombotic infarction (atherosclerotic, disseminated intravascular coagulation, superior sagittal sinus occlusion)
Treatment related (chemotherapy, radiotherapy, spontaneous intraparenchymal hemorrhage)
Syndromes due to central nervous system infections
Paraneoplastic syndromes associated with malignancy with unknown mechanism

nins, and various catecholamines. The diagnosis is usually established by relating symptoms to elevated levels of 5-hydroxyindoleacetic acid in the urine.[102]

Gynecomastia

In lung cancer, gynecomastia is usually due to ectopic gonadotropin production, although unilateral swelling may result from a breast metastasis.[103] Gynecomastia appears more commonly in large cell carcinomas and adenocarcinomas of the lung than in squamous or small cell cancers.[104] Gynecomastia may be unilateral or bilateral; if the condition is unilateral, it is usually on the same side as the lung cancer.[9] Elevated levels of the beta subunit of human chorionic gonadotropin or human placental lactogen may sometimes be associated with tender gynecomastia as well as with testicular atrophy.[105] Metastases to the breast can often be confused with primary breast cancer.[106]

Rarely, estrogen production by a gonadotropin-secreting tumor can cause uterine bleeding.[107]

Neurologic and Myopathic Syndromes

Carcinomatous neuromyopathies are the most frequent extrathoracic, nonmetastatic manifestation of lung cancer and are a source of major disability and discomfort for patients (Table 3–8). In one series, 16% of lung cancer patients showed evidence of neuromuscular dysfunction; 56% of those had small cell lung cancer, 22% had squamous cell lung cancer, 16% had large cell lung cancer, and 5% had adenocarcinomas.[108] Carcinomatous neuromyopathies are generally more common late in the disease than at presentation and are most common in patients who experience more than a 15% loss of body weight.[109] However, some neuromyopathies can present clinically months or even years before primary tumor symptoms occur and, in contrast to most paraneoplastic syndromes, may run a course independent of the status of the underlying tumor. The neurologic symptoms can present difficulties in initially staging some lung cancer patients, but some characteristic features are helpful in distinguishing metastatic from paraneoplastic syndromes. Paraneoplastic processes usually manifest as several different neurologic deficits, such as cerebellar findings in conjunction with a peripheral neuropathy or myopathy.[110] Other differential points are that the neurologic deficits are usually symmetric with paraneoplastic syndromes and the CT scan of the head produces negative findings.

Paraneoplastic neurologic syndromes may relate to the CNS or to peripheral nerves or muscles (Table 3–9). Carcinomatous myopathies are divided into myo-

TABLE 3–9. Paraneoplastic Syndromes of the Nervous System Associated with Lung Cancer

SYNDROME	CLINICAL FEATURES
Subacute cerebellar degeneration	Subacute, progressive bilateral, symmetric cerebellar failure often with dementia, dysarthria, cerebrospinal fluid (CSF) lymphocytosis, and elevated protein. Some reports of improvements with removal of primary tumor
Dementia	Variable presentation, acute to slowly progressive. Often associated with abnormalities in other areas of the neuraxis. EEG shows slowing. CSF pleocytosis sometimes seen
Limbic encephalitis	Dementia with degenerative changes in the hippocampus and amygdaloid nuclei. Often associated with inflammatory and degenerative lesions in other areas of the neuraxis. May or may not improve with removal of primary tumor (Ophelia syndrome)
Optic neuritis	Decrease in visual acuity, papilledema; unilateral or bilateral. Rare
Subacute necrotic myelopathy	Rapidly ascending motor and sensory paralysis to thoracic level. Elevated CSF protein. Severe tissue destruction of gray and white matter
Sensory neuropathy	Subacute onset of sensory loss including deep tendon reflexes, with normal strength and normal motor conduction velocity. Elevated CSF protein. Uncommon. Also called dorsal root ganglionitis
Sensorimotor peripheral neuropathy	Distal weakness and wasting, areflexia, distal sensory loss. Elevated CSF protein. Quite common. Recovery rare even with removal of primary tumor
Autonomic and gastrointestinal neuropathy	Orthostatic hypotension, neurogenic bladder, intestinal pseudo-obstruction. Many cases of Ogilvie's syndrome (colonic pseudo-obstruction) may be paraneoplastic
Dermatomyositis and polymyositis	Progressive muscle weakness developing gradually over weeks to months (proximal to distal). Usually not disabling. Elevated muscle enzymes and sedimentation rate. Stringent association in older males
Myasthenic syndrome (Eaton-Lambert syndrome)	Weakness and fatigability of proximal muscles, especially pelvic girdle and thigh. Dryness of mouth, dysphagia, dysarthria, and peripheral paresthesias common. EMGs show a facilitated response in active muscles. Poor response to edrophonium chloride (Tensilon). Should respond to therapy of primary tumor. Guanidine may also be useful

Modified from Bunn PA, Minna JD: Paraneoplastic syndromes. *In* DeVita VT, Hellman S, Rosenberg SA (eds): Cancer: Principles and Practice of Oncology, 4th Ed. Philadelphia, J. B. Lippincott, 1993.

sitis or primary degeneration of muscle fibers and myasthenia-like syndromes, in which the primary defect is in neuromuscular transmission. The myasthenia-like syndromes are characteristic of small cell lung cancer, whereas myositis is seen with all forms of lung cancer.[111] In a series of 100 lung cancer patients, 99 had abnormal muscle histology and 86 demonstrated atrophy of type II muscle fibers, although only 18 were classified as having a cachexic myopathy.[112] In most cases, proximal muscles of the thigh and pelvic girdle show the most prominent weakness.

Some of the neurologic paraneoplastic syndromes may be caused by ectopic secretion of brain-gut peptides.[97] In other cases, tumors with amine precursor uptake and decarboxylation properties such as small cell lung cancer share antigens with neural tissue.[113] In one large series, highly specific antineuronal antibodies were found in 38% of patients with paraneoplastic syndromes.[114] For example, antineural antibodies are frequently found in the serum and spinal fluid of patients with small cell lung cancer who have sensory neuropathies.[115] Whether these cross-reacting antibodies or other antitumor cellular immune responses can cause paraneoplastic syndromes is under active investigation.

Eaton-Lambert Syndrome

This myasthenic syndrome is seen in approximately 6% of small cell lung cancer patients (see Chapter 12).[116–123]

Peripheral Neuropathies

Neuropathies associated with lung cancer may develop in an acute or subacute time frame. Although they are generally combined sensorimotor neuropathies, pure sensory neuropathies are occasionally seen.[124] Combined sensorimotor peripheral neuropathies are common and are associated with distal weakness, especially of the lower extremities, and with areflexia, distal sensory loss, and elevated CSF protein.[125] Sometimes, there is an associated ataxia. The neuropathy may progress to paralysis before other signs of malignancy appear. The neurologic symptoms wax and wane and may respond to steroids but not to lung resection.

Occasionally, lung cancer patients with isolated sensory neuritides are seen. The pathologic lesion is a degeneration of the dorsal root ganglia. Patients have the subacute development of distal sensory loss, especially of proprioception, and loss of deep tendon reflexes with normal muscle strength. Motor nerve conduction velocities are normal. Patients rarely may have paresthesias in the distribution of a single nerve. CSF protein levels are usually increased. Pure sensory neuropathies often precede the diagnosis of cancer, are disabling, and rarely improve. An immune mechanism is postulated because organ-specific antibrain antibodies have been found in the sera and CSF of these patients.[126] Type 1 antineuronal nuclear antibody (ANNA-1), also known as anti-Hu, is a serologic marker for peripheral neuropathy in small cell lung cancer.[127] ANNAs are distinguished from the antinuclear antibodies found in immune disorders such as systemic lupus erythematosus by their selective binding to neuronal elements.

Subacute necrotic myelopathy is a rare paraneoplastic syndrome characterized by a rapidly ascending motor and sensory paralysis to the thoracic level, most often reported in association with lung cancer.[128] Severe tissue destruction of gray and white matter is seen pathologically, and CSF protein levels are elevated. ANNA-1 antibodies have also been noted in patients with necrotizing myelopathy.[129] This condition is usually lethal within days to weeks after its onset.

Cortical Cerebellar Degeneration

Cortical cerebellar degeneration, manifested by vertigo and ataxia and accompanied by marked mental changes, usually develops over the course of several weeks. Both the upper and lower extremities are affected, and the patient may have trouble walking or standing. A severe intention tremor and dysarthria are seen, but nystagmus is uncommon. Predominant ataxia of the upper extremity may occur. Bilateral and symmetric abnormalities and normal CSF are keys to the diagnosis.[15] Pathologically, degeneration of cerebellar Purkinje's cells, often accompanied by degeneration of brain stem nuclei, is the dominant finding.[130] Anti-Purkinje cell antibodies have been found in patients with paraneoplastic cerebellar degeneration.[131] The anti-Yo antibody in this syndrome reacts with a 34 kDa antigen. The gene encoding this antigen has been cloned and demonstrated to be a leucine zipper DNA–binding protein.[132]

Spinal cerebellar degeneration, another paraneoplastic syndrome, is a subacute or chronic development of marked weakness, muscle wasting, paresthesias, and evidence of cerebellar dysfunction, with no abnormalities of higher cortical functions.[133] The etiology is unknown.

Encephalopathy

Lung cancer patients frequently exhibit varying degrees of dementia, psychosis, or organic brain syndrome.[134] The encephalopathy may be acute or slowly progressive and is often associated with abnormalities in other areas of the neuraxis. The electroencephalogram is characteristically slowed, and there may be pleocytosis in the CSF.[135] Treatable causes of CNS dysfunction such as hypoglycemia, hyponatremia, hypoxemia, or hypercalcemia must be ruled out, and CNS metastases must also be excluded. Dementia may also be found associated with marantic emboli, thrombotic infarction with disseminated intravascular coagulation (DIC), and superior sagittal sinus occlusion in cancer patients. Paraneoplastic encephalopathy therefore must be a diagnosis of exclusion.

Limbic encephalitis is characterized by dementia, inappropriate affect, bizarre behavior, and in many cases, seizure disorders.[136] A loss of short- and long-term memory, hallucinations, depression, anxiety, and agitation are usual. Focal neurologic findings are uncommon. The CSF may be normal, but in most cases, there is an increased cell count and elevated protein levels so that leptomeningeal carcinomatosis must be excluded. An intense inflammatory reaction and degenerative changes are found, primarily in the limbic system (e.g., in the hippocampal gyrus, hippocampus, and amygdaloid nucleus), and often involve the temporal lobe.[137] ANNA-1 antibodies are usually detectable in patients who have limbic encephalitis and small cell lung cancer.[131] Limbic encephalitis usually does not improve with removal of the primary lung cancer, but it has been noted to respond after chemotherapy of small cell lung cancer.

Polymyositis

Polymyositis and serositis can occur with all cancers, but they are most often seen with lung cancers. Polymyositis presents with progressive muscle weakness, which is often most pronounced in the extensor muscles of the arm.[138] The weakness develops over a period ranging from weeks to months and may precede the tumor diagnosis by more than a year. Reflexes are decreased but present, and there is little initial muscle wasting. The process usually stabilizes short of disabling the patient. The sedimentation rate and aldolase levels are elevated, and muscle biopsy shows necrosis of muscle fibers with minimal inflammatory changes. In some cases, the disease course may be improved by steroids or androgens.

Autonomic and Gastrointestinal Neuropathy

Lung cancer patients, especially patients with small cell lung cancer, may present with symptoms of autonomic dysfunction, such as orthostatic hypotension or neurogenic bladder.[139] Ogilvie's syndrome is an intestinal pseudo-obstruction with midabdominal pain, nausea, vomiting, and gastric dilatation.[140] Radiographic studies reveal delayed transit of markers throughout the small bowel. Pathologic study of the gut shows widespread degeneration of the myenteric plexus, which is infiltrated by plasma cells and lymphocytes and contains a significantly reduced number of neurons.[141] Associated neuronal losses and lymphocytic infiltrations are seen in dorsal root ganglia. Patients with Ogilvie's syndrome have been found to have autoantibodies of an ANNA-1 specificity reactive with myenteric and submucosal neural plexuses of the jejunum and stomach.[142] Treatment of the underlying malignancy may not be successful in palliating symptoms of gastrointestinal dysmobility, even though tumor shrinkage is achieved.

The presence of historical features, such as postural dizziness, sweating abnormalities, bladder dysfunction, and ejaculatory difficulty, should alert the physician to the need to thoroughly assess the patient's autonomic function. These studies include a thermoregulatory sweat test, a screen of autonomic vagal and sympathetic reflex responses, and measurement of plasma fractionated catecholamine levels in the supine and standing positions.[143] These tests often indicate whether the neural lesion is preganglionic or postganglionic. This factor can be confirmed by using an intravenous edrophonium test.[144] Normal norepinephrine levels suggest normal postganglionic sympathetic fibers, although abnormalities in supine levels and responses to edrophonium may only be detected when there is widespread postganglionic degeneration. If autonomic function testing is abnormal, with evidence suggesting a preganglionic or central lesion, imaging of the brain and spinal cord is indicated. Magnetic resonance imaging is preferred in this situation because it provides excellent views of structures in the posterior cranial fossa and spinal cord.

Internuclear Ophthalmoplegia and Optic Neuritis

Visual deficits are occasionally described as remote effects of a bronchial carcinoma.[145] An acute loss of vision has been described in two small cell lung cancer patients whose sera contained antibodies to a determinant found both on cultured small cell lung cancer cells and on large retinal ganglion cells.[146] The optic neuritis is characterized by binocular loss of vision, with photosensitivity, ring scotomata, visual field loss, and attenuated arteriole caliber. Lung cancer patients with vision loss and no evidence of brain metastases have also been described who have secondary demyelination of the medial longitudinal fasciculus or round cell infiltration and adhesive arachnoiditis of the optic nerve.[147] The CSF in these patients was found to have increased protein but no inflammatory cells.

Hematologic Abnormalities in Lung Cancer Patients

Hematologic abnormalities are frequent in lung cancer patients and many can be considered as paraneoplastic syndromes. These abnormalities usually occur late in the course of disease in the setting of widespread or recurrent lung cancer. A series of three patients with idiopathic pancytopenia and hypercellular bone marrow who developed cancer of the lung within 2 years of diagnosis has been reported.[148] Pancytopenia may also be associated with myelophthisis, which is the replacement of marrow elements with cancer cells.[149] Leukoerythroblastic anemia from cancerous infiltration of the bone marrow is characterized by the occurrence of immature white and red cells in the peripheral blood.

Red Blood Cell Abnormalities

A normochromic, normocytic anemia with a moderate shortening of red blood cell survival is found in approximately 20% of lung cancer patients.[150] This anemia of chronic disease is most commonly due to dyserythropoiesis with decreased iron utilization and an associated block of reticuloendothelial iron release. A second population of hypochromic, microcytic cells may coexist. The anemia is characterized by decreased serum iron levels, decreased total iron-binding capacity, and increased marrow iron stores. Rarely, sideroblastic anemia occurs with increased serum iron levels, increased saturation of iron-binding proteins, and ringed sideroblasts in the marrow.[151] Secondary erythrocytosis rarely has been associated with lung cancer. It is usually mild and requires no treatment. Pure red cell aplasia with severe anemia occasionally has been reported with squamous cell lung cancer.[152] Rarely, acute hemolytic anemias occur in lung cancer, usually in association with disseminated intravascular coagulation (DIC).[153]

White Blood Cell Abnormalities

Lung cancer patients may develop a leukoerythroblastic picture with myeloblasts or neutrophilic myelocytes in the circulating blood, indicating malignant infiltration of the marrow.[154] Peripheral blood leukocytosis or leukemoid reaction resembling chronic myelogenous leukemia may occur rarely in lung cancer.[155] A granulocytic leukemoid reaction with a shift to the left is most common, but eosinophilic leukemoid reactions have also been associated with lung cancer. The leukemoid reactions differ from leukemia in that the cell counts are usually less than 100,000/μl, no blasts or progranulocytes are seen in peripheral blood, platelet and basophil counts are usually normal, there is no splenomegaly, leukocyte alkaline phosphatase is increased, serum vitamin B_{12} is normal, and there is no Philadelphia chromosome. There is no clear relationship between survival and the degree of elevation of the granulocyte count. Leukemoid reactions in lung cancers are thought to be related to tumor production of colony-stimulating factors. Lung cancer cell line supernatants and the urine and serum from lung cancer patients have been found to contain a component similar to colony-stimulating factor.[155] When lung cancer cells producing such factors are heterotransplanted, they can cause neutrophilia in athymic nude mice.[156]

Lung cancer may rarely be associated with either tissue or blood eosinophilia. Blood eosinophilia usually occurs with extensive metastatic disease. Serum and tumor extracts from a patient with large cell bronchogenic carcinoma and eosinophilia markedly stimulated the growth of eosinophil colonies from human bone marrow.[157] A 45 kDa eosinophilotactic factor has been isolated from lung cancer cells that was identical with eosinophil chemotactic factor of anaphylaxis.[158]

Platelet Abnormalities

Thrombocytosis was found by Silvis and colleagues in 60% of 153 lung cancer patients.[159] The differential diagnosis of thrombocytosis in a lung cancer patient includes coexistent myeloproliferative disorders, acute and chronic inflammatory disorders, acute hemorrhage, iron deficiency, and hemolytic anemias.

Thrombocytosis may also occur with drugs, especially steroids and vincristine. Platelet counts above $10^6/\mu$l, which might lead to thrombosis or hemorrhage, are rare in lung cancer.

Digital gangrene, associated with spontaneous platelet aggregation, has been reported in a patient with small cell lung cancer.[160] This patient responded dramatically after starting aspirin treatment. Other cases of digital ischemia associated with lung cancer have been attributed to vasospasm and tumor emboli.

Thrombocytopenia was noted in only 2.6% of lung cancer patients in the series of Silvis and colleagues.[159] Idiopathic thrombocytopenic purpura is occasionally seen, presenting with platelet counts generally less than 30,000/μl, a normal hematocrit, normal to increased megakaryocytes in the marrow, and no evidence of DIC or drug-induced thrombocytopenia.[161] About 80% of the patients have symptoms of bleeding, petechiae, or purpura. A rapid fall in the platelet count after platelet transfusion is noted. Severely affected patients may require splenectomy, which leads to an improvement in platelet counts in the majority of these patients.

Disseminated Intravascular Coagulation

DIC may be seen in all lung cancer subtypes, either alone or in association with migratory thrombophlebitis, or with thrombotic nonbacterial endocarditis.[162] DIC is thought to reflect the release of thromboplastic and proteolytic substances from tumor, as well as vascular damage and increased platelet adhesiveness. Abnormalities in blood coagulation studies reflect the rate of DIC and the effects of secondary activation of the fibrinolytic system. Lung cancers are often associated with thrombotic disturbances ascribed to alterations in coagulation factors, thrombocytosis, increased fibrinogen deposition, and decreased fibrinolysis.[163–164]

Migratory Venous Thrombosis (Trousseau's Syndrome)

Trousseau's syndrome has a characteristic migratory pattern of thrombosis or involvement of two or more venous sites simultaneously. The thrombosis can occur in patients without obvious predisposing causes and may occur in unusual distributions involving arm veins, the inferior vena cava, or the jugular venous system. In one series, the average time between the onset of phlebitis and the histologic confirmation of malignancy was 4 months.[165] The potential mechanisms involved in hypercoagulability are incompletely understood and include platelet activation, thrombocytosis, release of procoagulant substances by the tumor cell or from monocyte-macrophage stimulation, and dysfibrinogenemia.[166]

Thrombophlebitis occurs in about 1% of cases of lung cancer. Approximately 3% of all cases of thrombophlebitis are related to malignancy, and in men, lung cancer is the underlying malignancy most often observed.[167] In one-third of cases, thrombophlebitis occurs before the diagnosis of cancer is established.

TABLE 3–10. Dermatologic Lesions Seen in Lung Cancer

DISORDER	DESCRIPTION	COMMENTS
Acanthosis nigricans	Hyperkeratosis and pigmentation, especially of axillae, neck, flexures, and anogenital region	Most important to distinguish benign forms present from birth and benign forms associated with various syndromes
Acquired ichthyosis	Generalized dry, cracking skin, hyperkeratotic palms and soles, rhomboidal scales	Should be distinguished from hereditary form, which occurs before age 20
Bazex's disease	Erythema, hyperkeratosis with scales and pruritus predominantly on palms and soles	Males only
Dermatomyositis	Purplish pink erythema, especially of eyelids, neck, and hands	Malignant disease reported in 7% to 50%. Precedes carcinoma by days to years with an average of 6 months
Erythema gyratum	Rapidly changing and advancing gyri with scaling and pruritus	Almost always associated with malignancy
Lanuginosa acquisita (malignant down)	Rapid development of fine, long, silky hair, especially on ears and forehead, and possibly involving the entire body	High association with cancer
Leser-Trélat syndrome	Sudden appearance of large numbers of seborrheic (wartlike) keratoses	Must be distinguished from multiple seborrheic keratoses, which are common and may not be associated with malignancy. Occasionally associated with acanthosis
Pachydermoperiostitis	Thickening of skin and creation of new folds; thickened lips, ears, and lids; macroglossia; thick forehead and scalp; clubbing; excessive sweating	Occurs also in lung abscess, benign tumors

Modified from Bunn PA, Minna JD: Paraneoplastic syndromes. *In* DeVita VT, Hellman S, Rosenberg SA (eds): Cancer: Principles and Practice of Oncology, 4th Ed. Philadelphia, J. B. Lippincott, 1993.

Thrombophlebitis associated with malignancy is resistant to sodium warfarin and is best treated with heparin.[164] Patients with recurrent or migratory phlebitis, without apparent cause and with poor response to anticoagulant therapy, should be suspected of having a malignancy.

Lung cancer patients may rarely develop idiopathic thrombosis of the dural sinuses or cerebral veins that is not related to invasion or compression of these vessels by tumor metastases.[168] The syndrome is often misdiagnosed as metastatic disease, and digital subtraction angiography provides the only sure method of diagnosis.

Nonbacterial Thrombotic Endocarditis (Marantic Endocarditis)

Marantic endocarditis is the result of deposition of sterile, verrucous, bland, fibrin-platelet lesions on the heart valves, usually on the left side. The patients present with the sequelae of arterial emboli to the brain, spleen, kidney, and heart.[169] Neurologic symptoms may be abrupt or insidious; the patients may develop focal neurologic symptoms or diffuse abnormalities such as confusion, disorientation, seizures, or a change in the level of consciousness. Emboli to the coronary arteries may cause a myocardial infarction. The patients may demonstrate bleeding in the skin, CNS, genitourinary tract, pharynx, gastrointestinal tract, or lungs. Less than one-third of the patients have systolic heart murmurs, and the majority are afebrile. Most of the valvular lesions are smaller than 2 mm in size, so they are not readily detectable by echocardiography. Occlusion of large and small vessels in the brain is noted.[170] Marantic endocarditis is particularly common in adenocarcinoma of the lung, with a 7.5% prevalence at necropsy (twice that of adenocarcinomas of the pancreas or prostate).[171] Although the condition is usually seen in advanced disease, marantic endocarditis does not imply unresectability of the tumor.[172]

Dermatologic Lesions Associated with Lung Cancer

Various cutaneous manifestations of malignancy are well recognized (Table 3–10). Some are nonspecific, whereas others are almost always associated with underlying cancer. Dermatologic conditions associated with lung cancer include dermatomyositis, acanthosis nigricans, pruritus, tylosis, urticaria, angioedema, herpes zoster, scleroderma, acquired ichthyosis, hyperpigmentation, and an exfoliative dermatitis. The onset of symptoms in the paraneoplastic skin lesions is often more rapid than when the lesion is associated with a benign or hereditary cause.

Dermatomyositis

Dermatomyositis is the most common collagen-vascular manifestation of malignancy, although systemic lupus erythematosus and scleroderma have also been associated with lung cancer.[173] Between 14% and 20% of patients with dermatomyositis have a malignancy, and cancer should always be suspected in such patients older than 40 years of age. Dermatomyositis is more common in patients with adenocarcinoma of the lung than it is in patients with the other subtypes. A lilac-colored rash in a heliotrope-like pattern around the eyes is associated with symmetric muscle weakness, particularly of pelvic girdle muscles. The diagnosis is made by elevations of aspartate aminotransferase, alanine aminotransferase, and aldolase (but not creatine phosphokinase), as well as by electromyography and muscle biopsy.[174] In some cases, corticosteroids or antitumor therapy may improve the weakness and skin lesions.[175]

Hyperkeratosis

Patients with lung cancer, particularly those who have squamous cell histologic findings, may develop tylosis, a hyperkeratosis of the palms and soles.[176–177] There was a greater incidence of keratoses in males of both groups and in controls who smoked. The keratoses often appeared to antedate the appearance of the lung cancer, but they may be associated with smoking, because smoking and squamous cell lung cancer are closely associated. Pachydermoperiostosis is a thickening of skin and creation of new folds, leading to thickened lips, ears, eyelids, and skin of the forehead and scalp.[178] Macroglossia, clubbing, and excessive sweating are also seen.

Acanthosis nigricans is a symmetric epidermoid thickening, with hyperkeratosis and acanthosis, which is occasionally found in lung cancer but more often seen in gastrointestinal and breast cancers.[179] There is hyperpigmentation in the axilla and other flexural surfaces. The lesions may involve the oral mucous membranes, palms, and soles and may precede the appearance of any cancer. Tripe palms, which are part of the syndrome, have a thickened appearance, exaggerated ridges and furrows, and brown hyperpigmentation. Acanthosis nigricans appearing in patients older than 50 years of age is very suggestive of malignancy.

Leser-Trélat sign is the sudden appearance of a large crop of hyperpigmented seborrheic (wartlike) keratoses, which is often associated with various malignancies. The acuteness of the presentation helps distinguish Leser-Trélat syndrome from benign multiple seborrheic keratoses. The patient may have pruritus, and the syndrome can be associated with acanthosis nigricans. Leser-Trélat syndrome is more often seen with lung adenocarcinomas, but the condition has been reported with small cell lung cancer.[180] Both the Leser-Trélat syndrome and acanthosis nigricans have been associated with the production of transforming growth factor-alpha by malignant cells.[181]

Hyperpigmentation

Generalized hyperpigmentation secondary to ectopic adrenocorticotropic hormone and melanocyte-stimulating hormone production is occasionally seen in patients with small cell lung cancer.[182] The hyperpigmentation is particularly obvious on exposed portions of the body, nipples, lips, buccal mucous membranes, genitalia, skin creases, and recent scars. Other manifestations of Cushing's disease are absent.

Other Dermatologic Lesions

Erythema gyratum repens is a syndrome of rapidly changing and advancing gyri with scaling and pruritus, and the condition is occasionally seen with lung cancer.[183] This lesion is almost always associated with a malignancy.

Hypertrichosis lanuginosa acquisita (malignant down) is the rapid development of long, fine, silky hair, especially on the ears and forehead, but sometimes involving the entire body.[184] This finding is almost always associated with cancer. High urinary levels of free cortisol are found, and the lesion is hypothesized to be due to a corticotropin-like intermediate lobe peptide that is split off from the precursor molecule of ACTH.

Hypertrophic Pulmonary Osteoarthropathy

One of the most common remote effects of lung cancer is the development of hypertrophic pulmonary osteoarthropathy (HPO), also known as Bamberger-Marie disease. HPO is found in up to 5% of patients with lung cancer, is particularly common in patients with adenocarcinoma (12%), and is rare in mesothelioma and small cell lung cancer.[185] This may be a reflection of the speed of cancer growth. The dominant clinical findings are clubbing of the fingers and toes, loose nails, and symmetric, proliferating periostitis of the distal ends of long bones, particularly the tibia, fibula, radius, and ulna. Clubbing alone may be found in 21% of lung cancer patients at the time of diagnosis, and it usually develops rapidly.[186] The periostitis presents with pain, tenderness, and swelling over the affected bones, and the condition may progress to involve the metacarpals, metatarsals, femora, humeri, and other bones. The pain is often most prominent in the distal leg bones and characteristically improves when the patient is placed in a Trendelenburg position. There may be an associated polyarthritis and chronic synovitis similar to rheumatoid arthritis in the knees, ankles, and wrists.[187] The joints are often hyperemic and may show pannus formation. The synovial fluid in patients with HPO is noninflammatory and produces a good mucin clot. HPO can be associated with peripheral neurovascular changes such as cyanosis, hyperhidrosis, paresthesia, and erythema.[48] Bone roentgenograms show an ossifying periostitis, and the bone scan is positive in affected bones, reflecting ongoing deposition of osteoid and new bone formation along the inner aspect of the periosteum.[188] High uptake of radioactive material into areas of periosteal hypertrophy is seen on ^{99m}Tc diphosphonate bone scanning.

HPO may precede the diagnosis of tumor by several months and may respond promptly to surgical treatment of the lung cancer.[189] The etiology of HPO is unknown, and estrogens, growth hormone, and neurally transmitted signals are suggested inconclusively as playing roles in the etiology.[190] Reflex stimulation of afferent fibers of the vagus nerve has been suggested in the pathogenesis of HPO, and vagotomy proximal to the hilum may provide relief from the pain of HPO in some cases.[191] Elevated estrogen levels and gynecomastia are sometimes found associated with HPO.

HPO can also occur in chronic lung diseases such as tuberculosis, abscesses, and bronchiectasis. In these cases, the lesions develop more slowly and are less painful. Benign chest tumors and cancers metastatic to the chest can also result in HPO. The bone changes of hyperparathyroidism can simulate HPO.

Acromegaly

Acromegaly has been well-documented in patients with bronchial carcinoid tumors.[192] Acromegaly in these patients has been associated with secretion of growth hormone–releasing hormone by the tumors.[193] Although elevated growth hormone–releasing hormone levels have been found in other bronchogenic carcinomas, clinical acromegaly has not been evident, possibly because of the more rapid rate of development of these tumors.

Renal Paraneoplastic Syndromes

The most common remote effect of lung cancer on kidneys is the development of nephrotic syndrome.[194] Possible causes of nephrotic syndrome in these circumstances include immune complex glomerulopathy, diffuse glomerular fibrin deposition, renal amyloidosis, and renal vein thrombosis (Table 3–11).

The most frequently observed glomerular lesion in patients with carcinoma (in contrast to those with Hodgkin's disease) is membranous glomerulonephritis, characterized by subepithelial electron-dense deposits and granular capillary deposits of IgG.[195] This lesion is present in 80% to 90% of patients who have carcinoma and nephrotic syndrome. Occasional lung cancer patients have been documented to have lipoid nephrosis or a proliferative glomerulonephritis.[196] Tumor-specific antibodies have been eluted from the kidneys of two patients with lung cancer and nephrotic syndrome, suggesting that there was glomerular deposition of circulating antigen-antibody complexes. Lung cancer patients with nephrotic syndrome

TABLE 3–11. Differential Diagnosis of Renal Abnormalities in Patients with Lung Cancer

Direct infiltration of the kidney tumor
Obstruction of the urinary tract by tumor
Electrolyte imbalances, many of which are caused by the tumor or its treatment (e.g., calcium, uric acid, potassium)
Fluid imbalances induced by the tumor or its treatment (prerenal)
Infection
Toxicity of therapy (chemotherapy, radiotherapy, immunotherapy, antibiotics)
Glomerular lesions of uncertain etiology (usually associated with nephrotic syndrome), paraneoplastic
Obstruction by tumor products

Modified from Bunn PA, Minna JD: Paraneoplastic syndromes. *In* DeVita VT, Hellman S, Rosenberg SA (eds): Cancer: Principles and Practice of Oncology, 4th Ed. Philadelphia, J. B. Lippincott, 1993.

and either minimal change glomerular disease or mesangial proliferative glomerulonephritis have been documented to have marked improvements in or resolution of the nephrotic syndrome with effective treatment of their lung cancer.[197]

Two cases of small cell lung cancer associated with an IgA nephropathy have been reported.[198] The patients had hematuria, a purpuric leg rash resembling Henoch-Schönlein purpura, and proteinuria. Immunofluorescence with anti-IgA antisera was positive in the glomeruli in each case. IgA nephropathy is normally very rare in patients older than 60 years of age.

Gastrointestinal Paraneoplastic Syndromes

Gastrointestinal remote effects of lung cancer are relatively rare. A profuse watery diarrhea with hypokalemia and hypochlorhydria can be found in lung cancer patients.[199] This presentation is similar to a syndrome seen in patients with pancreatic non-B islet cell tumors or villous adenomas of the rectum. The cause of this syndrome is unknown.

LABORATORY FINDINGS IN LUNG CANCER

Although no laboratory findings are specific for lung cancer, some tests may document metabolic derangements owing to the tumor, and others act as markers for disease progression. Routine serum chemistry findings often show hyperglycemia and hypoalbuminemia.[200] Patients with liver or bone metastases have elevations in serum alkaline phosphatase levels. Ferritin is usually elevated in lung cancer, but alpha-fetoprotein is not.[201] Zinc levels are decreased.[202] Urine chemistries show increased excretion of hydroxyproline in patients with bone metastases. The most common finding in the urine is mild to moderate proteinuria (100 to 1000 mg/day). The urine protein is predominantly composed of low-molecular-weight glycoproteins.[194]

About 70% of lung cancer patients have elevations in carcinoembryonic antigen (CEA).[203] CEA is not specific enough to be used as a marker in routine cancer screening, but it can be used as a tumor marker to monitor therapy. If the CEA level is elevated above 15 to 20 mg/ml, then the prognosis is poor (in one series, 3 months was the median survival). High CEA levels often correlate with the development of hepatic metastases.[204]

ProACTH, or big ACTH, is a prohormone found in elevated serum concentrations in all histologic subtypes of lung cancer; it is immunologically identifiable but biochemically nonfunctional. In one series, 74% of 74 patients with lung cancer had elevations in proACTH, whereas all 26 control patients with benign diseases had normal plasma ACTH levels.[205] More recent reports, however, cast doubt on the specificity of proACTH for lung cancer diagnosis.[206] At present, a number of other markers are under investigation for their ability to mark or track lung cancer. Included among these markers are neuron-specific enolase and bombesin.[207] In general, most of these biomarkers are no more sensitive for purposes of disease evaluation than are careful clinical imaging and routine laboratory studies.

OTHER MEDICAL PROBLEMS OF LUNG CANCER PATIENTS

Many patients with lung cancer have underlying medical problems that affect the prognosis of the cancer as well as their options for treatment.[208] During the initial evaluation of a patient with lung cancer, it is important to determine the individual's physiologic status, degree of weight loss, and current performance status in order to decide among treatment options. In one study of 700 lung cancer patients, 36% had a history of significant cardiovascular disease.[15] Lung cancer patients commonly have chronic obstructive pulmonary disease related to smoking, and liver damage resulting from alcohol abuse. Sometimes, the exacerbation of a chronic, nonmalignant medical problem can be confused with the progression of cancer. Treatment of the cancer with either surgery, radiation therapy, or chemotherapy may aggravate such underlying medical problems. The results of the various treatments are closely correlated with the types of pretreatment factors and comorbid diseases.

Of the entire population of patients with lung cancer, 0.5% will develop a second primary cancer before death, which may be either synchronous or metachronous with the lung cancer. Common second primary tumors include other lung cancers, head and neck cancers, esophageal cancers, bladder cancers, and pancreatic cancers.[209] As would be expected, most of these other tumors have a common smoking-related etiology.

Development of a new primary cancer in a patient with lung cancer may simulate metastatic disease. Therefore, it is important to document the nature of such lesions with a biopsy, especially if each primary lesion is otherwise potentially curable. Two per cent of lung cancer patients undergoing resection and 10% of long-term survivors also develop second primary lung cancers, most within the first 5 years.[210] Therefore, patients should have frequent physical examinations, including annual head and neck examinations, after undergoing a resection of lung cancer for cure, and the discontinuation of smoking is essential. If a patient who was treated curatively for one lung cancer develops a second primary lung cancer, there is a good basis for aggressive treatment. In one series of 58 patients with metachronous primaries, a 36% cumulative survival rate at 5 years was found with aggressive surgery for the second primary, although there was a 9.3% postoperative mortality rate.[211]

SUMMARY

The rising incidence in lung cancer has made it an important and prevalent disease, which all clinicians should recognize. The many presentations that are possible for the various lung cancers should make the consideration of lung cancer a standard item on lists of differential diagnosis, especially among smokers and those with industrial exposures such as nickel, chromium, uranium, and asbestos. Lung cancer is particularly common among industrially exposed individuals who also smoke cigarettes. The evaluation of the course of the disease after treatment has developed in recent years largely owing to more effective therapies that allow patients to live long enough to develop new disease sequelae. It is critical both to patient care and to our understanding of these diseases that new sequelae be carefully studied in order to improve symptomatic care as well as to modify treatments earlier and achieve a higher percentage of long-term disease-free survivors.

SELECTED REFERENCES

Bunn PA, Minna JD: Paraneoplastic syndromes. *In* DeVita VT, Hellman S, Rosenberg SA (eds): Cancer: Principles and Practice of Oncology. 4th Ed. Philadelphia, J. B. Lippincott, 1993.
A comprehensive treatise on paraneoplastic syndromes with special reference to lung cancer. A superb integration of clinical and laboratory medicine that is extensively referenced. Much of the work cited derives from studies conducted by the authors and their colleagues.
Cohen MH: Lung cancer: Diagnosis, staging and therapy. *In* Harris CC (ed): Pathogenesis and Therapy of Lung Cancer. New York, Marcel Dekker, 1978, pp 653–700.
A well-referenced and coherently organized discussion of the clinical presentations of lung cancer. The chapter is beautifully written and contains numerous interesting clinical observations, reflecting the author's depth of experience in treating lung cancer.
Hyde L, Hyde CI: Clinical manifestations of lung cancer. Chest 65:299–306, 1974.
One of the best analyzed of the large group studies of lung cancer. This paper discusses the presenting signs and symptoms of bronchogenic carcinoma and contains short discussions of the pathophysiology of each finding.
Patel AM, Peters SG: Clinical manifestations of lung cancer. Mayo Clin Proc 68:273–277, 1993.
A succinct and well-written review of the presenting signs of lung cancer and the pathophysiology underlying the symptoms.

REFERENCES

1. Carbone PP, Frost JK, Feinstein AR, et al: Lung cancer: Perspective and prospects. Ann Intern Med 73:1024–1033, 1970.
2. Cromartie RS, Parker EF, May JE, et al: Carcinoma of the lung: A clinical review. Ann Thorac Surg 30:30–35, 1980.
3. Kreyberg L: WHO: The World Health Organization histologic typing of lung tumors. Am J Clin Pathol 77:123–136, 1982.
4. Weiss W, Boucot KR: The Philadelphia pulmonary neoplasm research project, early roentgenographic appearance of bronchogenic carcinoma. Arch Intern Med 134:306–311, 1974.
5. Benfield JR, Juillard GJF, Pilch YH, et al: Current and future concepts of lung cancer. Ann Intern Med 83:93–106, 1975.
6. Harley HRS: Cancer of the lung in women. Thorax 31:254–264, 1976.
7. Meigs JW: Epidemic lung cancer in women. JAMA 238:1055, 1977.
8. Green N, Kurohara SS, George FW, et al: The biologic behavior of lung cancer according to histologic type. Radiol Clin Biol 41:160–170, 1972.
9. Cohen MH: Signs and symptoms of bronchogenic carcinoma. Semin Oncol 1:183–189, 1974.

10. Tao LC, Delarue NC, Sanders D, et al: Bronchioalveolar carcinoma: A correlative clinical and cytologic study. Cancer 42:2759–2767, 1978.
11. Daly RC, Trastek VF, Pairolero PC, et al: Bronchoalveolar carcinoma: Factors affecting survival. Ann Thorac Surg 51:368–376, 1991.
12. Donaldson JC, Kaminsky DB, Elliot RC: Bronchiolar carcinoma: Report of 11 cases and review of the literature. Cancer 41:250–258, 1978.
13. Oels HC, Harrison EG, Carr DT, et al: Diffuse malignant mesothelioma of the pleura: A review of 37 cases. Chest 60:564–570, 1972.
14. Aisner J, Wiernik PH: Malignant mesothelioma: Current status and future prospects. Chest 74:438–443, 1978.
15. Hyde L, Hyde Cl: Clinical manifestations of lung cancer. Chest 65:299–306, 1974.
16. Loudon RG, Shaw GB: Mechanics of cough in normal subjects and in patients with obstructive respiratory disease. Am Rev Respir Dis 96:666, 1967.
17. Coy P, Kennally GM: The role of curative radiotherapy in the treatment of lung cancer. Cancer 45:698–702, 1980.
18. Wolfe JD, Simmons DH: Hemoptysis: Diagnosis and management (medical progress). West J Med 127:383, 1977.
19. Mahler DA, Snyder PE, Virgilto JA, et al: Positional dyspnea and oxygen desaturation related to carcinoma of the lung. Chest 83:826–827, 1983.
20. Gacad G, Akhtar N, Cohn JN: Orthostatic hypotension in a patient with lung carcinoma. Arch Intern Med 134:1113–1115, 1974.
21. Hardy JD, Ewing HP, Neely WA, et al: Lung carcinoma: Survey of 2280 cases with emphasis on small cell types. Ann Surg 193:539–548, 1981.
22. Baird JA: The pathways of lymphatic spread of carcinoma of the lung. Br J Surg 52:868–875, 1965.
23. Reingold IN, Ottoman RE, Konwaler BE: Bronchogenic carcinoma: A study of 60 necropsies. Am J Clin Pathol 20:515, 1950.
24. Gondos B, Reingold IM: Pathology of scalene lymph nodes. Cancer 18:84, 1965.
25. Agliozzo CM, Reingold IM: Scalene lymph nodes in necropsies of malignant tumors: Analysis of 166 cases. Cancer 20:2148, 1967.
26. Brantigan JW, Brantigan CO, Brantigan OC: Biopsy of non palpable scalene lymph nodes in carcinoma of the lung. Am Rev Respir Dis 107:962–974, 1973.
27. Cohen MH: Lung cancer: diagnosis, staging and therapy. In Harris CC (ed): Pathogenesis and Therapy of Lung Cancer. New York, Marcel Dekker, 1978, pp 653–700.
28. Tandon RK: The significance of pleural effusion associated with bronchial carcinoma. Br J Dis Chest 60:49, 1966.
29. Livingston RB, McCracken JD, Trauft CJ, et al: Isolated pleural effusion in small cell lung carcinoma: Favorable prognosis. Chest 81:208–215, 1982.
30. Kabnick EM, Sobo S, Steinbaum S, et al: Spontaneous pneumothorax from bronchogenic carcinoma. J Natl Med Assoc 74:478–479, 1982.
31. O'Connor BM, Ziegler P, Spaulding MB: Spontaneous pneumothorax in small cell lung cancer. Chest 102:628–629, 1992.
32. Farber SM, Mardel W, Spain DM: Diagnosis and Treatment of Tumors of the Chest. New York, Grune and Stratton, 1966.
33. Hansburg WS, Cureton RJR, Simon G: Pulmonary infarcts associated with bronchogenic carcinoma. Thorax 9:304–312, 1954.
34. Peihler JM, Pariolero PC, Weiland LH, et al: Bronchogenic carcinoma with chest wall invasion: Factors affecting survival following en bloc resection. Ann Thorac Surg 34:684–691, 1982.
35. Wall EW: The blood vascular and lymphatic systems. In Romains GS (ed): Cunningham's Textbook of Anatomy. 12th Ed. Oxford, Oxford University Press, 1964, pp 962–963.
36. Strauss BL, Matthews MJ, Cohen MH, et al: Cardiac metastases in lung cancer. Chest 71:607–610, 1977.
37. Al-Hillawi A, Hayward R, Johnson Nl, et al: Lung cancer masquerading as atrial myxoma. Thorax 38:870, 1983.
38. Katzir D, Klinovsky E, Kent V, et al: Spontaneous pneumopericardium: case report and review of the literature. Cardiology 76:305–308, 1989.
39. Lochridge SK, Knibbe WP, Doty DB: Obstruction of the superior vena cava. Surgery 85:14–24, 1979.
40. Lokich J, Goodman R: Superior vena cava syndrome: Clinical management. JAMA 231:58–61, 1975.
41. Salgali M, Clifton EE: Superior vena caval obstruction with lung cancer. Ann Thorac Surg 6:437–442, 1968.
42. Nogeire C, Mincer F, Botstein C: Long survival in patients with bronchogenic carcinoma complicated by superior vena caval obstruction. Chest 75:325–329, 1979.
43. Rubin P, Hicks GL: Biassociation of superior vena cava obstruction and spinal cord compression. N Y State J Med 73:2176–2182, 1973.
44. Mason BA: Axillary-subclavian vein occlusion in patients with lung neoplasms. Cancer 48:1886–1889, 1981.
45. Miller JI, Mansour KA, Hatcher JR: Carcinoma of the superior pulmonary sulcus. Ann Thorac Surg 28:44–47, 1979.
46. Paulson DL: Carcinomas in the superior pulmonary sulcus. J Thorac Cardiovasc Surg 70:1095–1102, 1975.
47. Doury, P: Review of algodystrophy: Reflex sympathetic dystrophy. Clin Rheumatol 7:173–180, 1988.
48. Thomas CR, Rest EB, Brown CR: Rheumatologic manifestations of malignancy. Med Pediatr Oncol 18:146–158, 1990.
49. Paulson DL: Carcinoma in the superior pulmonary sulcus. Ann Thorac Surg 29:3–4, 1979.
50. McCoy BP: Apical pulmonary adenocarcinoma with contra lateral hyperhidrosis. Arch Dermatol 117:659–661, 1981.
51. Chan P: Pulmonary carcinoma and provocative sweat testing. Arch Dermatol 119:185, 1983.
52. Alexander C: Diaphragm movements and the diagnosis of diaphragmatic paralysis. Clin Radiol 17:79–83, 1966.
53. Bongers KM, Willegers HMM, Koehler PJ: Referred facial pain from lung cancer. Neurology 42:1841–1842, 1982.
54. Henderson RD, Boszko A, Van Nostrand AWP: Pharyngoesophageal dysphagia and recurrent laryngeal nerve palsy. J Thorac Cardiovasc Surg 68:507–512, 1974.
55. Newman SJ, Hansen HH: Frequency, diagnosis and treatment of brain metastases in 247 consecutive patients with bronchogenic carcinoma. Cancer 33:492–496, 1974.
56. Jacobs L, Kinkel WR, Vincent RG: "Silent" brain metastasis from lung carcinoma determined by computerized tomography. Arch Neurol 34:690–693, 1977.
57. Cox JD, Komaki R, Byhardt RW, et al: Results of whole brain irradiation for metastases from small cell carcinoma of the lung. Cancer Treat Rep 64:957–961, 1980.
58. Nugent JL, Bunn PA, Matthews MJ, et al: CNS metastases in small cell lung carcinoma: Increasing frequency and changing pattern with lengthening survival. Cancer 44:1885–1893, 1979.
59. Bunn PA, Nugent JL, Matthews MJ: Central nervous system metastases in small cell bronchogenic carcinoma. Semin Oncol 5:314–322, 1978.
60. Rodichok LD, Harper GR, Ruckdeschel JC, et al: Early diagnosis of spinal epidural metastases. Am J Med 70:1181–1187, 1981.
61. Rodichok LD, Ruckdeschel JC, Harper GR, et al: Early detection and treatment of spinal epidural metastases: The role of myelography. Ann Neurol 20:696–702, 1986.
62. Rosen ST, Aisner J, Makuch RW, et al: Carcinomatous leptomeningitis in small cell lung cancer. Medicine 61:45–53, 1982.
63. Aisner J, Aisner SC, Ostrow S, et al: Meningeal carcinomatosis from small cell cancer of the lung. Acta Cytol 23:292–296, 1979.
64. Karten I, Bartfield H: Bronchogenic carcinoma simulating early rheumatoid arthritis. JAMA 179:160–161, 1962.
65. Beer OT, Dubowy J, Jimenez FA: Osteoblastic metastases from bronchogenic carcinoma. Am J Roentgenol Radium Ther Nucl Med 91:161, 1964.
66. Murray GC, Persellin RH: Metastatic carcinoma presenting as monoarticular arthritis: A case report and review of the literature. Arthritis Rheum 23:95–100, 1980.
67. Khan FA, Garterhouse W, Khan A: Metastatic bronchogenic carcinoma: An unusual cause of localized arthritis. Chest 67:738–739, 1975.
68. Covelli HD, Zaloznick AJ, Shekifka KM: Evaluation of bone pain in carcinoma of the lung. JAMA 244:2625–2627, 1980.
69. Rodichok LD, Harper GR, Ruckdeschel JC, et al: Early diagnosis of spinal epidural metastases. Am J Med 72:1181–1188, 1981.
70. Raju RN, Kardinal CG: Lactic acidosis in lung cancer. South Med J 6:397–398, 1983.

71. Dunnick NR, Ihde DC, Johnston-Early A: Abdominal CT in the evaluation of small cell carcinoma of the lung. Am J Roentgenol Radium Ther Nucl Med 133:1085–1088, 1979.

72. Burbige EJ, Radigan N, Belber JP: Metastatic lung carcinoma involving the gastrointestinal tract. Am J Gastroenterol 74:504–506, 1980.

73. Winchester DP, Merril JR, Victor TA, et al: Small bowel perforation secondary to metastatic carcinoma of the lung. Cancer 40:410–415, 1977.

74. Morton WJ, Tedesco FJ: Metastatic bronchogenic carcinoma seen as a gastric ulcer. Am J Dig Dis 19:766–770, 1974.

75. Matthews MJ: Problems in morphology and behavior of bronchopulmonary malignant disease. In Israel B, Chahinian AP (eds): Lung Cancer: Natural History, Prognosis and Therapy. New York, Academic Press, 1976, pp 23–62.

76. Yeung K, Haidak DJ, Brown JA, et al: Metastasis-induced acute pancreatitis in small cell bronchogenic carcinoma. Arch Intern Med 139:552–554, 1979.

77. Reingold IM: Cutaneous metastases from internal carcinoma. Cancer 19:162, 1966.

78. Kim RY, Perry SR, Levy DS: Metastatic carcinoma to the tongue: A report of two cases and a review of the literature. Cancer 43:386–389, 1979.

79. Carney DN, Cuttitta FC, Gazdar AF, et al: Autocrine clonogenic factors are produced by cell lines of small cell lung cancer. Proc Am Soc Clin Oncol 2:14, 1983.

80. Rassam JW, Anderson G: Incidence of paramalignant disorders in bronchogenic carcinoma. Thorax 30:86–90, 1975.

81. Heber D, Chlebowski RT, Ishibashi DE, et al: Abnormalities in glucose and protein metabolism in noncachectic lung cancer patients. Cancer Res 42:4815–4819, 1982.

82. Anthony HM, Schorah CJ: Severe hypovitaminosis C in lung cancer patients. Br J Cancer 46:354–367, 1982.

83. Costa G: Cachexia, the metabolic component of neoplastic diseases. Cancer Res 37:2327–2335, 1977.

84. Anderson G: The incidence of paramalignant syndromes. In Anderson G (ed): Paramalignant syndromes in lung cancer. London, William Heinemann, 1973, p 4.

85. Cryer PE, Kissaine JM: Clinicopathologic conference: Malignant hypercalcemia. Am J Med 65:486–494, 1979.

86. Mosely JM, Kubota M, Diefenbach-Jagger H, et al: Parathyroid hormone–related protein purified from a human lung cancer cell line. Proc Natl Acad Sci U S A 84:5048–5052, 1987.

87. Hayward ML, Howell DA, O'Donnell JF, et al: Hypercalcemia complicating small cell carcinoma. Cancer 48:1643–1646, 1981.

88. Hegie G, Carpenter JT: Hypercalcemia of malignancy. Int Med 6:71–79, 1985.

89. Myers WPL: Differential diagnosis of hypercalcemia and cancer. CA Cancer J Clin 27:258–272, 1977.

90. Hansen M: Clinical implications of ectopic hormone production in small cell carcinoma of the lung. Dan Med Bull 28:221–236, 1981.

91. Lees LH: The biosynthesis of hormones by nonendocrine tumors—a review. J Endocrinol 67:143–175, 1975.

92. Bliss DP, Battey JF, Linnoila RI, et al: Expression of the atrial natriuretic factor gene in small cell lung cancer tumors and tumor cell lines. J Natl Cancer Inst 82:305–310, 1990.

93. Odell WD, Wolfsen AR: Humoral syndromes associated with cancer. Annu Rev Med 29:379–406, 1978.

94. Fichman M, Bethune J: Effects of neoplasms on renal electrolyte function. Ann N Y Acad Sci 230:448–472, 1974.

95. Jeffcoate WJ, Rees LH: Adrenocorticotropin and related peptides in nonendocrine tumors. Curr Top Exp Endocrinol 3:57–74, 1978.

96. Richardson Rl, Greco FA, Oldham RK: Tumor products and potential markers in small cell lung cancer. Semin Oncol 5:253–262, 1978.

97. Gropp C, Havemann K, Scheuer A: Ectopic hormones in lung cancer patients at diagnosis and during therapy. Cancer 46:347–354, 1980.

98. Jex RK, van Heerden JA, Carpenter PC, Grant CS: Ectopic ACTH syndrome; diagnostic and therapeutic aspects. Am J Surg 149:276–282, 1985.

99. Howlett TA, Drury PL, Perry L, et al: Diagnosis and management of ACTH-dependent Cushing's syndrome: Comparison of the features in ectopic and pituitary ACTH production. Clin Endocrinol (Oxf) 24:699–713, 1986.

100. Hansen M, Hansen HH, Hirsch FR, et al: Hormonal polypeptides and amine metabolites in small cell carcinoma of the lung with special reference to stage and subtypes. Cancer 45:1432–1437, 1980.

101. Melmon KL, Sjoerdsma A, Mason DT: Distinctive clinical and therapeutic aspects of the syndrome associated with bronchial carcinoid tumors. Am J Med 39:568–581, 1965.

102. Mengel CE, Shaffer RD: The carcinoid syndrome. In Holland JF, Frei E (eds): Cancer Medicine. Philadelphia, Lea and Febiger, 1973, pp 1584–1594.

103. Blackman MR, Rosen SW, Weintraub BD: Ectopic hormones. Adv Intern Med 23:85–113, 1978.

104. Ayvazian LF: Extrapulmonary manifestations of tumors of the lung. Postgrad Med 63:93–99, 1978.

105. Vaitukaitis JL, Ross GT, Braunstein GD, et al: Gonadotropins and their subunits: Basic and clinical studies. Recent Prog Horm Res 32:289–321, 1976.

106. Palgon NM, Novetsky AD, Fogler RJ, et al: Lung carcinoma presenting as a breast tumor. N Y State J Med 61:1188–1189, 1983.

107. Smith LG, Lyubsky SL, Carlson HE: Postmenopausal uterine bleeding due to estrogen production by gonadotropin-secreting lung tumors. Am J Med 92:327–330, 1992.

108. Croft PB, Wilkinson M: Carcinomatous neuromyopathy: Its incidence in patients with carcinoma of the lung and breast. Lancet 1:184–188, 1965.

109. Hawley RJ, Cohen MH, Saini N, et al: The carcinomatous neuromyopathy of oat cell lung cancer. Ann Neurol 7:65–72, 1980.

110. Tyler HR: Paraneoplastic syndromes of nerve, muscle and neuromuscular junction. Ann N Y Acad Sci 230:348–357, 1974.

111. Trojaborg W, Frantzen E, Anderson I: Peripheral neuropathy and myopathy associated with carcinoma of the lung. Brain 92:71–82, 1969.

112. Gomm SA, Thatcher N, Barber PV, Cumming WJK: A clinicopathological study of the paraneoplastic neuromuscular syndromes associated with lung cancer. Q J Med 75:577–595, 1990.

113. Bell CE, Seetharam S: Expression of endodermally derived and neural crest–derived differentiation antigens by human lung and colon tumors. Cancer 44:12–18, 1979.

114. Moll JWR, Henzen-Logmans SC, Splinter TAW, et al: Diagnostic value of anti-neuronal antibodies for paraneoplastic disorders of the nervous system. J Neurol Neurosurg Psychiatry 53:940–943, 1990.

115. Wilkinson PC, Zeroniski J: Immunofluorescent detection of antibodies against neurones in sensory carcinomatous neuropathy. Brain 88:529–538, 1965.

116. Lambert EH, Eaton LM, Rooke ED: Defect of neuromuscular conduction associated with malignant neoplasms. Am J Physiol 187:612, 1956.

117. Lambert EH, Elmquist D: Quantal components of end plate potentials in the myasthenic syndrome. Ann N Y Acad Sci 183–199, 1971.

118. Oh SJ, Kim KW: Guanidine hydrochloride in Eaton-Lambert syndrome. Neurology (Minneap) 23:1084–1090, 1973.

119. Jenkyn LR, Brooks PL, Forder RJ, et al: Remission of the Lambert-Eaton syndrome and small cell anaplastic carcinoma of the lung induced by chemotherapy and radiotherapy. Cancer 46:1123–1127, 1980.

120. Fukunaga H, Engel AG, Osame M, et al: Paucity and disorganization of presynaptic membrane active zones in the Lambert-Eaton myasthenic syndrome. Muscle Nerve 5:686–697, 1982.

121. Oguro-Okano M, Griesmann GE, Wieben ED, et al: Molecular diversity of neuronal-type calcium channels identified in small cell lung carcinoma. Mayo Clin Proc 67:1150–1159, 1992.

122. Fukunaga H, Engel AG, Lang B: Passive transfer of Lambert-Eaton myasthenic syndrome with IgG from man to mouse depletes the presynaptic membrane active zones. Proc Natl Acad Sci U S A 80:7636–7640, 1983.

123. Roberts A, Perera S, Lang B, et al: Paraneoplastic myasthenic syndrome IgG inhibits Ca²⁺ flux in a human small cell carcinoma line. Nature 317:737–739, 1985.

124. Horwich MS, Cho L, Porro RS, et al: Subacute sensory neuropathy: A remote effect of cancer. Ann Neurol 1:7–19, 1977.

125. Croft PB, Urich H, Wilkinson M: Peripheral neuropathy of sensorimotor type associated with malignant disease. Brain 90:31–66, 1977.

126. Schuller-Petrovic S, Gebhart W, Lassmann H, et al: A shared antigenic determinant between natural killer cells and nervous tissue. Nature 306:179–181, 1983.

127. Dalmau J, Furneaux HM, Gralla RJ, et al: Detection of anti-Hu antibody in the serum of patients with small cell lung cancer—a quantitative Western blot analysis. Ann Neurol 27:544–552, 1990.

128. Mancall EL, Rosales RK: Necrotizing myelopathy associated with visceral carcinoma. Brain 87:636–639, 1964.

129. Altermatt HJ, Rodriguez M, Scheithauer BW, Lennon VA: Paraneoplastic anti-Purkinje and type 1 anti-neuronal nuclear autoantibodies bind selectively to central, peripheral, and autonomic nervous system cells. Lab Invest 65:412–420, 1991.

130. Morton DL, Itabashi HH, Gromes OF: Nonmetastatic neurological complications of bronchogenic carcinoma: The carcinomatous myopathies. J Thorac Cardiovasc Surg 51:14–29, 1966.

131. Anderson NE: Anti-neuronal autoantibodies and neurological paraneoplastic syndromes. Aust N Z J Med 19:379–387, 1989.

132. Fathallah-Shaykh H, Wang E, Posner JB, Furneaux HM: Cloning of a leucine zipper protein recognized by the sera of patients with antibody-associated paraneoplastic cerebellar degeneration. Proc Natl Acad Sci U S A 88:3451–3454, 1991.

133. Brain L, Wilkinson M: Subacute cerebellar degeneration associated with neoplasms. Brain 88:465, 1965.

134. Shapiro WR: Remote effects of neoplasm on the central nervous system: Encephalopathy. Adv Neurol 15:101–117, 1976.

135. Dorfman LH, Forno LS: Paraneoplastic encephalomyelitis. Acta Neurol Scand 48:556–574, 1972.

136. Brennan LV, Craddock PR: Limbic encephalopathy as nonmetastatic complication of oat cell lung cancer. Am J Med 75:518–520, 1983.

137. Corsellis JAN, Goldberg GJ, Norton AR: Limbic encephalitis and its association with carcinoma. Brain 91:481–497, 1968.

138. DeVere R, Bradley WG: Polymyositis: Its presentation, morbidity and mortality. Brain 98:637–666, 1976.

139. Ahmed MN, Carpenter S: Autonomic neuropathy and carcinoma of the lung. Can Med Assoc J 113:410–412, 1975.

140. Ogilvie H: Large intestine colic due to sympathetic deprivation. BMJ 2:671–673, 1948.

141. Schuffler MD, Baird HW, Fleming CR: Intestinal pseudo-obstruction as the presenting manifestation of small cell carcinoma of the lung. Ann Intern Med 98:129–134, 1983.

142. Lennon VA, Sas DF, Busk MF, et al: Enteric neuronal autoantibodies in pseudoobstruction with small cell lung carcinoma. Gastroenterology 100:137–142, 1991.

143. Ziegler MG, Lake CR, Kopin IJ: The sympathetic nervous system defect in primary orthostatic hypotension. N Engl J Med 296:293–297, 1977.

144. Leveston SA, Shah SD, Cryer PE: Cholinergic stimulation of norepinephrine release in man. J Clin Invest 64:374–380, 1979.

145. Sawyer RA: Blindness caused by photoreceptor degeneration as a remote effect of cancer. Am J Ophthalmol 81:606–613, 1976.

146. Grunwald GB, Klein R, Simmonds MA, et al: Autoimmune basis for visual paraneoplastic syndrome in patients with small-cell lung carcinoma. Lancet 23:658–661, 1985.

147. Pilay N, Gilbert JJ, Ebers GC, et al: Internuclear ophthalmoplegia and optic neuritis: Paraneoplastic effects of bronchial carcinoma. Neurology 34:788–791, 1984.

148. Raz I, Shinar E, Polliack A: Pancytopenia with hypercellular bone marrow—a possible paraneoplastic syndrome in carcinoma of the lung. Am J Hematol 16:403–408, 1984.

149. Berlin NI: Anemia of cancer. Ann N Y Acad Sci 230:211, 1974.

150. Zucker S, Friedman S, Lysik RM: Bone marrow erythropoiesis in the anemia of infection, inflammation and malignancy. J Clin Invest 53:1132–1138, 1974.

151. Waterburg L: Hematologic problems. *In* Abeloff MD (ed): Complications of Cancer: Diagnosis and Management. Baltimore, Johns Hopkins Press, 1979, pp 121–145.

152. Guthrie TH, Thronton RM: Pure red cell aplasia obscured by a diagnosis of carcinoma. South Med J 76:632–634, 1983.

153. Spira MA, Lynch EC: Autoimmune hemolytic anemia and carcinoma: an unusual association. Am J Med 67:753–758, 1979.

154. Ihde DC, Simms EB, Matthews MJ, et al: Bone marrow metastases in small cell carcinoma of the lung: Frequency, descrip-

155. Robinson WA: Granulocytosis in neoplasia. Ann N Y Acad Sci 230:212–218, 1974.

156. Asano S, Urabe A, Okabe T: Demonstration of granulopoietic factor(s) in the plasma of nude mice transplanted with a human lung cancer and in the tumor tissue. Blood 49:845–852, 1977.

157. Shungaard A, Ascensao J, Zanjani E, Jacob HS: Pulmonary carcinoma with eosinophilia: Demonstration of a tumor-derived eosinophilopoietic factor. N Engl J Med 309:778–781, 1983.

158. Ramaiah RS, Biagi RW: Eosinophilia: An unusual presentation of carcinoma of the lung. Practitioner 226:1805–1806, 1982.

159. Silvis SE, Turkbas N, Doscherhdmen A: Thrombocytosis in patients with lung cancer. JAMA 211:1852–1853, 1970.

160. Arrowsmith JE, Woodhead MA, Bevan DH, et al: Digital gangrene in small cell lung cancer: Response to aspirin treatment. Thorax 45:978–979, 1990.

161. Kim HD, Boggs DR: A syndrome resembling idiopathic thrombocytopenic purpura in 10 patients with diverse forms of cancer. Am J Med 67:371–377, 1979.

162. Rickles FR, Edwards RL: Activation of blood coagulation in cancer: Trousseau's syndrome revisited. Blood 63:14–31, 1983.

163. Owen CA, Bowie EJ: Chronic intravascular coagulation syndromes: A summary. Mayo Clin Proc 49:673–679, 1974.

164. Colman RW, Robboy SJ, Minna JD: Disseminated intravascular coagulation: A reappraisal. Annu Rev Med 30:359–374, 1979.

165. Byrd RB, Divertie MB, Spittell JA: Bronchogenic carcinoma and thromboembolic disease. JAMA 202:1019–1022, 1967.

166. Patterson WP: Coagulation and cancer. Semin Oncol 17:137–237, 1990.

167. Sack GH, Levin J, Bell WR: Trousseau's syndrome and other manifestations of chronic disseminated coagulopathy in patients with neoplasms. Medicine 56:1–37, 1977.

168. Hickey WF, Garnick MB, Henderson IC, et al: Primary cerebral venous thrombosis in patients with cancer—a rarely diagnosed paraneoplastic syndrome. Am J Med 73:740–749, 1982.

169. Rosen P, Armstrong D: Nonbacterial thrombotic endocarditis in patients with malignant neoplastic diseases. Am J Med 54:23–33, 1973.

170. McDonald RA, Robbins SG: The significance of nonbacterial thrombotic endocarditis: Autopsy and clinical study of 78 patients. Ann Intern Med 46:255–273, 1957.

171. Foyemi AO, Deppisch LM: Nonbacterial thrombotic endocarditis and myocardial infarction. Am Heart J 97:405–406, 1979.

172. Studdy P, Willoughby JMT: Non-bacterial thrombotic endocarditis in early cancer. BMJ 1:752, 1976.

173. Barnes BE: Dermatomyositis and malignancy: A review of the literature. Ann Intern Med 84:68–76, 1976.

174. Williams RC: Dermatomyositis and malignancy: A review of the literature. Ann Intern Med 50:1174–1181, 1959.

175. Arundell FD, Wilkinson RD, Haserick JR: Dermatomyositis and malignant neoplasms in adults. Arch Dermatol 82:772–775, 1960.

176. Schmidt WD, Bernhardt LC, Johnson SA: Tylosis and intrathoracic neoplasms. Chest 57:590–591, 1970.

177. Cuzick J, Harris R, Mortimer PS: Palmar keratoses and cancers of the bladder and lung. Lancet 8376:530–533, 1984.

178. Vogl A, Goldfischer S: Pachydermoperiostosis: Primary or idiopathic hypertrophic osteoarthropathy. Am J Med 33:166–187, 1962.

179. Ellenbogen BK: Acanthosis nigricans associated with bronchial carcinoma: Report of two cases. Br J Dermatol 61:251–254, 1949.

180. Hattori A, Umegae Y, Kataki S, et al: Small cell carcinoma of the lung with Leser-Trelat sign. Arch Dermatol 118:1017–1018, 1982.

181. Ellis DL, Kafka SP, Chow JC: Melanoma, growth factors, acanthosis nigricans, the sign of Leser-Trelat, and multiple acrochordons: A possible role of alpha-transforming growth factor in cutaneous paraneoplastic syndromes. N Engl J Med 317:1582–1587, 1987.

182. Odell WD, Wolfsen AR: Humoral syndromes associated with cancer. Annu Rev Med 29:379–406, 1978.

183. Summerly R: The figurate erythemas and neoplasia. Br J Dermatol 76:370–373, 1964.

184. Knowling MA, Meakin JW, Hradsky NS, et al: Hypertrichosis lanuginosa acquisita associated with adenocarcinoma of the lung. CMA Journal 126:1308–1309, 1982.

185. Green N, Kurohara SS, George FW, et al: The biologic behavior of lung cancer according to histologic type. Radiol Clin Biol 41:160–190, 1972.

186. LeRoux BT: Bronchial carcinoma with hypertrophic pulmonary osteoarthropathy. S Afr Med J 42:1074–1075, 1968.

187. Schumacher HR: Articular manifestations of hypertrophic pulmonary osteoarthropathy in bronchogenic carcinoma. Arthritis Rheum 19:629–636, 1976.

188. Freeman MH, Tonkin AK: Manifestations of hypertrophic pulmonary osteoarthropathy in patients with carcinoma of the lung. Radiology 120:363–365, 1976.

189. Knowles JH, Smith LH: Extrapulmonary manifestations of bronchogenic carcinoma. N Engl J Med 263:506–510, 1960.

190. Epstein O, Ajdukiewicz AB, Dick R, et al: Hypertrophic pulmonary osteoarthropathy: Clinical, roentgenologic, biochemical, hormonal and cardiorespiratory studies and review of the literature. Am J Med 67:88–99, 1979.

191. Carroll KB, Doyle L: A common factor in hypertrophic osteoarthropathy. Thorax 29:262–264, 1974.

192. Sonksen PH, Ayres AB, Braimbridge M: Acromegaly caused by pulmonary carcinoid tumors. Clin Endocrinol 5:505–513, 1976.

193. Scheithauer BW, Bloch B, Carpenter PC, Brazeau P: Ectopic secretion of a growth hormone–releasing factor: Report of a case of acromegaly with bronchial carcinoid tumor. Am J Med 76:605–616, 1984.

194. Rudman D, Chawla RK, Nixon DW, et al: Proteinuria with disseminated neoplastic disease. Cancer Res 39:699–703, 1979.

195. Richard-Mendes da Costa C, Dupont E, Hamers R, et al: Nephrotic syndromes in bronchogenic carcinoma: Report of two cases with immunochemical studies. Clin Nephrol 2:245–251, 1974.

196. Jermanovich NB, Giammarco R, Ginsberg SJ, et al: Small cell bronchogenic carcinoma of the lung with mesangial proliferative glomerulonephritis. Arch Intern Med 142:397–399, 1982.

197. Moorthy AV: Minimal change glomerular disease: A paraneoplastic syndrome in two patients with bronchogenic carcinoma. Am J Kidney Dis 3:58–61, 1983.

198. Mustonen J, Helin H, Pasternack A: IgA nephropathy associated with bronchial small-cell carcinoma. Am J Clin Pathol 76:652–656, 1981.

199. Smith J: Watery diarrhea (WDHA) syndrome associated with carcinoma of the lung. Aust N Z J Med 6:490–491, 1976.

200. Payan HM, Gilbert EF, Mattson M: Hematological and biochemical paraneoplastic disorders. Arch Pathol Lab Med 102:19–21, 1978.

201. Abelev Gl: Alpha-fetoprotein in oncogenesis and its association with malignant tumors. Adv Cancer Res 14:295–358, 1971.

202. Davies IJ, Musa M, Dormandy TL: Measurements of plasma zinc. II: In malignant disease. J Clin Pathol 21:363–365, 1968.

203. Dent PB, McCulloch PB, Wesley-James O: Measurement of carcinoembryonic antigen in patients with bronchogenic carcinoma. Cancer 42:1484–1491, 1978.

204. Lowenstein MS, Zaimcheck N: Carcinoembryonic antigen and the liver. Gastroenterology 72:161–166, 1977.

205. Wolfsen AR, Odell WD: ProACTH: Use for early detection of lung cancer. Am J Med 66:765–772, 1979.

206. Torstensson S, Thoren M, Hall K: Plasma ACTH in patients with bronchogenic carcinoma. Acta Med Scand 107:353–357, 1980.

207. Carney DN, Marangos PJ, Ihde DC, et al: Serum neuron–specific enolase: A marker for disease extent and response to therapy of small-cell lung cancer. Lancet 1:583–585, 1982.

208. Stanley KE: Prognostic factors for survival in patients with inoperable lung cancer. J Natl Cancer Inst 65:25–32, 1980.

209. Cahan WG: Multiple primary cancers of the lung, esophagus and other sites. Cancer 40:1954, 1977.

210. Shields TW: Multiple primary bronchial carcinomas (editorial). Ann Thorac Cardiovasc Surg 27:1–2, 1979.

211. Jensik RJ, Faber LP, Kittle CF: Segmental resection for bronchogenic carcinoma. Ann Thorac Surg 28:475–483, 1979.

4 EPITHELIAL NEOPLASMS OF THE LUNG

Victor E. Gould and William H. Warren

In recent years, the discovery of significant markers of cellular differentiation and the development of effective immunohistochemical, biochemical, and molecular studies to determine their expression in normal and neoplastic populations have resulted in a veritable revolution in our understanding of neoplasms and in the concepts and criteria applicable to their classification. At present, epithelial tumors are perhaps most accurately defined as those composed of cells whose exclusive or predominant intermediate filament cytoskeletal proteins are composed of cytokeratin polypeptides, which, in most instances, if not invariably, are coexpressed with desmosomal plaque proteins.[1] Malignant epithelial tumors are, by definition, carcinomas. The term carcinoma is often used synonymously with cancer; strictly speaking, this is not correct because the term cancer encompasses all malignant neoplasms, many of which are not epithelial.

The traditional term bronchogenic carcinoma is still often used to designate all forms of malignant epithelial tumors of the lung. This term is evidently misleading because a significant number of carcinomas of the lung are neither related to, nor do they arise from, bronchi. Worse yet, the term bronchogenic carcinoma includes types of lung carcinoma that vary very significantly not merely in their morphology but in their prognosis and response to therapy. Therefore, clinical and epidemiologic studies based on such umbrella designations encompassing heterogeneous groups of tumors may yield results and lead to conclusions of very questionable validity. For these and other reasons, it is our contention that the designation bronchogenic carcinoma should be abandoned.

More recently, the indiscriminate categorization of lung carcinomas into small cell and non–small cell types has become popular. The first group encompasses well-differentiated and small cell variants of neuroendocrine carcinomas, whereas the second group includes adenocarcinomas and squamous, bronchioloalveolar, large cell, and giant cell carcinomas, among others. We suggest that the demonstrable diversity of these tumors with regard to their pathologic and clinical characteristics makes such categorization unwarranted.

CLASSIFICATION

The clinical frequency and epidemiologic significance of bronchopulmonary carcinomas are matters of serious concern.[2] Given these facts, it is noteworthy that the basic classification scheme of bronchopulmonary carcinomas appears not to have changed appreciably in several decades. These observations become even more paradoxical as we note that our knowledge and understanding of the pathobiology of these tumors have grown very appreciably during the same period.

The first modern histologic classifications of epithelial lung neoplasms were almost simultaneously published by Kreyberg[3] and Foot[4] in 1952. Kreyberg continued his investigations,[5, 6] which culminated in the now classic monograph "Histological Lung Cancer Types" published in 1962.[7] Many features of this article, in turn, formed the basis of the first World Health Organization (WHO) publication entitled "Histological Typing of Lung Tumors" issued in 1967.[8] The second WHO-sponsored classification of lung tumors differs comparatively little from the first, although they are separated by 1½ decades.[9] But, as mentioned earlier, classifications are based on definitions and criteria that may or may not be accurate and readily reproducible. Not surprisingly, it is precisely the variability and inherent difficulties in applying many traditional definitions and criteria that account, to a large extent, for the confusing state of the classification of bronchopulmonary tumors.[10]

It should be mentioned that all current histologic classifications of lung epithelial tumors are based on the apparent feature(s) of differentiation displayed by the cells that comprise them, and not, as often stated, on their presumed histogenesis. Indeed the validity of the concept of histogenesis as a basic criterion for the pathologic classification of tumors is, at least, highly debatable.[11] Histogenesis and differentiation are notions derived from classic embryology. Histogenesis refers to processes whereby cells acquire structural and functional characteristics that permit us to predict their destiny in the mature embryo; these phenomena are frequently associated with cell migration. Differentiation, on the other hand, refers only to the acqui-

49

sition or the mere presence of those cellular characteristics; moreover, it does not necessarily imply migration and is not restricted to prenatal life. In the realm of diagnostic pathology, however, histogenesis means the putative cell of origin of a given neoplasm and is often further confused by demonstrably obsolete notions of embryology, whereas differentiation means the degree of similarity between a neoplastic cell population and its nontransformed presumed counterpart. A fundamental flaw in the prevalent notion of tumor histogenesis is that we truly know very little about the cell of origin of many, if not most, neoplasms. Conversely, our capability to objectively determine features of differentiation has improved considerably and continues to improve. It is therefore on the latter concept that our classifications of neoplasms are actually based (for review, see reference 11).

In this brief overview of epithelial lung neoplasms, we retain the major categories of epithelial tumors of the WHO classification,[9] although we depart from it with regard to certain traditional definitions and points of nomenclature. We attempt to clarify those instances in which currently accepted conventional definitions and traditional taxonomy should, in our opinion, be altered. And we will emphasize the contributions and impact of the modern tumor markers while outlining areas of uncertainty and current trends in research.

SQUAMOUS CELL CARCINOMA

Given the aforementioned problems of definition, it is not possible at present to give an accurate figure on the relative incidence of this type of carcinoma (figures ranging from 35% to 50% have been mentioned[12]); the need for a precise definition of these tumors has been emphasized for some time.[13] It has also been stated that squamous cell carcinoma is probably the most frequent form of lung carcinoma and the one most frequently found in men; it is also said to be the most closely correlated with smoking.[14] More recent observations, on the other hand, have suggested that adenocarcinomas may in fact be more frequent than their squamous cell counterparts. These changes may represent a true change in the relative incidence of these tumor types, reflect the outlined problems of definition, or both.

Theoretically, it may be possible to offer a molecular definition of squamous cell carcinoma related to the expression of those cytokeratin polypeptides associated with squamous cell differentiation. However, the application of such criteria would be impractical or practically impossible in most diagnostic laboratories. In addition, the problem of classifying neoplasms including only a minority of demonstrably squamous cells would remain unsolved. In our laboratory, we classify as squamous carcinomas those malignant epithelial neoplasms whose majority cell population show, by conventional light microscopy, convincing pearl formation, distinct intercellular bridges, or readily identifiable keratinization of single cells (dyskeratotic cells). These carcinomas are readily immunostained with antibodies to cytokeratin polypeptides of the epidermal type (see later). We exclude from the group of squamous carcinomas those tumors that merely show a pavement-like architectural pattern with or without prominent cell borders. Repeated studies have shown that few of these carcinomas can be immunostained with the aforementioned cytokeratin antibodies, whereas, conversely, the majority of them can be shown to express antigens related to exocrine (e.g., glandular) differentiation (see the sections on adenocarcinoma and large cell carcinoma).

Squamous cell carcinomas occur most frequently in major bronchi; therefore, they are predominantly central lung tumors. Peripheral squamous cell carcinomas occur far less frequently; squamous carcinomas arising in association with pulmonary scars rarely have been reported. Also in rare instances, squamous cell carcinomas have been reported to develop in the wall of bronchiectatic and other abscesses.

Grossly, squamous cell carcinomas may appear as foci of roughening of the bronchial mucosa, from which the tumor extends directly through the bronchial wall into the lung parenchyma, to the local lymph nodes and the soft tissues of the mediastinum. A predominantly polypoid growth form is uncommon; occasionally, well-differentiated squamous cell carcinomas of major bronchi may show a complex verrucous pattern similar to that described in certain verrucous carcinomas of the skin and some mucosal surfaces. Squamous cell carcinomas may develop extensive central necrosis. In such cases, the gross appearance of the tumor may be similar to, or even indistinguishable from, that of an abscess. In these cases, microscopic examination of samples of the wall of such abscesses readily discloses clusters of malignant squamous epithelium, thus proving their neoplastic character.

Microscopically, the classic well-differentiated squamous cell carcinomas display clusters of rather large round cells with abundant mildly to intensely eosinophilic cytoplasm. The nuclei are large, and although nucleoli are readily found, they are not prominent; mitoses tend to be abundant. Many neoplastic clusters display concentric aggregates of eosinophilic lamellate material (keratin pearls) (Fig. 4–1). Foci of necrosis at the center of large cellular aggregates are not unusual. Less well-differentiated squamous cell carcinomas lack keratin pearls but still display prominent intercellular bridges (that correspond to well-defined desmosomes by electron microcopy and to desmoplakin immunostaining), individual cell keratinization (dyskeratosis), or both. The uninvolved bronchial mucosa in the vicinity of squamous cell carcinomas often shows variable degrees of epithelial atypia ranging from mild dysplasia to carcinoma in situ.

By immunohistochemistry, squamous cell carcinomas are richly stained with widely available, commercial antibodies against epidermal-type cytokeratin, indicating the presence of high-molecular-weight cytokeratin polypeptides. The latter point has actually

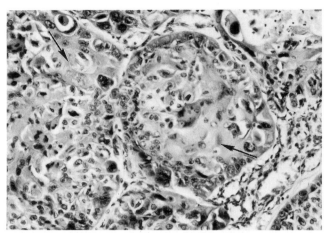

FIGURE 4–1. Squamous carcinoma. Note neoplastic clusters with prominent pleomorphism and irregular areas of keratinization *(arrows).* Hematoxylin and eosin, × 450. Unless otherwise specified, all tissues were conventionally fixed and embedded.

been proved with immunohistochemical studies using well-characterized specific antibodies, and by two-dimensional gel electrophoresis.[15, 16] The latter studies have in fact shown that pulmonary squamous cell carcinomas express a very complex array of cytokeratin polypeptides, including those of stratified epithelium type as well as those of the simple epithelium type (5, 6, 8, 13, 17, 18 and 19, and in some cases, also 4, 14 and 15).[15, 16] The consistent presence of the high-molecular-weight cytokeratins explains the fact that conventionally fixed and paraffin-embedded sections of squamous cell carcinomas can be readily immunostained for keratin given the known resilience of those proteins to conventional fixation and embedding processes, whereas other epithelial lung neoplasms that express sets of low-molecular-weight cytokeratin polypeptides often cannot be immunostained with similar ease (see later). Not surprisingly, squamous cell carcinomas are readily and consistently immunostained with desmosomal plaque proteins, confirming the presence of abundant desmosomes (Fig. 4–2).[15, 16]

A number of immunohistochemical studies are available that are helpful in discriminating between poorly differentiated squamous cell carcinomas and subsets of large cell carcinomas that may imitate them by conventional microscopy. As stated earlier, immunostaining with epidermal-type cytokeratin antibodies establishes the diagnosis of squamous cell carcinoma. Conversely, except for occasional cells, large cell carcinomas should not show that pattern of immunoreaction with such antibodies.[16] In addition, monoclonal antibodies to mucinous proteins, glycoproteins, and glycolipid-associated molecules (e.g., 44-3A6, 624-A12, A-80, CSLEX-1) related to exocrine differentiation (e.g., adenocarcinoma) have been described[17, 18]; not surprisingly, these antibodies do not immunostain squamous cell carcinomas, and in the case of positive reactions, only minority subpopulations are recognized.[18–23]

The most notable electron microscopic features of squamous cell carcinomas are prominent, undulating

bundles of closely packed intermediate filaments. These are often arranged concentrically around the nucleus, but they should also be seen converging toward the characteristically abundant, well-developed desmosomes.

ADENOCARCINOMA

In contrast with squamous cell carcinomas, pulmonary adenocarcinomas occur with approximately equal frequency in males and females, and they are more often than not peripheral rather than central neoplasms. Adenocarcinomas are said to be less frequently associated with smoking than their squamous counterparts. The precise relative incidence of adenocarcinoma vis a vis other lung carcinomas is reportedly variable; at present, it may be estimated to be at least in the 25% range[12, 13] but may in fact be far more frequent. This presumed variability in incidence is in part attributable to problems of definition (see section on large cell carcinoma) but may also reflect variability in the populations at risk.

Grossly, lung adenocarcinomas are irregularly round masses whose cut surfaces occasionally have a myxoid appearance. Peripherally located adenocarcinomas are often associated with a characteristic puckering of the overlying pleura. Adenocarcinomas often include significant amounts of fibroconnective tissue stroma. The latter may at times dominate the picture particularly in the tumor's center. These tumors are often referred to as scar carcinomas. Early studies suggested that the carcinomas arose as the result of the scarring often ascribed to tuberculosis. Although not totally excluding that early concept, it should be pointed out that more recent work has suggested that the prominent fibrous scarring observed in some lung adenocarcinomas may in fact be a response to or result from the tumor rather than being its cause.[24]

Microscopically, adenocarcinomas show variable degrees of glandular differentiation that may or may

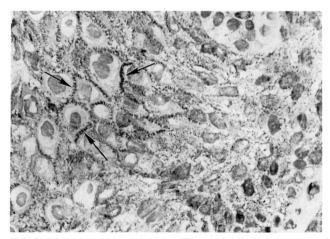

FIGURE 4–2. Squamous carcinoma. Frozen section immunostained with desmoplakin antibody. Dark dots at the periphery of cells represent desmosomes *(arrows).* Avidin-biotin complex technique, × 1050.

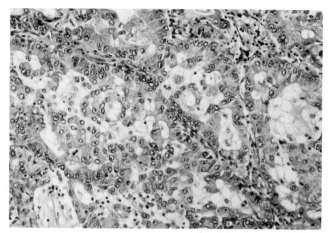

FIGURE 4–3. Adenocarcinoma. Note irregularly shaped glands and moderate cellular pleomorphism. Hematoxylin and eosin, × 450.

not include papillae. The individual cells are comparatively large with amphophilic or pale cytoplasm (Fig. 4–3). The nuclei often show prominent nucleoli. Mitotic activity is variable.

By conventional histochemistry, the majority of adenocarcinomas described earlier can be shown to produce mucosubstances that appear as pools in the glandular lumina, as intracytoplasmic droplets, or both. Less well-differentiated adenocarcinomas may predominantly display a solid histologic pattern with only occasional or even absent glandular structures but still comprise cells containing mucosubstance droplets.

In our experience, lung adenocarcinomas that are recognizable as such by conventional histology can be readily immunostained with monoclonal antibodies that recognize either a membrane-associated glycoprotein molecule (44-3A6)[18] (Fig. 4–4), the specific sugar sequence found in lacto-N-fucopentose III (624-A12)[19] or other mucin-like proteins and glycoproteins.[20–23] All of these molecules appear related to

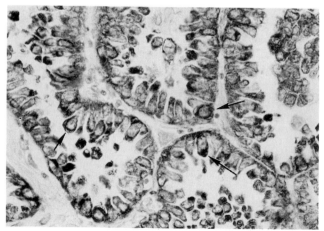

FIGURE 4–4. Adenocarcinoma immunostained with monoclonal antibody 44-3A6. The majority of neoplastic cells show immunoreactivity which is most marked at the cells' periphery *(arrows)*. Avidin-biotin complex technique, × 1050.

incompletely defined features of exocrine differentiation, and they are demonstrable in some but not all primary adenocarcinomas in sites other than the lung. Significantly, these antigens are well preserved and can be readily demonstrated in conventionally fixed and paraffin-embedded tissue sections.

Of additional significance for pathologic differential diagnosis is that the antigens disclosed by the aforementioned monoclonal antibodies are either absent or very weakly expressed in pleural mesotheliomas even when the latter display well-defined glandular and papillary structures. These mutually exclusive patterns of immunoreaction are reminiscent of those obtained with carcinoembyonic antigen (CEA) antibodies; the latter, however, are somewhat less specific.[25] Consistent application of these effective immunoprobes should result in an improved differential histodiagnosis between lung adenocarcinomas and pleural mesotheliomas, particularly if used in combination with the appropriate intermediate filaments studies (see later).

Lung adenocarcinomas can be readily immunostained with desmoplakin antibodies; in this context, they do not differ from other pulmonary epithelial neoplasms or from pleural mesotheliomas. However, the intermediate filament complement of lung adenocarcinomas is significantly different from those of squamous carcinomas (see earlier) and of mesotheliomas.[15, 16, 26] Adenocarcinomas express cytokeratin polypeptides of the simple epithelium type, i.e., Nrs 7, 8, 18, and 19 of the Moll catalog.[27] Pleural mesotheliomas, on the other hand, express a far more complex array of cytokeratin polypeptides, including the aforementioned plus the basic polypeptide 5 and, in some cases, polypeptides 4, 6, 14, and 17; moreover, mesotheliomas frequently coexpress vimentin.[28] These remarkable differences are demonstrable by immunohistochemistry as well as by two-dimensional gel electrophoresis, but for reliable results, these techniques require very well characterized antibodies and well preserved freshly frozen tumor samples.[28] Lacking those elements, however, it should be remembered that conventionally fixed and paraffin-embedded sections of squamous cell carcinomas can be readily and diffusely immunostained with antibodies to epidermal cytokeratins, whereas adenocarcinomas cannot be thus stained.

By electron microscopy, adenocarcinomas display the expected glands with more or less well-defined lumina and variably prominent microvilli. Intracytoplasmic lumina may also be noted. The glands may be encompassed by basal lamina that may show various abnormalities including gaps and focal reduplication. All these features are in fact displayed by numerous other types of adenocarcinomas, including mesotheliomas. Numerous investigators have attempted to establish criteria for discriminating between adenocarcinomas and mesotheliomas, underscoring the abundant, delicate, and often intertwining microvilli prominent in mesotheliomas.[29] And, although electron microscopy is occasionally useful in this regard, it has been largely replaced by immunohistochemistry.

BRONCHIOLOALVEOLAR-ALVEOLAR CELL CARCINOMA

These tumors may be regarded as variants of adenocarcinomas in that they display glandular features. However, they are a heterogeneous group that may differ considerably from adenocarcinomas in their conventional histologic and ultrastructural appearance, as well as in their clinical presentation, evolution, and prognosis. The relative incidence of these carcinomas compared with that of other lung carcinomas depends again on matters of definition; if narrowly defined, alveolar carcinomas may be said to be uncommon and probably represent less than 5% of lung carcinomas.

Characteristically, bronchioloalveolar carcinomas appear grossly either as multiple nodules, an infiltrate, or a single mass of variable size; some of the small foci are truly microscopic and thus are only incidentally found. The majority of these tumors are located peripherally and show no evident connection with a bronchus. Cut surfaces of the large tumors may be indistinguishable from those of other carcinomas. Some bronchioalveolar carcinomas present clinically with a profuse mucoid expectoration; these tumors display histologically abundant mucus production and their gross cut surfaces are predictably myxoid.

Histologically, alveolar carcinomas show a characteristic growth pattern consisting of cuboidal or cylindric cells lining the alveolar septa; the basic pulmonary architecture is thereby preserved (Fig. 4–5). The microscopic foci often blend imperceptibly with the surrounding normal alveoli; a number of these carcinomas display focal piling up of cells and variably defined papillary structures.[13, 30] These tumors are generally not associated with prominent fibrous stroma. Many of the aforementioned features may be imitated by primary lung adenocarcinomas or by adenocarcinomas of other sites metastasizing to the lung. Primary lung adenocarcinomas often show greater cellular pleomorphism and more prominent fibrous

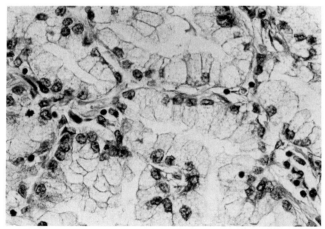

FIGURE 4–5. Bronchioloalveolar carcinoma. The alveolar architecture is preserved; note tall cylindrical cells with basal, moderately pleomorphic nuclei. The pale, abundant cytoplasm is rich in mucosubstance. Hematoxylin and eosin, × 1050.

stroma, whereas adenocarcinomas of other sites metastasizing to the lung are also pleomorphic and may, in addition, show a more clear-cut delineation from the surrounding parenchyma.

The degree of cytologic atypicality displayed by alveolar carcinomas is variable. Some cases display minimal atypicality and therefore may be difficult to differentiate from reactive or reparative alveolar hyperplasias associated with various inflammatory and infectious processes. These features may complicate the differential diagnosis, particularly given limited tissue or cytologic samples. A reportedly benign form (e.g., pulmonary adenomatosis) has been described[30]; the latter, however, is now acknowledged to be indeed a neoplasm. By light microscopy, a subset of alveolar carcinomas is composed of mucin-producing cells; these tumors, if sufficiently large and if draining into bronchi, may present clinically with a characteristic, profuse mucous expectoration. By electron microscopy, other bronchioloalveolar carcinomas have been shown to be composed of Clara-type cells or of recognizable Type II granular pneumocytes with their characteristic cytoplasmic inclusions. More recently, by using combined immunohistochemistry and electron microscopy, it has been shown that at least occasional alveolar carcinomas contain cellular subpopulations that simultaneously produce mucosubstances and neuroendocrine products, e.g., amphicrine carcinomas.[31] It remains to be determined whether or not the separation of these diverse and complex varieties of bronchioloalveolar carcinoma have clinical significance.

By immunohistochemistry, a group of bronchioloalveolar carcinomas analyzed with the 44-3A6 antibody was not immunostained despite their obvious glandular features. Interestingly, those tumors were all of the mucin-producing variety, whereby it may be argued that the protein epitopes were masked or otherwise rendered unavailable to the antibody, thus resulting in a negative reaction.[18] To reinforce this notion, one may advance the observation that other antibodies used to detect exocrine features that, however, do not depend on protein but rather on sugar or glycolipid epitopes readily immunostain most if not all alveolar carcinomas regardless of mucin production.[19–21] It is evident from these observations that subsets of bronchioloalveolar carcinomas may also be defined immunohistochemically as well as by electron microscopy. Again, the possible clinical significance of these subsets of carcinomas remains to be determined.

Comparatively few bronchioalveolar carcinomas have been analyzed to determine their complement of intermediate filaments. Our preliminary studies indicate that these tumors express the simple epithelium type of cytokeratin polypeptides 8, 18, and 19 of the Moll catalogue, thus paralleling conventional adenocarcinomas.[15, 16]

LARGE CELL CARCINOMA

At present, there is considerable confusion about the precise definition of these carcinomas; this confusion is reflected in the wide range of the figures (10% to 20%) representing their relative incidence. The WHO classification underscores that they lack "characteristic features of squamous cell, small cell or adenocarcinoma."[9] Yet, concomitantly, evidence has been accruing to the effect that so-called large cell carcinomas of the lung are not a homogeneous group but comprise carcinomas with diverse features of differentiation.

Grossly, large cell lung carcinomas have no characteristic or distinguishing feature. They may be related to major or intermediate-sized bronchi or arise in the periphery. Microscopically, they are composed of comparatively large cells ranging from 30 to 50 μm in diameter and are arranged in solid, often pavement-like clusters that may show central necrosis. The cytoplasm is abundant and pale to slightly eosinophilic; the nuclei are central and display rather prominent nucleoli (Fig. 4–6). Mitoses are frequent.

As stated earlier, the fundamental points in the conventional definition of large cell carcinomas are essentially negative, e.g., the absence of detectable glands and of overt keratinization.[9] Electron microscopic study of some of these carcinomas have shown slitlike lumina with delicate microvilli, which led to the notion that some large cell carcinomas are in fact poorly differentiated adenocarcinomas. Immunohistochemical studies using the above-mentioned monoclonal antibodies (Fig. 4–7) (44-3A6, 624-A12, A-80, B72.3, CSLEX-1) that detect features of exocrine differentiation have not only confirmed but broadened those earlier observations and have greatly simplified their determination.[18–23] At present, we can tentatively suggest that approximately 50% of large cell lung carcinomas could be regarded as poorly differentiated adenocarcinomas, given their expression of exocrine phenotype antigens.[32]

Also significant is that electron microscopic studies and immunohistochemical analyses with antibodies against neuroendocrine materials have suggested that a subset of large cell carcinomas (20% to 40%) have variable proportions of cells with demonstrable fea-

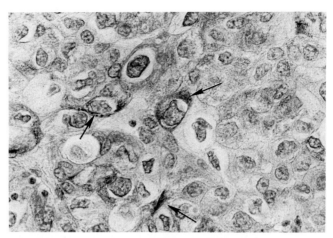

FIGURE 4–7. Large cell carcinoma, same case as previous figure. Immunostaining with monoclonal antibody 44-3A6 reveals several reactive cells *(arrows)*. Avidin-biotin complex technique, × 1050.

tures of neuroendocrine differentiation.[22, 32] The latter are particularly predictable in those carcinomas composed of elongated cells with pronounced peripheral palisading and central necrosis in their clusters.[33–36] There is little doubt that the overall group of large cell lung carcinomas include tumors with predominantly neuroendocrine differentiation. The aforementioned figure of 40% was obtained with polyclonal antisera, and it is therefore subject to revision (which is likely to be downward) as more precisely defined and increasingly specific immunoprobes are applied to the immunohistochemical analysis of these tumors.

Immunohistochemical and biochemical studies of the cytoskeletal proteins of large cell carcinomas have also provided significant data indicating that the majority of these tumors express cytokeratin polypeptides of the simple epithelium type (i.e., those shown by adenocarcinomas and neuroendocrine neoplasms), whereas a small subset displayed the cytokeratin polypeptide complement of the epidermal type characteristic of squamous cell carcinomas.[16] Interestingly, and to an extent predictably, a few cases of the latter subset could not be immunostained with antibodies 44-3A6, 624-A12, A-80, and others, nor did they seem to express neuroendocrine features. These diverse studies confirmed the heterogeneity of this class of lung carcinomas and suggest the need to undertake further, systematic investigations to clarify and quantify those points and establish or exclude their possible clinical significance. Yet, our studies suggest that those large cell carcinomas with extensive neuroendocrine differentiation behave essentially as neuroendocrine carcinomas.[34, 35] On the other hand, the finding that many and possibly the majority of large cell carcinomas share differentiation features with adenocarcinomas should not result in the elimination of large cell carcinoma as a distinct clinicopathologic group, because recent data indicate that stage I large cell carcinomas with predominant exocrine phenotype behave more aggressively than their conventional adenocarcinoma counterparts.[37]

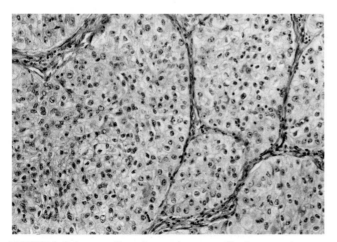

FIGURE 4–6. Large cell carcinoma. Low magnification reveals uniformly solid architecture; neither gland formation nor keratinization is noted. Hematoxylin and eosin, × 350.

CARCINOID, NEUROENDOCRINE CARCINOMAS, AND RELATED LESIONS

These are fundamentally epithelial tumors whose common denominator is that they are composed of epithelial cells that are simultaneously capable of expressing neuroendocrine markers (see later). This capability is reflected in the synthesis and/or release of substances of the neuroamine-neuropeptide and related groups. These substances can act as neurotransmitters, paracrine regulators or modulators, or true hormones. The term neuroendocrine reflects the fact that many of those materials (e.g., common peptides) are also synthesized and used in a similar manner by true neurons in the central and peripheral nervous systems, including the paraganglia, and may also be produced by truly neural neoplasms (e.g., neuroblastomas, pheochromocytomas, paragangliomas). We believe that, at present, the designation neuroendocrine is preferable to the acronym APUD (*a*mine, *p*recursor, *r*euptake, and *d*ecarboxylation), and to endocrine, which is simply too broad in this context.

The recognition of neuroendocrine features as frequent differentiation characteristics and the diagnosis of neuroendocrine neoplasms in general have been greatly facilitated by the development of numerous antisera and antibodies and of rather simple immunohistochemical techniques applicable to freshly frozen or conventionally fixed, paraffin-embedded sections. Commercial antisera and antibodies to serotonin and to numerous neuropeptides are readily available. In addition, there are significant antibodies to various other components of neuroendocrine cells that indicate their basic differentiation pattern but give no clue as to the particular neuropeptide(s) or other biologically active substances they may produce. The latter are termed pan-neuroendocrine markers.

Significant pan-neuroendocrine markers include (1) neuron-specific enolase (NSE), which is a cytoplasmic glycolytic enzyme; (2) chromogranin(s), which is a protein component originally isolated from the matrix of adrenal medulla neurosecretory granules and is, in fact, one member of a family of secretory granules' proteins; and (3) synaptophysin, a more recently isolated, integral membrane glycoprotein of presynaptic vesicles of bovine neurons that is highly conserved in numerous epithelial and other neuroendocrine cells and neoplasms (for comparative reviews on the relative advantages and limitations of these markers, see references 38 to 41).

Carcinoids

Carcinoids are neuroendocrine neoplasms that for the most part behave in a benign fashion. They were originally encompassed within the broad definition of bronchial adenomas, which are now understood to have included other distinct epithelial neoplasms that, at present, would be classified as adenoid cystic and mucoepidermoid carcinomas. Thus, the designation bronchial adenoma should be regarded as only of historical significance and should be abandoned.

Carcinoids arise predominantly in major bronchi and, for the most part, are therefore central tumors. Carcinoids tend to occur in a relatively younger group (fourth decade) than that affected by carcinomas, and they occur in males and females with similar frequency. Grossly, they appear as nodular or even polypoid elevations of the mucosa, which, if the tumor is small and not traumatized, remains uninvolved. Carcinoids are highly vascularized tumors; thus, fresh cut surfaces may appear hemorrhagic. However, when drained of blood, cut surfaces are gray to pale tan.

By light microscopy, carcinoids exhibit one or two patterns and often a combination of both (i.e., solid clusters or delicate cords and ribbons). If extensively sampled, some carcinoids may display glandular structures; this finding should not distract us from the essentially endocrine character of these tumors. Regardless of their architecture, carcinoids display a rich fibrovascular stroma. The individual cells are round to polygonal and are of moderate and rather uniform size and shape. The cytoplasm may range from clear to eosinophilic. The central nuclei have irregularly distributed chromatin, and nucleoli are not prominent (Fig. 4–8). If carcinoids are thus narrowly defined, cellular pleomorphism is minimal, mitoses are sporadic, and necrosis is absent, artifactual, or minimal. On the other hand, carcinoids are not encapsulated, and depending on their size and stage of evolution, they may be seen to infiltrate through the bronchial wall into the lung parenchyma and may also infiltrate mediastinal soft tissues.

We consider that the detection at the time of initial diagnosis of distant metastases, the presence of vascular invasion, or both would preclude the diagnosis of carcinoid and would mandate the diagnosis of neuroendocrine carcinoma regardless of the cytologic features. Local infiltration and metastasis to local lymph nodes appears to have little long-term implications, at least in adults. There is no question, however, that rare carcinoids that fit even the strictest aforemen-

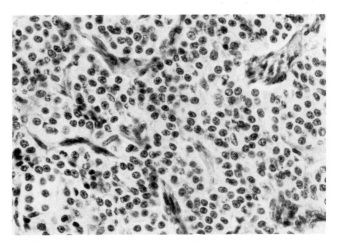

FIGURE 4–8. Carcinoid. Note solid organoid architecture, relative cellular uniformity and delicate fibrovascular stroma. Hematoxylin and eosin, × 1050.

tioned definition may be capable of true distant metastases.

In our experience with over 120 carcinoids followed clinically from 3 to 25 years, metastases occurred in nine instances. In seven of those patients, microscopic tumor foci were noted in local lymph nodes resected with the original specimen; these patients remain alive and well with no evidence of tumor. In the two additional patients, distant metastases to liver and bone developed, although, interestingly, neither patient had mediastinal lymph node metastases. One remains alive with documented bone metastases 19 years after the original resection and 11 years after the discovery of his bone metastases. The second patient died 10 years after the original resection and 5 years after the appearance of bone metastases. However, this patient was also severely debilitated with advanced rheumatoid arthritis. The precise cause of death was not determined, and no autopsy was performed.[42]

It should be emphasized that the clinical evolution of the rare case of true bronchial carcinoid with metastases is remarkably slow; and, partly because of it, we believe that the designation and the concept of carcinoid should be retained. We have not been able to detect any structural or functional feature in these metastasizing carcinoids that would set them apart from the majority of nonmetastasizing counterparts. Only one of the aforementioned 120 bronchial carcinoids was associated with a comparatively mild carcinoid syndrome.

By electron microscopy, carcinoids reveal a rich complement of neurosecretory granules that consist of a central core of variable electron density, a pale surrounding halo, and a single encompassing membrane; the granules' diameters range from 80 to 250 nm.[34–36] Often, within a single tumor or even within a single cell, the granule population is heterogeneous. In addition to the neurosecretory granules, carcinoids consistently display desmosomes. Ultrastructural features noted in bronchial carcinoids with variable frequency include abundant mitochondria (oncocytic carcinoids); aggregates of intermediate filaments, often in a paranuclear position; and the presence of glandular lumina with typical microvilli. Clusters of neoplastic cells are invariably surrounded by a basal lamina, which occasionally may show focal gaps; reduplication of the basal lamina may also be noted. In addition, in at least some carcinoids, the neoplastic aggregates are surrounded by slender sustentacular, Schwann-like cells akin to those observed in paragangliomas.

Immunohistochemical study of carcinoids with broad range or pan-neuroendocrine antibodies show them to express NSE (Fig. 4–9), chromogranin, and synaptophysin virtually without exception. Bronchial carcinoids also express very frequently the hormonal materials traditionally viewed as eutopic in non-neoplastic bronchial neuroendocrine cells (e.g., serotonin, bombesin, calcitonin, and leu-enkephalin). Frequently expressed are neuropeptides such as gastrin, somatostatin, and substance P. Only occasional true carci-

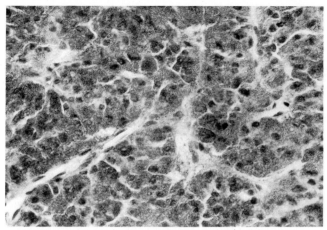

FIGURE 4–9. Carcinoid. Note diffuse and rather uniform immunostaining with anti-NSE antibody. Peroxidase–antiperoxidase technique, × 1050.

noids express adrenocorticotropic hormone (ACTH) (Fig. 4–10). Some of these materials should not necessarily be regarded as ectopic because knowledge of the materials normally expressed by bronchopulmonary solitary neuroendocrine cells and neuroepithelial bodies continues to expand (for overview, see reference 43), and the very notion of what constitutes ectopic expression has been challenged.[35]

As is the case with virtually all neuroendocrine neoplasms regardless of their primary site, bronchial carcinoids tend to express multiple hormonal substances; double immunostaining or immunostaining of adjacent step sections with different antibodies may show coexpression of more than one substance within single cells.[34–36, 44] A proportion of carcinoids studied with antibodies that detect exocrine features have shown immunostaining of variable extent and intensity (Fig. 4–11). This observation confirms the fact these tumors may display more than one differentiation characteristic; however, as mentioned earlier, and

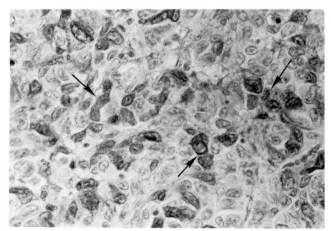

FIGURE 4–10. Carcinoid immunostained with anti-ACTH antibody; note intense staining of some cells *(arrows)*, whereas other cells show no reaction. Peroxidase–anti-peridoxidase technique, × 1050.

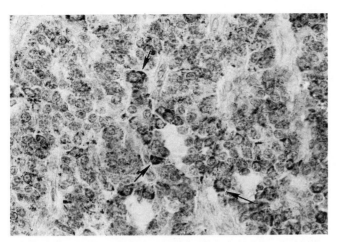

FIGURE 4–11. Carcinoid immunostained with monoclonal antibody 44-3A6. Note scattered cells with peripheral immunostaining *(arrows).* Avidin-biotin complex technique, × 1050.

for clinical purposes, these carcinoids should still be regarded as neuroendocrine neoplasms.

Early reports suggested that the cytoskeletal intermediate filaments of bronchial carcinoids were composed not of cytokeratin polypeptides but of neurofilament proteins.[45] However, subsequent studies by immunohistochemistry and two-dimensional gel electrophoresis provided unequivocal evidence that carcinoids express predominantly cytokeratin polypeptides of the simple epithelial type, together with desmoplakin.[46] Thus, carcinoids are constitutively epithelial neoplasms. Nevertheless, a certain proportion of bronchial carcinoids can be shown to coexpress cytokeratin and neurofilament proteins.[16] When immunostained with antibodies to vimentin, many carcinoids show the aforementioned sustentacular cells, which not surprisingly also react with antibodies to S-100 protein.

Neuroendocrine Carcinomas, Well-Differentiated Type

These carcinomas may be defined as those bronchopulmonary neuroendocrine neoplasms that retain many architectural features of true carcinoids but nevertheless display unmistakable albeit variable features of malignancy. This designation is meant to replace the unnecessarily vague designation of atypical carcinoid. Perhaps more important, well-differentiated neuroendocrine carcinomas should also serve to designate occasional neoplasms that have been regarded by some observers as (peripheral or Stage I) small cell carcinomas but that, on close examination, differ morphologically from the small cell carcinomas, and that, to a very significant extent, do not behave clinically as the small cell carcinomas would be expected to behave.

In contrast with true carcinoids, the majority of well-differentiated neuroendocrine carcinomas are not centrally located tumors. They may or may not be demonstrably related to the bronchial tree. They appear simply as irregularly nodular masses that may

have prominent central scarring. In addition, a surprising proportion of these tumors are incidentally detected.

Histologically, well-differentiated neuroendocrine carcinomas retain a distinct albeit variable organoid pattern; the predominant arrangement is one of solid clusters that may display focal necrosis. Well-differentiated neuroendocrine carcinomas do not exhibit the frequently extensive, if not massive, necrosis, crushing artifact, and linear, deeply basophilic staining that are so characteristic of small cell neuroendocrine carcinomas. The individual cells range from polygonal to fusiform; the fusiform shape may predominate in some cases. The degree of pleomorphism varies, but it may be pronounced. The number of mitoses also varies, but the rate may be brisk (Fig. 4–12); vascular invasion may be detected. Scarring is noted in at least a third of these carcinomas.

Metastatic well-differentiated neuroendocrine carcinoma in mediastinal lymph nodes or even in distant sites may be present at the time of initial diagnosis or may develop within 1 to 3 years thereafter. Nevertheless, survival of 3 to 5 years with metastases is not unusual, even with variable regimens of radiotherapy, chemotherapy, or no therapy. Our studies including 22 patients with completely resected stage I, II, and III well-differentiated neuroendocrine carcinoma showed that 18:22 survived for 2 years or longer,[47] whereas of 11 patients with completely resected stage I small cell neuroendocrine carcinoma, none survived.[48]

By electron microscopy, well-differentiated neuroendocrine carcinomas differ from typical carcinoids in that their complement of neurosecretory granules is less conspicuous. Also, granules tend to aggregate in dendrite-like cytoplasmic processes. Well-developed desmosomes are readily demonstrable; intermediate filaments may also be found but show less of a tendency to aggregate in paranuclear balls than is the case with carcinoids. Evidence of glandular differentiation may occasionally be noted in the usual sam-

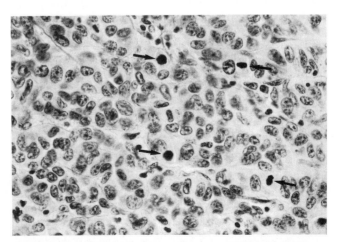

FIGURE 4–12. Neuroendocrine carcinoma, well-differentiated type. An organoid architecture is discernible. Note cellular and nuclear pleomorphism and mitoses *(arrows).* Compare this figure with Figure 4–8 at identical magnification. Hematoxylin and eosin, × 1050.

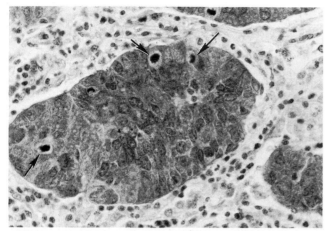

FIGURE 4–13. Neuroendocrine carcinoma, well-differentiated type. Neoplastic cluster is uniformly immunostained with anti-synaptophysin antibody; mitoses are noted *(arrows)*. ABC technique, × 1050.

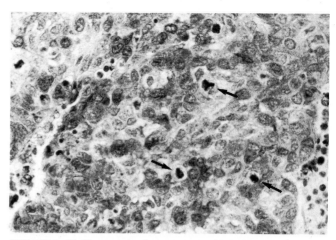

FIGURE 4–14. Neuroendocrine carcinoma, well-differentiated type. Most cells are immunostained with calcitonin; note also prominent mitoses *(arrows)*. Peroxidase–anti-peroxidase technique, × 1050.

ples. The basal lamina layer surrounding tumor cell clusters shows frequent discontinuities. Sustentacular cells are also less frequent than in typical carcinoids.

Immunohistochemical studies for neuroendocrine markers indicate that virtually without exception, well-differentiated neuroendocrine carcinomas express NSE and synaptophysin (Fig. 4–13); if monoclonal antibodies rather than polyclonal NSE antisera are applied, the number of NSE immunoreactive tumors decreases, as does the intensity and diffuseness of the reaction. Serotonin, bombesin, calcitonin (Fig. 4–14), and leu-enkephalin are often demonstrable in these tumors, as are other neuropeptide materials (Fig. 4–15). ACTH is more frequently expressed by these tumors than by carcinoids.[34–36, 49] A small but distinct proportion of these carcinomas is associated with clinically evident hormonal syndromes particularly related to overproduction of ACTH. A small series of these carcinomas have been studied immunohistochemically with antibodies that detect exocrine features, revealing occasional immunoreactive cells in some cases.[18–21] This observation is of interest and should be pursued; it remains, however, that the dominant differentiation pattern in these neoplasms is neuroendocrine, and they should be so classified.

Immunohistochemical and biochemical studies of the complement of intermediate filament and junctional proteins of these carcinomas have shown that they invariably express cytokeratin polypeptides of the simple epithelial type and desmoplakin.[16, 46] More recent studies have demonstrated that a subset of these carcinomas coexpress cytokeratin polypeptides and neurofilament proteins. Vimentin reactions are rare and are generally limited to the peripheral sustentacular elements.

At present, it is agreed that bronchopulmonary carcinoids and neuroendocrine carcinomas as a group are essentially epithelial neoplasms, as determined by their constitutive expression of cytokeratin polypeptides, although a subset of them have been shown to coexpress cytokeratins and neurofilament proteins.[16, 46, 50]

Neuroendocrine Carcinomas, Intermediate Cell Type

In this context, we use the word intermediate only to denote cellular size because the cells comprising these tumors clearly differ from small cells. At present, we regard these carcinomas essentially as variants of the classic small cell neuroendocrine carcinomas from which they do not seem to differ clinically. By the above mentioned designation we merely wish to emphasize their morphologic distinctness and to stress the fact that some of these carcinomas may still be inadvertently bypassed by pathologists as well as clinicians and classified as undifferentiated (large cell) carcinomas if pertinent immunostudies are not performed.

These carcinomas may be centrally or peripherally located; grossly, they exhibit no distinctive characteristic feature, although occasionally they may display central scarring. Histologically, they are composed of polygonal cells but, more frequently, they are com-

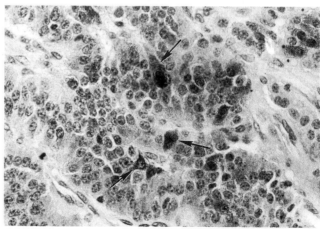

FIGURE 4–15. Neuroendocrine carcinoma, well-differentiated type, same case as in previous figure. Scattered cells show variable immunostaining for vasoactive intestinal polypeptide (VIP) *(arrows)*. Peroxidase–anti-peroxidase technique, × 1050.

posed of fusiform cells ranging from 25 to 40 μm in major diameter. The neoplastic cells are organized in large, solid clusters, which characteristically show peripheral palisading and often central necrosis. The cytoplasm is comparatively abundant and pale to slightly amphophilic. The central nuclei may show peripheral aggregation of their chromatin; nucleoli are discernible but are not prominent. Pleomorphism is marked and the mitotic activity is brisk; atypical mitoses may be readily found (Fig. 4–16).

As noted on electron microscopy, these carcinomas consist of cells with moderately abundant cytoplasm often displaying prominent arrays of intertwined cytoplasmic processes. Basal lamina deposition is inconsistent and often absent. The cytoplasmic matrix is of low density, and the complement of organelles variable. Microtubules and intermediate filaments may be noted. Neurosecretory granules are not abundant, and they tend to concentrate in the aforementioned cytoplasmic processes. Generally, the granules are small, ranging from 80 to 140 nm in diameter. Well-developed desmosomes can be found. In occasional cases, the above-mentioned features, which are characteristic for neuroendocrine differentiation, coexist with bundles of tonofilaments and lumina formation that indicate differentiation toward squamous cell carcinoma and adenocarcinoma, respectively (multidirectional differentiation).[34, 36]

Immunohistochemical studies of these carcinomas with a battery of antibodies to various neuroendocrine markers have shown that the majority express NSE (Fig. 4–17) and synaptophysin; chromogranin expression is somewhat less consistently demonstrable. Serotonin expression may be noted in some cases. With regard to the neuropeptides, bombesin, ACTH, calcitonin, and leu-enkephalin (Fig. 4–18) appear to be frequently expressed. However, it should be noted that these immunohistochemical findings may differ when poorly characterized polyclonal antisera are applied. A small but distinct minority of these neuroendocrine carcinomas are associated with clinical hormonal syndromes.

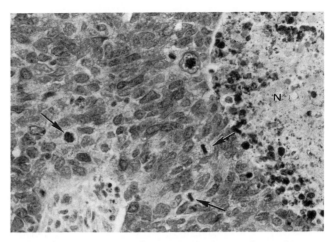

FIGURE 4–17. Neuroendocrine carcinoma, intermediate cell type. Mitoses *(arrows)* and prominent necrosis (N) are noted. Most tumor cells are diffusely immunostained for NSE. Peroxidase–antiperoxidase technique, × 1050.

Not surprisingly a small but distinct proportion of these predominantly neuroendocrine carcinomas can be, at least focally, immunostained with monoclonal antibodies capable of detecting features of exocrine differentiation.[23] This multidirectional character is retained by some of these carcinomas in culture and in nude mice xenografts.[19]

Immunohistochemical and biochemical studies with well-characterized antibodies have indicated that these carcinomas consistently express predominantly, if not exclusively, cytokeratin polypeptides of the simple epithelial type, as well as desmosomal plaque proteins.[46] A certain probably small but as yet undefined proportion of these carcinomas may focally coexpress neurofilament proteins.

Neuroendocrine Carcinoma, Small Cell Type

This is the classic small cell carcinoma. We regard the designation of small cell carcinoma as unnecessarily

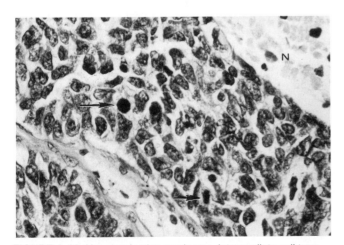

FIGURE 4–16. Neuroendocrine carcinoma, intermediate cell type. Portion of neoplastic cluster. Note irregular peripheral palisading, pleomorphism, mitoses *(arrows)*, and central necrosis (N). Hematoxylin and eosin, × 1050.

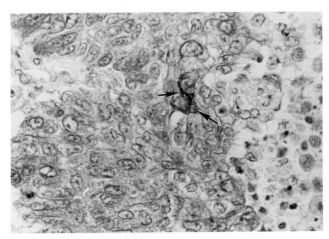

FIGURE 4–18. Neuroendocrine carcinoma, intermediate cell type, same case as in previous figure. The majority of cells are weakly immunostained for leu-enkephalin; a single cell shows prominently stained processes *(arrows)*. Peroxidase–anti-peroxidase, × 1050.

vague and suggest further that these carcinomas should no longer be classified as undifferentiated or anaplastic because their neuroendocrine characteristics can be readily demonstrated in the vast majority of cases. A small but significant proportion of these carcinomas is associated with a clinical hormonal syndrome related to overproduction of ACTH, adrenocortical hormone (ADH), or other materials. These carcinomas may or may not appear related to a grossly detectable bronchus. Histologically, they are composed of very small round to slightly fusiform cells in the 10 to 20 μm diameter range. These cells are often compared with lymphocytes, although they are in fact larger than lymphocytes. Characteristically, these cells have exceedingly scanty cytoplasm and display very pleomorphic and distinctly hyperchromatic nuclei. As a rule, mitoses are abundant. Also characteristic of these neuroendocrine carcinomas are the absence of a defined architectural pattern (Fig. 4–19), the conspicuous, often massive areas of necrosis, the crushing artifact, and the frequently prominent basophilic linear staining of stromal and vascular components.

Electron microscopic analysis of these carcinomas provided the initial clue to their endocrine character.[51] As could be predicted by light microscopy, the ultrastructural appearance of these tumors is dominated by their nuclei. The cytoplasm is scanty and its matrix is of low density. Irregularly intertwined cytoplasmic processes linked by rudimentary junctions, well-defined desmosomes, or both are recognized. These processes often contain small neurosecretory granules 80 to 140 nm in diameter; as a rule, the complement of granules is very limited. Indeed extensive sampling may be required in order to locate these granules. In addition, inconspicuous arrays of intermediate filaments may be found, as well as parallel groups of microtubules. Basal lamina deposition may be focally present; most cell clusters are, however, devoid of detectable basal laminae. In rare cases, neurosecretory granules are not identified despite extensive sampling.[34, 35]

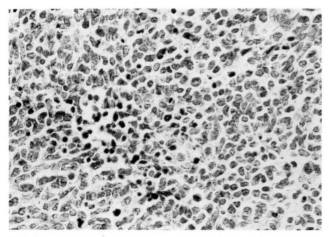

FIGURE 4–19. Neuroendocrine carcinoma, small cell type; this field is almost entirely composed of round cells. Note lack of distinct architecture, and compare the cell's size with that of Figure 4–16 at identical magnification. Hematoxylin and eosin, × 1050.

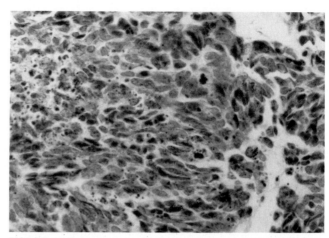

FIGURE 4–20. Neuroendocrine carcinoma, small cell type. Same case as in previous figure, but field displays numerous fusiform cells. The scanty cytoplasm shows immunostaining for bombesin; note also evidence of necrosis. Peroxidase–anti-peroxidase technique, × 1050.

By immunohistochemistry, small cell neuroendocrine carcinomas can be shown to express NSE and synaptophysin; chromogranin may also be demonstrated, albeit less frequently. In our experience to date, bombesin (Fig. 4–20) is the most frequently expressed neuropeptide, followed by ACTH and calcitonin; leu-enkephalin, vasoactive intestinal polypeptide, substance P, and somatostatin may occasionally be shown in scattered cells. As a rule, the expression of these hormonal materials is uneven in extent and intensity. Most small cell neuroendocrine carcinomas can be immunostained with one or more antibodies to neuroendocrine markers. A small number of conventional-appearing small cell carcinomas, however, cannot be immunostained with the currently available antibodies to neuroendocrine markers. This apparent negativity may be attributed to very limited sampling, poor tissue preservation, or both. However, we cannot exclude the possibility that a rare small cell carcinoma of the bronchopulmonary tract may not express neuroendocrine markers, or alternatively, that it may in fact express them but in such minute amounts that they escape detection by our current methods.

Immunohistochemical study of classic small cell neuroendocrine carcinomas with antibodies (e.g., 44-3A6, 624-A12, A-80) detecting features of exocrine differentiation as described earlier, have shown these tumors to be either negative or to include only very occasional, scattered cells that expressed those molecules.[18, 19, 23] Early studies of the intermediate filament complement of these carcinomas suggested that they exclusively expressed neurofilament proteins.[52] Subsequent immunohistochemical and biochemical investigations on frozen tissue samples, however, indicated that small cell carcinomas express cytokeratin polypeptides 8, 18, and 19.[16, 46] Desmoplakin proteins may be difficult to demonstrate, perhaps paralleling the relatively scanty well-defined desmosomes revealed by electron microscopy in many cases. These observations have been confirmed by two-dimensional gel electrophoretic analysis of tumor-rich frozen samples.[16, 46] In occasional small cell carcinomas, we have been unable to demonstrate intermediate filaments; this may be explained either by poor sample preservation or by a very low level expression of those proteins that our current methods fail to reveal. Alternatively, we cannot exclude the possibility that some of these tumors do not express intermediate filament proteins, as has been demonstrated in an experimental rat hepatoma model.[53] To date, we have not been able to show neurofilament proteins coexpressed in classic small cell neuroendocrine carcinomas. We have, however, shown neurofilament protein coexpression in cases with mixed small and intermediate cell populations; in these cases, neurofilament proteins were noted only in the intermediate cells.

It merits emphasis that the aforementioned cytoskeletal markers can be readily demonstrated in well-preserved freshly frozen tumor samples, whereas they often cannot be readily shown in conventionally fixed, paraffin-embedded samples. This apparent discrepancy may be explained by the fact that diverse antibodies are used in different laboratories; however, it should again be stressed that preservation of the tumor samples is most significant.[16, 28, 46] The demonstration of intermediate filaments in conventionally processed tissue samples can be improved to a certain extent by pretreating sections with one of various proteases prior to exposure to the primary antibody; alternative methods such as exposure of the sections to microwaves may improve results in some cases.

It should be stressed that a proportion of small cell neuroendocrine carcinomas include subpopulations of intermediate cells and vice versa. These cases behave with similar aggressiveness to that of both types individually; thus, the designation of poorly differentiated neuroendocrine carcinoma would be justified because it would emphasize that it retains the neuroendocrine qualifier while still separating these tumors from their less aggressive well-differentiated counterparts.[54]

Tumorlets

Tumorlets may be defined as microscopic foci composed of irregular aggregates of neuroendocrine cells often associated with a certain amount of scar tissue. The cells tend to be small and round to fusiform, and they display comparatively little cytoplasm. The nuclei are rather deeply basophilic, but pleomorphism is minimal. The neuroendocrine features of these cells can be readily demonstrated by electron microscopy, immunohistochemistry or both. NSE, synaptophysin, and bombesin, among other neuroendocrine markers, can be readily detected. Hasty examination of a tumorlet, particularly in microscopic sections of poor quality may lead to the erroneous diagnosis of small cell carcinoma. This may be avoided by considering that, by definition, tumorlets are microscopic and virtually without exception incidental findings. Tumorlets are also often multiple and may be found in association with various forms of chronic pulmonary

injury, particularly bronchiectasis, and with all types of tumors. If a lesion presents some histologic features of tumorlet but was detected clinically or radiologically or, alternatively, became evident macroscopically, the diagnosis of tumorlet becomes, in our view, highly questionable if not altogether untenable. Thus, clinically or grossly detected large or giant tumorlets are essentially neuroendocrine neoplasms and should be classified as per their pertinent features.

Microcarcinoids

Microcarcinoids are, as the term denotes, microscopic carcinoids occasionally found incidentally either at autopsy or in surgical specimens resected for other reasons. These minute tumors are also associated with chronic injury, particularly bronchiectasis. Their neuroendocrine features can be readily demonstrated by immunohistochemistry.[35]

Neuroendocrine Hyperplasias and Dysplasias

Neuroendocrine hyperplasias and dysplasias of variable severity have been described in the bronchopulmonary tract. These abnormal neuroendocrine cells may be noted as irregular aggregates, suggesting unduly large and prominent neuroepithelial bodies, or they may be seen arranged as long, irregular rows (linear hyperplasia) (Fig. 4–21). Not surprisingly, these lesions are also more often than not found in association with chronic bronchopulmonary diseases, particularly bronchiectasis[34, 35, 55] and with all tumor types. They may also be conspicuous in small or premature infants with idiopathic respiratory distress syndrome who survive their early problem and subsequently develop various degrees of bronchopulmonary dysplasia (Fig. 4–22).[56] They are not easily detected by conventional light microscopy but are readily revealed by immunohistochemistry as they express neuroendocrine markers, including presumably ectopic peptide hormones such as ACTH.[35, 55] The clin-

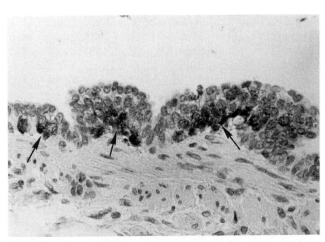

FIGURE 4–21. Bronchiectasis. Focally hyperplastic epithelium; note scattered rows of bombesin immunoreactive cells *(arrows).* Peroxidase–anti-peroxidase technique, × 1050.

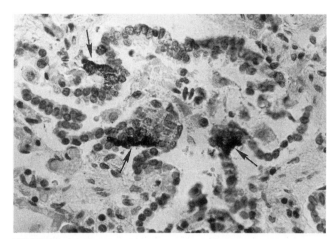

FIGURE 4–22. Specimen from premature infant, 850 g at birth, who was diagnosed as having idiopathic respiratory distress syndrome and was treated at postnatal age 30 days. Note abnormal airway architecture and prominent clusters of bombesin-immunoreactive cells *(arrows)*. Peroxidase–anti-peroxidase technique, × 1050.

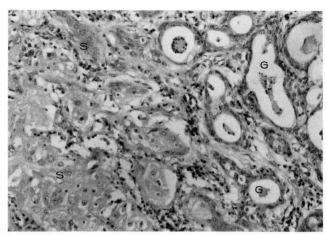

FIGURE 4–23. Adenosquamous carcinoma. Note coexistence of solid squamous areas (S) with well-defined glands (G). Hematoxylin and eosin, × 450.

ical significance of these lesions and their possible role as precursors of other conditions including neoplasms remain speculative.

MISCELLANEOUS NEOPLASMS

Giant Cell Carcinomas

As the designation indicates, these neoplasms are composed entirely or very predominantly of giant cells. Some observers have noted similarities with adenocarcinoma or squamous cell carcinomas, whereas others have regarded them as variants of large cell carcinomas (for a recent overview, see reference 57). Yet, clinically and histologically, these tumors comprise a distinct group. Clinically, these carcinomas behave aggressively. Grossly, they display no outstanding feature. Histologically, the absence of a distinct architectural pattern is characteristic. Bizarre, often multinucleated large cells are noted often coexisting with fusiform elements, large cells with clear cytoplasm, or both. Typical and atypical mitoses are abundant. Frequently noted in these carcinomas is phagocytosis by neoplastic giant cells of other neoplastic cells (cannibalism) or of inflammatory cells. It is possible that some lymphocytes that may be detected within neoplastic cells are not in the process of being phagocytosed but rather reflect the phenomenon of emperipolesis. Electron microscopic analysis of giant cell carcinomas has suggested that at least some of them display exocrine features; these observations are paralleled by light microscopy in that some giant cell carcinomas may be seen to blend with areas of glandular architecture; deeply eosinophilic cells, suggestive of keratinization may also be seen. Immunohistochemical studies with monoclonal antibodies to the 44-3A6 and particularly to the A-80 molecules have shown that the overwhelming majority of giant cell carcinomas have significant cell populations with exocrine phenotypic features.[57] However, the intermedi-

ate filament profile of these tumors is distinct in that low-molecular-weight cytokeratin polypeptides and, less frequently, their high-molecular-weight counterparts are almost invariably coexpressed with vimentin. Based on these structural and clinical characteristics, we believe that giant cell carcinomas constitute a distinct entity and merit being considered as such.[57]

Adenosquamous Carcinomas

Adenosquamous carcinomas display histologically variable admixtures of glands and solid clusters with either individual cell keratinization or keratin pearl formation (Fig. 4–23). Accordingly, they may be regarded as variants of either squamous cell carcinomas or adenocarcinomas. This is a morphologically striking and comparatively frequent form of multidirectional differentiation in lung carcinomas but by no means the only one (see later). Not surprisingly, when adenosquamous carcinomas are studied with monoclonal antibodies that detect exocrine features, their

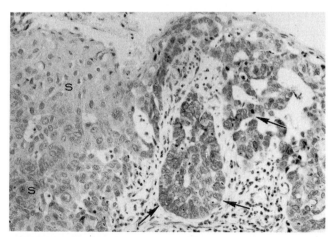

FIGURE 4–24. Adenosquamous carcinoma, same case as previous figure. Immunostaining with monoclonal antibody 44-3A6. Focus of glandular formation is stained *(arrows)*, whereas solid squamous area (S) is not. Avidin-biotin complex technique, × 450.

glandular component is readily immunostained, whereas their squamous areas are not (Fig. 4–24).[18, 23]

Spindle Cell Carcinomas

Spindle cell carcinomas are rare neoplasms that histologically may resemble various types of sarcoma and have often been classified as such. They are composed predominantly of fascicles and nests of fusiform cells often lacking a convincing organoid architecture. This architectural feature is significant because some neuroendocrine neoplasms may be either composed entirely of fusiform cells or include significant fusiform cell subpopulations. Electron microscopic study may reveal bundles of tonofilaments and desmosomes. The essentially epithelial character of these malignant neoplasms may be further demonstrated by immunostaining with anticytokeratin antibodies; however, vimentin coexpression may also be shown.

Carcinosarcoma

Carcinosarcoma of the lung is a rather distinct albeit uncommon entity.[13, 30] The tumor characteristically but not invariably occurs in elderly males, and it may appear grossly as a polypoid mass protruding into the lumen of a major bronchus. Histologically, carcinomatous nests coexist with a cellular stroma composed of variably atypical fusiform cells. By immunohistochemistry, cytokeratin can be shown in the aforementioned nests and in some of the fusiform cell population; the fusiform cells may be shown to express vimentin exclusively or to coexpress cytokeratin and vimentin. The latter cytokeratin-vimentin coexpression has been described in a number of carcinomas of the kidney, female genital tract, thyroid, and breast, and therefore may not be considered sufficient ground for the designation of carcinosarcoma. However, taking into account the basic histologic pattern of these tumors and the fact that electron microscopic study may show that at least some of the aforementioned fusiform cells display convincing features of smooth muscle differentiation, the designation of carcinosarcoma appears justified.

Salivary Gland Type Tumors

The entire spectrum of salivary gland type tumors may develop in major bronchi and occasionally within the lung parenchyma. Thus, pleomorphic adenomas (mixed tumors), mucoepidermoid carcinomas of various grades, adenoid cystic carcinomas, acinic cell tumors and oncocytomas may be encountered[13, 30]; these tumors are histologically indistinguishable from their counterparts in the salivary glands and other sites.

Mucous Gland Adenomas

Mucous gland adenomas are extremely rare bronchial tumors, appearing grossly as polypoid mucosal outgrowths that may cause obstruction.[13, 30] Microscopi-

cally, mucous gland adenomas share some features of adenomatous and inflammatory polyps of the gastrointestinal tract. They are composed of dilated glandular structures containing pools of mucosubstance; the individual cells are only minimally pleomorphic.

Chest Wall Tumors

A quantitatively small but clinically significant group of tumors composed of apparently undifferentiated small cells occur in the chest wall. Initially they were described in children and adolescents,[58] but they also occur in adults. Early studies showed that these chest wall tumors had neural features on electron microscopy and immunohistochemistry[58, 59]; thus, they parallel small cell lung carcinomas. However, clinicopathologic and cytogenetic data indicate even closer similarities to peripheral neuroepitheliomas or peripheral neuroectodermal tumors (see later).

These tumors may arise anywhere in the chest wall, infiltrate soft tissues (Fig. 4–25), may extend into the pleural cavity and fuse the pleurae, and may extend into lung parenchyma. On light microscopy, they consist of small cells, which are often arranged in poorly cohesive clusters and separated by variable amounts of stroma (Fig. 4–26); necrosis is generally not conspicuous, mitoses are readily found, and occasional rosettes may be seen. We have studied a series of these tumors in adults by electron microscopy and immunohistochemistry and found that small complements of convincing neurosecretory granules are demonstrable,[60] and synaptophysin was consistently shown. Notably, these tumors predominantly express vimentin (Fig. 4–27), often associated with neurofilament proteins and cytokeratin polypeptides, but they seemingly lack desmoplakins[60]; therefore, they appear to be the peripheral counterparts of central nervous system primitive neuroectodermal tumors.[61] The neuroendocrine character of these tumors is evident;

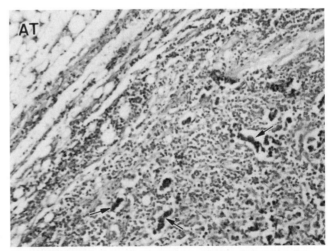

FIGURE 4–25. Primitive neuroectodermal tumors (PNET) of the chest wall; very low magnification depicts tumor in fibroconnective and adipose tissues (AT). Infiltrating edge shows abundant lymphocytes and scanty neoplastic aggregates *(arrows).* Hematoxylin and eosin, × 90.

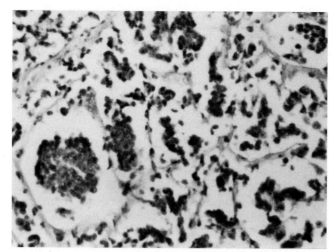

FIGURE 4–26. PNET of chest wall; note poorly cohesive tumor clusters composed of small dark cells. Hematoxylin and eosin, × 450.

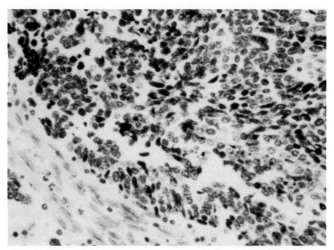

FIGURE 4–27. PNET of chest wall immunostained for vimentin; the majority of cells (dark) are reactive while a minority of cells (pale) show only the faintly counterstained nuclei. Avidin-biotin complex technique, × 920.

however, their distinct cytoskeletal profile distinguishes them from the constitutively epithelial pulmonary small cell neuroendocrine carcinomas. The differential diagnosis may indeed arise when small cell lung carcinomas rarely invade the chest wall and, relatively more frequently, when primitive neuroectodermal tumors (PNET) of the chest wall extend into the lung. An additional differential diagnosis may arise between PNET and variants of Ewing's sarcoma. Both may coexpress vimentin with cytokeratins and neurofilaments; however, PNETs consistently express synaptophysin while lacking desmoplakins, whereas the reverse is the case with Ewing's sarcoma.[61, 62] In our experience restricted to a small series, some patients with chest wall PNET seem to benefit from en block resections plus adjunct radiotherapy and chemotherapy, and although the prognosis of patients with this condition is guarded, as a group, PNETs behave less aggressively than the classic small cell neuroendocrine carcinomas of the lung.[61]

Carcinomas Limited to Lymph Nodes

Significant problems for clinicians, surgeons, and pathologists are posed when carcinoma is found in lymph nodes without an evident visceral primary tumor. In most instances, a primary tumor is either subsequently found or strongly suspected. However, there are instances of carcinoma-containing lymph nodes in which even the most thorough, refined, and repeated studies, including surgical procedures, fail to reveal a primary visceral tumor. Several explanations have been advanced to clarify such a phenomenon (for overview and further references, see reference 63).

We have reported on three patients with carcinoma of the thoracic lymph nodes in which no pulmonary or any other primary site could be found. In addition to clinical, radiographic, and laboratory studies, these patients were surgically explored and pulmonary tissue was obtained; one patient also had a pneumonec-

tomy. The carcinoma cells were organized in clusters, anastomosing cords, or both; they reacted for multiple cytokeratin polypeptides (Fig. 4–28), and coexpressed vimentin frequently and desmin occasionally; in one patient, a neuroendocrine subpopulation was noted.[63] We suggested the possibility that these and similar carcinomas may arise in the lymph nodes themselves[63] from the recently reported cytokeratin-positive (i.e., epithelial) extrafollicular reticulum cells in lymphoid organs, as described by Franke and Moll[64] and independently confirmed by others.[65] We have since studied several additional cases of carcinoma of variable phenotypes in lymph nodes of other chains in which, again, no primary site could be found; moreover, an independent report on similar cases has

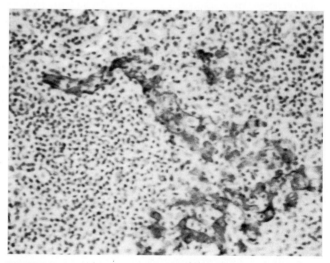

FIGURE 4–28. Carcinoma limited to thoracic lymph node(s) immunostained with a so-called cocktail of antibodies recognizing several low- and high-molecular-weight cytokeratins. An irregular cord of carcinoma cells, as well as some isolated cells, are strongly reactive; lymphoid cells in the background show only nuclear staining. Avidin-biotin complex technique, × 320.

been published.[66] We believe these data may help explain some puzzling cases, and merit follow-up studies.

CONCLUSIONS AND OUTLOOK

There is no doubt that our knowledge and understanding of the neoplasms arising in the bronchopulmonary tract have grown remarkably during the last decade. We are now in a position to characterize phenotypically by immunohistochemistry and by other techniques many of the aforementioned neoplasms with far greater precision than has previously been possible. These enhanced capabilities are reflected by the relative frequency with which the phenomenon of multidirectional differentiation (phenotypic heterogeneity) can be demonstrated. The occasional adenosquamous carcinoma or adenocarcinoma with a small cell carcinoma component were known to traditional light microscopic pathologists. But, by applying currently available, finely tuned markers, we can now show that conventional adenocarcinomas may contain occasional, unmistakable neuroendocrine cells. Conversely, exocrine differentiation may be readily demonstrated in at least some predominantly neuroendocrine neoplasms, and other combinations have been noted. We may therefore state that the phenomenon of multidirectional differentiation may be shown with comparative frequency, although it may be manifested in a qualitatively and quantitatively inconspicuous fashion. Moreover, it has become increasingly evident that differentiation of neoplastic populations may not only be multidirectional but may prove to be unstable, (i.e., variable within the natural or therapeutically altered life span of a given carcinoma).[67–70]

These techniques and observations should not be regarded as mere curiosities, because they have enabled us to establish the basically neuroendocrine characteristics of a considerable proportion of bronchopulmonary and other neoplasms. In the case of the nebulous group of large cell pulmonary carcinomas, subsets with exocrine and neuroendocrine differentiation can now be isolated, and these findings may have very significant clinical implications.[22, 37] The proven applicability of at least some of these immunomarkers to conventional cytologic smears is certain to broaden their impact.[71]

In a more speculative vein, even the finding of a quantitatively unimpressive neuroendocrine subpopulation in an otherwise non-neuroendocrine carcinoma may have important implications, given that some neuropeptides (e.g., bombesin) have been shown to be tumor growth factors in vitro[72] and in vivo.[73] Also noteworthy is the variability in the expression of oncogene products in lung neoplasms as determined by immunocytochemical methods.[74] Most recently, a group of dimeric molecules, designated as integrins, that function as receptors to extracellular matrix proteins have been characterized and effective antibodies that recognize them have been generated (for an overview, see reference 75). Immunohistochemical studies on lung tumors showed three groups with distinct integrin profiles (i.e., squamous-adenocarcinoma, bronchioloalveolar carcinomas, and carcinoid-neuroendocrine carcinomas).[76] In addition, the integrin profiles of pulmonary and other visceral adenocarcinomas differ substantially from those of pleural mesotheliomas, including those with marked glandular differentiation.[77] And, although the proximate applicability and possible clinical significance of these and related findings remain undetermined, they add to our understanding and deserve further investigation.

We should also consider that many aspects of recently acquired knowledge cannot be readily or effectively grafted on long-held traditional designations and classifications. Therefore, we may expect that the taxonomy of pulmonary epithelial neoplasms will undergo some changes. One may argue that the ideal would be to develop a classification scheme with a solid molecular basis. However, it does not necessarily follow that such a classification would prove to be superior to more conventional ones, because other indispensable ingredients of a superior classification (in this context, relative simplicity, reproducibility, and clinical significance) would have to be demonstrated. These issues merit thoughtful exploration and discussion.[11]

This is an exciting period for oncologically inclined clinicians and pathologists. Molecular markers and studies have opened and will continue to open new and often unsuspected horizons for tumor evaluation, diagnosis, and possibly, therapy. These developments should be received with cautious optimism and deliberation by pathologists and clinicians alike, for we should consider that new methods and concepts have, of necessity, their own limitations. Given those caveats, we may expect that progress will continue.

Acknowledgments

The desmoplakin and synaptophysin antibodies were generously provided by Prof. WW Franke, Heidelberg, Germany.

The pediatric tissues were kindly provided by Dr. NS Gould, Chicago, IL.

SELECTED REFERENCES

Dail DH, Hammar SP: Pulmonary Pathology. 2nd edition, Springer-Verlag, New York, 1993.
   Extensive discussion of common and uncommon bronchopulmonary tumors and an excellent background on general lung pathology.
Gould VE, Moll R, Chejfec G, et al: Cytoskeletal characteristics of epithelial neoplasms of the lung. *In* Lenfant C, Abrams PG, Cuttita F, Rosen, ST (eds): Biology of Lung Cancer. New York, Marcel Dekker, 1988, pp 121–154.
   An overview with immunohistochemical and biochemical data on the expression of intermediate filaments and desmosomal proteins in epithelial neoplasms of the lung. The discussion touches on significant technical issues including that of characterization of antibodies that clarify some aspects of this rapidly evolving field.
Gould, VE, Warren WH: The Bronchopulmonary Tract. *In* Lechago

J, Gould VE (eds): Endocrine Pathology. Baltimore, Williams & Wilkins, 1995.
Thorough and up-to-date discussion on pulmonary neuroendocrine cells, neuroepithelial bodies, and corresponding pathology; it includes current as well as historical references.

Lee I, Radosevich JA, Chejfec, G, et al: Malignant mesotheliomas. Improved differential diagnosis from lung carcinomas using monoclonal antibodies 44-3A6 and 624-A12. Am J Pathol 123:497–507, 1986.
Detailed discussion of the application of immunoprobes that detect features of exocrine differentiation; differential expression between lung adenocarcinomas and pleural mesotheliomas is emphasized.

Warren WH, Memoli VA, Jordan AG, et al: Reevaluation of pulmonary neoplasms resected as small cell carcinomas. Significance of distinguishing between well differentiated and small cell neuroendocrine carcinomas. Cancer 65:1003–1010, 1990.
Clinical, histologic and cytologic discussion emphasizing the differential diagnosis between well-differentiated and small cell neuroendocrine carcinomas.

REFERENCES

1. Moll R, Cowin P, Kapprell HP, et al: Desmosomal proteins: New markers for the identification and classification of tumors. Lab Invest 54:4–25, 1986.
2. Silverberg E: Cancer statistics. CA 31:13–28, 1981.
3. Kreyberg L: One hundred consecutive primary epithelial lung tumors. Brit J Cancer 6:112–119, 1952.
4. Foot NC: The identification of types of pulmonary cancer in cytologic smears. Am J Pathol 28:963–983, 1952.
5. Kreyberg L: The significance of histological typing in the study of the epidemiology of primary epithelial lung tumors. Br J Cancer 8:199–208, 1954.
6. Kreyberg L: Main histologic types of primary epithelial lung tumors. Br J Cancer 15:206–214, 1961.
7. Kreyberg L: Histological lung cancer types. Acta Pathol Microbiol Scand 157 (suppl), Oslo, 1962.
8. World Health Organization: Histological Typing of Lung Tumors. WHO Geneva, 1967.
9. World Health Organization: Histological typing of lung tumors. Am J Clin Pathol 77:123–136, 1982.
10. Kreyberg L: Cancer epidemiology. Some methodological reflections. Acta Pathol Microbiol Immunol Scand (A) 92 (suppl 285); 1–16, 1984.
11. Gould VE: Histogenesis and differentiation: A re-evaluation of these concepts as criteria for the classification of tumors. Hum Pathol 17:212–215, 1986.
12. Yesner R, Carter D: Pathology of carcinoma of the lung: Changing patterns. Clin Chest Med 3:257–289, 1982.
13. Carter D, Eggleston JC: Tumors of the Lower Respiratory Tract. Atlas of Tumor Pathology, 2nd Series, Fasc. 17. Washington, DC, Armed Forces Institute of Pathology, 1980.
14. Cotran RS, Kumar V, Robbins SL: Pathologic Basis of Disease. 4th ed. Philadelphia, W.B. Saunders, 1989, pp 797–803.
15. Blobel GA, Moll R, Franke WW, et al: Cytokeratins in normal lung and lung carcinomas: I. Adenocarcinomas, squamous cell carcinomas, and cultured cell lines. Virchows Arch (Cell Pathol) 45:407–429, 1984.
16. Gould VE, Moll R, Chejfec G, et al: Cytoskeletal characteristics of epithelial neoplasms of the lung. *In* Lenfant C, Abrams PG, Cuttita F, Rosen ST (eds): Biology of Lung Cancer. New York, Marcel Dekker, 1988, pp 121–154.
17. Radosevich JA, Ma Y, Lee I, et al: Monoclonal antibody 44-3A6 as a probe for a novel antigen found in human lung carcinomas with glandular differentiation. Cancer Res 45:5808–5812, 1985.
18. Lee I, Radosevich JA, Combs SG, et al: Immunohistochemical analysis of pulmonary carcinomas using monoclonal antibody 44-3A6. Cancer Res 45;5813–5817, 1985.
19. Lee I, Warren WH, Gould VE, et al: Immunohistochemical demonstration of lacto-N-fucopentose III in lung carcinomas with monoclonal antibody 624-A12. Pathol Res Pract 182:40–47, 1987.
20. Gould VE, Shin SS, Manderino GL, et al: Selective expression of a mucin-type glycoprotein in human tumors. Hum Pathol 19:623–627, 1988.
21. Shin SS, Gould VE, Gould JE, et al: Expression of a mucin-type glycoprotein in select epithelial dysplasias and neoplasms detected immunocytochemically with Mab A-80. APMIS 96:1129–1139, 1988.
22. Piehl MR, Gould VE, Warren WH, Lee I: Immunohistochemical identification of exocrine and neuroendocrine subsets of large cell lung carcinomas. Path Res Pract 183:675–682, 1988.
23. Koukoulis GK, Radosevich JA, Warren WH, et al: Immunohistochemical analysis of pulmonary and pleural neoplasms with monoclonal antibodies B72.3 and CSLEX-1. Virchows Arch Cell Pathol 58:427–433, 1990.
24. Barsky SH, Huang SJ, Bhuta S: The extracellular matrix of pulmonary scar carcinoma is suggestive of a desmoplastic origin. Am J Pathol 124:412–419, 1986.
25. Lee I, Radosevich JA, Chejfec G, et al: Malignant mesotheliomas. Improved differential diagnosis from lung carcinomas using monoclonal antibodies 44-3A6 and 624-A12. Am J Pathol 123:497–507, 1986.
26. Walts AE, Said JW, Shintaku IP, et al: Keratins of different molecular weight in exfoliated mesothelioma and adenocarcinoma cells: An aid to cell differentiation. Am J Clin Pathol 81:442–446, 1983.
27. Moll R, Franke WW, Schiller DL, et al: The catalog of human cytokeratin polypeptides: Patterns of expression of specific keratins in normal epithelia, tumors and cultured cells. Cell 31:11–24, 1982.
28. Blobel RA, Moll R, Franke WW, et al: The intermediate filament cytoskeleton of malignant mesotheliomas and its diagnostic significance. Am J Pathol 121:235–247, 1985.
29. Warhol MJ, Hickey WF, Corson JM: Malignant mesothelioma. Ultrastructural distinction from adenocarcinoma. Am J Surg Pathol 6:307–314, 1982.
30. Spencer H: Pathology of the Lung, Vol 2. 2nd Ed. Oxford, United Kingdom, Pergamon Press, 1985, pp 892–900.
31. Chejfec G, Capella C, Solcia E, et al: Amphicrine cells, dysplasias and neoplasias. Cancer 56:2683–2690, 1985.
32. Piehl MR, Lee I, Ma Y, et al: Subsets of pulmonary large cell undifferentiated carcinomas defined immunohistochemically. Lab Invest 55:60-A, 1987.
33. Warren WH, Memoli VA, Kittle CF, et al: The biological implications of bronchial tumors. J Thorac Cardiovasc Surg 87:274–282, 1984.
34. Gould VE, Linnoila RI, Memoli VA, et al: Neuroendocrine cells and neuroendocrine neoplasms of the lung. Pathol Annu 18(I):287–330, 1983.
35. Gould VE, Linnoila RI, Memoli VA, et al: Neuroendocrine components of the bronchopulmonary tract: Hyperplasias, dysplasias and neoplasms. Lab Invest 49:519–537, 1983.
36. Gould VE, Warren WH, Memoli VA: Neuroendocrine cells and neuroendocrine neoplasms of the lung. *In* Becker KL, Gazdar AF (eds): The Endocrine Lung. Philadelphia, W.B. Saunders, 1984, pp 406–445.
37. Gould VE, Tomanova R, Monson R, et al: Immunophenotypic subsets of large cell pulmonary carcinomas. Lab Invest 70:150-A, 1994.
38. Wiedenmann B, Franke WW, Kuhn C, et al: Synaptophysin: A marker protein for neuroendocrine cells and neoplasms. Proc Natl Acad Sci USA 83:3500–3504, 1986.
39. Gould VE, Lee I, Wiedenmann B, et al: Synaptophysin: A novel marker for neurons, certain neuroendocrine cells and their neoplasms. Hum Pathol 17:979–983, 1986.
40. Gould VE, Wiedenmann B, Lee I, et al: Synaptophysin expression in neuroendocrine neoplasms as determined by immunocytochemistry. Am J Pathol 126:243–257, 1987.
41. Gould VE: Synaptophysin: A new and promising pan-neuroendocrine marker. Arch Pathol Lab Med 111:791–794, 1987.
42. Warren WH, Gould VE: Long-term follow-up of classical bronchial carcinoid tumors. Scand J Thorac Cardiovasc Surg 24:125–130, 1990.
43. Lee I, Gould VE, Moll R, et al: Synaptophysin expression in the bronchopulmonary tract: Neuroendocrine cells, neuroepithelial bodies, and neuroendocrine neoplasms. Differentiation 34:115–125, 1987.
44. Warren, WH, Memoli, VA, Gould, VE: Immunohistochemical

and ultrastructural analysis of bronchopulmonary neuroendocrine neoplasms. I. Carcinoids. Ultrastruct Pathol 6:15–27, 1985.

45. Lehto VP, Miettinen M, Dahl D, Virtanen I: Bronchial carcinoid cells contain neural-type of intermediate filaments. Cancer 54:624–628, 1984.

46. Blobel GA, Gould VE, Moll R, et al: Coexpression of neuroendocrine markers and epithelial cytoskeletal proteins in bronchopulmonary neuroendocrine neoplasms. Lab Invest 52:39–52, 1985.

47. Warren WH, Memoli VA, Gould VE: Well differentiated and small cell neuroendocrine carcinomas of the lung. Two related but distinct clinicopathologic entities. Virchows Arch B Cell Pathol 55:299–310, 1988.

48. Warren WH, Memoli VA, Jordan AG, Gould VE: Reevaluation of pulmonary neoplasms resected as small cell carcinomas. Significance of distinguishing between well differentiated and small cell neuroendocrine carcinomas. Cancer 65:1003–1010, 1990.

49. Warren WH, Memoli VA, Gould VE: Immunohistochemical and ultrastructural analysis of bronchopulmonary neuroendocrine neoplasms. II. Well differentiated neuroendocrine carcinomas. Ultrastruct Pathol 7:185–199, 1984.

50. Lehto V-P, Bergh J, Virtanen I: Immunohistology in the classification of lung tumors. In Hansen, HH (ed): Lung Cancer; Basic and Clinical Aspects. Boston, Martinus Nijhoff Publishers, 1986, pp 1–30.

51. Bensch KG, Corrin B, Pariente R, et al: Oat-cell carcinoma of the lung: Its origin and relationship to bronchial carcinoid. Cancer 22:1163–1172, 1968.

52. Lehto VP, Stenman S, Miettinen M, et al: Expression of a neural type of intermediate filament as a distinguishing feature between oat cell carcinoma and other lung cancers. Am J Pathol 110:113–118, 1983.

53. Venetianer A, Schiller DL, Magin T, et al: Cessation of cytokeratin expression in the rat hepatoma cell line lacking differentiated functions. Nature 305:730–733, 1983.

54. Warren WH, Gould VE: Neuroendocrine neoplasms of the lung: A 10-year perspective on their classification. Zentrabl Pathol 139:107–113, 1993.

55. Tsutsumi, Y, Osamura, RY, Watanabe, K, et al: Immunohistochemical studies on gastrin-releasing peptide and adrenocorticotropic hormone-containing cells in the human lung. Lab Invest 48:623–632, 1983.

56. Stahlman MT, Kasselberg AG, Orth DN, et al: Ontogeny of neuroendocrine cells in human fetal lung. II. An immunohistochemical study. Lab Invest 52:52–60, 1985.

57. Chejfec G, Candel A, Jansson DS, et al: Immunohistochemical features of giant cell carcinoma of the lung: Patterns of expression of cytokeratins, vimentin and the mucinous glycoprotein recognized by Mab A-80. Ultrastruct Pathol 15:131–138, 1991.

58. Askin FB, Rosai J, Sibley RK, et al: Malignant small cell tumor of the thoracopulmonary region in childhood. A distinctive clinicopathologic entity of uncertain histogenesis. Cancer 43:2438–2451, 1979.

59. Gonzalez-Crussi F, Wolson SL, Misugi K, et al: Peripheral neuroectodermal tumors of the chest wall in childhood. Cancer 54:2519–2527, 1984.

60. Gould VE, Jansson DS, Warren WH: Primitive neuroectodermal tumors of the chest wall in adults. Lab Invest 64:115A, 1991.

61. Gould VE, Jansson DS, Molenaar WM, et al: Primitive neuroectodermal tumors of the central nervous system. Patterns of expression of neuroendocrine markers, and all classes of intermediate filament proteins. Lab Invest 62:498–509, 1990.

62. Moll R, Lee I, Gould VE, et al: Immunocytochemical analysis of Ewing's tumors. Patterns of expression of intermediate filaments and desmosomal proteins indicate cell type heterogeneity and pluripotential differentiation. Am J Pathol 127:288–304, 1987.

63. Gould VE, Warren WH, Faber LP, et al: Malignant cells of epithelial phenotype limited to thoracic lymph nodes. Eur J Cancer 26:1121–1126, 1990.

64. Franke WW, Moll R: Cytoskeletal components of lymphoid organs. I. Synthesis of cytokeratins 8 and 18 and desmin in extrafollicular reticulum cells of human lymph nodes, tonsils, and spleen. Differentiation 36:145–163, 1987.

65. Coggi G, Dell'Orto P, Braidotti P, et al: Coexpression of intermediate filaments in normal and neoplastic tissues: A reappraisal. Ultrastruct Pathol 13:501–514, 1989.

66. Eusebi V, Capella C, Cossu A, et al: Neuroendocrine carcinoma within lymph nodes in the absence of a primary tumor, with special reference to Merkel cell carcinoma. Am J Surg Pathol 16:658–666, 1992.

67. Abeloff, MD, Eggleston, JC: Morphologic changes following therapy. In Greco FA, Oldham RK, Bunn PA (eds): Small Cell Lung Cancer. New York, Grune & Stratton, 1981, pp 235–259.

68. Abeloff MD, Eggleston JC, Mendelsohn G, et al: Changes in morphologic and biochemical characteristics of small cell carcinomas of the lung: A clinicopathologic study. Am J Med 66:757–764, 1979.

69. Gazdar AF, Carney DN, Guccion JG, et al: Small cell carcinoma of the lung: Cellular origin and relationship to other pulmonary tumors. In Greco FA, Oldham RK, Bunn PA (eds): Small Cell Lung Cancer. New York, Grune & Stratton, 1981, pp 145–175.

70. Gould VE, Memoli VA, Dardi LE: Multidirectional differentiation in human epithelial cancers. J Submicroscop Cytol 13:97–113, 1981.

71. Banner BF, Gould VE, Radosevich JA, et al: Application of monoclonal antibody 44-3A6 in the diagnosis and classification of pulmonary carcinomas. Diagn Cytopathol 1:300–305, 1985.

72. Minna JD, Bunn PA, Carney DN, et al: Experience of the National Cancer Institute (USA) in the treatment and biology of small cell lung cancer. Bull Cancer 69:83–93, 1982.

73. Cuttitta F, Carney DN, Mulshine J, et al: Bombesin-like peptides can function as autocrine growth factors in human small cell lung cancer. Nature 316:823–826, 1985.

74. Lee I, Gould VE, Radosevich JA, et al: Immunohistochemical evaluation of ras oncogene expression in pulmonary and pleural neoplasms. Virchows Arch Cell Pathol 53:146–152, 1987.

75. Ruoslahti, E: Integrins. J Clin Invest 87:1–5, 1991.

76. Koukoulis GK, Virtanen I, Howeedy A, et al: Immunolocalization of integrins in the normal and neoplastic lung epithelium. Lab Invest 70:152-A, 1994.

77. Shen J, Koukoulis GK, Virtanen I: Immunolocalization of integrins in pleural mesotheliomas. Lab Invest 70:154-A, 1994.

5 FUNDAMENTALS OF DIAGNOSTIC IMAGING

Robert A. Clark

Lung cancer is the leading cause of cancer deaths in the United States.[1] Although the incidence of lung cancer in men peaked in 1982, the incidence of lung cancer in women continues to increase at a significant rate.[2, 3] Lung cancer now exceeds breast cancer as the leading cause of cancer deaths among women, and accounts for over one-fifth of female cancer-related mortality.[1, 3]

Primary thoracic neoplasms are a heterogeneous group of lesions with significant overlap in their anatomic-pathologic characteristics that affect imaging strategies.[4, 5] For example, squamous cell carcinomas and small cell carcinomas most frequently arise as masses in the central bronchi, whereas adenocarcinomas and large cell cancers arise more often in the periphery of the lung. Bronchoalveolar cell carcinoma behaves most often as a type of adenocarcinoma, and appears as a peripheral pulmonary nodule rather than its less common alveolar infiltrate appearance.

Certain lung cancers also have very different biologic behaviors that may determine the choice of the diagnostic imaging method to be used.[5, 6] Small cell anaplastic carcinomas are very aggressive, and systemic extrathoracic disease is present frequently at the time of initial diagnosis. Therefore, staging strategies using imaging techniques used for this neoplasm are different from those used for non–small cell cancers. Adenocarcinoma has a propensity to spread to the brain early in its metastatic course, suggesting that brain imaging, even in asymptomatic patients, may have some value.

Although the low overall survival of patients with lung cancer is discouraging, small improvements in diagnosis, staging, and treatment may help many patients with this devastating illness. Progress in diagnostic imaging technology and its use offers greater accuracy in diagnosis, staging, and monitoring therapy than was once possible. This chapter reviews the current principles of diagnostic imaging in thoracic oncology; it presents the fundamentals of chest radiographs, computed tomography (CT), magnetic resonance imaging (MRI), and image-guided percutaneous needle biopsy. More important, it attempts to clarify the clinical uses of these techniques in the areas of screening, detection, diagnosis, and staging.

IMAGING MODALITIES

Chest Radiography

Despite the impressive advances of computerized cross-sectional imaging techniques, the chest radiograph retains a central role in the evaluation of thoracic neoplasms. The standard chest examination consists of posteroanterior (PA) and lateral chest films obtained using high kilovoltage (120 to 150 kVp) technique to improve pulmonary nodule detection by increasing penetration through the mediastinum. The high kilovoltage technique sacrifices imaging detail of the ribs and diminishes visualization of calcium within lesions. In selected instances, low kilovoltage radiographs (60–80 kVp) may be helpful in imaging ribs or demonstrating calcium in a pulmonary nodule.

Most asymptomatic lung cancers are detected on conventional chest radiographs.[7] The radiographic signs of lung cancer are a pulmonary nodule, a central mass, segmental or lobar collapse, and postobstructive pneumonia. Signs of intrathoracic spread of neoplasm include pleural thickening or effusion, hilar metastasis, rib erosion, and interstitial markings due to lymphangitic neoplasm (e.g., Kerley's lines).[8, 9]

The differentiation of malignant lesions from benign lesions on chest radiographs is unreliable. General features of malignancy are a spiculated margin, documented growth on chest radiographs 1 to 24 months apart, and size greater than 3 cm.[4] For lesions smaller than 3 cm in diameter, assessment is more difficult. Central or concentric calcifications are typical for the diagnosis of benign granuloma, but uncommon presentations of malignancy include central calcification, as well as a thin-walled cystic cavity and air-space consolidation.

Central lesions may be visible only as an abnormal convexity in the hilum (Fig. 5–1), or they may be obscured by associated segmental or lobar collapse (Fig. 5–2). In the presence of collapse, the obstructing mass may often remain visible as a central bulge in the contour. Less often, obstructing neoplasm may also present as a consolidated, expanded lobe or segment, or as mucous plugging with inspissated secretions allowing visualization of the plugged bronchus itself.

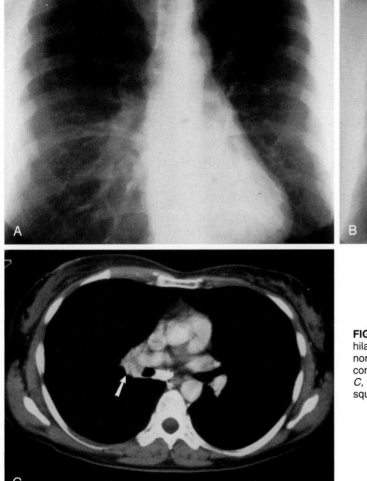
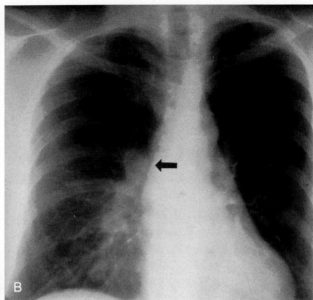

FIGURE 5–1. Primary squamous cell carcinoma, seen as a hilar mass. *A,* On a baseline chest radiograph, the hila are normal. *B,* Six months after A was taken, an abnormal convexity in the superior right hilum *(arrow)* has developed. *C,* CT confirms the right hilar mass *(arrow)* that was due to squamous cell carcinoma.

Although certain cell types of neoplasm have characteristic anatomic presentations, it is not reliable to predict cell type by radiographic appearance or location. Nevertheless, each interpretation of radiographic lesions should include a description of the primary lesion as central or peripheral; its size, shape, and anatomic location (if possible); any mediastinal abnormalities; and types of pleural or chest wall abnormalities. A peripheral lung lesion is usually detectable when its diameter exceeds 1 centimeter,[4, 10] but central lesions of this size may be obscured by hilar structures.

Upper lobe carcinomas are common, yet right upper lobe carcinomas are those most frequently undetected by chest radiographs.[4, 11] The upper ribs and clavicles project closely together and overlie the upper lobes, making it more difficult to visualize lesions radiographically. Therefore, one must have a high level of suspicion for any vague abnormality recognized in the upper lungs and supplement standard radiographs with additional oblique or lordotic views that may resolve an area of concern. The use of CT for such cases is also appropriate if conventional films remain equivocal.

The sensitivity of chest radiography for detection of pulmonary nodules is limited by both technical factors and problems resulting from subjective interpretation.[8–10] Missed nodules result from perceptual errors; a radiologist may not identify 30% to 50% of small nodules recognized in retrospect on chest radiographs.

Mediastinal or hilar contour abnormalities are often the only signs of adenopathy on chest films. The chest radiograph is less sensitive, but more specific, than CT for the detection of adenopathy. In certain cases, and especially in small cell carcinomas, mediastinal adenopathy may be the predominant radiographic feature, with a less conspicuous or unidentified primary lesion. Pleural and chest wall findings are ancillary abnormalities that may affect staging and prog-

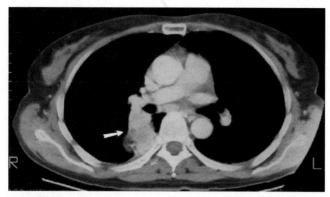

FIGURE 5–2. Central mass obscured by segmental pulmonary consolidation. CT shows consolidation of the superior segment of the right upper lobe *(arrow)*, secondary to obstructing bronchogenic carcinoma. The central mass cannot be seen.

nosis. The chest radiograph is relatively sensitive for effusion but does not reveal chest wall invasion unless bone destruction is evident.

Conventional film tomography of the chest is rarely used now that CT is widely available. However, in certain selected cases, conventional tomography may remain helpful. The axial cross-sectional orientation of CT may limit evaluation of lesions near the apex of the lung or near the diaphragm. Although MRI is useful in such cases, conventional tomography may be cheaper and more easily available for a given case. Moreover, confirmation of central calcification within a small pulmonary nodule may be more cheaply and easily accomplished with conventional tomography than with CT. Use of conventional tomography in the oblique position (approximately 55 degrees contralateral posterior oblique) is more accurate than standard chest radiography for evaluation of hilar masses and adenopathy, but the skill required for this technique has withered in most clinical departments with the availability of CT and MRI.

In recent years, there have been promising developments in the field of digital radiography applied to chest radiographs. These developments have used new techniques for acquiring direct digital recording of the radiographic beam that traverses the thorax, rather than recording this radiation on film. Such systems may use either conventional fixed x-ray tubes or moving slot-scan technology tubes to radiograph the chest, and either special storage phosphor cassettes or photomultiplier tubes to transfer the digital data directly to an electronic imaging system that permits viewing and recording from high-resolution television screens. These digital radiographic systems allow manipulation of image region, density, contrast, and other parameters much like CT or other computerized graphic systems. Although this technology remains investigational, it appears to be at least as accurate as standard radiography for the detection of lung nodules and mediastinal abnormalities.[12, 13] Moreover, it offers promising potential for more sensitive recognition of abnormalities owing to its ability to enhance contrast of equivocal lesions and to improve visualization in anatomic regions that may be overexposed or underexposed by conventional techniques.

Computed Tomography

CT has become widely accepted as the primary cross-sectional modality for evaluation of the thorax. It is critical to remember, however, that a histologic diagnosis is usually required to confirm an abnormal radiographic finding in the potentially curable patient. Therefore, CT is best used as a complement to other diagnostic and staging techniques such as bronchoscopy, mediastinoscopy, thoracoscopy, and percutaneous needle biopsy.

The standard chest CT examination consists of multiple contiguous 8- to 10-mm thick axial images obtained from the level of the lung apices to below the level of the adrenal glands. Some institutions routinely use 5-mm thick scans through the level of the hila and central bronchi, and others image the entire liver in the examination.

CT depicts more pulmonary nodules of a smaller size at an earlier time than conventional tomography or standard radiographs.[14–16] Intravenous contrast material is usually administered to more clearly delineate the vascular structures of the hila and mediastinum. Thinner, 5-mm thick, sections are useful for detection of calcium or fat within lesions, which usually suggest granuloma or hamartoma. Thin sections are also more sensitive in detecting pulmonary nodules smaller than 5 mm in diameter. Despite its high sensitivity, false-negative lung CT examinations may occur owing to technical difficulties, such as partial volume averaging, respiratory motion artifacts, and variations in the degree of respiration between sections.[17, 18]

Recent advances in CT technology have created the ability to perform helical, or spiral, volumetric CT during a single breath-hold.[18] This technique obviates problems such as respiratory motion artifacts, volume averaging, and respiratory variations. Moreover, volumetric acquisition allows subsequent reconstruction at thin slice equivalents, improving spatial resolution and detection of small nodules,[19, 20] when compared with conventional CT. This advance in CT technology offers improved detection capabilities in all anatomic areas of the body.

Magnetic Resonance Imaging

CT is the primary cross-sectional imaging modality in the thorax because of its superiority in spatial resolution compared with MRI. This superiority in spatial resolution permits better visualization of lung parenchyma and bronchial structures than MRI. Other advantages of CT over MRI are its lower cost, greater availability, and ability to detect calcification.

Both CT and MRI are tomographic techniques that allow separation of superimposed structures on chest radiographs. Both techniques are excellent for imaging the vascular structures of the mediastinum and hila, as well as for differentiating between benign

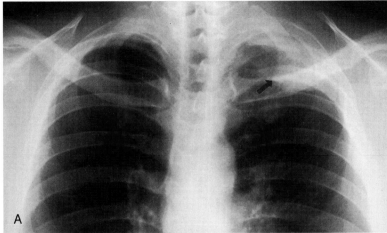

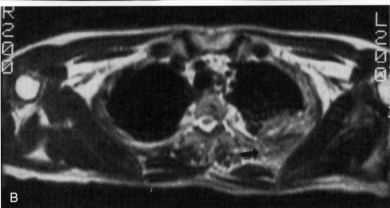

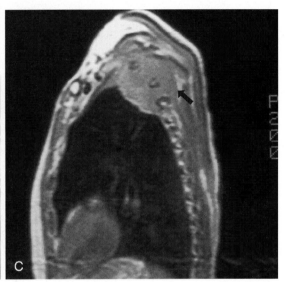

FIGURE 5–3. MRI evaluation of superior sulcus neoplasm. *A,* The chest film shows a superior sulcus mass *(arrow)* and apical pleural thickening. No rib destruction or extrapleural mass is seen. *B,* The axial MRI demonstrates the tumor mass extending into the posterior chest wall *(arrow). C,* The sagittal MRI shows extension of tumor into the posterior chest wall *(arrow)* and encasement of the ribs.

causes of mediastinal enlargement, such as vascular ectasia and lipomatosis.

MRI offers at least two advantages over CT: (1) the ability to image in planes other than axial, and (2) improved contrast resolution. Anatomic areas with a more vertical orientation, such as the lung apices, thoracocervical junction, aortopulmonic window, subcarinal region, and peridiaphragmatic areas, are often better imaged with MRI in coronal or sagittal planes than with axial CT. Therefore, MRI is useful for evaluating patients with Pancoast's tumors (Fig. 5–3) or mediastinal neoplasms and equivocal CT studies. The improved contrast resolution with MRI permits better detection of chest wall invasion, bone invasion, and direct mediastinal invasion than does CT (Fig. 5–4).

MRI relies on the ability of hydrogen protons to emit a radio wave after being exposed to a radiofrequency pulse while aligned within a magnetic field. The radio wave emitted is characteristic for the tissue in which the proton resides, and it can be precisely located anatomically using three-dimensional magnetic field gradients. The image created is usually identified according to parameters called relaxation times, so-called T1- or T2-weighted images. Specific tissues, such as fat, muscle, tumors, vessels, and fibrosis have characteristic appearances on T1- or T2-weighted images.

There is no standard MRI examination. The technique that is used for MRI varies, because the examination is most often used to evaluate a very specific and limited clinical-radiologic question. Typically, images are performed using 5- to 10-mm thick slices in axial and coronal planes, with both T1- and T2-weighted images obtained. The examination may be tailored to the specific need with thinner sections or with nonorthogonal imaging planes. Intravenous contrast material is rarely required, because vascular enhancement and magnetic resonance angiography (MRA) can be performed with technical manipulations to accentuate or minimize the signal from flowing blood.

CLINICAL USES OF DIAGNOSTIC IMAGING

Screening

The use of chest radiography to screen high-risk patients for lung cancer was evaluated in three large-scale, randomized controlled trials sponsored by the National Cancer Institute and conducted at Johns Hopkins Medical Institute, Memorial Sloan-Kettering Cancer Center, and Mayo Clinic.[21, 22] The participants,

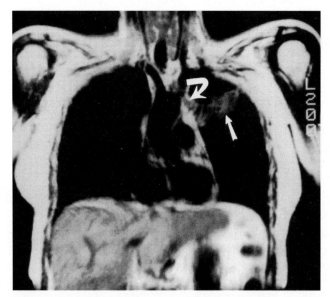

FIGURE 5–4. Direct mediastinal invasion by lung cancer, demonstrated by MRI. The coronal MRI demonstrates the primary tumor mass *(arrow)* and direct extension into the mediastinal fat *(curved arrow).*

middle-aged and older men who were chronic heavy cigarette smokers, were screened with chest radiography and sputum cytology every 4 months. The screening trial detected more cancers, more resectable cancers, and more early stage cancers than those detected in controls; the 5-year survival rate was higher for the screened group than the control group. However, the mortality rates in the screened and control groups were virtually the same. Because no benefit was demonstrated in the mortality rate, the results did not justify recommending large-scale radiologic or cytologic screening for lung cancer.[21]

However, recent reinterpretation of the Mayo Lung Project has renewed interest in the potential for lung cancer screening.[23, 24] Compared with controls, in the screened group of men, more lung cancers were detected, more cancers were resectable, and survival rate was greater; however, there were more lung cancer deaths in the screened group, so that mortality rates were not significantly different between groups. Previous analyses had suggested that overdiagnosis had accounted for the increased number of lung cancers detected in the screened group. The more recent alternative hypothesis is that chance alone might have accounted for the observed difference. If this were the case, additional cancers would have been detected in the control group had this chance event not occurred. Under this assumption, the mortality benefit of screening would approach statistical significance.[23] A simulation study[24] estimates that the benefit could be as high as 13%; the Mayo trial as conducted could not detect a benefit of less than 20%. For these reasons, these reanalyses have concluded that there is insufficient evidence to recommend *against* lung cancer screening. At present, another clinical trial of lung cancer screening with chest radiography is being conducted within the Prostate-Lung-Colon-Ovary Screening trials by the National Cancer Institute.

It remains problematic if and when the individual physician and asymptomatic high-risk patient should use chest radiography. Primary prevention, through cessation of smoking, remains the key to the control of lung cancer; high-risk patients and their physicians should decide when chest radiography is appropriate for individual cancer checkups.

Detection: The Pulmonary Mass or Nodule

The discovery of a pulmonary mass or nodule on the chest radiograph represents the best opportunity for early diagnosis of lung cancer at a curable stage. Calcifications are typically a sign of benign lesions, but they may be seen in malignant tumors. Calcification in malignant tumors may occur owing to tumor production, dystrophic calcification in tumor necrosis, or engulfment of pre-existing benign calcifications by tumor (Fig. 5–5). Characteristic benign calcifications are described as diffuse punctate, central dense, popcorn, or laminar (bull's-eye) types within the nodule. Stability of the mass size on sequential chest radiographs for at least 2 years is necessary to ensure benignity without biopsy. All solitary pulmonary nodules without such characteristic calcifications or demonstrated stability in size require a tissue diagnosis. As many as 40% of indeterminate nodules prove to be malignant at biopsy.[25]

Although there is controversy about the use of CT in T1N0M0 lesions, CT is probably indicated in each case of a newly discovered pulmonary nodule. CT is superior to chest radiography in defining the morphology of the lesion and is more sensitive in detecting calcifications. Additionally, it may detect the presence of mediastinal disease or other unsuspected pulmonary nodules in up to 30% of cases.[26] When additional nodules are detected, over 80% represent metastatic disease.[27] On occasion, CT helps identify the segmental location of a nodule prior to bronchoscopy or surgery.

In 1980, Siegelman and colleagues described the use of CT to identify benign pulmonary nodules.[28] These authors stated that if the CT numbers of the nodule exceeded 164 Hounsfield units (HU), the lesion contained calcification and was benign. They suggested that nonsurgical follow-up of such lesions could be performed, obviating surgical resection. However, other authors were unable to confirm these findings, because of differences in types of equipment, section thickness, and other technical variations among different brands of scanners. A subsequent multi-institutional trial modified the initial results and used a standardized reference phantom to confirm nodule density.[29] Although the technique can be useful in certain instances, few centers are using this technique at present, with its costly reference phantom, the variability demonstrated with various brands of equipment, and the need to standardize and calibrate each new CT machine acquired.

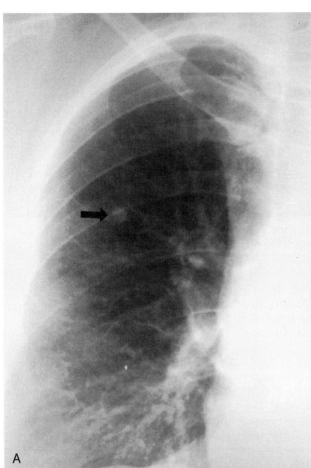

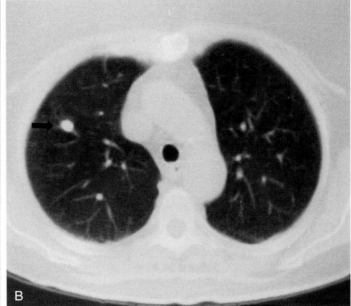

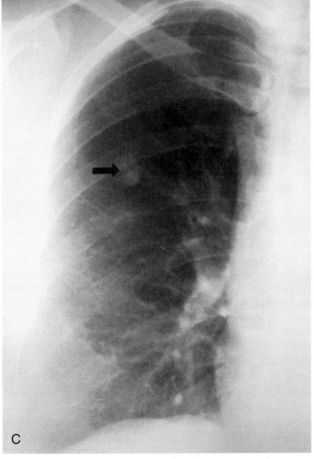

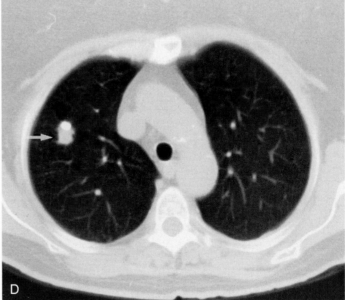

FIGURE 5–5. Incorporation of benign granulomatous calcification within lung malignancy. *A,* Baseline chest radiograph shows a typically benign nodule in the right lung with dense central calcification *(arrow).* *B,* CT confirms a densely calcified benign granuloma *(arrow)* with no soft-tissue component. *C,* Three years later, a new pulmonary nodule *(arrow)* is seen adjacent to the calcification on the chest film. *D,* CT now confirms the new neoplastic growth *(arrow)* that has engulfed the previous calcification.

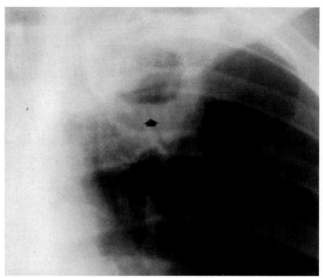

FIGURE 5–6. Cavitation in a primary squamous cell carcinoma of the lung. The tumor is seen as a thick-walled mass with central cavitation *(arrow)*.

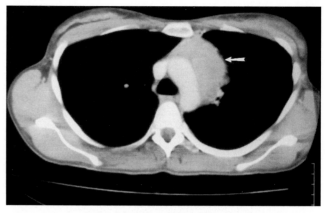

FIGURE 5–7. Small cell carcinoma presenting as a central mediastinal mass. The CT shows an abnormal mass *(arrow)* adjacent to the aortic arch. No peripheral lesion could be identified.

Radiographic Characteristics of Specific Lung Cancer Cell Types

Squamous cell carcinomas represent about one-third of all lung cancers.[10] They usually originate in the epithelium of the larger central bronchi and tend to invade locally. Therefore, these tumors are often occult until they generate obstructive pulmonary collapse. The degree of collapse is usually segmental, but it may be lobar or involve the entire hemithorax. When collapse occurs, it often obscures the radiographic visualization of the obstructing mass. Squamous cell carcinomas are more prone to central necrosis than other lung cancers; cavitation of a pulmonary nodule may be evident on plain films or CT (Fig. 5–6). Superior sulcus tumors, so-called Pancoast's tu-

mors, are usually squamous cell carcinomas (see Fig. 5–3). Peripherally located tumors account for about one-third of all squamous cell carcinomas.

Small cell carcinomas represent about one-fourth of all lung cancers.[10] Most occur centrally in the submucosa of the larger bronchi and spread rapidly to blood vessels and regional lymph nodes. The typical presentation is that of a large central mass or bulky adenopathy, often without a peripheral lesion (Fig. 5–7). The primary lesion does not tend to obstruct bronchi, but bulky metastatic adenopathy may cause extrinsic compression of major airways. Small cell carcinoma is rarely a peripheral nodule and does not cavitate. Over 70% of patients with this tumor have disease outside the thorax at the time of diagnosis.

Adenocarcinoma accounts for one-fourth to one-third of primary lung cancers.[10] It occurs most often as a peripheral pulmonary nodule, unrelated to bronchi (Fig. 5–8). Adenocarcinoma is more aggressive than squamous cell carcinoma, more frequently involving regional lymph nodes, pleura, and the contra-

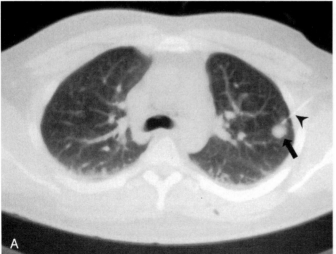

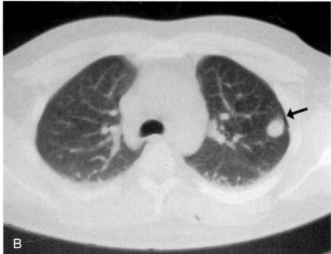

FIGURE 5–8. Adenocarcinoma of the lung presenting as a small peripheral pulmonary nodule. *A,* A 1.5-cm pulmonary nodule is seen in the peripheral left upper lobe *(arrow)*. Adenocarcinoma was confirmed by percutaneous fine-needle aspiration biopsy (FNAB) *(arrowhead)*. *B,* CT following biopsy shows a small pneumothorax *(arrow)* complicating the procedure.

lateral lung at presentation. Because of this biologic aggressiveness, adenocarcinoma often presents with mediastinal enlargement on the chest radiograph, the peripheral lesion being relatively small and over-looked. On the other hand, the peripheral lesions of adenocarcinomas tend to be larger than other cancers when discovered on chest radiographs.

The bronchoalveolar subtype of adenocarcinoma accounts for less than 15% of all lung cancers.[10] It appears as a diffuse multinodular type of lesion and tends to grow along alveolar walls in a low-grade fashion. Its radiographic manifestations are varied: a solitary nodule, multiple nodules of differing sizes, air-space consolidation (Fig. 5–9), or interstitial infil-trate. The lesions may be small, large, solitary, multi-ple, unilateral, or bilateral.

Large cell, undifferentiated, carcinoma represents about one-fifth of all lung cancers,[10] and occurs as a peripheral lesion twice as often as a central lesion (Fig. 5–10). These tumors tend to be large, bulky masses with occasional cavitation, often associated with me-diastinal adenopathy at presentation.

Diagnosis: Percutaneous Needle Biopsy

Percutaneous fine-needle aspiration biopsy (FNAB) of the lung and mediastinum has been used for decades and is now widely accepted as an excellent method for obtaining pathologic tissue diagnoses. This tech-nique has gained acceptance in the last 10 to 15 years in this country owing to more widespread acceptance of cytologic diagnosis, and improved radiologic im-aging with fluoroscopy and CT to guide needle place-ment.[30]

FNAB was developed in the 1960s, when Dahlgren and Nordenstrom introduced thin-walled 18-gauge or 20-gauge needles, biplane fluoroscopic guidance, and improved cytologic diagnostic techniques.[31] The FNAB technique offered fewer complications and equivalent diagnostic capability when compared with percutaneous lung biopsy using larger cutting needles. Multiple types of FNAB needles are commer-cially available, differing in gauge thickness, tip shape, and cutting ability of the tip edge. It probably does not matter what type of needle is used for FNAB; the choice of needle is dictated by the personal pref-erences of the radiologist and pathologist. All avail-able needles are efficacious, provided the procedure is performed properly and the cytologic material is prepared and examined properly.[30]

FNAB may be performed using guidance of any imaging modality. Fluoroscopy has been used most often for guidance, but as more and smaller lesions are detected only by CT, CT has become a more fre-quent guidance modality for FNAB (see Figs. 5–8 and 5–10).[32] Occasionally, sonography may be useful for FNAB of peripheral or pleural lesions.[33] In each in-stance, the imaging modality is used to identify and localize the lesion, as well as to document placement of the needle tip within the lesion prior to aspiration.

FNAB is indicated for tissue diagnosis of any lesion suspected of neoplasm, either primary or metastatic. However, FNAB should not be used for endobron-chial lesions associated with collapse, atelectasis, or consolidation when the mass itself is not clearly de-marcated. In such instances, false-negative results are likely due to aspiration of obstructed lung tissue; bronchoscopy is more accurate in evaluating such le-

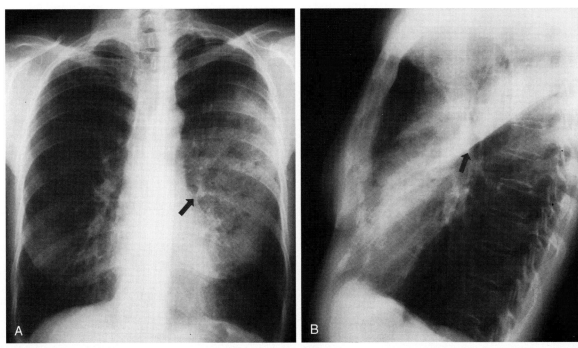

FIGURE 5–9. Bronchoalveolar cell carcinoma presenting as an alveolar infiltrate. *A,* The PA chest film shows diffuse air-space (alveolar) infiltrate in the left upper lobe *(arrow). B,* The lateral chest film shows the tumor/consolidation to be delimited posteriorly by the major fissure *(arrow).*

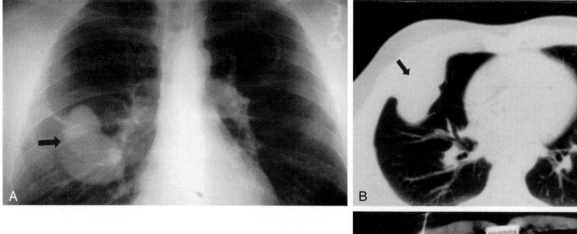

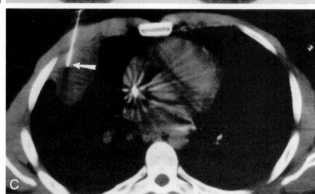

FIGURE 5–10. Large cell carcinoma. *A*, The PA chest radiograph shows a large, bulky mass in the right lower lobe *(arrow)*. *B*, CT confirms the large lesion *(arrow)*, located anteriorly adjacent to the pleura. *C*, Percutaneous FNAB *(arrow)* confirmed the diagnosis of large cell carcinoma.

sions. Central or mediastinal lesions that are clearly imaged, however, are candidates for biopsy, especially using CT guidance (Fig. 5–11).

One controversial indication for FNAB is the solitary pulmonary nodule with no contraindication to surgery. One may argue that all such lesions require excision, unless a specific benign diagnosis is obtained by FNAB. Because a nonspecific negative FNAB result is more common and is a potential false-negative result, many physicians would recommend excision of any nodule that is not clearly benign. Such a recommendation makes FNAB unnecessary in the evalua-

tion of solitary pulmonary nodules. On the other hand, some surgeons prefer to have a cytologic diagnosis prior to thoracotomy in order to discuss the diagnosis and treatment plans with the patient, as well as to obviate frozen section diagnosis at the time of surgery. Moreover, certain diagnoses arrived at by FNAB (e.g., small cell carcinoma) may preclude immediate thoracotomy in favor of nonsurgical therapy. The use of FNAB for the diagnosis of the solitary pulmonary nodule remains a common problem, which is often resolved by local practice and judgment.

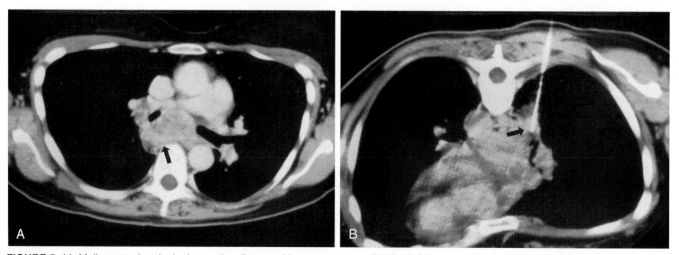

FIGURE 5–11. Malignant subcarinal adenopathy, diagnosed by percutaneous FNAB. *A*, CT shows subcarinal adenopathy *(arrow)*. *B*, FNAB performed with the patient prone from the right posterior percutaneous approach *(arrow)* confirmed neoplastic adenopathy.

FNAB is performed with local anesthesia, usually without intravenous sedation or premedication. The procedure may be performed on an inpatient or outpatient basis.[34] Potential complications are few. Pneumothorax following FNAB is the most common complication, occurring in 20% to 35% of patients (see Fig. 5–8). Following biopsy, chest radiographs are obtained immediately and at delayed intervals of 4 and 24 hours. A small proportion of pneumothoraces are detected only on delayed radiographs, but clinically significant pneumothoraces requiring intervention rarely occur after 4 hours.[30] Less than half of the pneumothoraces induced by FNAB require tube decompression; those that do require drainage may be managed with small, percutaneously placed catheters. Hemoptysis may occur infrequently and is usually self-limited; more severe complications are very rare.

The sensitivity of FNAB in diagnosing malignancy varies from 64% to 97%.[30] Most contemporary large series report sensitivities of at least 85%. The accuracy in diagnosis of squamous cell carcinoma is greater than that of other lung neoplasms. Differentiation of adenocarcinoma, bronchoalveolar carcinoma, and large cell carcinoma can be difficult.[30]

An increasing use of thoracoscopy has spawned a new CT-guided needle procedure: needle localization of a pulmonary nodule prior to thoracoscopy.[35] A small peripheral pulmonary nodule may be visualized only by CT and be too small a target for percutaneous needle biopsy. Thoracoscopic resection of such nodules has a lower rate of morbidity and postoperative rehabilitation than does open thoracotomy; however, the nodule is not easily identified for resection at thoracotomy. Recently, the technique of preoperative needle localization of nonpalpable breast lesions has been modified to address this thoracoscopic problem. Prior to thoracoscopy, a thin wire localization device may be placed percutaneously through a needle under CT guidance, using techniques similar to those used with FNAB. The surgeon then uses the localization wire to direct the thoracoscopic resection of lung parenchyma, removing the nodule adjacent to the localization wire.

Staging

There are two major issues in the use of diagnostic imaging for staging lung cancer patients: (1) the appropriate goal of any imaging strategy, and (2) which imaging modality(ies) to use to achieve that goal. The primary goal of the preoperative staging process is the identification of nonresectable patients, thereby avoiding unnecessary surgery. However, this goal is valid only for non–small cell carcinomas. Small cell carcinoma not only produces bulky mediastinal disease in the majority of patients but has a predilection for early and widespread metastases. Moreover, because chemotherapy is usually the primary therapy, the question of surgical resectability in small cell carcinoma is usually moot. The prognosis in small cell carcinoma is better in those patients with disease limited to the thorax, and treatment may differ if disease

is identified outside the chest. Imaging examinations for staging patients with small cell carcinoma then may include CT of the chest, liver, and adrenal glands, as well as CT or MRI of the brain and a radioisotope bone scan.

Non–small cell lung cancer is treated with surgery whenever possible. To identify unresectability, patients should undergo CT of the chest including the liver and adrenal glands. Findings of particular concern are enlarged mediastinal lymph nodes, chest wall invasion, rib destruction, pleural or parenchymal masses, and liver or adrenal masses. Preoperative imaging of the brain in asymptomatic patients with non–small cell lung cancer is probably not indicated,[26] although some authors cite a 5% to 10% incidence of brain metastases in patients with asymptomatic adenocarcinoma[36] and recommend CT or MRI of the brain in this tissue diagnosis. Preoperative bone scans in asymptomatic patients are similarly not routinely indicated.

Primary Tumor (T) Staging in the TNM System

Anatomic Location and Size

Up to 15% of newly diagnosed lung cancers may be occult, i.e., TX.[37] For the TX stage tumors detected by sputum cytology, bronchoscopy is the procedure of choice if the plain radiograph is negative. However, in certain instances, CT may be useful when bronchoscopic findings are negative. Occult carcinoma may be identified with CT using thin section scanning, and they are usually seen as a focal peribronchial thickening.[38]

Most solitary pulmonary nodules are T1 or T2 lesions. Unfortunately, no imaging modality adequately distinguishes tumor from postobstructive or consolidated lung. With contrast-enhanced CT, atelectatic lung may enhance more than its obstructing tumor; with T2-weighted MRI, consolidation may demonstrate brighter signal than the central mass.[39–41] However, neither CT nor MRI has been shown to improve the T-staging accuracy of lesions obscured on the plain radiograph by collapse or consolidation.

CT is more accurate than chest radiography for identifying the lobar position of a pulmonary nodule; tumor invasion through the pleural fissures is well visualized.[4] Moreover, additional or unsuspected lesions are better detected by CT.

Chest Wall Invasion

Invasion of the chest wall or mediastinum elevates the primary tumor stage to T3 or T4. Neither CT nor MRI accurately predicts chest wall invasion unless there is bone destruction or penetration of the chest wall.[4, 5] For example, CT is less accurate than the clinical finding of focal chest pain for the detection of chest wall invasion.[4] In the patient with a superior sulcus tumor, a combination of CT and MRI allows definition of bone destruction and soft tissue invasion (see Fig. 5–3). The direct coronal and sagittal images obtained by

MRI provide better evaluation of structures adjacent to the superior sulcus, such as the brachial plexus, vertebral bodies, and neural foramina.

Mediastinal Invasion

Gross mediastinal invasion by lung cancer elevates the primary tumor stage to T4. Gross invasion is evident on CT, but contiguity of the tumor with the mediastinum cannot be easily differentiated from subtle invasion. Fortunately, minimal invasion does not always preclude resection. The CT findings of mediastinal invasion are protrusion of tumor into the mediastinal fat or encasement of mediastinal structures by tumor mass. Most studies have found that CT and MRI are essentially equal for the detection of mediastinal invasion (see Fig. 5–4).[42] However, a recent prospective multi-institutional trial showed a significantly better accuracy for MRI than CT in the detection of mediastinal invasion by lung cancer.[43]

Superior vena cava invasion by tumor can be identified by either MRI or CT (Fig. 5–12). CT evaluation of vascular invasion requires intravenous injection of contrast material, whereas the MRI examination needs no contrast media. MRI is more accurate than CT for detecting tumor invasion of the heart or pericardium.[4] Tumor invasion of the pericardium (T3 stage) is recognized by tumor disruption of the normal low-signal pericardial stripe. Cardiac involvement (T4 stage) may be recognized by tumor infiltration of the cardiac muscle on T2-weighted images or by tumor growth into the cardiac chambers, which are normally very low signal on T1-weighted images.

Central Airway Invasion

The proximal extent of central airway invasion determines the resectability of lung cancer. T3 tumors, those that extend to within 2 cm of the carina without involvement of the carina, are usually resectable, whereas T4 lesions, those tumors that invade the carina or trachea, are not. CT is better than MRI for detection of central airway invasion because of its superior spatial resolution (Fig. 5–13).[4] However, CT is relatively insensitive in detecting airway invasion, and it has not been useful for predicting the need for pneumonectomy versus lobectomy.[44]

Pleural Effusion

A malignant pleural effusion connotes unresectability (T4 disease), whereas a benign pleural effusion does not affect staging or prognosis. Most effusions may be detected with plain chest radiographs, in the standard upright position, or in the decubitus (affected side down) position, which allows fluid to layer in the dependent lateral pleural space. The minimum effusion detectable by chest radiography is estimated to be about 200 ml, about 10 times the normal amount present.[45] CT, MRI, and sonography are all more sensitive than standard radiography for detection of pleural fluid. No imaging modality can distinguish benign from malignant pleural fluid. However, effusions are very likely to be malignant if they are associated with pleural masses that may be seen with any of the cross-sectional imaging modalities.[4, 45] Most patients require aspiration of fluid for cytologic diagnosis; sonography is particularly useful to guide aspiration of small effusions or loculated fluid collections, or it may be used in patients in whom unguided aspiration has failed. Sonography or CT may be used to guide biopsy of pleural soft tissue masses.[45]

Nodal Staging (N) in the TNM System

Cross-sectional imaging has improved the evaluation of nodal involvement by lung cancer compared with plain chest radiographs. Most studies have concentrated on detection of N2 and N3 disease, with fewer reports evaluating ipsilateral hilar node involvement (N1). Neoplastic involvement of lymph nodes has important staging implications. The presence of ipsilateral hilar adenopathy elevates a T1 or T2 lung cancer to Stage II; involvement of subcarinal or ipsilateral mediastinal nodes denotes a Stage III tumor. Stage IIIB disease, involvement of contralateral lymph nodes, is generally accepted as unresectable for surgical cure, although Stage IIIA disease may be unresectable as well.

Hilar Adenopathy

Plain chest films retain an important role in the evaluation of hilar adenopathy. A hilar mass is usually first suspected or diagnosed on standard radiographs. Lymphadenopathy is suggested when the hilar contour is enlarged with lobular margins; smooth margins are more likely to result from pulmonary artery enlargement. Unfortunately unilateral hilar enlargement is often overlooked because of the wide variation in the normal symmetry of the hila. However, when hilar enlargement is recognized, it has a high predictive value; abnormal chest radiographs correctly predicted hilar pathology in over 75% of patients with malignant lymphadenopathy.[46, 47]

CT has effectively replaced conventional tomography for evaluation of the pulmonary hila.[46, 47] CT aids in identifying individual nodes accurately, whereas conventional tomography interpretation relies on indirect signs of hilar contour abnormalities. Therefore, CT is more sensitive and more specific than conventional tomography for detection of enlarged hilar nodes.[46, 47] CT is also preferred because it simultaneously identifies mediastinal adenopathy and other significant extrahilar lesions, which may occur in up to 20% of patients with suspected hilar abnormalities.[46]

The pulmonary hila are best evaluated by CT, enhanced with a bolus of intravenous contrast material. With the dynamic, rapid imaging techniques of modern CT equipment and the use of mechanical injectors to deliver the contrast medium, excellent vascular enhancement can be obtained in virtually all patients. The CT criteria for the diagnosis of hilar malignancy

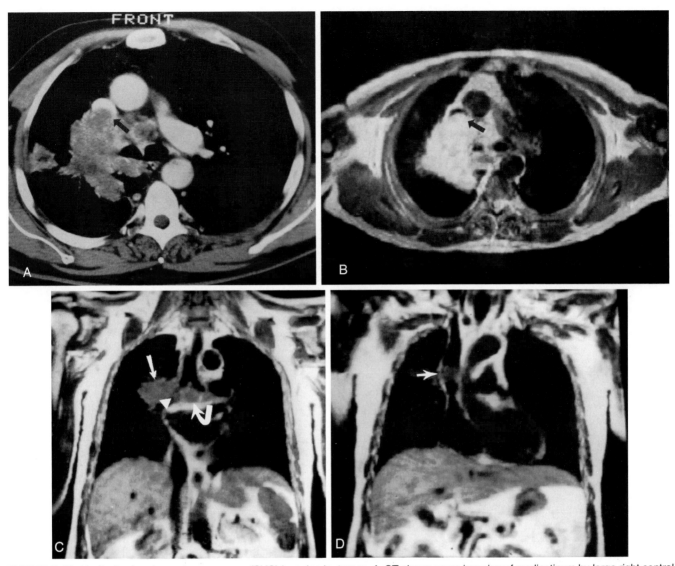

FIGURE 5–12. Mediastinal and superior vena cava (SVC) invasion by tumor. *A,* CT shows gross invasion of mediastinum by large right central neoplasm, with invasion of the posterior wall of the SVC *(arrow). B,* Axial MRI at the same level as *A* shows similar findings, with invasion of the SVC *(arrow). C,* Coronal MRI at the level of the carina, shows the large central mass *(arrow).* Encasement of the right main-stem bronchus *(arrowhead)* and subcarinal adenopathy *(curved arrow). D,* Coronal MRI at the level of the SVC shows tumor invasion of the mediastinum and SVC *(arrow).*

are (1) an avascular mass in the hilum; (2) hilar adenopathy larger than 1 cm in diameter; (3) thickened posterior wall of the bronchus intermedius, distal upper lobe bronchi, or both (Fig. 5–14); and (4) bronchial displacement, compression, or obstruction.[46–49]

These CT criteria have been extended to MRI of the hila; MRI is equivalent to CT for detection of abnormal hilar nodes.[50, 51] However, there are no MRI characteristics that offer advantages over CT; significant overlap of T1 and T2 values exists for benign and malignant conditions. As long as MRI detects only node enlargement, as does CT, it is not likely that MRI will offer any advantage over CT for evaluation of adenopathy.

The use of 1 cm as the upper limit of normal-sized nodes is controversial. Most lymph nodes smaller than 1 cm are normal, but normal-sized nodes may contain metastatic disease (false-negative examina-

tions) in at least 7% of patients.[52] Conversely, lymph node enlargement may be due to benign or malignant causes. Enlarged benign lymph nodes (false-positive examinations) occur in 20% to 30% of cases.[52] One should always remember that CT identifies abnormal anatomy, not histologic diagnoses; CT is best used to direct tissue biopsy confirmation of disease and to guide the choice of biopsy technique based on the anatomic nodal group involved.

Mediastinal Adenopathy

A recent survey[53] of thoracic surgeons regarding the preoperative assessment of lung cancer with CT revealed that 98% used CT preoperatively: 36% used it routinely, while 62% used it selectively. Uses included assessment of node size, feasibility of resection, and guidance of surgical node sampling. The survey dem-

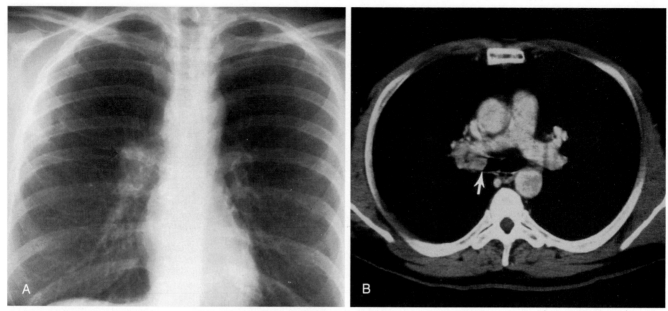

FIGURE 5–13. Central airway invasion by bronchogenic tumor, detected by CT. *A,* The chest radiograph shows a right hilar mass *(arrow). B,* The CT shows the central extent of neoplasm *(arrow)* to be 1.5 cm from the carina.

onstrated that the contribution of CT staging varied, depending on the usual practice or philosophy of surgeons and institutions.

The variability of use of CT in this survey is not surprising, given the wide range of results of CT studies reported in the literature. Aronchick[54] recently reviewed this "virtual sea of literature" and found the statistics of many studies to be contradictory and no uniformity among final conclusions of the authors. In a chronologic review of sensitivity rates for detection of mediastinal metastases, she found a trend in earlier studies to report high sensitivity rates; authors recommended CT to direct mediastinal biopsy and suggested that patients with negative CT studies could undergo thoracotomy directly without mediastinoscopy. In more recent studies, she found that, as investigators subjected patients to more extensive mediastinal exploration at surgery, more cases of metastases in normal-sized lymph nodes were found, thus decreasing the reported sensitivity rates in these studies. The sensitivity rates ranged from 24% to 94%. The discrepancies among studies were due mostly to two factors: (1) variances in the size criteria used to denote abnormal nodes, and (2) the variability of surgical and pathologic correlative proof.

The size criteria used for classifying mediastinal lymph nodes as abnormal vary from study to study.[54] Most authors agree that nodes smaller than 1 cm in diameter are normal, recognizing a small chance of metastases in these nodes. Most authors also agree that nodes larger than 1.5 cm are abnormal. The variability in reported data stems from the classification of equivocal nodes in the 11- to 15-mm range (Fig. 5–15). In patients who live in geographic regions where granulomatous disease is prevalent, or in patients who have migrated from such regions, enlarged nodes in the 11- to 15-mm range are more likely to be benign than those in patients who have not been exposed to endemic granulomatous disease.

The statistics for sensitivity and specificity rates are based on surgical and pathologic proof. However, most studies have not included complete mediastinal exploration at each surgical procedure and cannot confirm that a specific node identified by CT has been evaluated surgically and pathologically. If a prospective thorough mediastinal exploration is not performed in every patient in the study, normal-sized nodes containing microscopic metastatic disease could be overlooked at surgery, cloaking false-negative nodes and artificially elevating the sensitivity rates. The few studies that have performed more extensive nodal sampling have reported lower sensitivity rates for detection of metastatic adenopathy.[54]

Another area of controversy is the use of CT in the evaluation of the T1N0M0 lesion, the pulmonary nodule smaller than 3 cm in diameter.[52, 54] Some authors suggest that the incidence of mediastinal node metastases is so low (<5% to 10%) that patients with such lesions should not be evaluated with CT or invasive staging procedures but should undergo thoracotomy directly. Others argue that CT staging is cost effective and that it plays a role in directing biopsy and in confirming that a lesion is indeed solitary.[50] At our institution, we tend to follow the philosophy of the group that advocates the use of CT.

Despite all this controversy and debate, it seems reasonable to state several basic tenets. First, CT is useful in identifying macroscopic mediastinal nodal enlargement; such enlarged nodes should be confirmed as metastases with appropriate invasive staging procedures. Second, if the mediastinal CT is normal, it may be adequate to proceed directly to thoracotomy, if a thorough mediastinal nodal exploration is performed to accurately stage the patient.

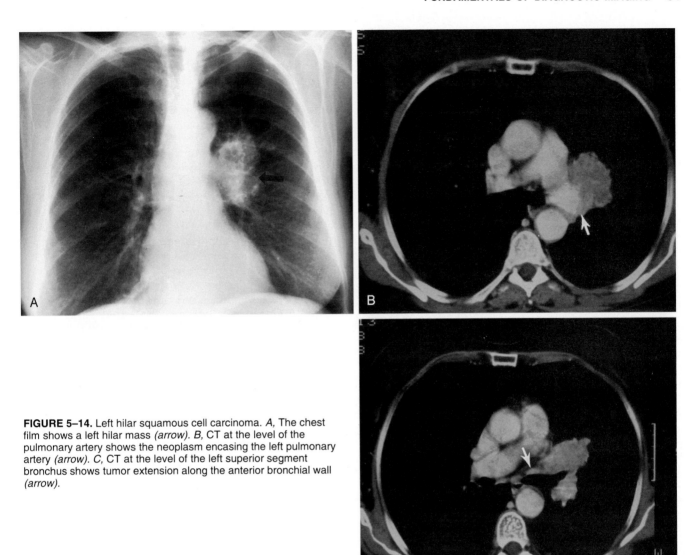

FIGURE 5–14. Left hilar squamous cell carcinoma. *A,* The chest film shows a left hilar mass *(arrow). B,* CT at the level of the pulmonary artery shows the neoplasm encasing the left pulmonary artery *(arrow). C,* CT at the level of the left superior segment bronchus shows tumor extension along the anterior bronchial wall *(arrow).*

Moreover, recent studies have suggested that patients with only microscopic mediastinal metastases discovered at surgery may have improved survival rates if the primary tumor and all metastases are resected.[54] Third, if extensive mediastinal exploration is not anticipated, invasive staging procedures, such as mediastinoscopy, should be employed following a normal mediastinal CT examination. At many institutions, the mediastinoscopy can be performed along with a planned definitive thoracotomy (the thoracotomy to follow only if the mediastinoscopy confirms no metastatic disease), combining these procedures with only one anesthetic event.

Distant Metastasis Staging (M) in the TNM System

Extrathoracic metastasis denotes Stage IV disease and implies surgical unresectability. The common sites of hematogenous metastases from primary lung cancer include lung, brain, skeleton, liver, and adrenal glands. The standard staging CT of the thorax should routinely include complete visualization of the adrenal glands and the superior portion of the liver. Some institutions choose to include the entire liver in the examination. Adrenal imaging is important, because up to 10% of patients who undergo staging CT will have an adrenal mass identified[4] and, at autopsy, up to one-fourth of cancer patients will have an adrenal metastasis.[55] However, it has been noted that benign adrenal adenomas of at least 1 cm in size can be found in about 1% of the adult population.[55] Therefore, the overall high prevalence of benign adrenal adenomas in the general population ensures that, even in patients with malignancy, most adrenal masses are benign. To avoid withholding surgery from otherwise operable patients, histologic confirmation of metastasis is required before classifying a patient as unresectable.

Several studies have demonstrated that benign adrenal adenomas may have a characteristic appearance on T2-weighted MRI, implying that MRI may be use-

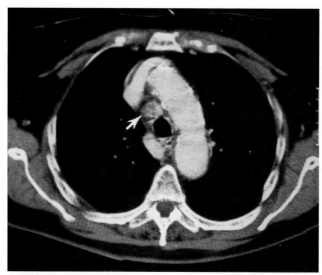

FIGURE 5–15. Enlarged benign mediastinal lymph node. CT at the level of the aortic arch shows a pretracheal node measuring 15 mm in diameter *(arrow)*. This node was enlarged owing to healed granulomatous disease.

ful in the diagnosis of adrenal lesions.[56, 57] However, with additional clinical experience, it became apparent that it was difficult to characterize a specific lesion.[58–60] MRI cannot differentiate benign from malignant adrenal masses. MRI may be able to identify benign adrenal adenomas if they meet specific MRI criteria: (1) on multiecho, T2-weighted images, the adrenal lesion remains isointense compared with the liver (the ratio of T2 values of adrenal mass-to-liver is 1.0 ± 0.2); (2) at 1.5 Tesla, the T2 value of the adrenal mass is < 60 msec[61]; and (3) the adrenal mass contains lipid on chemical-shift MRI.[62] Approximately 70% to 80% of benign adrenal adenomas fulfill the first two MRI criteria for adenoma; lesions that do not fulfill the criteria may be benign or malignant masses, cysts, hemorrhage, inflammatory masses, or primary or secondary tumors. The third criterion (i.e., demonstration of lipid with an adrenal mass) may be the most accurate sign of benignity[55, 62] and increases the specificity of the examination when combined with the first two criteria. However, there are no criteria to diagnose malignant adrenal masses. Therefore, MRI is useful only if it demonstrates benign criteria for the mass. If the mass does not fulfill benign criteria, it still requires histologic confirmation of malignancy to accurately stage lung cancer.

The precise role of MRI in the evaluation of the lung cancer patient with a newly discovered adrenal mass is undefined at present. The error rate of characterization of masses as benign by MRI is not known, and few clinicians are comfortable classifying an otherwise resectable patient as one who has Stage IV disease without pathologic confirmation of metastasis. In patients with known lung cancer who have a higher a priori probability of adrenal metastasis, it may be more efficient, specific, and cost effective to perform percutaneous FNAB of the adrenal mass directly without prior MRI. MRI is more useful for the evalu-

ation of the adrenal mass discovered incidentally in the patient without known malignancy, in whom the a priori probability of adrenal malignancy is small.

Most studies have demonstrated that the routine use of bone, brain, and liver imaging in all patients with lung cancer is unnecessary and potentially misleading.[63, 64] However, the staging of small cell lung cancer dictates detection of extrathoracic disease, because spread may occur early in this aggressive tumor, and primary therapy includes systemic chemotherapy. The most efficacious imaging protocol for small cell carcinoma has not been described, and the use of imaging strategies varies with different clinicians. However, typical regimens incorporate CT of the liver, radioisotope bone scan, and CT or MRI of the brain. Preoperative imaging of the brain in asymptomatic patients with non–small cell lung cancer is probably not indicated,[26] although some authors cite a 5% to 10% incidence of brain metastases in patients with asymptomatic adenocarcinoma[36] and recommend CT or MRI of the brain in this tissue diagnosis.

SELECTED REFERENCES

Bragg DG: The applications of imaging in lung cancer. Cancer 67(suppl):1165–1168, 1991.

Webb WR, Gatsonis C, Zerhouni EA, et al: CT and MR imaging in staging non–small cell bronchogenic carcinoma: Report of the Radiology Diagnostic Oncology Group. Radiology 178:705–713, 1991.

Woodring JH (ed): Lung cancer. Radiol Clin North Am 28(3):489–664, 1990.

White CS, Templeton PA, Belani CP: Imaging in lung cancer. Semin Oncol 20:142–152, 1993.

REFERENCES

1. Boring CC, Squires TS, Tong T: Cancer statistics, 1993. CA 43:1, 1993.
2. Horm JWW, Lessler LG: Falling rates of lung cancer in men in the United States. Lancet i:425–428, 1986.
3. Aronchik JM: Lung cancer: Epidemiology and risk factors. Semin Roentgenol 25:73–80, 1990.
4. White CS, Templeton PA, Belani CP: Imaging in lung cancer. Semin Oncol 20:142–152, 1993.
5. Bragg DG: The applications of imaging in lung cancer. Cancer 67(suppl):1165–1168, 1991.
6. Bragg DG: Imaging in primary lung cancer: The role for detection, staging, and follow-up. Semin Ultrasound CT MR 10:453–466, 1989.
7. Bragg DG: Advances in tumor imaging (review). Hosp Pract (Off) 19:83–92, 95–98, 1984.
8. Muhm JR, Miller WE, Fontana RS, et al: Lung cancer detected during a screening program using four-month chest radiographs. Radiology 148:609–615, 1983.
9. Theros EG: 1976 Caldwell Lecture: varying manifestations of peripheral pulmonary neoplasms: A radiologic-pathologic correlative study. Am J Roentgenol 128:893–914, 1977.
10. Sorenson JA, Mitchell CR, Armstrong JD, et al: Effects of improved contrast on lung nodule detection: A clinical ROC study. Invest Radiol 122:772–780, 1987.
11. Austin JHM, Tomney BM, Soldsmith LS: Missed bronchogenic carcinoma: Radiographic findings in 27 patients with a potentially resectable lesion evident in retrospect. Radiology 182:115–122, 1992.
12. Schaefer CM, Greene R, Oestmann JW, et al: Digital storage

phosphor imaging versus conventional film radiography in CT-documented chest disease. Radiology 174:207–210, 1990.

13. Schaefer CM, Greene R, Hall DA, et al: Mediastinal abnormalities: Detection with storage phosphor digital radiography. Radiology 178:169–173, 1991.

14. Peuchot M, Libshitz H: Pulmonary metastatic disease: Radiologic-surgical correlation. Radiology 164:719–722, 1987.

15. Muhm JR, Brown LR, Crowe JK: Detection of pulmonary nodules by computed tomography. AJR Am J Roentgenol 128:267–270, 1977.

16. Gross BH, Glazer GM, Bookstein FL: Multiple pulmonary nodules detected by computed tomography: Diagnostic implications. J Comput Assist Tomogr 9:880–885, 1985.

17. Krudy AG, Doppman JL, Herdt JR: Failure to detect a 1.5 centimeter lung nodule by chest computed tomography. J Comput Assist Tomogr 6:1178–1180, 1982.

18. Remy-Jardin M, Remy J, Giraud F, Marquette C-H: Pulmonary nodules: Detection with thick-section spiral CT versus conventional CT. Radiology 187:513–518, 1993.

19. Bock P, Soucek M, Daepp M, Kalender WA: Lung: Spiral volumetric CT with single breath-hold technique. Radiology 176:864–867, 1990.

20. Costello P, Anderson W, Blume D: Pulmonary nodule: Evaluation with spiral volumetric CT. Radiology 179:875–876, 1991.

21. Fontana RS, Sanderson DR, Woolner LB, et al: Screening for lung cancer: A critique of the Mayo Lung Project. Cancer 67(suppl):1155–1164, 1991.

22. National Cancer Institute Cooperative Early Lung Cancer Detection Program: Summary and conclusions. Am Rev Respir Dis 130:565–567, 1984.

23. Strauss GM, Gleason RE, Sugarbaker DJ: Screening for lung cancer re-examined: A reinterpretation of the Mayo Lung Project randomized trial on lung cancer screening. Chest 103:337s–341s, 1993.

24. Flehinger BJ, Kimmel M, Polyak T, Melamed MR: Screening for lung cancer: The Mayo Lung Project revisited. Cancer 72:1573–1580, 1993.

25. Trunk K, Gracey DR, Byrd RB: The management and evaluation of the solitary pulmonary nodule. Chest 66:236–239, 1974.

26. Berman CG, Clark RA: Diagnostic imaging in cancer. Prim Care 19:677–713, 1992.

27. Peuchol M, Libshitz HI: Pulmonary metastatic disease: Radiologic-surgical correlation. Radiology 164:719–722, 1987.

28. Siegelman SS, Zerhouni EA, Leo FP, et al: CT of the solitary pulmonary nodule. AJR Am J Roentgenol 135:1–13, 1980.

29. Zerhouni EA, Stitik FP, Siegelman SS, et al: CT of the pulmonary nodule: A cooperative study. Radiology 160:319–327, 1986.

30. Weisbrod GL: Transthoracic percutaneous lung biopsy. Radiol Clin North Am 28:647–655, 1990.

31. Dahlgren SE, Nordenstrom B: Transthoracic Needle Biopsy. Chicago, Year Book Medical Publishers, 1966, pp 1–132.

32. vanSonnenberg E, Casola G, Ho M, et al: Difficult thoracic lesions: CT-guided biopsy experience in 150 cases. Radiology 167:457–461, 1988.

33. Yang PC, Luh KT, Sheu JC, et al: Peripheral pulmonary lesions: Ultrasonography and ultrasonically guided aspiration biopsy. Radiology 155:451–456, 1985.

34. Stevens GM, Jackman RJ: Outpatient needle biopsy of the lung: Its safety and utility. Radiology 151:301–304, 1984.

35. Plunkett MB, Peterson MS, Landrenneau RJ, et al: Peripheral pulmonary nodules: Preoperative percutaneous needle localization with CT guidance. Radiology 185:274–275, 1992.

36. Mintz BJ, Tuhrim S, Alexander S, et al: Intracranial metastases in the initial staging of bronchogenic carcinoma. Chest 86:850–853, 1984.

37. Melamed MR, Flehinger BJ, Zaman MD, et al: Detection of true pathologic stage I lung cancer in a screening program and the effect on survival. Cancer 47:1182–1187, 1981.

38. Webb WR, Gamsu G, Speakman JM: Computed tomography of the pulmonary hilum in patients with bronchogenic carcinoma. J Comput Assist Tomogr 7:219–225, 1983.

39. Tobler J, Levitt RG, Glazer HS, et al: Differentiation of proximal bronchogenic carcinoma from postobstructive lobar collapse by magnetic resonance imaging: Comparison with computed tomography. Invest Radiol 22:538–543, 1987.

40. Herold CJ, Kuhlman JE, Zerhouni EA: Pulmonary atelectasis: Signal patterns with MR imaging. Radiology 178:715–718, 1991.

41. Mayr B, Heywang SH, Ingrisch H, et al: Comparison of CT with MR imaging of endobronchial tumors. J Comput Assist Tomogr 11:43–48, 1987.

42. Martini N, Heelen R, Westcott J, et al: Comparative merits of conventional, computed tomographic and magnetic resonance imaging in assessing mediastinal involvement in surgically confirmed lung carcinoma. J Thorac Cardiovasc Surg 90:639–648, 1985.

43. Webb WR, Gatsonis C, Zerhouni EA, et al: CT and MR imaging in staging non–small cell bronchogenic carcinoma: Report of the Radiology Diagnostic Oncology Group. Radiology 178:705–713, 1991.

44. Quint LE, Glazer GM, Orringer MB: Central lung masses: Prediction with CT of the need for pneumonectomy versus lobectomy. Radiology 165:735–738, 1987.

45. Miles DW, Knight RK: Diagnosis and management of malignant pleural effusions. Cancer Treat Rev 19:151–168, 1993.

46. Glazer GM, Francis IR, Shirazi KK, et al: Evaluation of the pulmonary hilum: Comparison of conventional radiography, 55 degree posterior oblique tomography, and dynamic computed tomography. J Comput Assist Tomogr 7:983–989, 1983.

47. Osborne DR, Korobkin M, Ravin CE, et al: Comparison of plain radiography, conventional tomography, and computed tomography in detecting intrathoracic lymph node metastases from lung carcinoma. Radiology 142:156–161, 1982.

48. Webb WR, Glazer GM, Gamsu G: Computed tomography of the normal pulmonary hilum. J Comput Assist Tomogr 5:467–484, 1981.

49. Webb WR, Gamsu G, Glazer GM: Computed tomography of the abnormal pulmonary hilum. J Comput Assist Tomogr 5:485–490, 1981.

50. Glazer GM, Gross BM, Asien AM, et al: Imaging of the pulmonary hilum: A prospective comparative study in patients with lung cancer. AJR Am J Roentgenol 145:245–248, 1985.

51. Levitt RG, Glazer HS, Roper CL, et al: Magnetic resonance imaging of mediastinal and hilar masses: Comparison with CT. AJR Am J Roentgenol 145:9–14, 1985.

52. Templeton PA, Caskey CI, Zerhouni EA: Current uses of CT and MR imaging in the staging of lung cancer. Radiol Clin North Am 28:631–646, 1990.

53. Epstein DM, Stephenson LW, Gefter WB, et al: Value of CT in the perioperative assessment of lung cancer: A survey of thoracic surgeons. Radiology 161:423–427, 1986.

54. Aronchick JM: CT of mediastinal lymph nodes in patients with non–small cell lung carcinoma. Radiol Clin North Am 28:573–581, 1990.

55. Reinig JW: MR imaging differentiation of adrenal masses: Has the time finally come? Radiology 185:339–340, 1992.

56. Reinig JW, Doppman JL, Dwyer AJ, et al: Distinction between adrenal adenomas and adrenal metastases using MR imaging. J Comput Assist Tomogr 9:898–901, 1985.

57. Francis IR, Gross MD, Shapiro B, et al: Integrated imaging of adrenal disease. Radiology 184:1–9, 1992.

58. Chuang A, Glazer HS, Lee JKT, et al: Adrenal gland: MR imaging. Radiology 163:123–128, 1987.

59. Chezmar JL, Robbins SM, Nelson RC, et al: Adrenal masses: characterization with T2-weighted MR imaging. Radiology 166:357–359, 1988.

60. Reinig JW, Doppman JL, Dwyer AJ, et al: MRI of indeterminate adrenal masses. AJR Am J Roentgenol 147:493–496, 1986.

61. Baker ME, Blinder R, Spritzer C, et al: MR evaluation of adrenal masses at 1.5 T. AJR Am J Roentgenol 153:307–312, 1989.

62. Mitchell DG, Crovello M, Matteucci T, et al: Benign adrenocortical masses: Diagnosis with chemical shift MR imaging. Radiology 185:345–351, 1992.

63. Turner P, Haggith JW: Preoperative radionuclide scanning in bronchogenic carcinoma. Br J Dis Chest 75:291–294, 1981.

64. Hooper RG, Beechler CR, Johnson MC: Radioisotope scanning in the initial staging of bronchogenic carcinoma. Am Rev Respir Dis 118:279–286, 1978.

6 STAGING OF LUNG CANCER

Jonathan C. Nesbitt and Darroch W. O. Moores

Staging is the determination of the extent of disease in an individual with the intent of grouping patients with similar levels of disease for analytic, therapeutic, and prognostic purposes. The staging of lung cancer provides a scale of relative disease that can be assigned to all patients with primary lung malignancies. Accurate staging of lung cancer is essential for defining operability, selecting treatment regimens, predicting survival, and reporting comparable end results. Several different staging systems for lung cancer have been developed since the 1950s, and each one is subtly different from the others. The evolution of staging systems has paralleled technologic advances in the documentation and measurement of both the extent of disease and its impact on survival. The commonly used systems have been merged, establishing a single system that is now universally accepted. The focus of this chapter is to explain the development of this universal system (called the International Staging System), describe the specifics of the system, and discuss some of the staging problems and controversies that remain.

HISTORY OF STAGING

Each staging system used in the diagnosis of lung cancer has been based primarily on anatomic criteria. The TNM system developed by Pierre Denoix in 1946 for staging of malignant tumors has remained the fundamental scheme for the classification of primary lung carcinoma.[1] The letters T, N, and M are individual descriptors of the tumor, the regional lymph nodes, and the distant metastases, respectively. Numbers are paired with each letter to denote the magnitude of pathologic involvement. The TNM designation always refers to the greatest anatomic extent of disease. It has been the basis of the staging systems used by both the American Joint Committee for Cancer (AJCC) and the International Union Against Cancer (UICC), as well as of the International Staging System, which has replaced the two earlier systems.

American Joint Committee for Cancer Staging and End Results Reporting

The AJCC was first organized in 1959 to develop systems of staging cancer by primary sites of the disease that would be acceptable to the American medical profession.[2] Sponsoring organizations included the American College of Surgeons, American College of Radiology, American College of Pathologists, American College of Physicians, American Cancer Society, and National Cancer Institute. In 1973, an AJCC Task Force on Lung Cancer developed a lung cancer staging system based on the anatomic extent of disease and adapted from the TNM system of the UICC Committee on Clinical Stage Classification and Applied Statistics.[3] The data, collected from 2155 cases of lung cancer, included the size, location, and extent of each primary tumor; the presence of complications such as obstructive pneumonitis, atelectasis, and pleural effusion; the presence and extent of lymph node metastasis; and the presence of distant metastatic disease. Only information obtained before thoracotomy was used in developing the AJCC staging system. Data on each of the four major cell types of lung cancer were analyzed separately. Survival curves were based on the extent of the primary tumor, regional lymph node involvement, and the presence of distant metastases, as defined by the TNM descriptor system of the UICC. These curves were used to classify TNM groups with similar survival rates into three stages of disease (subsequently changed to four stages of disease in 1986).[4]

Realizing that the accuracy of staging relies on available clinical information, the AJCC developed a TNM staging system based on preoperative and subsequent evaluations at different times during the course of the disease: clinical-diagnostic staging (c), surgical-evaluative staging (s), postsurgical resection-pathologic staging (p), retreatment staging (r), and autopsy staging (a). One of these letters is sometimes used as a prefix to the TNM descriptors to identify the point during the course of the disease at which the stage was established (e.g., cTNM for clinical-diagnostic staging).

Clinical-diagnostic staging is based on the anatomic extent of disease, which can be determined by any diagnostic testing short of thoracotomy. Such an evaluation may include findings from the history, physical examination, routine and special roentgenograms, bronchoscopy, esophagoscopy, mediastinoscopy, mediastinotomy, thoracentesis, thoracoscopy, and any other examinations, including those used to demonstrate the presence of extrathoracic metastases. This may be the final staging of disease in patients who do not undergo a thoracotomy.

Surgical-evaluative staging, sTNM, is based on information obtained at the time of exploratory thoracotomy, including biopsy results but excluding information obtained from complete examination of a therapeutically resected specimen. With proper preoperative evaluation, few patients should undergo exploratory thoracotomy without resection and the number of patients for whom this is the final staging should be small (less than 5%).[5] Surgical-evaluative staging is rarely used now.

Postsurgical resection-pathologic staging, pTNM, is based on findings at thoracotomy and at pathologic examination of the resected specimen. To ensure accuracy, all other available data are considered as well. Retreatment staging, rTNM, refers to the restaging of a patient with progressive disease when the primary treatment has failed. Before further treatment is initiated, all available evidence is used to restage the patient. Autopsy staging, aTNM, uses data from the postmortem examination.

International Union Against Cancer

The UICC, an international nongovernmental organization composed of over 200 member organizations, has developed effective methods of cancer staging through its various committees. The UICC Committee on Tumor Nomenclature and Statistics adopted the general definitions of local extension of malignant tumors suggested by the World Health Organization (WHO) Subcommittee on the Registration of Cases of Cancer.[6] In 1953, this committee held a joint meeting with the International Commission on Stage Grouping in Cancer and Presentation of the Results of Treatment of Cancer appointed by the International Congress of Radiology. At this meeting, the TNM system, previously developed by Denoix, was adopted for all tumors.

In 1954, the Research Commission of the UICC organized the Committee on Clinical Stage Classification and Applied Statistics. This committee, known as the Committee on TNM Classification, published its first recommendation for the staging of lung cancer in 1966.[7] The T, N, and M definitions used in the UICC classification system are identical to those used by the AJCC.

In 1973, stage groupings based on TNM subsets were introduced by the AJCC and adopted by the UICC.[8] Subsequent revision of the groupings system has been based on pretreatment clinical data and postsurgical histologic findings.[4] Change has been necessary in recognition of the heterogeneity of the affected subgroups and the significant differences in their survival rates.

International Staging System

The AJCC and UICC systems served well for approximately 15 years and achieved wide popularity and usage. As time passed, significant differences in survival were noted among certain TNM subsets that had been grouped prospectively into the same clinical stage. To achieve uniformity in the descriptors of the TNM system and to heighten accuracy in predicting stage-specific survival, the AJCC and the UICC in 1985 developed a single system that has become the primary system used internationally today: the International Lung Cancer Staging System, or International Staging System. It was presented at the Fourth World Conference on Lung Cancer by Clifton F. Mountain, Chairman of the Task Force on Lung Cancer of the AJCC as a cooperative effort of the AJCC and the UICC.[4] Intended to unify the many systems used throughout the world and to correct some of the inherent deficiencies of these systems, the International Staging System was approved by the AJCC and the UICC and supported by the TNM Study Committees from Japan and Germany. The International Staging System has gained worldwide acceptance and remains the predominant system for the staging of lung cancer.

The TNM Classification (Table 6–1) and Stage Groupings (Table 6–2) outline the International Staging System. Each stage is illustrated in Figures 6–1 through 6–4.

TNM DESCRIPTORS

T Factor

The primary tumor descriptor, T, derives its classification based on size, location, and extent of local invasion. T0 indicates no evidence of a primary tumor and is used primarily during retreatment staging. TX describes tumors that are identified cytologically by malignant cells in sputum samples or bronchial washings, but no specific site of origin can be recognized radiographically or bronchoscopically. TX also is used to describe tumors that cannot be adequately assessed during retreatment staging.

Carcinoma in situ usually can be assessed bronchoscopically and represents the earliest stage of disease. Accordingly, those malignancies that are confined to the bronchial mucosa are labeled Tis. T1 tumors are invasive lesions 3.0 cm or less in greatest dimension, surrounded entirely by pulmonary parenchyma or intact visceral pleura, and without evidence of invasion proximal to or including a lobar bronchial orifice. Uncommonly, superficial tumors that are confined to the bronchial wall are classified as T1 tumors; the invasive component is limited to the bronchial submucosa. Such superficial tumors are defined histopathologically, not clinically, and may be located in the main bronchus, within 2 cm from the carina.

T2 tumors are more than 3.0 cm in greatest dimension, invade visceral pleura, or have associated atelectasis or pneumonitis extending to the hilum. Associated atelectasis must involve less than the entire lung. The proximal extent of the tumor may include the lobar bronchial orifice, bronchus intermedius, or main-stem bronchus but must be at least 2 cm distal to the carina.

Tumors that have grown beyond the confines of the pulmonary parenchyma are classified as T3 or T4 lesions. These tumors may be of any size. T3 tumors

TABLE 6–1. International Staging System TNM Classification

PRIMARY TUMOR (T)

T0	No evidence of primary tumor
TX	The tumor is identified cytologically by malignant cells in sputum samplings or bronchial washings. No specific site of origin can be recognized radiographically or bronchoscopically. Tumors that cannot be adequately assessed in retreatment staging are identified with this descriptor
Tis	Carcinoma in situ
T1	The tumor is an invasive lesion 3.0 cm or less in greatest dimension, surrounded by lung or intact visceral pleura and without evidence of invasion proximal to or including a lobar bronchial orifice*
T2	The tumor is more than 3.0 cm in greatest dimension, invades the visceral pleura, or has associated atelectasis or pneumonitis extending to the hilum. The proximal extent may include the lobar bronchial orifice, bronchus intermedius, or main-stem bronchus but must be at least 2 cm distal to the carina. Any associated atelectasis must involve less than an entire lung
T3	The tumor is any size and involves the parietal pleura, chest wall, diaphragm, mediastinal pleura, mediastinal fat, parietal pericardium, phrenic nerve, or vagus nerve; or a tumor in the main bronchus within 2 cm of the carina* without involving the carina; or a tumor-associated atelectasis or obstructive pneumonitis of the entire lung
T4	The tumor is any size and invades the structures of the deep mediastinum including heart, great vessels, trachea, esophagus, vertebral body, or carina; or a tumor associated with a pleural effusion containing malignant cells

NODAL INVOLVEMENT (N)

N0	No demonstrable metastasis to regional lymph nodes
N1	Metastases to lymph nodes in the peribronchial or the ipsilateral hilar region, including nodes affected by direct extension of the tumor
N2	Metastases to lymph nodes in the ipsilateral mediastinum or subcarina, including nodes affected by direct extension
N3	Metastases to lymph nodes in the contralateral mediastinum, contralateral hilum, ipsilateral or contralateral scalene or supraclavicular regions

DISTANT METASTASIS (M)

M0	No known distant metastasis
M1	Metastases to distant organs or other lymph node sites

*Note: The uncommon superficial tumor of any size with its invasive component limited to the bronchial wall, which may extend proximal to the main bronchus, is also classified T1.

TABLE 6–2. International Staging System Stage Grouping

Occult carcinoma:	
TX N0 M.	Bronchial secretions or bronchoalveolar lavage contain malignant cells, but there is no other evidence of a primary tumor, nodal disease, or metastatic spread
Stage 0:	
Tis N0 M0.	Carcinoma in situ
Stage I:	
T1 N0 M0.	Tumors designated as T1 or T2 without evidence
T2 N0 M0.	of nodal or metastatic disease
Stage II:	
T1 N1 M0.	Tumors designated as T1 or T2 with evidence of
T2 N1 M0.	ipsilateral nodal spread to peribronchial, lobar or hilar nodes without metastatic disease
Stage IIIA:	
T1-3 N2 M0.	Tumors with T3 status without or with nodal
T3 N0 M0.	disease involving hilar or ipsilateral mediastinal
T3 N1 M0.	nodes. This category includes ipsilateral mediastinal nodal disease with a primary tumor of T1-T3 status
Stage IIIB:	
T4 N0-3 M0.	Tumors with T4 status with or without nodal
AnyT N3 M0.	disease involving hilar or contralateral mediastinal nodes. This category includes contralateral nodes with a primary tumor of any T status
Stage IV:	
AnyT, Any N, M1:	All combinations of T and N status with metastatic disease

N Factor

Regional lymph node involvement is classified using the descriptor, N. When no demonstrable metastases exist in regional lymph nodes, the N0 descriptor is given. Metastatic disease to hilar lymph nodes is classified as N1 disease, whereas metastases to ipsilateral mediastinal lymph nodes or subcarinal lymph nodes are classified as N2 disease. The specific locations of hilar and mediastinal lymph nodes are important to staging and are discussed later. Metastatic disease located in lymph nodes in the contralateral mediastinum, contralateral hilum, ipsilateral scalene region, ipsilateral supraclavicular region, contralateral scalene region, or contralateral supraclavicular region is classified as N3 disease.

M Factor

Metastases to distant organs or to other lymph node sites beyond the N3 locations are identified by the M1 descriptor. Within this grouping are several issues regarding intrathoracic metastases that also are designated as M1. These topics are addressed later.

STAGE GROUPINGS AND SURVIVAL BY STAGE

Figures 6–5 through 6–11 illustrate cumulative 5-year survival curves based on clinical and surgical stage and nodal involvement.

involve structures that are amenable to resection and include the parietal pleura, chest wall, diaphragm, mediastinal pleura, mediastinal fat, pericardium, phrenic nerve, and sympathetic chain. The T3 descriptor also describes invasive tumors that reside within 2 cm of the carina without involving the carina. Atelectasis of the entire lung is considered to be consistent with T3 status. T4 tumors invade the structures of the deep mediastinum, including the heart, great vessels, trachea, esophagus, vertebral body, and carina, or are associated with a pleural effusion containing malignant cells. The implication of a pleural effusion in conjunction with lung cancer is addressed later in the chapter.

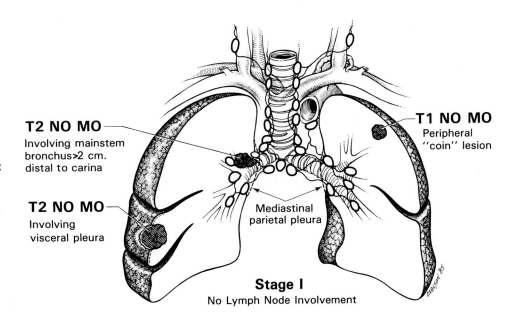

T2 NO MO

Involving mainstem bronchus>2 cm. distal to carina

T2 NO MO

Involving visceral pleura

T1 NO MO

Peripheral "coin" lesion

Mediastinal parietal pleura

Stage I

No Lymph Node Involvement

FIGURE 6–1. New International Staging System Stage I. (From Mountain CF: A new international staging system for lung cancer. Chest 89[Suppl]:225S–233S, 1986, with permission.)

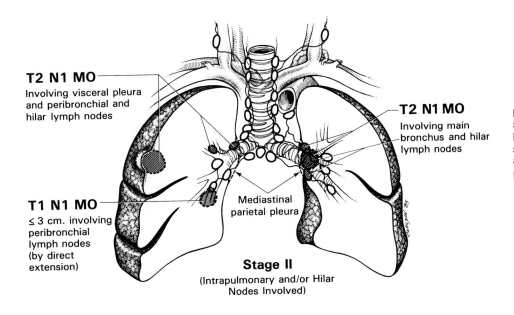

T2 N1 MO

Involving visceral pleura and peribronchial and hilar lymph nodes

T2 N1 MO

Involving main bronchus and hilar lymph nodes

T1 N1 MO

≤ 3 cm. involving peribronchial lymph nodes (by direct extension)

Mediastinal parietal pleura

Stage II

(Intrapulmonary and/or Hilar Nodes Involved)

FIGURE 6–2. New International Staging System Stage II. (From Mountain CF: A new international staging system for lung cancer. Chest 89[Suppl]:225S–233S, 1986, with permission.)

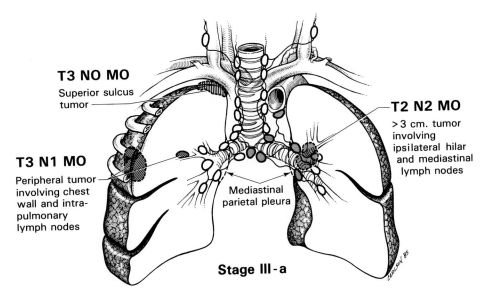

T3 NO MO

Superior sulcus tumor

T2 N2 MO

> 3 cm. tumor involving ipsilateral hilar and mediastinal lymph nodes

T3 N1 MO

Peripheral tumor involving chest wall and intra-pulmonary lymph nodes

Mediastinal parietal pleura

Stage III-a

FIGURE 6–3. New International Staging System Stage IIIA. (From Mountain CF: A new international staging system for lung cancer. Chest 89[Suppl]:225S–233S, 1986, with permission.)

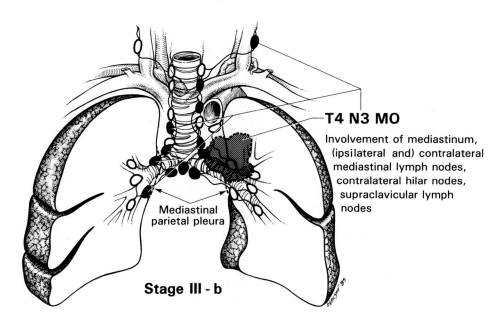

T4 N3 MO

Involvement of mediastinum, (ipsilateral and) contralateral mediastinal lymph nodes, contralateral hilar nodes, supraclavicular lymph nodes

Mediastinal parietal pleura

Stage III - b

FIGURE 6–4. New International Staging System Stage IIIB. (From Mountain CF: A new international staging system for lung cancer. Chest 89[Suppl]:225S–233S, 1986, with permission.)

Patients with Stage I disease (T1 N0, T2 N0) have survival rates approaching 60% to 70% at 5 years.[4, 9–12] Within the group several factors appear to influence survival: T status, size independent of T status, and histology. The more favorable tumors are T1 squamous cell and T1 localized bronchoalveolar cell carcinomas.

Stage II disease (T1 N1, T2 N1) indicates metastatic disease in hilar nodes or other intrapulmonary nodes and predicts an overall 5-year survival rate of 39% to 43%.[13, 14] Several studies have evaluated this group of patients to identify tumor characteristics that have an impact on survival. The Lung Cancer Study Group reported significant survival differences between patients with squamous carcinoma and adenocarcinoma and between patients with T1 and T2 lesions.[10, 15] More specifically, patients with T1 squamous carcinoma had a 5-year survival rate of 75% in comparison to those with T2 adenocarcinoma, who had a 5-year survival

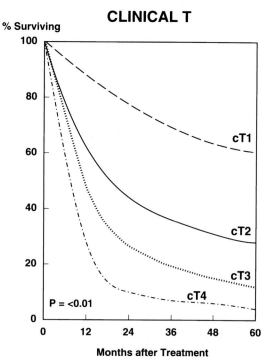

FIGURE 6–5. Cumulative survival according to clinical estimates of the extent of the primary tumor, the cT classification (non–small cell lung cancer, M0 disease). (From Mountain CF: Lung cancer staging classification. Clin Chest Med 14:43, 1993, with permission.)

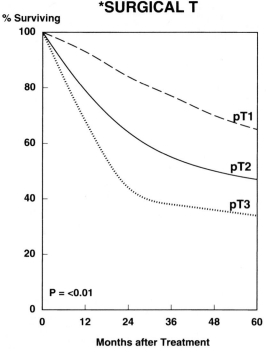

FIGURE 6–6. Cumulative survival according to the extent of the primary tumor. Determined from pathologic examination of resected specimens, the pT classification (non–small cell lung cancer, M0 disease). (From Mountain CF: Lung cancer staging classification. Clin Chest Med 14:43, 1993, with permission.)

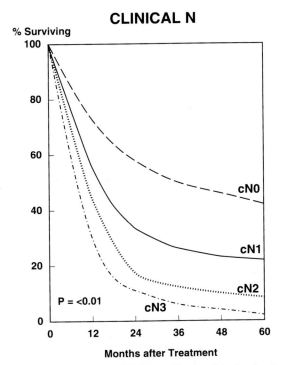

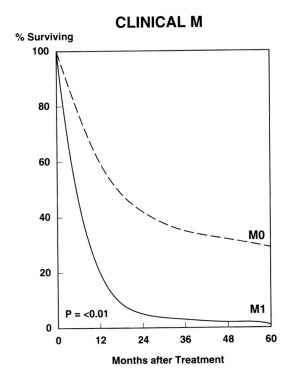

FIGURE 6–7. Cumulative survival according to clinical estimates of the extent of regional lymph node involvement, the cN classification. (From Mountain CF: Lung cancer staging classification. Clin Chest Med 14:43, 1993, with permission.)

FIGURE 6–9. Cumulative survival according to clinical estimates of the absence or presence of distant metastasis, the cM classification. (From Mountain CF: Lung cancer staging classification. Clin Chest Med 14:43, 1993, with permission.)

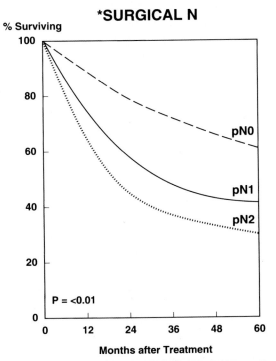

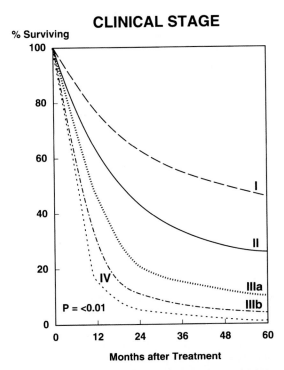

FIGURE 6–8. Cumulative survival according to the extent of regional lymph node involvement. Determined from pathologic examination of resected specimens, the pN classification. (From Mountain CF: Lung cancer staging classification. Clin Chest Med 14:43, 1993, with permission.)

FIGURE 6–10. Cumulative survival according to clinical stage of disease. (From Mountain CF: Lung cancer staging classification. Clin Chest Med 14:43, 1993, with permission.)

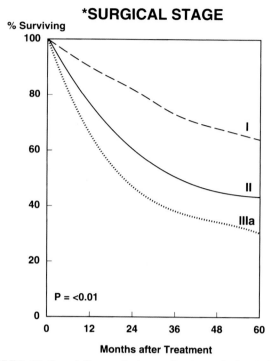

*SURGICAL STAGE

P = <0.01

Months after Treatment

FIGURE 6–11. Cumulative survival according to surgical-pathologic stage of disease. This evaluation of disease extent is based on pathologic examination of resected specimens. (From Mountain CF: Lung cancer staging classification. Clin Chest Med 14:43, 1993, with permission.)

rate of 25%. The Ludwig Lung Cancer Study Group studied 253 patients with Stage II disease and also noted better survival for patients with T1 lesions than for those with T2 lesions.[16] A review from Memorial Sloan-Kettering of 214 patients found no differences in survival based on histology or T status.[13] However, tumor size and number of involved N1 nodes were identified as prognostic factors. Naruke and associates also found no difference in survival by histology in 221 patients with Stage II disease; but the 5-year survival rate was significantly different at 52% for T1 lesions and 38% for T2 lesions.[14] Mountain reported similar 5-year survival rate in 317 patients: 54% for T1 lesions and 40% for T2 lesions.[4]

Approximately 25% to 40% of patients with non–small cell lung cancer have Stage III disease.[17, 18] Of these patients, approximately one-third will present with potentially resectable disease, Stage IIIA, (T1-3 N2, T3 N0, T3 N1). The median survival for all patients with Stage IIIA (clinical or surgical stage) disease is 12 months and the 5-year survival rate is 9% to 15%.[4, 19] Within the Stage IIIA subset, however, survival rates vary widely:

- Patients with T3 N0 tumors, based on chest wall invasion only, have a favorable 5-year survival rate that can approach 50% to 60%, whereas those with T3 N2 disease have a 5-year survival rate ranging from 16% to less than 5%.[20, 21]
- Patients with clinical (preoperative) N0 or N1 disease but pathologic (postresection) N2 disease survive longer than patients with clinical N2 disease.

Martini and Flehinger noted 3- and 5-year survival rates of 47% and 34% for such patients.[22] Pearson and colleagues noted that patients with negative mediastinoscopic findings who were found to have N2 disease following resection had a 24% 5-year survival rate; the 5-year survival rate was only 9% for those who underwent resection after positive mediastinoscopy.[23]

- Patients with completely resected N2 disease have a median 5-year survival rate approaching 22%.[22, 24–27]
- Patients with tumors of the left upper lobe and nodal metastases to the superior mediastinum or subaortic region survive comparatively longer than patients with other combinations of N2 disease.[22, 28–30]
- Patients with a single level of nodal involvement survive longer than those with multiple levels.[28, 31, 32]

The median survival for Stage IIIB patients is 8 months, and the 5-year survival rate is 5% or less.[4, 19] There is, however, one subset of patients that can be considered for surgical resection: the group with Stage IIIB disease based on a T4 tumor involving the carina. With increased but acceptable operative morbidity and mortality rates, resection and reconstruction techniques can be undertaken.[33–36] Three-year survival is directly related to nodal status, and the survival rate ranges from 0% to 43%.[36, 37] Mathisen has reported an overall 5-year survival of 19%.[33] This topic is discussed later.

Approximately 25% to 30% of all patients who present with non–small cell lung carcinoma have Stage IV disease (Any T Any N M1). These patients, who have M1 (metastatic) disease, usually are treated with systemic therapy or palliative radiotherapy; their 5-year survival rate is generally less than 5%.[38] There is one subset of patients that can be considered for surgical intervention; those with resectable lung carcinoma and a resectable solitary brain metastasis. In this select group, surgery seems to prolong life and improve quality of life better than nonsurgical treatment.[39] The 5-year survival rate has been shown to range from 13% to 21%, and the reported median survival is 14 months.[39–41]

METHODS OF STAGING

As with any medical evaluation, a thorough history and physical examination is essential. Because 70% of patients with lung cancer present with advanced disease, clues to clinical stage often are evident on examination. Signs, symptoms, and physical findings may suggest a preliminary stage assessment and should direct appropriate testing. Accurate clinical staging includes a combination of noninvasive and invasive procedures.

Noninvasive Studies

Radiography

At the time of presentation, clinical T1 tumors may have a 22% prevalence of mediastinal lymph node metastases.[42] Thirty-two per cent of patients with a centrally located lesion and a normal mediastinum by a standard chest radiograph have mediastinal metastases whereas fewer than 15% of patients with peripheral T1 tumors and a normal mediastinum have mediastinal metastases.[43]

Computed tomography (CT) is the most effective noninvasive technique for evaluating primary lung carcinomas and mediastinal lymph nodes. Unfortunately, the accuracy of CT scanning in identifying metastatic disease in mediastinal lymph nodes is highly variable, with sensitivity ranging from 51% to 95%.[24, 30, 44–67] This variation in accuracy is secondary to variations in criteria of nodal abnormality that are based on the size and shape of the node, CT scanner differences, and nonuniformity in nodal mapping. A lymph node size of 1 cm or greater in transverse diameter has been used as the criterion of abnormal nodal enlargement. Approximately 8% to 15% of patients considered to have a negative CT scan for mediastinal nodal enlargement ultimately are found to have mediastinal nodal involvement at the time of operation.[44–46, 48–54, 56, 60]

The negative predictive accuracy of CT (the probability of negative disease given a negative test) is 85% to 92% for mediastinal lymph node metastases.[52, 60, 68] Therefore patients with no evidence of mediastinal lymph node enlargement by CT usually do not need to undergo invasive staging prior to thoracotomy. Patients who have nodal enlargement of greater than 1 cm should be considered to have potential N2 disease. Further invasive investigation, such as mediastinoscopy, is warranted to obtain a histologic diagnosis, because approximately one-third of these patients prove not to have metastatic involvement of the mediastinal nodes.[22, 62]

Magnetic Resonance Imaging

Magnetic resonance imaging (MRI) is not used for the routine evaluation of patients with lung cancer (see Chapter 5).

Gallium Scintigraphy

Gallium scanning is a simple and inexpensive test. Its role in the evaluation of patients with lung carcinoma has met with mixed reviews. If a chest CT has been performed, gallium scanning provides very little additional information. Gallium scanning is clearly inferior to CT for the identification of brain metastases and is less sensitive than bone scans in detecting osseous metastases[69]; therefore, it has few indications for use in evaluating patients with lung carcinoma.

Invasive Studies

Invasive procedures that directly assess the extent of disease include bronchoscopy, transbronchial or transthoracic fine-needle aspiration biopsy, scalene node biopsy, mediastinoscopy, anterior mediastinotomy, and thoracoscopy. Patients who present with clinical or radiographic evidence of extensive disease usually require the least invasive procedure to establish inoperability. Cytologic or histologic confirmation through fine-needle aspiration biopsy usually is sufficient to confirm suspicion of N3 or M1 disease. Other patients with less extensive disease often present with subtle radiographic findings that require more invasive techniques for adequate staging, particularly when mediastinal lymph node involvement is suspected.

Bronchoscopy

Bronchoscopy remains the most important procedure for determining the endobronchial extent of disease. T status can be defined by measuring tumor proximity to the carina and various bronchi and by identifying unsuspected occult lesions that indicate multiplicity of disease. Bronchoscopy also provides access for transtracheal or transbronchial biopsy of parenchymal masses or mediastinal adenopathy.

Mediastinoscopy

In 1954, Harken and colleagues introduced the use of the Jackson laryngoscope to explore the mediastinum through a supraclavicular incision.[70] They promoted the concept of inoperability of lung tumors with associated mediastinal involvement. For similar purposes, cervical mediastinoscopy was developed by Carlens in 1959, and it remains the most accurate method for evaluating middle mediastinal, peritracheal, and subcarinal lymph nodes.[71]

Mediastinoscopy is useful in determining which patients with positive mediastinal nodes will benefit from resection. This is illustrated by the work of Pearson and colleagues based on a series of patients who underwent resection after a positive mediastinoscopy.[23] Resection was restricted to patients with non–small cell carcinoma who had ipsilateral superior mediastinal node involvement in whom a completely or potentially curative resection was thought to be possible. Of 79 patients with positive mediastinoscopy who were selected for thoracotomy, 51 underwent potentially curative resections. The overall 5-year survival rate was 9%, and it was 15% for those patients who underwent complete resection. It should be emphasized that these patients represented a select subset of those who had a positive mediastinoscopy. Of 62 patients with negative mediastinoscopies in whom N2 metastases were found at thoracotomy, the overall 5-year survival was 24% following resection; it was 41% in those patients who underwent complete resection.

Several large series have noted morbidity rates for mediastinoscopy ranging from 0.9% to 3.39% and mortality rates ranging from 0% to 0.08%.[72–76] The accuracy of cervical mediastinoscopy has ranged from 80%[77, 78] to 90%.[79] The level most commonly missed is the subcarinal region. The subaortic and aortopulmonary window regions are inaccessible by standard cervical mediastinoscopy and add to the overall inaccuracy of the procedure.

Extended cervical mediastinoscopy, a variation of standard mediastinoscopy, has been useful for staging lesions in the left upper lobe. The standard mediastinoscopy incision is used with the plane of dissection extending anterior to the innominate artery and aorta anterolaterally to the level of the aortopulmonary window. Direct tumor invasion into the mediastinum or nodal disease within the prevascular space and aortopulmonary window can be assessed with this technique. Accuracy rates are higher than 91%.[80, 81]

Mediastinotomy

Anterior mediastinotomy, originally described by McNeil and Chamberlain,[82] permits direct visual access of the anterior mediastinum through the second, third, or fourth anterior interspace with or without removal of a short portion of the adjacent cartilage. For right-sided lesions, the procedure provides access to the proximal pulmonary artery and superior vena cava. The procedure is used on the left to evaluate disease in the subaortic and lateral aortic regions.

Scalene and Supraclavicular Lymph Node Biopsy

Scalene node biopsy was one of the first invasive techniques used to determine nodal involvement in patients with lung cancer. The procedure is now reserved for patients with potentially resectable N2 disease to rule out scalene or supraclavicular N3 disease, which precludes resection. Anywhere from 3.5% to 22% of nonpalpable ipsilateral scalene and supraclavicular lymph node biopsies are positive[83–86]; the incidence of positives is highest in patients with nonsquamous tumors[84] and centrally located tumors.[83, 84, 86]

Thoracoscopy

Thoracoscopy has been a valuable tool since it was first described by the Swedish internist Jacobaeus in 1910.[87] Although the technique initially was limited primarily to lysing of adhesions to create a pneumothorax for the treatment of tuberculosis, thoracic surgeons retained the procedure as a valuable part of the surgical armamentarium for evaluating pleural diseases. Thoracoscopy permits visualization of the entire visceral, parietal, and mediastinal pleural surfaces. Excisional or incisional biopsies for establishing N and M status can be performed safely under direct vision. Advances in technology and therapy have enabled broader applications for this technique. Thoracoscopy has recently been used both diagnostically and therapeutically in the staging and treatment of lung cancer. With the introduction of video technology and the refinement of endoscopic stapling devices, video-assisted thoracoscopy has enabled a broader range of applications, including resectional techniques. Although the role of video-assisted thoracic surgery for the treatment of lung cancer has not been defined, several reports indicate that the accuracy of diagnosis and staging may be enhanced by using such minimally invasive procedures.[88–93]

Thoracoscopy is very helpful for staging lung cancer in the presence of associated pleural disease. Pleural effusions in patients with lung cancer require further evaluation of the pleural surface before thoracotomy. Discontinuous foci of tumor on the pleural surface or positive fluid cytology are indicative of T4 disease and preclude resection. Thoracoscopy affords the potential for more complete staging of patients with suspected mediastinal nodal spread and has become a valuable adjunct to cervical mediastinoscopy and anterior mediastinotomy.[88, 91] Through separate thoracoscopic incisional sites, the posterior mediastinum as well as the paratracheal, subazygous, hilar, and aortopulmonary window nodal regions can be reached.[94] Precarinal and high subcarinal nodes are usually inaccessible. Low subcarinal nodes can be reached, but they are more easily removed from the right side than the left side. Thoracoscopy can be used to assess contralateral or ipsilateral parenchymal disease remote from the primary tumor, mediastinal masses, and pericardial disease that may represent T4 or M1 disease. With more experience, improved instrumentation, and refinement in operative techniques, surgeons will continue to improve the accuracy of histologic staging using thoracoscopy.

Operative Staging

Operative staging provides the opportunity to histologically verify the extent of gross and microscopic disease. The surgeon is responsible for performing a complete nodal dissection or nodal sampling as an integral part of the thoracotomy. Lymph nodes are removed and labeled according to the location of the station on the regional station map (Figs. 6–12 and 6–13). Lymph node maps were introduced in the 1970s, when nodal dissection was recognized as an important component of surgical staging.[95] In 1983, the American Thoracic Society, using transverse section anatomy as defined by CT and viewed at thoracotomy, developed a regional lymph node staging map,[96] which was further revised by the Lung Cancer Study Group of North America (see Fig. 6–12). Another map that is commonly used was developed by Naruke,[95] proposed by the Japan Lung Cancer Society (see Fig. 6–13), and recommended by the AJCC.[97] The important difference between the two classifications exists in recognizing the location of station 10. In the ATS/LCSG map, station 10 represents mediastinal lymph nodes. In the AJCC/JLCS map, station 10 represents hilar lymph nodes. Therefore, when labeling station 10 lymph nodes, it is important to specify whether the ATS/LCSG map or the AJCC/JLCS map is being used.

Hilar lymph nodes reside adjacent to bronchi and are enclosed within the visceral pleura. Lymph nodes that lie within the mediastinal pleural envelope are mediastinal lymph nodes. Within the mediastinum, a phantom midline exists to differentiate N2 and N3 nodes. Ipsilateral positive lymph nodes are N2 nodes,

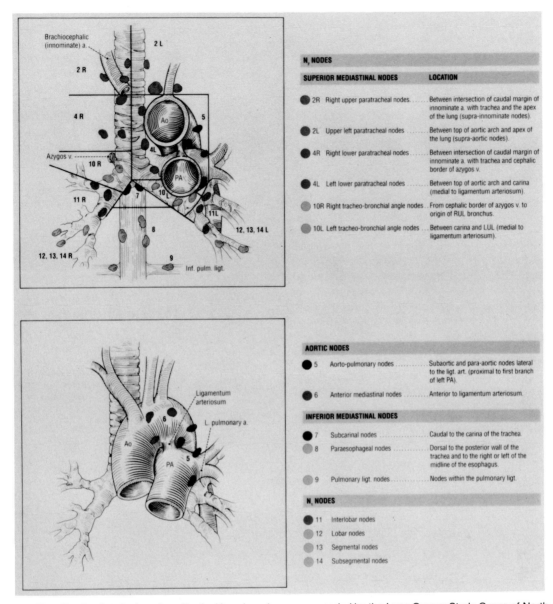

N₂ NODES

SUPERIOR MEDIASTINAL NODES	LOCATION
● 2R Right upper paratracheal nodes	Between intersection of caudal margin of innominate a. with trachea and the apex of the lung (supra-innominate nodes).
● 2L Upper left paratracheal nodes	Between top of aortic arch and apex of the lung (supra-aortic nodes).
● 4R Right lower paratracheal nodes	Between intersection of caudal margin of innominate a. with trachea and cephalic border of azygos v.
● 4L Left lower paratracheal nodes	Between top of aortic arch and carina (medial to ligamentum arteriosum).
● 10R Right tracheo-bronchial angle nodes	From cephalic border of azygos v. to origin of RUL bronchus.
● 10L Left tracheo-bronchial angle nodes	Between carina and LUL (medial to ligamentum arteriosum).

AORTIC NODES

● 5 Aorto-pulmonary nodes	Subaortic and para-aortic nodes lateral to the ligt. art. (proximal to first branch of left PA).
● 6 Anterior mediastinal nodes	Anterior to ligamentum arteriosum.

INFERIOR MEDIASTINAL NODES

● 7 Subcarinal nodes	Caudal to the carina of the trachea.
● 8 Paraesophageal nodes	Dorsal to the posterior wall of the trachea and to the right or left of the midline of the esophagus.
● 9 Pulmonary ligt. nodes	Nodes within the pulmonary ligt.

N₁ NODES

● 11   Interlobar nodes
● 12   Lobar nodes
● 13   Segmental nodes
● 14   Subsegmental nodes

FIGURE 6–12. Classification for staging of mediastinal lymph nodes recommended by the Lung Cancer Study Group of North America.

whereas contralateral positive lymph nodes are N3 nodes. If a lymph node straddles the midline and has its major component residing on one side, the nodal station is labeled according to the site of predominant location. Subcarinal nodes always bridge the midline, but are classified as N2 nodes. If nodes within the subcarinal region obviously reside on the contralateral side, they should be labeled as N3 nodes. The surgeon ultimately is responsible for determining the boundary of the mediastinal and visceral pleura, as well as for documenting the precise location of all lymph nodes prior to submitting them to the pathologist for examination.

The technique of mediastinal nodal removal is standard. On the right side, the mediastinal pleura is incised longitudinally along the trachea and esophagus from the apex to the base of the right hemithorax. Often, the azygous vein must be divided to allow adequate access to the trachea. All accessible lymph nodes in the superior mediastinum are removed, usually with adjacent fat; these include the superior mediastinal, upper paratracheal, pretracheal, lower paratracheal, and those of the tracheobronchial angle. In the inferior mediastinum, the posterior mediastinal pleura is reflected and the inferior pulmonary ligament is divided. The tracheal bifurcation is exposed. Within the compartment bordered by the carina superiorly, the pericardium anteriorly, and the esophagus posteriorly, all nodes and adjacent fat are removed. Lymph node stations in this region include the subcarinal, paraesophageal, and inferior pulmonary ligament. The inferior mediastinum is approached on the left side in a fashion similar to that on the right. Exposure of the subcarinal region is slightly more difficult and requires slight posterior retraction of the great vessels with gentle anterolateral

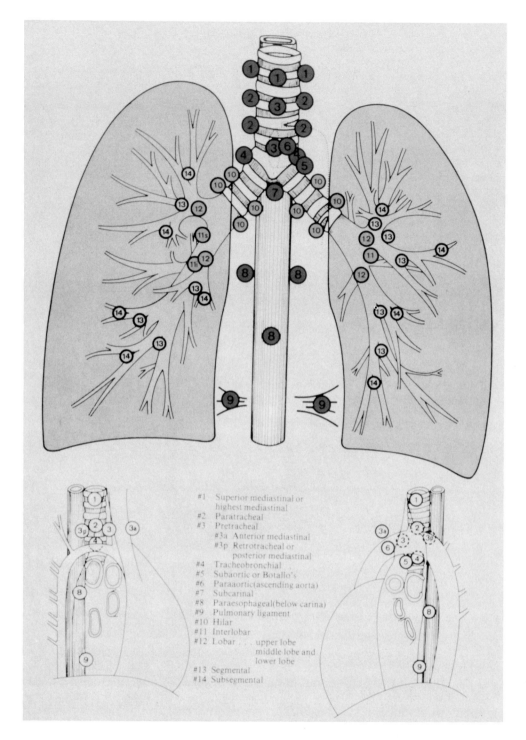

FIGURE 6–13. Lymph node stations recommended by the American Joint Committee on Cancer. (From Naruke T, Suemasu K, Ishikawa S: Lymph node mapping and curability at various levels of metastasis in resected lung cancer. J Thorac Cardiovasc Surg 76:832, 1978, with permission.)

#1 Superior mediastinal or highest mediastinal
#2 Paratracheal
#3 Pretracheal
     #3a Anterior mediastinal
     #3p Retrotracheal or posterior mediastinal
#4 Tracheobronchial
#5 Subaortic or Botallo's
#6 Paraaortic(ascending aorta)
#7 Subcarinal
#8 Paraesophageal(below carina)
#9 Pulmonary ligament
#10 Hilar
#11 Interlobar
#12 Lobar . . . . upper lobe
                middle lobe and
                lower lobe
#13 Segmental
#14 Subsegmental

retraction of the left main-stem bronchus. The superior mediastinal pleura is incised from the apex to the subaortic region. All accessible nodes are removed, including the upper paratracheal, pretracheal, subaortic, para-aortic, and those of the tracheobronchial angle. The lower paratracheal nodes usually are inaccessible. Mobilizing the aorta to remove lymph nodes under the aortic arch by sacrificing several intercostal arteries has been advocated,[28] but its possible associated morbidity make it ill-advised for conventional staging.

PROBLEMS AND CONTROVERSIES

The prognosis implied by T, N, and M status has been determined partly by retrospective analysis of historical data. Yet not all tumors conform to the International Staging System nor to the prognosis implied within each category. Several staging problems are incompletely addressed by the staging system and remain ambiguous. Mountain and associates stated that "in the absence of a body of data that describes the prognostic implications of tumors with no applicable specific staging rule, the TNM and stage classifications must be assigned according to logic or convention."[98] The following section discusses common questions and sources of confusion for each of the staging parameters.

The Primary Tumor

T3 and T4 Tumors

Most tumors that invade the parietal pleura, chest wall, diaphragm, pericardium, superior sulcus, or specific structures within the superficial mediastinum and the proximal main-stem bronchus are considered T3 tumors. T3 tumors also may invade the mediastinal pleura, mediastinal fat, pericardium, and nerves without involving organs or major vascular structures. Such tumors usually are readily resectable, and adjacent tissues are usually included to ensure a complete resection.[99] Tumors that involve major structures or organs (trachea, esophagus, heart, aorta, aortic branch vessels, vena cava, brachial plexus, or vertebral body), are considered to be T4. If a tumor bridges T categories, it should be staged at the higher level.

Proximal Airway

Tumors located within 2 cm of the carina are classified as T3 lesions. Tumors directly involving the carina are T4 lesions. The carina includes the most distal trachea, the orifices of the main-stem bronchi, and the inferior ridge or septum that separates the proximal and medial main-stem bronchial walls. If any portion of the carina or proximal 2 cm of the main stem is histologically involved (including a tumor involving the right upper lobe orifice that originates within 2 cm of the carina) or if any portion of them is included within the resection, the tumor should be assigned the higher tumor descriptor.

Resection can be undertaken in patients with tumors involving the proximal airway and carina. For patients with adequate pulmonary reserve, pneumonectomy may be required to completely encompass the tumor mass. In selected patients, bronchial sleeve resection has proved to be a safe and effective method for pulmonary preservation with mortality and survival rates comparable to those following pneumonectomy.[100–102] In selected patients with tumors confined to the carina or tracheobronchial angle, sleeve pneumonectomy can achieve a complete resection; however, the significant 30-day mortality risk of 8% to 20.9% indicates that caution must be used in recommending such a procedure.[33–36]

A 5-year survival rate of 38% has been reported following sleeve resection of T3 lesions[103]; the survival rate appears to be directly related to the extent of N2 nodal involvement.[104] The overall 5-year survival rate in Stage III disease patients who undergo sleeve lobectomy is 21%.[105] Survival after resection of T4 tumors that involve the carina is directly related to the extent of nodal disease; 3-year survival rates range from 43% for N1 disease, 34% for disease involving

only the subcarinal node, and 0% for that involving upper mediastinal nodes.[36, 37]

Early Lung Cancer Within the Proximal Main Bronchus

Naruke and colleagues have identified a subset of patients who have tumors confined to the bronchial mucosa yet residing within 2 cm from the carina.[106, 107] Technically, these tumors should be staged as T3 tumors by International Staging System criteria. However, Naruke showed that these patients who also have no lymph node metastasis or distant metastasis may have a 5-year survival of over 80%. Accordingly, in 1987, the International Staging System recognized this select group of patients and classified their tumors as T1.

Visceral Pleura

The T2 descriptor includes a subset of tumors of any size that invade the visceral pleura. In one study, Brewer found that tumors with subpleural involvement were associated with an 8% 5-year survival rate, although lymph node status was not assessed.[108] Merlier and colleagues reported a similarly poor prognosis for patients with these tumors regardless of the degree of lymph node involvement.[109] Inchonise and associates analyzed a group of patients with Stage I disease and found a significant adverse prognostic influence when the tumor was exposed on the pleural surface.[110] Martini's series of patients with Stage II disease showed a trend toward a difference in 5-year survival from 41% in patients without visceral pleural involvement to 33% when tumors extended into the visceral pleura. Though the trend was not significant, there was significance when tumor size was greater than 3 cm (5-year survival 25%) suggesting that the subset of T2 tumors with visceral pleural involvement have a worse prognosis than other T2 tumors.[13] Tumors that extend through the pulmonary parenchymal envelope may seed the pleural cavity and may use this route for systemic spread, resulting in decreased survival.

Parietal Pleura and Chest Wall

Tumors that reside within the peripheral pulmonary parenchyma may have associated inflammatory adhesions to the parietal pleura, especially if there is pneumonia distal to an obstructed bronchus. The presence of loose attachments between the visceral and parietal pleura should not be considered neoplastic invasion; usually they can be lysed with ease or taken down in an extrapleural plane. If parietal pleural infiltration is identified histologically, T3 status is appropriate. Tumors that extend into the chest wall musculature and ribs should also be considered T3 lesions.

Overall 5-year survival rates for patients with surgically resected T3 tumors have ranged from 12% to 40%.[20, 21, 85, 111–119] The primary factor affecting survival in patients with T3 tumors is nodal status. In patients with tumors considered T3N0 because of chest wall invasion, 5-year survival rates approach 33% to 60%.[20, 21, 111, 113, 115, 116] In patients with T3N2 tumors, on the other hand, the 5-year survival rate is less than 5%,[118] although Martini has reported a 5-year survival rate of 21% for patients with regional lymph node involvement.[120] Other factors adversely influencing survival are incompleteness of resection and depth of invasion of the tumor into the chest wall.[112, 116, 119–121] The role of radiotherapy and its influence on survival of patients with these types of tumors are unknown.

Vertebral Body

Tumors that invade the cortex of the vertebral body are considered T4 lesions. Costotransverse foramen invasion also confers T4 status, because complete resectability is precluded by the inability to achieve a negative margin of resection lateral to the spinal cord. If a tumor is adherent to the vertebral body with no radiologic evidence of erosion, the tumor probably involves the overlying soft tissues (pleura, prevertebral fascia, and periosteum). In such instances, the tumor should be designated as clinical T3.[122] Such tumors can be resected by including a portion of the vertebral body as part of the en bloc resection. If pathologic interpretation of the resected specimen shows tumor involvement of the bony cortex, the tumor is a postsurgical resection-pathologic T4.

Superior Sulcus Tumors

Tumors originating in the apex of the lung and invading the parietal pleural cupula may extend deeply into the adjacent chest wall and neurovascular structures. The T3 descriptor is appropriate when rib, intercostal muscle, sympathetic chain, stellate ganglion, or the lowest cord of the brachial plexus is involved. In most cases, such tumors can be completely resected, including the lowest cord of the brachial plexus, the sacrifice of which causes minimal neurologic compromise.

Superior sulcus tumors with associated Pancoast's syndrome (Horner's syndrome, pain in the C8-T1 distribution, and atrophy of the intrinsic muscles of the hand) usually have extensive involvement of the brachial plexus. Irrespective of vertebral body or vascular invasion, tumors with Pancoast's syndrome (true Pancoast tumors) carry a poor prognosis and should be classified as T4 lesions. Tumors that involve the vertebral body, subclavian vessels, or deep aspects of the brachial plexus are usually inoperable and are associated with a poor prognosis. In circumstances of limited invasion, the subclavian artery can be resected and reconstructed.[123, 124] When the tumor is adherent to the vertebral body, a portion can be removed with the en bloc resection without altering long-term survival.[123] If radiologic studies indicate vertebral body invasion, the tumor is considered T4 and incurable. In the majority of patients, vascular and vertebral body invasion signify a poor prognosis and preclude complete resectability.

The overall five-year survival rate for patients with resected superior sulcus tumors ranges from 28% to 56%.[115, 117, 124–133] The presence of nodal disease significantly shortens survival.[24, 55, 126, 134] For all patients who receive radiotherapy alone, the 5-year survival rate ranges from 1.6% to 23%.[125, 135, 136]

Pulmonary Artery or Pulmonary Vein

Tumors involving the right or left main pulmonary artery or the pulmonary veins can preclude resection because of their proximity to the heart. Resection can be accomplished distal to the bifurcation of the main pulmonary arterial trunk. Likewise, a portion of the left atrium can sometimes be included with the pulmonary veins to accomplish a complete resection. If tumor extends into the intrapericardial portion of the vessel, the tumor should be considered T4. Vascular involvement outside the pericardium indicates a T3 lesion. The situation is similar for tumors that extend to the level of the confluence of the pulmonary veins and the left atrium. The surgeon must use intraoperative findings to differentiate between T3 and T4 tumors.

Superior and Inferior Vena Cava

Tumors that involve the vena cava are considered T4 tumors. If the vena cava becomes directly involved by the primary pulmonary neoplasm, the effect is compression or wall invasion. Compression or obstruction of the vena cava is manifested by distal venous engorgement, which most frequently compromises the superior vena cava, causing superior vena cava syndrome. Although the more common cause of superior vena cava syndrome is compression from metastatic disease to lymph nodes in the superior mediastinum, direct tumor compression can cause the same process. In most instances such tumors represent extensive disease and carry a poor prognosis. Treatment is usually nonsurgical, although in a few cases of localized disease with vena caval involvement, the tumor can be resected by including a portion of the vessel wall.[37, 137, 138]

Diaphragm

Tumors that invade the diaphragm are considered to be T3 lesions. These lesions are encompassable within a resection that must be followed by diaphragmatic closure or reconstruction. If underlying abdominal structures are involved, that is, peritoneum, liver, spleen, omentum, colon, stomach, or small bowel, such structures may be included with the resection. Under such circumstances, the tumor should be upgraded to T4 status. Discontinuous foci of tumor that involve the diaphragm represent distant sites of disease and are classified M1.

Synchronous Tumors

Synchronous Primary Tumors

Multiple synchronous cancers may represent synchronous primary lung cancers or primary lung cancer with parenchymal metastases (satellite lesions). Synchronous primary lung cancers occur in 0.26% to 1.7% of all patients with lung cancer.[139–142] Practical pathologic and clinical criteria have been proposed as guidelines to distinguish primary and metastatic tumors.[77, 139–141, 143–148] Probable or definite synchronous lung cancers are physically separate and are located in a different segment, lobe, or lung with no regions of common lymphatic involvement and have a different histologic type or are proved to arise from different endobronchial lesions by bronchoscopy or from separate foci of carcinoma in situ at pathologic examination. Patients with unilateral tumors and hilar or mediastinal lymph node metastases are not considered to have synchronous tumors.

When synchronous tumors are confirmed as individual primary tumors, they should be staged separately and independently according to standard TNM definitions. The patient's overall tumor stage should be determined by the higher staged lesion.

Survival rates after complete resection of synchronous lung cancers are worse than those for isolated lesions of similar stage.[77, 139, 145, 146] The overall 5-year survival rate for all patients with synchronous lesions ranges from 0% to 44%, and the median survival ranges from 11 to 43 months; patients with no hilar or mediastinal node metastases generally survive longer.[77, 139, 142, 143, 145]

Satellite Lesions

Histologically identical tumors that arise within the same lobe without definite endobronchial foci of origin can be considered satellite metastases.[144] Satellite pulmonary nodules (intrapulmonary metastases) are well-circumscribed accessory carcinomatous foci clearly separated from the main tumor; they occur in 7.6% to 19% of lobectomy specimens.[144, 149] The nodules are smaller than the primary tumor and are usually located within the same lobe. The existence of such nodules indicates locally advanced disease; the 5-year survival rates by stage are 32% (Stage I), 12.5% (Stage II), and 5.6% (Stage III).[144] Watanabe and colleagues also have identified the poor prognostic implication of satellite lesions in Stage I and Stage II disease, noting survival rates similar to those in patients with Stage IIIA disease.[150] Deslauriers and associates have proposed that a tumor accompanied by satellite nodules be considered a T3 tumor.[144] Mountain has recommended upgrading the T status because of the poor survival rate of patients with multiple intraparenchymal lesions. If all lesions are present within the same lobe, the T status of the primary tumor is raised one level. If tumors reside within separate ipsilateral lobes and are considered to originate from the primary lesion because of anatomic and histologic characteristics, the tumors are considered to be T4.[98] This method classifies satellite nodules more completely than that of Deslauriers and appears to correlate more appropriately with survival groupings.

Metachronous Tumors

In a patient who has previously been treated for a malignant lung tumor, a new lesion may represent a new primary tumor (metachronous tumor), a metastatic lesion from the previously treated tumor, a local recurrence, or a benign lesion. Metachronous (asynchronous) lesions comprise distinct tumors that arise in separate anatomic sites and are of different histologic types; they may be of the same histologic type if there had been complete resection of the initial primary lung cancer without stump involvement, the tumors originated in separate lobes or lungs, there is no cancer in the common lymphatics or extrapulmonary disease at the time of diagnosis, and the site of origin of the second primary can be identified (or, if the original site is unknown, there is a 2- to 3-year interval between the two tumors).[140, 143, 145] Shields has reported that approximately 0.5% of the entire population with lung carcinoma will have a second primary lung tumor diagnosed before death.[151] As the number of patients successfully treated for lung cancer increases, the incidence of second primaries will also increase.[148] Multiple lung cancers occur in 10% to 25% of patients who survive longer than 3 years.[145, 151, 152] Patients in whom the multiple lesions are metachronous survive significantly longer (10-year survival rates reported at 42% for survival from time of diagnosis of the original tumor) than those in whom the multiple lesions are synchronous. This survival rate is strongly influenced by the interval to recurrence and the stage of the second primary tumor.[45] The time interval between the development of asynchronous primary lesions may exceed 10 years.[145, 147]

Staging for metachronous tumors is the same as that for the initial primary tumor. Although second primary tumors occur after the initial treatment phase of the original tumor, the prefix r (rTNM), indicating recurrence, should not be used for second primary tumors, because a separate stage classification is assigned to the new tumor. Staging procedures should proceed in the same fashion as for the first tumor.

Survival rates after treatment for synchronous or metachronous primary lung lesions are better than those for metastatic or locally recurrent disease. (Locally recurrent disease has been reported to develop at a median time interval of 13 months and to have a 4-year survival rate of 5% to 23%.[145, 153]) Using the criteria outlined previously for identifying and differentiating multiple lung cancers, the prognostic significance of new disease can be reliably assessed. This factor becomes important for predicting patient survival and for selecting appropriate treatment.

Discontiguous Pleural Seed

When a parietal or visceral pleural implant occurs, the tumor becomes T4, as with a malignant pleural effusion. Discontinuous tumor foci beyond the parietal pleural envelope, within the chest wall, or in the diaphragm are classified as M1.

Pleural Effusion

Approximately 8% to 25% of patients with lung cancer will present with a pleural effusion, which confers a poor prognosis regardless of its cytologic characteristics.[154, 155] In a review of 702 patients with carcinoma of the lung, Parker noted that 25% presented with pleural effusions, and of those evaluated (77), 41% contained malignancy with no 5-year survivors.[154] Tumor-related pleural fluid accumulation usually occurs secondary to impaired lymphatic drainage, which may occur as a consequence of mediastinal lymphatic metastases, pleural implants, superior vena cava syndrome, or malignant pericarditis. Reactive effusions may occur from obstructive atelectasis that is accompanied by pneumonitis and parapneumonic processes. A malignant effusion (one that contains malignant cells) represents a noncurative situation, for which chemotherapy and radiotherapy are the treatments used. It is imperative that a coexistent pleural effusion, which may contain malignant cells, undergoes evaluation, because such effusions are considered T4 and are not amenable to surgical or radiation therapy. A bloody or exudative effusion should raise the suspicion of malignancy even if the cytologic evaluation is nonconfirmatory. In the minority of patients, the fluid is nonmalignant and is associated with a potentially resectable tumor. If the fluid is cytologically negative on at least two consecutive taps, nonexudative, and nonbloody, the effusion should be disregarded in staging and the tumor should be staged according to other indicators. If suspicion of malignancy remains high, the patient should undergo thoracoscopy with direct parietal pleural biopsy before surgical resection.

Pericardial Effusion

If a malignant pericardial effusion exists, T4 status is established.

Phrenic Nerve

Diaphragmatic paralysis usually represents phrenic nerve involvement. Most commonly, this is caused by invasion from the adjacent tumor. The nerve can usually be easily included in the surgical resection. Such tumors are considered to be T3 lesions.

Vagus and Recurrent Laryngeal Nerve

Direct neoplastic invasion of the vagus nerve usually evades clinical detection unless the nerve is involved above the takeoff of the recurrent laryngeal nerve; this is a rare problem that is more likely to occur with left rather than right apical malignancies. Tumors that arise superiorly and medially may cause such a problem by direct extension, and patients with such lesions present with hoarseness. Below the level of the takeoff of the recurrent laryngeal nerve, the tumor may invade the vagus nerve and produce no clinical signs. In either location, the tumor represents a T3 lesion unless T4 criteria pertain, and the vagus nerve can be sacrificed to permit a complete surgical resection. Permanent vocal cord paralysis may result with apical lesions, but patients usually compensate well without significant sequelae.

In most instances, recurrent laryngeal nerve symptoms occur secondary to metastases to the lymph nodes within the aortopulmonary window. The tumor may also directly invade the nerve in this region. Importantly, nerve paralysis from lesions in this region, resulting from nodal metastases or primary tumor, usually indicates incurability and poor survival.[98] For this reason, recurrent nerve invasion by tumors in the region of the aortopulmonary window should be classified as T4 tumors.

Sympathetic Chain and Stellate Ganglion

Tumors that involve the sympathetic chain or stellate ganglion usually are readily encompassable within a resection; they are considered T3 tumors unless other factors exist that would upgrade the tumor.

Atelectasis and Obstructive Pneumonitis

Atelectasis or some degree of obstructive pneumonitis was found in 44% of the patients with lung cancer evaluated by Mountain and colleagues in the 1973 report of the Task Force on Carcinoma of the Lung of the AJCC.[3] Analysis of the survival of selected subgroups of patients with parenchymal changes led to the addition of pneumonitis and atelectasis to the list of factors considered when assigning T status. It appears that the finding of atelectasis, determined by standard chest radiographs alone, was fortuitous as a predictor of survival. With subsequent radiologic refinement and the universal use of CT scans, varying degrees of atelectasis and pneumonitis are more accurately detected. Many tumors have an associated bronchial obstructive component. CT has enhanced recognition of such changes irrespective of tumor size or local spread.

Atelectasis is considered to be a relative predictor of more advanced disease. When surrounding pulmonary parenchyma is so affected, the likelihood of a more advanced tumor is higher. The greater the degree of involvement, the worse the prognosis. Atelectasis has been shown to influence the T status and remains a key staging element.

Regional Lymph Nodes

Mediastinal Nodal Disease

The frequency of mediastinal lymph node involvement in patients with resectable non–small cell carcinoma of the lung ranges from 22% to 33%.[156] Approximately 33% of patients with Stage IIIA disease (based on N2 nodal metastases) present with a single positive node, whereas the remainder present with multiple nodes involved at a single station or at multiple stations.[22, 28] Patients with multiple station involvement have a significantly worse prognosis than patients with single node involvement.[28, 32] For patients with multiple level nodal disease, the effect of subcarinal lymph node metastases on survival is controversial. Watanabe and associates have shown that subcarinal lymph node involvement makes no significant difference in survival in patients with multiple levels of involvement following surgical resection.[28] On the other hand, Naruke and colleagues,[95] Kirsh and Sloan,[27] and the Lung Cancer Study Group[157] have shown that patients with multiple-level involvement that includes subcarinal nodes have a poorer prognosis.

The prognostic implication of the location of single-level metastases remains unclear. Watanabe and colleagues reported that patients who underwent resection with single-level metastases at locations other than the subcarina survived longer than those whose single-level metastases affected the subcarinal region, although there was no statistical difference in survival between the two groups.[28] Others have noted that the presence of subcarinal nodal metastasis alone does not connote a significantly worse prognosis than that in single-level metastases in other N2 nodal groups.[32, 157]

Some surgeons believe that patients with metastases to the highest mediastinal node have undergone an incomplete resection and have a high probability for further disease.[117, 157] Others have not accepted this interpretation and believe that a complete resection can be accomplished even if the most distal node is involved by metastatic disease.[24, 28, 32] No international agreement has been reached. A prospective, randomized study by the Lung Cancer Study Group reported that recurrence and survival rates are not significantly different between patients with N2 metastases in high mediastinal nodes and those with disease in subcarinal lymph nodes.[157] In their study, metastasis to resected subcarinal lymph nodes was considered a complete resection, whereas metastasis to the highest mediastinal lymph nodes was arbitrarily chosen to represent an incomplete resection. Because there was no difference in survival, this study suggests the lack of sufficient data to support the distinction of an incomplete resection if based on highest nodal involvement alone.

The relevance of the extent of N2 disease on subsequent survival or postresection survival requires further study, but some observations can be made. Patients with metastases involving multiple nodal stations have a worse prognosis than patients whose metastases involve only a single nodal station. In patients with metastases involving a single station, a significant survival difference has not been demonstrated between those with subcarinal metastases and those with metastases to other stations. In patients with multiple station metastases, the significance of subcarinal involvement is uncertain. The significance

of metastases to the highest mediastinal lymph node and the definition of an incomplete resection based on N2 lymph node metastases are unclear.

Extranodal Disease

Patients with intranodal disease have a significant survival advantage in comparison to those patients with extranodal extension.[78, 158, 159] Lymph nodes that extend beyond the confines of the nodal capsule have an increased propensity to involve adjacent tissue, reducing the chances of a complete resection. Such gross perinodal spread confers the possibility of microscopic residual disease, which may account for increased local recurrence rates and carry a worse prognosis.[117]

Small Cell and Bronchioloalveolar Carcinoma

Small Cell Carcinoma

Because of the propensity for systemic spread of small cell carcinoma at presentation, treatment usually consists of chemotherapy with or without radiotherapy. These tumors are staged as limited and extensive; approximately 60% to 70% of patients present with extensive disease.[160, 161] This simple two-stage system, conceived by the Veterans Administration Lung Cancer Study Group (VALG), has evolved as the different prognostic significances of intrathoracic and extrathoracic disease have been recognized.[161–163] Furthermore, it has facilitated the comparison of clinical trials and has helped clarify their results. Limited disease is confined to the hemithorax and may contain metastases to ipsilateral or contralateral mediastinal or supraclavicular nodes. Ipsilateral malignant effusion and superior vena cava syndrome are considered limited disease. All of these areas are encompassable within a tolerable radiotherapy portal. If pericardial disease is present or if extrathoracic disease spreads beyond the sites defined as limited disease, the tumor requires too wide a radiotherapy portal for treatment and is labeled as extensive disease.

Other staging systems have been proposed for small cell carcinoma, including a version of the TNM system, but their value is unproven.[161, 163] Specific anatomic staging is unneccessary except in those few patients with very limited disease for whom surgical resection is considered.[164–166] The infrequent case of very limited small cell carcinoma (tumor suspected to be confined only to the lung) should be staged with the TNM system and may be treated initially by surgery alone or in combination with chemotherapy. Actuarial and projected 5-year survival rates for postresectional Stages I to IIIA small cell lung cancer have ranged as high as 36% to 39%.[164–166]

Bronchioloalveolar Carcinoma

Bronchioloalveolar carcinoma is an extremely confusing pulmonary malignancy because of its wide variability in presentation and behavior. Classification of this tumor into two groups, solitary and multicentric, and three subgroups, secretory, nonsecretory, and poorly differentiated, has been based on radiologic, surgical, and cytopathologic findings. Approximately 60% appear as solitary lesions, which can be staged satisfactorily by the TNM system. The remaining 40% appear as multicentric or diffuse processes, which may present within a lobe or lung or bilaterally. The multicentric pattern confounds standard T assessment and should be designated TX. If disease is bilateral, it should be considered M1. Solitary lesions carry a favorable prognosis, but multicentric and poorly differentiated lesions have a uniformly poor prognosis.[167]

SUMMARY

Lung cancer staging organizes the cohort of patients with lung cancer by assigning each patient to a category that is commensurate with the level of disease. In the TNM system, staging categories are based on anatomic criteria that measure the extent of disease as an indicator of prognosis. Staging facilitates the selection of treatment, allows accurate predictability of survival, permits international uniformity for comparative research, and provides a valuable resource for reporting of end results. Owing to the biologic heterogeneity and unpredictability of lung cancer growth and spread, there can be no perfect staging system. The International Staging System, which has replaced the AJCC and the UICC systems, has heightened the accuracy of staging and has been responsive to the needs of the treatment disciplines involved with lung cancer. It serves well as a framework on which to classify lung tumors.

SELECTED REFERENCES

Mountain CF: A new international staging system for lung cancer. Chest 89:225S, 1986.
This landmark article proposes the International Staging System. Dr. Mountain's monograph is the product of many years of research and attendance at international meetings that results in unified agreement and global acceptance for this single system to stage lung cancer.
Naruke T, Suemasu K, Ishikawa S: Lymph node mapping and curability at various levels of metastases in resected lung cancer. J Thorac Cardiovasc Surg 76:832, 1978.
This article discusses a 10-year study of patients with metastatic disease to hilar and mediastinal lymph nodes. Dr. Naruke shows the importance and prognostic value of lymph node mapping. The specific map that was developed remains the current map used by the AJCC.

REFERENCES

1. Denoix PF: Enquete permanent dans les centres anticancereaux. Bull Inst Nat Hyg Paris 1:70–75, 1946.
2. Copeland MM: Committee on Cancer Staging and End Results reporting: Origin, objectives, and program. Bull Am Coll Surg 47(part 1):235, 1962.
3. Mountain CF, Carr DT, Anderson WAD: A system for the clinical staging of lung cancer. Am J Roentgen Radium Ther Nucl Med 120:130, 1974.
4. Mountain CF: A new international staging system for lung cancer. Chest 89:225S–233S, 1986.
5. Maassen W: The staging issue—problems: Accuracy of mediastinoscopy. *In* Delarue NC, Eschapasse H (eds): International Trends in General Thoracic Surgery. 1st Ed. Philadelphia, W.B. Saunders, 1985, pp 42–53.
6. Anonymous: WHO Technical Report Series. No. 53. 1952, pp. 45–54.
7. Committee on TNM Classification: Malignant tumors of the lung: Clinical stage classification and presentation of results. *In* Anonymous (ed): International Union Against Cancer (UICC). Geneva, 1966.
8. Anonymous: Supplement to TNM classification of malignant tumors. *In* Anonymous (ed): Interntional Union Against Cancer and American Joint Committee for Cancer Staging and End Results Reporting. Geneva, 1973.
9. Martini N, McCaughan BC, McCormack PM, et al: The extent of resection for localized lung cancer: Lobectomy. *In* Kittle CF (ed): Current Controversies in Thoracic Surgery. Philadelphia, W.B. Saunders, 1986, pp 171–174.
10. Mountain CF, Lukeman JM, Hammar SP: Lung cancer classification: The relationship of disease extent and cell type to survival in a clinical trials population. J Surg Oncol 35:147–156, 1987.
11. Flehinger BJ, Kimmel M, Melamed MR: The effect of survival from early lung cancer. Chest 101:1013, 1992.
12. Prestidge BR, Cox RS, Johnson DW: Non–small cell lung cancer: Treatment results at a USAF referral center. Mil Med 156:479, 1991.
13. Martini N, Burt ME, Bains MS, et al: Survival after resection of stage II non–small cell lung cancer. Ann Thorac Surg 54:460–466, 1992.
14. Naruke T, Goya T, Tsuchiya R, et al: Prognosis and survival in resected lung carcinoma based on the new international staging system. J Thorac Cardiovasc Surg 96:440, 1988.
15. Holmes EC: Treatment of stage II lung cancer (T1N1 and T2N1). Surg Clin North Am 67(5):945, 1987.
16. Ludwig Lung Cancer Study Group: Patterns of failure in patients with resected stage I and II non–small cell carcinoma of the lung. Ann Surg 205:67, 1987.
17. Anonymous: Rational integration of radiation and chemotherapy in patients with unresectable stage IIIA or IIIB NSCLC: Results from the Lung Cancer Study Group, Eastern Cooperative Oncology Group, and Radiation Therapy Oncology Group. Chest 103(1):35S, 1993.
18. Mountain CF: Prognostic implications of the international staging system for lung cancer. Semin Oncol 3:236, 1988.
19. Ihde DC, Minna JD: Non–small cell lung cancer, I: Biology, diagnosis, and staging. Curr Probl Cancer 15:63, 1991.
20. Nakahashi H, Yasumoto K, Ishida T, et al: Results of surgical treatment of patients with T3 non–small cell lung cancer. Ann Thorac Surg 46:178, 1988.
21. Albertucci M, DeMeester TR, Rothberg M, et al: Surgery and the management of peripheral lung tumors adherent to the parietal pleura. J Thorac Cardiovasc Surg 103:8, 1992.
22. Martini N, Flehinger BJ: The role of surgery in N2 lung cancer. Surg Clin North Am 67(5):1037, 1987.
23. Pearson FG, DeLarue NC, Ilves R, et al: Significance of positive superior mediastinal nodes identified at mediastinoscopy in patients with resectable cancer of the lung. J Thorac Cardiovasc Surg 83:1, 1982.
24. Watanabe Y, Shimizu J, Oda M, et al: Aggressive surgical intervention in N2 non–small cell cancer of the lung. Ann Thorac Surg 51:253, 1991.
25. Naruke T, Goya T, Tsuchiya R, et al: The importance of surgery to non–small cell carcinoma of lung with mediastinal lymph node metastasis. Ann Thorac Surg 46:603, 1988.
26. Regnard JF, Magdeleinat P, Azoulay D, et al: Results of resection for bronchogenic carcinoma with mediastinal lymph node metastases in selected patients. Eur J Cardiothorac Surg 5:583, 1991.
27. Kirsh MM, Sloan H: Mediastinal metastases in bronchogenic carcinoma: Influence of postoperative irradiation, cell type, and location. Ann Thorac Surg 33:459, 1982.
28. Watanabe Y, Hayashi Y, Shimizu J, et al: Mediastinal nodal involvement and the prognosis of non–small cell lung cancer. Chest 100:422, 1991.
29. Patterson GA, Piazza D, Pearson FG, et al: Significance of

metastatic disease in subaortic lymph nodes. Ann Thorac Surg 43:155, 1987.

30. Cybulsky IJ, Lanza LA, Ryan MB, et al: Prognostic significance of computed tomography in resected N2 lung cancer. Ann Thorac Surg 54:533, 1992.

31. Naruke T, Suemasu K, Ishikawa S: Mediastinal lymph node dissection and its significance in surgery of lung cancer. Lung Cancer 2:96, 1986.

32. Martini N, Flehinger BJ, Zaman MB, et al: Prospective study of 445 lung carcinomas with mediastinal lymph node metastases. J Thorac Cardiovasc Surg 80:390, 1980.

33. Mathisen DJ, Grillo HC: Carinal resection for bronchogenic carcinoma. J Thorac Cardiovasc Surg 102:16, 1991.

34. Watanabe Y, Shimizu N, Oda M, et al: Results in 104 patients undergoing bronchoplastic procedures for bronchial lesions. Ann Thorac Surg 50:607, 1990.

35. Tsuchiya R, Goya T, Naruke T, et al: Resection of tracheal carina for lung cancer. J Thorac Cardiovasc Surg 99:779, 1990.

36. Dartevelle PG, Khalife J, Chapelier A, et al: Tracheal sleeve pneumonectomy for bronchogenic carcinoma: Report of 55 cases. Ann Thorac Surg 46:68, 1988.

37. Dartevelle P, Marzelle J, Chapelier A, et al: Extended operations for T3-T4 primary lung cancers: Indications and results. Chest 96(1):51S, 1989.

38. Mountain CF: Lung cancer staging classification. Clin Chest Med 14:43, 1993.

39. Magilligan DJ: Treatment of lung cancer metastatic to the brain. Surg Clin North Am 67(5):1073, 1987.

40. Magilligan DJ, Duvernoy C, Malik G, et al: Surgical approach to lung cancer with solitary cerebral metastasis: Twenty-five years' experience. Ann Thorac Surg 42:360, 1986.

41. Burt M, Wronski M, Arbit E, et al: Resection of brain metastases from non-small cell lung carcinoma. J Thorac Cardiovasc Surg 103:399, 1992.

42. Seely JM, Mayo JR, Miller RR, Müller NL: T1 Lung cancer: Prevalence of mediastinal nodal metastases and diagnostic accuracy of CT. Radiology 186:129–132, 1993.

43. McKenna RJ, Libshitz HI, Mountain CF, et al: Roentgenographic evaluation of mediastinal nodes for preoperative assessment in lung cancer. Chest 88:206, 1985.

44. Khan A, Gersten KC, Garvey J, et al: Oblique hilar tomography, computed tomography and mediastinoscopy for prethoracotomy staging of bronchogenic carcinoma. Radiology 156:295, 1985.

45. Osborne DR, Korobkin M, Ravin CE, et al: Comparison of plain radiography, conventional tomography, and computed tomography in detecting intrathoracic lymph node metastases from lung carcinoma. Radiology 142:157, 1982.

46. Rea HH, Shevland JE, House AJS: Accuracy of computed tomographic scanning in assessment of the mediastinum in bronchial carcinoma. J Thor Cardiovasc Surg 81:825, 1981.

47. Lewis JW, Madrazo BL, Gross SC, et al: The value of radiographic and computed tomography in the staging of lung carcinoma. Ann Thorac Surg 34:553, 1982.

48. Baron RL, Levitt RG, Sagel SS, et al: Computed tomography in the preoperative evaluation of bronchogenic carcinoma. Radiology 145:727, 1982.

49. Goldstraw P, Kurzer M, Edwards D: Preoperative staging of lung cancer: Accuracy of computed tomography versus mediastinoscopy. Thorax 38:10, 1983.

50. Richey HM, Matthews JI, Helsel RA, et al: Thoracic CT scanning in the staging of bronchogenic carcinoma. Chest 85:218, 1984.

51. Breyer RH, Karstaedt N, Mills SA, et al: Computed tomography for evaluation of mediastinal lymph nodes in lung cancer: Correlation with surgical staging. Ann Thorac Surg 38:215, 1984.

52. Daly BDT, Faling LJ, Pugatch RD, et al: Computed tomography: An effective technique for mediastinal staging in lung cancer. J Thorac Cardiovasc Surg 88:486, 1984.

53. Brion JP, DePauw L, Kuhn G, et al: Role of computed tomography and mediastinoscopy in preoperative staging of lung carcinoma. J Comput Assist Tomogr 9:480, 1985.

54. Daly BDT, Faling LJ, Bite G, et al: Mediastinal lymph node evaluation by computed tomography in lung cancer: An analysis of 345 patients grouped by TNM staging, tumor size, and tumor location. J Thorac Cardiovasc Surg 94:664, 1987.

55. Friedman PJ, Feigin DS, Liston SE, et al: Sensitivity of chest radiography, computed tomography, and gallium scanning to metastasis of lung carcinoma. Cancer 54:1300, 1984.

56. Izbicki JR, Thetter O, Karg O, et al: Accuracy of computed tomographic scan and surgical assessment for staging of bronchial carcinoma. J Thorac Cardiovasc Surg 104:413, 1992.

57. Grant D, Edwards D, Goldstraw P: Computed tomography of the brain, chest, and abdomen in the preoperative assessment of non-small cell lung cancer. Thorax 43:883, 1988.

58. Patterson GA, Ginsberg RJ, Poon PY, et al: A prospective evaluation of magnetic resonance imaging, computed tomography, and mediastinoscopy in the preoperative assessment of mediastinal node status in bronchogenic carcinoma. J Thorac Cardiovasc Surg 94:679, 1987.

59. Sider L, Horejs D: Frequency of extrathoracic metastases from bronchogenic carcinoma in patients with normal-sized hilar and mediastinal lymph nodes on CT. Am J Radiol 151:893, 1988.

60. Lewis JW, Pearlberg JL, Beute GH, et al: Can computed tomography of the chest stage lung cancer? Yes and no. Ann Thorac Surg 49:591, 1990.

61. Wittens CHA, Bollen ECM, van Duin CJ, et al.: Accuracy of computed tomography of the mediastinum in bronchogenic carcinoma. Neth J Surg 43(6):240, 1991.

62. Whittlesey D: Prospective computed tomographic scanning in the staging of bronchogenic cancer. J Thorac Cardiovasc Surg 95:876, 1988.

63. Gefter WB: Magnetic resonance imaging in the evaluation of lung cancer. Semin Roentgenol 25:73, 1990.

64. Libshitz HI, McKenna RJ, Haynie TP, et al: Mediastinal evaluation in lung cancer. Radiology 151:295, 1984.

65. Staples CA, Muller NL, et al: Mediastinal nodes in bronchogenic carcinoma: Comparison between CT and mediastinoscopy. Radiology 167:367, 1988.

66. McLoud TC, Bourgouin PM, Greenberg RW, et al: Bronchogenic carcinoma: Analysis of staging in the mediastinum with CT by correlative lymph node mapping and sampling. Radiology 182:319, 1992.

67. Glazer GM: Radiologic staging of lung cancer using CT and MRI. Chest 96:44S, 1989.

68. Daly BDT: N2 lung cancer: Outcome in patients with false-negative computed tomographic scans of the chest. J Thorac Cardiovasc Surg 105:904, 1993.

69. Bekerman C, Caride VJ, Hoffer PB, et al: Noninvasive staging of lung cancer: Indications and limitations of gallium-67 citrate imaging. Radiol Clin North Am 28:497, 1990.

70. Harken DE, Black H, Clauss R: A simple cervicomediastinal exploration for tissue diagnosis of intrathoracic disease: With comments on the recognition of inoperable carcinoma of the lung. N Engl J Med 251:1041, 1954.

71. Carlens E: Mediastinoscopy: A method for inspection and tissue biopsy in the superior mediastinum. Dis Chest 36:343, 1959.

72. Luke WP, Pearson FG, Todd TRJ, et al: Prospective evaluation of mediastinoscopy for assessment of carcinoma of the lung. J Thorac Cardiovasc Surg 91:53, 1986.

73. Japssen O: Mediastinoscopy. Copenhagen, Munksgaard, 1966.

74. Foster ED, Munro DD, Deboll ARC: Mediastinoscopy: A review of anatomical relationships and complications. Ann Thorac Surg 13:273, 1972.

75. Coughlin M, Deslauries J, Beaulieu M, et al: Role of mediastinoscopy in pretreatment staging of patients with primary lung cancer. Ann Thorac Surg 40:556, 1985.

76. Jolly PC, Hill LD, Lawless PA, et al: Parasternal mediastinotomy and mediastinoscopy: Adjuncts in the diagnosis of chest disease. J Thorac Cardiovasc Surg 66:549, 1973.

77. DeMeester TR: The staging issue: Unification of criteria; discussion. *In* Delarue NC, Eschapasse H (eds): Lung Cancer. Philadelphia, W.B. Saunders, 1985, pp 37–41.

78. Bergh NP, Larsson S: The significance of various types of mediastinal lymph node metastases in lung cancer. *In* Jepssen O, Ruhbek-Sorenson H (eds): Mediastinoscopy: Proceedings of an International Symposium. Odense, Denmark, Odense University Press, 1971, pp 36–39.

79. Ginsberg RJ: Evaluation of the mediastinum by invasive techniques. Surg Clin North Am 67(5):1025, 1987.

80. Lopez L, Varela A: Extended cervical mediastinoscopy: Prospective study of 50 patients. Ann Thorac Surg, 57(3):555–558, 1994.

81. Ginsberg RJ, Rice TW, Goldberg M, et al: Extended cervical mediastinoscopy: A single stage procedure for bronchogenic carcinoma of the left upper lobe. J Thorac Cardiovasc Surg 94:673, 1987.

82. McNeill TM, Chamberlain JM: Diagnostic anterior mediastinotomy. Ann Thorac Surg 2:532, 1966.

83. Yee J, Llewellyn GA, Williams PA, et al: Scalene lymph node dissection: A study of 354 consecutive dissections. Am J Surg 118:596, 1969.

84. Schatzlein MH, McAuliffe S, Orringer MB, et al: Scalene node biopsy in pulmonary carcinoma: When is it indicated? Ann Thorac Surg 31:322, 1981.

85. Cromartie RS, Parker EF, May JE, et al: Carcinoma of the lung: A clinical review. Ann Thorac Surg 30:30, 1980.

86. Bernstein MP, Ferrara JJ, Brown L: Effectiveness of scalene node biopsy for staging of lung cancer in the absence of palpable adenopathy. J Surg Oncol 29:46, 1985.

87. Jacobaeus HC: Über die moglichkeit, die zystoskopie bei untersuchung seroser hohlungen anzuwenden. Munch Med Wsch 57:2090–2092, 1910.

88. Mack MJ, Aronoff RJ, Acuff TE, et al: Present role of thoracoscopy in the diagnosis and treatment of diseases of the chest. Ann Thorac Surg 54:403, 1992.

89. Hazelrigg SR, Nunchuck S, LoCicero J, III: The video-assisted thoracic surgery study group data. Ann Thorac Surg 56(5):1039–1044, 1993.

90. Rusch VW, Ginsberg RJ, Bains MS, et al.: The contribution of videothoracoscopy to the management of the cancer patient. Ann Surg Oncol 1:94–98, 1994.

91. Rice TW: Thoracoscopy in the staging of thoracic malignancies. In Kaiser LR, Daniel TM (eds): Thoracoscopic Surgery. Boston, Little, Brown & Co., 1993, pp 153–162.

92. Landreneau RJ, Hazelrigg SR, Mack MJ: Thoracoscopic mediastinal lymph node sampling: Useful for mediastinal lymph node stations unaccessible by cervical mediastinoscopy. J Thorac Cardiovasc Surg 106:554, 1993.

93. Wain JC: Video-assisted thoracoscopy and the staging of lung cancer. Ann Thorac Surg 56:776, 1993.

94. Landreneau RJ, Mack MJ, Hazelrigg SR, et al: Video-assisted thoracic surgery: Basic technical concepts and intercostal approach strategies. Ann Thorac Surg 54:800, 1992.

95. Naruke T, Suemasu K, Ishikawa S: Lymph node mapping and curability at various levels of metastases in resected lung cancer. J Thorac Cardiovasc Surg 76:832, 1978.

96. Tisi GM, Friedman PJ, Peters RM, et al: American Thoracic Society: Clinical staging of primary lung cancer. Am Rev Respir Dis 127:659, 1983.

97. American Joint Committee on Cancer (AJCC): Lung. In Beahrs OH, Hensen DE, Hutter RVP, Myers MH (eds): Manual for Staging of Cancer. 4th Ed. Philadelphia, J.B. Lippincott, 1992, pp. 115–121.

98. Mountain CF, Libshitz HI, Hermes KE: Lung Cancer: A Handbook for Staging and Imaging. Houston, Charles P. Young, 1992, p 37.

99. Trastek VF, Paierolero PC, Piehler JM: En bloc (non-chest wall) resection for bronchogenic carcinoma with parietal fixation. J Thorac Cardiovasc Surg 87:352, 1984.

100. Weisel RD, Cooper JD, DeLarue NC, et al: Sleeve lobectomy for carcinoma of the lung. J Thorac Cardiovasc Surg 78:839, 1979.

101. Deslauriers J, Gaulin P, Beaulieu M, et al: Long-term clinical and functional results of sleeve lobectomy for primary lung cancer. J Thorac Cardiovasc Surg 92:871, 1986.

102. Faber LP: Sleeve resections for lung cancer. Semin Thorac Cardiovasc Surg 5:238, 1993.

103. Frist WH, Mathisen DJ, Hilgenberg AD, et al: Bronchial sleeve resection with and without pulmonary resection. J Thorac Cardiovasc Surg 93:350, 1987.

104. Naruke T: Bronchoplastic and bronchovascular procedures of the tracheobronchial tree in the management of primary lung cancer. Chest 96(1):53S, 1989.

105. Tedder M, Anstadt MP, Tedder SD, et al: Current morbidity, mortality and survival after bronchoplastic procedures for malignancy. Ann Thorac Surg 54:387, 1992.

106. Naruke T, Goya T, Tsuchiya R, et al: Prognosis and survival in resected lung carcinoma based on the new international staging system. J Thorac Cardiovasc Surg 96:440–447, 1988.

107. Naruke T: Analysis of early lung cancer. In Ikeda S (ed): Practice of Mass Screening. 1st Ed. Tokyo, Igaku Shoin, 1986, pp 49–50.

108. Brewer LA, III: Patterns of survival in lung cancer. Chest 71:644, 1977.

109. Merlier M, Miranda AR, Gharbi N, et al: The staging issue: Unification of criteria. In Delarue NC, Eschapasse H (eds): International Trends in General Thoracic Surgery. 1st Ed. Philadelphia, W.B. Saunders, 1985, pp 27–36.

110. Ichinose Y, Hara N, Ohta M, et al: Is T factor of the TNM staging system a predominant prognostic factor in pathologic stage I non–small cell lung cancer? A multivariate prognostic factor analysis of 151 patients. J Thorac Cardiovasc Surg 106(1):90–94, 1993.

111. Piehler JM, Pairoler PC, Weiland LH, et al: Bronchogenic carcinoma with chest wall invasion: Factors affecting survival following en bloc resection. Ann Thorac Surg 34:684, 1982.

112. Patterson GA, Ilves R, Ginsberg RJ, et al: The value of adjuvant radiotherapy in pulmonary and chest wall resection for bronchogenic carcinoma. Ann Thorac Surg 34(6):692, 1982.

113. McCaughan BC, Martini N, Bains MS, et al: Chest wall invasion in carcinoma of the lung. J Thorac Cardiovasc Surg 89:836, 1985.

114. Van de Wal HJCM, Lacquet LK, Jongerius CM: En bloc resection for bronchogenic carcinoma with chest wall invasion. Acta Chir Belg 85:89, 1985.

115. Carrel T, Nachbur B, Bleher A: Is radiotherapy prior to surgical resection indicated for bronchogenic carcinoma with chest wall infiltration and for Pancoast tumors? Lung Cancer 4:A80, 1988.

116. Ratto GB, Piacenza G, Frola C, et al: Chest wall involvement by lung cancer: Computed tomographic detection and results of operation. Ann Thorac Surg 51:182, 1991.

117. Mountain CF: Expanded possibilities for surgical treatment of lung cancer: Survival in stage IIIa disease. Chest 97(5):1045, 1990.

118. Van Raemdonck DE, Schneider A, Ginsberg RJ: Surgical treatment for higher stage non–small cell lung cancer. Ann Thorac Surg 54:999, 1992.

119. Paone JF, Spees EK, Newton CG, et al: An appraisal of en bloc resection of peripheral bronchogenic carcinoma involving the thoracic wall. Chest 81:203, 1982.

120. Martini N: Surgical treatment of non–small cell lung cancer by stage. Semin Surg Oncol 6:248, 1990.

121. Allen MS, Mathisen DJ, Grillo HC, et al: Bronchogenic carcinoma with chest wall invasion. Ann Thorac Surg 51:948, 1991.

122. DeMeester TR, Albertucci M, Dawson PJ, et al: Management of tumor adherent to the vertebral column. J Thorac Cardiovasc Surg 97:373, 1989.

123. Wright CD, Moncure AC, Shepard JAO, et al: Superior sulcus lung tumors: Results of combined treatment (irradiation and radical resection). J Thorac Cardiovasc Surg 94:69, 1987.

124. Dartevelle PG, Chapelier AR, Macchiarini A, et al: Anterior transcervical-thoracic approach for radical resection of lung tumors invading the thoracic inlet. J Thorac Cardiovasc Surg 105:1025, 1993.

125. Rice TW, Pringle JF, Sinclair JE, et al: Superior sulcus tumours—Results of treatment. Lung Cancer 2:156, 1986.

126. Stanford W, Barnes RP, Tucker AR: Influence of staging in superior sulcus (Pancoast) tumors of the lung. Ann Thorac Surg 29:406, 1980.

127. Paulson DL: Technical considerations in stage III disease: The "superior sulcus" lesion. In Delarue NC, Eschapasse H (eds): International Trends in General Thoracic Surgery, Vol. 1: Lung Cancer. Philadelphia, W.B. Saunders, 1985, pp 121–131.

128. Anderson TM, Moy PM, Holmes EC: Factors affecting survival in superior sulcus tumors. J Clin Oncol 4:1598, 1986.

129. Beyer DC, Weisenburger T: Superior sulcus tumors. Am J Clin Oncol 9(2):156, 1986.

130. Shahian DM, Neptune WB, Ellis FH: Pancoast tumors: Improved survival with preoperative and postoperative radiotherapy. Ann Thorac Surg 43:32, 1987.

131. Miller JI, Discussion of Shahian DM, Neptune WB, Ellis FH:

Pancoast tumors: Improved survival with preoperative and postoperative radiotherapy. Ann Thorac Surg 43:37, 1987.

132. McKneally M, Discussion of Shahian DM, Neptune WB, Ellis FH: Pancoast tumors: Improved survival with preoperative and postoperative radiotherapy. Ann Thorac Surg 43:37, 1987.

133. Ricci C, Rendina EA, Venuta F: Surgical treatment of superior sulcus tumors. Lung Cancer 4(suppl):A95, 1988.

134. Hilaris BS, Martini N, Wong GY: Treatment of superior sulcus tumor (Pancoast tumor). Surg Clin North Am 67:965, 1987.

135. Komaki R, Roh J, Cox JD, et al: Superior sulcus tumors: Results of irradiation of 36 patients. Cancer 48:1563, 1981.

136. Van Houtte P, MacLennan I, Poulter C, et al: External radiation in the management of superior sulcus tumor. Cancer 54:223, 1984.

137. Dartevelle PG, Chapelier AR, Pastorino U, et al: Long-term follow-up after prosthetic replacement of the superior vena cava combined with resection of mediastinal-pulmonary malignant tumors. J Thorac Cardiovasc Surg 102:259–265, 1991.

138. Nakahara K, Ohno K, Mastumura A, et al: Extended operation for lung cancer invading the aortic arch and superior vena cava. J Thorac Cardiovasc Surg 97:428–433, 1989.

139. Ferguson MK, DeMeester TR, Deslauriers J, et al: Diagnosis and management of synchronous lung cancers. J Thorac Cardiovasc Surg 89:378, 1985.

140. Wu SC, Lin ZQ, Xu CW, et al: Multiple primary lung cancers. Chest 92(5):892, 1987.

141. Sugimura R, Watanabe S: Case-control study on histologically determined multiple primary lung cancer. J Natl Cancer Inst 79(3):435, 1987.

142. Ferguson MK: Synchronous primary lung cancers. Chest 103S:398S, 1993.

143. Martini N, Melamed MR: Multiple primary lung cancers. J Thorac Cardiovasc Surg 70:606, 1975.

144. Deslauriers J, Brisson J, Cartier R, et al: Carcinoma of the lung: Evaluation of satellite nodules as a factor influencing prognosis after resection. J Thorac Cardiovasc Surg 97:504, 1989.

145. Rosengart TK, Martini N, Ghosn P, et al: Multiple primary lung carcinomas: Prognosis and treatment. Ann Thorac Surg 52:773, 1991.

146. Deschamps C, Pairolero PC, Trastek VF, et al: Multiple primary lung cancers: Results of surgical treatment. J Thorac Cardiovasc Surg 99:769, 1990.

147. Christensen ES: Diagnosis and treatment of bilateral primary bronchogenic carcinoma. J Thorac Cardiovasc Surg 61(4):501, 1971.

148. Mathisen DJ, Jensik RJ, Faber LP, et al: Survival following resection for second and third primary lung cancers. J Thorac Cardiovasc Surg 88:502, 1984.

149. Miller RR, Nelems B, Evans KG, et al: Glandular neoplasia of the lung: A proposed analogy to colonic tumors. Cancer 61:1009, 1988.

150. Watanabe Y, Shimizu J, Oda M, et al: Proposals regarding some deficiencies in the new international staging system for non–small cell lung cancer. Jpn J Clin Oncol 21(3):160–168, 1991.

151. Shields TW: Multiple primary bronchial carcinomas. Ann Thorac Surg 27:1, 1979.

152. Van Bodegom PC, Wagenaar SS, Corrin B, et al: Second primary lung cancer: Importance of long term follow up. Thorax 44:788, 1989.

153. Green N, Kern W: The clinical course and treatment results of patients with postresection locally recurrent lung cancer. Cancer 42:2478, 1978.

154. Parker EF, Martini N, Flehinger BJ, et al: Prospective study of 445 lung carcinomas with mediastinal lymph node metastases. J Thorac Cardiovasc Surg 80:49, 1980.

155. Tandon RK: The significance of pleural effusions associated with bronchial carcinoma. Br J Dis Chest 60:49, 1966.

156. Rocmans P: Surgery in non–small cell lung cancer. J Belge Radiol 68:217, 1985.

157. Thomas PA, Piantadosi S, Mountain CF: Should subcarinal lymph nodes be routinely examined in patients with non–small lung cancer? J Thorac Cardiovasc Surg 95:883, 1988.

158. Bergh NP, Schersten T: Bronchogenic carcinoma: A follow-up study of a surgically treated series with special reference to the prognostic significance of lymph node metastases. Acta Chir Scand 347(suppl):1–42, 1965.

159. Larsson S: Pretreatment classification and staging of bronchogenic carcinoma. Scand J Thorac Cardiovasc Surg Suppl 10:1, 1973.

160. Minna JD, Pass H, Glatstein E, et al: Cancer of the lung. In DeVita VT, Hellman S, Rosenberg SA (eds): Cancer: Principles and Practice of Oncology. 3rd Ed. Philadelphia, J.B. Lippincott, 1989, pp 591–636.

161. Aisner J, Whitley NO: Staging of small cell lung cancer: Do we need a new staging system? Lung Cancer 5:163, 1989.

162. Zelen M: Keynote address on biostatistics and data retrieval. Cancer Chemother Rep 4(2)(part 3):31, 1973.

163. Chauvin F, Trillet V, Court-Fortune I, et al: Pretreatment staging evaluation in small cell lung carcinoma: A new approach to medical decision making. Chest 102:497, 1992.

164. Ginsberg RJ: Operation for small cell lung cancer—Where are we? Ann Thorac Surg 49:692, 1990.

165. Shepherd FA, Ginsberg RJ, Feld R, et al: Surgical treatment for limited small-cell lung cancer. J Thorac Cardiovasc Surg 101(3):385–393, 1991.

166. Muller LC, Salzer GM, Huber H, et al: Multimodal therapy of small cell lung cancer in TNM stages I through IIIa. Ann Thorac Surg 54:493, 1992.

167. Blaha HM, Weber N, Hellmann A: Bronchioloalveolar carcinoma. In Delarue NC, Eschapasse H (eds): International Trends in General Thoracic Surgery. Philadelphia, W.B. Saunders, 1985, pp 249–264.

7 PREOPERATIVE ASSESSMENT OF PATIENTS UNDERGOING LUNG RESECTION FOR CANCER

Jorge A. Wernly and Tom R. DeMeester

Analysis of the complications and deaths occurring after lung resection for cancer permits the identification of the following four incremental risk factors that are major predictors of postoperative outcome: age, status of the respiratory system, presence of cardiovascular disease, and the extent of resection. These risk factors, frequently interacting with each other, are of paramount importance in guiding the surgeon's selection of the appropriate procedure and in predicting patient survival after surgery. Further, preoperative assessment permits the identification of reversible abnormalities, which, if controlled perioperatively, can decrease the incidence of postoperative complications or death. In this regard, it establishes priorities for perioperative management. It is pointless to identify high-risk patients unless there is an opportunity to select the level of care delivered and the availability of high-quality perioperative management.

INCREMENTAL RISK FACTORS IN PATIENTS

Older age[1-4]; the presence of respiratory disease, restricted pulmonary function, or both[3, 5-8]; the presence of cardiovascular disease[1, 4, 9]; the need for pneumonectomy[1-3, 10]; and several general risk factors have been identified as incremental risk factors for pulmonary resections. The vast majority of the complications and nearly all the postoperative deaths after lung resection for cancer are cardiorespiratory in nature.[1, 3, 8, 10] Complications affecting other systems are few.

Age

For patients with a normal cardiorespiratory system, understanding the effect of age on the surgical risk is one of the most important aspects of the preoperative assessment. Advancing age is associated with decreased overall physiologic function of different systems, regardless of the clinical presence or absence of associated diseases. Aging causes a progressive decrease in maximum heart rate, oxygen consumption, stroke output, and overall cardiovascular performance.[11] The effects of aging on pulmonary function include decreases in static lung volumes, maximal expiratory flow, and activities of upper airway reflexes.[12] An increase in closing volume and a reduction in strength of the respiratory muscles also occurs, and favors the development of postoperative atelectasis. This overall reduction of cardiopulmonary function is associated with increased operative morbidity and mortality. A study of 15,930 surgical patients showed a steady increase in mortality with advancing age, and the rate climbed precipitously for patients over the age of 75. Risks at 90 to 94 years of age were nearly twice those at 75 to 84, which, in turn, were nearly twice those of 0 to 69 years.[13] Despite these findings, age per se is not a contraindication to operation. Although on one hand, several series have demonstrated that patients older than 70 years of age have a higher incidence of operative mortality after lung resection, other studies have shown that better patient selection, improved preoperative preparation, and advances in critical care have resulted in a decreased operative risk for carefully selected elderly patients.[2, 3, 8]

Presence of Respiratory Disease and Abnormal Pulmonary Function

The case against *smoking* is clear. Smokers, as a group, are more likely to have increased respiratory secretions and decreased ability to clear them, a higher prevalence of chronic lung disease, and reduced performance on pulmonary function testing.[12, 14] Postoperatively, smokers have an increased risk of atelectasis, pneumonia, and respiratory complications.[12, 15]

It is generally accepted that patients with *acute or chronic pre-existing respiratory diseases* have an increased incidence of postoperative pulmonary complications and death following upper abdominal or thoracic surgery.[5, 7, 8, 16] Fowkes and colleagues, reviewing a large number of patients undergoing general anesthesia, found that a history of chronic lung disease increased the postoperative mortality rate from all causes almost tenfold in patients under 45 years of age but less markedly in those over 65 years of age.[17] In other series, the risk of respiratory disease in ages over 65 years of age appeared to be additive.[16]

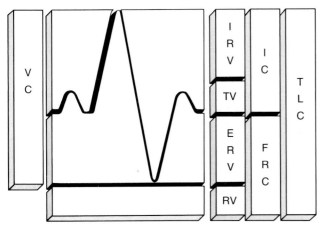

FIGURE 7–1. The volumes and capacities of the lung. The vital capacity (VC) includes the inspiratory (IRV) and expiratory (ERV) reserve volumes. Inspiratory capacity (IC) includes tidal volume (TV) and IRV. The functional residual capacity (FRC) includes the residual volume (RV) and the ERV. Total lung capacity (TLC) includes both VC and RV. (From Weber KT, Janicki JS: Cardiopulmonary Exercise Testing. Philadelphia, W.B. Saunders, 1986.)

A number of studies of patients undergoing operations for lung cancer showed that postoperative morbidity and mortality are correlated with preoperative *abnormal pulmonary function.*[5, 7, 18–22] Most authors agree that simple spirometry can identify patients who are at increased risk for postoperative morbidity and mortality owing to pulmonary complications. Standard spirometric nomenclature is provided in Figure 7–1. As early as 1955, Gaensler and colleagues used spirometry to identify patients at high risk of developing complications. Although a positive statistical association has been demonstrated between the frequency of postoperative complications and preoperative functional abnormalities, no single pulmonary function test exists that can absolutely contraindicate surgery.[23] Enough variation has been demonstrated in the so-called prohibitive values that, as a concept, the pursuit of an isolated measure that would contraindicate surgery is no longer warranted. Pulmonary function test (PFT) criteria from the literature suggesting increased surgical risk are listed in Table 7–1.

Presence of Cardiovascular Disease

The operative risk of pulmonary resection is clearly increased in patients with preoperative cardiovascular disease.[4, 9, 24] Such patients are five times more likely to suffer postoperative mortality[1] and twice as likely to develop major complications.[8]

Significant *coronary disease* is found frequently in a lung cancer population. The presence of ischemic heart disease has been reported to correlate with an increased risk of infarction and death following noncardiac operations.[4, 24–27] Unstable angina appears to be of grave prognostic significance,[10] whereas stable angina appears to be much less dangerous; some studies suggest that it is an unimportant risk factor.[4]

Three classic studies have shown that a major non-

TABLE 7–1. Interpretation of Spirometry in Relation to Operative Risk

	High Risk	Moderate Risk	Low Risk
VC[7, 18]	<1.8 L	1.8–3.0 L	>3.0 L
FEV$_1$[7, 10]	<1.2 L	1.2–2.0 L	>2.0 L
FEV$_1$ (% Predicted)[9, 23, 53]	<35%	35–70%	>70%
MBC[7]	<28 L/min	30–80 L/min	>80 L/min
MBC (% Predicted)[21]	<50%	>50%	

cardiac surgical procedure performed after a *recent myocardial infarction* is associated with a significantly increased incidence of perioperative infarction (Fig. 7–2).[25, 27] The shorter the interval between the previous myocardial infarction and operation, the greater the risk. Tarhan and colleagues reported that patients on whom surgery was performed within 3 months of the infarction had a 37% reinfarction rate.[26] The incidence of reinfarction dropped to 16% within 3 to 6 months and stabilized at 5% after 6 months. Recurrent infarction after a major operation is more serious and lethal than an isolated myocardial infarction. A mortality rate from such a reinfarction is reported to be 50% to 70% in such patients,[25–27] and this rate has been confirmed in a more recent review.[28]

It should be noted that a history of an *old myocardial infarction* (occurring more than 6 months before the op-

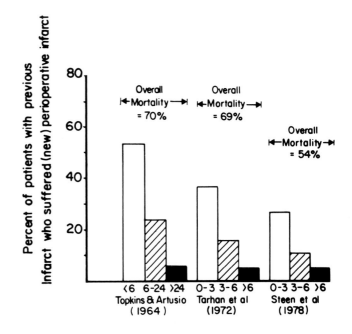

FIGURE 7–2. The influence of a recent myocardial infarction on the postoperative rate of myocardial infarction following noncardiac surgery. (Reproduced with permission from Salem DN, Homas DC, Isner JM: Management of cardiac disease in the general surgical patient. *In* Harvey WP [ed]: Current Problems in Cardiology, Vol. V, No. 2. Copyright © 1980 by Year Book Medical Publishers, Inc., Chicago.)

eration) is also associated with an increased cardiac risk. Tarhan and colleagues found that the chances of a postoperative infarction rose from 0.13% to 5% when a history of an old infarction was present.[26] Another study showed a threefold increase in all types of cardiovascular complications.[29]

Cardiac arrhythmias are frequently discovered during preoperative evaluation. The presence of frequent premature ventricular contractions correlates with increased perioperative complications and death.[2, 4, 5] Although many patients with premature contractions died for reasons other than ventricular arrhythmias, the premature ventricular contractions should be considered important because they can be a marker for more severe heart disease.[4, 24]

Clinical evidence of *heart failure* suggests that cardiac reserve is very limited and an increased incidence of postoperative complications is to be expected in such patients.[4] A recent report has assessed the operative mortality and cardiac morbidity following noncardiac operations in a population of patients in whom the existence of coronary disease had been defined by cardiac catheterization.[30] The analysis was performed on a data base of 1600 patients from the Coronary Artery Surgery Study (CASS) registry who underwent noncardiac operations. The study showed that signs and symptoms of congestive heart failure, specifically, angiographic evidence of *left ventricular dysfunction*, were strong prognostic indicators of increased surgical risk.

These findings seem to imply that the degree of ventricular impairment[30] and the severity of ventricular arrhythmias[2, 4, 5] produced by the myocardial infarction are the significant factors in relation to the surgical risk, rather than simply the history of a previous infarction or other symptoms of ischemic heart disease.

Further, *hypertension* has been identified as a significant risk factor in relationship to both surgical morbidity and mortality.[30] Although hypertension was not recognized as an independent risk factor in the classic review of Goldman and colleagues,[4] other investigators[27, 29] have confirmed the observation that patients with hypertension do experience increased surgical morbidity and mortality. Steen and colleagues showed that if the preoperative diagnosis of hypertension was made, the incidence of perioperative myocardial infarction was approximately twice that in patients without hypertension.[27]

Limited available evidence suggests that *peripheral vascular disease* does not add significantly to the postoperative risk.[4] The presence of *cerebrovascular disease,* on the other hand, seems to be correlated with an increase in postoperative cardiovascular complications and, in some studies, has been identified as an independent predictor of cardiovascular risk.[29] Contrary to common belief, there appears to be *no* evidence that patients undergoing noncardiac surgery with a history of an old cerebrovascular accident have a higher risk of postoperative stroke.[14] It is also generally accepted that the presence of an asymptomatic carotid bruit does not increase the risk of a postoperative stroke.[31]

Extent of Resection

Although no particular difference in the morbidity or mortality rates exists between lobectomy and lesser resections,[2, 3] both rates are significantly increased in patients undergoing pneumonectomy.[2, 3, 8, 32] Furthermore, the combination of performing a pneumonectomy in an older patient with cardiopulmonary disease results in significantly higher rates of operative morbidity and mortality than for pneumonectomy alone. This factor should be taken into account when recommending surgical treatment to older patients.[1, 3]

General Risk Factors

Besides age, several other general risk factors are known to increase the surgical risk.

Nutrition. The nutritional status of the patient is important in determining the outcome of surgery. Poor nutrition affects the host's resistance and the rate at which anastomoses and wounds are healed.[32, 33] Further, several clinical studies have found a direct relationship between hypoalbuminemia and the incidence of respiratory complications and survival after surgery.[32, 34]

Obesity. This condition constitutes a major general risk factor for increased postoperative complications.[12] Population studies have demonstrated that obese patients show a decrease in functional reserve capacity (FRC) and residual volume (RV), proportional to their weight and are particularly prone to develop basilar atelectasis and infections.[12, 19]

Other Associated Conditions. Conditions that directly affect pulmonary function, such as thoracic deformities and neuromuscular diseases, as well as systemic diseases, such as diabetes and renal insufficiency, adversely affect the postoperative course.[12, 14] Careful medical evaluation of these associated problems should be performed in an attempt to correct potentially reversible abnormalities.

COMMON PRE-EXISTING PHYSIOLOGIC DISTURBANCES OF THE RESPIRATORY SYSTEM

An understanding of some of the common physiologic disturbances of the respiratory apparatus that contribute to respiratory insufficiency is basic to the assessment of the respiratory system and is of paramount importance in the interpretation of pulmonary function data. The error of deciding that a patient cannot undergo an operation simply on the basis of test results must be avoided. Some of the common disturbances are as follows:

1. Increased pulmonary arterial venous shunting.
2. Increased pulmonary dead space.
3. Increased work of breathing.

4. Decreased oxygen transport in the blood.
5. Decreased resistance to infection.

Increased Pulmonary Arterial Venous Shunting. Pulmonary shunting is defined as that part of the cardiac output that does not participate in the pulmonary gas exchange and is returned, nonoxygenated, to the left side of the heart as a venous admixture to the arterial blood. A fixed anatomic shunt and an intrapulmonary shunt, which may be caused by atelectasis, uneven distribution of ventilation and perfusion, or a diffusion block, contribute to the total pulmonary shunting. The anatomic shunt caused by the drainage of the bronchial veins into the pulmonary veins is normally 2% of the cardiac output. Anatomic shunts cause hypoxemia only in the presence of abnormal communications between the pulmonary arteries and veins or an intracardiac right-to-left shunt.

Atelectasis. Atelectasis resulting from bronchial occlusion produces a situation in which a portion of the lung is perfused but not ventilated, causing hypoxemia. This situation is only of temporary importance because perfusion of the atelectatic area of the lung also decreases. In most chronic situations, the atelectasis acts as a silent pulmonary unit, with neither ventilation nor perfusion occurring.

Uneven Distribution of Ventilation and Perfusion. This is the mechanism most frequently found to produce intrapulmonary shunting. Under these conditions, a portion of the lung is ventilated less than it is perfused. This results in a decrease in the partial pressure of oxygen and an increase in the partial pressure of carbon dioxide within the alveoli and the capillary blood. Local hypercapnia is corrected by the increase of alveolar ventilation in the unaffected lung. However, because of the flattened configuration of the upper portion of the oxygen hemoglobin dissociation curve, hyperventilation of the unaffected lung does not compensate for hypoxemia. Uneven ventilation can be a source of pulmonary shunting only when the patient is breathing room air, and it is usually obliterated when the patient is breathing 100% oxygen. Measuring a pulmonary shunt while the patient is breathing 100% oxygen and room air is the only way of distinguishing the contribution made to shunting by uneven distribution of ventilation and perfusion.

Increased Lung Water. Any process that increases lung water impairs oxygenation. Evidence suggests that the initial mechanisms of hypoxia found in pulmonary edema do not involve impaired diffusion of gases per se. It appears that perialveolar interstitial edema acutely reduces FRC and that peribronchiolar edema increases closing volume (CV).[35, 36] These processes create ventilation perfusion abnormalities with increased shunting rather than imposing a barrier to diffusion.

Diffusion Block. If the alveolar oxygen tension remains between 80 and 100 mm Hg, diffusion block is rarely a cause of increased shunting. However, one factor that affects diffusion is the time allowed for diffusion to take place. Although it is apparent that a normal lung at sea level has sufficient time to carry out the diffusion of oxygen, it has become apparent that the time allowed for diffusion may be a factor in producing pulmonary shunt in the following circumstances: when the ambient oxygen tension is low, such as at an altitude of 1000 feet or more above sea level; when the lung is not uniform in structure, owing to destruction from disease processes leading to abnormal transit times in some part of the capillary bed; or when diffuse fibrosis results in a decreased capillary alveolar interface at which O_2 diffusion takes place.

If a patient has a sizable shunt present preoperatively, attempts should be made to determine the cause and location of the shunt. In some cases, the mechanisms of the shunt can be modified preoperatively. In others, the shunt is due to a localized disease process in the lung that is planned to be removed when the shunt cannot be corrected preoperatively or is not going to be affected by the operation. Then careful assessment of the magnitude of the shunt should be determined before proceeding with the operation.

Increased Pulmonary Dead Space. Only that portion of the ventilation that enters the perfused alveoli is effective in delivering oxygen to the blood. A part of each breath remains within the upper airway and tracheobronchial tree and does not reach the gas-exchanging surface of the alveoli. An increase in dead space is produced by several mechanisms. The most classic example is an acute pulmonary embolus. Other causes are pulmonary artery occlusion secondary to carcinoma or diffuse chronic fibrosis of the lung with a resulting decrease in perfusion while ventilation is maintained. As a result of increased dead space, either the tidal volume or the respiratory frequency must be increased in order to maintain adequate alveolar ventilation. This increase in respiratory effort reduces pulmonary reserve, resulting in dyspnea and fatigue.

Patients who are expected to have surgery to remove areas of the lung that are ventilated but are not being perfused will experience a reduction in their dead space with a resultant increase in the efficiency of the respiratory function. On the other hand, if the proposed operation does not decrease the abnormal amount of dead space present, one can expect that the borderline patients will be unable to tolerate additional respiratory effort placed on them as a result of the operation.

Increased Work of Breathing. Assessment of the mechanics of ventilation is an important aspect of the preoperative evaluation of pulmonary function. Ventilation requires an intact neuromuscular system. Factors that disrupt the mechanical function of the chest are listed in Table 7–2. The presence of chronic obstructive pulmonary disease (COPD) is the most significant factor predisposing patients to postoperative respiratory complications.[12, 37] The defective mechanism in COPD is a diffuse increase in airway resistance that greatly increases the work of breathing. This pathologic process accounts for the following

TABLE 7–2. Factors That Impair Ventilation

Restriction of Lung	Obstruction to Flow
Entrapped lung	COPD—asthma
Pulmonary edema	Stenosis
Pulmonary fibrosis	Aspiration
Surfactant failure	Trauma
Mechanical Uncoupling	Increased Work of Breathing
Effusion	Pregnancy
Hemorrhage	Ascites
Pneumothorax	Obesity
Muscular Weakness	Structural Defects
Malnutrition—cachexia	Scoliosis
Deconditioning of muscles	Kyphosis
Myasthenia—paralysis	Flail chest

two alterations of the respiratory system in the postoperative period that contribute directly to operative morbidity and mortality: (1) an ineffective cough to clear secretions and (2) respiratory fatigue, secondary to increased work of respiration.

A second, and less important, type of mechanical impairment to ventilation is restrictive lung disease. In patients with this impairment, the inspiratory volume is decreased owing to muscular weakness, the presence of interstitial fibrosis secondary to interstitial disease or radiation, or direct compression of the lungs by an extrapulmonary neoplasm or a restrictive fibrous pleural peel. Restrictive pulmonary disease, unless very severe, does not greatly increase the work of breathing and therefore is rarely disabling. Patients with this condition usually do not have problems after surgery, primarily because their cough is adequate. It should be recognized, however, that if restriction is severe, for example in patients with diffuse interstitial fibrosis, further loss of pulmonary tissue must be avoided or the loss in the pulmonary vascular bed already compromised by the restrictive disease may lead to acute or subacute pulmonary hypertension and right-sided heart failure.

Decreased Oxygen Transport in the Blood. Normally, 97% of the oxygen transported from the lungs to the tissues is carried in combination with hemoglobin in the red blood cells, and the remaining 3% is carried in the dissolved state in the water of the plasma and cells. Different conditions that reduce oxygen transport from the lungs to the tissues include anemia; carbon monoxide poisoning, in which a large proportion of the hemoglobin becomes unable to transport oxygen; and decreased blood flow to the tissues, as in shock. Obviously, all these abnormalities should be corrected before the preoperative evaluation is completed.

Decreased Resistance to Infection. Pulmonary defense mechanisms protect the lung against inhaled particulate matter and microorganisms. Cough is a primary function defense for clearance of the upper airways, whereas the distal airways and the alveoli depend on the mucociliary system, alveolar macro-

phages, and lymphatic drainage.[38, 39] These mechanisms can be impaired preoperatively from local factors such as aspiration, inhalation injury, radiation, contusion, and atelectasis or from systemic processes such as steroid therapy, autoimmune disorders, or acquired immune deficiency syndrome. Particularly interesting is the observation that recent respiratory viral infection can depress bacteria clearance from the lung for several weeks.[39]

THE SURGICAL PROCEDURE: RISK FACTORS DEPENDENT ON THE NATURE, CONDUCT, AND EXTENT OF THE OPERATION

Normal Alterations of Pulmonary Function in the Postoperative Period

In addition to the loss of pulmonary function, which occurs as a direct consequence of the lung resection, there are identifiable postoperative changes that affect pulmonary function after any surgery and that can be seen in otherwise normal patients.[12, 15] There are three main areas in which these changes in pulmonary function occur: (1) lung volumes and ventilatory patterns, (2) gas exchange, and (3) pulmonary defense mechanisms.

Lung Volumes and Ventilatory Patterns. The most significant effect of an operation on respiratory function is reduced ventilation, which is caused by pain, instability of the chest wall, mediastinal shift, and a decrease in diaphragmatic function that seems to have a neuroreflex basis rather than local, irritative causes.[40] The tidal volume, vital capacity (VC), FEV_1, RV, and FRC usually fall between 35% to 50% of preoperative values in the immediate postoperative period and gradually return to normal over the next 10 days (Fig. 7–3).[12, 15, 41] The loss in VC and tidal volume is compensated by an increase in respiratory rate, which causes a decrease in the efficiency of ventilation owing to the fact that the same amount of dead space must be ventilated, or in other words, the ratio of VC or tidal volume to dead space has increased. Of extreme importance in this regard are the decreases in FRC and RV that occur because their loss promotes postoperative airway closure and the development of atelectasis.[12]

These changes in static lung volumes are associated with an abnormal pattern of ventilation. Normal adults breathe with a tidal volume that alternates with spontaneous deep breaths every 5 to 10 minutes.[42, 43] This normal breathing pattern disappears during the early phase of the postoperative period after abdominal and thoracic surgery. It has been shown that abolition of normal rhythmic hyperinflation (sighing) after the operation, combined with the decrease in FRC, leads to closure of airways and gradual collapse of alveoli in dependent lung areas.[42, 43]

Gas Exchange. Arterial hypoxemia is a common

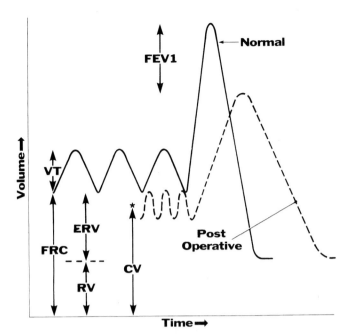

FIGURE 7–3. Postoperative changes in pulmonary function. VT = Tidal volume. FRC = Functional residual capacity. ERV = Expiratory reserve volume. RV = Residual volume. CV = Closing volume. FEV$_1$ = Forced expiratory volume in first second. See text for explanation. (Modified from Pett SB, Wernly JA: Respiratory function in surgical patients. *In* Nyhus LM [ed]: Surgery Annual. East Norwalk, Appleton-Crofts, 1988.)

finding in the immediate postoperative period.[37, 44, 45] This condition is a function of the effects of position, immobilization, and changes in the ventilatory pattern, leading to an abnormal relationship between ventilation and perfusion and to the development of diffuse microatelectasis.[46]

Pulmonary Defense Mechanisms. All the mechanisms that protect the lung against inhaled particulate matter and microorganisms are altered in the postoperative period. A reduction in the cough reflex due to combined effects of anesthesia and sedation impairs the clearance of the upper airway.[12] The mucociliary system, alveolar macrophages, and lymphatic drainage have been shown to be depressed after the operation.[38]

The extent and duration of these postoperative changes in pulmonary function are frequently related to the magnitude of the operative procedure. In general, all these alterations reach their maximum level 48 to 72 hours after the operation and usually return to normal within 7 days[12, 41, 45, 47] without ever being clinically apparent. In some patients, however, these changes progress.

Risk Factors Dependent on the Conduct of the Procedure

Although the preoperative status of the patient sets the stage, it is often the conduct of the surgical procedure that determines who will actually suffer respiratory complications. Anesthetic management is ex-

tremely important. During general anesthesia, all protective reflexes are lost, and the patient's ability to directly communicate distress is largely abolished. Every potential mechanism of respiratory embarrassment must be considered during the operation. Monitoring capabilities should be used liberally and should include end tidal CO_2, in-line anesthetics gas analysis, pulse oximeters, and pulmonary and radial arterial catheters. Fluid management during surgery has a significant impact on respiratory function. The probability of adult respiratory distress syndrome is related to the quantity of blood products administered. Pulmonary edema is related to the volume of fluid administered.[48] Fluid management based on pulmonary capillary wedge pressure may be difficult in patients intraoperatively while receiving single lung anesthesia or postoperatively after a pneumonectomy because inflation of a Swan-Ganz balloon in the wedge position may acutely decrease cardiac output by impeding blood flow from the right ventricle.[49]

Particularly after a pneumonectomy, the remaining lung should be treated with all possible care. Attention should be directed to the control of secretions and prevention of aspiration. The use of double-lumen endotracheal intubation and single lung anesthesia makes the resection easier, avoids retraction on the remaining lung when lobectomy is performed, and permits the use of a smaller incision.[37, 50] It is important to avoid periods of ventilation at a low volume, which can cause airway closure with the subsequent need for reopening, leading to alveolar damage and surfactant depletion.[50]

Risk Factors Dependent on the Extent of the Operation

Pulmonary Function Loss Due to the Pulmonary Resection. In order to refine our ability to determine which patients with poor pulmonary function can safely undergo resection, we must be able to predict accurately the loss of pulmonary function, if any, that will be caused by the resection. Radionuclide ventilation and perfusion lung scans permit accurate prediction regarding pulmonary function after pneumonectomy or lobectomy by combining the results of the spirometry with the quantitative measurement of differential function. The lung function that is predicted to remain is determined by multiplying the preoperative spirometry data by the percentage of perfusion, ventilation, or both in the remaining lung. Several studies have demonstrated that this method can be used to predict postoperative forced vital capacity (FVC), FEV$_1$, diffusing capacity of the lungs for carbon dioxide (DL$_{CO}$), and even maximal breathing capacity (MBC) with a high degree of accuracy.[18, 22, 51–53]

The following theoretical case provides an example of the use of lung scans to calculate the lung function loss that will result from a proposed resection: The chest radiograph showed a mass in the right upper lobe that was demonstrated by bronchoscopy and biopsy to be a squamous cell carcinoma. The overall FEV$_1$ was 1.3 L. The perfusion scan showed that 45%

of the function was in the right lung, but there was virtually no function in the upper lobe. It is unlikely that resection of the right upper lobe in this patient will significantly change his measured preoperative lung function.

Calculation of Pulmonary Function After Pneumonectomy. The postoperative FEV_1 after pneumonectomy can be calculated from the preoperative FEV_1 value and the percentage of ventilation and/or perfusion in the remaining lung according to the following equation:

Postop FEV_1 = preop FEV_1 × % of function in the remaining lung.

Although we recommend the use of the perfusion value, in our experience, no significant difference between the accuracy of the ventilation or perfusion values to predict postoperative FEV_1 was observed.[53] The following example illustrates the application of this simple formula, using the values of our hypothetical patient whose tumor at operation required a pneumonectomy for removal:

Postop FEV_1 = 1.3 L × 0.55 = 0.65 L

Calculation of Pulmonary Function After Lobectomy. The remaining function after a lobectomy can be calculated by two different methods. The first method, which was described by Ali and associates,[51] is based on the function of the affected lung from which the lobe is to be removed and is expressed by the following equation:

Expected loss of function = preop FEV_1 × number of segments in the lobe to be resected ÷ total number of segments of that lung × % of function of the affected lung.

The postoperative function = preop FEV_1 − the expected loss of function.

For example, using the values of our hypothetical patient just discussed, the loss of function after lobectomy is calculated as follows:

Expected loss of function = 1.3 L × 3/10 × 0.45 = 0.17 L.

Postoperative function = 1.3 L − 0.17 L = 1.13 L.

The second method that we have described is based on the regional function of the lobe to be resected, as estimated from a direct reading of the scans.[53] The function of the affected lobe is scored as follows: normal—1.0, mild impairment—0.75, moderate impairment—0.5, severe impairment—0.25, and absent—0. For the purpose of reading the scans, the lungs are divided into functional segments, which differ slightly from the anatomic segments. There are 10 functional segments in the right lung (upper lobe, three; middle lobe, two; lower lobe, five) and nine in

the left lung (upper lobe, five; lower lobe, four), resulting in a total of 19 segments for the two lungs. The contribution of the lobe to the overall pulmonary function is expressed by the following equation:

Expected loss of function = preop FEV_1 × number of segments to be resected ÷ total number of segments (both lungs) × The score for the regional function of the lobe to be resected.

For example, the expected loss of function after the resection of a *normal* right upper lobe would be as follows:

Expected loss of function = 1.3 L × 3/19 × 1.0 = 0.20 L

However, in the hypothetical patient described earlier, the expected loss of function after the resection of a *severely impaired* lobe would be the following:

Expected loss of function = 1.3 L × 3/19 × 0.25 = 0.05 L

Based on these methodologies for the predictions of postoperative pulmonary function and using an FEV_1 value of 0.8 L or greater as the acceptable level of postoperative function favoring resection, one would conclude that a lobectomy in this patient would be very well tolerated, whereas a pneumonectomy would be associated with a great operative risk and a high likelihood of postoperative chronic respiratory insufficiency. It is important, however, to use normal values adjusted for body size, sex, and age rather than absolute numbers in determining the lower limits of predicted FEV_1 values to decide on the patient's operability.[50] (See the section entitled Evaluation of the Respiratory System in this chapter.)

The accuracy of such calculation has been established by a number of studies[18, 51, 52] and confirmed by our own experience.[53] The predictive value of the radionuclide scans was analyzed in 85 patients undergoing lung resection for tumor. Our results showed that calculations based on quantitative perfusion were as accurate as those based on ventilation or combined ventilation and perfusion values (Fig. 7–4). Although the difference was not statistically significant, the perfusion scan seemed to be a slightly better predictor.[53] The greater accuracy of the perfusion scan as a predictor of postoperative function was also confirmed in the group of patients who had a significant disparity in the degree of ventilation and perfusion of the lung bearing the tumor. It was our conclusion that "the simple quantitative perfusion scan is the best method of predicting postoperative function and that its accuracy was not augmented by the ventilation study."[53] These observations support previous experience showing that oxygen uptake of a lung measured by bronchospirometry correlates better with the results of perfusion radionuclide studies than with ventilation values.[54]

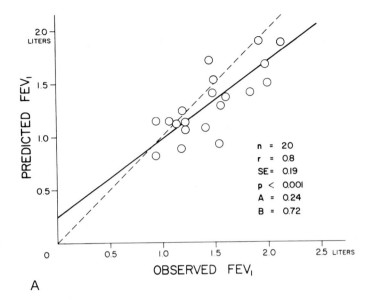

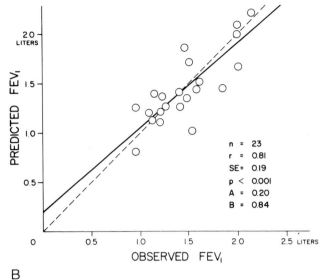

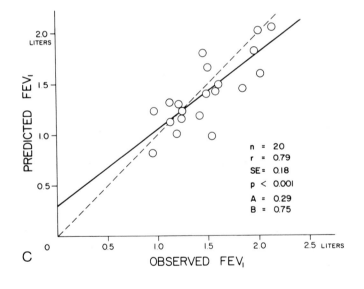

FIGURE 7–4. *A, B, C,* Correlation between predicted postpneumonectomy FEV_1 and observed FEV_1 after pneumonectomy. *Open circles* = Individual patient values. *Solid straight line* = Derived line of regression from the individual values. *Broken line* = Line of identity. n = Number of patients. r = Coefficient of correlation. SE = Standard error of the estimate. p = Level of significance. A = Intercept. B = Slope. (From Wernly JA, DeMeester TR, Krichner PT, et al: Clinical value of qualitative ventilation perfusion lung scans in the surgical management of bronchogenic carcinoma. J Thorac Cardiovasc Surg 80:533–543, 1980.)

Postoperative function after lobectomy can be accurately calculated from the ventilation and perfusion scans by assessment of the unilateral function of the tumor-bearing lung[51] or the regional pulmonary function of the affected lobe.[53] Although we postulated that assessment of the regional pulmonary function of the involved lobe permitted a more accurate prediction,[53] our study of 45 patients undergoing lobectomy showed that postoperative function could be effectively calculated by either of these two methods, with an error of less than 10% (Fig. 7–5).

CONCOMITANT CARDIAC AND PULMONARY OPERATIONS: THE RATIONALE, INDICATIONS, AND RISKS OF COMBINED PROCEDURES

The presence of ischemic heart disease correlates with an increased risk of perioperative cardiac complications and death following noncardiac operations.[1, 4, 18, 24, 26, 30] Identification of significant coronary disease by angiography constitutes an incremental risk factor as

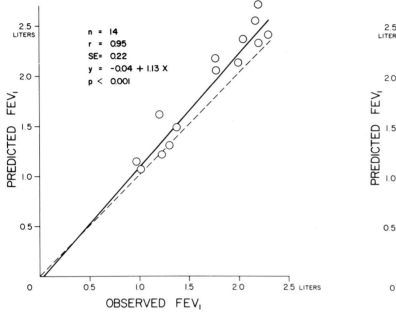

POST OP FEV₁ PREDICTED FROM PERFUSION
SCAN AFTER LOBECTOMY

BASED ON REGIONAL PULMONARY FUNCTION

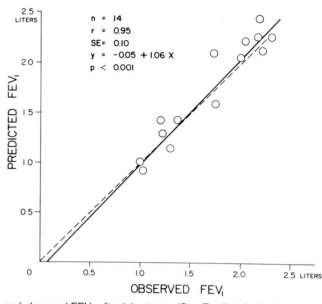

POST OP FEV₁ PREDICTED FROM PERFUSION
SCAN AFTER LOBECTOMY

BASED ON UNILATERAL PULMONARY FUNCTION

FIGURE 7–5. *A, B,* Correlation between predicted postoperative FEV₁ and observed FEV₁ after lobectomy. (See Fig. 7–4 for key.)

great as the occurrence of a previous myocardial infarction.[55] If significant left main coronary artery stenosis, severe triple vessel disease or critical narrowing in dominant vessels is found in a patient with lung cancer, myocardial revascularization should be performed prior to or concurrent with pulmonary resection.[30, 37, 55] Data from the CASS registry of patients undergoing noncardiac operations support the concept that myocardial revascularization should be performed prior to a major noncardiac operation on patients with severe coronary artery disease, particularly when impaired ventricular function exists.[30]

The decision to perform concomitant cardiac and pulmonary procedures should be individualized after a careful assessment. Traditionally, there has been general reluctance to perform a pulmonary resection at the time of a cardiac operation because of potential bleeding related to heparinization and limited exposure through the median sternotomy. Definitive correction of both diseases at one operation without the need for a second procedure is preferred in selected patients. Unfortunately, a review of the literature reveals that only a few groups of patients have been treated with a combined approach, and firm conclusions cannot be reached.[56–59] Some authors have recommended performing the lung resection on cardiopulmonary bypass while the lungs are deflated and the heart is decompressed. This improves the exposure and permits resections of areas otherwise not easily approached.[60]

In our opinion, pulmonary resection should not be performed during anticoagulation because of the in-

creased risk of bleeding.[59] In favorable anatomic situations, if the tumor can be excised by a wedge resection or a lobectomy, the resection should be performed at the completion of the open heart procedure, if the patient is stable with good cardiac function and hemostasis after heparin reversal is satisfactory. The patient should be anesthetized using a double-lumen tube because it facilitates the lung resection through a median sternotomy. For many patients who have extensive pleural adhesions tumors with parietal fixation, tumors localized in the left lower lobe, or central tumors requiring pneumonectomy for removal, the pulmonary resection should be delayed because the combined procedure may increase the operative risk.[61] For these patients, in our opinion, a delay of 4 to 6 weeks is advisable.[37] The operative risk of the lung resection at this time is similar to that of patients without coronary artery disease.[29, 55]

Although several series suggest that combined cardiac operations and adequate pulmonary resections can safely be performed in selected patients, there are no data to assess the long-term survival of these patients. The possibility that cardiopulmonary bypass has a transient effect on the immune system that could have an adverse impact on long-term survival needs to be addressed in the future. Some series have reported a disquieting short survival after combined procedures performed during bypass.[60]

A different but highly debatable and frequently occurring question pertains to the indication for resection of nodules of unknown etiology at the time of cardiac operations.[59] If the lesion is benign, the need for a second operation is eliminated with a simultaneous excision. If the lesion proves to be malignant, one has the option of performing a concomitant or delayed definitive resection. Some authors have recommended that undiagnosed pulmonary nodules not be resected at the time of a cardiac operation because of the potential risk of disseminating infections from infectious granulomas or fungal infiltrates while the patient is temporarily immunologically compromised.[37] Other reports have shown that safe excision of peripheral lesions can be performed at the time of a cardiac operation in carefully selected patients.[56–59] It should be remembered that these recommendations are based on data and experience obtained before the advent of video-assisted thoracic surgery. Although the role of video-assisted thoracic surgery in this setting has not been completely defined, there is no doubt that this less stressful method of diagnosis for pulmonary nodules and infiltrates, mediastinal masses, and pleural effusions will affect our approach to the patient who requires a combined procedure.

PREOPERATIVE EVALUATION

General Evaluation

The patient undergoing lung resection requires a detailed history, a thorough physical examination, routine laboratory studies, and a chest x-ray examination. This initial evaluation permits the identification of symptoms, signs, and abnormalities that will direct the clinician to a more precise and objective assessment of other organ systems. Several general risk factors that are known to increase surgical risk should be assessed, including age, nutritional status, use of alcohol, and other pathologic conditions, such as diabetes and renal disease.

Evaluation of the Cardiovascular System

The assessment of the cardiovascular system rests on the identification of recognized cardiac risk factors. This requires a careful history and physical examination to evaluate the presence of angina, heart failure, previous myocardial infarction, serious cardiac arrhythmias or conduction abnormalities, valvular heart disease, systemic hypertension, and significant peripheral arterial disease.[9]

Theoretically, individual risk factors associated with an adverse postoperative outcome can be combined into a single multivariate index of risk. This has a more predictive power than any of the factors taken alone. In 1977, Goldman and associates introduced the Cardiac Risk Index for the assessment of noncardiac surgery patients.[4] Although the Cardiac Risk Index has been criticized on clinical and statistical grounds, the concept it embodies will most likely be employed more frequently in the future. Multifactorial assessment of risk is more reliable than estimates based on just one factor. For example, patients with a recent myocardial infarction can be subdivided into high-risk and moderate-risk groups based on the presence or absence of other major cardiac risk factors.[24] Other multivariate indices of cardiac risk for the surgical patient have been proposed,[29] but none of them has been developed sufficiently to be applied to routine clinical use to evaluate patients undergoing pulmonary surgery.

When the history, physical examination, or electrocardiogram (EKG) suggests the presence of *coronary artery disease,* exercise stress testing should be the first step. Stress testing is useful in estimating the presence and severity of coronary disease and helps provide guidelines for selecting patients who need more extensive diagnostic investigations. Patients suspected of having significant ischemic disease based on either the clinical history or the stress test may be referred for radionuclide examination of cardiac muscle profusion or coronary angiography.[9, 37]

Patients with *congestive heart failure* should be objectively evaluated and optimally treated before the operation. Patients with borderline compensation can develop frank cardiac failure as a response to the surgical stress. Studies have documented that patients whose congestive heart failure is well controlled before surgery have a substantially lower risk than those whose heart failure is not adequately controlled.[24] Radionuclide ventriculography and two-dimensional echocardiography provide objective information regarding ventricular performance noninvasively, and studies using the Swan-Ganz catheter permit assessment of cardiac reserve at the bedside.

Patients with *chronic valvular heart disease* should be initially investigated with echocardiography. They may require cardiac catheterization in order for the presence of a hemodynamically significant lesion to be confirmed. If cardiac catheterization reveals the presence of critical aortic or mitral stenosis, valve replacement should be considered before lung resection is performed.[4, 24] Patients who have other forms of valve heart disease should be assessed noninvasively and, in most situations, will be able to tolerate a noncardiac procedure. Patients with prosthetic heart valves and those who are undergoing chronic anticoagulant therapy should be placed on intravenous heparin, after which the anticoagulant can be discontinued. After surgery, the anticoagulant therapy should be restarted as soon as possible in order to minimize thromboembolic complications.[62]

Cardiac arrhythmias are frequently discovered during the preoperative evaluation, and ambulatory EKG monitoring is often required to assess their significance. Patients with atrial fibrillation should be treated to prevent a rapid ventricular response and should be mildly heparinized to reduce the risk of stroke and peripheral or pulmonary embolism. Patients with symptomatic premature ventricular contractions should be treated before operation.[9] Patients with nonsustained ventricular tachycardia should undergo electrophysiologic testing, and if ventricular tachycardia is induced, the response to antiarrhythmia drugs can be tested. From this, the decision can be made to proceed with surgery while the patient is under medication.[63] Temporary pacing is used to manage patients with preoperative conduction abnormalities.[24, 30] In *hypertensive* patients, optimal control of blood pressure is necessary before the operation is performed.[9]

Patients with syncope (i.e., the transient loss of consciousness with spontaneous recovery) should be evaluated to determine if the cause is cardiovascular, noncardiovascular, or idiopathic because the prognosis differs significantly, with cardiovascular causes faring worse. The cardiovascular causes are usually reduced left ventricular function (LVEF ≤ 40%), bundle branch block, or coronary artery disease. In patients with a normal heart, a tilt test should be performed to provoke an unrecognized neurocardiogenic syncope.

Radionuclide Examination of the Heart. Two different scanning techniques, radionuclide ventriculography and myocardial perfusion scanning, have been recommended for the assessment of coronary artery disease and ventricular function. They should be used judiciously, either alone or in combination, in the evaluation of candidates for lung resection.[64]

Radionuclide ventriculography, or gated cardiac blood pool imaging, provides dynamic visualization of the cardiac chambers by detection of gamma radiation from the blood. The technique permits accurate evaluation of ventricular function by allowing calculation of an ejection fraction ratio and measurement of several other objective parameters. This procedure is also an excellent means of evaluating regional wall motion, at rest or during exercise. With exercise, radionuclide ventriculography permits the identification of stress-induced ischemic wall motion abnormalities and can be used effectively as a means of diagnosing significant coronary disease.[64] Several studies have suggested exercise radionuclide ventriculography to be superior to conventional stress electrocardiographic testing in diagnosing coronary disease.

Whereas radionuclide ventriculography identifies the functional effect of ischemia, myocardial perfusion scanning with thallium-201 directly analyzes the distribution of myocardial blood flow. This technique is most frequently used in conjunction with stress electrocardiography testing and is a valuable tool for evaluating patients with a suspicion of coronary artery disease.[63] The value of combining these two diagnostic tests has been demonstrated on several studies. Although thallium-201 imaging is not as definitive as coronary arteriography in identifying patients with and without coronary disease, a negative scan is very reassuring and usually obviates the need for coronary angiography.[65]

Several studies have compared the accuracy of these two imaging techniques. Although each has proponents, it appears that both tests have similar sensitivity for detecting coronary disease, but thallium-201 is more specific. Some studies suggest that thallium stress imaging is able to detect perfusion abnormalities before they are severe enough to cause abnormal wall motion.[66] More recently, dipyridamole-induced

coronary dilatation has been introduced as an alternative to stress testing during thallium imaging because of the difficulty of achieving adequate levels of exercise in some patients. This technique has been shown to have a sensitivity and specificity for the detection of coronary disease similar to that of thallium stress imaging.[67] Using this technique to predict postoperative and long-term myocardial infarction and cardiac death after noncardiac surgery, Lette and associates[68] showed that cardiac event rates were 1% and 3.5%, respectively, in patients with normal scans or fixed perfusion defects, and 17.5% and 22% in patients with reversible defects. Figure 7–6 shows the chances of remaining cardiac event–free after noncardiac surgery for patients with normal scans or fixed defects, reversible perfusion defect(s), and transient dipyridamole-induced left ventricular dilatation.[68]

Gated cardiac blood pool imaging, on the other hand, is useful in diagnosing right ventricular dysfunction in patients with right ventricular overload due to pulmonary artery hypertension secondary to severe obstructive pulmonary disease.[69] Methods of assessing pulmonary artery pressure based on imaging of the right atrium and ventricle have been developed.[70] They may prove to be helpful in selecting pa-

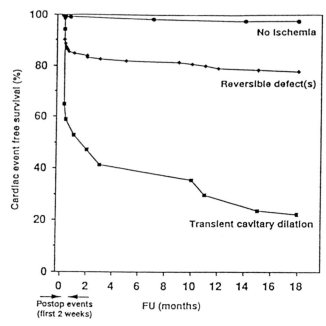

FIGURE 7–6. Proportion of patients who remained cardiac event–free with normal scans or fixed defects *(upper curve)*, reversible perfusion defect(s) *(middle curve)*, and transient dipyridamole-induced left ventricular cavitary dilatation *(lower curve)*. Patients with normal scans or fixed defects have an excellent prognosis. Patients with reversible defect(s) are at an increased risk but clearly cannot be labeled as high risk. For patients with transient dipyridamole-induced left ventricular cavitary dilatation, the postoperative cardiac event rate is high, and most patients who survive the surgery eventually sustain a cardiac event on long-term follow-up, usually within the first 3 months after the surgery. (From Lette J, Waters D, Bernier H, et al: Preoperative and long-term cardiac risk assessment. Predictive value of 23 clinical descriptors, 7 multivariate scoring systems, and qualitative dipyridamole imaging in 360 patients. Ann Surg 216:192–204, 1992.)

tients for invasive studies to further evaluate the unsuspected presence of pulmonary hypertension.

Coronary Angiogram. The most frequent indication for cardiac catheterization is the presence of significant symptoms of coronary disease. However, as delineated earlier, patients with incidental positive findings on a stress test confirmed by a radionuclide study, patients with recent myocardial infarction, and patients with atypical chest pain in whom noninvasive testing has been inconclusive should be evaluated by coronary angiography. Myocardial revascularization should be performed before a major noncardiac operation on patients with severe coronary artery disease, particularly when impaired ventricular function exists.[29] Determining the most appropriate course of action would depend on the magnitude of the planned resection and the availability of histologic diagnosis, as discussed earlier in this chapter.

Theoretical Screening for Assessing Cardiac Risk. The logical course in evaluating a patient is to use the clinical history, physical examination, and simple tests for screening patients to determine who should undergo more specialized second-line testing. Those with abnormal results could then be studied by more invasive and expensive techniques. Although no consensus exists as to which tests should be performed in which patients, a logical (theoretical) screening procedure is suggested in Figure 7–7.

Evaluation of the Respiratory System

Probably the most important evaluation a thoracic surgeon performs in the patient with lung cancer is the objective assessment of the overall pulmonary function and the estimation of the loss of function that will be caused by the resection. Surgical therapy is often predicated on these results. Methods for assessing pulmonary function and predicting pulmonary status after the operation range from purely subjective[71] to highly scientific.[51, 53, 72, 73] Although methods that reliably predict pulmonary function after resection are available, the surgeon must not underestimate the value of a physical examination and the observation of the patient during exercise.

Clinical Evaluation. The first step in the evaluation of pulmonary function is to obtain an accurate history with emphasis on the respiratory symptoms. A history of chronic respiratory disease is a risk factor for the development of postoperative respiratory complications and death. Specific questions relating to exercise tolerance should be asked, such as the number of stairs that can be negotiated and the level of activity at which dyspnea occurs. If the patient is generally sedentary, it is important to conduct an informal exercise tolerance test by accompanying the patient while climbing stairs or walking rapidly in a corridor.[72] Observing of the degree of dyspnea and changes in cardiac and respiratory rates yields valuable, if imprecise, information about the patient's cardiopulmonary reserve and general neuromuscular conditioning.[72]

Exercise Capacity. Accurate measurement of the patient's exercise capacity, which determines the combined performance level of both the circulatory and respiratory systems, is a sensitive predictor of operative morbidity and mortality after thoracotomy.[72] Ex-

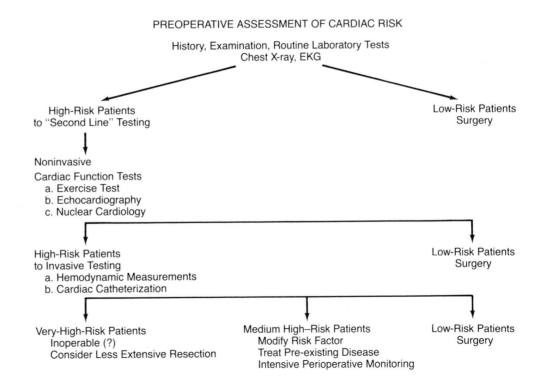

PREOPERATIVE ASSESSMENT OF CARDIAC RISK

History, Examination, Routine Laboratory Tests
Chest X-ray, EKG

High-Risk Patients to "Second Line" Testing

Low-Risk Patients Surgery

Noninvasive
Cardiac Function Tests
  a. Exercise Test
  b. Echocardiography
  c. Nuclear Cardiology

High-Risk Patients to Invasive Testing
  a. Hemodynamic Measurements
  b. Cardiac Catheterization

Low-Risk Patients Surgery

Very-High-Risk Patients Inoperable (?) Consider Less Extensive Resection

Medium High–Risk Patients Modify Risk Factor Treat Pre-existing Disease Intensive Perioperative Monitoring

Low-Risk Patients Surgery

FIGURE 7–7. Preoperative assessment of cardiac risk. (Modified from Seymour G: Medical Assessment of the Elderly Surgical Patient. Rockville, Maryland, Aspen Publishers, Inc., p 123, 1986.)

ercise capacity, however, does not help to determine the function of the lung to be resected or predict the postoperative pulmonary function of the patients. Exercise capacity does have a strong correlation with the incidence of postoperative cardiopulmonary complications and can be quantitated by measuring maximum oxygen consumption (V_{O_2} max).[73, 74] A V_{O_2} max during exercise greater than 20 ml/min/kg of body weight indicates a low risk, whereas volumes below 15 ml/min/kg are associated with high risk. There is some evidence that a V_{O_2} max less than 10 ml/kg/min indicates a prohibitive risk, even if spirometry is within acceptable limits.[75] A potentially curable resection should not be denied to a patient solely on the basis of poor results on the exercise capacity test. On the contrary, the most useful contribution of exercise testing is to identify surgical candidates who might otherwise be denied a thoracotomy on the basis of borderline pulmonary function tests.

Spirometry. Simple spirometry serves as an excellent screening test to identify those patients who are at increased risk of developing postoperative cardiopulmonary complications. Table 7–1 lists a sample of values from the literature that suggest increased risk. VC and FEV_1, because of their proven value and ease of measurement, should be determined in virtually all patients. The measurement can be performed at the bedside by a physiotherapist who prepares the patient for the operation. If the test is abnormal, a more comprehensive measurement should be conducted in the pulmonary function laboratory.

It should be remembered that spirometric testing depends not only on the state of the lungs and pleura but also on the function of the chest cage and neuromuscular control. The measurement is dependent on the patient's understanding and cooperation. The person performing the test must assess these factors in order to evaluate the results properly.[37] Tests should not be performed when the patient is fatigued or after lengthy roentgenographic procedures, bronchoscopy, or other diagnostic studies. To detect increased airway resistance and bronchospasm, which are of crucial importance in the postoperative course, spirometry should be repeated after the administration of bronchodilators. Changes suggestive of reversible airway obstruction should result in intensive preoperative treatment.

The assessment of VC provides information about restrictive lung disease and the patient's ability to expand and inflate the lungs and the chest cage. VC appears to be a poor predictor of postoperative morbidity, because it is not related to flow rate and does not provide an estimate of the degree of obstruction.

A number of values that are related to the rate of air flow can be derived from the FVC curve. The first of these is the FEV, which is a measurement of the volume that is expired within a specific period of time. Usually this is confined to the first second and is termed FEV_1 (see discussion presented earlier in this chapter). It is usually expressed as the absolute volume of gas expelled in 1 second or as a percentage

of the predicted normal value for an individual of the same age. The FEV_1 is reduced in patients with obstructive pulmonary disease but not in those who have restrictive pulmonary disease. The use of the FEV_1 is helpful in identifying high-risk patients for pulmonary resection. It gives information about potential ventilatory exchange and an estimate of the actual loss of function that has resulted from the obstructive pulmonary disease. Burrows and colleagues have shown that an FEV_1 between 0.8 and 1.0 L is necessary to avoid chronic respiratory insufficiency.[76] This is based on the observation that when the FEV_1 falls below these values, the incidence of CO_2 retention increases,[77] the exercise tolerance decreases, and the mortality resulting from chronic respiratory failure increases to 10% per year (Fig. 7–8).[78] An FEV_1 of 0.8 to 1.0 L after the pulmonary resection has proved to be a reasonable, although arbitrary, lower limit for determining operability.[10, 12, 18, 19, 37] However, age, sex, and height are important factors to take into account when considering whether an FEV_1 value implies an increased risk. Undoubtedly, a small elderly female does not need the same postpneumonectomy FEV_1 as a tall young male.[22] Several authors have suggested that using a percentage of the predicted normal value as a cutoff would be better than using the same arbitrary FEV_1 volume for all patients (see Table 7–1).[22, 50]

Miller and associates, using the VC and the FEV in 0.5 sec, developed a quadrant system (Fig. 7–9) for the identification of normal, restrictive, obstructive, and combined ventilatory defects.[79] They plotted the ventilatory parameters of patients who showed CO_2 retention and who would represent the ultimate in high surgical risk. A line was fitted so as to develop a

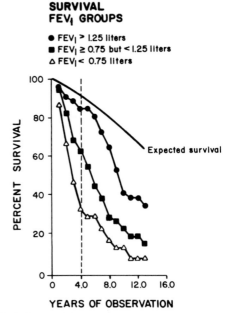

**SURVIVAL
FEV_1 GROUPS**

● FEV_1 > 1.25 liters
■ FEV_1 ≥ 0.75 but < 1.25 liters
△ FEV_1 < 0.75 liters

FIGURE 7–8. Survival of groups of patients distinguished on the basis of their FEV_1 at the time of enrollment in the study. (From Diener CR, Burrows B: Further observations on the course and prognosis of chronic obstructive lung disease. Am Rev Respir Dis 111:719–724, 1975.)

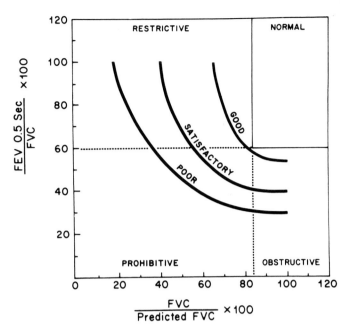

FIGURE 7–9. Miller's quadrant of postoperative risk based on pulmonary function test. (From Williams CD, Brenowitz JB: "Prohibitive" lung function and major surgical procedures. Am J Surg 132:763–766, 1976.)

theoretical limiting curve. Those patients with values plotted to the left of this line were considered to be at a prohibitive risk for surgery. However, in the clinical use of the quadrant system, patients falling into the prohibitive range were found to tolerate major surgical procedures with a reasonable rate of complications (20% major pulmonary complications and 6% mortality).[80] It was suggested that the prohibitive range should be called increased risk instead. Obviously, postoperative problems should be expected in this group of patients, and every effort should be made to prevent them.

A number of other values have been used to recognize patients with obstructive pulmonary disease. Two of these are the maximal expiratory flow rate and the maximal mid-expiratory flow rate. Stein and Cassara have shown that a maximal expiratory flow rate below 200 L/min correlates even better with an increased incidence of respiratory complication than does the FEV_1.[6] Although this test may well be the best way to assess small airway disease, the technology involved is expensive and, until recently, was usually found in specialized laboratories. This explains why it has not been used widely in surgical patients.

The concept of the CV was introduced more recently.[81] In adults who are breathing normally, the small airways and alveoli remain open at all times. Near the end of a maximal expiration, however, distal airways may begin to close. The lung volume at which airway closure begins is the CV. Under certain medical and surgical circumstances, small airway closure may occur not just at the end of forced expiration but during normal quiet breathing (see Fig. 7–3). This

means that the CV exceeds the FRC, and when this occurs, the risk for atelectasis is very high. Any condition likely to increase the CV, reduce the FRC, or both tends to favor the development of atelectasis and respiratory complications. Factors increasing CV include age, smoking, and COPD. Among the factors causing FRC to fall are thoracic and upper abdominal incisions, supine position, and obesity. Although the predictive value of CV in identifying patients at greater risk from postoperative complications has been confirmed,[12] this test is seldom used because it is technically more demanding than simple spirometry.

The MBC, now more frequently referred to as maximum voluntary ventilation (MVV), antedates the use of the FVC curve and is often used as an alternative to the FEV_1 and other expiratory flow measurements (see Table 7–1).[20, 21] MBC is performed by having the patient breathe as hard and as fast as possible for 15 seconds. The expired gas is collected and then expressed in liters per minute. Results are often reported as a percentage of normal value for the individual of the same age. Unlike the single breath maneuvers, the MBC measures the integrated performance of the respiratory pump per unit of time, including such factors as respiratory muscle blood supply, fatigue, and progressive air trapping. The disadvantages of the MBC are that it is a more difficult test for the patient to perform, and more importantly, that the estimation of unilateral pulmonary function cannot be accurately calculated from it (see the section entitled Pulmonary Function Loss Due to Resection earlier in this chapter).

Arterial Blood Gas Analysis. Proper interpretation of data from arterial blood gas analysis may be altered by patient reactions to the arterial puncture such as restricted or increased breathing due to fear or pain. The ideal evaluation for the patient with borderline pulmonary function includes the insertion of a radial artery catheter and obtaining samples when the patient is in supine and upright positions and, if necessary, after exercise.

The carbon dioxide partial pressure (Pco_2) provides the most useful information because it is an indication of adequacy of alveolar ventilation. A minimal elevation of the Pco_2 indicates a significant dysfunction of the gas exchange system. Some patients with advanced COPD still have satisfactory regulation of Pco_2, whereas others who are prone to let hypercapnia develop have a greater postoperative risk. Some carefully selected patients may tolerate lung resection in spite of an elevated Pco_2. In these patients, the response to exercise and the level of exercise tolerance are important factors in determining operative risk.[19, 37, 74] Conversely, if blood gas analysis after exercise reveals further increase in Pco_2, pulmonary resection is contraindicated.

The interpretation of the Po_2 is more complex. There is no specific study relating the Po_2 and the feasibility of surgery.[19] Depression of the Po_2 to as low as 60 mm Hg in patients breathing room air without hypercapnia does not contraindicate resection in and of itself.

The interpretation of hypoxemia, like the interpretation of the spirometry, requires knowledge of regional pulmonary function. If abnormal areas of the lung will be removed when the cancer is resected, one can anticipate that the Po_2 will actually improve after resection. However, in the absence of atelectasis or obvious shunting, a Po_2 of less than 50 mm Hg is usually associated with such severe restriction that lung resection is not feasible.

Regional Pulmonary Studies. Regional lung function studies are critical to the process of estimating the loss of function caused by the proposed resection (see the section entitled Pulmonary Function Loss Due to Resection earlier in this chapter). All other tests of lung function assess overall pulmonary function. Judgment of the ability of a patient to undergo a resection based on these measurements is often misleading. If the function of both lungs is assumed to be equal, it is possible for a patient with borderline pulmonary function to be incorrectly considered unsuitable for surgery. Regional pulmonary function can be determined by means of bronchospirometry, the lateral position test, or radionuclide ventilation perfusion studies.

Bronchospirometry measures the individual contribution of each lung to total pulmonary function. It consists of placing a double-lumen endotracheal tube at the carina and connecting each lumen to a separate spirometer.

Quantitative radionuclide ventilation and perfusion scans have replaced bronchospirometry and the lateral position test as the means of determining regional lung function and providing the most practical and least invasive method of making such estimates.[51, 52, 54] The technique of quantitative radionuclide ventilation and perfusion scans is similar to that used for the detection of pulmonary emboli. Using computer techniques, the radioactive counts composing the different images are quantified in order to express the contribution of specific areas of the lung to overall pulmonary function. From a *qualitative* point of view, lung scans permit the recognition of the following patterns of regional ventilation and perfusion:

1. The area to be removed has the same distribution of ventilation and perfusion as the rest of the lung. The loss of function will be proportionate to the magnitude of the resection.

2. The area to be removed has no appreciable function because of limited or no ventilation and perfusion. The resection, therefore, will not appreciably affect postoperative function.

3. The area to be removed is the site of an abnormal ventilation and perfusion relationship. In a patient with arterial hypoxemia, it may be the site of a right-to-left shunt. In this instance, resection will correct the cause of hypoxemia.

4. A distribution of ventilation and perfusion contrary to the normal effect of gravity is suggestive of pulmonary artery hypertension. If confirmed by direct evaluation, the presence of severe pulmonary hyper-

tension usually contraindicates further loss of the capillary bed.[9, 18]

From a *quantitative* point of view, ventilation and perfusion lung scans permit accurate prediction of the level of pulmonary function after pneumonectomy or lobectomy by combining the results of the spirometry with the quantitative measurement of differential function (see earlier discussion in this chapter). Several studies have demonstrated that this method can be used to predict postoperative VC, FEV_1, DL_{CO}, and even MBC with a high degree of accuracy.[18, 52, 53] We chose FEV_1 as the most important variable because it has been shown to be one of the most reliable indices of pulmonary insufficiency.[76–78]

Assessment of differential pulmonary function becomes particularly important in patients with a preoperative FEV_1 of less than 2.0 L if pneumonectomy is contemplated because of the risk of reducing the FEV_1 postoperatively to below the critical values of 0.8 to 1.0 L. Lobectomy causes a smaller loss of pulmonary function and consequently is well tolerated by most patients. There are, however, some borderline patients (i.e., whose FEV_1 is less than 1.5 L) for whom the prediction of postoperative function after lobectomy is needed. In some borderline patients, knowledge of the regional pulmonary function allows identification of those patients who have little or no function in the lobe to be resected and who, as a consequence of resection, would suffer little loss of overall pulmonary reserve.[53] Although controversial, the more frequent use of video-assisted thoracic surgery with minimal incisions for anatomic resections and the more liberal use of segmentectomy and wedge resection for lung cancer has reshaped previously defined thresholds of operability. Several authors have reported using a preoperative FEV_1 as low as 600 ml as a spirometric criteria for wedge resection.[82]

Assessment of the Pulmonary Circulation. Although radionuclide scans can detect pulmonary hypertension from indices such as the right ventricular ejection fraction and atrial emptying rate,[70] the pulmonary circulation can be objectively assessed only with invasive procedures. Measurement of pulmonary artery pressure (PAP) and resistance (PVR) with[18, 83] and without[84] balloon occlusion of the artery to the diseased lung is rarely indicated in the preoperative evaluation and then only to assess the operability of patients suspected of having severe pulmonary hypertension.[19, 22] In such patients, objective measurement of PAP will help to determine whether or not the patient would have an adequate pulmonary vascular bed after pulmonary resection.[12, 18, 84]

The technique of temporary unilateral pulmonary artery occlusion involves measurement of pulmonary artery pressure and arterial blood gas at rest and during exercise while the pulmonary artery to the lung to be resected is temporarily occluded with a special balloon-tipped catheter.[83] Patients with a mean PAP greater than 35 mm Hg and arterial hypoxemia (Pao_2 <45 mm Hg) were defined as not being surgical can-

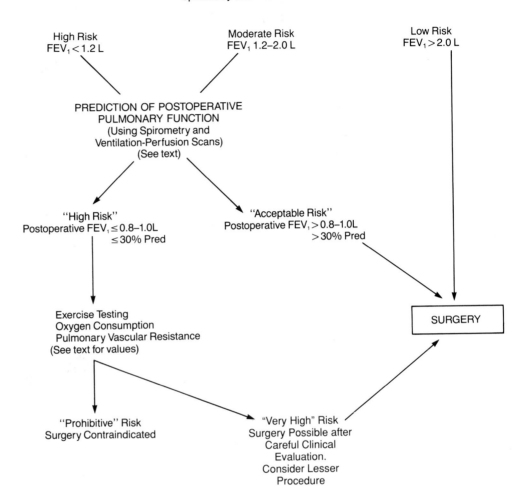

PREOPERATIVE ASSESSMENT OF RESPIRATORY RISK

History, Examination, Chest X-Ray,
Spirometry and Arterial Blood Gases

High Risk
FEV$_1$ < 1.2 L

Moderate Risk
FEV$_1$ 1.2–2.0 L

Low Risk
FEV$_1$ > 2.0 L

PREDICTION OF POSTOPERATIVE
PULMONARY FUNCTION
(Using Spirometry and
Ventilation-Perfusion Scans)
(See text)

"High Risk"
Postoperative FEV$_1$ ≤ 0.8–1.0L
≤ 30% Pred

"Acceptable Risk"
Postoperative FEV$_1$ > 0.8–1.0L
> 30% Pred

Exercise Testing
Oxygen Consumption
Pulmonary Vascular Resistance
(See text for values)

SURGERY

"Prohibitive" Risk
Surgery Contraindicated

"Very High" Risk
Surgery Possible after
Careful Clinical
Evaluation.
Consider Lesser
Procedure

FIGURE 7–10. Preoperative assessment of respiratory risk.

didates. Olsen and colleagues found that this assessment of the cardiopulmonary reserve is an accurate means to evaluate tolerance to pulmonary resection.[18] A high technical failure rate of the procedure itself and the lack of these specialized catheters have relegated this technique to historic value only.[22]

Fee and colleagues determined PVR at rest and during exercise, using a flow-directed thermodilution balloon catheter.[84] The procedure requires minimal technical expertise and is associated with virtually no complications. PVR varies with age but is usually less than 80 dynes-sec-cm^{-5} and it should decrease with exercise. In this study, a PVR of 190 dynes-sec-cm^{-5} during exercise was associated with a high surgical risk, even in patients who were considered low risk on the basis of spirometric and arterial blood gas criteria. The study supports the contention that the loss of vascular compliance, not the loss of diffusion surface, determines postoperative function and suggests that patients with an elevated PVR do not tolerate thoracotomy, regardless of the amount of lung resected. Although the usefulness of PAP measurement in predicting morbidity and mortality has been veri-

fied by several investigators, studies have failed to show that a single value consistently predicts postoperative outcome.[22]

More recently, PAP and the function of the right ventricle has been accurately assessed noninvasively with two-dimensional echocardiography. Although the role of echocardiography for the evaluation of the pulmonary circulation in borderline patients has not yet been defined, there is little doubt that its contribution to the preoperative evaluation for the cardiovascular system will be substantial.

A screening procedure for the preoperative assessment of respiratory risk is delineated in Figure 7–10.

OTHER PERIOPERATIVE THERAPEUTIC CONSIDERATIONS

Besides identifying the patients who are at increased risk, one of the goals of the preoperative assessment is to institute appropriate interventions designed to decrease that risk. The validity of this concept is intuitively obvious but is difficult to prove clinically. A discussion of the large number of interrelated patient and procedural factors that can modify the surgical risk and prevent postoperative complications is beyond the scope of this review. However, some recommended guidelines concerning the prevention of respiratory and cardiovascular complications follow.

Prevention of Cardiovascular Complications

Much of the improvement in the outcome of surgery for high-risk patients is attributable to careful preoperative therapy of pre-existing conditions and precise intraoperative and postoperative patient management reflecting the state of the art. Guidelines for patients with *ischemic heart disease* and indications for myocardial revascularization have been discussed earlier in this chapter.

The timing of pulmonary resection following a *recent myocardial infarction* is of considerable importance. Each case should be considered on its own merits. A delay should be considered if this is thought to be prudent after objective assessment of the significance of the coronary artery disease. In this situation, we believe that an interval of only 4 weeks is acceptable when the relative urgency of lung cancer is considered. Proper monitoring and meticulous perioperative management minimizes the well-known risk of a surgical procedure after a recent infarction.[85]

Preoperative *heart failure* should be controlled with diuretics, inotropic drugs, and afterload reduction agents. Infrequently, a patient who has severe ventricular dysfunction can be supported with an intra-aortic balloon pump during the perioperative period.

Although most authors discourage the prophylactic use of digoxin for its inotropic action in patients without congestive heart failure, its prophylactic use to prevent supraventricular arrhythmias is recommended.[86] Routinely, we preoperatively digitalize patients who are candidates for a pneumonectomy or who otherwise have a prior history of supraventricular arrhythmias. Criteria for temporary pacing in patients with arrhythmias, conduction abnormalities, and severe heart failure have been recently reviewed.[23]

Prevention of Respiratory Complications

Attention to preoperative preparation and careful intraoperative and postoperative care are essential in order to reduce the incidence of respiratory complications. Available data support the contention that prophylactic measures decrease the incidence of both fatal and nonfatal complications and justify the prolongation of the preoperative hospitalization, which is compensated by an earlier discharge and a lower cost of patient care.[6, 45, 47, 80] A description of some of the essential features of preoperative preparation follows.

Smoking should be discontinued for as long as possible before the operation. Although a short abstention may improve the mucociliary transport mechanism and mobilization of secretions, recent information suggests that smokers need to stop at least 8 weeks prior to an operative procedure before a significant reduction of respiratory complications is observed.[87]

The patient must be educated to the importance of coughing and deep breathing maneuvers. Preoperative teaching with the incentive spirometer encourages and trains the patient to perform hyperinflation maneuvers.[6, 45, 47] In patients with COPD, it is important to identify the presence of reversible factors such as bronchial edema and increased bronchial muscle tone. Repeated spirometric testing after the use of bronchodilators permits identifying those patients who would benefit from preoperative bronchodilators.[6] Patients with chronic bronchitis should receive special preoperative attention, including nebulization, chest physiotherapy, and postural drainage, to promote mobilization of secretions. If infection is present, proper antibiotic treatment should be added to the above-mentioned measures. In at least one study, failure of spirometric values to improve significantly after preoperative therapy has been shown to be correlated with an increased risk of developing pulmonary complications.[47]

Other programs such as *weight reduction, proper nutrition, exercise,* and *abstention from alcohol* benefit borderline patients[37] and should be attempted when a temporary delay is possible.

Pain is one of the most important considerations in the postoperative period. Narcotics administration should be minimized. Use of effective forms of a regional analgesic allows early mobilization of the patient and, most importantly, permits an effective cough. Postoperative intercostal nerve blocks result in less reduction in FVC and FEV_1 after thoracotomy than conventional analgesic treatments.[88, 89] The use of epidural, intrathecal, and subpleural narcotics has received renewed enthusiasm over the past 10 years.

The amount of *intravenous fluids* administered should be carefully monitored. Patients undergoing pulmonary resection are very sensitive to an excessive amount of fluids and are prone to develop interstitial and alveolar pulmonary edema.[48] On the other hand, dehydration and the risk of inspissated secretions should also be avoided. Table 7–3 summarizes the prophylactic measures for perioperative care.

CONCLUSIONS

Surgeons who restrict patient selection to the most fit can achieve low morbidity and mortality rates. This should not necessarily be equated with higher quality patient care because borderline and high-risk patients may be deprived of the potential benefits of surgery. Although it is impossible to ignore the fact that the government, third-party carriers, consumer groups, and the media are focusing on mortality rates as a measure of patient care, patients with a disease that is virtually fatal without surgery (i.e., lung cancer) should not be denied resection because the operative risk is above some arbitrary limit. To do so will im-

TABLE 7–3. Prophylactic Measures Recommended to Decrease Postoperative Complications

Preoperative: Patient education to ensure optimal postoperative compliance and performance, cessation of smoking, training in proper breathing (incentive spirometry), bronchodilation and control of infection and secretions when indicated, and weight reduction when appropriate

Intraoperative: Decrease in time under anesthesia, double-lumen endotracheal intubation control of secretions, prevention of aspiration, maintenance of optimal bronchodilation, and intermittent hyperinflations

Postoperative: Continuation of preoperative measures, with particular attention to hyperinflation, mobilization of secretions, early ambulation, encouragement to cough, and control of pain focusing on the effects of analgesia on the pattern of breathing

Modified from Tisi GM: Preoperative evaluation of pulmonary function. Am Rev Respir Dis 119:303, 1979.

prove survival rates of surgery patients at the expense of the patients who do not undergo surgery; the survival of the total patient population, however, will decrease.

At the present time, the quantitative lung scan combined with spirometry is an accurate and readily available test to predict postoperative pulmonary function that correlates well with actual measured postoperative values. The previously established minimal FEV_1 values for determining operability, although associated with an acceptable incidence of complications, need to be questioned and re-examined. Considering the poor prognosis for nonresected lung cancer, it seems reasonable to push the lower limit of operability to still lower values. Using percentage of normal values seems to be more useful than an arbitrary FEV_1.

The state of knowledge in cardiopulmonary testing in patients being considered for lung resection is constantly changing. As yet, in borderline cases, no single test or combination of tests can predict with certainty the ability of a given patient to withstand surgical resection. Statistics apply to groups but often not to the individual patient. In the final assessment, there will be no substitute for clinical judgment that, in addition to objective tests, takes into account subjective factors such as patient attitude and motivation.

SELECTED REFERENCES

Gass GD, Olsen GN: Preoperative pulmonary function testing to predict postoperative morbidity and mortality. Chest 89:127–135, 1986.
This is a well-presented, concise review of the clinical significance of pulmonary function tests. Different pulmonary function techniques available and recent work on exercise testing, oxygen consumption, and pulmonary vascular resistance measurement are critically assessed. The review is supported by an extensive bibliography.
Goldman L: Cardiac risk and complications of non-cardiac surgery. Ann Intern Med 98:504–513, 1983.
This well-presented review is probably the most comprehensive monograph on cardiac risks for noncardiac surgery patients. Largely based on Goldman's original article entitled "Multifactorial Index of Cardiac Risk in Noncardiac Surgical Procedures," it discusses all

known preoperative risk factors that affect the development of postoperative cardiac complications. It emphasizes the concept that in order to improve the outcome of surgery for high-risk patients, the preoperative estimation of cardiac risk should be accompanied by effective treatment of pre-existing conditions and careful perioperative monitoring and management.
Peters RM: Special problems in preoperative and postoperative management. *In* Delarue NC, Eschapasse H: International Trends in General Thoracic Surgery, Vol. 1: Lung Cancer. Philadelphia, W.B. Saunders, 1985, pp 67–75.
This excellent review of the preoperative and postoperative management of the lung cancer patient is written by an author who has written extensively on the subject. Multiple issues related to the evaluation of both respiratory and cardiovascular systems are carefully discussed. The review is nicely complemented by an authoritative discussion by Bjorn Jonson that emphasizes the need for using FEV_1 values adjusted for age and sex of the patient in assessing the lower limits of operability.
Tisi GM: Preoperative evaluation of pulmonary function. Am Rev Respir Dis 119:293–310, 1979
This is a classic and comprehensive review of the literature. The validity, indications, and benefits of preoperative evaluation of pulmonary function for both general and thoracic surgery patients are extensively discussed. Although the article is almost 15 years old now, it serves as a good reference source for the reader interested in pursuing certain areas in greater depth.
Wernly JA, DeMeester TR, Kirchner PT, et al: Clinical value of quantitative ventilation-perfusion lung scans in the surgical management of bronchogenic carcinoma. J Thorac Cardiovasc Surg 80:533–543, 1980.
This is a summary of our clinical experience comparing the value of ventilation and perfusion lung scans combined with spirometry in the evaluation of patients undergoing pulmonary resection for lung cancer. It validates previous work on the subject and suggests the superiority of the perfusion scan as a simpler technique and a more accurate predictor. This review emphasizes the value of assessing regional function within the affected lung when predicting the loss of function that will be caused by lobectomy.

REFERENCES

1. Pastorino U, Valente M, Bedini V, et al: Effect of chronic cardiopulmonary disease on survival after resection for stage Ia lung cancer. Thorax 37:680–683, 1982.
2. Kohman LJ, Meyer JA, Ikins PM, et al: Random versus predictable risks of mortality after thoracotomy for lung cancer. J Thorac Cardiovasc Surg 91:551–554, 1986.
3. Ginsberg RJ, Hill LD, Eagan RT, et al: Modern thirty-day operative mortality for surgical resections in lung cancer. J Thorac Cardiovasc Surg 86:654–658, 1983.
4. Goldman L, Caldera DL, Nussbaum SR, et al: Multifactorial index of cardiac risk in noncardiac surgical procedures. N Engl J Med 197:845–850, 1977.
5. Boushy SF, Billig DM, North LB, et al: Clinical course related to preoperative and postoperative pulmonary function in patients with bronchogenic carcinoma. Chest 59:383, 1971.
6. Stein M, Cassara E: Preoperative pulmonary evaluation and therapy for surgery patients. JAMA 211:787–790, 1970.
7. Lockwood P: Lung function test results and the risk of postthoracotomy complications. Respiration 30:529–542, 1973.
8. Nagasaki F, Flehinger BJ, Martini N: Complications of surgery in the treatment of carcinoma of the lung. Chest 82:25–29, 1982.
9. Ali MK, Ewer MS: Preoperative cardiopulmonary evaluation of patients undergoing surgery for lung cancer. Cancer Bull 32:100–104, 1980.
10. Miller JI, Grossman GD, Hatcher CR: Pulmonary function test: Criteria for operability and pulmonary resection. Surg Gynecol Obstet 153:893–895, 1981.
11. Weisfeldt ML: Aging of the cardiovascular system. N Engl J Med 303:1172–1174, 1980.
12. Tisi GM: Preoperative evaluation of pulmonary function. Am Rev Respir Dis 119:293–310, 1979.
13. Sikes ED, Detmer DE: Aging and surgical risk in older citizens of Wisconsin. Wis Med J 78:27–30, 1979.

14. Seymour G: Medical Assessment of the Elderly Surgical Patient. Rockville, Maryland, Aspen Publishers, Inc., 1986.

15. Latimer G, Dickman M, Day CW, et al: Ventilatory patterns and pulmonary complications after upper abdominal surgery determined by preoperative and postoperative computerized spirometry and blood gas analysis. Am J Surg 122:622–632, 1971.

16. Tarhan S, Moffit EA, Sessler AD, et al: Risk of anesthesia and surgery in patients with chronic bronchitis and chronic obstructive pulmonary disease. Surgery 74:720–726, 1973.

17. Fowkes FG, Lumm JN, Farrow SC, et al: Epidemiology in anesthesia. III: Mortality risk in patients with coexisting physical disease. Br J Anaesth 54:819–825, 1982.

18. Olsen GN, Block AJ, Swenson EW, et al: Pulmonary function evaluation of the lung resection candidate: A prospective study. Am Rev Respir Dis 111:379–387, 1975.

19. Kanarek DJ: Assessment of pulmonary function in lung cancer. In Choi NC, Grillo H (eds): Thoracic Oncology. New York, Raven Press, 1983, pp 103–113.

20. Gaensler EA, Cugell DW, Lingren L, et al: The role of pulmonary insufficiency in mortality and invalidism following surgery for pulmonary tuberculosis. J Thorac Surg 29:163, 1955.

21. Mittman C: Assessment of operative risk in thoracic surgery. Am Rev Respir Dis 84:197–207, 1961.

22. Ferguson MK, Little L, Rizzo L, et al: Diffusing capacity predicts morbidity and mortality after pulmonary resection. J Thorac Cardiovasc Surg 96:894–900, 1988.

23. Gass GD, Olsen GN: Preoperative pulmonary function testing to predict postoperative morbidity and mortality. Chest 89:127–135, 1986.

24. Goldman L: Cardiac risk and complications of noncardiac surgery. Ann Intern Med 98:504–513, 1983.

25. Topkins MJ, Artusio JF: Myocardial infarction and surgery: A five year study. Anesth Analg 43:716–720, 1964.

26. Tarhan S, Moffit EA, Taylor WF, et al: Myocardial infarction after general anesthesia. JAMA 220:1451–1454, 1972.

27. Steen PA, Tinker JH, Tarhan S: Myocardial reinfarction after anesthesia surgery. JAMA 239:2566–2570, 1978.

28. Becker RC, Underwood DA: Myocardial infarction in patients undergoing noncardiac surgery. Cleve Clin J Med 54:25–28, 1987.

29. Detsky AS, Abrams HB, Forbath N, et al: Cardiac assessment for patients undergoing noncardiac surgery: A multifactorial clinical risk index. Arch Intern Med 146:2131–2134, 1986.

30. Foster ED, Davis KB, Carpenter J, et al: Risk of noncardiac operation in patients with defined coronary disease: The Coronary Artery Surgery Study (CASS) registry experience. Ann Thorac Surg 41:42–50, 1986.

31. Corman LC: The preoperative patient with an asymptomatic cervical bruit. Med Clin North Am 63:1335–1340, 1979.

32. Putnam JB, Lammermeier DE, Colon R, et al: Predicted pulmonary function and survival after pneumonectomy for primary lung carcinoma. Ann Thorac Surg 49:909–915, 1990.

33. Bashir Y, Graham TR, Torrance A, et al: Nutritional state of patients with lung cancer undergoing thoracotomy. Thorax 45:183–186, 1990.

34. Fatzinger P, DeMeester TR, Darakjian H, et al: The use of serum albumin for further classification of stage III non–oat cell lung cancer and its therapeutic implications. Ann Thorac Surg 37:115–122, 1984.

35. Biddle TL, Uy PN, Hodges M, et al: Hypoxemia and lung water in acute myocardial infarction. Am Heart J 92:692, 1976.

36. Mahafan VK, Simon M, Huber GL: Re-expansion pulmonary edema. Chest 75:192, 1979.

37. Peters RM: Special problems in preoperative and postoperative management. In Delarue NC, Eschapasse H (eds): International Trends in General Thoracic Surgery, Vol 1: Lung Cancer. Philadelphia, W.B. Saunders, 1985, pp 67–75.

38. Newhouse M, Sanchis J, Brenenstock J: Lung defense mechanisms. N Engl J Med 295:990, 1976.

39. Green GM, Jakab GJ, Low RB, et al: Defense mechanisms of the respiratory membrane. Am Rev Resir Dis 115:479, 1977.

40. Ford GT, Whitelaw WA, Rosenal TW, et al: Diaphragm function after upper abdominal surgery in humans. Am Rev Respir Dis 127:431, 1983.

41. Beecher HK: Effect of laparotomy on lung volume: Demonstration of a new type of pulmonary collapse. J Clin Invest 12:651, 1933.

42. Mead J, Collier C: Relation of volume history of lungs to respiratory mechanics in dogs. J Appl Physiol 14:669, 1959.

43. Bendixen HH, Smith GM, Mead J: Pattern of ventilation in young adults. J Appl Physiol 19:195, 1964.

44. Bjork VD, Hilty HJ: The arterial oxygen and carbon dioxide tension during the postoperative period in cases of pulmonary resections and thoracoplastics. Surgery 27:155, 1953.

45. Bartlett RH, Gazzaniga AB, Geraghty T: Respiratory maneuvers to prevent postoperative pulmonary complications: A critical review. JAMA 224:1017, 1973.

46. Prys-Roberts C, Nunn JF, Dobson RH, et al: Radiographically undetectable pulmonary collapse in the supine position. Lancet ii:399, 1967.

47. Gracey DR, Divertie MB, Didier EP: Preoperative pulmonary preparation of patients with chronic obstructive pulmonary disease. Chest 76:123–129, 1979.

48. Zeldin RA, Normandin D, Landtwing D, et al: Postpneumonectomy pulmonary edema. J Thorac Cardiovasc Surg 87:35969, 1984.

49. Wittnich C, Trudel J, Zidulka A, et al: Misleading "pulmonary wedge" pressure after pneumonectomy: Its importance in postoperative fluid therapy. Ann Thorac Surg 42:192–196, 1986.

50. Jonson B: Discussion of Peters RM: Special problems in preoperative and postoperative management. In Delarue NC, Eschapasse H (eds): International Trends in General Thoracic Surgery, Vol. 1: Lung Cancer. Philadelphia, W.B. Saunders, 1985, pp 76–79.

51. Ali MK, Ewer MS, Atallah MR, et al: Regional and overall pulmonary function changes in lung cancer. J Thorac Cardiovasc Surg 86:1–8, 1983.

52. Kristersson S, Lindell S, Sranbert L: Prediction of pulmonary function loss due to pneumonectomy using 133Xe-radiospirometry. Chest 62:694–698, 1972.

53. Wernly JA, DeMeester TR, Kirchner PT, et al: Clinical value of quantitative ventilation-perfusion lung scans in the surgical management of bronchogenic carcinoma. J Thorac Cardiovasc Surg 80:533–543, 1980.

54. DeMeester TR, VanHeertum Rl, Kallas JR, et al: Preoperative evaluation with differential pulmonary function. Ann Thorac Surg 18:61–70, 1974.

55. Mahar LJ, Steen PA, Tinker JH, at al: Perioperative myocardial infarction in patients with coronary artery disease with and without aorta-coronary artery bypass grafts. J Thorac Cardiovasc Surg 76:533–537, 1978.

56. Girardet RE, Masri ZH, Lansing AM: Pulmonary lesions in patients undergoing open heart surgery: Approach and management. J Ky Med Assoc 79:645–648, 1981.

57. Bricker DL, Parker TM, Dalton ML Jr, Mistrot JJ: Open heart surgery with concomitant pulmonary resection. Cardiovasc Dis Bull Tex Heart Inst 7:411–419, 1980.

58. Dalton ML Jr, Parker TM, Mistrot JJ, Bricker DL: Concomitant coronary artery bypass and major noncardiac surgery. J Thorac Cardiovasc Surg 75:621–624, 1978.

59. Piehler JM, Trastek VF, Pairolero PC, et al: Concomitant cardiac and pulmonary operations. J Thorac Cardiovasc Surg 90:662–667, 1985.

60. Yokoyama T, Derrick MJ, Lee AW: Cardiac operation with associated pulmonary resection. J Thorac Cardiovasc Surg 105:912–917, 1993.

61. Urschel HC Jr: Discussion in Piehler JM, Trastek VF, Pairolero PC, et al: Concomitant cardiac and pulmonary operations. J Thorac Cardiovasc Surg 90:667, 1985.

62. Katholi RE, Nolan SP, McGuire LB: The management of coagulation during noncardiac operations in patients with prosthetic heart valves: A prospective study. Am Heart J 96:163, 1978.

63. Stanton MS, Heger JJ: Recurrent ventricular arrhythmias: Which may signal sudden death? J Crit Illn 4:17–32, 1989.

64. Berger JH, Zaret BL: Nuclear cardiology. N Engl J Med 305: Part 1, 799–807; Part 11, 855–865, 1981.

65. Brown KA, Boucher CA, Okada RO, et al: Prognostic value of exercise Thallium 201 imaging in patients presenting for evaluation of chest pain. J Am Coll Cardiol 1:944, 1983.

66. Jengo JA, Freeman R, Brizandine M, et al: Detection of coronary artery disease: Comparison of exercise stress radionuclide angiography and thallium stress perfusion scanning. Am J Cardiol 45:535–541, 1980.

67. Boucher CA, Brewster DC, Darling RC, et al: Determination of cardiac risk by dipyridamole-thallium imaging before peripheral vascular surgery. N Engl J Med 312:389–394, 1985.
68. Lette J, Waters D, Bernier H: Preoperative and long-term cardiac risk assessment. Ann Surg 216:192–204, 1992.
69. Berger H, Matthay RA, Loke J, et al: Assessment of cardiac performance with quantitative radionuclide angiocardiography: Right ventricular ejection fraction with reference to findings in chronic obstructive pulmonary disease. Am J Cardiol 41:897, 1978.
70. Marmor AT, Mijiritsky Y, Plich M, et al: Improved radionuclide method for assessment of pulmonary artery pressure in COPD. Chest 99:64–69, 1986.
71. Abby-Smith R: Evaluation of the long-term results of surgery for bronchial carcinoma. J Thorac Cardiovasc Surg 82:325–333, 1981.
72. Reichel J: Assessment of operative risk of pneumonectomy. Chest 62:570–576, 1972.
73. Eugene J, Brown SE, Light RW, et al: Maximum oxygen consumption: a physiology guide to pulmonary resection. Surg Forum 33:260–262, 1982.
74. Smith TP, Kinasewitz GT, Tucker WY, et al: Exercise capacity as a predictor of post-thoracotomy morbidity. Am Rev Respir Dis 129:730–734, 1984.
75. Morice RC, Peters EJ, Ryan MB, et al: Exercise testing in the evaluation of patients at high risk for complications from lung resection. Chest 101(2):356–361, 1992.
76. Burrows B, Strauss RN, Niden AH: Chronic obstructive lung disease. III. Interrelationships of pulmonary function data. Am Rev Respir Dis 91:861–868, 1965.
77. Segall JJ, Butterworth BA: Ventilatory capacity in chronic bronchitis in relation to carbon dioxide retention. Scand J Respir Dis 47:215, 1966.
78. Diner CF, Burrows B: Further observations on the course and prognosis of chronic obstructive lung disease. Am Rev Respir Dis 111:719–724, 1975.
79. Miller WF, Wu N, Johnson RL Jr: Convenient method of evaluating pulmonary ventilatory function with a single breath test. Anesthesiology 17:480, 1956.
80. Williams CD, Brenowitz JB: Prohibitive lung function and major surgical procedures. Am J Surg 132:763–766, 1976.
81. McCarthy DS, Spencer R, Green R, Milic-Emili J: Measurement of "closing volume" as a single and sensitive test for early detection of small airway disease. Am J Med 52:747, 1972.
82. Miller JI: Physiologic evaluation of pulmonary function in the candidate for lung resection. J Thorac Cardiovasc Surg 105:347–352, 1993.
83. Laros CD, Swierenga J: Temporary unilateral pulmonary artery occlusion in the preoperative evaluation of patients with bronchial carcinoma. Med Thorac 24:269, 1967.
84. Fee HJ, Holmes EL, Gewirtz H, et al: Role of pulmonary vascular measurements in preoperative evaluation of candidates for pulmonary resection. J Thorac Cardiovasc Surg 75:519–523, 1978.
85. Rao TLK, Jacobs KH, El-Etr AA: Reinfarction following anesthesia in patients with myocardial infarction. Anesthesiology 59:499–505, 1983.
86. Shields TW, Vjiki GT: Digitalization for prevention of arrhythmias following pulmonary surgery. Surg Gynecol Obstet 126:743–746, 1968.
87. Warner MA, Tinker JH, Divertie MB: Preoperative cessation of smoking and pulmonary complications in pulmonary dysfunction. Anesthesiology 59:A60, 1983.
88. Toledo-Pereyra LH, DeMeester TR: Prospective randomized evaluation of intrathoracic intercostal nerve block with bupivacaine on postoperative ventilatory function. Ann Thorac Surg 27:203–205, 1979.
89. de la Rocha AG, Chambers K: Pain amelioration after thoracotomy: A prospective, randomized study. Ann Thorac Surg 37:239, 1984.

THERAPY

8 SURGERY FOR NON–SMALL CELL LUNG CANCER

Robert J. Ginsberg, Melvyn Goldberg, and Paul F. Waters

HISTORICAL CONSIDERATIONS

Surgical removal of lung malignancies dates back to the middle of the last century. Initially, nonanatomic portions of the lung were removed by gross cautery dissection.

Nonanatomic Resection. Heidenhain was the first to perform such a partial resection for lung cancer, with a survival of 2 months, according to Sauerbruch.[1] In 1895, Pean reported the successful removal, about 30 years earlier, of a portion of the lung and chest wall that had been invaded by a primary lung cancer.[2] That very primitive operation included exteriorization of the tumor, suturing together the visceral and parietal pleura, and, finally, cauterizing the eviscerated mass.

Lobectomy. The first lobectomy for lung cancer was described by Davies in 1912.[3] Prophetically, he wrote

Cancer of the lung is in some varieties, in its earlier stages, now accessible to surgical intervention and complete removal, but until this fact is more fully recognized, and all pulmonary cases are subjected to routine radiologic examination, the growths will not be recognized until they have extended beyond the possibility of all treatment. In all doubtful cases, at least an exploratory thoracotomy should be undertaken.

Apparently the first operation in which hilar ligation of the vessels and lobectomy were performed, his procedure was successful, but unfortunately the patient died of an empyema 8 days after the operation.

Despite this technical success, for almost 20 more years surgeons continued to attempt to remove tumors by nonanatomic methods.[4] In 1929, Brunn again reported a one-stage lobectomy that represented a major advance because he used an intercostal drain with an underwater seal in anticipation of a broncho-pleural fistula.[5] The removal of air and exudates and the expansion of the remaining lobe therefore were ensured.

The first long-term survival from lobectomy was reported by Allan and Smith[6] in 1930. This was a two-stage resection, involving first adhesions between the upper and middle lobe and the parietal pleura and, subsequently, 12 days later, a lower lobectomy using mass ligature and cautery division. The patient recovered and was well 2 years later. By the time Churchill performed a right middle and lower lobectomy for bronchogenic carcinoma in 1933,[7] only 35 patients with the diagnosis of malignant lung disease had survived their pulmonary resection and seven had had a long period of freedom from recurrence.

Pneumonectomy. Although it was not until 1932 that Graham performed his historic pneumonectomy for carcinoma on a physician, using mass ligation followed by thoracoplasty,[8] experimental pneumonectomy had been performed for the preceding 50 years. Gluck in 1881[9] and Biondi in 1882[10] had successfully performed pneumonectomies on rabbits and dogs. Problems related to bronchial closure and the remaining pneumonectomy space were identified frequently. Kummel did perform a pneumonectomy for lung cancer in 1910, clamping the pedicle and leaving the clamps in situ, but the patient survived only 6 days.[11] In 1922, Hinz accomplished the first individual hilar ligation of vessels with pneumonectomy.[12] Unfortunately, the patient died of heart failure on the third day. Churchill in 1930 also performed a pneumonectomy with individual ligation of the vessels in the hilum.[7] A tube was placed in the residual bronchus and brought out through the chest wall. The patient died within 3 days. Archibald[13] in 1931 and Ivanissevich[14] in 1933 also reported having performed pneumonectomies. Unfortunately, both patients died in the early postoperative period. It was not until Rienhoff, in the year of Graham's classic operation, successfully performed a pneumonectomy with individual ligation of the three main vessels and suturing of the main bronchus that the technique of modern pneumonectomy was instituted.[15] By the 1940s, standard pneumonectomy became the accepted operation for resectable lung cancer.

Advanced Techniques. Surgeons applied the techniques of individual ligation to lobectomy and to segmentectomy in 1939, as described by Churchill and Belsey.[16] Allison described his "radical" pneumonectomy in 1946, advocating en bloc removal of all mediastinal nodes and intrapericardial ligation of the hilar vessels and recognizing that incomplete resection of lung cancer inevitably led to recurrence.[17]

In 1947, Price-Thomas performed the first sleeve resection for a right main-stem bronchial adenoma.[18] He credited Allison with the first sleeve resection for carcinoma, which was carried out in 1952. The technique of carinal resection for proximal bronchial tumors was first reported by Mathey and colleagues[19] and by Thompson[20] in 1966.

En bloc resection of lung cancer invading the chest wall was described by Coleman in 1947.[21] Chardak and MacCallun in 1956 reported a successful en bloc resection of a superior sulcus tumor.[22] In 1961 Shaw and colleagues popularized the management of superior sulcus tumors with preoperative radiation followed by en bloc surgical removal.[23]

By the middle 1950s, pneumonectomy was no longer the standard treatment for lung cancer. Lung-conserving operations (lobectomies) became the standard approach for peripheral tumors.

Lesser resections (segmentectomy and wedge resection) for peripheral lung cancer have always been reserved for compromised patients who could not tolerate more extensive procedures such as lobectomy or pneumonectomy. Jensik began performing segmental resection for cure in peripheral tumors in the 1960s.[24] Recently, there has been increased interest in segmental and lesser resections for treating T1N0 tumors.[25–27]

SURGERY AND THE NATURAL HISTORY OF NON–SMALL CELL LUNG CANCER

Does surgery alter the natural history of lung cancer? It is easy to understand that earlier diagnosis and treatment will certainly increase length of survival. Whether this occurs because early diagnosis leads to curative therapeutic intervention or because it simply starts the "survival clock" running sooner (i.e., increases lead time) is a moot point. Despite some arguments to the contrary, most investigators agree that complete surgical resection offers real hope for total cure of this disease.[28] This has been confirmed by the recent analysis of long-term follow-up of patients found to have an early lung cancer in the National Screening Study and treated by methods other than surgery. There were no survivors at 5 years despite the early diagnosis. The authors conclude that surgical intervention is necessary for survival.[29]

Approximately 95% of lung cancers arise in the bronchial or bronchoalveolar surface epithelium or from bronchial mucous glands. A sequential change occurs during the development from metaplasia through dysplasia to carcinoma in situ and ultimately to invasive carcinoma.[30] The life of a tumor has three phases: an in situ phase, a preclinical or asymptomatic phase, and a final clinical or symptomatic phase. The detailed natural history of lung cancer is provided in Chapter 3. Most symptomatic patients have advanced lung cancer when diagnosed; only 20% to 30% have localized, potentially curable disease.

Only 5% of all lung cancers are detected in the asymptomatic phase. These are usually Stage I tumors and are highly curable. Most present as asymptomatic peripheral nodules on chest radiography. Endobronchial tumors detected in the "occult" state by sputum cytologic examination are frequently found to be only "in situ" (Tis) or locally invasive T1N0 tumors. At this "x-ray negative" stage, they are virtually all curable by surgical excision. These tumors are almost always squamous cell carcinomas and most arise within the proximal lobar or segmental bronchi. Further growth may produce local symptoms due to bronchial obstruction or tumor erosion that leads to hemoptysis.

Tumors arising in the distal bronchial tree and presenting as peripheral nodules tend to be adenocarcinomas. The doubling time may be slow for the tumors, which remain asymptomatic for long periods of time.[31] Peripheral tumors not arising from bronchial or bronchoalveolar epithelium may arise directly from the subpleura or within previous scars. Eventually, locally invasive T1 tumors will spread via the lymphatics or the blood stream, producing regional (N) or metastatic (M) disease with resulting local systemic symptoms and a greatly diminished chance of cure.

Role of Surgery

Because surgical treatment is usually limited to tumors identified as being completely resectable at the time of diagnosis, it is sometimes difficult to predict the impact of surgery on lung cancer in general. This is even more difficult to evaluate considering that most patients with lung cancer have inoperable tumors. In the classic study by Buchberg and colleagues, only 2% of untreated individuals survived beyond 5 years.[32] Presently, it is predicted that 13% of patients diagnosed as having lung cancer will survive 5 years or longer.[33] Virtually all of these surviving patients will have been treated by surgery. Presumably, therefore, surgery does have an impact on the overall survival among patients with lung cancer. However, lung cancer is being diagnosed earlier than it was 40 years ago. This increased "lead time" also will have impact on the overall rate of survival.

THE SOLITARY PULMONARY NODULE
(Fig. 8–1)

The small, solitary pulmonary nodule (SPN)[34] deserves separate discussion because it frequently represents a diagnostic and therapeutic dilemma as well as an opportunity to "cure" early lung cancer. Many refined diagnostic techniques such as fine-cut tomography, computed tomography (CT) scanning with CT number determination,[35, 36] transthoracic needle aspiration biopsy,[37] and transbronchial biopsy[38] or cytology have increased the ability to accurately diagnose these lesions without thoracotomy. For purposes of this discussion, we will define the SPN as having the following characteristics:

1. Diameter between 1 and 4 cm.
2. Well-circumscribed lesion.
3. Lesion surrounded by lung.
4. No evidence of major bronchial obstruction.
5. Approximately round.

Most frequently, these lesions will present on a routine chest radiograph as an unexpected finding. Although there are usually no symptoms, if present, they may point to a diagnosis. Obtaining a careful history, which should include information about the patient regarding smoking and previous malignancy, and conducting a thorough physical examination are essential but may not be helpful. Previous chest x-ray results should be sought for comparison if they are available.

If the lesion has not changed for 2 years or more, one can confidently ascribe a benign diagnosis.[39] No further investigation other than follow-up chest x-ray examinations is required in this situation. Unfortunately, this is rarely the case.

Without the benefit of previous x-ray results, attempts to further characterize the nature of the lesion should be made. Conventional tomography may identify features suggesting a benign lesion such as dense, central, "popcorn" or lamellar calcification. Tomography can also help to accurately localize the nodule for needle or transbronchial biopsy, if indicated.

In more recent years, CT scanning, especially with third- and fourth-generation machines, has proved to be useful. Theoretically, the chances of a highly dense (calcified) lesion being malignant are slight, whereas a low-density lesion is more ominous. Unfortunately, determining a threshold number is difficult, and there is disagreement in the literature because the results of the technique vary, depending on the machine and the operator.[35, 36] Nevertheless, a single lesion with a

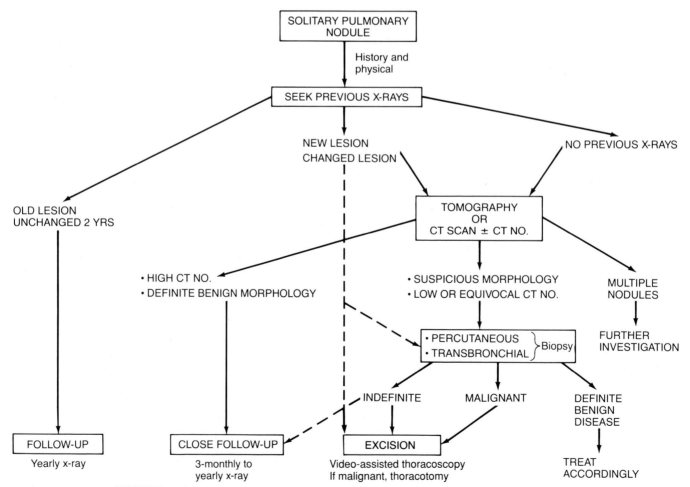

FIGURE 8–1. Algorithm for decision making in patients presenting with solitary pulmonary nodules.

high CT number will be of less concern and may, in the right setting, be treated by careful follow-up x-ray examinations at frequent intervals.

Not uncommonly, following these radiologic investigations, doubt remains about the diagnosis. Further investigations such as percutaneous fine-needle aspiration biopsy or transbronchial biopsy are indicated in the hope that diagnosis can be made before surgery is considered. It is important to be aware of the "track record" of the personnel involved in endoscopic, radiologic, and cytologic procedures to interpret the significance of a "negative" biopsy. In experienced hands, two "negative" biopsies can virtually confirm the lesion as benign.

Despite complete investigations, a number of patients always remain whose lesions continue to elude a diagnosis and in whom malignant disease cannot be excluded. This occurs most frequently with SPNs. It is in this situation that a more invasive technique of obtaining tissue is indicated for diagnosis and ultimate management. In the past few years, a minimally invasive approach using video-assisted thoracic surgery (VATS) has been applied.[40] This technique has capitalized on the improved technology, optics, and instrumentation resulting from the rapidly increasing field of laparoscopic surgery. Although the final role for VATS in therapeutic interventions is not yet established, there is little doubt that because of its relative simplicity it will be used with increasing frequency in establishing the diagnosis of a SPN. This is especially true when tiny nodules, less than 1 cm, are identified serendipitously on routine chest x-ray or CT scans performed for another reason. These tiny nodules are difficult to localize. Preoperative percutaneous needle localization or intraoperative ultrasonography before a VATS excision may be of help.[41, 42]

If still undiagnosed, at thoracotomy, intraoperative aspiration cytology, core needle biopsy, wedge or segmental resection, and, occasionally, lobectomy may be required before diagnosis can be made. Rapid intraoperative cytologic examination or frozen-section analysis of the tissue is required for confirmation at the time of thoracotomy. It is our belief that pneumonectomy should not be performed without definite evidence of malignancy, unless a destroyed, irretrievable lung requires this procedure, no matter what the diagnosis. For this reason, in most cases every attempt should be made to obtain tissue diagnosis before thoracotomy.

INDICATIONS FOR SURGERY (Fig. 8–2)

Curative Surgery

Surgical resection is generally accepted as the treatment of choice when attempting to cure localized lung cancer. It must be applied on a selective basis, taking into account the quality as well as the length of survival. The age of the patient, extent and cell type of the lesion (tumor, nodes, and metastases [TNM] stage and histology), type of resection necessary for complete removal, and patient's cardiac and pulmonary functional status are all important considerations.

Before surgery is recommended, the clinical stage of the disease and its potential for complete cure by surgery must be assessed (see Chapter 9). The benefits likely to be gained by resection are weighed against the risks of operation, which include early and late morbidity as well as mortality. Also, in assessing the role of surgery, one must always keep in mind that clinical staging frequently understages vis-à-vis the final pathologic stage (Table 8–1).

Stage I and II Disease. Patients with non–small cell lung cancer determined to be clinical Stage I or II disease should always be considered for possible surgical resection if warranted by their functional status. These tumors usually can be completely resected and are highly curable.

Stage III Disease. Patients with clinical Stage III disease usually have a much poorer prognosis and should be considered for surgery only on a selective basis, depending on the TNM status of the lesion and the ability of the surgeon to completely resect the tumor. In general, Stage IIIa (T3 or N2) is potentially resectable, whereas Stage IIIb (T4 or N3) is unresectable.

T3 Tumors (Table 8–2). T3N0 tumors have the best prognosis of any Stage III lung cancer. Those involving the chest wall, especially the rib cage, have a 50% 5-year survival rate if completely resected and no nodal involvement is present.[43] Tumors involving mainstem bronchi without nodal involvement that are treated by sleeve lobectomy or pneumonectomy have a similar prognosis.[44] Tumors invading the pericardium can be resected, as can tumors involving the mediastinal pleura or fat. However, the prognosis of this type of T3 tumor appears much less frequently in any reported retrospective series.[45] There is no information on tumors invading the diaphragm. It is our experience that most tumors with local invasion of diaphragm have diffuse involvement of the diaphragm and almost always in reality are T4 tumors. Also, the majority of these tumors are found at surgery to have associated N2 disease—a very ominous combination.

Tumors of the superior sulcus are considered T3. Most series report a 30% to 40% 5-year survival rate for completely resected lesions. In a recent analysis at Memorial Sloan-Kettering Cancer Center, patients with these tumors, treated by lobectomy and en bloc resection, when completely resected have a 60% 5-year survival rate. The overall 5-year survival rate of all patients treated by surgical resection was 30%. Incomplete resection and wedge resection of the pulmonary component (versus lobectomy) were adverse prognostic factors.[46]

T4 Tumors. Tumors involving organs of the mediastinum (superior vena cava, esophagus, vagus nerve, major vessels) or those invading a vertebral body are rarely cured by surgical resection. An occasional patient may benefit from this approach. The absolute contraindications

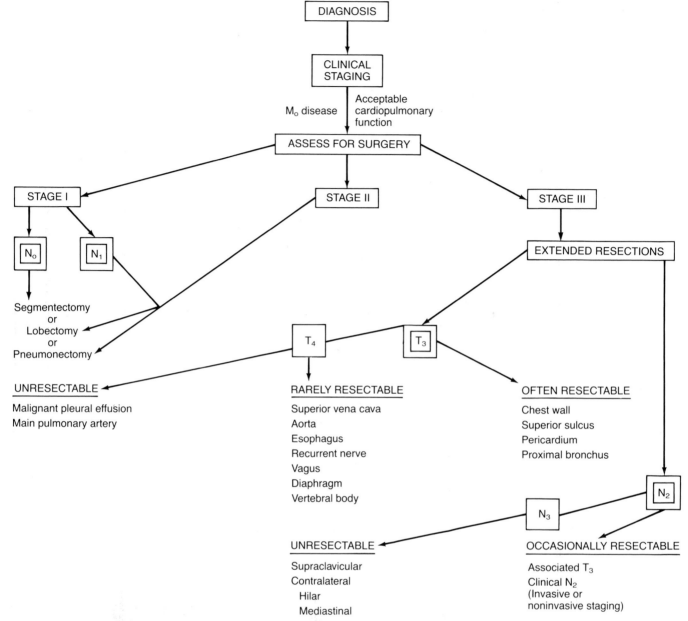

FIGURE 8–2. Schema for resectability and types of resection indicated in operable non–small cell lung cancer.

to complete resection with extrapulmonary intrathoracic invasion include involvement of the left recurrent laryngeal nerve, main pulmonary artery, aorta or superior vena cava, and esophagus when these organs are invaded to any significant extent. Tumors with malignant pleural effusion are also considered to be inoperable and incurable. The designation provided by the American Joint Committee on Cancer Staging (AJCC) and The International Union Against Cancer (UICC) Staging Classification of a T4 tumor denotes incurability and, except for the occasional unusual case, is accurate in this designation.[47]

N2 Disease (Tables 8–3 and 8–4). Only N2 disease that can be completely resected will result in a significant 5-year survival rate (up to 30%) after surgery.[48–50] This survival rate decreases if more than one N2 nodal station is involved with tumor, if there is extracapsular involvement of the lymph nodes (less likely to yield a complete resection), or if N2 disease is associated with a T3 tumor.[51]

Tumors most likely to be completely resected will be those that are clinically staged before surgery to be less than N2 (clinical N0 or N1) by imaging or mediastinoscopy. Those tumors identified at mediastinoscopy to have even single station ipsilateral intranodal involvement have an increased likelihood of incurability. Most series have suggested a 10% or less chance of long-term cure with surgical resection.

N3 Disease. Contralateral mediastinal lymph nodes or supraclavicular lymph nodes indicate an extremely poor prognosis with primary surgical resection. Many investigators are exploring the use of extended lymphadenectomy for this group of patients.[52, 53] A

TABLE 8–1. Survival Rate According to Final Pathologic Staging After Surgical Resection

STAGE	TNM	NO. OF PATIENTS	FIVE-YEAR SURVIVAL RATE (%)
I	T1N0M0	245	75.5
	T2N0M0	291	57.0
II	T1N1M0	66	52.5
	T2N1M0	153	38.4
IIIA	T3N0M0	106	33.3
	T3N1M0	85	39.0
	T1-3N2M0	368	15.1
IIIB	T1-3N3M0	55	0
	T4 any N > M0	104	8.2
IV	any T any N > M1	258	7.5

Adapted from Naruke T, Goya T, Tsuchiya R, Suemasu K: Prognosis and survival in resected lung carcinoma based on the new international staging system. J Thorac Cardiovasc Surg 96:440–447, 1988.

TABLE 8–2. Results of Surgical Resection for T3 Tumors

STUDY	YEAR	NO. OF RESECTIONS	ESTIMATED 5-YEAR SURVIVAL
CHEST WALL			
Patterson et al[93]	1982	35	38
Piehler et al[43]	1982	93	33
McCaughan[126]	1985	125	40
Allen et al[123]	1991	52	26
SUPERIOR SULCUS			
Paulson[127]	1985	79	31
Rice[128]	1986	36	28
Ricci[129]	1988	41	34
Ginsberg et al[46]	1994	100	
PROXIMAL AIRWAY*			
Ungar[133]	1981	99	54
Eschapasse[134]	1985	31	42
Naruke[135]	1989	62	39
Vogt-Moykopf[136]	1986	97	12

*Reports detailing proximal airway involvement treated by sleeve resection.

recent report from the Southwest Oncology Group reported the results of induction chemotherapy and radiotherapy for this stage of disease. Median survival times have been prolonged, and ultimate survival appears to be more promising than with a direct surgical approach and to be similar to that of patients determined before surgery as having N2 disease.[54]

M1 Disease. A select group of patients with solitary metastasis to the brain and completely resectable primary lung carcinoma can be treated surgically for both the primary and solitary metastatic focus with an expectation of a significant 5-year survival rate. Burt and colleagues recently reported results suggesting a 17% 5-year survival rate with this aggressive surgical approach.[55] MacGilligan and colleagues and Brent and colleagues previously reported results suggesting a 25% 5-year survival rate.[56]

Palliative Resections

Occasionally, there is an indication to remove a tumor, albeit incompletely, to afford palliation of debilitating symptoms. However, in most instances other therapeutic modalities can be used as effectively.

Infection and Hemoptysis. Occasionally, a tumor that is causing distal obstruction and abscess formation or one that is producing massive hemoptysis, uncontrollable by other means, may require resection, even though it is anticipated that an incomplete resection will be performed. Other therapeutic interventions such as endoscopic laser therapy or radiotherapy can frequently afford the same type of palliation.

Osteoarthropathy. Severe hypertrophic osteoarthropathy may warrant a palliative resection. Proximal ipsilateral vagotomy, however, appears to produce the same degree of symptom relief.[57]

Pain. We have not been impressed with the palliation afforded by incompletely resecting tumors invading the chest wall, including those in the superior sulcus. However, the value of incompletely resecting these tumors, combined with high-dose postoperative radiotherapy, by either afterloading techniques, implantation, or external beam irradiation, has not been evaluated in a prospective way.

TABLE 8–3. Results of Surgery for N2 Disease: Preoperatively Identified N2 Disease Has an Extremely Poor Prognosis After Surgical Resection

STUDY	YEAR	NO. OF RESECTIONS	ESTIMATED 5-YEAR SURVIVAL (%)
ALL N2			
Naruke[130]	1988	426	14
Levasseur and Regnard[124]	1990	254	18
Watanabe et al[125]	1991	153	17
COMPLETELY RESECTED			
Martini[131]	1987	151	30
Naruke[130]	1988	242	19
Levasseur and Regnard[124]	1990	191	23
Watanabe et al[125]	1991	84	24
MEDIASTINOSCOPY-POSITIVE (+ ve) N2			
Pearson[132]	1982	79	9
McCaughan[126]	1985	28	18

TABLE 8–4. Factors Adversely Affecting Survival in Resected N2 Disease

T3 tumors
Adenocarcinomas
High mediastinal nodes
Multiple involved N2 sites
Incomplete resections
Clinical N2 disease

Debulking. At thoracotomy, if a tumor is deemed unresectable, it is frequently difficult for the surgeon to decide not to attempt an incomplete resection, hoping (despite usually disappointing results) that resection and postoperative adjuvant therapy may yield some associated benefit. Whether one should intentionally incompletely resect a tumor at thoracotomy is still unknown. Retrospective analyses of these approaches do not provide an answer as to which is more beneficial to the patient.[51]

It is known that when an incomplete resection is performed, either as a planned procedure or when curative resection had been attempted, there is an associated high perioperative mortality and morbidity rate as well as an extremely poor (less than 5%) 5-year survival rate. Quality of survival is usually poor in our experience.

For all of the above reasons, "debulking" procedures have not become standard in the armamentarium of the thoracic surgeon managing lung cancer. More information is required before this type of procedure can be recommended for palliation or as part of an overall multimodality program.

Induction Therapy (Neoadjuvant, Preoperative)

Recently, there has been significant interest in the use of preoperative chemotherapy with or without concomitant radiotherapy in locally advanced Stage IIIA and B disease that otherwise would be considered unresectable. This approach theoretically should reduce local tumor bulk, enabling complete resection at the time of surgery, as well as eliminate micrometastatic disease elsewhere, the most common site of failure following resection (see Chapter 9). Whether these previously "unresectable" tumors are better treated by induction followed by surgery than by standard radiotherapy or chemoradiotherapy without surgery awaits the results of Phase III randomized trials now being carried out in the United States and Canada.[58, 59]

ANATOMIC CONSIDERATIONS

The surgical treatment of lung cancer depends on a detailed knowledge of the surgical anatomy of the lung and the biologic behavior of those tumors arising within the lung. Lung cancer usually arises within lobar or segmental bronchi. Initially, local growth occurs and eventually spreads to the regional lymphatics. Since the surgical management of non–small cell lung cancer may involve a range of procedures, from a very limited wedge resection to a sleeve pneumonectomy, it is important that the surgeon have a detailed knowledge of the segmental anatomy of the lung as well as the lymphatic drainage so complete excision can be performed.

Segmental Anatomy

The segmental anatomy as proposed by Jackson and Huber[60] in 1943 is generally accepted, as is the numeric designation developed by these authors (Figs. 8–3, 8–4). It is important to remember that the pulmonary artery follows the branching of the bronchial tree within a segment. More important for the surgeon is the fact that the pulmonary veins drain intersegmentally, demarcating the segments at the time of resection.

It is not within the scope of this chapter to provide a more detailed description of the segmental anatomy or the technique of segmental resection. Suffice it to say that with an accurate knowledge of segmental anatomy a surgeon can anatomically resect any of the 18 segments, although certain segments (apical, apical-posterior, lingular, and superior) are more amenable to segmental resection than others.

Lymphatic Drainage of the Lung (Fig. 8–5)

Once lung cancer spreads to lymph nodes, the ultimate prognosis becomes much worse. Before a surgeon contemplates resection of a tumor, it is important to anticipate complete removal of all involved lymph nodes. For this reason, a detailed knowledge of the lymphatic drainage of the lung is of prime importance.

The lymphatic drainage of the tracheobronchial tree and mediastinum is complex, with great variation. In general the patterns remain as described in the classic treatises by Rouviere,[61] Drinker,[62] Borrie,[63] and Nohl-Oser.[64] The introduction of mediastinoscopy by Carlens has made possible further study of the lymphatic spread of lung cancer.[65]

Microscopic Lymphatics

Electron microscopy has demonstrated that lymphatic capillaries are not present in the interalveolar septa. However, within the interlobular, pleural, peribronchial, and perivascular connective tissue sheaths, lymphatic capillaries can be identified, abutting closely onto the alveolar wall. These microscopic vessels are called "juxta-alveolar lymphatic capillaries," which have great permeability and are involved with active transport. The absorption of fluid into the interalveolar connective tissue takes place through these lymphatic channels, which then coalesce into larger channels in the peribronchial regions. Intrapulmonary lymph nodes are the first lymphoid aggregates to drain these channels. These intrapulmonary nodes are in juxtaposition to divisions of segmental and smaller bronchi, often lying in the bifurcation of the branches

Nomenclature for Peripheral Bronchi

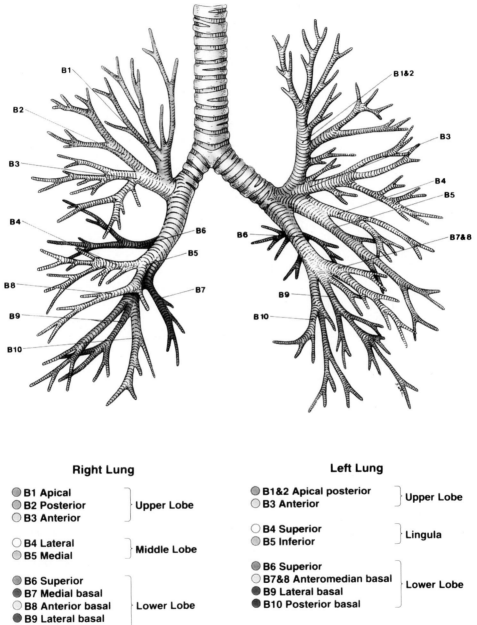

Right Lung

- ⬤ B1 Apical
- ⬤ B2 Posterior } Upper Lobe
- ◯ B3 Anterior

- ◯ B4 Lateral
- ⬤ B5 Medial } Middle Lobe

- ⬤ B6 Superior
- ⬤ B7 Medial basal
- ◯ B8 Anterior basal } Lower Lobe
- ⬤ B9 Lateral basal
- ⬤ B10 Posterior basal

Left Lung

- ⬤ B1&2 Apical posterior } Upper Lobe
- ◯ B3 Anterior

- ◯ B4 Superior } Lingula
- ⬤ B5 Inferior

- ⬤ B6 Superior
- ◯ B7&8 Anteromedian basal } Lower Lobe
- ⬤ B9 Lateral basal
- ⬤ B10 Posterior basal

FIGURE 8–3. The segmental anatomy of the bronchial tree with the universally adopted descriptive and numeric identification.

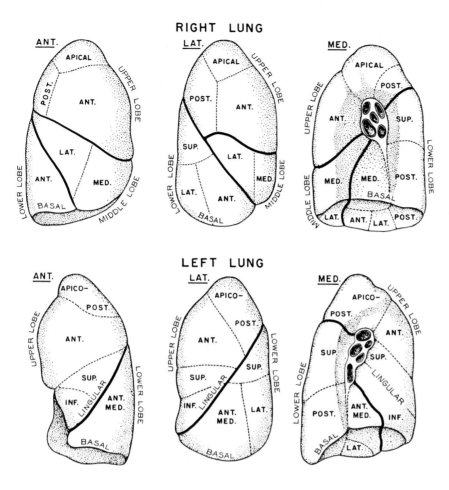

FIGURE 8–4. The segmental anatomy of the lung. (From Warehin EE, Huse WM: Surgical anatomy of the lung. Surgical Clinics of North America 44:1191–1200, 1964.)

of the pulmonary artery. More proximally, broncho-pulmonary lymph nodes are situated in the angles formed by the bifurcation of lobar bronchi (interlobar nodes) and along the main branches of the main bronchi (hilar nodes).

Lymphatic drainage proximal to hilar nodes occurs within the mediastinum into nodes that can be divided into three groups: anterior mediastinal, posterior mediastinal, and superior mediastinal (tracheobronchial and paratracheal) nodes.

SURGICAL-PATHOLOGIC CONSIDERATIONS

Peribronchial Spread of Lung Cancer

Cotton demonstrated that peribronchial lymphatic spread is far more common than submucosal extension.[66] In an analysis of 100 resected specimens, Lange-Cordes found submucosal malignant infiltration at the point of resection in more than 25% of cases.[67] Because of these findings, it has been recommended that a 2-cm resection margin be obtained in every case. Practically, it appears less important to have this relatively long resection margin in cases where lymphatic spread is absent. However, a generous resection margin is advised if peribronchial lymphatic spread is identified in the resected specimen.

Sump Nodes

In his classic article, Borrie described the "lymphatic sump."[63] This term is used by surgeons to refer to the interlobar nodes found in the depths of the major fissure that drain all lobes of each lung and that, if involved by the tumor, often determine the extent of resection.

Right Sump Nodes (Fig. 8–6). These nodes are found in the depths of the right major fissure and drain all three lobes of the right lung. They lie in relation to the bronchus intermedius near the angle of the right upper lobe and along the pulmonary artery from the superior segmental branch of the lower lobe to the middle lobe branches.

With tumors arising in the right lower lobe, a right lower and middle lobectomy is usually required for complete ablation of the disease if these nodes are involved. A simple lower lobectomy would not achieve this result. Tumors of the right upper lobe rarely spread to lymph nodes lying below the origin of the middle lobe bronchus. Therefore, an upper lobectomy can usually provide complete anatomic extirpation of disease. The nodes of the right sump, however, will have to be dissected from the pulmonary artery and its branches during this procedure to identify any spread within them.

The Left Sump (Fig. 8–7). The nodes that form the

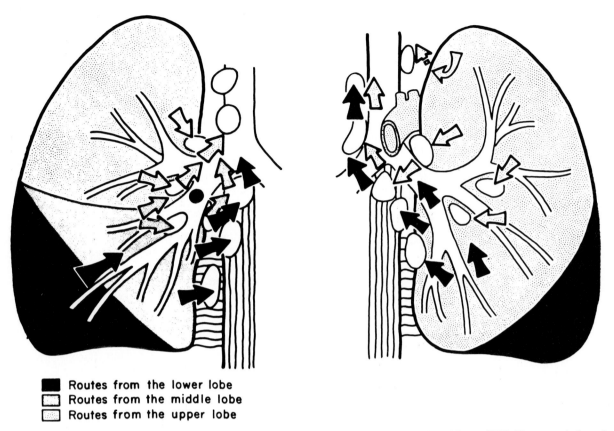

Routes from the lower lobe
Routes from the middle lobe
Routes from the upper lobe

FIGURE 8–5. Schematic illustration of lymphatic drainage from the various lung zones. (Modified from Hinson KFW: The spread of carcinoma of the lung. *In* Bignall JR [ed]: Edinburgh, E & S Livingstone, Ltd, 1958; and reproduced with permission from Paulson DL: Carcinoma of the lung. *In* Ravitch MM et al [eds]: Current Problems in Surgery. Copyright © 1967 by Year Book Medical Publishers, Chicago.)

FIGURE 8–6. The collection of lymph nodes constituting the right lymphatic sump along the bronchus intermedius. The tangential straight lines indicate the lowest retrograde flow of lymph nodes from the upper lobes. (From Nohl-Oser HC: An investigation of the anatomy of the lymphatic drainage of the lungs as shown by the lymphatic spread of bronchial carcinoma. Ann R Coll Surg Engl 51:157–176, 1972.)

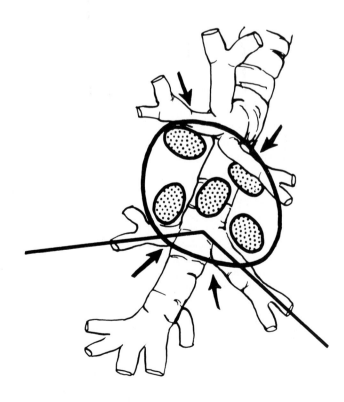

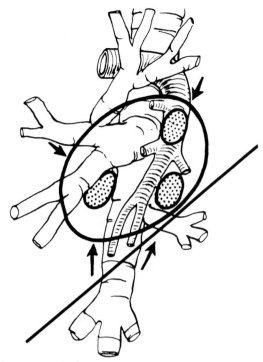

FIGURE 8–7. The collection of lymph nodes constituting the left lymphatic sump. The tangential line indicates the lowest retrograde flow from the left upper lobe. (From Nohl-Oser HC: An investigation of the anatomy of the lymphatic drainage of the lungs as shown by the lymphatic spread of bronchial carcinoma. Ann R Coll Surg Engl 51:157–176, 1972.)

left sump lie between the upper and lower lobes in the main fissure. A constant node is present in the bifurcation between the upper and lower lobe bronchi, in close proximity to the origins of the lingular and basal bronchi. In patients with N1 disease involving the left sump, since there is no bronchus intermedius as on the right, it may difficult to clear these nodes by upper or lower lobectomy alone, and a pneumonectomy may be necessary.

Mediastinal Lymph Nodes. The prognosis is significantly altered if the lung cancer involves the mediastinal lymph nodes. Even in the most favorable cases, in which all N2 disease can be completely resected, the cure rate rarely exceeds 30%. The site of mediastinal lymph node spread depends on the location of the primary tumor. The advent of mediastinoscopy has allowed a much better understanding of the drainage of mediastinal lymph nodes. In 1972, Nohl-Oser undertook an analysis of 749 persons with bronchogenic carcinoma in whom mediastinoscopy and/or scalene node biopsy had been performed.[68] Since that time, several monographs and papers have confirmed his concept of lymphatic drainage from the lung to the mediastinum.

Right Lung (Fig. 8–8)

Lower Lobe. Drainage to the mediastinum from right lower lobe tumors can be directly toward the inferior

pulmonary ligament and periesophageal nodes from medial and posterior basal tumors. Tumors of the superior segment or other basal segments will frequently drain via intrapulmonary nodes to the right sump and then to either subcarinal nodes or tracheobronchial angle nodes via hilar nodes.

Middle Lobe. Drainage from the middle lobe is directly to the anterior mediastinum via the middle lobe vein or to the right sump and, therefore, to tracheobronchial angle nodes or along the bronchus intermedius to the subcarinal nodes.

Right Upper Lobe. Most frequently, these tumors drain to the tracheobronchial angle nodes directly via hilar nodes or indirectly through the right sump. Occasionally, nodes will be involved in the anterior mediastinum in the region of the superior vena cava and main pulmonary artery. Rarely, malignancy spreads to subcarinal nodes.

Left Lung (Fig. 8–9)

Lower Lobe. As in right-sided disease, tumors in the left lower lobe may drain to the mediastinum along nodes near the inferior pulmonary vein or via the sump to the subcarinal space. Contralateral spread to right tracheobronchial angle nodes (N3) from the left

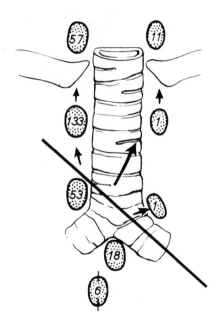

SUPERIOR MEDIASTINAL SPREAD

Ipsilateral —— 190 cases —— 45%

Contralateral — 13 cases —— 3%

FIGURE 8–8. Lymphatic drainage to the superior mediastinum from the right lung: an analysis of 423 cases. Subcarinal and tracheobronchial angle nodes were excluded from the analysis but are considered to be mediastinal nodes. (From Nohl-Oser HC: An investigation of the anatomy of the lymphatic drainage of the lungs as shown by the lymphatic spread of bronchial carcinoma. Ann R Coll Surg Engl 51:157–176, 1972.)

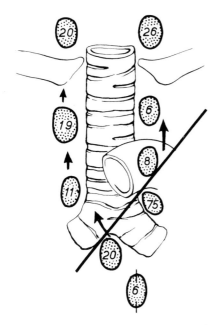

SUPERIOR MEDIASTINAL SPREAD

Ipsilateral —— 40 cases — 12·2 %•

Contralateral — 50 cases — 15·3 %•

FIGURE 8–9. Analysis of lymphatic spread from 326 cases of carcinoma of the left lung. Subaortic and subcarinal nodes were excluded from the analysis but are mediastinal nodes. (From Nohl-Oser HC: An investigation of the anatomy of the lymphatic drainage of the lungs as shown by the lymphatic spread of bronchial carcinoma. Ann R Coll Surg Engl 51:157–176, 1972.)

lower lobe can occur once the subcarinal nodes are involved with tumor.

Left Upper Lobe. Left upper lobe tumors frequently drain to subaortic nodes and then to anterior mediastinal nodes lateral to the aorta and subclavian artery, eventually reaching the left scalene node area. However, approximately 50% of lymphatic spread beyond the subaortic region occurs along the left main-stem bronchus to the ipsilateral tracheobronchial and paratracheal lymph nodes. Contralateral mediastinal spread by left upper lobe tumors is rare indeed.

Complete resection of left upper lobe tumors involved with N2 disease is limited by the extent of spread into the superior mediastinum via the tracheobronchial angle nodes. Spread beyond low tracheobronchial nodes virtually precludes the possibility of a complete surgical resection unless a median sternotomy approach is used and should be heeded by the surgeon before considering the option of resection in such a patient.

The prognosis following surgical resection for lung cancer is most affected by lymph node involvement and decreases remarkably once mediastinal lymphatics harbor tumor.

SURGICAL TECHNIQUES

It is not the purpose of this chapter to describe surgical techniques in detail. The reader is referred to the

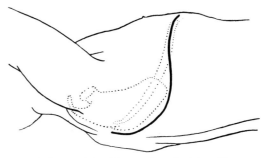

FIGURE 8–10. Posterolateral thoracotomy incision. (From Waldhausen JA, Pierce WS [eds]: Johnson's Surgery of the Chest. 5th Ed. Chicago, Year Book Medical Publishers, 1985.)

standard textbooks and monographs dealing with this subject.[69–72] However, it is important to indicate the advantages, disadvantages, and problems encountered in thoracic approaches, standard resections, and extended resections.

Thoracic Approaches

Posterolateral Thoracotomy (Fig. 8–10). This is the incision of choice for the majority of intrathoracic operations, especially surgical resection of lung cancer. It is usually made through the fifth or sixth intercostal space or through the bed of the resected fifth rib. This posterolateral approach offers the optimum exposure to all aspects of the ipsilateral mediastinum, the chest wall, the diaphragm, and lung, compared with any other type of thoracic approach.

Anterolateral Thoracotomy (Fig. 8–11). Although used less frequently, the standard anterolateral thoracotomy, with the patient in the supine position, provides quick entry into the chest, minimal disturbances of respiratory and circulatory function, ease of closure, and less pain after the thoracotomy. The pleural space can be entered through the bed of the resected fourth, fifth, or sixth rib or, more commonly, through one of the intercostal spaces without rib resection. This approach provides more than adequate exposure to the anterior hemimediastinum, the middle lobe,

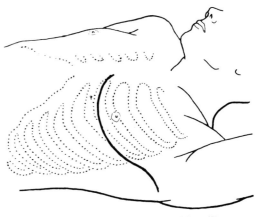

FIGURE 8–11. Anterolateral thoracotomy incision. (From Waldhausen JA, Pierce WS [eds]: Johnson's Surgery of the Chest. 5th Ed. Chicago, Year Book Medical Publishers, 1985.)

and the upper lobes. Lower lobe segments may be difficult to expose with this incision, especially on the left side where retraction of the heart can lead to repeated episodes of decreased venous return, hypotension, and cardiac arrhythmias during the surgical procedure.

Posterior Thoracotomy (Fig. 8–12). A posterior thoracotomy, performed with the patient in the prone position, is rarely used today, although it was the approach of choice for many of the pioneer thoracic surgeons. The procedure had the following advantages over posterolateral thoracotomy when one-lung anesthesia was not available: (1) better ventilation of the contralateral lung, (2) excellent drainage of both lungs, reducing the possibility of aspiration of infected secretions into the contralateral lung, and (3) availability of thoracic anesthesia with spontaneous ventilation, without intubation. This approach is still used by some surgeons, especially when managing tumors invading the posterior chest wall, including superior sulcus tumors.

Sternotomy (Fig. 8–13). Although median sternotomy is the approach of choice for exposure of the anterior mediastinum, heart, and great vessels, until recently it was rarely used in the treatment of primary malignancies of the lung. However, median sternotomy is gaining increased popularity as an alternative approach for malignant pulmonary processes,[73] especially when bilateral synchronous malignancies are present.[74] Some surgeons have advocated that this be considered the approach of choice for virtually all bronchogenic carcinomas.[75]

Median sternotomy has the advantage of significantly less postoperative pain as well as the distinct advantage of allowing complete superior mediastinal node dissection in left upper lobe tumors. However, disadvantages exist, including difficulty in managing adhesions in the posterior pleural space, poor exposure of the left lower lobe (especially if cardiac enlargement is present), and increased difficulty excising posterior mediastinal nodes.

In the treatment of lung cancer, we personally reserve this approach for bilateral synchronous primary disease and for patients undergoing combined cardiac

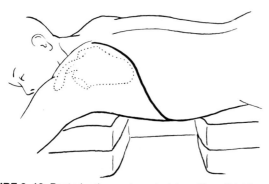

FIGURE 8–12. Posterior thoracotomy incision. (From Waldhausen JA, Pierce WS [eds]: Johnson's Surgery of the Chest. 5th Ed. Chicago, Year Book Medical Publishers, 1985.)

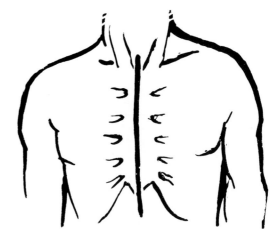

FIGURE 8–13. Sternotomy incision. (From Waldhausen JA, Pierce WS [eds]: Johnson's Surgery of the Chest. 5th Ed. Chicago, Year Book Medical Publishers, 1985.)

and pulmonary operations. On occasion, we have used it to facilitate mediastinal lymph node dissection in left upper lobe tumors or in patients with very poor pulmonary reserve, anticipating postoperative pain and associated morbidity.

Clamshell Incision (Transverse Sternotomy Plus Bilateral Anterior Thoracotomy). This incision affords greater exposure to lower lobes and has been used more recently for the indications for which sternotomy is used. A recent report from the Memorial Sloan-Kettering Cancer Center suggests its use in bilateral synchronous tumors. The postoperative pain is similar to that of the median sternotomy. We have found it to be especially useful in dealing with lower lobe tumors and pulmonary metastases when bilateral exploration is required.[77]

Muscle-Sparing Incisions. There has been renewed interest in smaller incisions, such that the larger muscles of the chest wall are not divided to obtain access to the chest. Advocates of these incisions claim there is less pain and better early function for the patient. However, comparison with standard incision has failed to demonstrate any significant benefit for either early postoperative pain or late pulmonary function. Proponents of this approach suggest that these parameters are extremely difficult to measure.[78, 79]

Video-Assisted Thoracic Surgery. VATS has created international interest. This technique, an extension of thoracoscopy, has been used mainly for diagnostic purposes.[29, 40–42] Improved equipment has allowed surgeons to visualize the thoracic cavity extremely well and dissect hilar structures (Fig. 8–14). Used mainly for diagnostic wedge resections of lung, this technique is also being explored in major resectional surgery (Fig. 8–14). Lobectomies, pneumonectomies, and lymph node dissections have been accomplished. Whether this approach will replace standard thoracotomies as the approach of choice awaits further development of this technique. Appropriately controlled trials are needed to define the role of VATS in patients with lung cancer.

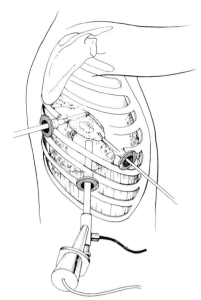

FIGURE 8–14. The three-stick approach to thoracoscopic pulmonary wedge resection. (From Brandt H-J, Loddenkemper R, Mai J, et al [eds]: Atlas of Diagnostic Thoroscopy. Indications–Techniques. New York, Thieme Medical Publishers, Inc., 1985. Copyright 1985, Thieme Medical Publishers.)

Surgical Staging

The prognosis of resected non–small cell carcinoma is dependent on TNM staging and histology. Before advising surgical removal of lung cancer, the surgeon is obligated to have clinically staged the disease (cTNM) by noninvasive methods, as outlined in previous chapters. To determine ultimate prognosis and perhaps consider adjuvant therapy is important at the time of surgery and at the pathologic examination to complete the surgical stage and ultimately arrive at the final pTNM stage. The surgeon and pathologist must work together to accurately assess the final pathologic staging of the tumor.

T Status. Although pathologists can easily measure the size of the tumor and determine whether the visceral or parietal pleura has been invaded, they cannot estimate the distance of the tumor from the carina, the presence or absence of pleural fluid, or the presence or absence of mediastinal invasion unless it is pointed out by the surgeon. Because the status depends not only on size, the surgeon must indicate to the pathologist before final pathological staging whether there are extenuating circumstances that place the tumor in a T3 category. Otherwise, we have found that tumors are frequently downgraded. For example, a 1-cm tumor arising in the right upper lobe but extending into the right main-stem bronchi is actually a T2 tumor and should be designated as such by the combined efforts of the surgeon and pathologist.

N Status. The identification of mediastinal nodes cannot be the province of the pathologist. At the time of thoracotomy (or at mediastinoscopy if performed before surgery), the lymph nodes of the mediastinum must be labeled by the surgeon before being sent to the pathologist. It has been our practice to label every node obtained at mediastinoscopy and subsequently every node obtained at thoracotomy as to its site. This can be facilitated by using the lymph node staging maps of either Naruke and colleagues[76] or the American Thoracic Society (ATS) (see Chapter 6).

Our own practice includes either a complete mediastinal lymph node dissection for improved staging (RJG) or sampling to obtain biopsy specimens of lymph nodes from all the various sites accessible at the time of thoracotomy (MG and PW). Minimal lymph node sampling requirements, as defined by the Lung Cancer Study Group, include specimens from the subcarinal (7), paratracheal (4R) or aortopulmonary (5), hilar and tracheobronchial angle (10) nodes. Frozen-section examination of hilar nodes is included in these biopsies. If hilar nodes are involved, a more radical mediastinal lymph node dissection must be performed even if mediastinal nodes are uninvolved at biopsy. On occasion, "skip" lesions with involvement of a solitary mediastinal lymph node can occur even from peripherally placed T1N0 tumors, emphasizing the need for extensive mediastinal node examination and the possible value of complete mediastinal lymph node dissection in all patients not only for accurate staging but also for improved survival.

To completely stage a tumor, bronchopulmonary lymph nodes from the lobar, segmental, and more peripheral sites must also be examined. We find it best if the surgeon takes the responsibility to sample lobar and segmental nodes, especially if a lobectomy is being performed. It is the responsibility of the pathologist to dissect more distally into the lung to examine bronchopulmonary nodes at the time of surgical prosection.

Unless all nodal stations are sampled, the final pathologic TNM staging will not be accurate. This entire process can be expedited if a node map is available in the operating room and in the surgical pathology room for reference during node sampling. In this way, the nodes can be correctly labeled according to site and identified accurately.

Surgical Resections

Pneumonectomy

Standard Pneumonectomy. Although at one time the procedure of choice for all resections, pneumonectomy presently is used only when required and accounts for approximately 20% of pulmonary resections for lung cancer. More careful surgical techniques with high division of the main-stem bronchus, the use of surgical staples, and perioperative prophylactic antibiotics have helped to reduce the incidence of the morbid complications of empyema and bronchopleural fistula. Pneumonectomy is required when the tumor or lymph nodes involve proximal structures such that a lung-conserving operation will not allow complete resection. This procedure permits a wide local resection of the tumor and accomplishes a more complete removal of the lymphatic drainage of the lung. Its major disadvantages include a higher mortality rate and an increased incidence of major complications. A relatively large volume of functioning lung is removed, especially after right pneumonectomy, which may lead to the late development of pulmonary hypertension and chronic respiratory failure.

Radical Pneumonectomy. Not infrequently, because of proximal involvement of the pulmonary vessels, intrapericardial dissection[17, 80, 81] is required with ligation of one or more of the vessels in the pericardial sac. This is also required if there is involvement of the pericardium either by the tumor itself or lymph nodes in the area of the pulmonary veins or main pulmonary artery.

Sleeve Pneumonectomy. Sleeve pneumonectomy, with resection of the carina for T3 tumors that involve the proximal main-stem bronchus or carina itself (T4) can be performed without difficulty. High-frequency jet ventilation has facilitated this technique. This extension of pneumonectomy has been used most frequently with right-sided disease, because the right main-stem bronchus is short and it, or the carina, may be involved with tumor. A right posterolateral approach or median sternotomy provides excellent exposure. Similarly, a tumor of the proximal left main-stem bronchus can be resected along with the carina either through a left posterolateral thoracotomy with mobilization of the arch of the aorta by means of a median sternotomy or as a staged procedure with a left thoracotomy for pneumonectomy followed by carinal resection through a subsequent right posterolateral thoracotomy.

The results of sleeve pneumonectomy depend on the N status. Recent reports by Deslauriers and colleagues,[82] Jensik and colleagues,[83] and Darteville and colleagues[84] indicate that one can expect a 5-year survival rate in patients who have had complete resections. Although the mortality rate for this operation can be high, with experience, it should be in the range of pneumonectomy.

Lobectomy

Standard Lobectomy. Lobectomy is the most commonly used resection for lung cancer, especially in N0 and N1 disease in which complete resection can be performed without removing the complete lung.

Sleeve Lobectomy. Sleeve lobectomy, first used in the treatment of bronchial carcinoids, has become a standard part of the armamentarium of thoracic surgeons. Most frequently, this is applicable to tumors of the right upper lobe involving the right main-stem bronchus. Preservation of the middle and lower lobes will still allow complete excision of the tumor. With N0 tumors, one can expect 5-year survival rates as high as with any other procedure for the same stage; however, with N1 or N2 disease, less optimistic 5-year survival rates naturally will occur, but they will be no poorer than those associated with pneumonectomy. Although sleeve resection is most frequently used with right upper lobe tumors, any variety of sleeve resections can be performed as long as resection mar-

gins are negative. On occasion, sleeve resection of the bronchus with concomitant sleeve resection of the pulmonary artery can be performed in upper lobe tumors. This approach is rarely indicated and its results are unknown, although 5-year survival rates have been described by Toomes and Vogt-Moykopf.[85]

Segmentectomy. Segmentectomy is usually reserved for patients with peripherally placed N0 tumors and compromised pulmonary function such that it is believed that they cannot tolerate any more extensive resection. Jensik[86] and, more recently, Kulka and Forrail[87] have suggested that these lesser pulmonary resections may be as adequate as lobectomy in the treatment of T1N0 tumors. A recent randomized trial by the Lung Cancer Study Group has demonstrated an increased local recurrence rate and poorer 5-year survival using limited resection versus lobectomy despite sampling of bronchopulmonary lymph nodes draining the segment to ensure that resection was complete and no occult N1 disease existed beyond the limited resection. In this study, there was no difference in morbidity and mortality between patients receiving the segmentectomy or lobectomy and no detectable difference in right pulmonary function, suggesting that lobectomy remains the treatment of choice for patients with T1N0 tumors.[88] A recent analysis by Warren and Faber of the original Rush Presbyterian (Jensik) approach confirms this high incidence of local recurrence compared with that for lobectomy. These authors also conclude that lobectomy should remain the treatment of choice, even for early-stage lung cancer peripherally placed.[89]

Bronchoscopically visible tumors should rarely be considered for segmentectomy, although in a compromised patient, this may be all that is possible and, if a complete resection can be performed, this would be acceptable. In these situations, the surgeon must be aware of the proximity of the tumor to the intersegmental plane. Frequently, wedge excision of adjacent segments will provide a wider margin of safety to ensure a complete resection.

Lesser Resections. Very limited resection in the treatment of lung cancer has been reserved for patients with extremely poor pulmonary function who could tolerate no more than a very limited resection because of their underlying medical condition or low pulmonary reserve. Two types of limited resections have been advocated: wedge excision and lumpectomy.

Wedge Resection. A wedge excision in peripherally placed T1 or T2 tumors has been successfully used in compromised patients. The introduction of stapling devices has made this a much simpler procedure. Care must be taken not to transgress the tumor during the application of the stapling devices or clamps before suturing the lung. Recently, Errett and colleagues retrospectively reviewed their experience and found a surprisingly high 5-year survival rate with this type of resection, quite comparable to the 5-year survival rate found with lobectomy in similar patients.[27] However, in most reported series this operation has been a compromise, with a higher incidence of local recurrence than lobectomy. There was a 3.5-fold increase in local recurrence after wedge resection (versus lobectomy) in the Lung Cancer Study Group Trial.[88]

STAPLING DEVICES. As mentioned previously, this chapter is not intended to be a treatise on surgical methods. However, it is worthwhile to indicate the advances in surgical technique that have occurred with the use of the mechanical automatic stapling devices. The use of these devices for closure of the bronchus, pulmonary arteries, and veins, as well as lung parenchyma, has become prevalent. This technique was evaluated objectively in 349 consecutive patients undergoing various types of pulmonary resection.[90] In this series, bronchopleural fistulae occurred only twice in 60 patients undergoing pneumonectomy. In both patients, recurrence of carcinoma was demonstrated as the cause. No bronchopleural fistulae occurred after 136 lobectomies. There were only five significant parenchymal air leaks in 289 patients after staples were used to divide fissures. No complications resulted from the stapled closure of pulmonary vessels. The careful use of stapling devices is at least equal in risk and effectiveness to the careful suture closure of bronchi and major arteries and veins. As in the use of any other surgical technique, care must be taken to avoid catastrophic complications. These stapling devices can greatly reduce anesthetic and operating times. There is no doubt that parenchymal closures performed even by experienced surgeons are greatly facilitated by the use of surgical staples.[90] For procedures other than suturing parenchyma, careful suture and ligature techniques should be at least as effective as mechanical staplers.

Lumpectomy. Although lumpectomy is rarely used in the treatment of bronchogenic carcinoma, Perelman has described a technique of precision cautery dissection that allows a wide excision of T1 or T2N0 tumors.[25] This can be applied to more deeply seated tumors using a combination of electrocautery and ligation of larger vessels and airways. With this technique more proximal T1 or T2N0 tumors can be widely excised, preserving the remaining lung in patients with severely compromised pulmonary function. If the procedure is performed with care, postoperative air leaks will be minimal, and in selected high-risk patients this can result in curative resections.

The general consensus continues that all of these limited resections in the treatment of T1 or T2N0 lung cancer should be reserved for the high-risk patient with minimal pulmonary reserve.

Extended Operations

Pulmonary resection can be combined with resection of other structures. In the case of T3 tumors, contiguous involvement of the chest wall, mediastinal structures, or the carina may require an extended procedure. Similarly, with N2 disease, en bloc mediastinal lymph node dissection will be required for complete extirpation of the tumor.

Chest Wall Resection. A carcinoma involving the parietal pleura, intercostal muscle, and/or ribs (T3) can still be totally resected for cure by en bloc resection of the involved structure. The survival rate will be as high as 50% if only the parietal pleura is involved without lymph node disease.[28] Extension of the tumor into the chest wall will increase the risk of failure. Associated N2 disease is an ominous prognostic sign; we have never been able to cure a patient with this condition. If N2 disease is identified before surgery, we do not advise surgery. However, if it is identified at thoracotomy and can be completely removed, we proceed with the resection, even though the prognosis is poor.

Most authors believe that for tumors involving the parietal pleura, resection with only parietal pleurectomy (extrapleural resection) and without concomitant resection of the chest wall (ribs and intercostal muscle) decreases the chance of complete removal of the tumor and increases the risk of local recurrence.[91] However, Martini and colleagues have reported equal survival rates regardless of whether the tumor was resected extrapleurally or en bloc with the chest wall.[92]

If the tumor involves intercostal muscle or ribs, a chest wall excision is required. A wide excision is necessary, at least 2 cm of healthy tissue being removed beyond the involved area. Frozen-section guidance is helpful. Smaller chest wall defects, especially those covered posteriorly by the scapula, may not require plastic reconstruction. However, large chest wall defects (three or more ribs) or anterior chest wall defects (two or more ribs) should be reconstructed with a plastic mesh (e.g., Marlex mesh), woven fabric (e.g., Gortex), or a combination of a plastic mesh and methylmethacrylate to provide thoracic wall rigidity (see Chapter 38).

Any incomplete resection of a tumor invading the chest wall almost inevitably results in local recurrence. Even completely resected tumors frequently recur locally. The value of postoperative adjuvant radiotherapy, with either local implantation or external beam irradiation, has not been assessed in a prospective manner. Some authors believe that this may decrease the chance of local recurrence.[93]

Resection of Vertebra. Invasion of the rib and subjacent transverse process does not necessarily eliminate the possibility of total resection for cure by partial or complete removal of these structures. However, involvement of the vertebral body usually portends an incomplete resection and ultimate recurrence. Attempts have been made recently to completely excise the vertebral body, replacing the structure with methylmethacrylate. The result of this more aggressive resection is not known.

Carinal Resection. As mentioned previously, carinal resection may be required and is indicated for tumors involving the carina that can be completely resected. In some instances of very localized disease, this procedure may be accomplished without pulmonary resection or with preservation of one or more lobes. Lung preservation should be attempted whenever possible, with the understanding that a complete resection of the tumor is required. There have been many reports of the results of sleeve pneumonectomy that include carinal resection and ipsilateral pneumonectomy. Most authors have found that this approach is valuable for T3N0 or T4N0 tumors. Tumors with associated nodal disease frequently recur after this approach, with a very poor 5-year survival rate.

All of these extended resections increase morbidity and mortality. Care must be taken in proper selection of patients when considering these more extensive surgical approaches.

Mediastinal Lymph Node Dissection (Radical Resection)

Whether complete mediastinal lymph node dissection is required in every resection performed for lung cancer is a controversial issue. Certainly, complete mediastinal lymph node staging using frozen-section identification of metastatic disease, carried out either before surgery by mediastinoscopy or at the time of surgery, is necessary for accurate staging and treatment of the patient. If hilar (N1) or mediastinal (N2) disease is identified before surgery or at the time of surgery, the surgeon is obligated to perform a lymph node dissection that is as complete as necessary, keeping in mind the drainage areas of the various lobes. There are no data to suggest that complete mediastinal lymph node dissection is required in N0 or bronchopulmonary N1 disease, as long as hilar or N2 disease has been excluded by frozen-section analysis.

In instances of lower lobe tumors draining to the nodes of the posterior mediastinum, that area can be easily dissected, especially if a posterolateral thoracotomy is used. The pleura should be opened from the inferior pulmonary vein to the subcarinal space, and all lymph nodes should be dissected, including those in the inferior pulmonary ligament, along the esophagus, and in the subcarinal space; preferably they should be dissected en bloc with the specimen.

In left upper lobe tumors, when mediastinal lymph nodes involve only the subaortic and anterior mediastinal regions, a complete en bloc dissection can be performed without difficulty. Attempts should be made to preserve the recurrent and phrenic nerves, excising all lymphatic tissue in the region. If there is adherence to the aorta, the subadventitial plane can be used. The pericardium can and should be removed if lymphatic tissue is adherent to it.

In left upper lobe tumors involving superior mediastinal lymph nodes, dissection under the aortic arch along the left main-stem bronchus can reach only the tracheobronchial angle. Attempts at dissection above this point require opening the mediastinal pleura between the subclavian and carotid arteries. Radical mediastinal lymph node dissection for left upper lobe tumors is most easily performed using a median sternotomy approach.

In right upper lobe tumors, the superior mediastinal lymph nodes can easily be resected en bloc with the right upper lobe. The arch of the azygos vein should be divided proximally at its entrance to the superior vena cava and distally at the level of the hemiazygos confluence. The complete superior mediastinal lymph node "package" should be removed from the area bounded superiorly by the innominate artery, medially by the aorta, posteriorly by the tracheoesophageal groove, and anteriorly by the superior vena cava, and the right mediastinal pleura is removed en bloc. Care must be taken not to injure the right recurrent nerve near the right subclavian artery or the left recurrent nerve along the left tracheoesophageal groove. In all upper lobe tumors requiring node dissection, a concomitant subcarinal lymph node dissection should also be performed.

After mediastinal lymph node dissection, the most proximal nodes excised should be submitted for frozen section to confirm total clearance of disease. It is our policy to identify superior mediastinal lymph node disease at preoperative mediastinoscopy and to perform complete nodal staging with frozen section at the time of surgery. Mediastinal lymph node dissection is the best and most accurate type of staging and occasionally may benefit a patient with occult mediastinal disease found in a single node only because of the complete nodal dissection.

The Positive Resection Line. It is appropriate to confirm complete clearance of the tumor at the time of resection by submitting the bronchial resection margin to frozen section prior to completing the operation.

A tumor may involve the bronchial resection area by virtue of continuity of the primary tumor, submucosal spread beyond the obvious tumor margin, peribronchial lymphatic spread, and focal areas of dysplasia or carcinoma in situ at the resection margin. In analyses by Griess and colleagues[94] and Cotton,[66] significant spread of tumor beyond the palpable mass occurred in only 12% of patients. The maximum distance of spread was 2 cm.

Despite a positive resection margin at the time of surgery, it is apparent that these patients will have a higher survival rate than those having an incomplete resection of T3 disease elsewhere. Soorae and Stevenson[95] identified 64 of 434 consecutive patients with positive resection margins due to microscopic residual tumor. Twenty-four per cent of patients survived 5 years or longer. Most of these patients had small squamous cell carcinomas with areas of in situ disease at the resection margin. Submucosal or peribronchial lymphatic involvement was an ominous sign; no patients in this category survived beyond 3 years. Jeffrey[96] and Shields[97] have also reported 5-year survivors among patients with residual tumor on the bronchial stump. Kaiser has confirmed the favorable result of in situ disease at the resection line versus submucosa or peribronchial lymphatic involvement.[98]

It is unlikely that the survival of patients with positive resection margins is due to spontaneous regression of the tumor. It has been postulated that other factors may be operating: local mechanical trauma to residual neoplastic cells, interference with nutrition of the residual cells, or a positive immunologic response by the patient to the microscopic residual foci.

All reasonable attempts should be made to convert a positive resection margin to a negative resection margin at the time of surgery. No direct relationship has been found between the distance of the resection from the tumor margin and survival. In treating the patient, consideration should be given to converting a lobectomy to a sleeve lobectomy or pneumonectomy and a pneumonectomy to a sleeve pneumonectomy if simple re-resection of the bronchial stump fails to clear all tumor. It has been our practice, however, not to perform additional surgery with a negative resection margin, even if it is millimeters from the primary tumor. Obviously, the prognosis is more favorable if only the mucosa and not the lymphatics in the submucosa or peribronchial region are involved near the resection margin.

It has been suggested that postoperative radiotherapy in patients with residual tumor at the bronchial resection margin may favorably alter the prognosis. This has not been proved conclusively.[97] There can be no definite recommendation for the role of either chemotherapy or radiotherapy in patients with proven positive resection margins, although most authorities recommend the latter modality.

Synchronous Primary Lung Carcinomas

Synchronous primary lung carcinomas present a special problem. Preoperative assessment of other possible primary sites should be made to determine that lesions are in fact primary lung tumors and not metastatic lesions. Patients with synchronous primary mucosal squamous cell carcinomas should be suspected of having multiple areas of squamous carcinoma, and a search must be made to rule out further primary squamous cell tumors in the aero-digestive tract.[99] This would include nasopharyngoscopy, laryngoscopy, complete bronchoscopic examination with multiple biopsies of all segments, and esophagoscopy.[100]

In patients with peripheral tumors, evaluation for other pulmonary parenchymal lesions should be exhaustive and is best carried out with thoracic CT examination.

The usual criteria of operability should be applied using procedures including mediastinoscopy to assess N2 disease; selective studies to rule out metastatic foci in the brain, bone, liver, and adrenals; and preoperative estimation of pulmonary function after the resections.

These tumors may be approached synchronously through a median sternotomy or transverse sternotomy and bilateral anterior thoracotomies (clamshell incision), attempting to preserve as much pulmonary tissue as possible. Many surgeons prefer a staged resection, using sequential bilateral thoracotomies, delaying the second surgery until the patient recovers from the first.

Although bilateral lobectomies certainly can be used without major pulmonary compromise for synchronous primary tumors, if one tumor happens to be placed peripherally and is staged T1N0, a limited resection, although somewhat of a compromise, is frequently used. The most extensive resection of pulmonary tissue that can be performed safely would be a pneumonectomy with a contralateral limited resection (wedge or segment).

At the time of surgery the proper staging procedures with nodal biopsies should be performed, as in any operation for primary lung cancer.

Sometimes it is difficult to assess whether the "second primary" is not really a solitary contralateral pulmonary metastasis. It has been our approach to consider these as second primaries, unless definitely proved otherwise, and to treat the patient accordingly.

The Lung as a Second Primary Site. The lung frequently is the second site of a cancer, especially in patients who have previously experienced other aero-digestive tumors. Frequently, in these cases as well, it is difficult to determine whether the new lesion is a metastatic focus or a second primary carcinoma. Two analyses have demonstrated that in two-thirds of patients, the new lesion within the lung is indeed a second primary lung cancer.[101, 102] These patients, if their first primary carcinoma is controlled, should be investigated and treated as if they had a primary lung cancer. Unfortunately, the ultimate survival rate is only about 25 per cent in most series. It is very rare for patients to present with simultaneous malignancies of the head, neck, and lung. In these patients, the most urgent problems should be addressed first, usually those involving the lung. Resectional surgery for the lung cancer should be offered only if both malignancies can be cured.

RESULTS OF TREATMENT

Postoperative Complications

The major improvements in postoperative management of patients that have occurred over the past few decades represent the most significant advance in the surgical treatment of lung cancer. These improvements have resulted in decreased operative and postoperative mortality as well as morbidity. The tremendous advances in the understanding of cardiopulmonary physiology and the advent of intensive care units as well as assisted mechanical ventilation and cardiorespiratory monitoring in the postoperative period have all contributed to this improvement.

Postoperative Mortality (Table 8–5). Retrospective analyses of work done in the 1950s and 1960s and published in the early 1970s suggested that postoperative mortality could be as high as 20% for pneumonectomy and as high as 5% to 10% for lobectomy.[103, 104] However, more recent analyses have indicated that the true 30-day postoperative mortality for pulmo-

TABLE 8–5. Postoperative Mortality After 2220 Pulmonary Resections for Lung Cancer

TYPE OF RESECTION AND AGE OF PATIENT	NO. OF RESECTIONS	30-DAY MORTALITY (%)
All resections	2220	3.7
Pneumonectomy	569	6.2
Lobectomy	1508	2.9
Segmentectomy or wedge resection	143	1.4
60 years	847	1.3
60–69 years	920	4.1
70 years	443	7.2

Modified from Ginsberg RJ, Hill LD, Eagan RT, et al: Modern 30 day operative mortality for surgical resections in lung cancer. J Thorac Cardiovasc Surg 86:654–657, 1983.

nary resectional surgery in the treatment of lung cancer should be less than 4%.[105, 106] Lobectomies and lesser resections are relatively safe, with fewer than 3% of patients failing to survive the postoperative period. Unfortunately, pneumonectomy still has a 6% to 7% mortality rate. The mortality rate increases with age, associated diseases, and the extent of resection. The Lung Cancer Study Group analyzed more than 2000 resections. In patients aged 70 and over, the mortality rate was 7% for both lobectomy and pneumonectomy. The most common postoperative complications leading to death include cardiovascular and respiratory problems. There is still a small but significant effect on mortality rates that is related to surgical technical problems, including hemorrhage, postoperative bronchopleural fistula, and empyema. The estimate of perioperative risk for an individual patient must be tempered by the consideration of all of these variables. Recent single-institution retrospective analyses have demonstrated even more improved postoperative mortality with proper patient selection.[107]

Postoperative Morbidity

The most common complication following pulmonary resection is supraventricular arrhythmia, especially atrial fibrillation. In a recent analysis of more than 1000 consecutive pulmonary resections, we found that 70% of patients had a normal postoperative course without complication.[108] Minor complications occurred in 20% of patients. Half of these were uneventful supraventricular arrhythmias, and one-fourth were postoperative atelectasis. Nonfatal major complications occurred in 10% of patients. In this consecutive group, the 30-day surgical mortality was 3.2%. Significant risk factors for major complications included the following: age greater than 60 years, FEV_1 less than 2 L, weight loss of 10%, associated systemic disease, stage of cancer greater than Stage I, and extent of resection (pneumonectomy and extended resections).

Postoperative pulmonary complications should and can be minimized with appropriate preoperative attention to these patients, most of whom are suffering from cardiovascular and chronic obstructive pulmo-

nary disease. Whether or not preoperative digitalization will prevent supraventricular arrhythmias has not been addressed in a prospective fashion. With the isotope techniques now available to preoperatively estimate pulmonary reserve after surgery, it is rare for a patient to be left a respiratory cripple. After a pneumonectomy, most patients have sufficient pulmonary reserve to manage normal daily activities. However, in long-term surviving patients after pneumonectomy, especially right pneumonectomy, the development of slowly progressive cor pulmonale and ultimate respiratory failure are occasionally observed.

The postoperative complications related to surgical technique have been minimized by preventing bronchopleural fistula with meticulous attention to bronchial closure, avoidance of long bronchial stumps, and prevention of sepsis with the use of perioperative antibiotics.

Prognosis Following Resection

The prognosis of surgically resected non–small cell lung cancer has been well analyzed.[109–111] Historically, it was known that patients with peripheral lesions fared better than central ones, patients undergoing lobectomy fared better than those requiring pneumonectomy, and patients with involved hilar lymph nodes had a much poorer prognosis than those without.

In 1988, the modern TNM staging was introduced by the American Joint Committee for Cancer (AJCC) Staging and End Results Reporting.[112] The definitions and rules were defined from analyses of data based on more than 2000 cases contributed by the AJCC. Subsequent to the introduction of the AJCC TNM staging, many analyses of results of surgically treated patients have appeared in the literature. The most recent analysis from the University of Texas and the Lung Cancer Study Group appears in Table 8–6[47] and forms the basis for the modern TNM staging for lung cancer introduced in 1986 by both the AJCC and UICC.

The prognosis following surgery depends on TNM staging,[110] histology,[111] and completeness of the resec-

TABLE 8–6. Postsurgical Survival of More Than 1400 Patients Analyzed by University of Texas and Lung Cancer Study Group*†

STAGE	TN SUBSET	NO. OF PATIENTS	5-YEAR SURVIVAL (%)
I	T1N0	429	69
	T2N0	436	59
	T1N1	67	54
II	T2N1	250	40
III	T3N0	57	44
	T3N1	29	18
	Any N2	168	28

*Postoperative mortality is excluded
†T3N2 disease was not analyzed separately because the numbers were small, but it carries the poorest prognoses (<10%).
Modified from Mountain CF: A new international staging system for lung cancer. Chest 89(suppl):225–233, 1986.

tion.[113] The 5-year survival following surgery is best analyzed according to TNM stage. The Lung Cancer Study Group has further analyzed the prognosis according to TN stage and histology (Table 8–7).[114, 115] For non–small cell lung cancer, the tumor with the best prognosis is T1N0 squamous cell (greater than 70% 5-year survival), the poorest prognosis occurs with T3N2 adenocarcinoma (less than 10% 5-year survival). In most series, 15% to 20% of all deaths occurring in the 5-year period are non-cancer related. The actual "cure" rate of T1N0 squamous cell cancer appears to be about 85% with surgical resection. Our Japanese colleagues have reported extensive analyses of the results of surgical resection stage by stage and node status by node status. Their results are similar to those in the U.S. literature (see Table 8–1).

The Mayo Clinic has analyzed late recurrence rates in Stage I carcinoma.[116] Beyond 5 years, primary tumors recur rarely. However, the incidence of second primary carcinomas remains stable throughout the follow-up of the patient.

Sites of Recurrence

It is becoming increasingly evident that the first site of recurrence following resection for lung cancer is most commonly in distant organs.[117, 118] The brain is a common single organ site of first recurrence and is found to be the first site in over 10% of patients. Other common sites include bone, liver, adrenal, and contralateral lung. In about two-thirds of patients distant metastases will appear without evidence of local recurrence. In one-third of patients they will recur locally as the initial site of failure, including ipsilateral lung and mediastinum. There is some variability of site of recurrence according to initial stage. In those patients with Stage III disease cancer will tend to first recur distantly somewhat more frequently than in patients with Stage I disease.[115]

Postsurgical Follow-up

The fact that only 30% to 40% of all patients following curative surgery for lung cancer will survive 5 years without evidence of recurrent disease, and the fact that some of these patients will develop second pri-

TABLE 8–7. Analysis of Survival According to Stage and Histology from the Lung Cancer Study Group*†

STAGE	SUBSET	CELL TYPE	4-YEAR SURVIVAL (%)
I	T1N0	Squamous cell	85
		adenocarcinoma	72
	T1N1	Squamous cell	80
		adenocarcinoma	63
	T2N0	Squamous cell	65
		adenocarcinoma	60
II, III		Squamous cell	37
		adenocarcinoma	25

*Postoperative mortality is excluded.
†See reference 115.

mary tumors or local problems that can potentially be treated, suggests that follow-up on a regular basis is essential in the management of lung cancer.[119]

Early local recurrences and occasionally solitary brain or other distant metastases can be managed surgically, with the expectation of complete salvage in some patients. Early attention to other recurrences may decrease the morbidity associated with the recurrent cancer. For all these reasons, regular follow-up is mandatory. Since most recurrences present within the first 2 years, it is suggested the patient should be seen every 3 months during this period of time. A complete history, physical examination, and chest x-ray examination are the basis of follow-up. In patients with squamous cell carcinoma, it has been our practice to perform sputum cytologic examinations with each follow-up visit. These patients have a significant risk of developing other aerodigestive tract squamous cell cancers.[120–122] The sputum cytologic examination is facilitated by using a 3-day pooled specimen technique.

Although early recurrence can sometimes be identified by nonspecific blood markers (serum glutamic-oxaloacetic transaminase [SGOT], alkaline phosphatase, serum calcium, and white blood cell count [WBC]), whether or not any of these are required at each follow-up visit is a moot point. Often, a spurious elevation of one of these blood markers will lead to much fruitless investigation. Abnormal blood tests should be confirmed before other investigations are begun. Continued weight loss with each visit suggests recurrent disease.

Between the second and fifth years following the surgical resection, it is suggested that patients be seen every 6 months. Subsequently, only yearly examination is required, with the understanding that a second primary cancer may develop. The second primaries are most successfully treated if picked up early by chest x-ray examination or sputum cytology before symptoms develop.

Once a recurrence is suspected, further investigation may be useful. This type of investigation is dictated by the patient's symptoms or signs. Patients with symptoms suggesting locoregional recurrence but with a normal chest radiograph are often best investigated by repeat bronchoscopy and CT scan. This is especially helpful in identifying early recurrent mediastinal disease and recurrent disease at the location of a pneumonectomy.

FUTURE DIRECTIONS IN SURGERY

With biologic markers, further improvements in the preoperative identification of metastatic disease will occur, allowing surgeons to select more appropriately the patients who will benefit from surgical resection. Monoclonal antibody–labeled isotopes specific for lung cancer and PET scanning may improve preoperative staging techniques, allowing a more rational approach to treatment.

There is no doubt that in the future more sophisticated surgical techniques will reduce the risks associated with resection. Preoperative identification of high-risk patients has already reduced that risk. Further improvements in preoperative, intraoperative, and postoperative care will decrease perioperative morbidity and mortality. We hope in the future that with improved screening techniques, second primary tumors when they occur will be identified earlier and thus allow improved survival for this group of patients.

Minimally invasive techniques and improved perioperative pain control may allow patients a surgical approach without the morbidity due to pain. For the foreseeable future, surgery will continue to play a major role in the curative management of non–small cell lung cancer.

SELECTED REFERENCES

Delarue NC, Eschapasse H (eds): International Trends in General Thoracic Surgery, Vol 1: Lung Cancer. Philadelphia, W. B. Saunders, 1985.
 This first volume of a projected series of monographs on the topic of thoracic surgery presents controversial opinions regarding the management of lung cancer. It is well written by experts from around the world and remains current even today.
VanRaemdonck DE, Schneider A, Ginsberg RJ: Surgical treatment for higher stage non-small cell lung cancer: A collective review. Ann Thorac Surg 54:999–1013, 1992.
 This collective review summarizes the information from the world literature on surgical resection for higher stage lung cancer over a 10-year period.
Waldhausen JA, Pierce WS: Johnson's Surgery of the Chest, 5th ed. Chicago, Year Book Medical Publishers, 1985.
 This is an excellent reference for the standard surgical techniques used in the management of carcinoma of the lung.

REFERENCES

1. Sauerbruch F: Die Operation Entfernung von Lungengeschwulste. Zentralbl Chir 53:852–854, 1926.
2. Pean J: Chirurgie des poumons. Discussion Ranc Chir Proc Verh Paris 9:72–74, 1895.
3. Davies HM: Recent advances in the surgery of the lung and pleura. Br J Surg 1:228–231, 1913–1914.
4. Sauerbruch F: Die Chirurgie der Brustorgane, Vol 2. Berlin, J Springer, 1925.
5. Brunn HB: Surgical principles underlying one-stage lobectomy. Arch Surg 18:490–496, 1929.
6. Allan CI, Smith FJ: Primary carcinoma of the lung with report of case treated by operation. Surg Gynecol Obstet 55:151–155, 1932.
7. Churchill ED: The surgical treatment of carcinoma of the lung. J Thorac Surg 2:254–261, 1933.
8. Graham EA, Singer JJ: Successful removal of the entire lung for carcinoma of the bronchus. JAMA 101:1371–1374, 1933.
9. Gluck T: Experimenteller Beitrag zur Frage der Lungenexstirpation. Berl Klin Wochenschr 18:645–646, 1881.
10. Biondi D: Extirpazione del polmone. G Intern S Med 4:759–760, 1882.
11. Kummel H: Proceedings of the 40th Congress, Berlin, April 19–22, 1911. Verh Dtsch Ges Chir 40:147, 1911.
12. Hinz R: Totale extirpation der linken Lunge wegen Bronchial Carcinoma. Arch Klin Chir 124:104–107, 1923.
13. Archibald E: Discussed in Churchill ED: The surgical treatment of carcinoma of the lung. J Thorac Surg 2:254–261, 1933.
14. Ivanissevich O, Ferrari RC: La Neumectomia en el Hombre. Boll Trab Soc Cirug Buenos Aires 17:553, 1933.
15. Rienhoff WF: Pneumonectomy: A preliminary report of operative technique in two successful cases. Bull Johns Hopkins Hosp 53:390–392, 1933.
16. Churchill E, Belsey HR: Segmental pneumonectomy in bronchiectasis. Ann Surg 109:481–485, 1939.
17. Allison PR: Intrapericardial approach to the lung root in the treatment of bronchial carcinoma by dissection pneumonectomy. J Thorac Surg 15:99–104, 1946.
18. Price-Thomas C: Conservative resection of the bronchial tree. J R Coll Surg Edinb 1:169–171, 1956.
19. Mathey J, Binet JP, Galey JJ, et al: Tracheal and tracheobronchial resections: Technique and results in 20 cases. J Thorac Cardiovasc Surg 51:1–13, 1966.
20. Thompson DT: Tracheal resection with left lung anastomosis following right pneumonectomy. Thorax 21:560–563, 1966.
21. Coleman FP: Primary carcinoma of the lung with invasion of ribs: Pneumonectomy and simultaneous block resection of chest wall. Ann Surg 126:156–158, 1947.
22. Chardak WM, MacCallun JD: Pancoast tumor (5 yr survival without recurrence or metastases following radical resection and postoperative irradiation). J Thorac Surg 31:535–542, 1956.
23. Shaw RR, Paulson DL, Kee JL Jr: Treatment of the superior sulcus tumor by irradiation followed by resection. Ann Surg 154:29–40, 1961.
24. Jensik RJ, Faber LP, Milloy FJ, et al: Segmental resection for lung cancer: A fifteen year experience. J Thorac Cardiovasc Surg 66:563–572, 1973.
25. Perelman MI: Lumpectomy for lung cancer. Chest 89(suppl):336S–337S, 1986.
26. Kouka S, Forai I: The segmental and atypical resection of primary lung cancer. Proc IV World Conference on Lung Cancer, 48, 1985.
27. Errett LE, Wilson J, Chin RC, Munroe D: Wedge resection as an alternative procedure for peripheral bronchogenic carcinoma in poor-risk patients. J Thorac Cardiovasc Surg 90:656–661, 1985.
28. Wright JL, Coppin C, Mullen BJ, et al: Surgical treatment of early lung cancer: Promise and problems of early diagnosis. Can J Surg 29:205–208, 1986.
29. Flehinger BJ, Melamed MR: Current status of screening for lung cancer. Chest Surg Clin North Am 4:1–15, 1994.
30. Auerbuch O, Stout AP, Hammond EC, et al: Changes in the bronchial epithelia in relation to cigarette smoking and in relation to lung cancer. N Engl J Med 265:253, 1961.
31. Weiss W: Tumor doubling time and survival of men with bronchogenic carcinoma. Chest 65:3–8, 1974.
32. Buchberg GA, Lubliner R, Rubin EH: Carcinoma of the lung: Duration of life of individuals not treated surgically. Dis Chest 20:257–276, 1951.
33. Silverberg E, Lubera J: Cancer statistics 1986. CA Cancer J Clin 36:9–25, 1986.
34. Taylor RR, Rivkin LN, Salyer JM: The solitary pulmonary nodule: A review of 236 consecutive cases, 1944–1956. Ann Surg 147:197–202, 1958.
35. Siegelman SS, Zerhouni EA, Leo FP, Khouri NF, Stitik FP: CT of the solitary pulmonary nodule. AJR Am J Roentgenol 135:1–13, 1980.
36. Proto AU, Thomas SR: Pulmonary nodules studied by computed tomography. Radiology 156:149–153, 1985.
37. Todd TR, Weisbrod GH, Tao LC, Sanders DE, et al: Aspiration needle biopsy of thoracic lesions. Ann Thorac Surg 32:1981.
38. Cortese DA, McDougall JC: Biopsy and brushing of peripheral lung cancer with fluoroscopic guidance. Chest 75:141–145, 1979.
39. Nathan MH, Collins VP, Adams RA: Differentiation of benign and malignant pulmonary nodules by growth rate. Radiology 79:221–231, 1962.
40. Velasco FT, Rusch VW, Ginsberg RJ: Thoracoscopic management of chest neoplasms. Semin Laparoscopic Surg 1:43–51, 1994.
41. Mack MJ, Gordon M, Postma TW, et al: Percutaneous localization of pulmonary modules for thoracoscopic resection. Ann Thorac Surg 53:1123–1124, 1992.

42. Shennib H: Intraoperative localization techniques for pulmonary nodules. Ann Thorac Surg 56:745–748, 1993.

43. Piehler JM, Pairolero PC, Weiland LH, et al: Bronchogenic carcinoma with chest wall invasion: Factors affecting survival following en bloc resection. Ann Thor Surg 34:684–691, 1982.

44. Eschapasse H, Gaillar DJ, DaHan M, et al: Sleeve lobectomy for carcinoma of the lung. Chest 89(suppl):335S–336S, 1986.

45. Burt ME, Pomerantz AH, Bains MS, et al: Results of surgical treatment of stage III lung cancer invading the mediastinum. Surg Clin North Am 67:987–100, 1987.

46. Ginsberg RJ, Martini N, Armstrong J: The influence of surgical resection and brachytherapy in superior sulcus tumor. Presented at the 30th Annual Meeting of the Society of Thoracic Surgeons Meeting, January 31–February 2, 1994, New Orleans.

47. Mountain CF: Prognostic implications of the international staging system for lung cancer. Semin Oncol 1988;15:236–45.

48. Pearson FG: Mediastinal adenopathy—the N2 lesion. In Delarue NC, Eschapasse H (eds): International Trends in General Thoracic Surgery, Vol 1: Lung Cancer. Philadelphia, W. B. Saunders, 1985, pp 104–107.

49. Sawamura K, Mori T, Hashimoto S, et al: Results of surgical treatment for N2 disease. Lung Cancer 2:96, 1986.

50. Naruke T, Suemasu K, Ishikawa S, et al: Mediastinal lymph node dissection and its significance in surgery of lung cancer. Lung Cancer 2:96, 1986.

51. Martini N, Flehinger B, Zaman M, Beattie EJ Jr, et al: Prospective study of 445 lung carcinomas with mediastinal lymph node metastases. J Thorac Cardiovasc Surg 80:390–397, 1980.

52. Hata E, Hayakawa H, Miyamoto H, et al: The incidence and the prognosis of the contralateral mediastinal node involvement of the left lung cancer patients who underwent bilateral mediastinal dissection and pulmonary resection through the median sternotomy. Lung Cancer 4(suppl):A87, 1988.

53. Watanabe Y, Ichihashi T, Iwa T: Mediansternotomy as an approach for pulmonary surgery. Thorac Cardiovasc Surg 36:227–231, 1988.

54. Rusch VW, Albain KS, Crowley JJ, et al: Surgical resection of stage IIIa and IIIb non-small cell lung cancer after concurrent induction chemotherapy: A Southwest Oncology Group Trial. J Thorac Cardiovasc Surg 105:97–106, 1993.

55. Burt M, Wronski M, Arbit E, Galicich JH, and the Memorial Sloan-Kettering Cancer Center Thoracic Surgical Staff: Resection of brain metastasis from non-small cell lung cancer: Results of therapy. J Thorac Cardiovasc Surg 1103:399–411, 1992.

56. MacGilligan DJ, Duvenory C, Malik G, et al: Surgical application to lung cancer with cerebral metastases: 25 years experience. Ann Thorac Surg 42:360–364, 1986.

57. Yacoub MH: Relation between the history of bronchial carcinoma and hypertrophic pulmonary osteoarthropathy. Thorax 20:537, 1965.

58. Roth JA, Fossella F, Komaki R, et al: A randomized trial comparing perioperative chemotherapy and surgery with surgery alone in resectable stage III non-small cell lung cancer. J Natl Cancer Inst 86:673–680, 1994.

59. Rosell R, Gomez-Codina J, Camps C, et al: A randomized trial comparing preoperative chemotherapy plus surgery with surgery alone in patients with non-small cell lung cancer. N Engl J Med 330:153–158, 1994.

60. Jackson OL, Huber CL: Correlated applied anatomy of bronchial tree and lungs with system nomenclature. Dis Chest 9:319–326, 1943.

61. Rouviere EH: Anatomy of the human lymphatic system. Ann Arbor, Edwards, 1938.

62. Drinker EK: The lymphatic system. Lane Medical Lectures. Palo Alto, Stanford University Press, 1942.

63. Borrie J: Primary carcinoma of the bronchus: Prognoses following surgical resection. A clinical pathological study of 200 patients. Ann R Coll Surg Engl 10:165–168, 1952.

64. Nohl-Oser HC: An investigation into the lymphatic and vascular spread of carcinoma of the bronchus. Thorax 11:172, 1956.

65. Carlens E: Mediastinoscopy. Dis Chest 36:343–542, 1959.

66. Cotton RE: The bronchial spread of lung cancer. Br J Dis Chest 53:142–150, 1959.

67. Lange-Cordes E: Uber die Intramukose Ausbreitrung der Bronchial Carcinome. Thorax Chir 4:327–333, 1956.

68. Nohl-Oser HC: An investigation of the anatomy of the lymphatic drainage of the lungs as shown by the lymphatic spread of bronchial carcinoma. Ann R Coll Surg Engl 51:157–176, 1972.

69. Shields TW (ed): General Thoracic Surgery. Philadelphia, Lea & Febiger, 1983.

70. Sabiston DC, Spencer FC (eds): Gibbon's Surgery of the Chest. Philadelphia, W. B. Saunders, 1983.

71. Waldhausen JA, Pierce WS (eds): Johnson's Surgery of the Chest, 5th Ed. Chicago, Year Book Medical Publishers, 1985.

72. Hood RM: Techniques in General Thoracic Surgery. Philadelphia, W. B. Saunders, 1985.

73. Cooper JD, Nelems JM, Pearson FG, et al: Extended indications for a median sternotomy in patients requiring pulmonary resections. Ann Thorac Surg 26:413, 1978.

74. Takita H, Merrin C, Didolkar MS, et al: The surgical management of multiple lung metastases. Ann Thorac Surg 24:359–364, 1977.

75. Urschel HC Jr: Discussed in Cooper JD, Nelems JM, Pearson FG, et al: Extended indications for a median sternotomy in patients requiring pulmonary resections. Ann Thorac Surg 26:413, 1978.

76. Naruke T, Suemasu K, Ishikawa S, et al: Lymph node mapping and curability at various levels of metastasis in resective lung cancer. J Thorac Cardiovasc Surg 76:832–839, 1978.

77. Bains MS, Ginsberg RJ, Jones WGH, et al: The clamshell incision: An improved approach to bilateral pulmonary and mediastinal tumor. Ann Thorac Surg 58:30–33, 1994.

78. Ginsberg RJ: Alternative (muscle-sparing) incisions in thoracic surgery. Ann Thorac Surg 56:752–754, 1993.

79. Hazelrigg SR, Landreneau RJ, Boley TM, et al: The effect of muscle-sparing versus standard posterolateral thoracotomy on pulmonary function, muscle strength, and postoperative pain. J Thorac Cardiovasc Surg 101:394–401, 1991.

80. Brock R, Whytehead LL: Radical pneumonectomy for bronchial carcinoma. Br J Surg 43:8–24, 1955.

81. Cahan WG, Watson WL, Pool JL, et al: Radical pneumonectomy. J Thorac Surg 22:449–473, 1951.

82. Deslauriers J, Beaulieu M, Benazera A, et al: Sleeve pneumonectomy for bronchogenic carcinoma. Ann Thorac Surg 28:465–474, 1978.

83. Jensik RJ, Faber LB, Kittle CF, et al: Survival in patients undergoing tracheal sleeve pneumonectomy for bronchogenic carcinoma. J Thorac Cardiovasc Surg 84:489–496, 1982.

84. Darteville PG, Khilife J, Levasseur A, et al: Tracheal sleeve pneumonectomy for bronchogenic carcinoma: Report of 46 cases in results according to node invasion. Lung Cancer 2:102, 1986.

85. Toomes SH, Vogt-Moykopf FI: Conservative resection for lung cancer. In Delarue NC, Eschapasse H (eds): International Trends in General Thoracic Surgery. Philadelphia, W. B. Saunders, 1985, pp 88–99.

86. Jensik RJ: The role of segmental resection in lung cancer. Chest 89(suppl):335S, 1986.

87. Kulka F, Forrai I: The segmental and atypical resection of primary lung cancer. Lung Cancer 2:99, 1986.

88. Ginsberg RJ, Rubinstein L, for the Lung Cancer Study Group: A randomized comparative trial of lobectomy vs limited resection for patients with T1 N0 non-small cell lung cancer. Lung Cancer 7(suppl):83, 1991.

89. Warren WH, Faber LP: Segmentectomy vs lobectomy in patients with stage I pulmonary carcinoma: Five year survival and patterns of intrathoracic recurrence. J Cardiovasc Surg 107:1087–1094, 1994.

90. Hood RM, Kirksey TD, Calhoon JH, et al: The use of automatic stapling devices and pulmonary resection. Ann Thorac Surg 16:85–98, 1973.

91. Trastek VF, Pairolero PC, Piehler J, et al: En bloc (non-chest wall) resection for bronchogenic carcinoma with parietal fixation. J Thorac Cardiovasc Surg 87:352–358, 1984.

92. Martini N, McCaughan B, Bains M, McCormick PM, et al: Improved survival in resection for selected Stage III lung cancer. Lung Cancer 2:97, 1986.

93. Patterson GA, Ilves R, Ginsberg RJ, et al: The value of adjuvant radiotherapy and pulmonary and chest wall resection for bronchogenic carcinoma. Ann Thorac Surg 34:692–697, 1982.

94. Griess DF, McDonald JR, Claggett OT, et al: The proximal extension of carcinoma of the lung and the bronchial wall. J Thorac Surg 14:362–368, 1945.
95. Soorae AS, Stevenson HM: Survival with residual tumor on a bronchial margin after resection for bronchogenic carcinoma. J Thorac Cardiovasc Surg 78:175–180, 1979.
96. Jeffrey RM: Survival in bronchial carcinoma: Tumor remaining in bronchial stump following resection. Ann R Coll Surg Engl 51:55–59, 1972.
97. Shields TW: The fate of patients after incomplete resection of bronchial carcinoma. Surg Gynecol Obstet 139:569–572, 1974.
98. Kaiser LR, Fleshner P, Keller S, Martini N: The significance of extramucosal residual tumor at the bronchial resection margin. Ann Thorac Surg 47:265–269, 1989.
99. Marks P, Schecter S: Multiple primary carcinomas of the head, neck, and lung. Ann Thorac Surg 33:324–332, 1982.
100. Auerbach O, Stout AP, Hammond EC, et al: Multiple primary bronchial carcinoma. Cancer 20:699–705, 1967.
101. Yellin A, Hill LR, Benfield JR: Bronchogenic carcinoma associated with upper aerodigestive cancers. J Thorac Cardiovasc Surg 91:674–683, 1986.
102. Lefor AT, Bredenberg CE, Kellman RM, Aust JC: Multiple malignancies of the lung and head and neck. Arch Surg 121:265–269, 1986.
103. Weiss W: Operative mortality and 5 year survival rates in men with bronchogenic carcinoma. Chest 66:483–487, 1974.
104. Mittman C, Brukerman I: Lung cancer: To operate or not? Ann Rev Resp Dis 116:477–496, 1977.
105. Ginsberg RJ, Hill LD, Eagan RT, et al: Modern 30 day operative mortality for surgical resections in lung cancer. J Thorac Cardiovasc Surg 86:654–657, 1983.
106. Nagasaki F, Flehinger B, Martini N, et al: Complications of surgery in the treatment of carcinoma of the lung. Chest 82:25–29, 1982.
107. Miller JI: Thallium imaging in preoperative evaluation of the pulmonary resection candidate. Ann Thorac Surg 54:249–252, 1992.
108. Deslauriers J, Ginsberg RJ: Unpublished data.
109. Williams DE, Pairolero PC, Davis CS, et al: Survival of patients surgically treated for Stage I lung cancer. J Thorac Cardiovasc Surg 82:70–76, 1981.
110. Shields TW, Humphrey EW, Matthews M, et al: Pathological stage grouping of patients with resected carcinoma of the lung. J Thorac Cardiovasc Surg 80:400–405, 1980.
111. Shields TW, Yee J, Conn JH, et al: Relationship of cell type and lymph node metastases to survival after resection of bronchial carcinoma. Ann Thorac Surg 20:501–510, 1975.
112. American Joint Committee for Cancer Staging and End Results Reporting. Task Force on the Lung. Anderson WAD, Carr DT, Cochairmen: Clinical staging of lung cancer. Chicago, 1973.
113. Freise G, Gabler A, Liebig S: Bronchial carcinoma and long term survival: Retrospective study of 433 patients who underwent resection. Thorax 33:228–234, 1978.
114. Gail MH, Eagan RT, Feld R, Ginsberg RJ, et al: Prognostic factors in patients with resected Stage I non-small cell lung cancer—a report from the Lung Cancer Study Group. Cancer 54:1802–1813, 1984.
115. Lung Cancer Study Group: Unpublished data.
116. Pairolero PC, Williams DE, Bergsterahl MS: Post-surgical Stage I bronchogenic carcinoma: morbid implications of recurrent disease. Ann Thorac Surg 38:331–338, 1984.
117. Immerman SC, Vanecko RM, Fry W, et al: Site of recurrence of patients with Stages I and II carcinoma of the lung resected for cure. Ann Thorac Surg 32:23–27, 1981.
118. Feld R, Rubenstein L, Weisenburger T, et al: Sites of recurrence in resected Stage I non-small cell lung cancer: A guide for future studies. J Clin Oncol 2:1352–1358, 1984.
119. Ginsberg RJ: Follow-up supervision after resection for lung cancer. In Delarue NC, Eschapasse H (eds): International Trends in General Thoracic Surgery, Vol 1: Lung Cancer. Philadelphia, W. B. Saunders, 1985.
120. Olsen JH: Second Cancer Following Cancer of the Respiratory System in Denmark, 1943–1980. National Cancer Institute Monograph No 68, 1985.
121. Boyce JD, Fraumeni JF: Second Cancer Following Cancer of the Respiratory System in Connecticut, 1935–1982. National Cancer Institute Monograph No 68, 1985.
122. Lefor AT, Bredenberg CE, Kellam RM, Aust JC: Multiple malignancies of the lung and head and neck. Arch Surg 121:265–270, 1986.
123. Allen MS, Mathisen DJ, Grillo HC, et al: Bronchogenic carcinoma with chest wall invasion. Ann Thorac Surg 51:948–951, 1991.
124. Levasseur PH, Regnard JF: Long term results after surgery for N2 non small cell lung cancer. Presented at the IASLC workshop, June 17–21, 1990, Bruges, Belgium.
125. Watanabe Y, Shimizu J, Oda M, et al: Aggressive surgical intervention in N2 non-small cell cancer of the lung. Ann Thorac Surg 51:253–261, 1991.
126. McCaughan BC, Martini N, Bains MS, McCormack PM: Chest wall invasion in carcinoma of the lung. Therapeutic and prognostic implications. J Thorac Cardiovasc Surg 89:836–841, 1985.
127. Paulson DL: The "superior sulcus" lesion. In Delarue NC, Eschapasse H. International Trends In General Thoracic Surgery, Vol 1: Lung Cancer. Philadelphia: W.B. Saunders Company, 121–131, 1985.
128. Rice TW, Pringle JF, Sinclair JE, et al: Superior sulcus tumors; results of treatment. Lung Cancer 2:156–157, 1986. (Abstract.)
129. Ricci C, Rendina EA, Venuta F: Surgical treatment of superior sulcus tumors. Lung Cancer 4(suppl):A95, 1988. (Abstract.)
130. Naruke T, Goya T, Tsuchiya R, Suemasu K: Prognosis and survival in resected lung carcinoma based on the new international staging system. J Thorac Cardiovasc Surg 96:440–447, 1988.
131. Martini N, Flehinger BJ: The role of surgery in N2 lung cancer. Surg Clin N Am 67:1037–1049, 1987.
132. Pearson FG, Delarue NC, Ilves R, et al: Significance of positive superior mediastinal nodes identified at mediastinoscopy in patients with resectable cancer of the lung. J Thorac Cardiovasc Surg 83:1–11, 1982.
133. Ungar I, Gyeney I, Scherer E, Szarvas I: Sleeve lobectomy: an alternative to pneumonectomy in the treatment of bronchial carcinoma. Thorac Cardiovasc Surg 29:41–46, 1981.
134. Eschapasse H: Proceedings of the minisymposia of the IV world conference on lung cancer. Toronto 1985, pp 52–53.
135. Naruke T: Bronchoplastic and bronchovascular procedures of the tracheobronchial tree in the management of primary lung cancer. Chest 96:53S–56S, 1989.
136. Vogt-Moykopf I, Fritz T, Meyer G, et al: Bronchoplastic and angioplastic operation in bronchial carcinoma: long term results of a retrospective analysis from 73-83. Int Surg 71:211–220, 1986.

PREOPERATIVE AND POSTOPERATIVE THERAPY FOR NON–SMALL CELL LUNG CANCER

Henry Wagner, Jr. and Philip Bonomi

RATIONALE AND DEFINITIONS OF ADJUVANT THERAPY

Adjuvant therapy may be defined as treatment given when all known tumor has been removed surgically (or controlled radiotherapeutically) in hope of reducing the risk of or delaying the time to clinical manifestation of subclinical residual disease. Its therapeutic niche is defined, in part, by the inadequacies of our present diagnostic and therapeutic tools. If we had better tools for detecting minimal disease burdens, fewer patients would appear to be disease free, and we would speak less of adjuvant therapy and more of therapy for detectable but preclinical disease. If our therapies for recurrent disease were more effective, we could consider strategies of observing patients at risk for relapse and treating only those who actually did relapse.

In the few malignancies for which early detection and treatment of systemic relapse are usually curative (e.g., embryonal carcinoma of the testis), this efficacy of salvage therapy blunts the relative benefit of adjuvant treatment. A randomized trial comparing adjuvant therapy of patients with pathologic Stage II non-seminomatous testicular cancer to a policy of close observation (including frequent CT scan and determination of alpha-fetoprotein and beta-hCG) failed to show a survival benefit for the use of adjuvant chemotherapy despite a substantial relapse rate in the group not given adjuvant therapy. Testicular cancer is a relatively unique adult solid tumor in both its ease of detection at a time of minimal disease burden and the curability of systemic metastatic disease, but the general principle remains that the main role of adjuvant therapy is in situations of intermediate therapeutic efficacy. Unfortunately, in the treatment of non–small cell cancer (non–SCLC), we are far from this point.

It is important also to consider the impact of sites of relapse on the patient's subsequent survival time and quality of life. If a particular category of disease recurrence is poorly palliated, its prevention by appropriate adjuvant therapy may be desirable, even in the absence of any gain in survival time for this approach.

REVIEW OF FAILURE RATES AND PATTERNS OF FAILURE FOLLOWING TREATMENT WITH SURGERY ALONE FOR PATIENTS WITH STAGE I to IIIA DISEASE

Surgery is the most effective treatment for patients with localized non–SCLC. The outcome of patients following resection of all known disease in the thorax depends on anatomic and biologic prognostic factors, and ranges from an 80% or better 5-year survival for patients with T1N0M0 squamous cell carcinoma to less than 15% for patients with T3N2M0 disease.[1–5] Selection of patients for adjuvant therapy requires the ability to predict which patients are at high risk for relapse and the sites of these relapses. If we had nontoxic systemically effective therapy, this would not be a major concern. With the limitations of presently available therapies, the ability to select those patients who may potentially most benefit from adjuvant therapy is essential.

Data on patterns of persistent or recurrent disease, or both, date back to the pioneering work of Mary Matthews, who in 1973 reported a series of autopsies on patients who had undergone potentially curative resections for non–SCLC but died within 30 days of surgery.[6] She found that a high percentage of these patients could be demonstrated to have remaining foci of malignancy consistent with the clinical observation of high relapse rates despite so-called curative resection. For patients with large cell carcinoma and adenocarcinoma, these sites were overwhelmingly systemic, with or without intrathoracic disease, whereas for patients with squamous cell carcinoma, half of those found to have disease at autopsy had remaining disease demonstrable only in the chest. These patients, or about 15% of all patients with resected squamous cell carcinoma, would appear to have the potential for improved survival with the addition of local postoperative adjuvant treatment, such as irradiation of the hilar and mediastinal structures and possibly the tumor bed, while systemic adjuvant therapy would play the greater role for the other histologic types and also benefit patients with squamous histology.

TABLE 9–1. Rates and Patterns of Relapse Following Resection of Non–SCLC

SERIES	STAGE	HISTOLOGY	NO. OF PATIENTS	SURVIVAL (YEAR)	CHEST ONLY (%)	DISTANT ONLY (%)
Feld*[99]	T1N0	Non–SCLC	162	ns	9	17
Feld*	T2N0	Non–SCLC	196	ns	11	30
Feld*	T1N1	Non–SCLC	32	ns	9	22
Pairolero[100]	T1N0	Non–SCLC	170	71% (5)	6	15
Pairolero	T2N0	Non–SCLC	158	59% (5)	6	23
Pairolero	T1N1	Non–SCLC	18	33% (5)	28	39
Thomas*‡[101]	T1N0	Squamous	226	~85%	5	7
Thomas*‡	T1N0	Nonsquamous	346	~65%	9	17
Martini‡[102]	T1–2N1	Squamous	93	44%	16	31
Martini‡	T1–2N1	Adenocarcinoma	114	34%	8	54
Martini†	T2–3N2	Squamous	46	~30% (5)	13	52
Martini†	T2–3N2	Nonsquamous	103	~30% (5)	17	61

*First site of relapse only.
†Some patients received postoperative radiation and/or chemotherapy.
‡Relapse rates include patients relapsing in multiple sites.

These autopsy observations have been confirmed in several careful analyses of clinical patterns of relapse following resection. Recurrence rates increase with the stage of disease involved and are greater for patients with nonsquamous histologies than for those with squamous cell histologies. Table 9–1 summarizes data on rates and patterns of failure following resection with curative intent in several recent series and provides a basis for rational planning of adjuvant therapy. Recurrence of disease in extrathoracic sites is the most common mode of relapse for all non–SCLC histologies. Intrathoracic relapse is more common in patients with squamous cell carcinoma, and brain metastases are more common in patients with adenocarcinoma; however, nonlocalized systemic disease (contralateral lung, bone, liver, adrenal) is frequent for all histologies. This places a high burden on the effectiveness of any proposed systemic adjuvant therapy and limits the improvements in survival that can be ex-

pected from local adjuvant modalities such as mediastinal irradiation.

It is essential in planning trials of adjuvant therapy to use care in estimating the relapse rate for the control group based on well-staged patients. The use of overly high estimates of relapse rates, based on older surgical series in which patients may not have been thoroughly staged, results in small trials with little power to detect modest but clinically important differences in outcome.

In addition to the classic prognostic factors of histology and stage, the burgeoning understanding of the molecular biology of lung cancer has added several new factors that may help predict those patients at high risk of relapse and thus with greatest potential for gain with adjuvant therapy. At present, these factors fall into three broad categories: assays of tumor proliferation rate; evaluation of abnormalities of oncogene structure or expression, or both; and evaluation of expression of antigens on the cell surface. A wide variety of prognostic factors have been proposed, and there is a great need both for standardization of assay techniques for many of these, as well as for prospective trials to better evaluate the significance and independence of many of these factors. Table 9–2 lists a number of the known and proposed prognostic factors in patients with resected non–SCLC. These include factors reflecting the proliferative activity of the tumor such as DNA content and S-phase fraction[7-9] (Ki67 staining,[10] bromodeoxyuracil [BRDU] labeling[11]); mutational activation or overexpression of oncogenes or tumor suppressor genes, or both (e.g., k-ras,[12-14] p53,[15-18] epidermal growth factor receptor [EGFR]–receptor-like molecules[19]), or molecularly less well-characterized genetic alterations (deletions of material on 3p[17]); and altered expression of cell surface antigens that may be related to adhesion molecules (blood group antigens and their precursors,[20, 21] tumor angiogenesis,[19] and perioperative transfusions).[22] It should also be kept in mind that prognostic factors do not exist in isolation but depend on the efficacy of treatment. One is reminded of the lengthy debates about such prognostic factors as his-

TABLE 9–2. Proposed Prognostic Factors in Resected Non–SCLC

FACTOR	REFERENCE
Stage	Mountain[3]
Number of nodal sites	Martini[116]
Extranodal extension	Cybulski[115]
Histology	Feld[5]
Grade	Rosenthal[120]
Ploidy	Zimmerman[7], Dazzi[9]
PCNA Staining	Landberg[119]
Ki67 Staining	Scagliotti[10]
BRDU Labeling	Teodori[117]
k-ras Mutation	Slebos[13]
3p Deletion	Horio[17]
p53 Mutation	Horio[17]
p53 Overexpression	Carbone[16]
Angiogenesis	Machiarini[19]
Epidermoid growth factor receptor expression	Scagliotti[10]
neu Oncogene expression	Scagliotti[10]
Blood group A expression	Lee[21]
H/Ley/Leb Antigen expression	Miyake[20]
MoAb Detection of nodal metastases	Chen[118]

tologic subtype in radiation therapy for Hodgkin's disease and the blunting of the impact of these factors with the development of effective chemotherapy. Although we are far from this point in the treatment of lung cancer, we should be cautious both in our adoption of new prognostic factors and in their retrospective use in claiming benefit for newly identified subgroups of patients in clinical trials that may show little difference when the entire population is analyzed.

STATISTICAL CONSIDERATIONS IN ADJUVANT TRIALS: COMPETING RISKS OF MULTIPLE SITES OF FAILURE, DEATH FROM INTERCURRENT DISEASE, AND SECOND PRIMARY TUMORS

The analyst of a trial of adjuvant therapy must be mindful of a number of factors that can influence the presentation and interpretation of the data. These factors include the manner of detecting and reporting sites of relapse, statistical calculation of relapse rates when there are several competing patterns of relapse, death from second primary tumors and intercurrent disease, and the possibility that therapy given to patients at the time of relapse may prolong survival, possibly more for patients who did not receive adjuvant therapy than for those who did, as has been reported for patients with adenocarcinoma of the breast. Each of these factors can strikingly alter the apparent results of an adjuvant trial, and their combined effects may introduce unpredictable distortions.

In some series, only the sites of first relapse are reported. This approach has the advantages of speed in reporting and greater simplicity and uniformity in data collection, but it may underestimate the ultimate extent of involvement of a specific site. It does give an estimate of the maximum increment in survival that might accrue if relapses in this site were completely prevented. For such considerations, however, it is important to require a uniform and thorough search for relapse in other sites that is not yet clinically evident. Although such a policy may be reasonable at the time of initial relapse, it will be difficult to justify at a later time after relapse, and the use of additional therapy at the time of relapse may well alter patterns of subsequent relapse.

In addition to the logistical and ethical difficulties of continued surveillance of patients who are dying of progressive disease, such analyses are also impaired by the assumption that relapses are independent events. It seems more likely that there exist subgroups of patients who are at high risk for relapse in all sites as well as low-risk groups. Both the long follow-up period of the low-risk group and the short survival time following distant relapse may reduce the apparent rate of local relapse.

Gelman and associates have proposed an alternate analytic methodology for looking at competing sites of relapse that does not require the assumption of their independence.[23] The time to first failure (at any site) is analyzed first, and the patterns of failure analyzed second. An improvement in local control with the addition of a local adjuvant treatment could then be manifested as an overall increase in time to first failure or an unchanged time to first failure but a decrease in the proportion of local failures:

Note that in comparing two treatments (A and B), A could improve time to local failure in three ways. (1) If A increases true time to local failure and does not change true time to distant failure, then A will be associated with longer time to first failure. (2) If A increases both true time to local failure and true time to distant failure, then A will be associated with longer time to first failure. (3) If A increases true time to local failure and decreases true time to distant failure (by an equivalent amount), then patients receiving either A or B will have a similar time to first failure, but a smaller percentage of patients on A will fail first locally.[23]

Cumulative listing of involvement of various sites by recurrent disease gives a better estimate of the relative importance of each site in the overall disease process but is subject to interference by the effects of additional therapy given following relapse and variations in patient evaluation and survival following relapse. Rigor in documenting sites of secondary failure is rarely optimal patient care.

Arriagada and colleagues have reviewed the influence of the methodology used in determining relapse rates in patients with small cell lung cancer (SCLC) treated with combinations of chemotherapy and chest irradiation.[24] Rates of local and distant recurrence were calculated according to three different methodologies: censoring secondary events, ignoring secondary events, and assuming competing events. The relative magnitude of the different classes of relapse differed markedly by the analytic methodology used. Explicit statement of methodologies used for investigating and reporting patterns of initial and subsequent failure is critical to adjuvant trials.

POSTOPERATIVE RADIATION THERAPY: HISTORICAL SERIES AND PROSPECTIVE CONTROLLED TRIALS

The observation of local recurrence prompted a number of institutions to deliver adjuvant postoperative radiation therapy. By the early 1980s, several of these experiences had been reported, with results suggesting benefits for survival and local control.[25–27] No randomized prospective trials had been performed. Two cooperative groups, the Lung Cancer Study Group (LCSG) and the European Organization for Research and Treatment of Cancer (EORTC), conducted randomized prospective trials comparing adjuvant postoperative radiation with observation in completely resected patients to better define the risks and benefits of such therapy (Table 9–3).

The LCSG trial (LCSG 773) was designed to include patients with Stage II and III disease.[28] Patients were required to have undergone complete resection, and the highest resected mediastinal node could not be

TABLE 9–3. Adjuvant Thoracic Irradiation Following Resection of Non–SCLC

SERIES	STAGE	HISTOLOGY	RANDOMIZED	RADIATION DOSE	LOCAL FAILURE (%)	SURVIVAL (%)
Green[103]	TxN0	All	No	None	—	22 at 5 yr
		All		44 Gy*	—	27 at 5 yr
	TxN1–2	All	No	None	—	3 at 5 yr
		All		44 Gy*	—	35 at 5 yr
Kirsch[104]	TxN2		No	None	—	0 at 5 yr
				50–55 Gy	—	23 at 5 yr
Choi[25]	TxN1–2	Adenocarcinoma	No	None	—	8 at 5 yr
		Adenocarcinoma		40–50 Gy	—	43 at 5 yr
	TxN1–2	Squamous	No	None	—	33 at 4 yr
		All		40–50 Gy	—	42 at 4 yr
Chung[105]	TxN2	All	No	None	—	10 at 3 yr
				46 Gy median	—	40 at 3 yr
Israel for EORTC[30]	TxN1–2	Squamous	Yes	None	44	50 at 3 yr†
				45–55 Gy	26	70 at 3 yr†
Van Houtte for EORTC[29]		All (including SCLC)	Yes	None	—	45 at 5 yr
		All (including SCLC)		60 Gy	—	20 at 5 yr
LCSG[28]	II-III (mostly N1)	Squamous	Yes	None	20	~35 at 5 yr
				50 Gy	1	~35 at 5 yr

*Range 30 to 60 Gy.
†Disease-free survival.
~ = Value interpolated or extrapolated from published survival curve.

positive. Because of the data of Matthews and associates that indicated that local recurrence was most common in patients with squamous cell carcinoma, this trial was limited to patients with this histology. Patients were randomized between 50 Gy in 25 daily fractions of 2 Gy over 5 weeks, to start within 6 weeks of surgery, and observation. Over an 8-year period, 230 patients were randomized in this trial. The majority were Stage II, with about 25% of patients at Stage III (N2) and about 10% at Stage III (T3N0).

The results of this trial were strongly positive in demonstrating a marked and statistically significant reduction of the rate of local recurrence in the irradiated patients. The crude local recurrence rates (as first recurrence) were 20/108 for the unirradiated group and 1/102 for the irradiated group. The high effectiveness of radiation therapy as a local modality, however, did not translate to any difference in overall survival, which was about 35% at 5 years for both groups.

The EORTC conducted two prospective trials of postoperative radiation therapy. The first, conducted between 1966 and 1975, enrolled 224 patients (of whom 175 were eligible) who had undergone potentially curative resection and did not have evidence of nodal metastatic disease.[29] This trial included 14 patients with SCLC and two with pulmonary sarcoma. They were randomized between observation and 60 Gy in 6 weeks to the mediastinum. Treatment was given using ^{60}Co and a three-field technique (anterior and two posterior obliques), with a standard field size of 15×9 cm. For all patients, the 5-year survival rate was 24% for the irradiated patients and 43% for the control group (NS). For subsets of patients (e.g., those with T2 lesions) the detrimental effect of radiation was statistically significant. Irradiated patients had a lower rate of regional recurrence (4/83 versus 19/92), these figures include regional-only and regional plus distant relapse) but also a high rate of serious complications (9/83) and clearly no survival advantage.

The second EORTC trial was limited to patients with squamous cell carcinoma who had undergone complete resection.[30] Patients were stratified by nodal status (N+ versus N−) and randomized first to those receiving radiotherapy (45–55 Gy every 4 1/2 weeks) versus those receiving no radiotherapy and, within each of these groups, randomized again to those receiving no further treatment, those receiving chemotherapy with CCNU/CTX/MTX or intradermal bacille Calmette-Guérin (BCG), or both. Only a preliminary analysis of the first 230 patients on this trial has been published. Overall time to failure was not significantly different for the irradiated versus the nonirradiated patients; a local component at the time of first failure appeared to be decreased (11.5% versus 20.6%), although this difference did not reach statistical significance.

All of the trials of postoperative radiation therapy have been flawed in design or execution. The most striking difficulty is the heterogeneity of stage and the inability to make firm conclusions for each stage. The LCSG trial has been criticized by Choi and colleagues on several grounds: inadequate control of the quality of the radiation therapy, with 26% of patients receiving less than 95% of the prescribed radiation dose; absence of adequate cardiorespiratory screening prior to randomization and a corresponding higher rate of deaths from cardiorespiratory disease in those patients receiving radiation therapy; limited requirements for evaluation for distant metastatic disease; delays of up to 8 weeks between surgery and the start

TABLE 9–4. Trials of Adjuvant Systemic Chemotherapy in Resected Non–SCLC

SERIES	PATIENTS	STAGE	HISTOLOGY	REGIMEN	MEDIAN SURVIVAL TIME (mo)	SIGNIFI-CANCE	5-YEAR SURVIVAL (%)	SIGNIFICANCE
LCSG 772[106]	—	II–III	A,L	CAP i.p. BCG				
LCSG 791[34]	—	Incomp. resected	A,L,S	RT/CAP RT				
LCSG 801[35]	—	T1N1, T2N0	A,L,S	CAP None	~72 ~72	ns	~55 ~58	ns
Niiranen[107]	—	I–III	A,L,S	CAP None	n/a n/a		67 56	p = 0.05
Teramatsu[108]	—	?	A,L,S	None DDP/VDS then UFT UFT			62.6 3yr 72.5 3yr 75.1 3yr	p = 0.082 p = 0.038
Kimura[109]	11 13 12	Curative	NSC	None DDP/VDS DDP/VDS/LAK/IL2	— — —	— — —	34.1 4yr 34.2 4yr 70.9 4yr	
	35 33	Noncurative	NSC	DDP/VDS DDP/VDS/LAK/IL2	— —	— —	29.3 4yr 43.1 4yr	
Tsuchiya[110]	91 90	III	NSC	None DDP/VDS	No benefit		No benefit	

A = Adenocarcinoma; CAP = cyclophosphamide, doxorubicin, and cisplatin; DPP = cisplatin; IL2 = interleukin-2; L = large cell carcinoma; LAK = lymphakine-activated killer cells; NSC = non–small cell carcinoma; RT = radiotherapy; S = squamous cell carcinoma; UFT = tegafur plus uracil; V = vindesine.

of radiation therapy; and the planned radiation dose of 50 Gy/25 fractions/5 weeks as allegedly inadequate.[31] It is important to remember, however, that whatever its flaws in design or execution, the radiation therapy as given in this trial was highly successful in achieving a dramatic improvement in local control of disease. Choi's arguments would suggest either an imbalance in undetected distant disease between the two arms or would postulate that there exists a brief period after surgery in which adjuvant radiation can both achieve local control and prevent distant dissemination but beyond which only local control is improved. Occam's razor would likely cut off such speculation in favor of the simpler hypothesis that resected lung cancer, when it has metastasized to regional (N1 or N2) nodes, will have a relapse pattern with sufficient distant failures to reduce the survival impact on any additional treatment that reduces only local failure rates.[32] It is entirely possible, were systemic therapy to affect only extrathoracic relapse and not chest or brain failure, that a much more substantial survival benefit would be seen with adjuvant mediastinal irradiation. This hypothesis forms part of the basis of several ongoing randomized trials.

Postoperative Chemotherapy: Historical Series and Prospective Controlled Trials

The need for effective systemic adjuvant therapy is clear from the high distant relapse rates. Efforts to combine systemic chemotherapy and local treatment with surgery or radiation therapy began shortly after the discovery of chemotherapeutic agents. A number of nonrandomized trials of single-agent chemotherapy and combinations of agents were carried out in the 1950s and 1960s without evidence of benefit (Table 9–4).

In the mid-1970s, the identification of cisplatin as a modestly active single agent and cisplatin-containing

regimens that would produce response rates of 20% to 30% in patients with metastatic non–SCLC regenerated interest in adjuvant chemotherapy. There was also the realization that proper studies would need to be relatively large to detect the small expected benefits and would require scrupulous attention to the details of surgical staging. With these considerations in mind, the LCSG began a series of trials of adjuvant chemotherapy in 1977 that continued through the next decade.

The first of these, LCSG 772, was for patients with completely resected Stage II and III adenocarcinoma and large cell carcinoma of the lung.[33] At the same time, LCSG 773 addressed the question of adjuvant mediastinal irradiation in patients with squamous histology. When this trial was designed, there was concern about the use of an untreated control arm, so the randomization was between chemotherapy with cyclophosphamide, doxorubicin, and cisplatin (CAP) and intrapleural BCG. With the subsequent demonstration of lack of activity of adjuvant BCG in patients with Stage I disease, the trial has been analyzed as one of CAP versus inactive placebo, although questions have been raised as to whether the patients receiving intrapleural BCG may have impaired survival times. Both time to recurrence and survival time were significantly longer in the CAP-treated group (Gehan p = 0.003 for recurrence, 0.047 for survival).

While this trial was being completed, a second trial (LCSG 791) was begun for patients with adenocarcinoma, large cell carcinoma, and squamous cell carcinoma who had been thought to be resectable preoperatively but turned out have had gross or microscopic residual disease or involvement of the highest resected mediastinal lymph node group.[34] Patients were randomized to receive treatment with mediastinal irradiation alone or combined with CAP chemotherapy. There was a statistically significant improve-

TABLE 9–5. Selected Trials of Adjuvant Immunotherapy in Resected Non–SCLC

SERIES	STUDY	PATIENTS	RESULTS
McKneally[111]	Intrapleural BCG	169	Trend favoring BCG for Stage I
Mountain[39]	Intrapleural BCG	425	No benefit
Edwards	Subdermal BCG	500	No benefit
Amery[112]	Preoperative and postoperative levamisole	211	Decrease in cancer deaths in levamisole group; suggestion of dose response
Anthony[113]	Preoperative and postoperative levamisole	318	Excess noncancer deaths in levamisole group
Study Group for Lung Carcinoma	Preoperative and postoperative levamisole	111	Improved recurrence-free survival with levamisole
Wright	Intrapleural BCG + / − levamisole	100	No benefit with levamisole

Adapted from Fishbein G: Immunotherapy of lung cancer. Semin Oncol 20:351–358, 1993.
BCG = Bacille Calmette-Guérin vaccine.

ment in time to relapse and in 1-year survival for the arm receiving both CAP and radiation therapy compared with the arm receiving radiation alone, and the addition of chemotherapy reduced the rate of extra-thoracic non–central nervous system (non–CNS) relapse.

Because of the suggestion of survival benefits seen in these studies, the LCSG instituted a third trial of adjuvant chemotherapy in a more favorable patient population—those with resected Stage I (T1N1M0 or T2N0M0) disease (LCSG 801). The most favorable group of patients, those with T1N0M0, were excluded. This study included patients with both squamous and nonsquamous histologies. Randomization was between observation and CAP for four cycles. This trial has been reported and disappointingly showed no benefits for recurrence-free or overall survival.[35] The overall relapse rates for the control group patients, particularly those with nonsquamous histologies, was only 65% of that which had been anticipated based on prior studies, suggesting more rigorous staging in this trial.

A large trial was instituted in Canada, randomizing 339 patients postoperatively to one of four regimens, depending on the patient's lymph node status.[36] Patients with negative nodes were randomized between no additional therapy and adjuvant chemotherapy with vindesine and cisplatin. Node-positive patients (stratified as N1 versus N2) received postoperative radiation therapy with or without vindesine and cisplatin. To date, the overall trial results have not been reported. An abstract in 1991 noted that, for the groups of patients randomized to receive adjuvant chemotherapy, patients who received more than 50% of the predicted drug doses had a significantly longer disease-free interval (29 versus 17 months, p = 0.02) and overall median survival time (31 versus 19 months, p = 0.01) than those receiving smaller doses. The authors interpreted this finding as suggestive of a dose-response relation for the adjuvant chemotherapy. Such retrospective analyses of received dose, when the dose levels were not randomized, is highly dubious, and the lack of data regarding an overall survival difference between the groups receiving any chemotherapy and no chemotherapy is suspect.

Postoperative Immunotherapy

Many patients with lung cancer have significant defects in the humoral and cellular effector limbs of the immune system when they are diagnosed.[37] The role of these immunologic deficits in the virulence of their disease remains somewhat speculative, with uncertainty as to the role of the immune system in regulating the pace of overt disease with the immune deficits being a reflection rather than a cause of advanced disease. Definition of tumor-associated and specific antigens, and assessment of basal and inducible immunologic reactivity to these antigens may better illustrate the causal role of immunologic deficits in lung cancer development and progression.

The observation by Ruckdeschel and McKneally that a group of patients who developed postoperative empyemas had a better survival time than patients without this postoperative event sparked interest in adjuvant immunotherapy.[38] At the time, our understanding of the immune system, as well as our ability to manipulate it in any specific fashion, was primitive, so the trials begun at that time look almost quaint in retrospect.

The first LCSG immunotherapy trial (LCSG 771) randomized patients with stage I (T1N0, T2N0) to groups receiving intrapleural saline or those receiving adjuvant therapy with intrapleural BCG and systemic isoniazid.[39] This study accrued 473 patients with Stage I disease. There was no difference in time to recurrence or length of survival between the two arms or for subgroups by T stage. An important additional finding was that in this well-staged group of patients, all of whom had careful sampling of mediastinal nodes, the 5-year survival rate was 75% for T1N0M0 and 50% for T2N0M0. The definition of this favorable survival rate for T1N0M0 patients makes them a difficult group to study in subsequent trials, both in terms of the required sample size and in the limitations of acceptable toxicity of an adjuvant regimen. Table 9–5 summarizes several other larger randomized trials of adjuvant immunotherapy, using BCG by several routes, the nonspecific immunostimulant levamisole, or active immunization with tumor vaccines. With the exception of the Hollinshead vaccination study, which has not been replicated, these trials fail to show substantial evidence for the benefits of adjuvant immunotherapy.

At present, no immunologically based therapy has convincingly been shown to alter patterns of failure, time to relapse, or overall survival time in patients with resected non–SCLC. Its use outside the context of a prospective clinical trial is not warranted. This negative assessment is not meant to suggest that such therapies may not have a role in the future as the nature both of specific immune deficits in patients with lung cancer and the distinctive antigenic properties of lung cancer cell lines become better understood. Recent reports have indicated that, at least for SCLC, many patients develop antibodies that cross react against their own tumor antigens as well as common antigens found in other patients with SCLC.[40] These antigens include oncogene products such as p53. The survival time of patients who have developed such antibodies is superior to that of patients without them. Whether this represents a lead to the development of specific antitumor immunotherapy or merely indicates that the presence of these antibodies is reflective but not causal of improved survival awaits further study.

Is There a Role for Prophylactic Cranial Irradiation in Non–SCLC?

Brain metastases are common in patients with lung cancer, particularly small cell carcinoma, adenocarcinoma, and large cell undifferentiated carcinoma.[41–43] Because the realization that prophylactic (or more properly pre-emptive) cranial irradiation (PCI) could effectively reduce the rate of CNS relapse and improve cure rates in pediatric acute lymphoblastic leukemia, there have been efforts to extend its use to lung cancer. Most of these trials have been in patients with SCLC, and despite its incorporation into dozens of treatment programs and several randomized trials specifically addressed to the role of PCI, its value remains controversial and the subject of several current large randomized trial in the United States and Europe. For patients with non–SCLC, there have been three randomized trials of PCI, although none of these trials has included operable and resected patients.[44–46] These trials have not studied patients whose intrathoracic disease was controlled, and they have failed to show any survival benefits. An analysis of LCSG patterns of failure data in resected patients suggests little potential benefit for this approach because few patients of any stage or histology failed exclusively in the brain.[47] Finally, attempts to combine PCI with systemic adjuvant therapy face the problems of CNS toxicity that have been noted in patients with SCLC.[48] At present, PCI cannot be recommended as routine practice for any patients with non–SCLC.

CURRENT PROSPECTIVE TRIALS: EASTERN COOPERATIVE ONCOLOGY GROUP (ECOB)–COORDINATED INTERGROUP AND OTHERS

A current United States Intergroup trial is addressing the question of adjuvant chemotherapy in resected node-positive patients and is attempting to resolve some of the difficulties of past trials. Patients will undergo complete resection with either a complete mediastinal dissection or a thorough sampling of mediastinal nodes, including, at a minimum, the subcarinal, tracheobronchial, level 4 on the right, and level 5 or 7 on the left. Patients with N1 and N2 disease are eligible, and there is stratification for nodal level, weight loss, and histology (squamous versus nonsquamous). After extensive discussions as to the best question to ask from the standpoint of science and the standpoint of accruing patients to the trial, it was decided to compare postoperative mediastinal irradiation with a regimen on concurrent irradiation and chemotherapy with cisplatin and etoposide. The inclusion of postoperative mediastinal irradiation in both arms of the study will give optimal local tumor control, which may increase the ability to detect a benefit in distant relapse rates from the addition of chemotherapy. The primary study endpoint is survival, and in looking for a 40% increase in median survival time and a one-sided statistical test, the required number of patients is 462. This may be compared with most of the trials listed in Tables 9–3 to 9–6, in which vastly smaller numbers of patients were entered. It is likely that many past trials have been underpowered to detect small differences in long-term survival (e.g., a 20% improvement in 3-year survival), which would be clinically valuable. The situation in the study of breast cancer, in which there has been recent consensus on the need for large, broadly constructed trials with good statistical power to allow these questions to be answered directly rather than

TABLE 9–6. Summary of Preoperative MVP Trials

INVESTIGATORS	PATIENTS	RESPONSE RATE (%)	HISTOLOGIC COMPLETE RESPONSE (%)	MEDIAN SURVIVAL (mo)	2-YEAR SURVIVAL (%)	TREATMENT MORTALITY (%)
MSKCC[76]	73	76	12	19	36	3
Toronto[77]	39	64	7.7	18.6	40	20
LCSG[57]	30	46	0	12	n/a	23
Spain[114]	53	68	n/a	>15	n/a	n/a

MSKCC = Memorial Sloan-Kettering Cancer Center; LCSG = Lung Cancer Study Group; n/a = not available.

hinted at by meta-analyses, has been noted in several recent reviews.[49, 50]

An alternate design for adjuvant postoperative combined modality therapy, as proposed by the Cancer and Leukemia Group B (CALGB), is to deliver several cycles of chemotherapy first and then to deliver mediastinal irradiation after the completion of chemotherapy.[50, 51] This sequence will be compared with a standard postoperative arm of mediastinal irradiation alone. Possible advantages of this sequence will be the ability to deliver somewhat higher doses of cisplatin and etoposide using granulocyte colony stimulating factor (G-CSF) support, which will be possible because there is no concurrent radiation therapy. It should be noted that there are no convincing data for a dose-response relationship for cisplatin or etoposide in treating overt metastatic disease in the dose levels being used in these two studies (cisplatin [DDP] 60 mg/M2 d1 and etoposide [VP16] 120 mg/M2 d1-3 in the ECOG study, DDP 33 mg/M2 d1-3, VP16 200 mg/M2 d1-3 in the CALGB trial). The delay in the start of mediastinal irradiation is another possible drawback to this design. It may be relevant that the Radiation Therapy Oncology Group (RTOG) adjuvant trial for advanced head and neck cancer, which compared immediate postoperative RT versus three cycles of cisplatin and 5-fluorouracil followed by RT, failed to show a benefit in survival for the combined adjuvant approach.[52] Also, it may be shown that concurrent radiation therapy and chemotherapy are more beneficial so long as their increased acute toxicities, primarily hematologic and mucosal, can be supported and late toxicities are acceptable. The designs of both the ECOG/RTOG trial and the CALBG trial have merit, and because they are to accrue similar patients and share a common control arm with adjuvant radiation alone, comparison of their outcomes should prove interesting.

PATTERNS OF FAILURE IN UNRESECTED STAGE III NON–SMALL CELL LUNG CANCER

About 35% to 40% of non–SCLC patients present with clinically apparent, locally advanced disease (Stage III). Nonsurgical trials in which these patients were treated with radiation therapy alone[53] or with radiation therapy combined with cisplatin[54, 55] have shown virtually equivalent rates of local and distant failure, with the possible exception of lower local recurrence rates in patients who received 6000 Gy of radiation therapy delivered on a continuous schedule[56] or in those who received daily cisplatin with radiation.[55] There are at least three potential explanations for the high local failure rate in patients with Stage III non–SCLC. First, pulmonary resection is not performed in the majority of these patients. Second, patients with Stage III disease tend to have bulky primary tumors and extensive mediastinal lymph node metastases. In sequential Phase II trials evaluating combined modality therapy in 211 patients with Stage III non–SCLC,

the median cross-sectional tumor area was 25 cm^2 and 53% of patients had mediastinal lymph node metastases.[54] Third, trials of preoperative radiation alone[57] or preoperative chemoradiation therapy have shown that complete histologic clearance of tumor occurs in only 10% to 20% of patients with Stage III disease who were considered eligible for resection.[58] The group of Stage III patients that is classified as ineligible for surgery has even more extensive local disease and probably has a lower rate of tumor clearance with radiation or with chemoradiation. Based on these considerations, it is not surprising to observe local recurrence in a high percentage of patients with Stage III disease.

It seems unlikely that a high rate of local control will be achieved using radiation alone or radiation combined with chemotherapy. In a Phase II trial of preoperative 5-fluorouracil, cisplatin, and concurrent radiation therapy, local recurrence was observed in only 17% of patients who had complete resection. In contrast, local recurrence was observed in 51% of patients who had incomplete resection of tumor or who did not undergo thoracotomy.[59] In Phase II combined modality trials conducted at Rush University, 128 of 211 patients with Stage III disease were initially classified as eligible for surgery. Within the surgically eligible group, 99 patients (77%) had complete resection. The local failure rate in the surgically eligible patients (128 patients) was 34% compared with 59% for ineligible patients (83 patients).[54] The apparently lower local failure rates in patients who had complete tumor resection or who were classified as eligible for surgery may be due to less extensive local and regional disease. On the other hand, it is possible that tumor resection contributes significantly to local control in selected Stage III non–SCLC patients. A proposed intergroup study will address this question by randomizing patients to surgery or additional radiation after initial treatment with cisplatin, etoposide, and radiation. This study design will eliminate imbalances in pretreatment prognostic factors and will provide an answer regarding the role of surgery in patients with Stage III non–SCLC.

There are relatively few data regarding sites of failure in relation to the new international staging system that was introduced in 1986.[3] One group of investigators has applied the new staging system retrospectively to a group of patients that had received radiation therapy alone, and they observed virtually equal local failure rates in Stages IIIA and IIIB patients.[60, 61] In one of these studies, there was no difference in survival for Stage IIIA versus Stage IIIB,[60] whereas in the other trial, there was a significant survival difference in the 2-year survival rates, which were 20% for patients with Stage IIIA disease and 12% for patients with Stage IIIB disease.[61] In 211 patients treated with combined chemotherapy and radiation, with surgery being performed in selected patients, there was a significant difference in survival time for patients with Stage IIIA disease versus those with Stage IIIB disease.[54] Also, the overall failure rate was lower at 58% in patients with Stage IIIA disease versus 72% in those with Stage IIIB disease, and the local failure rate was 37% and 54% in patients with Stage IIIA and Stage IIIB disease, respectively.[62] The majority of Stage IIIA patients had undergone pulmonary resection, suggesting that the longer survival and the trend for lower local recurrence in patients with Stage IIIA disease resulted from resection of residual intrathoracic tumor. Certainly, this treatment approach should not be considered standard therapy for Stage IIIA disease unless this type of treatment is associated with significantly longer survival in a randomized trial.

Rationale for Neoadjuvant Therapy

The use of chemotherapy prior to resection of locally advanced cancer has been called neoadjuvant treatment, but some investigators prefer the term primary chemotherapy for this treatment sequence. There are potential advantages for this therapeutic approach. First, the extensive nature of the local-regional disease frequently precludes resection. Reducing the tumor burden could result in removal of a lesion that had been unresectable initially. Second, tumor reduction might enable the surgeon to reduce the extent of resection. Third, initial treatment with chemotherapy theoretically provides the earliest opportunity to treat distant micrometastases, which are present in a high percentage of patients. Potential disadvantages of incorporating chemotherapy as the initial treatment for Stage III non–SCLC are the concern that local disease might progress during preoperative treatment in patients whose tumor could have been resected initially. Also, the accompanying rates of morbidity and mortality from surgery following chemotherapy or chemoradiation therapy might be excessive.

Whether the theoretical advantages of neoadjuvant treatment will translate into improved survival for Stage III lung cancer patients will require a large, well-designed Phase III study. However, results of Phase II trials appear to have eliminated concerns about the possible major disadvantages from this treatment sequence. Tumor progression was infrequent among 128 patients who received preoperative chemotherapy and radiation in Phase II trials conducted at Rush.[63] Progressive disease was observed prior to surgery in only 6% of the patients, and local progression occurred in only 1% of the patients. Similarly, excessive morbidity and mortality rates have not been observed in most Phase II trials.[58] Certainly, surgery after chemotherapy or chemoradiation is difficult because of dense fibrosis and loss of surgical planes. However, in the hands of experienced thoracic surgeons, morbidity and mortality rates have not been excessive following preoperative treatment.

PREOPERATIVE RADIATION THERAPY

One of the theoretical reasons for giving preoperative radiation therapy included the hope that radiation would destroy areas of tumor that had extended into critical areas or into lymph nodes that could not be removed surgically initially. Potentially, reduction of nodal metastases or of tumor invading major structures would enable complete resection of local disease. The other theoretical consideration was that preoperative radiation might have a lethal effect on tumor cells that would have seeded the operative site or disseminated via the vascular or lymphatic systems. In several early nonrandomized trials that evaluated preoperative radiation therapy, no residual tumor was found in the resected specimens in more than 30% of the patients,[64, 65] and there appeared to be a higher rate of resection in these nonrandomized trials.[66] Also, nonrandomized trials testing preoperative radiation therapy in the superior sulcus had shown relatively high 5-year survival rates.[67]

The theoretical and empirical observations described earlier led to two large randomized trials in which immediate surgery was compared with radiation followed by pulmonary resection.[68, 69] In each trial, patients were randomized to surgery alone or to radiation (40–50 Gy) over 4 to 5 weeks followed by a 4- to 6-week rest period and subsequent surgery. Information regarding the stage of the patients in these randomized trials is not available because the TNM system had not been adopted at that time. The first study, which was conducted by the Veterans Association for the Study of Lung Cancer, showed that the long-term survival rate of patients who had immediate surgery was 20%, and for those who had preoperative radiation therapy, it was 12%.[68] This difference was not statistically significant. Analyzing the survival data in this trial revealed that there was an increased rate of deaths during the first 6 months in the patients who received preoperative radiation therapy. The reasons for this increase were not entirely clear, but the author speculated that it might have been related to a deleterious effect of preoperative radiation therapy on cardiopulmonary reserve.

In the other study, 560 operable patients were randomized to immediate surgery or to surgery following preoperative radiation therapy.[69] Similar to the veterans study, there was no significant difference in survival for immediate surgery versus surgery following radiation.

Although the exact staging data are not available for either trial, it is likely that there were a significant number of Stage I and II patients included in these studies. For this reason, the LCSG decided to conduct a randomized Phase II trial in which carefully staged patients with advanced non–SCLC were assigned either to preoperative radiation therapy (44 Gy) or chemotherapy consisting of mitomycin, vinblastine, and cisplatin (MVP).[57] The objective of this study was to assess the toxicity and efficacy of the preoperative treatment and to initiate a Phase III trial if results were promising. Unfortunately, the median survival time was only 12 months. Therefore, these investigators believed that a Phase III trial evaluating preoperative radiation therapy in patients with Stage III lung cancer was not warranted at this point.

PREOPERATIVE CHEMOTHERAPY

During the past decade, investigators observed response rates of approximately 50% in patients with Stage III non–SCLC compared with 25% in patients with Stage IV disease.[70] The apparently higher response rate in Stage III patients raised the possibility that chemotherapy might have a significant effect on distant micrometastases, and this hypothesis led to the initiation of at least four randomized, nonsurgical trials in which radiation therapy alone was compared with chemotherapy followed by radiation. In two of these trials, a modest improvement in survival was observed in patients who received chemotherapy and radiation,[71–73] whereas no difference in survival was noted in the other randomized trials.[74, 75] Almost simultaneously, investigators at Sloan-Kettering initiated a Phase II trial in which two to three courses of MVP were given prior to thoracotomy to Stage III non–SCLC patients.[76] Virtually all of these patients had histologically confirmed ipsilateral mediastinal lymph node metastases. These investigators observed a 76% clinical response rate in 73 patients. Histologically documented complete clearance of tumor was observed in 10% of the patients. The median survival time was 19 months, and 34% of the patients were alive at 2 years. In addition, treatment-related mortality was only 3%.

These encouraging results led three additional groups of investigators to conduct Phase II trials of preoperative MVP.[57, 77, 78] Response rates, survival data, and treatment-related mortality for Phase II trials of preoperative MVP are listed in Table 9–6. Two groups observed rates of treatment-related mortality of 20%[77] and 23%.[78] With preoperative MVP, the treatment-related deaths resulted from infections during periods of leukopenia; in particular, exacerbations of smoldering postobstructive pneumonia were observed. The appearance of adult respiratory distress syndrome during the immediate postoperative period was another case of treatment-related mortality in these studies. Despite the fact that the MVP regimen produces relatively high response rates in Stage III lung cancer patients, it is doubtful that this regimen will be successfully tested in a Phase III trial because of the concerns relating to lethal toxicity. In fact, a cooperative group Phase III trial that was designed to test induction MVP followed by radiation therapy or resection has been aborted because of low patient accrual.

Other chemotherapy regimens have not been tested as preoperative treatment, but more recent trials in which two courses of cisplatin-vinblastine[73] or of vindesine, lomustine, cisplatin, and cyclophosphamide[71] were given prior to definitive radiation have revealed chemotherapy response rates of 36% and 27%, respectively. Larger numbers of patients were treated in these more recent trials, and therefore, it is likely that these results are closer to the true response rate for cisplatin-containing combination regimens in patients with Stage III non–SCLC. On the other hand, it could be argued that these patients received only two

courses of chemotherapy before radiation or that more effective regimens are available. Certainly, it is possible that higher response rates might have been observed with three or four courses of chemotherapy, or with alternative regimens. However, the patients may experience higher rates of morbidity and mortality from thoracotomy following more courses of chemotherapy. Similarly, it seems unlikely that one of the chemotherapy regimens available at the present time will emerge as clearly superior in patients with Stage III non–SCLC because large Phase III trials in patients with Stage IV disease have failed to identify a more effective regimen.[70]

PHASE II TRIALS OF PREOPERATIVE CHEMORADIATION THERAPY

A variety of cisplatin-containing combination chemotherapy regimens and simultaneous thoracic radiation have been tested as preoperative treatment in patients with Stage III non–SCLC (Table 9–7).[66, 79–82] Interpreting the results of these trials is difficult because staging was not uniform. Some of these trials required the presence of N_2 disease, whereas others included patients whose stage was T3N0.[58] In addition, eligibility requirements included histologic documentation of nodal metastases in some studies, but radiologic evidence of lymph node enlargement was considered adequate proof of lymph node metastases in other trials. Despite these limitations, the Phase II trials have provided important information regarding toxicity and about the feasibility of pulmonary resection following simultaneous chemotherapy and radiation. In addition, data regarding clinical and surgical pathologic response rates and survival estimates have been obtained. The earliest studies tested 5-fluorouracil–cisplatin (FP)[83, 84] or CAP combined with radiation.[79, 85] More recent efforts have involved the study of plant alkaloids (etoposide[63, 81, 82] or vinblastine[86] combined with cisplatin and simultaneous radiation). The doses and schedules of chemoradiation are summarized in Table 9–8.

There have been two relatively large Phase II trials that tested FP and simultaneous thoracic irradiation.[59, 83] In a study focusing on a single institution, four courses of FP and simultaneous split course radiation therapy were administered to 64 patients prior to thoracotomy.[83] The clinical response rate was 56%; 39 patients (61%) underwent thoracotomy, and nine patients (14%) had no residual tumor in the resected specimen. Treatment complications included one death secondary to septicemia (1.6%) and two cases of operative mortality (5%). The median survival time for all patients was 16 months, and the 2-year survival rate was 35%. Similar results were observed by members of the LCSG when they tested two courses of FP given simultaneously with continuous radiation therapy in 85 patients.[59] The clinical and complete histologic response rates were 56% and 9%, respectively; the median survival time was 13 months, and the estimated 2-year survival rate was 25%. Toxicity dur-

TABLE 9–7. Preoperative Chemotherapy and Radiation Trial Treatment Regimens

INVESTIGATORS	DRUG	TOTAL DOSE	DOSE INTENSITY PER COURSE	COURSES	DAILY RT (Gy/Fx)	TOTAL RT (Gy)
Ruth[83]	Cisplatin	240 mg/m²	30 mg/m²/wk			
	5-FU	16 g/m²	2 g/m²/wk	4	2	40 S
LCSG[59]	Cisplatin	150 mg/m²	21 mg/m²/wk			
	5-FU	8 g/m²	8 g/m²	2	2	30 C
Harvard*[85]	Cisplatin	100 mg/m²	16 mg/m²/wk			
	Doxorubicin	100 mg/m²	16 mg/m²/wk			
	Cyclophosphamide	100 mg/m²	16 mg/m²/wk	2	2	30 C
LCSG[79]	Cisplatin	180 mg/m²	15 mg/m²/wk			
	Doxorubicin	120 mg/m²	10 mg/m²/wk			
	Cyclophosphamide	120 mg/m²	10 mg/m²/wk	3	3	30 S
CALGB[86]	Cisplatin	200 mg/m²	25 mg/m²/wk			
	5-FU	60 mg/kg	7.5 mg/kg/wk			
	Vinblastine	12 mg/m²	1.5 mg/m²/wk	2	2	45 C
Rush[63]	Cisplatin	240 mg/m²	20 mg/m²/wk	4	2	40 S
	5-FU	12.8 g/m²	1.1 g/m²/wk			
	Etoposide	960 mg/m²	80 mg/m²/wk			
Rush[63]	Cisplatin	240 mg/m²	20 mg/m²/wk	4	1.5 BID	39 S
	5-FU	12.8 g/m²	1.1 g/m²/wk			
	Etoposide	960 mg/m²	80 mg/m²/wk			
SWOG[82]	Cisplatin	200 mg/m²	25 mg/m²/wk	2	1.8	45 C
	Etoposide	500 mg/m²	62 mg/m²/wk			
Rhode Island[81]	Cisplatin	200 mg/m²	25 mg/m²/wk	2	?	51
	Etoposide	500 mg/m²	50 mg/m²/wk			

C = Continuous course radiation therapy; S = split course radiation therapy; 5-FU = 5-fluorouracil; SWOG = Southwestern Oncology Group.
*Additional radiation and chemotherapy were given postoperatively.

ing preoperative treatment was not excessive, and the surgical mortality rate was 7%.

Both of the FP and radiation studies showed that toxicity and surgical mortality rates were acceptable. However, the survival results in the multicenter trial (LCSG) did not appear to be appreciably better than results reported for so-called positive nonsurgical trials in which chemotherapy and radiation were used.[71, 72]

The CAP regimen has been given sequentially with radiation prior to thoracotomy in a single-institution trial[85] and simultaneously with split course radiation as preoperative treatment in a multi-institution LCSG study.[79] The median survival time was 32 months for 41 patients treated in the single-institution trial compared with a median survival time of 11 months and a 2-year survival rate of 8% in 39 LCSG patients. Both groups of investigators showed that pulmonary resection was feasible after treatment with CAP chemotherapy and radiation. However, the survival results from the multi-institution CAP, radiation, and surgery trial are similar to results reported for radiation

alone,[53] and further study of preoperative CAP and radiation has not been conducted.

Multiple institutions within CALGB tested cisplatin, 5-fluorouracil, and simultaneous radiation combined with vinblastine.[86] Forty-one patients received two courses of this regimen preoperatively, and the clinical and histologic response rates were 51% and 10%, respectively. Complete tumor resection was carried out in 61% of patients. There were six (15%) treatment-related deaths, with half of the lethal complications occurring during the preoperative period. The median survival time was 15.5 months, and the projected 5-year survival rate was 22%. Although the survival results with this combined modality treatment are relatively good, the lethal toxicity rate of 15% is higher than lethal toxicity rates of some other preoperative regimens (Table 9–7).

Etoposide has also been combined with FP and radiation.[63] Twenty-nine patients received four courses of chemotherapy and single daily fractions (2 Gy) of split course radiation for 5 days, and 45 patients were treated with three courses of chemotherapy and two

TABLE 9–8. Summary of Preoperative Cisplatin-Etoposide Radiation Trials

INVESTIGATORS	PATIENTS	RESPONSE RATE (%)	HISTOLOGIC COMPLETE RESPONSE (%)	MEDIAN SURVIVAL (mo)	2-YEAR SURVIVAL (%)	TREATMENT MORTALITY (%)
SWOG[82]	75	69	21	17	40	6
Rhode Island[81]	53	89	22	24	50	n/a

SWOG = Southwestern Oncology Group.

daily fractions (1.5 Gy/fraction) of radiation for 5 days. The histologic complete remission rate was 17%. Combining the results of these successive Phase II trials has shown that complete resection could be accomplished in 60 patients (81%) and that the median survival duration was 22 months. This relatively long median survival time is probably related to the fact that 42% of the patients were classified as showing Stage T3N0. Although many patients experienced fatigue and anorexia on this regimen, overall treatment-related lethal toxicity was 6% and surgical mortality was 5%.

Two relatively large Phase II trials have tested etoposide cisplatin and simultaneous radiation.[81, 82] Although there were some differences in the doses and schedules for chemotherapy and radiation, continuous radiation with concurrent chemotherapy during the first and last weeks of radiation was used in both studies. The results of these trials are summarized in Table 9–7. Both studies showed relatively high 2-year survival rates—40% and 50%. The fact that one of these studies was conducted as a Southwest Oncology Group multi-institute trial makes the 40% 2-year survival rate particularly impressive. The rates of overall lethal toxicity and of surgical mortality in the Southwestern Oncology Group trial were 5% and 6%, respectively, showing that this regimen is relatively safe to use as preoperative treatment in the setting of a multi-insitutional clinical trial.

PHASE III SURGICAL ADJUVANT TRIALS

Several institutions have recently reported the results of Phase III trials comparing surgery with neoadjuvant therapy followed by surgery, and the results appear to be positive. Trakhtenberg and associates compared surgery alone with surgery preceded by 20 Gy/ five fractions/1 week to the primary tumor and regional nodes.[87] Surgery followed preoperative radiation therapy within 5 days in 90% of the patients. Patients with Stage I to III disease were included, and details of the staging evaluation are not given. There were no outcome differences for patients with Stage I or II disease. In the 273 patients with Stage III disease, however, significant 5-year survival differences favoring preoperative radiotherapy were seen for Stage III squamous cell carcinoma (29.2% versus 15.8%, $p < 0.05$) and for all patients with intrathoracic nodal metastases (22.6% versus 14.9%, $p < 0.05$). No benefit for Stage III patients with adenocarcinoma was seen. Patterns of relapse were not reported.

Fleck and colleagues in Porto Allegre, Brazil, have given preliminary results of a randomized trial comparing preoperative chemotherapy using MVP with preoperative chemoradiotherapy using FP and 30 Gy of radiation in 3 weeks.[88] This trial was generated in part by the limited availability of radiation therapy facilities in Brazil, and it was the hope of the authors that the more widely available chemotherapy would be as effective as chemoradiotherapy. Current data clearly show superior response and resectability rates with the combined modality preoperative approach and suggest improved time to relapse and survival. This trial, if the results hold with maturation of data, strongly indicates an impact of improved local control on survival in patients with Stage IIIA non–SCLC treated with both local and systemic therapy.

Rosell and associates in Barcelona randomized patients with Stage IIIA non–SCLC to immediate surgery or to three cycles of preoperative mitomycin, ifosfamide, and cisplatin prior to resection.[89] All patients were to receive postoperative mediastinal irradiation. Sixty patients were entered on the trial before it was suspended when interim analysis at 24 months showed a significant difference in survival favoring the preoperative chemotherapy arm. At the time of publication, median survival in the surgery-only arm is 8 months versus 26 months in the preoperative chemotherapy arm ($p < 0.001$). Differences in survival were seen regardless of age, histologic subtype, tumor location and size, or number of N2 levels involved. These results are promising; however, the median survival of only 8 months in the surgery group, of whom 27 of 30 underwent complete resection, is unusually low and inferior to that seen in most series of patients with unresectable Stage IIIA non–SCLC. Although all patients in this series had Stage IIIA disease, 29 were N0 or N1, making this study somewhat different from series in which the majority of patients have N2 disease.

A recently completed trial from the M.D. Anderson Cancer Center compared surgery alone with preoperative chemotherapy with cyclophosphamide, etoposide, and cisplatin, with additional postoperative chemotherapy given to patients responding to the preoperative cycles.[90] Sixty patients were entered on this trial, 32 to surgery and 28 to perioperative chemotherapy plus surgery. As in the case of the Barcelona trial, this study was stopped short of its planned accrual when results of an interim analysis showed highly significant survival differences favoring the perioperative chemotherapy arm. At the time of final analysis, with a median time from randomization of 37 months, the median survival for the surgery patients was 11 months as compared with 64 months for patients who received perioperative chemotherapy ($p = 0.008$ by log rank, $p = 0.018$ Wilcoxon). Although the authors rightly pointed out that, in a small trial such as this, unknown imbalances in prognostic factors may distort and inflate outcome differences apparently due to treatment, both this and the Barcelona trial strongly suggest a benefit for the addition of chemotherapy to surgery for patients with resectable Stage IIIA non–SCLC. The present United States intergroup trial of postoperative radiation therapy alone or with concurrent cisplatin and etoposide should clarify the issue for postoperative chemotherapy, whereas a larger confirmatory trial will be needed to better define the indications for preoperative chemotherapy.

The Southwest Oncology Group has initiated a Phase III trial in which patients with Stage IIIA and IIIB non-SCLC are begun on therapy with etoposide, cisplatin, and concurrent thoracic radiation. The patients are randomly assigned to proceed to thoracotomy after receiving 45 Gy of radiation therapy to an additional cycle of chemotherapy and continuation of radiation to a total of 61.2 Gy. Many investigators are conducting Phase II trials in which preoperative chemotherapy or chemoradiation therapy is being evaluated. In addition, there are two Phase III cooperative group trials in which chemotherapy (cisplatin and vinblastine or carboplatin and etoposide) followed by radiation is being compared with chemotherapy followed by surgery.

If each group of investigators continues to pursue its own interests, it is unlikely that any single group will be able to complete one of these studies. Therefore, at the present time, investigators are planning to cooperate in a single intergroup trial in which the Southwest Oncology Group regimen will be tested. Unlike the current Southwest Oncology Group trial, patients with Stage IIIB disease will be excluded from the proposed intergroup study. Otherwise, the study design will remain the same—all patients will receive etoposide, cisplatin, and thoracic radiation with random assignment to surgery or to additional chemoradiation therapy. This approach assumes that simultaneous chemotherapy and radiation are superior to either modality alone. Having made this assumption, this study will provide important information about the role of surgery in Stage IIIA disease.

FUTURE PROSPECTS

The present finds oncologists in a period of rapid growth in their understanding of the molecular aspects of lung cancer genesis, clinical evolution, metastatic spread, and development of resistance to our present therapeutic modalities, yet in a time of modest and incremental progress in our therapy. For patients with resectable Stage I, II, and minimal IIIA disease, surgery alone or the combination of surgery and postoperative mediastinal irradiation gives a very high rate of local control. Improvements in local therapy for this patient population may derive from isolating subgroups of patients who remain at higher risk for local failure (possibly those with multiple involved nodes, extracapsular extension, or high proliferative rates) and treating them more aggressively. Conversely, another avenue of clinical improvement may be identification of subgroups of patients in whom resection alone gives a very high rate of local control and for whom the morbidity and occasional mortality associated with the cardiopulmonary toxicities of postoperative irradiation may be eliminated. Technical improvements in the delivery of radiation therapy and the delineation of the minimal volume to be irradiated will also be useful.

Improving survival of patients with resectable or marginally resectable non–SCLC requires more effective chemotherapeutic agents and optimal combination of these agents with surgery and radiation therapy. Several new chemotherapeutic agents with activity against non–SCLC have been identified. A number of these agents, such as the taxoids (Taxol, taxotere, and other analogues), the camptothecins (Topotecan, Irinotecan, and others), and antimetabolites such as gemcitabine have new mechanisms of action and may provide significant additions to our present therapeutic armamentarium.[91] They also present, however, the same general patterns of hematopoietic and gastrointestinal toxicities that have limited doses of most chemotherapeutic agents, and it is also clear that a number of mechanisms of resistance to their actions are present in lung cancer cell lines.[91, 92] Most fundamentally, they remain agents whose cytotoxicity is not specifically targeted against any of the specific aspects of tumor cell biology.

Past immunotherapeutic efforts at biologically based therapy of overt or occult non–SCLC have combined a worthy intent and a woeful lack of tools. With the better definition of the biologic specificities of lung cancer cells, including altered expression of structurally normal cell surface antigens, expression of structurally altered antigens such as mutated EGF receptors[93] and the alterations in DNA replication checkpoint control brought about by abnormalities in p53,[94] there is rational hope for therapies with greater biologic specificity. Several recent observations and trials are pointing in this direction.

Winter and colleagues have demonstrated that many patients with SCLC produce antibodies that react to antigens found on both their own tumor cells and tumor cells from many, but not all, other patients with SCLC.[40] These patients have an improved survival time compared with patients lacking such antibodies. It is appealing to think that these antitumor antibodies are the cause of the improved survival, but this factor remains to be demonstrated; they may merely reflect underlying performance status, immunocompetence, and like immunoreactivity to keyhole limpet hemocyanin, merely point to a yet undiscovered and more fundamental process.

The definition of truly tumor-specific antigens (as opposed to tumor-associated antigens) may afford more selective approaches to immunologically based detection and therapy strategies. The recent report by Garcia de Palazzo and colleagues[93] that a specific EGFR deletion mutant, which appears to be found only in malignancies, was present in 5 of 32 lung cancer specimens is promising in this regard. Overexpression of structurally normal EGFR is common in lung cancer, being reported in 38% to 83% of specimens, but antibodies directed against such a target would be expected to cross react extensively with normal tissue. The definition of molecular structures unique to the malignancy, often the product of a mutated oncogene, particularly when such structures are located in the extracellular regions of transmembrane proteins and thus accessible to monoclonal antibodies, suggests promising therapeutic targets for monoclonal antibody– or antibody fragment–directed therapy with radionuclides, cytotoxic agents, or toxins such as ricin.

The ability to block gene transcription by the introduction of specific antisense RNA constructs offers another opportunity for biologically based adjuvant therapy. Roth has shown that antisense constructs to k-*ras* were able to block expression of mutant k-*ras*, reduce but not abolish cell growth in vitro, and abolish tumorigenicity in nude mice of human H460a lung adenocarcinoma cells. Modulation of p53 gene expression, in this case incorporation of sense oriented cDNA by electroporation, was also able to modulate growth of cells lacking endogenous wild-type p53 production.[95]

One approach to block expression of mutant oncogenes is to introduce antisense constructs that will bind either to DNA or mRNA and interfere with transcription or translation. Such constructs have been effective in vitro and in experimental in vivo systems. Roth and his colleagues have targeted the mutation of the k-*ras* gene, which is seen in about 30% of patients with adenocarcinomas and is associated with a poor prognosis in resected patients. The sequence of the construct is specific for the mutated k-*ras*, thus allowing normal expression of the remaining *ras* genes in both tumor and normal tissues. This approach has been shown to decrease cell growth rate in vitro and reduce tumorigenicity of these cell lines in nude mice.[95]

The protein encoded by the *ras* oncogene forms part of the membrane-receptor signal transduction complex. It must be inserted in the cell membrane and requires farnesylation catalyzed by the enzyme farnesyl protein transferase, which recognizes a consensus CAAX sequence. Two groups have described synthesis of peptide or peptidomimetic analogues to this motif that potently inhibit this enzyme and that block the transforming activity of mutant *ras* constructs in vitro.[96, 97] Despite the rather widespread requirement for farnesylation of membrane proteins, other cellular processes seemed remarkably unimpaired, and it has been suggested that the presence of cytoplasmic non-farnesylated mutant *ras* may have direct effects on these cells. Such a strategy is not yet ready for clinical trial, and *ras* mutations represent only a portion of the spectrum of genetic abnormalities in lung cancer (they are present in about 30% of patients with adenocarcinoma, occasionally in patients with histologies other non–SCLC, and rarely, if ever, in patients with small cell carcinoma), but this represents the start of an exciting series of new agents for lung cancer and other malignancies.

Resources for clinical trials are limited, and therefore, it is essential that these efforts be coordinated in order to obtain sufficient data to answer a specific question, such as the effect of surgery on survival in the Stage IIIA patients. At the present time, there are multiple groups conducting Phase II trials testing preoperative regimens. It seems more reasonable for most investigators to participate in the intergroup Phase III trial testing preoperative etoposide, cisplatin, and concurrent radiation therapy. Then a limited number of investigators could conduct Phase II trials evaluating new regimens as preoperative treatment.

Identification of treatment-related prognostic factors that would enable early selection of promising neoadjuvant regimens would be useful. It is possible that the rate of histologically confirmed, complete tumor clearance following preoperative treatment might serve this purpose. Significantly longer survival times have been observed in the groups of patients who experience complete tumor clearance.[98] If this observation is confirmed, the rate of histologic complete remission could be used to limit the number of patients in Phase II trials and to choose a preoperative regimen for testing in a Phase III trial.

REFERENCES

1. Mountain C, McMurtrey M, Frazier O: Present status of postoperative adjuvant therapy for lung cancer. Cancer Bull 32:108–112, 1980.
2. Mountain C, McMurtry M, Frazier O: Current results of surgical treatment for lung cancer. Cancer Bull 32:105–108, 1980.
3. Mountain C: A new international staging system for lung cancer. Chest 89(suppl):225–233, 1986.
4. Mountain C: Value of the new TNM staging system for lung cancer. Chest 97:935–947, 1989.
5. Feld R, Rubinstein L, Weisenberg T, et al: Sites of recurrence in resected stage I non-small cell lung cancer: A guide for future studies. J Clin Oncol 2:1352–1358, 1985.
6. Matthews M, Kanhouwa S, Pickren J, et al: Frequency of residual and metastatic tumor in patients undergoing curative surgical resection for lung cancer. Cancer Chemother Rep [Part 3] 4:63–67, 1973.
7. Zimmerman P, Hawson G, Bint M: Ploidy as a prognostic determinant in surgically treated lung cancer. Lancet 2:530–533, 1987.
8. Carp N, Ellison D, Brophy P, et al: DNA content in correlation with postsurgical stage in non–small cell lung cancer. Ann Thorac Surg 53:680–683, 1992.
9. Dazzi H, Thatcher N, Haselton P, et al: DNA analysis by flow cytometry in non–small cell lung cancer: Relationship to epidermal growth factor receptor, histology, tumour stage and survival. Respir Med 84:217–223, 1990.
10. Scagliotti G, Micela R, Gubetta L, et al: Prognostic significance of Ki67 labeling in resected non small cell lung cancer. Eur J Cancer 29a:363–365, 1993.
11. Rice T, Bauer T, Gephardt G, et al: Prognostic significance of flow cytometry in non–small cell lung cancer. J Thorac Cardiovasc Surg 106:210–217, 1993.
12. Rodenhuis S, Van de Wetering M, Mooi W, et al: Mutational activation of the K-*ras* oncogene: A possible pathogenetic factor in adenocarcinoma of the lung. N Engl J Med 317:929–935, 1987.
13. Slebos R, Kibbelaar R, Dalesio O, et al: K-*ras* oncogene activation as a prognostic marker in adenocarcinoma of the lung. N Engl J Med 323:561–565, 1990.
14. Slebos R, Rodenhuis S: The *ras* gene family in human non–small cell lung cancer. J Natl Cancer Inst Monogr 13:23–29, 1992.
15. Carbone D, Minna J: The molecular genetics of lung cancer. Adv Intern Med 37:53–171, 1992.
16. Carbone DP, Mitsudomi T, Rusch V, et al: p53 Protein overexpression, but not gene mutation, is predictive of significantly shortened survival in resected non–small cell lung cancer (NSCLC) patients. Proc Am Soc Clin Oncol 12:334, 1993. (Abstract 1112.)
17. Horio Y, Takahashi T, Kuroishi T, et al: Prognostic significance of p53 mutations and 3p deletions in primary resected non–small cell lung cancer. Cancer Res 53:4, 1993.
18. Takahashi T, Nau MM, Chiba I: P53: A frequent target for genetic abnormalities in lung cancer. Science 246:491–494, 1989.
19. Macchiarini P, Dulmet E, Fontanini G, et al: Non–small cell

lung cancer (NSCLC) invading the thoracic inlet: A curable disease. Proc Am Soc Clin Oncol 12:326, 1993. (Abstract 1081.)

20. Miyake M, Taki Y, Hitomi D, et al: Correlation of expression of H/Le^y/Le^b antigens with survival in patients with carcinoma of the lung. N Engl J Med 327:14–18, 1992.
21. Lee J, Ro J, Sahin A, et al: Expression of blood-group antigen A: A favorable prognostic factor in non–small cell lung cancer. N Engl J Med 324:1084–1090, 1991.
22. Moores D, Piantadosi S, McKneally M: Effect of perioperative blood transfusion on outcome in patients with surgically resected lung cancer. Ann Thoracic Surg 47:346–351, 1989.
23. Gelman R, Gelber R, Henderson I, et al: Improved methodology for analyzing local and distant recurrence. J Clin Oncol 8:548–555, 1990.
24. Arriagada R, Kramar A, LeChevalier T, et al: Competing events determining relapse-free survival in limited small-cell lung carcinoma. J Clin Oncol 10:447–451, 1992.
25. Choi N, Grillo H, Gardiello M, et al: Basis of new strategies in postoperative radiotherapy of bronchogenic carcinoma. Int J Radiat Oncol Biol Phys 6:31–35, 1980.
26. Bangma P: Postoperative radiotherapy. *In* Deeley T (ed): Carcinoma of the Bronchus (Modern Radiotherapy). New York, Appleton-Century-Crofts, 1971, pp 163–170.
27. Emami B, Kim T, Roper C, et al: Postoperative radiation therapy in the management of lung cancer. Radiology 164:251–253, 1987.
28. Weisenburger T for the Lung Cancer Study Group: Effects of postoperative mediastinal radiation on completely resected stage II and stage III epidermoid carcinoma of the lung. N Engl J Med 315:1377–1381, 1986.
29. Van Houtte P, Rocmans P, Smets P, et al: Postoperative radiation therapy in lung cancer: A controlled trial after resection of curative design. Int J Radiat Oncol Biol 6:983–986, 1980.
30. Israel L, Bonadonna G, Sylvester R, et al: Controlled study with adjuvant radiotherapy, chemotherapy, immunotherapy, and chemoimmunotherapy in operable squamous carcinoma of the lung. *In* Muggia F, and Rozencweig M (eds): Lung Cancer: Progress in Therapeutic Research. New York, Raven Press, 1979, pp 443–455.
31. Choi N, Kanarek D, Grillo H: Effect of postoperative radiotherapy on changes in pulmonary function in patients with Stage II and IIIA lung carcinoma. Int J Radiat Oncol Biol Phys 18:95–99, 1990.
32. Turrisi A: The sound and fury about postoperative therapy for lung cancer. Mayo Clinic Proc 67:1197–1200, 1992.
33. Holmes E: Postoperative chemotherapy for non–small cell lung cancer. Chest 103:30s–34s, 1993.
34. Sadeghi A, Payne D, Rubenstein L, et al: Combined modality treatment for resected advanced non–small cell lung cancer: Local control and local recurrence. Int J Radiat Oncol Biol Phys 15:89–97, 1991.
35. Feld R, Rubenstin L, Thomas P, et al: Adjuvant chemotherapy with cyclophosphamide, doxorubicin, and cisplatin in patients with completely resected stage I non–small cell lung cancer. J Natl Cancer Inst 85:299–306, 1993.
36. Ayoub J, Vigneault E, Hanley J, et al: The Montreal multicenter trial in operable non–small cell lung cancer: A multivariate analysis of the predictors of relapse. Proc Am Soc Clin Oncol 10:247, 1991.
37. Fishbein G: Immunotherapy of lung cancer. Semin Oncol 20:351–358, 1993.
38. Ruckdeschela J, Codish S, Stranahan A, et al: Postoperative empyema improves survival in lung cancer: Documentation and analysis of a natural experiment. N Engl J Med 287:1013–1017, 1972.
39. Mountain C, Gail M: Surgical adjuvant intrapleural BCG treatment for stage I non–small cell lung cancer: Preliminary report of the Lung Cancer Study Group. J Thorac Cardiovasc Surg 82:649–657, 1981.
40. Winter S, Sekido Y, Minna J, et al: Antibodies against autologous tumor cell proteins in small cell lung cancer patients are associated with good performance status and improved survival. Proc Am Soc Clin Oncol 12:334, 1993. (Abstract 1113.)
41. Alexopoulos C, Vaslamatzis M, Patila E, et al: Incidence of CNS involvement and the role of prophylactic irradiation (PCI) in the small cell lung cancer (SCLC). Proc Am Soc Clin Oncol 12:356, 1993. (Abstract 1201.)

42. Sharma D, Krasnow S, Wadleigh R, et al: Outcome of brain metastases (BMS) from lung cancer. Proc Am Soc Clin Oncol 12:357, 1993. (Abstract 1206.)
43. Abner A: Prophylactic cranial irradiation in the treatment of small cell carcinoma of the lung. Chest 103:445s–448s, 1993.
44. Cox J, Petrovich Z, Paig C, et al: Prophylactic cranial irradiation in patients with inoperable carcinoma of the lung. Cancer 42:1135–1140, 1978.
45. Mira J, Taylor S, Stephens R, et al: Simultaneous chemotherapy-radiotherapy with prophylactic cranial irradiation for inoperable adeno and large cell lung carcinoma. Int J Radiat Oncol Biol Phys 15:757–761, 1988.
46. Russell A, Pajak T, Selim H, et al: Prophylactic cranial irradiation for lung cancer patients at high risk for development of cerebral metastases: Results of a prospective randomized trial conducted by the Radiation Therapy Oncology Group. Int J Radiat Oncol Biol Phys 21:637–643, 1991.
47. Figlin R, Piantadosi S, Feld F, et al: Intracranial recurrence of carcinoma after complete surgical resection of stage I, II and III non–small cell lung cancer. N Engl J Med 318:1300–1305, 1988.
48. Turrisi A: Brain irradiation and systemic chemotherapy for small cell lung cancer: Dangerous liaisons? J Clin Oncol 8:196–199, 1990.
49. Bonadonna G: Evolving concepts in the systemic adjuvant therapy of breast cancer. Cancer Res 52:2127–2137, 1992.
50. Green M: New adjuvant strategies for the management of resectable non–small cell lung cancer. Chest 103:352s–355s, 1993.
51. Green M: Chemotherapy and radiation in the nonoperative management of Stage III non–small cell lung cancer: The right chemotherapy works in the right setting. *In* DeVita V, Hellman S, Rosenberg S (ed): Important Advances in Oncology, Philadelphia, J.B. Lippincott, 1993, pp 125–137.
52. Laramore G, Scott C, Al-Sarraf M, et al: Adjuvant chemotherapy for resectable squamous cell carcinomas of the head and neck: Report on Intergroup study 0034. Int J Radiat Oncol Biol Phys 23:705–713, 1992.
53. Perez C, Pajak T, Rubin P, et al: Long-term observations of the patterns of failure in patients with unresectable non–oat cell carcinoma of the lung treated with definitive radiotherapy. Cancer 59:1874–1881, 1987.
54. Bonomi P, Gale M, Gaber L, et al: Implication of tumor size and stage group in locally advanced non-small cell lung cancer patients. Proc Am Soc Clin Oncol 12:338, 1993. (Abstract 1128.)
55. Schaake-Koning C, Van Den Bogert W, Dalesio O, et al: Effects of concomitant cisplatin and radiotherapy in inoperable non–small cell lung cancer. N Engl J Med 326:524–530, 1992.
56. Perez C, Stanley K, Grundy G, et al: Impact of irradiation technique and tumor extent in tumor control and survival of patients with unresectable non–oat cell carcinoma of the lung. Report by the Radiation Therapy Oncology Group. Cancer 50:1091–1099, 1987.
57. Wagner H Jr, Lad T, Piantadosi S: Randomized phase II evaluation of preoperative radiation therapy and preoperative chemotherapy with mitomycin-C, vinblastine, and cisplatin in patients with technically unresectable stage IIIa and IIIb non–small cell lung cancer. Lung Cancer 7(suppl):157, 1991.
58. Faber L, Bonomi P: Combined preoperative chemoradiation therapy. Chest Surg Clin North America 1:43–59, 1991.
59. Weiden P, Piantadosi S: Preoperative chemotherapy (cisplatin and fluorouracil) and radiation therapy in stage III non–small cell lung cancer: A phase II study of the Lung Cancer Study Group. Lung Cancer 83:266–273, 1991.
60. Curran W, Stafford P: Lack of apparent difference in outcome between clinically staged IIIa and IIIb non–small cell lung cancer treated with radiation therapy. J Clin Oncol 8:409–415, 1990.
61. Curran W, Cox J, Azarnia N, et al: Comparison of the radiation therapy oncology group and American Joint Committee on cancer staging systems among non–small lung cancer received hyperfractionated radiation therapy. Cancer 68:509–516, 1991.
62. Reddy S, Lee M, Bonomi P, et al: Combined modality therapy for stage III non–small cell lung carcinoma: Results of treatment and pattern of failure. Int J Radiat Oncol Biol Phys 24:17–23, 1992.

63. Bonomi P, Faber L: Neoadjuvant chemoradiation therapy in non–small cell lung cancer: The Rush University experience. Lung Cancer 9:383–390, 1993.

64. Bromley L, Szur L: Combined radiotherapy and resection for carcinoma of the bronchus. Lancet 5:937–941, 1955.

65. Bloedorn F, Cowley R, Cuccia C, et al: Combined therapy with irradiation and surgery in the treatment of bronchogenic carcinoma. Am J Roentgenol 85:875–885, 1961.

66. Komaki R: Preoperative radiation therapy for superior sulcus tumors. Chest Surg Clin North America 1:13–35, 1991.

67. Paulson D: Carcinoma of the superior pulmonary sulcus. J Thorac Cardiovasc Surg 70:1095–1104, 1975.

68. Shields T, Higgins G, Lawton R, et al: Preoperative x-ray therapy as an adjuvant in the treatment of bronchogenic carcinoma. J Thorac Cardiovasc Surg 59:49–61, 1970.

69. Warram J: Preoperative irradiation of cancer of the lung: Final report of a therapeutic trial. Cancer 36:914–925, 1975.

70. Bonomi P: Brief overview of combination chemotherapy in non–small cell lung cancer. Semin Oncol 13(suppl 3):89–91, 1986.

71. Arriagada R, LeChevalier T, Quoix E, et al: Effect of chemotherapy on locally advanced non–small cell lung carcinoma. Int J Radiat Oncol Biol Phys 20:1183–1190, 1991.

72. Dillman R, Seagren S, Propert K, et al: A randomized trial of induction chemotherapy plus high-dose radiation versus radiation alone in stage III non–small cell lung cancer. N Engl J Med 323:940–945, 1990.

73. Dillman R, Seagren S, Herndon J, et al: Randomized trial of induction chemotherapy plus radiation therapy vs RT alone in stage III non–small cell lung cancer (NSCLC): Five year follow-up of CALGB. Proc Am Soc Clin Oncol 12:329, 1993. (Abstract 1092.)

74. Holsti L: Inoperable non–small cell lung cancer: Radiation with or without chemotherapy: Final results of a randomized trial. Lung Cancer 7(suppl):162, 1991.

75. Morton R, Jett J, McGinnis W, et al: Thoracic radiation therapy alone compared with combined chemoradiotherapy for locally unresectable non–small cell lung cancer. Ann Intern Med 115:681–686, 1991.

76. Kris M, Martin N, Gralla R, et al: Primary chemotherapy in stage IIIa non–small cell lung cancer patients with clinically apparent mediastinal lymph node metastases: Focus on five-year summary. Lung Cancer 9:369–376, 1993.

77. Burkes R, Ginsberg R, Shepherd R, et al: Induction chemotherapy with MVP (mitomycin-C + vindesine + cisplatin) for stage III (T1-3, N2, M0) unresectable non–small cell lung cancer: The Toronto experience. Lung Cancer 9:377–382, 1993.

78. Henriquez I, Munoz-Galindo I, Rebollo J: Neoadjuvant chemotherapy with cisplatin, mitomycin-C and vindesine in locally advanced non–small cell lung cancer. Proc Am Soc Clin Oncol 9:227, 1990.

79. Eagan R, Ruud C, Lee R, et al: Pilot study of induction therapy with cyclophosphamide doxorubicin, and cisplatin (CAP) and chest irradiation prior to thoracotomy in initially inoperable stage III M0 non-small cell lung cancer. Cancer Treat Rep 71:895–900, 1987.

80. Strauss G, Sherman D, Goutsou M: Neoadjuvant chemotherapy and radiotherapy followed by surgery in stage IIIa non–small cell carcinoma of the lung: A phase II study of the cancer and leukemia group B. *In* Salmon S (ed): Adjuvant Therapy of Cancer VI. Proc of the Sixth International Conference on the Adjuvant Therapy of Cancer, 1990, pp 125–132.

81. Weitberg A, Yoshen L, Posner M, et al: Combined modality therapy for stage IIIa non–small cell lung cancer. Proc Am Soc Clin Oncol 12:293, 1993.

82. Rusch V, Albain K, Crowley J, et al: Surgical resection of stage IIIa and stage IIIb non–small cell lung cancer after concurrent induction chemoradiotherapy. J Thorac Cardiovasc Surg 105:97–106, 1993.

83. Taylor S, Trybula M, Bonomi P: Simultaneous cisplatin-fluorouracil infusion and radiation followed by surgical resection in regionally localized stage III, non–small cell lung cancer. Ann Thorac Surg 43:87–91, 1987.

84. Weiden P, Piantadosi S: Preoperative chemoradiotherapy in stage III non–small cell lung cancer (NSCLC): A phase II study of the lung study group (LCSG). Proc Am Soc Clin Oncol 7:197, 1988.

85. Skarin A, Jochelson M, Sheldon T, et al: Neoadjuvant chemotherapy in marginally resectable stage III Mo non–small cell lung cancer: Long-term follow-up in 41 patients. J Surg Oncol 40:266–274, 1989.

86. Strauss G, Herndon J, Sherman D, et al: Neoadjuvant chemotherapy and radiotherapy followed by surgery in stage IIIA non–small cell carcinoma of the lung: Report of a cancer and leukemia group B phase II study. J Clin Oncol 10:1237–1244, 1992.

87. Trakhtenberg AKH, Kiseleva ES, Pitskhelauri VG, et al: Preoperative radiotherapy in the combined treatment of lung cancer patients. Neoplasma 35:459–465, 1988.

88. Fleck J, Camargo J, Godoy D, et al: Chemoradiation therapy (CRT) versus chemotherapy (CT) alone as a neoadjuvant treatment for stage III non–small cell lung cancer (NSCLC). Preliminary report of a phase III prospective randomized trial. Proc Am Soc Clin Oncol 12:338, 1993. (Abstract 1108.)

89. Rosell R, Gomez-Codina J, Camps C, et al: A randomized trial comparing preoperative chemotherapy plus surgery alone in patients with non–small cell lung cancer. N Engl J Med 330:153–158, 1994.

90. Roth JA, Fossella F, Komaki R, et al: A randomized trial comparing perioperative chemotherapy and surgery with surgery alone in resectable stage III non–small cell lung cancer. J Natl Cancer Inst, 1994 (in press).

91. Feigal E, Christian M, Cheson B, et al: New chemotherapeutic agents in non–small cell lung cancer. Semin Oncol 20:185–201, 1993.

92. Slichenmyer W, Rowinski E, Donehower R, et al: The current status of camptothecin analogues as antitumor agents. J Nat Cancer Inst 85:271–291, 1993.

93. Garcia de Palazzo I, Adams G, Sundareshan P, et al: Expression of mutated epidermal growth factor receptor by non–small cell lung carcinomas. Cancer Res 53:3217–3220, 1993.

94. Kaston M, Onyine O, Sidransky D, et al: Participation of p53 protein in the cellular response to DNA damage. Cancer Res 51:6304–6311, 1991.

95. Roth J, Mukhopadhyay T, Tainsky M, et al: Molecular approaches to prevention and therapy of aerodigestive tract cancers. J Natl Cancer Inst Monogr 13:15–21, 1992.

96. James G, Goldstein J, Brown M, et al: Benzodiazepine peptidomimetics: Potent inhibitors of *ras* farnesylation in animal cells. Science 260:1937–1942, 1993.

97. Kohl N, Mosser S, deSolms S, et al: Selective inhibition of *ras*-dependent transformation by a farnesyltransferase inhibitor. Science 260:1934–1937, 1993.

98. Bonomi P, Gale M, Taylor SI: Prognostic significance of histologic complete remission in neoadjuvant trials in stage III non–small cell lung cancer. Proc Am Soc Clin Oncol 9:230, 1990.

99. Feld R, Rubenstein L, Weisenberger T, et al: Sites of recurrence in resected stage I non–small cell lung cancer: A guide for future studies. J Clin Oncol 2:1352–1358, 1984.

100. Pairolero P, Williams D, Bergstralh M, et al: Post-surgical stage I bronchogenic carcinoma: Morbid implications of recurrent disease. Ann Thorac Surg 38:331–338, 1984.

101. Thomas P, Rubenstein L: The Lung Cancer Study Group: Cancer recurrence after resection T1N0 non–small cell lung cancer. Ann Thorac Surg 48:242–247, 1990.

102. Martini N, Flehinger B, Zaman M, et al: Prospective study of 445 lung carcinomas with mediastinal lymph node metastases. J Thorac Cardiovasc Surg 80:390–397, 1980.

103. Green N, Kurohara S, George III FW, et al: Postresection irradiation of primary lung cancer. Radiology 116:405–407, 1975.

104. Kirsch M, Sloan H: Mediastinal metastasis in bronchogenic carcinoma: Influence of postoperative irradiation, cell type and location. Ann Thorac Surg 33:459–463, 1982.

105. Chung C, Stryker J, O'Neill M, et al: Evaluation of adjuvant postoperative radiotherapy for lung cancer. Int J Radiat Oncol Biol Phys 8:1877–1880, 1982.

106. Holmes E: Surgical adjuvant therapy of non–small cell lung cancer. J Surg Oncol 42(suppl 1):26–33, 1989.

107. Niiranen A, Niitamo-Korhonen S, Kouri M, et al: Adjuvant chemotherapy after radical surgery for non–small cell lung cancer: A randomized study. J Clin Oncol 10:1927–1932, 1992.

108. Teramatsu T, Iioka S, Nobohiro N, et al: Assessment of postoperative adjuvant chemotherapy on non–small cell lung cancer. Lung Cancer 7:124, 1991. (Abstract 462.)

109. Kimura H, Yamaguchi Y, Fujisawa T, et al: A randomized controlled trial of postoperative adjuvant chemoimmunotherapy of resected non–small cell lung cancer with IL2 and LAK cells. Lung Cancer 7:133, 1991. (Abstract 498.)
110. Tsuchiya R, Ohta M, Suemasu K, et al: Surgical adjuvant chemotherapy in stage III non–small cell lung cancer: Randomized controlled trial. Lung Cancer 7:155, 1991. (Abstract 578.)
111. McKneally M, Maver V, Lininger L, et al: Four year followup of the Albany experience with intrapleural BCG in lung cancer. J Thorac Cardiovasc Surg 81:485–492, 1981.
112. Amery W, Cosemans J, Gooszen H, et al: Four year results from double-blind study of adjuvant levamisole treatment in resectable lung cancer. *In* Terry W, Rosenberg S (eds): Immunotherapy of Human Cancer. New York, Elsevier North Holland, 1982, pp 123–133.
113. Anthony H, Mearns A, Mason M: Levamisole and surgery in bronchial carcinoma patients: Increase in deaths from cardiorespiratory failure. Thorax 34(1):4–12, 1979.
114. Spain R: Neoadjuvant mitomycin C, cisplatin, and infusion vinblastine in locally and regionally advanced non–small cell lung cancer: Problems and progress from the perspective of long-term follow-up. Semin Oncol 15:6–15, 1988.
115. Cybulski I, Lanza L, Ryan B, et al: Prognostic significance of computed tomography in resected N2 lung cancer. Ann Thorac Surg 54:533–537, 1992.
116. Martini N, Flehinger B: The role of surgery in N2 lung cancer. Surg Clin North Am 67:1037–1049, 1987.
117. Teodori L, Trinca M, Goehde W, et al: Cytokinetic investigation of lung tumors using the antibromodeoxyuridine (BUdR) monoclonal antibody method: Comparison with DNA flow cytometric data. Int J Cancer 45:995–1001, 1990.
118. Chen Z-L, Perez S, Holmes E, et al: Frequency and distribution of occult micrometastases in lymph nodes of patients with non-small cell carcinoma. J Natl Cancer Inst 85:493–498, 1993.
119. Landberg G, Roos G: Antibodies to proliferating cell nuclear antigen as S-phase probes in flow cytometric cell cycle analysis. Cancer Res 51:4570–4574, 1991.
120. Rosenthal SA, Curran WJ Jr: The significance of histology in non–small cell lung cancer. Cancer Treat Rev 17(4):409–425, 1990.

10 DEFINITIVE RADIOTHERAPY AND COMBINED MODALITY THERAPY FOR INOPERABLE NON–SMALL CELL LUNG CANCER

Thomas H. Weisenburger

It is estimated that 172,000 persons in the United States developed lung cancer in 1994.[1] Approximately 55% of these patients will be found to have distant metastases, 30% to have regional dissemination, and 15% to have the tumor confined to the lung.[2, 3] Only 15% of patients with lung cancer can be offered resection for cure,[4] and the remainder of the patients who present without clinically apparent distant metastatic disease (approximately 45,000 to 50,000 patients per year) form a population eligible to be considered for definitive and potentially curative radiation therapy. The overall rate of survival in this group of patients is discouragingly low, however, and therefore a debate has continued for a number of years about whether radiotherapy should be offered to all patients in this category.[5–13] Physicians caring for these patients must identify candidates for radiotherapy based on a sound clinical assessment of each individual and on their knowledge of each of the available treatment modalities and their associated benefits and morbidity. Because radical radiotherapy for lung cancer is not performed without some associated morbidity, it should not be considered a "soft alternative to surgery."[14]

> To cure sometimes,
> To relieve often,
> To comfort always.
> ANONYMOUS[15]

ANATOMIC AND CLINICAL CONSIDERATIONS

It is important to understand the lymphatic drainage of the lung when considering the use of radiotherapy to treat patients with lung cancer. The lymphatics of the right upper lobe drain to the mediastinal lymph nodes at the junction of the azygos vein and superior vena cava. The left upper lobe drains to the nodes near the ligamentum arteriosum located between the aortic arch and left pulmonary artery.[16] Involvement of these nodes may affect the recurrent laryngeal nerve. The lymphatics of the inferior portions of the lungs drain to the nodes in the corresponding anterior pulmonary ligaments. These nodes communicate with the subcarinal nodes[17] and inferiorly with nodes near the cisterna chyli,[18] allowing direct spread to the upper retroperitoneal area and perhaps explaining the poorer prognosis for lower lobe carcinoma reported by Deeley.[19] The remaining portion of the lungs drains to the hilar lymph nodes. There is crossover of lymph from the lingula of the left upper lobe and from the left lower lobe to the right side of the mediastinum via the subcarinal nodes. The lymph then flows from the right side to the right lymphatic duct. On the left side, the paratracheal bronchial nodes drain into the thoracic duct. Involvement of the parietal pleura allows direct spread to subdiaphragmatic, axillary, or supraclavicular lymphatics, depending on the location.

In selecting candidates for a radical course of radiotherapy, it is important to be aware of prognostic clinical factors. Komaki and colleagues[20] evaluated these factors in 45 3-year survivors from a series of 410 patients who had inoperable non–small cell lung cancer (non–SCLC) and small cell lung cancer (SCLC). Prognostic factors associated with increased survival were high performance status, an early stage of cancer, large cell carcinoma histologic findings, inoperability due to medical reasons, thoracotomy necessary to determine unresectability, and high total dose of radiation. Stanley[21] analyzed 5502 patients from seven studies by the Veterans Administration Lung Group. These patients had both small cell and non–small cell cancer and both limited and extensive disease. The three most important prognostic factors were the extent of disease, prior weight loss, and Karnofsky performance status. The group of patients with extensive disease, weight loss of more than 10%, and a performance status of less than 70 with scalene or supraclavicular nodal involvement had a median survival time of 3 weeks compared with 46 weeks for patients with limited disease, weight loss of less than 10%, and a performance status of 90 to 100. Caldwell and Bagshaw[22] noted that the presence of pain or hemoptysis or the requirement of treatment fields of more than 200

cm^2 made long-term control less likely. These differences, however, were not statistically significant. Hoarseness was a presenting symptom in 34 of their 269 patients (13%). None of these patients survived for 2 years.

In addition to clinical indicators, the inherent biologic nature of the malignancy may significantly affect the prognosis. Weiss and colleagues[23] evaluated the doubling time in 18 patients with solitary nodules, 10 of whom had resection. They noted a direct correlation between the doubling time of the tumor and survival. Macchiarini and colleagues[24] examined tumor tissue from 87 patients with T1N0M0 non–SCLC for neovascularization in the region adjacent to the tumor. At a median of 8 years, all patients with extensive neovascularization had relapsed, whereas only 10% of those with minimal neovascularization had relapsed. Zimmerman and others[25] analyzed the tumor ploidy in a group of 100 surgically treated patients by flow cytometry (45% aneuploid and 55% diploid) and noted that patients with aneuploid tumors had significantly shorter survival times than those with diploid tumors ($p < 0.0005$). Of 45 patients with diploid tumors without nodal involvement, 41 (91%) were alive at 2 years compared with only 16 of the 29 patients (55%) with aneuploid tumors ($p < 0.05$). Ploidy was independent of age, sex, type of operation, site of primary tumor, histology, or TNM category. A similar study by Yu and colleagues[26] confirmed these findings.

Although these parameters are useful in predicting survival rates in large groups of patients, they cannot be relied on as absolute indicators in the decision-making process for an individual patient. A significant effort is being made to develop predictive assays of radioresponse based on in vitro tumor properties to assist in treatment planning on an individual basis.[27, 28]

Patient selection criteria for radical radiotherapy have included, in addition to good performance status, evidence of adequate pulmonary reserve based on a forced expiratory volume at 1 sec (FEV_1) of more than 700 ml, the ability to climb one flight of stairs without severe dyspnea, no evidence of hypercapnia at rest, a maximal breathing capacity of at least 50% of that predicted,[15] diffusing capacity of carbon monoxide of 45, PaO_2 of at least 60 mm Hg, and a vital capacity of at least 45% of predicted.[29] If concurrent infection is present, including tuberculosis, appropriate antimicrobial therapy should be given, followed by radiotherapy as soon as the infection is under control.[15, 16, 30] The hemoglobin level should be more than 10 gm/dl.[16] Malignant pleural effusion is a contraindication to radical radiotherapy.[14]

The careful clinical evaluation of patients with an established diagnosis of non–SCLC is essential before making a decision regarding radical treatment[31] (Fig. 10–1). Computed tomography (CT) scanning of the upper abdomen should include the adrenals, which can harbor occult metastatic disease. Nielsen and colleagues[32] found asymptomatic adrenal masses in 15 of 84 patients, with four of these confirmed at biopsy. Oliver and associates[33] identified 32 adrenal masses in 330 patients with non–small cell bronchogenic carcinoma. Eight of the 25 patients (32%) who underwent biopsy had histologically proven metastatic disease. Although the rate of detection is low (3% to 5%), inclusion of the upper abdomen at the time of CT examination of the chest should be considered, since it would avoid unnecessarily aggressive treatment of the regional disease.[34] Biopsy of the suspicious area should be performed because of the high false-positive rate of CT scans. CT scans of the brain in patients who have normal laboratory studies and no symptoms of systemic disease are probably not warranted because of the low yield. Hooper and colleagues[35] observed that none of 28 patients had positive CT brain scans if they showed no symptoms or signs of bronchogenic carcinoma. The incidence of positive CT brain scans increased as the number of clinical and laboratory factors indicative of disease increased. Salvatierra and colleagues[36] reported the results of whole-body bone scanning and CT scans of the brain and upper abdomen in 146 patients with non–SCLC who had potentially resectable disease. Metastatic disease was found in 44 patients (30%). Brain metastases were found in 19 patients (13%), only four of whom (2.7%) were asymptomatic. Bone scans were positive in only 3.4% of asymptomatic patients. They found that if head CT scans in symptomatic patients with squamous cell and in all patients with adenocarcinoma and large cell carcinoma, bone scans in symptomatic patients, and abdominal CTs scans in all patients had been performed, only one patient would have been understaged, and 80% of bone scans and 53% of brain scans would have been avoided.

RADIOTHERAPY TECHNIQUES

Accurate localization of the tumor within the thoracic cavity before planning for radiotherapy is extremely important to optimize the effect of radiation on the tumor and to minimize the risk of normal tissue reaction. Although the benefit of CT treatment planning has not been demonstrated in a prospective trial, it has become established in the management of patients with lung cancer and should be considered when available in the treatment-planning process.[29]

Mira and associates[37] evaluated 45 chest CT scans in patients with lung cancer and compared them with treatment planning by conventional radiography examination. CT scans demonstrated greater tumor extension in 11 of 14 patients (78%) whose regular radiograph results were considered to show satisfactory tumor boundaries. In one patient, who had atelectasis demonstrated by CT, the tumor was smaller than reported by conventional radiography. In 21 of 31 patients (68%) whose radiographs did not show tumor localization, CT was able to demonstrate the tumor. CT scans showed anterior spread toward the sternum and posterior involvement around the vertebral bodies toward the spinal cord and costal pleura, both of which are important in regard to radiotherapy boost fields. There are limitations in the use of CT, however,

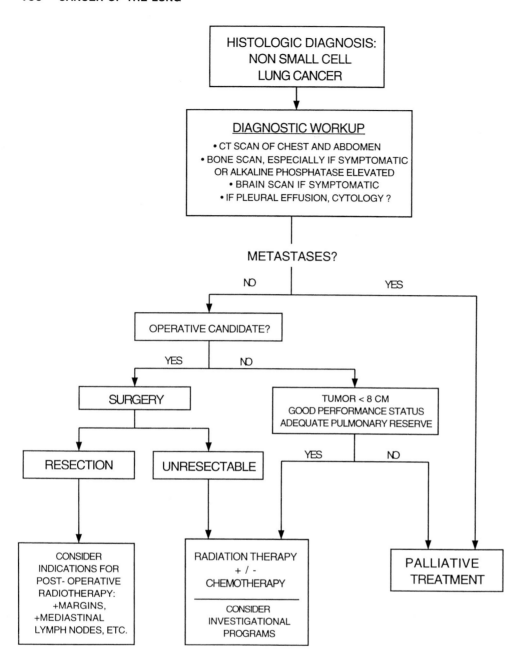

FIGURE 10–1. Flow chart for the diagnosis and treatment of non–small cell lung cancer.

because atalectasis is not always distinguishable from tumor and the resolution of the best scanners is no better than 0.5 mm, raising the possibility that there may be undetected subclinical involvement outside the proposed treatment fields.

Although CT imaging data are increasingly being integrated into the radiotherapy planning process,[38] care must be taken to perform treatment planning CT scans with the patient in the treatment position, using a flat couch similar to a treatment table. Also, external markers must be placed on the patient, usually at the time of pre-CT simulation, to translate the beams of radiation defined during treatment optimization to the patient, which is usually done during post-CT simulation to confirm the fields. In addition, the CT hard-copy image can have as much as 10% distortion.[39]

CT also provides the attenuation characteristics of the tissues being traversed by a radiotherapy beam. Orton and colleagues[40] evaluated four commonly used lung correction algorithms and showed them to be in agreement with data from a specially constructed phantom. Although cooperative groups are not using inhomogeneity corrections at this time, the authors contend that over the next several years these should be introduced into clinical trials. In another study, van't Riet and colleagues[41] examined 23 patients with carcinoma of the bronchus, comparing CT scan treatment planning, using electron densities obtained by the scans, with methods having no correction for lung density. The minimum tumor dose prescribed in this group of patients was 60 Gy. The corrected minimum dose using the CT scans varied between 63 and 77 Gy (105% to 128%). The clinical usefulness of these calculations has not yet been shown.[38] It is reasonable to gather data from the cooperative groups so that comparisons of corrected and uncorrected doses can be performed and the benefit of this method can be determined.

The recommendations for the radiotherapy fields generally include at least a 2-cm margin around the clinically appreciable tumor and the entire mediastinum[29] (Figs. 10–2A, 2B, and 10–3). The inferior border of the field should be at least 5 cm below the carina unless there is evidence of lower lobe involvement, in which case the inferior margin should extend to the diaphragm. The superior border should be at the suprasternal notch. The ipsilateral hilar region should be included, with a margin of at least 1 cm around the contralateral hilar region.[42] It is generally recommended that the ipsilateral supraclavicular region be included if the tumor is poorly differentiated or is in the upper lobes or if mediastinal lymph nodes are involved. Irradiation of the ipsilateral supraclavicular regions reduces the frequency of metastasis to lymph nodes in this area, but no data are available

concerning whether radiation of these regions is necessary with respect to survival.[43] One unresolved issue is elective nodal irradiation.[44] Curran and colleagues[44] have shown that increasing field sizes to include more elective fields decreases the predicted minimal FEV_1. Hazuka and coworkers[45] evaluated elective nodal irradiation in a retrospective series of 88 patients treated with high-dose thoracic irradiation incorporating beam's eye view display. There was no difference with respect to local progression-free survival or survival between large volume treatment (inclusion of supraclavicular and contralateral lymph nodes) and small volume treatment (exclusion of the elective nodal areas). Armstrong and Minsky[46] discussed field selection in Stage I and II non–SCLC and concluded that it is acceptable to confine the field of treatment to the primary alone in patients with N0 disease who have pulmonary compromise that would preclude safe delivery of elective mediastinal irradiation and that mediastinal irradiation is recommended for patients with N1 disease. Therefore, especially in patients with marginal pulmonary function and N0

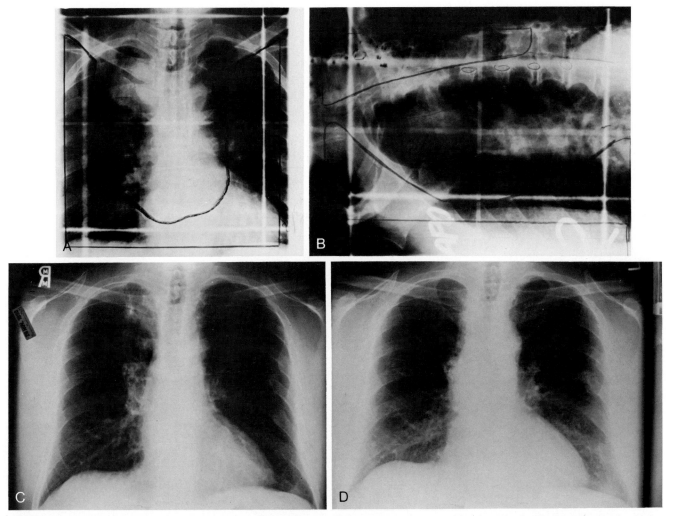

FIGURE 10–2. A 47-year-old man with Stage IIIB adenocarcinoma. *A*, *B*, Simulator films for the AP (*A*) and LAO (*B*) ports showing the design of custom-shaped blocks for each field (e.g., AP, PA, LAO, RPO). *C*, PA chest film taken 1 year after treatment showing radiographic radiation pneumonitis. The patient was asymptomatic. *D*, PA chest film taken 4 years later showing slight volume loss and paratracheal consolidation from the irradiation. The patient is free of disease.

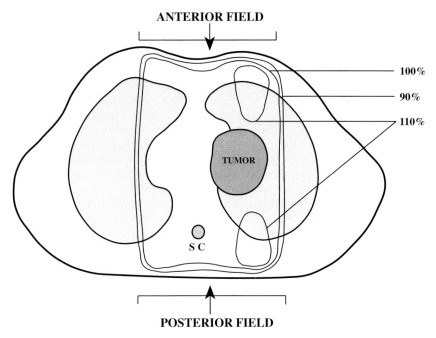

ANTERIOR FIELD

100%

90%

110%

TUMOR

S C

POSTERIOR FIELD

FIGURE 10–3. Idealized output from a computerized treatment plan that takes into account tissue inhomogeneities when isodose curves are calculated. This field arrangement could be utilized until the tolerance of the cord is reached, and then fields that avoid treating the spinal cord would be required (see Fig. 10–5). SC = Spinal cord.

disease, it may be reasonable to exclude the elective nodal sites.

When there is a significant slope to the chest wall, the superior portion of the field, including the spinal cord, may receive a substantially higher dose than is calculated at the field center.[47] It may be necessary to use a wedge or compensating filter to provide a more uniform distribution of radiation (Fig. 10–4).[16] Numerous studies have used posterior spinal cord blocks to limit the dose from posterior fields. This leads to an underdosage in the mediastinum in the tissues underlying this block. With the availability of simulators and CT scans to aid in treatment planning, it is possible to use combinations of oblique and lateral fields to avoid treating the spinal cord above the level of

tolerance without the aid of a posterior spinal cord block (Fig. 10–5).[43]

RESULTS OF RADIOTHERAPY AS A PRIMARY MODALITY

Leddy and Moersch in 1940[48] reported one of the first series to document long-term survival using radiotherapy to treat lung cancer. Of 250 patients proven to have primary lung cancer, 125 received radiotherapy and 125 control subjects received no treatment. None of the patients in the control group lived longer than 1 year after diagnosis: 25 of the 125 patients in whom radiotherapy was used survived 1 year, and five (4%)

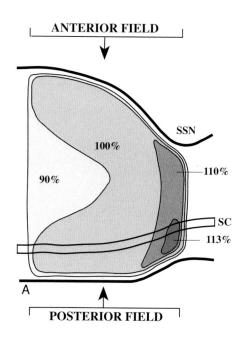

ANTERIOR FIELD

SSN

100%

90%

110%

SC

113%

A

POSTERIOR FIELD

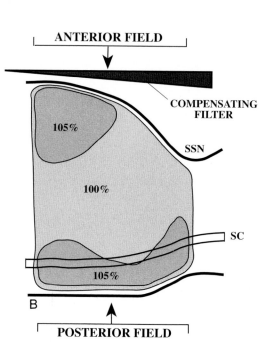

ANTERIOR FIELD

COMPENSATING FILTER

105%

SSN

100%

SC

105%

B

POSTERIOR FIELD

FIGURE 10–4. *A,* Because of the slope of the chest wall and the thinner diameter of the patient at the superior border of the field, the dose to the spinal cord may be as high as 13% above that dose measured at the midline when there is no wedge or compensating filter. *B,* A compensating filter or wedge can reduce this discrepancy and keep the dose to the spinal cord to only 5% above that measured in the central axis. SSN = Suprasternal notch. SC = Spinal cord.

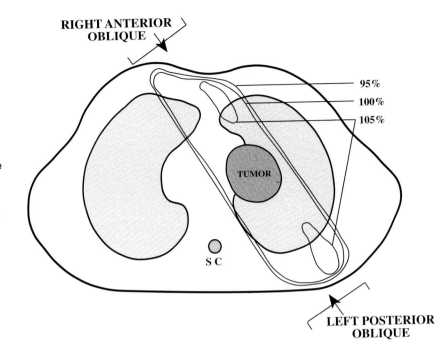

FIGURE 10–5. Opposed anterior and posterior fields provide a possible arrangement to boost the primary tumor beyond 45 Gy while avoiding the spinal cord (SC).

survived 5 years, with the longest survival being 12 years at the time of the report. Smart and Hilton[49] reported on 40 patients proved by biopsy to have cancer who were treated by radiotherapy alone. The patients selected were in good general condition and had localized, operable lesions with no clinical or radiographic evidence of lymph node involvement. At 5 years, nine patients were alive (22.5%), and three (7.5%) survived 10 years. This clearly established the role of radiotherapy as a potentially curative modality in the treatment of lung cancer. Morrison and colleagues[50] compared the use of radiotherapy with surgery in 58 patients, 37 of whom had epidermoid carcinoma and 19 of whom had anaplastic carcinomas. Patients received 45 Gy in 4 weeks using 8-MeV photons. For the patients with epidermoid carcinoma, the 4-year survival rate was 30% with resection and 6% with radiotherapy. These results establish that surgery is the treatment of choice for operable non–small cell tumors of the lung but also that irradiation can provide a small but real chance of cure.

As noted earlier, because of the modest long-term survival rates, there has been considerable discussion regarding whether all patients should be offered treatment.[5–13] Roswit and colleagues[51] compared the use of immediate irradiation (IRT) with supportive care in a randomized trial in which 308 patients received radiotherapy (40 to 50 Gy, principally with orthovoltage techniques) and 246 received only supportive care. All patients had local or regional inoperable (90%) or unresectable or recurrent (10%) lung cancer of all histologic types (14% had small cell histologic findings). With orthovoltage machines, most were treated with relatively low doses by current standards (33% received less than 40 Gy). The survival rate at 1 year was 18% in the treated group and 14% in the control group, a statistically significant ($p < 0.05$) but clinically small difference.

Several studies have investigated the benefit of radiotherapy added to chemotherapy in locally advanced disease. Niederle and colleagues[52] evaluated immediate radiotherapy (IRT) compared with IRT plus chemotherapy or radiotherapy delayed until palliation was needed in 47 patients with T1-2N2-3 non–SCLC. IRT consisted of 4 Gy given twice weekly to a total of 52 to 56 Gy. Median survival was 15, 19, and 11 months, respectively ($p = 0.06$). Johnson and colleagues[53] compared the use of chemotherapy (vindesine) with the same chemotherapy plus radiotherapy (60 Gy in 6 weeks) or radiotherapy alone in a three-armed randomized trial of patients with locally advanced nonmetastatic non–SCLC. The overall response rate was superior for patients who received radiotherapy compared with patients who received vindesine, but there was no difference in median or 5-year survival. Kubota and colleagues[54] reported on a series of patients who initially received chemotherapy and then were randomized to receive 50 to 60 Gy or no further treatment. They noted a prolonged time to progression and increased 2-year survival in the patients who received radiotherapy group (29% versus 6%).

Survival rates after treatment by irradiation alone have varied considerably depending on the population studied. The best results are obtained in patients who have early, potentially resectable disease but are inoperable for medical reasons.[49, 55–61] As expected, survival appears to decrease with increasing tumor size. Survival rates in this group range from 10% to 32% (Table 10–1). Cox and associates[62] reported a 13% (10 of 77) 5-year survival rate in a selected series of patients with unresectable disease who had a high Karnofsky performance status (90 or 100) and who

TABLE 10–1. Selected Studies of Primary Radiotherapy for Early Non–Small Cell Lung Cancer

STUDY	NO. OF PATIENTS	MEDIAN SURVIVAL	5-YR SURVIVAL (%)	STAGE	COMMENTS
Smart and Hilton[49]	40	NR	23	Operable	Presumed resectable
Haffty et al[55]	43	28 months	21	T1-2,N0	IMR
Noordijk et al[56]	50	27 months	16	T1-2,N0	IMR, SR, elderly (mean age = 74)
Zhang et al[57]	44	NR	32	Early	IMR
Talton et al[58]	77	18 months	17	T1-3,N0	IMR
Dosoretz et al[59]	152	17 months	10	T1-3,N0	IMR, increased survival with increased dose, decreased survival with increasing tumor size
Rosenthal et al[60]	62	18 months	12	T1-2,N1	NS, results comparable to Stage I patients
Sandler et al[61]	77	20 months	*17	T1-2,N0	IMR, SR, increased survival with better staging, decreased survival with increasing tumor size

SR = surgery refused, IMR = inoperable for medical reasons, NS = reason for selection for radiotherapy not stated, NR = not reported.
*3-year survival.

received 46 to 60 Gy continuous course therapy. For unselected patients who are unresectable because of tumor or nodal status, the 5-year survival for patients with locally advanced non–SCLC is usually approximately 5%.[63]

Fractionation

Because of the population diversity with respect to tumor and nodal stage, performance status, histology, adequacy of pretreatment evaluation, biologic diversity of the tumor, and various treatment factors, including total radiation dose, continuous versus split course, and treatment planning with and without simulators or CT scans, it is difficult to arrive at a consensus concerning standard radiotherapy recommendations for this disease.[12] A number of fractionation schemes have been used clinically, but the optimal fractionation schedule has yet to be determined.[63]

Split course irradiation has been used by many clinicians because of both radiobiologic and clinical considerations.[64–67] The potential biologic advantages of split course irradiation that have been postulated are (1) reoxygenation of initially hypoxic tumor cells through rapid initial destruction of sensitive cells, al-

lowing increased formation of vessels; (2) redistribution of cells from G0 to more sensitive phases of the cell cycle; and (3) greater repair capacity of normal tissues compared with tumor tissues. From a clinical standpoint, there are several advantages: (1) In a disease in which the survival is so short, the time spent in treatment is minimized, reducing costs and creating less disturbance of the patient's lifestyle; (2) some of the patients will develop metastatic disease or local progression during the rest period and therefore will not require a second course of therapy (approximately 20% of patients[68]); (3) treatment volume may be reduced in the second course, minimizing complications; and (4) pulses of radiation may be combined with chemotherapy.[63]

Split course treatments have been compared with continuous course radiotherapy in a number of randomized, prospective clinical trials. Levitt and colleagues[66] reported the results of a randomized, prospective trial comparing the use of 18 Gy delivered in three fractions on three consecutive days and repeated 28 days later in 15 patients with the use of 60 Gy given in a continuous manner over 6 to 8 weeks in 14 patients with epidermoid carcinoma. No difference was seen in survival or symptom relief between these

TABLE 10–2. Split Course vs Continuous Course Radiotherapy

RANDOMIZED STUDIES	DOSES IN GY	SURVIVAL	PALLIATION	CONCLUSIONS
Levitt et al[66]	3600 SC vs 6000 Cont	No difference	No difference	More side effects in SC
Lee et al[67]	5000 SC vs 5000 Cont	No difference	No difference	SC more practical
Holsti and Mattson[69]	5500 SC vs 5000 Cont	No difference	No difference	SC better tolerated
Perez et al[42]	4000 Cont 4000 SC 5000 Cont 6000 Cont	No difference*	Not assessed	More side effects in SC and 6000 Gy groups Local control better in 6000 Gy group

SC = split course, Cont = continuous course, 900 to 1000 Gy/wk.
*More complete responders in the 6000 Gy group and the survival was greater in complete responders compared with partial or nonresponders. Overall survival among groups was not different, however.

two regimens. There was a suggestion of a higher incidence of lung fibrosis in the patients undergoing split course therapy and a slightly higher incidence of local recurrence in the treated area. Split course technique was believed to be preferable in the treatment of these patients with advanced squamous cell carcinoma because of the fewer treatments required.

Lee and colleagues[67] compared the use of in 34 patients 50 Gy given in a split-course fashion with 50 Gy given continuously (25 Gy/2-week rest/25 Gy cycle/ versus 50 Gy in a continuous course; all fractions, 1.75 to 2 Gy). The randomization was stratified by cell type (31% of each group had small cell carcinoma), TNM stage, and prior surgery. No difference was observed in clinical or objective improvement between these two regimens. The authors maintained that split course radiotherapy was better tolerated and allowed re-evaluation of the patients before the second course of therapy, permitting the physician to avoid unnecessary treatment in patients whose disease had progressed.

Holsti and Mattson[69] randomly compared the use of 50 Gy in a 5-week continuous course with 55 Gy over 7 to 8 weeks with a mid-course rest period of 2 to 3 weeks. The 5-year survival rate was 7% (9 of 134 patients) in the continuous course group and 4% (7 of 180 patients) in the split course group. The authors stated that the end results achievable with split course therapy are similar to those of continuous course treatment, with the advantages of better tolerance and less marked or milder side effects in the split course group. Perez and colleagues[42] reported the results of the Radiation Therapy Oncology Group (RTOG) study 73-01 that compared regimens of 40-Gy continuous course, 40-Gy split course (20 Gy in 1 week followed by a 2-week rest, followed by an additional 20 Gy in 1 week), 50 Gy in 25 fractions over 5 weeks, and 60 Gy in 30 fractions over 6 weeks. A total of 376 patients who were randomized to evaluate these different schedules had stage T1-3, N0-2 non–oat cell lung cancers that were either unresectable or inoperable because of tumor location or the patient's medical status. The survival at 3 years following treatment was higher in patients treated with 60 Gy than in those treated with lower doses. No difference in survival was evident at 5 years, however. A 25% complete response rate was seen with 60-Gy continuous treatment, compared with 23% at 50-Gy course, 18% at 40-Gy continuous course, and 10% at 40-Gy split course (p ≤ 0.04). When the survival of patients was plotted versus their response to therapy at 3 years, the survival rate was 23% in complete responders, 10% in partial responders, and 5% in those who were stable, indicating that complete response is prognostically significant. There was a suggestion of increased complications with the split course technique that were related mainly to an increase in pulmonary fibrosis. Severe or life-threatening complications were more frequent in the split course patients and 60-Gy continuous course patients (approximately 14%) compared with the 40- and 50-Gy continuous irradiation regimen patients.

Considering these randomized, prospective studies collectively (Table 10–2), the only significant difference between treatment regimens appears to be a significantly lower complete response rate in the split course group compared with the other groups in the RTOG 73-01 study and a significant difference in intrathoracic failure rates (33% with 60-Gy continuous course, 42% with 50-Gy continuous course, 44% with 40-Gy split course, and 52% with 40-Gy continuous course at 3 years, p = 0.02). Because of the better control rates with 60-Gy continuous course, it was adopted as the standard schedule in the United States.[70] There is a theoretic disadvantage to split course therapy if it leads to a significant delay in completing the treatment course. Accelerated repopulation of the tumor, which appears to begin after approximately 4 weeks, may decrease the control rates.[71]

In addition to the studies mentioned earlier, a number of retrospective reviews have considered *dose response*, relating radiation dosages to both survival and local control. These are not randomized studies carried out in uniform populations for the purpose of establishing dosages, but they do suggest a dose-response curve with respect to survival and local control. Choi and Doucette[72] reported on a retrospective study of 162 patients with unresectable non–small cell bronchogenic carcinoma who were treated with definitive radiotherapy between 1972 and 1977. Patients were initially treated with 40 to 45 Gy administered in small volumes. Over the course of the study, this dose increased to 60 to 64 Gy administered using a large-volume en bloc approach, including the primary tumor, regional lymphatics, and both supraclavicular areas. The 3-year survival rate for the high-dose (60 to 64 Gy) en bloc approach was 10% versus 3% for the low-dose small-volume group (p < 0.05). The actuarial 5-year survival rate was 7.5% with doses equal to or greater than 50 Gy. None of the patients who were given less than 50 Gy survived 5 years. Local tumor control at 15 months was 76% for high-dose versus 29% for low-dose groups (p < 0.05).

Sherman and colleagues[73] reported on 66 patients with lung cancer who were treated primarily with radiation therapy. This group survived a minimum of 18 months after treatment, and the 5-year actuarial survival rate was 5.6%. Thirteen of these 66 patients failed with locally recurrent disease. The failure rate was higher in those who received lower doses (four of eight who received less than 50 Gy, six of 27 who received 50 to 55 Gy, two of 11 who received 55 to 59 Gy, and one of 20 who received more than 59 Gy). It was believed that six of these 13 local failures might have been eliminated with the use of careful treatment planning and simulation.

These retrospective studies indicate correlations between total dose and tumor response, tumor response and survival (similar to RTOG 73-01), and total dose and survival. The results of radiotherapy alone in unresectable disease remain disappointing. A recent French study incorporating routine post-treatment biopsies revealed a local control rate of only 15% in patients who received 65 Gy in 6½ weeks.[74] Attempts to increase the biologic effect of the treatment have included dose escalation, accelerated fractionation (including concurrent boost technique), hyperfractionation, and the addition of chemotherapy.

Retrospective *dose-escalation studies*[45, 75] using standard fractionation and CT-based treatment planning have established the feasibility of delivering doses up to 70 Gy. Prospective studies to evaluate the potential benefit of dose escalation are under way.[45]

The rationale for *accelerated fractionation* is to deliver a conventional number of dose fractions in a considerably shortened overall treatment time to reduce the opportunity for tumor cell regeneration during treatment.[76] *Hyperfractionation* is defined as the administration of multiple fractions of radiation per day, with each dose lower than usual, whereas the overall treatment time remains about the same. The theoretic advantages include (1) increased redistribution and reoxygenation between fractions, (2) possible lower oxygen enhancement ratio, and (3) decreased late complications in normal tissues.[76, 77]

The RTOG evaluated an *accelerated fractionation* scheme that included a concomitant boost for non–SCLC in a Phase I and II trial (RTOG 84-07).[78] A total of 355 patients were studied. In addition to the standard fields, which receive 50.4 Gy in 5½ weeks, there was a concomitant boost to the volume of gross disease of 1.8 Gy × 11, for a total of 70.2 Gy in 5½ weeks. They concluded that more Phase I and II testing was necessary to define this technique more precisely before considering Phase III testing. Saunders and Dische[79] reported on a series of 62 patients who received 50.4 to 54 Gy in 1.5-Gy fractions given three times a day (6 hours between fractions) for 12 consecutive days as part of an evaluation of continuous, hyperfractionated, accelerated radiotherapy (CHART). Complete response was noted in 46% of patients, and 34% survived 2 years, a substantial improvement over their historical control (p = 0.004). A randomized trial of CHART is ongoing.

The RTOG conducted a Phase I/II trial of hyperfractionated radiation therapy for non–SCLC.[80] Patients received 1.2-Gy fractions administered twice daily, with at least 4 hours between fractions. They were randomized to receive minimum total doses of 60.0, 64.8, 69.6, 74.4, and 79.2 Gy. There were no significant differences in the risks of acute or late effects in normal tissues among the 848 patients analyzed in the five arms. Analysis of a subgroup of 350 of the patients (41%) who had excellent performance status (Karnofsky performance status, 70 to 100) and minimal weight loss (less than 6%) revealed that the dose response for survival with 69.6 Gy (median, 13.0 months; 2 years, 29%) was significantly better than those for the lower total doses (p = 0.02). There were no differences in survival rates among the three arms with the highest total doses. Retrospective comparison with results in similar patients treated with 60 Gy over 6 weeks suggested a benefit from hyperfractionated radiation therapy with 69.6 Gy.

Radiotherapy and Chemotherapy

Chemotherapy has been combined with radiotherapy to increase local control and to control systemic micrometastatic disease. The two methods of treatment can be given sequentially, concurrently, or in an alternating fashion. The chemotherapy must demonstrate activity in measurable disease order to potentially benefit patients with occult metastases. Combination chemotherapy alone produces complete and partial responses of approximately 35% each when cisplatin-containing regimens are used in patients with Stage IV non–SCLC[73, 81, 82] and of 44% to 56%[83–86] in Stage III patients. Pisters and colleagues[87] reported a 12% pathologic complete response in patients with locally advanced non–SCLC treated with vindesine (or vinblastine), cisplatin, and mitomycin.

To increase local control, the combination of chemotherapy and irradiation must provide an increased tumor cell response without a corresponding increase in normal tissue toxicity. There is in vitro evidence that cisplatin given after irradiation results in increased tumor cell kill. Possible mechanisms are hypoxic sensitization, inhibition of cellular repair processes, depletion of endogenous radioprotectors, and production of intrastrand and interstrand cross links in DNA.[88] Kanazawa and associates[89] have shown in a mouse model that cisplatin demonstrated the most tumor enhancement with the least enhancement of normal tissue reaction when given daily with irradiation, suggesting that this may be the optimal schedule for an improved therapeutic ratio.[90]

There have been a number of randomized, prospective studies that have compared chemotherapy plus irradiation with irradiation alone for the treatment of non–SCLC (Tables 10–3 and 10–4). Considerable variation in treatment parameters exists, however, making firm conclusions as to the optimal combination tenuous at this time.[91]

Three of the trials using a sequential approach have produced a significant increase in survival (see Table 10–3). The Cancer and Leukemia Group B (CALGB) trial reported by Dillman and colleagues[92, 93] used cisplatin and vinblastine before 60 Gy in 6 weeks in a favorable population of patients with Stage III disease who had a performance status of 0 or 1 and minimal weight loss, and results showed a 4-month increase in median survival and a doubling of 2- and 5-year survival rates. The French multicenter trial reported by LeChevalier and colleagues[74, 94] compared 65 Gy in 6.5 weeks to induction therapy with three cycles of vindesine, cyclophosphamide, cisplatin, and lomustine (VCPC), followed by 65 Gy in 6.5 weeks and three more cycles of VCPC. With a median follow-up of 5 years, there is a significant increase in survival (p < 0.02) with the combined treatment. Bronchoscopy following treatment revealed only 15% and 17% histologic control rates, respectively. There was a significant reduction in distant metastases at 1 year from 67% to 45% with chemotherapy (p < 0.002). The preliminary results of a three-armed intergroup trial comparing hyperfractionated radiotherapy (69.6 Gy at

TABLE 10–3. Selected Randomized Studies of Sequential Chemotherapy and Radiotherapy for Locally Advanced Non–Small Cell Lung Cancer

STUDY	NO. OF PATIENTS	CHEMOTHERAPY*	RT (Gy/wk)†	SURVIVAL Median (mo)	2 Yr	5 Yr	p
Dillman et al[92, 93]	78	P/Vbl	60/6	13.7	26%	19%	0.01
	77	—	60/6	9.6	13%	7%	—
LeChevalier et al[74, 94]	176	VCPC	65/6.5	12	21%	12%	0.02
	177	—	65/6.5	10	14%	4%	—
Mattson et al[97]	119	CAP	55/7 (SC)	11	19%	—	NS
	119	—	55/7 (SC)	10.4	17%	—	—
Morton et al[98]	55	MACC	60/6	10.5	21%	5%	NS
	54	—	60/6	9.7	16%	7%	—
Mira et al[99]	109	FOMi/CAP	58/6	9.1	—	—	NS
	117	—	58/6	9.2	—	—	—
Trovo et al[100]	49	CAMP‡	45/3	10	16%	—	NS
	62	—	45/3	11.7	19%	—	—
Crino et al[101]	33	PE	56/NR	14	30%	10%	0.056
	33	—	56/NR	9	14%	0%	—
Sause et al[95]		P/Vbl	60/6	13.8	—	—	0.03
	452 total	—	69.6/5.8§	12.3	—	—	NS
		—	60/6	11.4	—	—	NS

P/Vbl = cisplatin, vinblastine, VCPC = vindesine, cyclophosphamide, cisplatin, CCNU, CAP = cyclophosphamide, Adriamycin, cisplatin, MACC = methotrexate, Adriamycin, cyclophosphamide, CCNU, FOMi/CAP = 5-FU, vincristine, mitomycin c/cyclophosphamide, Adriamycin, cisplatin, CAMP = cyclophosphamide, Adriamycin, methotrexate, procarbazine, PE = cisplatin, etoposide, * = given before RT unless specified otherwise, † = continuous unless specified otherwise, ‡ = given after RT, SC = split course, § = hyperfractionated, NR = not reported.

1.2 Gy BID), standard fraction radiotherapy (60 Gy in 6 weeks), and induction chemotherapy with cisplatin and vinblastine before 60 Gy in 6 weeks indicate a statistically significant increase (p = 0.03) in median survival in the combined modality arm.[95]

A number of studies have compared concurrent chemotherapy and radiotherapy (Table 10–4). The European Organization for Research and Treatment for Cancer (EORTC) compared the 55-Gy split course regimen with the 55-Gy split course regimen combined with either daily or weekly cisplatin in a three-armed study.[96] They reported an increased survival rate for the group receiving daily cisplatin plus radiotherapy compared with the group receiving radiotherapy alone (3-year survival, 16% versus 2%, respectively; p = 0.009). There was no difference in survival between the group receiving weekly cisplatin plus radiotherapy (3-year survival rate, 13%) and either of the other groups. Also noted was an increased survival rate without local recurrence in the group receiving daily cisplatin plus radiotherapy compared with the group receiving radiotherapy alone (p = 0.003), but there was no difference in time to distant metastasis, which is in contrast to the reports of LeChevalier and colleagues,[74, 93] who used sequential therapy. Other randomized trials of sequential or concurrent chemotherapy plus radiotherapy have not achieved statistical significance.[53, 97–104]

Alternating regimens have been suggested in the attempt to maximize the advantages of sequential and concurrent treatment and minimize toxicity by temporal separation of delivery of chemotherapy and radiotherapy.[105] There is a theoretic advantage to using radiotherapy initially to induce significant tumor regression and deplete the population of cells that might be resistant to the chemotherapy.[106, 107] To date,

TABLE 10–4. Selected Randomized Studies of Concurrent Chemotherapy and Radiotherapy for Locally Advanced Non–Small Cell Lung Cancer

STUDY	NO. OF PATIENTS	CHEMOTHERAPY*	RT (Gy/wk)*	SURVIVAL Median (mo)	2 Yr	3 Yr	p
Schaake-Koning et al[96]	102	P daily	55/7 SC	NR	26%	16%	0.009
	98	P weekly	55/7 SC	NR	19%	13%	—
	108	—	55/7 SC	NR	13%	2%	—
Johnson et al[53]	87	Vds	60/6	9.4	14%	7%	NS
	87	—	60/6	8.6	13%	5%	—
Trovo et al[104]	84	P daily	45/3	10.3	15%	—	NS
	83	—	45/3	10	15%	—	—
Ansari et al[102]	90	P q3wkX3	60/6	8.1	15%	5%	NS
	93	—	60/6	9.5	9%	7%	—
Soresi et al[103]	45	P weeklyX6	50/5.5	16	—	—	NS
	50	—	50/5.5	11	—	—	—

P = cisplatin, Vds = vindesine, * = continuous unless specified otherwise, SC = split course, NR = not reported.

there have been no studies that have demonstrated superiority of this treatment method.

A recent meta-analysis of 22 randomized clinical trials comparing radiotherapy with radiotherapy and chemotherapy, including 3033 patients (11 trials used platinum-based regimens, and five used long-term alkylating agents), was performed by the NSCLC Collaborators Group.[108] Trials using chemotherapy as a radiosensitizer were excluded. The hazard ratio was 0.91 when chemotherapy was used, with an estimated survival benefit at 2 years of 3% (p = 0.01). For cisplatin regimens, the hazard ratio was 0.87, or a benefit of 4% at 2 years. The addition of alkylating agents gave a hazard ratio of 1.02. The statistical significance of this analysis and the evidence from several of the individual randomized studies mentioned earlier indicate that it is possible to achieve a modest increase in the survival of patients with locally advanced non–SCLC by combining chemotherapy with radiotherapy. The optimal combination of chemotherapy agents and delivery schedules and the optimal dose and schedule of irradiation have not been determined.[91]

Endobronchial Brachytherapy

Delivery of high doses to the endobronchial component of a lung cancer is possible using radioactive sources placed bronchoscopically, most frequently using high-dose-rate remote afterloading techniques. This technique provides excellent palliation of symptoms caused by endobronchial disease such as hemoptysis (95% to 99,%), dyspnea (88% to 87%), cough (79% to 85%), and postobstructive pneumonia (88% to 99%).[109, 110] The relief of obstruction obtained allows volume sparing when endobronchial brachytherapy is used with external beam radiotherapy.[77] The parameters of treatment have varied significantly in the reported series.[111] Speiser and Spratling, who reported the largest series of patients treated with high-dose-rate brachytherapy,[110] recommend 7.5 Gy measured at 1 cm for three fractions given once a week for patients with recurrent disease. Complications include radiation bronchitis and stenosis (11%)[112] and fatal hemoptysis (7% in the report by Speiser and Spratling,[110] up to 32% in the series reported by Bedwinek et al[113]). The effect on survival in patients with potentially curable, localized non–SCLC must await randomized clinical trials.[114]

Hypoxic Cell Sensitizers

Hypoxic cells, which are resistant to radiation, undoubtedly exist in all lung cancers.[115] Attempts have been made to develop drugs that would replace oxygen in these hypoxic tumors. Misonidazole has been used in five randomized trials containing a total of 345 patients.[116–120] None of these studies demonstrated a benefit regarding palliation, tumor control, or survival. Because of the neurotoxicity of misonidazole, the dose is limited, and so far, the sensitizing efficiency has been small.[121] Newer sensitizers that may have less neurotoxicity may provide increased sensitization.[29]

Neutron Therapy

Efforts to overcome the resistance to radiation shown by the hypoxic cells that are present in most cancers have included high linear energy transfer radiation, such as a neutron beam, which is not as dependent on oxygen to produce a biologic effect.[122] Laramore and colleagues[123] reported on 102 patients in a randomized comparison of fast neutron radiotherapy versus mixed beam (neutron/photon) radiotherapy versus conventional radiotherapy. Patients had medically or technically inoperable non–SCLC. Patients received a dose equal to 60 Gy in each arm. There were no differences in local response rates or survival among the three arms of the study. Complications were higher in the fast neutron and the mixed beam arms, which included four patients with radiation myelitis. A prospective, multicenter, randomized study that compared fast neutron radiation therapy with conventional photon radiotherapy for patients with inoperable non–SCLC was reported by Koh and colleagues.[124] A total of 193 eligible patients (99 on the neutron arm and 94 on the photon arm) were randomized to receive 20.4 Gy in 12 fractions with neutrons versus 66 Gy in 33 fractions with photons. At a minimum follow-up of 16 months, no difference in overall survival was observed; however, for patients with squamous cell histology, there was a statistically significant improvement in survival (p = 0.02). There was a trend toward improved survival for those with favorable prognostic factors (i.e., patients who were not T4N3; had no pleural effusion; and had weight loss of less than 5% from baseline) (p = 0.15), favoring the neutron-treated group. With the exception of skin and subcutaneous changes, acute and late toxicity was similar in both arms of the study.

Hyperthermia

At this point there is no reproducible method of uniformly heating normal tissue and monitoring tumor temperatures in the thorax with regional techniques.[29] Systemic hyperthermia can produce temperatures in the range of 40°C to 42°C and is being evaluated in a pilot study combined with radiotherapy.[125]

Intraoperative Radiotherapy

Intraoperative radiotherapy with an electron beam has been evaluated by several investigators clinically[126–129] and in the laboratory setting.[130] The experience with intraoperative radiotherapy is too limited at this time to draw conclusions about its usefulness in combination with or instead of more conventional therapy.

Interstitial Radiation

It is possible to deliver a higher dose of irradiation to a tumor with either permanent or temporary interstitial sources of radiation than with an external beam. Hilaris and colleagues[131] reported on 318 patients with Stage III non–SCLC who underwent thoracotomy. One-third of the patients (100) were treated with a multimodality approach that consisted of resection and/or intraoperative brachytherapy followed by external radiation. These patients had either residual gross disease (47%) or close resection margins that were suspicious for involvement (53%). The mediastinum was treated with an iridium-192 implant for subclinical disease and a permanent iodine-125 implant if gross residual disease was present. All patients received postoperative external beam radiation of 30 to 40 Gy in 2 to 4 weeks. The local control rates were 53% and 89%, respectively, in those who had complete resections with and without tumor at the margins. When residual gross disease was present after thoracotomy, the local control rate was 72%. The 5-year survival rate was 30% in patients who had all gross disease removed and 13% in those who did not. This is a nonrandomized study containing two different populations of patients. The survival rate in the resected group is similar to that in published reports for patients who have had resections with postoperative radiation.[132–134] The 13% survival rate in patients with residual gross disease who received interstitial radiation is similar to the survival rate in patients with high performance status who have had unresectable non–small cell cancer treated with high-dose continuous radiation.[62] More experience is needed with this technique to establish its role in the management of this disease.

Hypofractionation

A reduced number of large-sized fractions (hypofractionation) has been used by some authors for patients with unresectable non–SCLC with the main aim of "convenience." Deely[135] compared the use of two fractions per week with the use of five and found no difference in survival, and Slawson and colleagues[136] reported on 120 patients with advanced locoregional lung cancer and compared the use of 5 Gy once a week for 12 weeks (60 Gy) with the use of 60 Gy in 30 fractions in 6 weeks. The complete response rates were similar (26% and 17%, respectively), as were the survival rates at 2 years (29% and 23%). No difference in late toxicity was noted. Increased late toxicity has been reported, however, by Pirtoli and colleagues,[137] who treated 86 patients with weekly fractions of 8.8, 5.5, and 7 Gy to total doses of 44 to 42 Gy. They reported severe late effects in the soft tissues of the chest wall (40%) and lungs (55.5%). Because of the possibility of increased toxicity, care must be exercised when using hypofractionation for locally advanced disease.

Partial Resection and Positive Margins

To study the value of partial resection before irradiation, Guttman[138] compared the 28% 2-year survival rate of 95 patients who had radiotherapy after biopsy only with the 11% 2-year survival rate of historical control subjects who had partial resection, and she concluded that partial resection was detrimental. In contrast, Caldwell and Bagshaw[22] reported a 29% 2-year survival rate (seven of 24) in patients who underwent partial resection followed by radical radiotherapy compared with 17% (12 of 69) in those who had biopsy only followed by radiotherapy. It does not appear that partial resection provides an advantage over biopsy alone before radical irradiation.[139] There have been no randomized, prospective trials to evaluate the benefit of postoperative radiotherapy in patients who have positive margins of resection. Although there have been reports of long-term survivors without further treatment among these patients, it is reasonable to consider radiotherapy the standard treatment in this situation.[12]

Complications of Radiotherapy

Because the esophagus is usually included in the treatment volume, many patients (50%)[16] experience a transient esophagitis, beginning after 2 weeks of therapy, lasting until 1 to 2 weeks after therapy is completed, and then subsiding. Radiation pneumonitis is present radiographically in almost all patients receiving radiotherapy for lung cancer. Hellman and colleagues[140] reported a 100% radiographic incidence but only a 5% clinical incidence of radiation pneumonitis in patients with lung cancer who were receiving radiotherapy. Severity of the symptoms associated with acute radiation pneumonitis depends on the volume of lung that is irradiated. Initially, a dry cough, dyspnea, a sense of chest fullness, and mild fever may be present. Symptoms may subside if a small volume is involved. If the reaction involves a larger volume, the cough may be productive of thick, white or orange-red to pink sputum (the color is uniformly distributed, unlike the color of the sputum in hemoptysis due to carcinoma), and progressive symptoms of fever, respiratory distress, cor pulmonale, and even death may result.[141]

The differential diagnosis includes viral or bacterial infectious pneumonitis, recurrent cancer, lymphangitic spread, or metastases.[141] Careful review of the chest films and radiation portals is necessary to determine whether the involved portion of lung was in the treatment volume (see Fig. 10–2C). Radiographically, a diffuse haziness appears in the treated lung in 7 to 10 days, coalescing to form patchy infiltrates. Over time, there is gradual consolidation of the irradiated region, with subsequent loss of lung volume[142] (see Fig. 10–2D). The combination of radiotherapy and radiosensitizing drugs, such as doxorubicin and actinomycin D, can increase the risk of pulmonary injury and must be used with caution.

Although radiation therapy that includes the heart can produce acute pericarditis, this is usually noted when massive tumors around the heart are treated. Delayed pericarditis with or without pericardial effusion is the most common reaction reported and usually resolves spontaneously.[143] Pancarditis and myocarditis have been reported with radiotherapy to the mediastinum[144] and are directly related to the volume of heart included in the radiation portals.[145] Lawson and colleagues[146] reported a 4% incidence when half of the heart volume received 45 to 50 Gy in 4 to 5 weeks. It is possible, however, that this figure underestimates the true incidence of pericarditis, because subclinical effusions may go undetected and spontaneously resolve and therefore will not be included in these statistics.[145] Acute effects included transient symptomless decrease in left ventricular function that resolved within 6 months and slight pericardial effusion in one-third of patients with breast cancer treated with an internal mammary field.[147]

The most devastating complication is radiation myelitis. Doses of 1.8 to 2 Gy per day administered to the spinal cord in 5 weeks of continuous radiation are considered safe.[148, 149] Because the incidence of neural injury increases substantially with increasing fraction size,[150, 151] the dose to the spinal cord must be minimized if large fractions are used. Dorfman and colleagues have reported on spinal somatosensory conduction velocity in patients who received therapeutic radiation to the spinal cord in the range of 20 to 43.8 Gy.[152] The velocity was significantly slower in the patients treated with radiation than in controls, suggesting that radiotherapy may produce some clinical spinal cord dysfunction, even at conventional dosage schedules.

Palliation of Symptoms

Slawson and Scott[153] reviewed 330 patients with lung cancer who had definite symptoms that could be evaluated at the time of radiotherapy. There was relief of hemoptysis in 84% (95 of 113), relief of chest pain in 61% (66 of 108), relief of superior vena cava syndrome in 86% (36 of 42), and relief of dyspnea in 60% (51 of 85), Vocal cord paralysis was relieved in only 6% (three of 54 patients), and atelectasis was relieved in 15% (three of 20) of patients with squamous cell carcinoma and 57% (four of 7) of patients with oat cell carcinoma. Overall, 61% (290 of 476) of symptoms were relieved. These response rates have been confirmed by others (Table 10–5).[154, 155]

FUTURE CONSIDERATIONS

There are newer chemotherapy agents, such as taxol, which may lead to accumulation of cells in the radio-

TABLE 10–5. Palliation of Symptoms in Patients Following Radiotherapy[81–83]

SYMPTOM	PERCENTAGE*
Hemoptysis	84 to 95
Chest pain	61 to 72
Dyspnea	60
Atelectasis	
SCLC	57
Non-SCLC	15

*Percentage of patients experiencing palliation.
SCLC = small cell lung cancer, non–SCLC = non–small cell lung cancer.

sensitive G2/M phase of cell division,[156] and topotecan, a topoisomerase I inhibitor that leads to DNA strand breaks that could possibly interact with irradiation.[157] However, further significant advancements must await agents with greater activity both as radiosensitizers (while sparing normal tissues) and as systemic agents to treat occult metastatic disease. Optimal chemotherapy combinations and radiotherapy delivery schedules remain to be defined. The optimal integration of chemotherapy and radiotherapy must await further study.

SUMMARY

Although the long-term survival rates from unresectable or inoperable local or regional non–SCLC remain a formidable therapeutic challenge, a small percentage of patients can be cured and the symptoms of many can be palliated with radiotherapy. Cisplatin-based chemotherapy combined with radiotherapy has produced encouraging results and is considered by many to be the standard treatment for selected patients. It is the responsibility of the physician to determine as carefully as possible, based on prognostic factors and the stage of the disease, the patients who are most likely to benefit, and to determine the most efficient method of delivering the treatment. Radical radiotherapy with or without chemotherapy should be considered for patients with the following characteristics:

- Resectable disease and classification as not suitable for operation for medical reasons.
- Inoperable tumors confined to the lung with ipsilateral hilar and mediastinal nodes.
- Positive margins after resection.
- Postsurgical recurrence involving one hemithorax.

Such radiotherapy is contraindicated when any of the following exists:

- Evidence of distant metastasis.
- Malignant pleural effusion.
- Inadequate pulmonary reserve.
- Uncontrolled pulmonary infection.
- Poor performance status.

The results of radical radiotherapy and the promising results of combined chemotherapy and radiotherapy remain modest, however, and patients should be considered candidates for investigational studies of newer therapeutic agents and fractionation schemes.

SELECTED REFERENCES

Perez CA, Stanley K, Grundy G, et al: Impact of irradiation technique and tumor extent in tumor control and survival of patients with unresectable non-oat cell carcinoma of the lung: Report of the Radiation Therapy Oncology Group. Cancer 50:1091, 1982. *Report of RTOG 73–01 comparing a variety of fractionation schemes.*
Hazuka MBO, Turrisi AT: The evolving role of radiation therapy in the treatment of locally advanced lung cancer. Semin Oncol 20:174, 1993.

Discusses current understanding of the role of radiotherapy in lung cancer alone and in combination with chemotherapy.

Wagner H: Rational integration of radiation and chemotherapy in patients with unresectable stage IIIA or IIIB NSCLC: Results from the Lung Cancer Study Group, Eastern Cooperative Oncology Group, and Radiation Therapy Oncology Group. Chest 103(1 suppl):35, 1993.

Discusses the recent trials from several cooperative groups and the rationale for various methods of integration.

Bleehen N, Cox J: Radiotherapy for lung cancer. Int J Radiat Oncol Biol Phys 11:1001, 1985.

Good discussion of selection factors for radical radiotherapy.

REFERENCES

1. Boring CC, Squires TS, Tong T, et al: Cancer statistics, 1994. CA Cancer J Clin 44:7, 1994.
2. Paulson D: A philosophy of treatment for bronchogenic carcinoma. Ann Thorac Surg 5:289, 1968.
3. LaRoux B: Bronchial carcinoma. Thorax 23:136, 1968.
4. Shields TW, Robinette C: Long term survivors after resection of bronchial carcinoma. Surg Gynecol Obstet, 136:759, 1973.
5. Krant M: The question of irradiation therapy in lung cancer. JAMA 195:177, 1966.
6. Rubin P, Ciccio S, Setisarn B: Controversial status of radiation therapy in lung cancer. *In* Proceedings of the Sixth National Cancer Conference. Philadelphia, JB Lippincott, 1970, p 655.
7. Phillips T, Miller R: Should asymptomatic patients with inoperable bronchogenic carcinoma receive immediate radiotherapy? Yes. Am Rev Respir Dis 117:405, 1975.
8. Brashear R: Should asymptomatic patients with inoperable bronchogenic carcinoma receive immediate radiotherapy? No. Am Rev Respir Dis 117:411, 1978.
9. Cox J, Komaki R, Byhardt R: Is immediate chest radiotherapy obligatory for any or all patients with limited-stage non-small cell carcinoma of the lung? Yes. Cancer Treat Rep 67:327, 1983.
10. Cohen M: Is immediate radiation therapy indicated for patients with unresectable non-small cell cancer? No. Cancer Treat Rep 67:33, 1983.
11. Berry R, Laing A, Newman C, et al: The role of radiotherapy in treatment of inoperable lung cancer. Int J Radiat Oncol Biol Phys 2:433, 1977.
12. Pett SJ, Wernly J, Aki B: Lung Cancer—Current concepts and controversies. West J Med 145:52, 1986.
13. Payne D: Should unresectable stage III patients routinely receive high-dose radiation therapy? J Clin Oncol 6:552, 1988.
14. Ash D: Role of radiotherapy: Recent results. Cancer Res 92:99, 1984.
15. Lee R: Radiotherapy of bronchogenic carcinoma. Semin Oncol 1:245, 1974.
16. Lee R: Radiotherapy for lung cancer. *In* Strauss MJ (ed): Lung Cancer: Clinical Diagnosis and Treatment. New York, Grune & Stratton, 1977, p 163.
17. Weinberg J: The intrathoracic lymphatics. *In* Haagensen C, Feind CR, Herter FP, et al (eds): The Lymphatics in Cancer. Philadelphia, WB Saunders, 1972.
18. Weinberg J: The intrathoracic lymphatics. *In* Haagensen C, Feind CR, Herter FP, et al (eds): The Lymphatics in Cancer. Philadelphia, WB Saunders, 1972, p 231.
19. Deeley T: Radiotherapy for carcinoma of the bronchus. Cancer Treat Rev 1:39, 1974.
20. Komaki R, Cox J, Hartz A, et al: Characteristics of long-term survivors after treatment for inoperable carcinoma of the lung. Am J Clin Oncol (CCT) 5:362, 1985.
21. Stanley K: Prognostic factors for survival in patients with inoperable lung cancer. J Natl Cancer Inst 65:25, 1980.
22. Caldwell W, Bagshaw M: Indications for end results of irradiation for carcinoma of the lung. Cancer 22:99, 1968.
23. Weiss W, Boucot K, Cooper D: Growth rate in the detection and prognosis of bronchogenic carcinoma. JAMA 198:108, 1966.
24. Macchiarini P, Fontanini G, Hardin MJ, et al: Relation of neovascularisation to metastasis of non-small-cell lung cancer. Lancet 340:145, 1992.
25. Zimmerman P, Bint M, Hawson G, et al: Ploidy as a prognostic determinant in surgically treated lung cancer. Lancet 2:530, 1987.
26. Yu J, Shaeffer J, Zhu A, et al: Flow cytometric DNA content and clinical outcome in patients with non-small cell lung cancer given postoperative radiation therapy. Cytometry 14:428, 1993.
27. Peters L, Brock W, Johnson T, et al: Potential methods for predicting tumor radiocurability. Int J Radiat Oncol Biol Phys 12:459, 1986.
28. Russo A, Mitchell J, Kinsella T, et al: Determinants of radiosensitivities. Semin Oncol 12:332, 1985.
29. Bleehen N, Cox J: Radiotherapy for lung cancer. Int J Radiat Oncol Biol Phys 11:1001, 1985.
30. Fulkerson L, Perlmutter G, Zack M, et al: Radiotherapy in chest malignant tumors associated with pulmonary tuberculosis. Radiology 106:645, 1973.
31. LeChevalier T: Do clinical and non-specific biologic data influence staging? Rev Mal Respir 9(suppl 4):R305, 1992.
32. Nielsen M, Heiston D, Dunnick N: Pre-operative CT evaluation of adrenal glands in non-small cell bronchogenic carcinoma. Am J Roentgenol 139:317, 1982.
33. Oliver TJ, Bernardino M, Miller J, et al: Isolated adrenal masses in non-small cell bronchogenic carcinoma. Radiology 153:217, 1984.
34. Newell J: Concepts in CT staging of lung cancer. Appl Radiol 103:108, 1986.
35. Hooper R, Tenholder M, Underwood G, et al: Computed tomographic scanning of the brain in the initial staging of bronchogenic carcinoma. Chest 85:774, 1984.
36. Salvatierra A, Baamonde C, Llamas J, et al: Extrathoracic staging of bronchogenic carcinoma. Chest 97:1052, 1990.
37. Mira J, Potter J, Thorton G, et al: Advantages and limitations of computed tomography scans for treatment planning of cancer. Int J Radiat Oncol Biol Phys 5:1617, 1982.
38. Glatstein E, Lichter AS, Fraass BA, et al: The imaging revolution in radiation oncology: Use of CT, ultrasound, and NMR for localization, treatment planning in treatment delivery. Int J Radiat Oncol Biol Phys 11:299, 1985.
39. Ibbott G: Radiation treatment planning and the distortion of CT images. Med Phys 7:261, 1980.
40. Orton CG, Mondalek PM, Spicka JT, et al: Lung corrections in photon beam treatment planning: Are we ready? Int J Radiat Oncol Biol Phys, 10:291, 1984.
41. van't Riet A, Stam HC, Mak A, et al., Implications of lung corrections for dose specification in radiotherapy. Int J Radiat Oncol Biol Phys 11:621, 1985.
42. Perez CA, Stanley K, Grundy G, et al: Impact of irradiation technique and tumor extent in tumor control and survival of patients with unresectable non-oat cell carcinoma of the lung: Report of the Radiation Therapy Oncology Group. Cancer 50:1091, 1982.
43. Cox J: Current role of radiation therapy for inoperable carcinoma of the lung. *In* Cox JD (ed): A Categorical Course in Radiation Therapy Lung Cancer. New York, Radiologic Society of North America, 1985, p 55.
44. Curran W, Modolfsky P, Solin L: Analysis of the influence of elective nodal irradiation on postirradiation pulmonary function. Cancer 65:2488, 1990.
45. Hazuka M, Turrisi A, Lutz S, et al: Results of high-dose thoracic irradiation incorporating beam's eye view display in non-small cell lung cancer: A retrospective analysis. Int J Radiat Oncol Biol Phys 27:273, 1993.
46. Armstrong J, Minsky B: Radiation therapy for medically inoperable stage I and II non-small cell lung cancer. Cancer Treat Rev 16:247, 1989.
47. Lambert P: Radiation myelopathy of the thoracic spinal cord in long-term survivors treated with radical radiotherapy using conventional fractionation. Cancer 41:1751, 1978.
48. Leddy E, Moersch H: Roentgen therapy for bronchiogenic carcinoma. JAMA 115:2239, 1940.
49. Smart J, Hilton G: Radiotherapy of cancer of the lung: Results in a selective group of cases. Lancet 1:880, 1956.
50. Morrison R, Deeley TJ, Cleland W: The treatment of carcinoma of the bronchus: A clinical trial to compare surgery and supervoltage radiotherapy. Lancet 1:683, 1963.

51. Roswit B, Patno ME, Rapp R, et al: The survival of patients with inoperable lung cancer: A large scale randomized study of radiation versus placebo. Radiology 90:688, 1968.

52. Niederle N, Alberti W, Stuschke M, et al: Prospective randomized study comparing immediate radiotherapy (RT), chemoplus radiotherapy (CT + RT) or delayed radiotherapy in limited disease non-small cell lung cancer (abstract). Proc Am Soc Clin Oncol 7:214, 1988.

53. Johnson DH, Einhorn LH, Bartolucci A, et al: Thoracic radiotherapy does not prolong survival in patients with locally advanced, unresectable non-small cell lung cancer. Ann Intern Med 113:33, 1990.

54. Kubota K, Furuse K, Kawahara M, et al: Randomized trial of chemotherapy with or without thoracic radiation therapy for treatment of local advanced non-small cell lung cancer. Proc Am Soc Clin Oncol 9:226, 1990.

55. Haffty BG, Goldberg MB, Gerstley J, et al: Results of radical radiation therapy in clinical stage I technically operable non-small cell lung cancer. Int J Radiat Oncol Biol Phys 15:69, 1988.

56. Noordijk EM, Clement E, Hermans J, et al: Radiotherapy as an alternative to surgery in elderly patients with resectable lung cancer. Radiother Oncol 13:83, 1988.

57. Zhang HX, Yin WB, Zhang LJ, et al: Curative radiotherapy of early operable non-small cell lung cancer. Radiother Oncol 14:89, 1989.

58. Talton B, Constable W, Kersh C: Curative radiotherapy in non-small cell carcinoma of the lung. Int J Radiat Oncol Biol Phys 19:1521, 1990.

59. Dosoretz DE, Katin M, Blitzer P, et al: Radiation therapy in the management of medically inoperable carcinoma of the lung: Results and implications for future treatment strategies. Int J Radiat Oncol Biol Phys 24:3, 1992.

60. Rosenthal SA, Curran W, Herbert S, et al: Clinical stage II non-small cell lung cancer treated with radiation therapy alone: The significance of clinically staged ipsilateral hilar adenopathy (N1 disease). Cancer 70:2410, 1992.

61. Sandler HM, Curran WJ, Turrisi A: The influence of tumor size and pre-treatment staging on outcome following radiation therapy alone for stage I non-small cell lung cancer. Int J Radiat Oncol Biol Phys 19:9, 1990.

62. Cox JD, Komaki R, Eisert DR: Irradiation for inoperable carcinoma of the lung and high performance status. JAMA 244:1931, 1980.

63. Perez C: Non-small cell carcinoma of the lung: Dose-time parameters. Cancer Treat Symp 2:131, 1985.

64. Scanlon P: The effect of mitotic suppression and recovery. Am J Roentgenol Rad Ther Nucl Med 81:433, 1955.

65. Holsti L: Clinical experience with split course radiotherapy: A randomized clinical trial. Radiology 92:591, 1969.

66. Levitt SH, Bogardus CR, Ladd G: Split dose intensive radiation therapy in the treatment of advanced lung cancer: A randomized study. Radiology 88:1159, 1967.

67. Lee RE, Carr DT, Childs D: Comparison of split course radiation therapy and continuous radiation therapy for unresectable bronchogenic carcinoma: Five year results. Am J Roentgenol Rad Ther Nucl Med 126:116, 1976.

68. Kjaer M: Radiotherapy of squamous, adeno- and large cell carcinoma of the lung. Cancer Treat Rev 9:1, 1982.

69. Holsti LR, Mattson K: A randomized study of split course radiotherapy of lung cancer: Long-term results. Int J Radiat Oncol Biol Phys 6:977, 1980.

70. Hazuka MB, Turrisi AT: The evolving role of radiation therapy in the treatment of locally advanced lung cancer. Semin Oncol 20:174, 1993.

71. Withers R: Treatment-induced accelerated human tumor growth. Semin Radiat Oncol 3:135, 1993.

72. Choi N, Doucette J: Improved survival of patients with unresectable non-small cell bronchogenic carcinoma by an innovative high-dose en bloc radiotherapeutic approach. Cancer 48:101, 1981.

73. Sherman OW, Weichselbaum R, Hellman S: The characteristics of long-term survivors of lung cancer treated with radiation. Cancer 47:2575, 1981.

74. LeChevalier T, Arriagada R, Quoix E, et al: Significant effect of adjuvant chemotherapy on survival in locally advanced non-small cell lung cancer. J Natl Cancer Inst 84:58, 1992.

75. Emami B, Graham M, Lockett M: High dose thoracic irradiation (RT) using computed tomography (CT)-based treatment planning and beam's eye view (BEV) display in non-small cell lung cancer (NSCLC): Patients with good prognostic factors. Lung Cancer 7:89, 1991.

76. Thames HD, Peters LJ, Withers HR, et al: Accelerated fractionation versus hyperfractionation: rationales for several treatments per day. Int J Radiat Oncol Biol Phys 9:127, 1983.

77. Bastin K, Mehta M, Kinsella T: Thoracic volume radiation sparing following endobronchial brachytherapy: A quantitative analysis. Int J Radiat Oncol Biol Phys 25:703, 1993.

78. Byhardt R, Pajak T, Emami B, et al: A phase I/II study to evaluate accelerated fractionation via concomitant boost for squamous, adeno, and large cell carcinoma of the lung: Report of Radiation Therapy Oncology Group 84-07. Int J Radiat Oncol Biol Phys 26:459, 1993.

79. Saunders M, Dische S: Continuous, hyperfractionated, accelerated radiotherapy (CHART) in non-small cell carcinoma of the bronchus. Int J Radiat Oncol Biol Phys 19:1211, 1990.

80. Cox JD, Azarnia N, Byhart RW, et al: A randomized phase I/II trial of hyperfractionated radiation therapy with total doses of 60.0 Gy to 79.2 Gy: Possible survival benefit with ≥69.6 Gy in favorable patients with Radiation Therapy Oncology Group stage III non-small-cell lung carcinoma: Report of Radiation Therapy Oncology Group 83-11. J Clin Oncol 8:1543, 1990.

81. Greco F: Rationale for chemotherapy for patients with advanced non-small cell lung cancer. Semin Oncol 13:92, 1986.

82. Wagner H, Ruckdeschel J, Bonomi P, et al: Treatment of locally advanced non-small cell lung cancer (NSCLC) with mitomycin-C, vinblastine and cis-DDP (MVP) followed by radiation therapy (RT): ECOG Pilot Study. Proc Am Soc Clin Oncol 4:183, 1985.

83. Bonomi P, Rowland K, Taylor SG, et al: Phase II trial of etoposide, cisplatin, continuous infusion 5-fluorouracil, and simultaneous split-course radiation therapy in stage III non-small cell bronchogenic carcinoma. Semin Oncol 13:115, 1986.

84. Longeval E, Klastersky J: Combination chemotherapy with cisplatin and etoposide in bronchogenic squamous cell carcinoma and adenocarcinoma. Cancer 50:2751, 1982.

85. Fram R, Skarin A, Balikian J, et al: Combination chemotherapy followed by radiation therapy in patients with regional stage III unresectable non-small cell cancer. Cancer Treat Rep 69:557, 1985.

86. Osoba D, Rusthoven JJ, Evans WK, et al: Combined chemotherapy and radiation therapy for non-small cell lung cancer. Semin Oncol 13:121, 1986.

87. Pisters K, Kris M, Gralla R, et al: Pathologic complete response in advanced non-small-cell lung cancer following preoperative chemotherapy: Implications for the design of future non-small-cell lung cancer combined modality trials. J Clin Oncol 11:1757, 1993.

88. Cox JD, Samson MK, Herskovic AM, et al: Cisplatin and etoposide before definitive radiation therapy for inoperable squamous carcinoma, adenocarcinoma, and large cell carcinoma of the lung: A phase I-II study of the Radiation Therapy Oncology Group. Cancer Treat Rep 70:1219, 1986.

89. Kanazawa H, Rappacchietta D, Kallman R: Schedule-dependent therapeutic gain from the combination of fractionated irradiation and cis-diaminedichloroplatinum (II) in C3H/Km mouse model systems. Cancer Res 48:3158, 1988.

90. Bonomi P: Radiation and simultaneous cisplatin in non-small cell lung cancer. Int J Radiat Oncol Biol Phys 27:739, 1993.

91. Sause W: Chemotherapy and radiation therapy for lung cancer. Semin Thor Cardiovasc Surg 5:268, 1993.

92. Dillman RO, Seagren S, Propert K, et al: A randomized trial of induction chemotherapy plus high-dose radiation versus radiation alone in stage III non-small-cell lung cancer. N Engl J Med 323:940, 1990.

93. Dillman R, Seagren S, Herndon J, et al: Randomized trial of induction chemotherapy plus radiation therapy vs RT alone in stage III non-small cell lung cancer (NSCLC): Five year follow up of CALGB 84-33. Proc Am Soc Clin Onc 12:329, 1993.

94. LeChevalier T, Arriagada R, Quoix E, et al: Radiotherapy alone versus combined chemotherapy and radiotherapy in nonresectable non-small-cell lung cancer: First analysis of a randomized trial in 353 patients. J Natl Cancer Inst 83:417, 1991.

95. Sause W, Scott C, Taylor S, et al: RTOG 8808 ECOG 4588: Preliminary analysis of a phase III trial in regionally advanced unresectable non-small cell lung cancer. Proc Am Soc Clin Oncol 13:325(A1072), 1994.

96. Schaake-Koning C, Van dan Bogaert W, Dalesio O, et al: Effects of concomitant cisplatin and radiotherapy on inoperable non-small-cell lung cancer. N Engl J Med 326:524, 1992.

97. Mattson K, Holsti L, Holsti P, et al: Inoperable non-small cell lung cancer: Radiation with or without chemotherapy. Eur J Cancer Clin Oncol 24:477, 1988.

98. Morton RF, Jett J, McGinnis WI, et al: Thoracic radiation therapy alone compared with combined chemoradiotherapy for locally unresectable non-small cell lung cancer. Ann Intern Med 115:681, 1991.

99. Mira J, Miller T, Crowley J: Chest irradiation (RT) vs chest RT + chemotherapy ± prophylactic brain RT in localized non small cell lung cancer: A Southwest Oncology Group randomized study. Proc ASTRO 19:145, 1990.

100. Trovo M, Minatel E, Veronesi A, et al: Combined radiotherapy and chemotherapy versus radiotherapy alone in locally advanced epidermoid bronchogenic carcinoma: A randomized study. Cancer 65:400, 1990.

101. Crino L, Meacci M, Corgna E, et al: Long-term results in locally advanced inoperable non-small cell lung cancer (NSCLC): A randomized trial of induction chemotherapy (CT) plus radiotherapy (RT) vs radiation alone (abstract). Lung Cancer 7:161, 1991.

102. Ansari R, Tokara R, Fisher W, et al: A phase III study of thoracic irradiation with and without concomitant cisplatin in locally advanced unresectable non-small cell lung cancer: A Hoosier Oncology Group study. Proc Am Soc Clin Oncol 10:241, 1991.

103. Soresi E, Clerici M, Grilli R, et al: A randomized clinical trial comparing radiation therapy versus radiation therapy plus cis-dichlorodiamine platinum in the treatment of locally advanced non-small cell lung cancer. Semin Oncol 15(suppl 7):20, 1988.

104. Trovo M, Minatel E, Franchin G, et al: Radiotherapy versus radiotherapy inhanced by cisplatin in stage III non-small cell lung cancer. Int J Radiat Oncol Biol Phys 24:11, 1992.

105. Looney W, Hopkins H: Rationale for different chemotherapeutic and radiation therapy strategies in cancer management. Cancer 67:1471, 1991.

106. Looney NB, Goldie J, Little JB, et al: Alternation of chemotherapy and radiotherapy in cancer management. I. Summary of the Division of Cancer Treatment Workshop. Cancer Treat Rep 69:769, 1985.

107. Goldie JH, Coldman AJ, Hopkins HA, et al: Experimental and theoretical basis for the concept of alternating chemotherapy and radiotherapy. Int J Radiat Oncol Biol Phys 10:148, 1984.

108. Pignon J-P, Stewart LA, Souhami RL, et al: A meta-analysis using individual patient data from randomized clinical trials (RCTS) of chemotherapy (CT) in non-small cell lung cancer (NSCLC): (2) Survival in the locally advanced (LA) setting. Proc Am Soc Clin Oncol 13:334(A1109), 1994.

109. Cheng LL, Horvath J, Peyton W, et al: High dose rate afterloading intraluminal brachytherapy in malignant airway obstruction of lung cancer. Int J Radiat Oncol Biol Phys 28:589, 1994.

110. Speiser B, Spratling L: Remote afterloading brachytherapy for local control of endobronchial carcinoma. Int J Radiat Oncol Biol Phys 25:579, 1993.

111. Speiser B: High dose rate endobronchial brachytherapy: Whither goest thou? Int J Radiat Oncol Biol Phys 23:249, 1992.

112. Speiser B, Spratling L: Radiation bronchitis and stenosis secondary to high dose rate endobronchial irradiation. Int J Radiat Oncol Biol Phys 25:589, 1993.

113. Bedwinek J, Petty A, Bruton C, et al: The use of high dose rate endobronchial brachytherapy to palliate symptomatic endobronchial recurrence of previously irradiated bronchogenis carcinoma. Int J Radiat Oncol Biol Phys 22:23, 1992.

114. Speiser B: High dose rate brachytherapy of lung cancer: Cure or palliation? Int J Radiat Oncol Biol Phys 28:781, 1994.

115. Thomlinson RH, Gray L: The histologic structure of some human lung cancers and the possible implications for radiotherapy. Br J Cancer 9:539, 1955.

116. Abe M, Oni K, Takahashi M, et al: Clinical studies of misonidazole in Japan. Cancer Treat Symp 1:103, 1983.

117. Basutti L: Clinical trials and preliminary results obtained by Association of Electronaffinic Hypoxic Cell Radiosensizing Drugs (misonidazole and metronidazole) with radiotherapy (telocobalt therapy) for the treatment of some types of neoplastic diseases at a locally advanced stage. In Breccia RC, Adams GE (eds): Advanced Topics on Radiosensitizers of Hypoxic Cells. New York, Plenum Press, 1982, pp 261–268.

118. Mantyla MJ, Nordman EN, Ruotsalainen PJ, et al: Misonidazole and radiotherapy in lung cancer: A randomized double-blind trial. Int J Radiat Oncol Biol Phys 8:1719, 1982.

119. Kjaer M, Panduro J, Hansen H: Misonidazole combined with radiotherapy in the treatment of inoperable squamous cell carcinoma of the lung: A double-blind randomized trial. Proc AACR 22:502, 1981.

120. Saunders MI, Anderson P, Dische S, et al: A controlled clinical trial of misonidazole in the radiotherapy of patients with carcinoma of the bronchus. Int J Radiat Oncol Biol Phys 8:347, 1982.

121. Dische S: A review of hypoxic cell radiosensitization. Int J Radiat Oncol Biol Phys 20:147, 1991.

122. Withers H: Biological basis for high LET radiotherapy. Radiology 105:131, 1973.

123. Laramore GE, Bauer M, Griffin TW, et al: Fast neutron and mixed beam radiotherapy for inoperable non-small cell carcinoma of the lung: Results of an RTOG randomized study. Am J Clin Oncol 9:233, 1986.

124. Koh W-J, Krall J, Peters L, et al: Neutron vs photon radiation therapy for inoperable regional non-small cell lung cancer: Results of a multicenter randomized trial. Int J Radiat Oncol Biol Phys 27:499, 1993.

125. Robbins HI, Hugander A, Steeves R, et al: Radiotherapy and hyperthermia for lung cancer. Int J Radiat Oncol Bioi Phys 12:147, 1986.

126. Abe M, Takehishi M, Yabumoto E, et al: Clinical experiences with intraoperative radiotherapy of locally advanced cancers. Cancer 45:40, 1980.

127. Calvo FA, Ortiz de Urbina D, Abuchaibe O, et al: Intraoperative radiotherapy during lung cancer surgery: Technical description and early clinical results. Int J Radiat Oncol Biol Phys 19:103, 1990.

128. Juettner F, Arian Schad K, Porsch G, et al: Intraoperative radiation therapy combined with external irradiation in non-resectable non-small cell lung cancer: Preliminary report. Int J Radiat Oncol Biol Phys 18:1143, 1990.

129. Pass HI, Sindelar WF, Kinsella TJ, et al: Delivery of intraoperative radiation therapy after pneumonectomy: Experimental observations and early clinical results. Ann Thorac Surg 44:14, 1987.

130. Tochner ZA, Pass HI, Sindelar WF, et al: Long term tolerance of thoracic organs to intraoperative radiotherapy. Int J Radiat Oncol Biol Phys 22:65, 1992.

131. Hilaris BS, Gomez J, Nori D, et al: Combined surgery, intraoperative brachytherapy, and postoperative external radiation in stage III non-small cell lung cancer. Cancer 55:1221, 1985.

132. Kirsh MM, Rotman H, Argenta L, et al: Carcinoma of the lung: Results of treatment over ten years. Ann Thorac Surg 21:371, 1976.

133. Green N, Kurohara SS, George FW, et al: Post resection irradiation for primary lung cancer. Radiology 116:405, 1975.

134. Choi N, Grillo NC, Gardiello M, et al: Basis for new strategies in postoperative radiotherapy of bronchogenic carcinoma. Int I Radiat Oncol Bioi Phys 6:31, 1980.

135. Deely T: The Chest: Monographs in Oncology. London, Butterworth, 1973.

136. Slawson R, Salazar O, Poussin-Rosillo H, et al: Once-a-week vs conventional daily radiation treatment for lung cancer: Final report. Int J Radiat Oncol Biol Phys 15:61, 1988.

137. Pirtoli L, Bindi M, Belezza A, et al: Unfavorable experience with hypofractionated radiotherapy in unresectable lung cancer. Tumori 78:305, 1992.

138. Guttman R: Results of radiation therapy in patients with inoperable carcinoma of the lung whose status was established at exploratory thoracotomy. Am J Roentgenol Rad Ther Nucl Med 93:99, 1965.

139. Gregor A: Radiotherapy for inoperable non-small cell carcinoma of the bronchus. In Smythe JF (ed): The Management of Lung Cancer. London, Arnold, 1984, p 91.

140. Hellman S, Kligerman MM, von EC, et al: Sequelae of radical radiotherapy of carcinoma of the lung. Radiology 82:1055, 1964.
141. Roswit B, White D: Severe radiation injuries of the lung. Am J Roentgenol 129:127, 1977.
142. Libshitz HI, Southard M: Complications of radiation therapy: The thorax. Semin Roentgenol 9:41, 1974.
143. Stewart J, Fajardo L: Radiation-induced heart disease: An update. Prog Cardiovasc Dis 27:173, 1984.
144. Fajardo LP, Stewart JR, Cohn K: Morphology of radiation induced heart disease. Arch Pathol 86:512, 1968.
145. Ruckdeschel JC, Chang P, Au M, et al: Radiation related pericardial effusions in patients with Hodgkin's disease. Medicine 54:245, 1975.
146. Lawson R, Ross WM, Gold RJ, et al: Post radiation pericarditis: Report on four more cases with special reference to bronchogenic carcinoma. J Thorac Cardiovasc Surg 63:841, 1972.
147. Ikaheimo M, Niemela K, Linnaluoto M, et al: Early cardiac changes related to radiation therapy. Am J Cardiol 56:943, 1985.
148. Phillips TL, Buschke F: Radiation tolerance of the thoracic spinal cord. Am J Roentgenol 105:59, 1969.
149. Wara WM, Phillips TL, Sheline GE, et al: Radiation tolerance of the spinal cord. Cancer 35:1558, 1975.
150. Hatlevoll R, Host H, Kaalhus O: Myelopathology following radiotherapy of bronchial carcinoma with large single fractions: A retrospective study. Int J Radiat Oncol Biol Phys 9:41, 1983.
151. Dische S, Martin W, Anderson P: Radiation myelopathy in patients treated for carcinoma of bronchus using a six fraction regimen of radiotherapy. Br J Radiol 54:29, 1981.
152. Dorfman LJ, Donaldson SS, Gupta PR, et al: Electrophysiologic evidence of subclinical injury to the posterior columns of the human spinal cord after therapeutic radiation. Cancer 50:2515, 1982.
153. Slawson RG, Scott R: Radiation therapy in bronchogenic carcinoma. Radiology 132:175, 1979.
154. Line D, Deeley T: Palliative therapy. *In* Deeley TJ (ed): Carcinoma of the Bronchus. New York, Appleton-Century-Crofts, 1972, p 298.
155. Mantell B: Superior sulcus pancoast tumours: Results of radiotherapy. Br J Dis Chest 67:315, 1973.
156. Tishler R, Schiff P, Geard C, et al: Taxol: A novel radiation sensitizer. Int J Radiat Oncol Biol Phys 22:613, 1992.
157. Wagner H: Rational integration of radiation and chemotherapy in patients with unresectable stage IIIA or IIIB NSCLC: Results from the Lung Cancer Study Group, Eastern Cooperative Oncology Group, and Radiation Therapy Oncology Group. Chest 103(1 suppl):35, 1993.

11 MANAGEMENT OF DISSEMINATED NON–SMALL CELL LUNG CANCER

Charles C. Williams, Jr., and John C. Ruckdeschel

OVERVIEW

The treatment of disseminated non–small cell lung cancer (SCLC) will continue to be a therapeutic problem for many years. In developed societies, it is the most lethal malignancy of adult men and women. It is estimated that there will be 94,000 and 59,000 deaths in men and women, respectively, from this disease in 1994 in the United States alone.[1] Only 13% of all persons with lung cancer will survive 5 or more yr.[2]

Non–SCLC is a heterogeneous entity that accounts for the majority of patients with lung cancer. One-third of these patients have true early-stage disease, which is confined to the thorax, for which surgery is the treatment of choice.[2-5] Adjuvant therapy for resected patients at high risk of relapse and combined-modality therapy for selected patients with advanced locoregional disease are discussed elsewhere in this text.

Most patients with non–SCLC present with a disseminated process. From 40% to 50% of all patients present initially with metastases, and relapses are common in early-stage patients believed to be cured by a local therapy.[3, 6] Systemic management therefore is the only therapeutically reasonable strategy for most patients. Nevertheless, chemotherapy for metastatic non–SCLC should be put into proper perspective for the individual patient given the marginal benefits for those treated with currently available agents.[7, 8]

Non–SCLC is distinctive from SCLC on morphologic and biologic grounds.[9, 10] Typically, non–SCLC is relatively resistant to chemotherapy and radiation compared with SCLC; there is, however, overlap of their biologic properties.[11] From 20% to 25% of non–small cell cancers have the neuroendocrine phenotype that is seen in more than 75% of small cell cancers.[12] In more than 90% of SCLC and 50% of non–SCLC, the short arm of chromosome 3 is deleted.[11] Conversely, data from the study of lung cancer cell lines indicate that *ras* family gene mutations are features of non–small cell cancers, whereas *myc* family mutations dominate in small cell cancers.[13]

The clinical application of chemotherapy for non–SCLC should be based on a combination of agents shown to be consistently effective in properly designed clinical trials.[14] Despite the limitations of the drug armamentarium for metastatic lung cancer, there is cause for continued optimism since the first writing of this chapter.[7] It is now clear that cisplatin-based combination regimens are the most active and form the basis for comparison of new therapies.[15] Etoposide plus cisplatin or carboplatin could be considered a standard therapy today for metastatic non-SCLC in the nonprotocol setting given the broad clinical experiences with these agents and the results of major trials.[7, 16, 17] The clinical outcome measures of toxicity and efficacy favor carboplatin in this circumstance.[17]

For the first time in many years, there are several new agents demonstrating activity in the Phase II evaluation process.[18] There also are more extensive data on the novel use of older agents in this disease that appear to hold promise of added therapeutic benefit.[19] These developments have occurred despite the imprecise stratification of patients into prognostic subgroups in clinical trials.[17]

The future of systemic therapy for non–SCLC lies in a better understanding of the biology of this disease. The multiple genetic lesions that occur in lung cancer could be used to develop specific novel therapies.[20] Human gene therapy protocols have recently been initiated with some enthusiasm for cancer and other genetic disorders.[21, 22] Also encouraging are data on new compounds that block the actions of mutated RAS oncogenes.[23] It appears that rational, less-toxic therapies may emerge from work in progress and recent developments.[24]

SINGLE AGENT CHEMOTHERAPY

The use of a single agent in the treatment of non–SCLC continues to evolve in the clinical trial process. Several new agents that appear to be promising have emerged.[25] As reviewed by Joss and colleagues[26] and Kris and associates,[27] five previously used agents have shown consistent activity in this disease of more than 15%. Carboplatin, an analogue of cisplatin, may be less active than the parent compound in non–SCLC,[28] but it is less neurotoxic, nephrotoxic, and emetogenic, as well as more convenient to administer.[29] In a large randomized trial of the Eastern Cooperative Oncology Group (ECOG), carboplatin resulted in superior sur-

TABLE 11–1. Selected Trials of New Agents

AGENT	NO. OF PATIENTS	MAJOR RESPONSE RATE (%)	MEDIAN SURVIVAL (mo)	PATIENTS WITH DISSEMINATED DISEASE (%)	STUDY
CPT-11 (camptothecin)	73	31.9	10	55	Fukuoka et al[41]
Gemcitabine	161	20.4	Not reported	60	Shepherd et al[50]
Epirubicin	24	25	10	42	Martoni et al[55]
Taxol	24	20.8	6	100	Chang et al[61]
Navelbine	117	12.8	7.25 (estimated)	100	Vokes et al[74]
Oral etoposide	25	20	4	60	Estape et al[81]

vival rates compared with other combinations.[16] Vindesine has a response rate of 18%[27] and appears to have no advantage over other vinca alkaloids. It is not generally available for use in the United States. Mitomycin C, with a response rate of 17%, is problematic because of the potential for significant pulmonary and hematologic toxicity.[27] Ifosfamide has been reported to have response rates of 21% to 25% in Phase II evaluation, but myelosuppression is dose limiting.[30, 31]

Bakowski and Creech[32] concluded in their review of single agents used in the treatment of non–SCLC that etoposide was sufficiently studied to be considered active with a response rate of 18%. This agent is schedule dependent and requires further clinical trial study to determine the optimal dose and administration schedule.[33]

Cisplatin is established as one of the most active agents for use in non–SCLC. A single agent response rate of 21% is considered by many to be an accurate reflection of its activity.[34] There is experimental evidence of a steep dose-response relationship in vitro for this agent in the treatment of non–SCLC.[35] Although the optimal dose of cisplatin is unknown, this relationship has not been confirmed in the clinical setting.[36]

New agents active in the treatment of non–SCLC include camptothecins, edatrexate, gemcitabine, epirubicin, taxanes, navelbine, and etoposide. Included in this list are agents that are old but have novel applications. There are sufficient data to suggest that these agents will improve the chemotherapy experience in this disease.[18]

Camptothecin (CPT) is the active agent in extracts from the stem wood of the Chinese tree *Camptotheca acuminata* isolated in 1966.[37] Its toxicity profile precluded further clinical testing until the 1980s, when its mechanism of action was identified. CPT is a specific inhibitor of topoisomerase I.[38] Topotecan and CPT-II are the two analogues of CPT that are undergoing clinical investigation for the treatment of non–SCLC.[39] The spectrum of activity of these agents, their mechanisms of action, and their toxicity merit further investigation in combination with other active agents (e.g., cisplatin).[40, 41]

Edatrexate is a substituted 4-aminofolate that is active in Phase I and II trials in the treatment of non–SCLC.[42] It is superior in activity to methotrexate and other antifolates, due in part to its cell flow characteristics.[43] This agent has been reported to have a major response rate of 16% in single-agent phase II trials of patients with advanced non–SCLC.[44] Combinations including edatrexate have been tested based on this preclinical and early clinical experience. In a small series of Stage IIIB/IV patients, a major objective response of 37% was reported to edatrexate, cisplatin, and cyclophosphamide.[45] The outcome of a recently completed randomized chemotherapy trial[46] and future results of investigations regarding the role of leucovorin[47] are awaited with interest.

Gemcitabine is a novel antimetabolite that has properties similar to cytarabine but superior activity when administered intermittently.[48] This agent causes dose-limiting thrombocytopenia, anemia, and occasional skin rashes.[49] A 20% single agent response rate in advanced non–SCLC has been confirmed.[50, 51]

Epirubicin was created by Arcamone and colleagues[52] in the 1970s by modifying the aminosugar moiety of doxorubicin. It is less cardiotoxic than the parent compound and has equivalent murine and human xenograft antitumor activities.[53] The activity of this agent in non–SCLC is noteworthy when it is given in high doses.[54] In the study by Martoni and coworkers[55] of 24 patients with advanced non–SCLC, myelosuppression was the dose-limiting toxicity at "optimal" doses of 120 to 135 mg/m^2 (Table 11–1).

The taxanes represent a new class of antimitotic agents that have a novel mechanism of action.[56] Taxol was first isolated from the bark of the Pacific yew, *Taxus brevifolia*.[57] Taxotere, also used in clinical trials, is a Taxol derivative prepared from extracts of the needles of the European yew, *Taxus baccata*.[58] Both agents stabilize microtubules, prolonging or blocking cells in the G2 or M phase of the cell cycle.[59, 60] The activity of paclitaxel (Taxol) in non–SCLC was demonstrated in the studies of Chang and associates[61] and Murphy and colleagues.[62] Response rates of 20.8% and 24% were reported, respectively, in patients with metastatic disease, and in the ECOG trial,[61] 40% of patients survived more than 1 yr. Myelosuppression is the dose-limiting toxicity reported consistently with both agents in the doses and schedules tested.[63] Taxol is being investigated in combination with other agents in patients with non–SCLC,[64] and Taxotere appears promising as a single agent in early Phase II trials.[65, 66] Taxotere also demonstrates a moderate degree of fluid retention, especially pleural effusions, in some patients.[65, 66]

Navelbine (vinorelbine) is the best studied analogue

TABLE 11–2. Representative Results of Major Trials Using Combination Chemotherapy

TYPE OF COMBINATION CHEMOTHERAPY	NO. OF PATIENTS	MAJOR RESPONSE RATE (%)	MEDIAN SURVIVAL (mo)	PATIENTS WITH DISSEMINATED DISEASE (%)	STUDY
FU/VCR/MI	127	26.0	5.0	100	Miller et al[89]
CTX/ADR/PLAT/CAP	132	17.0	6.0	100	
FU/VCR/MI (FOMI)/CAP	126	22.0	5.75	100	
CBP (CTX/BLEO/PLAT)	112	20.0	5.5	100	Ruckdeschel et al[90]
AFP (ADR/FU/PLAT)	109	17.0	5.25	100	
MVP (MI/VND/PLAT)	104	26.0	5.8	100	
CAP (CTX/ADR/PLAT)	107	23.0	5.8	100	
VP/PLAT	124	20.0	6.5	100	Ruckdeschel et al[91]
CAMP (CTX/ADR/MTX/PROC)	115	17.0	6.25	100	
MVP (MI/VBL/PLAT)	121	31.0	5.5	100	
	126	26.0	6.5	100	
MVP (MI/VBL/PLAT)	176	20.0	5.6	100	Bonomi et al[16]
VP (VBL/PLAT)	175	13.0	6.28	100	
MVP/CAMP	172	13.0	6.25	100	
VP/PLAT	81	26.0	6.5	66	Klastersky et al[92]
MI/IFOS	66	30.3	6.75	70	Gatzemeier et al[93]
MI/VND	66	22.7	5.75	83	
VP/PLAT	60	25	6.25	75	
VBL/PLAT	52	28.9	8.75	50	Mylonalis et al[94]
MVP (MI/VBL/PLAT)	51	15.6	8	53	

VP = etoposide (VP16–213), VND = vindesine, PLAT = cisplatin, ADR = doxorubicin, CTX = cyclophosphamide, VBL = vinblastine, BLEO = bleomycin, FU = 5-fluorouracil, VCR = vincristine, MI = mitomycin C, PROC = procarbazine, MTX = methotrexate, IFOS = ifosfamide.

of vinblastine that is least toxic to neural microtubules compared with other alkaloids.[67] This feature and its broad antitumor activity have accelerated its investigation in cancer therapy.[68, 69] As a single agent, Navelbine has activity in non–SCLC with a response rate of 29%.[70] Major toxicities with weekly doses of 30 mg/m^2 IV are neutropenia, alopecia, and phlebitis.[71] Although the optimal dose and schedule of administration are not known, the use of Navelbine represents an area of active investigation.[72, 73] The oral formulation of this agent, which allows for chronic dosing, merits further clinical study.[74]

Etoposide is an active antineoplastic agent in many malignant diseases[75] and is one of the standard agents in combination therapy for non–SCLC.[76] It is a cell-cycle–specific inhibitor of topoisimerase II with known schedule dependency in SCLC.[33, 77] This agent is available in an oral preparation and has undergone clinical trial evaluation for several cancers, including non–SCLC[78–81] (see Table 11–1). Although the optimal schedule and dose of oral etoposide are matters of continued study,[82, 83] this agent alone or in combination with carboplatin represents an appealing alternative palliative therapy in non–SCLC.[84]

COMBINATION CHEMOTHERAPY

The response rates to combination chemotherapy for non–SCLC are higher than those to single agents, and although a survival benefit has been demonstrated, it is sufficiently modest to warrant caution in the routine application of this treatment.[7, 15] Cisplatin-based regimens generally achieve higher responses than those that do not contain this agent, and responders survive longer than do treatment failures,[85] although there are concerns with this type of analysis.[86] It is heartening to observe the widening apparent gap between survival times for treated and nontreated patients; however, it is necessary to recognize that the benefits are modest at best.[87] In the absence of curative therapy, prolongation of survival with combination chemotherapy is a reasonable objective, but quality-of-life concerns should enter into the decision-making process.[88]

Several factors confound a clear-cut analysis of the value of combination chemotherapy in the treatment of non–SCLC. Often, the populations under study are not uniform. An inadequate sample size can undermine generalization of the results.[17]

Table 11–2 summarizes data from a selection of recently reported randomized and nonrandomized clinical trials using combination chemotherapy to treat patients with advanced non–SCLC. It includes the number of patients, major response rates (complete response and partial response), median survival in months, and the percentage of patients with Stage IV disease.[16, 89–94] The inclusion of Stage IIIA and IIIB patients in some series makes rational interpretation of the data more difficult; however, from a natural history point of view, regional supraclavicular or contralateral hilar or mediastinal node involvement portends distant dissemination.[95]

Recent clinical experience indicates that Stage IIIA and IIIB disease is more responsive to chemotherapy than true Stage IV cancer.[96, 97] However, Fukuoka et al[98] reported a 44% objective response rate to mitomycin, vindesine, and cisplatin in patients who had

Stage IIIB disease, and the response rate for Stage IV patients was 56%. Von Rohr and coworkers[99] treated 12 patients with Stage IIIB cancer with mitomycin, ifosfamide, and carboplatin and reported a response rate of 75%. The Stage IV patients (n = 22) in this series had a response rate of 13.8% with this combination. Despite conflicting results from Phase II trials with regard to the response of Stage IIIB versus Stage IV disease, a trend toward poorer response rates emerges for trials that include a larger percentage of patients with Stage IV disease. This highlights the problem of clinical trial analysis when the study population is ambiguous.[17]

The true response rates for patients with Stage IV non–SCLC are in the range of 20% and 40% and associated with a median survival time of 5 to 6 mo.[100] As shown in Table 11–3, the larger studies have poorer response and survival rates, reflecting what is achievable in realistic terms. A response to therapy usually portends an increase in survival; however, it is not possible to determine whether this is a result of the treatment itself. A response to chemotherapy is by itself of prognostic significance.[101] By virtue of the study design, these trials cannot resolve the issue of whether the prolongation of median survival is a result of treatment or whether treatment identifies a subset of patients with a more benign natural history.[86, 102] Careful attention to the methodologic issues in carrying out clinical trials is appropriate to accurately interpret their true importance.

Combination chemotherapy in patients with metastatic non–SCLC has the potential for improvement in the quality of life of those successfully treated.[103] Kris and associates[104] reported an improvement in performance status and weight gain in a substantial fraction of study patients treated with combination chemotherapy who rated the severity of their disease-related symptoms. Further study of this issue is needed given these reported clinical observations.[105, 106] However, quality-of-life measures are difficult to implement and assess.[87, 107]

PROGNOSTIC FACTORS

Analysis of the cumulative experience of large cooperative groups with combination chemotherapy for non–SCLC reveals that certain factors are of major importance in therapeutic outcome[89, 108, 109] (see Table 11–3). Performance status is the major determinant of response and survival. The impact of gender requires further study; however, higher response and survival rates for female patients undergoing combination chemotherapy are generally noted. Feld and colleagues[110] found that performance status and stage or extent of disease were of definite importance in non–SCLC and that gender, weight loss, and lactate dehydrogenase level were possibly important. The review by Finkelstein and coworkers[109] of the ECOG experience revealed that the absence of weight loss, absence of liver or bone metastases, and good performance status were associated with an increased probability of 1-year survival. The response to chemotherapy decreases as a function of increased disease extent, an observation consistently reported in several series.[100, 111] These data have provided a rationale for the aggressive application of neoadjuvant and adjuvant chemotherapy.[112]

Histology and age of the patient are important determinants of treatment outcome in chemotherapy trials of non–SCLC.[110] The fact that response to chemotherapy is a powerful prognostic indicator could be used to restrict subsequent chemotherapy to patients who demonstrate an initial response to treatment. An analysis of ECOG trials 2575 and 1581 revealed, however, that slower response to chemotherapy was associated with longer survival. This controversial matter requires further study.[85]

Performance status is a consistent predictor of treatment outcome in trials of chemotherapy for non–SCLC. It is instructive to consider the experience of the performance status of two patients treated with combination chemotherapy in ECOG trial 1581.[91] A lower response rate was not associated with performance status 2. However, performance status of 2 was associated with both shorter survival and more frequent near-fatal or fatal toxicity. Inferior performance status is associated with lower response rates in other studies.[89, 101] Based on the ECOG experience with symptomatic patients, chemotherapy should be withheld in this group as toxicity is excessive and survival is reduced. Treatment-related mortality, which can vary from 0% to 10%, could obscure the impact of combination chemotherapy on overall survival for patients with non–SCLC.

In general, a better outcome would be expected for

TABLE 11–3. Comparative Ranking of Major Prognostic Factors from Analysis of Large Clinical Experiences Using Combination Chemotherapy for Non–Small Cell Lung Cancer Patients

PATIENT CHARACTERISTIC	MSKI (N = 378; O'CONNELL ET AL[108])	ECOG (N = 893; FINKELSTEIN ET AL[109])	SWOG (N = 452; MILLER ET AL[89])
Performance status	1	1	2
Age	NS	—	NS
Sex	4	3	1
Histology	NS	5	NS
Disease extent	5	—	3
Site of metastasis	2	2	NS

MSKI = Memorial Sloan Kettering Institute Cancer Center, ECOG = Eastern Cooperative Oncology Group, SWOG = Southwestern Oncology Group.

a group of patients with good to excellent performance status. As indicated previously, patients with only intrathoracic disease have better responses to chemotherapy than those with metastases.[113] This may be due to generally better performance status, but it may also reflect the enhanced effect of chemotherapy on a small tumor burden.[114]

The majority of patients with Stage IV non–SCLC do not have meaningful benefits from chemotherapy. There are too few patients entering clinical trials that might be considered the "best" therapeutic option for those who qualify. The recent refinement of homogeneous treatment groups based on new prognostic information and the availability of more active drug combinations provide an impetus for re-evaluating the potential benefit of chemotherapy. Outside of a clinical trial, it is reasonable to use chemotherapy to treat patients with a good performance status who have disseminated non–SCLC.

CONCLUSIONS

The role of chemotherapy in disseminated non–SCLC is in the setting of treatment with noncurative intent.[115] Under these circumstances, cost[116] and toxicity assume a major importance in the equation, whereas cure or clinical efficacy is a tertiary consideration. These relationships are reversed when therapy with curative intent is considered (Fig. 11–1).

Although it is considered marginally effective, systemic therapy for non–SCLC does benefit selected patients. These patients have limited disease and a good performance status. It is anticipated that they would respond to combination chemotherapy, incur minimal toxicity, and enjoy prolonged survival. The characteristics of a reasonable candidate for combination chemotherapy outside of a clinical trial are as follows: no medical contraindication, performance status of 1 or better (ECOG), measurable or evaluable disease, no prior chemotherapy, and patient understands risk and desires treatment. Therapy should be individualized, and aggressive support (e.g., ondansetron, colony-stimulating factors) should be used as indicated.

Clinical trial studies are required to rigorously prove a beneficial outcome as a result of exposure to combination chemotherapy. All patients should initially be considered for enrollment into protocol studies exploring novel treatment options, if eligible. In situations in which protocols are unavailable, the administration of moderately intense combination chemotherapy to treat "fit"[117] patients with non–SCLC is

fully defensible but suboptimal. It is hoped that with a better understanding of the biology of lung cancer, insight for new treatment approaches will be gained.

SELECTED REFERENCES

Feigal EG, Christian M, Chason B, et al: New chemotherapeutic agents in non–small cell lung cancer. Semin Oncol 20:185, 1993.
A very complete review of the new generation of drugs that will form the focus of an entire series of Phase II and III trials, examining both responsiveness in metastatic disease and the ability to combine these agents with radiation.
Gandara DR, Crowley J, Livingston RB, et al: Evaluation of cisplatin intensity in metastatic non–small lung cancer. A phase III study of the Southwest Oncology Group. J Clin Oncol 2:873, 1993.
Although there is likely a threshold dose for the cisplatin activity, this paper refutes the idea that if we could just give truly higher doses we would do more. Most of the additive effects were toxic.
Ihde DC: Chemotherapy of lung cancer. N Engl J Med 327:1434, 1992.
A more conservative but well-balanced approach to the issues of who to treat and when to treat patients with metastatic non–SCLC. The article places chemotherapy for NSCLC in a context for the general internist, as well as for oncologists.
Mulshine JL, Glastein E, Ruckdeschel JC: Treatment of non–small cell lung cancer. J Clin Oncol 4:1704, 1986.
This was the earliest review of the modern era in the therapy of non–small cell lung cancer. It placed the role of chemotherapy in an appropriate context and predicted the later adoption of etopside-cisplatin as a standard therapy and the dramatic increase in the use of combined modality therapy.

REFERENCES

 1. Boring CC, Squires TS, Tong T, Montgomery S: Cancer statistics, 1994. CA Cancer J Clin 44:7, 1994.
 2. Ginsburg RJ, Kris MG, Armstrong JG: Cancer of the lung. *In* DeVita VT Jr, Hellman S, Rosenburg SA (eds): Cancer: Principles and Practice of Oncology. 4th Ed. Philadelphia, J. B. Lippincott, 1993, pp 673–723.
 3. Ihde DC, Minna JD: Non-small cell lung cancer. I. Biology, diagnosis, and staging. Curr Probl Cancer 15:61, 1991.
 4. Mulshine JL, Glastein E, Ruckdeschel JC: Treatment of non-small cell lung cancer. J Clin Oncol 4:1704, 1986.
 5. Mountain CF: A new international staging system for lung cancer. Chest 89:2255, 1986.
 6. Hazuka MB, Bunn PA: Controversies in the nonsurgical treatment of stage III non-small cell lung cancer. Am Rev Resp Dis 145:967, 1992.
 7. Mulshine JL, Ruckdeschel JC: The role of chemotherapy in the management of disseminated non-small cell lung cancer. *In* Roth JA, Ruckdeschel JC, Weisenburger TH (eds): Thoracic Oncology. 1st Ed. Philadelphia, W. B. Saunders, 1989, pp 220–228.
 8. Ihde DC: Chemotherapy of lung cancer. N Engl J Med 327:1434, 1992.
 9. Gazdar AF, Linnoila RI: The pathology of lung cancer—changing concepts and newer diagnostic techniques. Semin Oncol 15:215, 1988.
 10. Souhami R: Lung cancer. Br Med J 304:1298, 1992.
 11. Carney DN: Biology of small cell lung cancer. Lancet 339:843, 1992.
 12. McCue PA, Finkel GC: Small-cell lung carcinoma: An evolving histopathological spectrum. Semin Oncol 20:153, 1993.
 13. Richardson GE, Johnson BE: The biology of lung cancer. Semin Oncol 20:105, 1993.
 14. Gralla RJ: New directions in non-small cell lung cancer. Semin Oncol 17(suppl 7):14, 1990.
 15. Ihde DC, Minna JD: Non-small cell lung cancer. II. Treatment. Curr Probl Cancer 15:105, 1991.
 16. Bonomi PD, Finkelstein DM, Ruckdeschel JC, et al: Combina

FIGURE 11–1. Relative importance of treatment outcome measures in the curative and noncurative setting.

Curative intent

Clinical efficacy
Toxicity profile
Cost

Noncurative intent

tion chemotherapy versus single agents followed by combination chemotherapy in stage IV non-small cell lung cancer: A study of the Eastern Cooperative Oncology Group. J Clin Oncol 7:1602, 1989.

17. Ruckdeschel JC: Therapeutic options for the treatment of small cell and non-small cell lung cancer. Curr Opin Oncol 5:323, 1993.

18. Green MR: New directions for chemotherapy in non-small cell lung cancer. Chest 103:370S, 1993.

19. Lilenbaum RC, Green MR: Novel chemotherapeutic agents in the treatment of non-small cell lung cancer. J Clin Oncol 11:1391, 1993.

20. Tang DC, Carbone DP: Potential application of gene therapy to lung cancer. Semin Oncol 20:368, 1993.

21. Davies K, Williamson B: Gene therapy begins. Br Med J 306:1625, 1993.

22. Gutierrez AA, Lemoine NR, Sikora K: Gene therapy for cancer. Lancet 339:715, 1992.

23. Travis J: Novel anticancer agents move closer to reality. Science 260:1877, 1993.

24. Minna JD: The molecular biology of lung cancer pathogenesis. Chest 103:449S, 1993.

25. Feigal EG, Christian M, Chason B, et al: New chemotherapeutic agents in non-small cell lung cancer. Semin Oncol 20:185, 1993.

26. Joss RA, Cavalli F, Goldhirsch A, et al: New agents in non-small cell lung cancer. Cancer Treat Rev 11:205, 1984.

27. Kris M, Cohen E, Gralla R, et al: An analysis of 134 phase II trials in non-small cell lung cancer (NSCLC). Lung Cancer 2:119, 1986.

28. Bunn PA: Review of therapeutic trials of carboplatin in lung cancer. Semin Oncol 16(suppl 5):27, 1989.

29. Ozols R: Optimal dosing with carboplatin. Semin Oncol 16(suppl 5):14, 1989.

30. Johnson D: Overview of ifosfamide in small cell and non-small cell lung cancer. Semin Oncol 17(suppl 4):24, 1990.

31. Ettinger DS: Ifosfamide in the treatment of non-small cell lung cancer. Semin Oncol 16(suppl 3):31, 1989.

32. Bakowski MT, Creech JC: Chemotherapy of non-small cell lung cancer: A reappraisal and look to the future. Cancer Treat Rev 10:159, 1983.

33. Slevin ML, Clark PJ, Joel SP, et al: A randomized trial to evaluate the effect of schedule on the activity of etoposide in small cell lung cancer. J Clin Oncol 7:1333, 1989.

34. Bunn PA: The expanding role of cisplatin in the treatment of non-small cell lung cancer. Semin Oncol 16(suppl 6):10, 1989.

35. Perez EA, Putney JD, Gandara DR: In vitro dose-response relationship to cisplatin in human non-small cell lung cancer cell lines. Proc Am Assoc Cancer Res 30:459, 1989.

36. Gandara DR, Crowley J, Livingston RB, et al: Evaluation of cisplatin intensity in metastatic non-small cell lung cancer: A phase III study of the Southwest Oncology Group. J Clin Oncol 2:873, 1993.

37. Wall ME, Wani MC, Cook CE, et al: Plant antitumor agents: I. The isolation and structure of camptothecin, a novel alkaloidal leukemia and tumor inhibitor from Camptotheca acuminata. J Am Chem Soc 88:3888, 1966.

38. Hsiang YH, Hertberg R, Hecht S, et al: Camptothecin induces protein-linked DNA breaks via mammalian DNA topoisomerase I. J Biol Chem 260:14873, 1985.

39. Slichenmyer WJ, Rowinsky EK, Sonehower RC, Kaufman SH: The current status of camptothecin analogues as antitumor agents. J Natl Cancer Inst 85:271, 1993.

40. Burris HA, Rothenberg ML, Kuhn JG, Von Hoff DD: Clinical trials with topoisomerase I inhibitors. Semin Oncol 19:663, 1992.

41. Fukuoka M, Niitani H, Suzuki A, et al: A Phase II study of CPT-II, a new derivative of camptothecin for previously untreated non-small cell lung cancer. J Clin Oncol 10:16, 1992.

42. Grant SC, Kris MG, Young CW, Sirotnak FM: Edatrexate, an antifolate with antitumor activity: A review. Cancer Invest 11:36, 1993.

43. Sirotnak FM, DeGraw JI, Moccio DM, et al: New folate analogs of the 10-dozen-aminopterin series: Basis for structural design and biochemical and pharmacologic properties. Cancer Chemother Pharmacol 12:18, 1984.

44. Kris MG: Combination lung cancer therapy with edatrexate. Cancer Invest 2(suppl 1):56, 1993.

45. Lee JS, Libshitz HI, Fossella FV, et al: Edatrexate improves the antitumor effects of cyclophosphamide and cisplatin against non-small cell lung cancer. Cancer 68:959, 1991.

46. Grall RJ, Lee JS, Comis R, et al: Testing the role of edatrexate (EDAM) in non-small cell lung cancer: Preliminary results of a randomized combination chemotherapy trial in 277 patients. Lung Cancer 7(suppl):133, 1991.

47. Lee JS, Libshitz HI, Fossella FV, et al: Improved therapeutic index by leucovorin of edatrexate, cyclophosphamide, and cisplatin regimen for non-small cell lung cancer. J Natl Cancer Inst 84:1039, 1992.

48. Grunewald R, Kantarjian H, Keating MH: Pharmacologically directed design of the dose rate and schedule of 2',2'-difluorodeoxycytidine gemcitabine administration in leukemia. Cancer Res 50:6823, 1990.

49. Abbruzzese JL, Grunewald R, Weeks EA, et al: A phase I clinical, plasma, and cellular pharmacology study of gemcitabine. J Clin Oncol 9:491, 1991.

50. Shepherd F, Gatzemeier V, Gotfried M, et al: An extended phase II study of gemcitabine in non-small cell lung cancer (NSCLC). Proc Am Soc Clin Oncol 12:330, 1992.

51. Fossella FV, Lippman S, Pang A, et al: Phase I/II study of gemcitabine (G) by 30 minute weekly intravenous (IV) infusion × 3 weeks every 4 weeks for non-small cell lung cancer. Proc Am Soc Clin Oncol 12:326, 1993.

52. Arcamone F, Penco S, Vigevani A: Adriamycin (NSC-123127): New chemical developments and analogs. Cancer Chemother Rep 6(pt 3):123, 1975.

53. Goldin A, Venditti JM, Geran R: The effectiveness of the anthracycline analog 4'-epidoxorubicin in the treatment of experimental tumors: A review. Invest New Drugs 3:3, 1985.

54. Martoni A, Melotti B, Guaraldi M, et al: High dose epirubicin for untreated patients with advanced tumors: A phase I study. Eur J Cancer 26:1137, 1990.

55. Martoni A, Melotti B, Guaraldi M, et al: Activity of high-dose epirubicin on advanced non-small cell lung cancer. Eur J Cancer 27:1231, 1991.

56. Schiff PB, Fant J, Horwitz SB: Promotion of microtubule assembly in vitro by taxol. Nature 22:665, 1979.

57. Wani MC, Taylor HL, Wall ME, et al: Plant antitumor agents: VI. The isolation and structure of taxol, a novel antileukemic and antitumor agent from Taxus brevifolia. Am Chem Soc 93:2325, 1971.

58. Denis JN, Correa A, Greene AE: An improved synthesis of the taxol side chain and of RP56976. J Org Chem 55:1957, 1990.

59. Horwitz SB: Mechanism of action of taxol. Trends Pharmacol Sci 13:134, 1992.

60. Ringel I, Horwitz SB: Studies with RP56976 (taxotere): A semisynthetic analogue of taxol. J Natl Cancer Inst 83:288, 1991.

61. Chang A, Kim K, Glick J, et al: Phase II study of Taxol, Merbarone, and Piroxantrone in stage IV non-small cell lung cancer: The Eastern Cooperative Oncology Group Results. J Natl Cancer Inst 85:338, 1993.

62. Murphy WK, Fossella FV, Winn RJ, et al: Phase II study of taxol in patients with untreated advanced non-small cell lung cancer. J Natl Cancer Inst 85:384, 1993.

63. Rowinsky EK, Onetto N, Cannetta RM, et al: Taxol: The first of the taxanes, an important new class of antitumor agents. Semin Oncol 19:646, 1992.

64. Rowinsky EK, Gilbert MR, McGuire WP, et al: Sequence of taxol and cisplatin: A phase I and pharmacologic study. J Clin Oncol 9:1692, 1991.

65. Cerny T, Wanders J, Kaplan S, et al: Taxotere is an active drug in non-small cell lung (NSCLC) cancer: A phase II trial of the Early Clinical Trials Group (ECTG). Proc Am Soc Clin Oncol 12:331, 1993.

66. Rigas JR, Francis PA, Kris MG, et al: Phase II trial of taxotere in non-small cell lung cancer (NSCLC). Proc Am Soc Clin Oncol 12:336, 1993.

67. Binet S, Chaineau E, Fellous A, et al: Immunofluorescence study of the action of navelbine, vincristine, and vinblastine on mitotic and axonal microtubules. Int J Cancer 46:262, 1990.

68. Cros S, Wright M, Morimoto M, et al: Experimental antitumor activity of navelbine. Semin Oncol 2(suppl 4):15, 1989.

69. Armand JP, Marty M: Navelbine: A new step in cancer therapy? Semin Oncol 2(suppl 4):41, 1989.
70. DePierre A, Lemarie E, Dabouis G, et al: A phase II study of navelbine in the treatment of non-small cell lung cancer. Am J Clin Oncol 14:115, 1991.
71. Yokoyama A, Furuse K, Niitani H: Multi-institutional phase II study of navelbine (Vinorelbine) in non-small cell lung cancer. Proc Am Soc Clin Oncol 11:957, 1992.
72. Jacoulet P, Dubiez A, DePierre A, et al: One week versus 3-week intervals in the administration of cisplatin in combination with Vinorelbine: A randomized study in non-small cell lung cancer (NSCLC). Proc Am Soc Clin Oncol 11:301, 1992.
73. Gralla RJ, Kardinal CG, Clark RA, et al: Enhancing the safety, efficacy, and dose intensity of Vinorelbine (navelbine) in combination chemotherapy regimens. Proc Am Soc Clin Oncol 12:336, 1993.
74. Vokes E, Rosenberg R, Jahenzelo M, et al: Multicenter study of oral navelbine (NVB) in previously untreated stage IV non-small cell lung cancer (NSCLC). Proc Am Soc Clin Oncol 12:336, 1993.
75. O'Dwyer PJ, Leyland-Jones B, Alonso MT, et al: Etoposide (VP-16): Current status of an active anticancer drug. N Engl J Med 312:692, 1992.
76. Ruckdeschel JC: The role of standard-dose etoposide in the management of non-small cell lung cancer. Semin Oncol 19(suppl 13):39, 1992.
77. Osheroff N: Effect of antineoplastic agents on the DNA cleavage/religation reaction of eukaryotic topoisomerase II: Inhibition of DNA religation by etoposide. Biochemistry 28:6157, 1989.
78. Carney DN: The pharmacology of intravenous and oral etoposide. Cancer 67(suppl):299, 1991.
79. Splinter TAW, van der Gaast A, Kok TC: What is the optimal dose and duration of treatment with etoposide? I. Maximum tolerated duration of daily treatment with 50, 75, and 100 mg of oral etoposide. Semin Oncol 19(suppl 14):1, 1992.
80. DeVore R, Hainsworth J, Greco FA, et al: Chronic oral etoposide in the treatment of lung cancer. Semin Oncol 19(suppl 14):28, 1992.
81. Estape J, Palumbo H, Sanchez-Lloret, et al: Chronic oral etoposide in non-small cell lung carcinoma. Eur J Cancer 28A:835, 1992.
82. Hande KR, Krozely MG, Greco FA, et al: Bioavailability of low-dose oral etoposide. J Clin Oncol 11:374, 1993.
83. Thompson DS, Hainsworth JD, Hande KR, et al: Prolonged continuous infusion of low dose etoposide: Seeking the best dose and schedule. Proc Am Soc Clin Oncol 12:134, 1993.
84. Johnson DH, Hainsworth JD, Hand KR, Greco FA: Combination chemotherapy with oral etoposide. Semin Oncol 19(suppl 14):19, 1992.
85. Johnson D: Chemotherapy for unresectable non-small cell lung cancer. Semin Oncol 17(suppl 7):20, 1990.
86. Anderson JR, Cain KC, Gebber RD: Analysis of survival by tumor response. J Clin Oncol 1:710, 1983.
87. Evans WK: Rationale for the treatment of non-small cell lung cancer. Lung Cancer 9(suppl):S5, 1993.
88. Slevin ML: Quality of life: Philosophical question or clinical reality. Br Med J 305:466, 1992.
89. Miller TP, Chen T, Coltman CA, et al: Effect of alternating combination chemotherapy on survival of ambulatory patients with metastatic large cell and adenocarcinoma of the lung. J Clin Oncol 4:502, 1986.
90. Ruckdeschel JC, Finkelstein DM, Mason RA, et al: Chemotherapy for metastatic non-small cell brincetogenic carcinoma: EST 2575, generation V—A randomized comparison of four cisplatin-containing regimens. J Clin Oncol 3:72, 1985.
91. Ruckdeschel JC, Finkelstein DM, Ettinger DS, et al: A randomized trial of the four most active regimens for metastatic non-small cell lung cancer. J Clin Oncol 4:14, 1986.
92. Klastersky J, Sevlier JP, Bureau G, et al: Cisplatin versus cisplatin plus etoposide in the treatment of advanced non-small cell lung cancer. J Clin Oncol 7:1087, 1989.
93. Gatzemeier V, Heckmayr M, Hossfield D, et al: A randomized trial with mitomycin-C/ifosfamide versus mitomycin-C/vindesine versus cisplatin/etoposide in advanced non-small cell lung cancer. Am J Clin Oncol (CCT) 14:405, 1991.
94. Mylonalis N, Tsavaris N, Bacoyiannis C, et al: A randomized prospective study of cisplatin and vinblastine versus cisplatin, vinblastine and mitomycin in advanced non-small cell lung cancer. Ann Oncol 3:127, 1992.
95. Mountain CF: Prognostic implications of the International Staging System for lung cancer. Semin Oncol 15:236, 1988.
96. Belani CP: Multimodality management of regionally advanced non-small lung cancer. Semin Oncol 20:302, 1993.
97. Bonomi P: A brief overview of combination chemotherapy in non-small cell lung cancer. Semin Oncol 13(suppl 3):88, 1986.
98. Fukuoka M, Neoro S, Masuda N, et al: Mitomycin C, vindesine, and cisplatin in advanced non-small cell lung cancer. Am J Clin Oncol 15:18, 1992.
99. Von Rohr A, Anderson H, McIntosh R, Thatoher N: Phase II study with mitomycin, ifosfamide, and carboplatin in inoperable non-small cell lung cancer. Eur J Cancer 27:1106, 1991.
100. Longeval E, Klastersky J: Combination chemotherapy with cisplatin and etoposide in bronchogenic squamous cell and adenocarcinoma: A study for the EORTC Lung Cancer Working Party (Belgium). Cancer 50:2751, 1982.
101. Splinter TAW: Chemotherapy in advanced non-small cell lung cancer. Eur J Cancer 26:1093, 1990.
102. Vokes EE, Bitran JD, Vogelzang NJ: Chemotherapy for non-small cell lung cancer: The continuing challenge. Chest 99:1326, 1991.
103. Hardy JR, Noble T, Smith IE: Symptom relief with moderate dose chemotherapy (mitomycin-C, vinblastine, and cisplatin) in advanced non-small cell lung cancer. Br J Cancer 60:764, 1989.
104. Kris MG, Gralla RJ, Potanovich LM, et al: Assessment of pretreatment symptoms and improvement after EDAM and mitomycin and vinblastine (EMV) in patients with inoperable non-small cell lung cancer (NSCLC). Proc Am Soc Clin Oncol 9:229, 1990.
105. Osoba D, Rusthoven JJ, Turnbull KA, et al: Combination chemotherapy with bleomycin, etoposide, and cisplatin in metastatic non-small cell lung cancer. J Clin Oncol 3:1478, 1985.
106. Vinante O, Bari M, Segati R, et al: The combination of mitomycin, vinblastine, and cisplatin is active in the palliation of stage IIIB-IV non-small cell lung cancer. Oncology 50:1, 1993.
107. Johnson DH: Chemotherapy for metastatic non-small cell lung cancer—Can that dog hunt? J Natl Cancer Inst 85:766, 1993.
108. O'Connell JP, Kris MG, Gralla RJ, et al: Frequency and prognostic importance of pretreatment clinical characteristics in patients with advanced non-small cell lung cancer treated with combination chemotherapy. J Clin Oncol 4:1604, 1986.
109. Finkelstein DM, Ettinger DS, Ruckdeschel JC: Longterm survivors in metastatic non-small cell lung cancer: An Eastern Cooperative Oncology Group Study. J Clin Oncol 4:702, 1986.
110. Feld R, Arrigadea R, Ball DL, et al: Prognostic factors in non-small cell lung cancer: A consensus report. Lung Cancer 7:3, 1991.
111. Vokes EE, Vijayakumar S, Bitran JD, et al: Role of systemic therapy in advanced non-small cell lung cancer. Am J Med 89:777, 1990.
112. Dillman RO, Seagren SL, Propert KJ, et al: A randomized trial of induction chemotherapy plus high dose radiation versus radiation alone in stage III non-small cell lung cancer. N Engl J Med 323:940, 1990.
113. Splinter TAW: Therapy for small cell and non-small cell lung cancer. Curr Opin Oncol 4:315, 1992.
114. Miller TP: Rationale for the use of chemotherapy in non-small cell lung cancer. Semin Oncol 17(suppl 7):11, 1990.
115. Ruckdeschel JC: Current status and future role of carboplatin. Bristol-Myers Squibb Monograph. January 1994.
116. Evans WK: Management of metastatic non-small cell lung cancer and a consideration of cost. Chest 103:685, 1993.
117. Aisner J, Belani CP: Lung cancer: Recent changes and expectations of improvements. Semin Oncol 20:383, 1993.

SMALL CELL LUNG CANCER

12 CLINICAL PRESENTATION AND NATURAL HISTORY OF SMALL CELL LUNG CANCER

Per Dombernowsky and Heine H. Hansen

Small cell lung cancer (SCLC) has to be considered separately from other types of primary lung cancer because of its unique biologic and clinical features. The high rate of cell proliferation, the early and widespread dissemination, and the many paraneoplastic endocrine and neurologic syndromes are some of the characteristic biologic properties associated with SCLC.

Approximately 3% to 4% of all patients with SCLC present without an obvious pulmonary or mediastinal lesion on chest x-ray study or chest CT scan, and with normal bronchoscopy or sputum cytology. These primary extrapulmonary small cell carcinomas can arise in the esophagus, stomach, pancreas, larynx, hypopharynx, salivary glands, uterine cervix, breast, prostate, urinary bladder, and skin and resemble SCLC morphologically at microscopy, showing neuroendocrine features by immunochemistry and electron microscopy. The clinical behavior of these tumors often is aggressive, with a tendency to early dissemination, and they also can be associated with paraneoplastic syndromes. Extrapulmonary SCLC has recently been reviewed elsewhere,[1-3] and the following review focuses exclusively on small cell carcinoma of pulmonary origin.

When the diagnosis of SCLC is established, dissemination to distant organs has occurred in a high percentage of patients.[4] This finding is substantiated by autopsy data in patients dying from non–cancer-related causes within 30 days of complete surgical resection for lung cancer. Among 19 patients, 68% had persistent disease, including 63% with distant metastases and 5% with persistent local disease only. The sites of distant metastases included the liver (7 pa-

tients) adrenal glands (4 patients), and lymph nodes (6 patients). In contrast, in large cell carcinoma, epidermoid carcinoma, and adenocarcinoma, 14%, 33%, and 43%, respectively, had persistent disease at autopsy. Furthermore, the metastatic patterns at autopsy in patients with SCLC show lung cancer metastases in nearly every organ in the body.[5]

STAGING PROCEDURES

Nearly all therapeutic trials in SCLC have used the single two-stage classification of the Veterans Administration Lung Cancer Study Group (VALG), in which patients with inoperable lesions are divided into those with limited and those with extensive disease.[6] Limited disease is defined as a tumor confined to one hemithorax and its regional lymph nodes, with or without local extension or involvement of the ipsilateral supraclavicular nodes. In practice, there has not always been strict adherence to the VALG definition of limited disease, and minor variations have occurred in different studies.[6] The most recent international recommendations for staging procedures in SCLC according to the Third International Association for the Study of Lung Cancer (IASLC) Workshop on SCLC are given in Table 12–1.[7]

Some of the differences may be explained by the pretreatment staging performed at the time of diagnosis. Another potential source of variability is the sensitivity and specificity of the methods used to diagnose metastases in a particular site. The increased sensitivity of newer imaging techniques can identify additional patients with metastases at a given site.

TABLE 12–1. Recommendation of Staging Procedures in Small Cell Lung Cancer

	CLINICAL PRACTICE		
	Local Treatment Modality Under Consideration		
PROCEDURE	No	YES	CLINICAL TRIAL
GENERAL PROCEDURES			
Patient history	+	+	+
Physical examination	+	+	+
Blood counts	+	+	+
Serum biochemistry	+	+	+
Cytologic or histologic documentation of SCLC	+	+	+
PROCEDURES FOR LOCAL DISEASE			
Chest x-ray study	+	+	+
Chest CT	—	+§	+*
Fiberoptic bronchoscopy	—	—	+†
Mediastinoscopy	—	—	+‡
Cytology of effusion	—	+§	+
Cytology of supraclavicular node	—	—	+§
PROCEDURES FOR DISTANT DISEASE			
Bone			
Bone scan	—	+‖	+
Bone x-ray studies	—	+¶	+¶
Liver and retroperitoneal organs			
Ultrasound and abdominal CT	—	+‖	+
Fine-needle aspiration/biopsy	—	+‖	+§
Bone marrow			
Aspirate and biopsy	—	+‖	+
Brain			
CT	—	+‖	+

*Especially for trials of limited disease.
†If use of bronchoscopy is anticipated at restaging, surgery for limited disease is considered or diagnosis cannot be obtained otherwise.
‡Only if needed by surgeon for preoperative work-up.
§If the findings are doubtful and the establishment of a positive finding affects the treatment.
‖If one of tests is positive, further evaluation can be discontinued if not clinically indicated.
¶Only in areas of increased uptake on bone scan.
CT = Computed tomography, SCLC = small cell lung cancer.
From Stahel RA, Ginsberg R, Havemann K, et al: Staging and prognostic factors in small cell lung cancer: A consensus report. *In* Hansen HH, Kristjansen PEG (eds): Management of Small Cell Lung Cancer: Third IASLC Workshop on Small Cell Lung Cancer. Amsterdam, Elsevier, 1989, pp 1–8.

This factor has direct clinical implications as such patients survive longer than patients whose metastases are diagnosed with less sensitive techniques, resulting in so-called stage migration.[8]

The percentage of patients with limited disease varies from study to study. In a tabulation of eight trials including 1768 patients, 36% had limited disease and 64% had extensive disease.[9] In a more recent review including 1527 consecutive patients entered in nine controlled studies from 1973 to 1986 by one study group, 49% had limited disease and 51% had extensive disease.[10]

Table 12–2 gives an overview of the results of pretreatment staging procedures among systematically staged patients with SCLC.[6]

Among patients classified as having extensive stage disease, distant metastatic tumor is documented in only a single organ system in one-half to two-thirds of the patients, with multiple organs being involved in the remaining.[11, 12] The most common sites of isolated extensive disease are the bone, liver, and central nervous system (CNS).[11, 12]

CLINICAL COURSE

Signs and symptoms of SCLC are either related to the primary tumor and the presence or absence of re-gional or distant metastases. With the exception of the relatively uncommon paraneoplastic endocrine and neurologic syndromes, most clinical signs are no more specific for SCLC than for other histologic types of lung cancer. SCLC differs from other major histologic types of lung cancer in two major ways.

First, in most cases, it is disseminated from its outset, and the survival time is inferior to that of other histologic types of lung cancer.[13, 14] Studies by the American Joint Committee for Staging have shown that for cell types other than SCLC, there is a clear relationship between the clinical stage of the primary tumor and survival time. When the identical clinical staging system is applied to SCLC, no significant relationship between clinical stage and survival time is apparent. This indicates that the disease is generally disseminated beyond the apparent confines of clinical involvement and that local treatment modalities alone addressing the clinically apparent disease will be ineffective in controlling the overall disease process. A study performed by the Medical Research Council prior to the development of effective systemic chemotherapy verified this hypothesis.[15] In this study, patients who were thought to have potentially resectable disease were randomized to surgery or radiation therapy. Among 144 patients with apparently limited

TABLE 12–2. Sites and Frequency of Distant Metastases in Small Cell Lung Cancer at the Time of Diagnosis

	PATIENTS WITH POSITIVE FINDINGS (%)	REFERENCES
Chest Evaluation:		
Abnormal chest x-ray study	70–90	11, 27, 31, 32, 33
Mediastinal metastases (CT scan)	80–92	41, 52
Bronchoscopy		
Visual endobronchial tumor		
Cytology/biopsy positive	95	11
Pleural effusion	15–38	11, 12, 41
Supraclavicular lymph nodes	15–20	11, 12, 68
Bone (bone scan)	22–26	6, 11
Bone x-ray study	6	49
Bone marrow	17–23	11, 44, 45, 46, 47
Liver (biopsy proven)	21–25	6, 46, 57, 58
Central nervous system		
Brain	10 (range 4–23)	46, 66
Spinal	1–3	65, 78, 79
Leptomeninges	0.5	66, 74
Adrenal glands, retroperitoneal nodes and pancreas (CT scan)	14–22	52, 56

Modified from Ihde DC, Hansen HH: Staging procedures and prognostic factors in small cell carcinoma of the lung. *In* Greco FA, Oldham RK, Bunn PA (eds): Small Cell Lung Cancer. New York, Grune & Stratton, 1981, pp 261–283.

disease, 97% died within 5 years of metastatic disease.[15]

Second, studies have shown that, in most cases, SCLC is a rapidly proliferating tumor. Experimental and clinical studies have shown that SCLC has a relatively high 3H-thymidine labeling index, growth fraction, and shorter volume doubling time when compared with the other histologic types of lung cancer.[16–18]

NATURAL HISTORY

Information regarding the natural course of lung cancer is based on both retrospective and prospective randomized studies. In the studies of untreated cases of lung cancer from 1950 to 1970, the median survival time from the time of diagnosis was 3 to 6 months.[19–21] In a group of inoperable untreated patients, Elmendorff observed a median survival of 3.2 months in 128 patients with SCLC, compared with 4.5 months in 235 patients with epidermoid carcinoma and 4.2 months in 40 patients with adenocarcinoma.[22]

During the 1960s, the VALG performed a series of studies in male patients with lung cancer. After stratification for limited or extensive disease, patients with clinically inoperable lung cancer were allocated randomly to treatment with radiation therapy, chemotherapy, or placebo and best supportive care.[14, 23–25]

In these VALG studies, more than 7500 men with nonresectable lung cancer were included.[26] One thousand sixty-eight patients received placebo treatment alone, thus giving a valuable resource for studying the natural history of lung cancer.

In 630 male veterans with extensive lung cancer

included in different protocols and receiving only symptomatic nonspecific therapy, median survival rates for small cell, epidermoid, and large cell carcinomas and adenocarcinomas were found to be 1.2, 2.2, 1.6, and 2.6 months, respectively.[14] Based on the 231 patients with limited disease who were also only receiving symptomatic therapy, the median survival rates for small cell, epidermoid, and large cell carcinoma and adenocarcinoma were 2.7, 3.6, 3.5, and 5.2 months, respectively. In untreated patients, the survival was also shown to be related to Karnofsky's performance scale.[14] Details from two of the studies are given in the following section.

In a VALG study of chest radiation therapy, 31 patients with limited-stage SCLC treated with placebo were included. Their median survival time was 3.1 months, and 21% and 3.5% survived after 6 and 12 months, respectively.[23,24]

In a parallel study of patients with extensive SCLC, cyclophosphamide and placebo were compared. The median survival time in the 87 placebo treated patients was 1.4 months, and 10% and 2% survived after 6 and 12 months, respectively.[25]

In conclusion, in the natural history of SCLC, the median survival time for male veterans ranges from 2 to 4 months from inclusion in a treatment protocol. The VALG studies also show a difference between limited and extensive disease with regard to median survival time. However, these survival times observed during the 1960s cannot be directly applied to today's results among others owing to the more detailed staging procedures introduced in the last 2 decades.

CLINICAL PRESENTATION

With the onset of local tumor growth and invasion, SCLC can give rise to signs and symptoms as well as to abnormalities that appear on the chest radiograph. The findings may be the result of local tumor growth; invasion of adjacent structures; regional lymphatic spread with metastases to peribronchial, hilar, mediastinal, and supraclavicular nodes; growth in distant sites due to lymphatic or hematogenous dissemination; or a remote effect of the cancer (paraneoplastic syndromes).

The propensity for rapid growth and early dissemination is reflected in the clinical presentation of SCLC. In most series, the time interval from the onset of symptoms to diagnosis tends to be short and is less than 3 months in 66% to more than 80% of all cases.[27, 28] With the exception of the rare case found coincidentally by mass screening, 96% to 98% of patients with SCLC present with symptomatic disease.[27–30] The symptoms are most frequently due to the primary tumor and less frequently due to mediastinal tumor extension and metastatic disease.

SIGNS AND SYMPTOMS DUE TO PRIMARY TUMOR OR INTRATHORACIC SPREAD

On conventional chest x-ray study, SCLC presents with a central tumor mass, hilar node enlargement, or both in 70% to 90% of patients.[11, 27, 31–33] Superior mediastinal masses or widening are apparent in at least 15% to 20% of patients. Discrete peripheral masses can be appreciated in 20% to 30% of patients. About 40% of patients have obstructive pneumonitis or atelectasis, whereas pleural effusion, apical tumor, and multiple tumor masses are less common findings on conventional chest x-ray studies. Peripheral presentation of small cell carcinoma as a single nodule is observed in about 4% of all patients, but the frequency is higher in patients with SCLC detected on screening radiographs.[34, 35]

In SCLC, cavitation with lung abscess was found in 1.4% of patients prior to chemotherapy,[36] substantiating the data by Byrd and colleagues[32] and Chaudhuri.[37] In contrast, cavitation occurred in 22% of patients with squamous cell carcinoma, in 6% with large cell carcinomas, and in 2% with adenocarcinoma.[32]

Figure 12–1 shows the classic chest x-ray study of a patient with SCLC with bilateral mediastinal enlargement and minor central infiltration in the left lung.

Use of x-ray studies alone to diagnose one or the other form of lung cancer, however, is not sufficient because all histologic types of lung cancer can present as either peripheral or central lesions.

The main symptoms and signs related to the primary tumor in patients with SCLC include cough, chest pain, hemoptysis, dyspnea due to obstruction, postobstructive pneumonitis due to atelectasis with loss of lung volume, wheeze, and stridor.[38]

The major presenting symptoms and signs in SCLC compiled from 5 major series including 1134 patients are shown in Table 12–3.[27–29, 30, 39] The presentation of cough, chest pain, hemoptysis, dyspnea, and other manifestations of local spread in the chest are discussed in more detail in Chapter 3.

SIGNS AND SYMPTOMS FROM METASTATIC SPREAD

Autopsy studies have shown that extrathoracic metastases of SCLC occur earlier and more frequently compared with other histologic types of lung cancer.[5]

The most frequent extrathoracic sites of SCLC metastatic involvement at diagnosis are shown in Table 12–2. In the following sections, these extrathoracic metastatic presentations are discussed in more detail.

Pleural Effusion

At diagnosis, pleural effusions are present in about 12% of all lung cancer patients[40] and may be present in up to 35% of patients with SCLC.[11, 41] In most cases, the effusion is secondary to tumor involvement of the visceral pleura. Mediastinal lymphatic obstruction or obstructive atelectasis are other, more unusual explanations. Pleural effusions may also be due to coexistent congestive heart failure, pulmonary infarction, or infections, including tuberculosis.

In contrast to other types of lung cancer, an ipsilateral pleural effusion does not adversely affect the prognosis in patients with SCLC.[42]

Bone and Bone Marrow Metastases

Bone marrow metastases are observed in about 20% of patients with SCLC at diagnosis, based on unilateral bone marrow examination.[43, 44] The yield from bone marrow examination increases to 23% when bilateral bone marrow aspiration and biopsy are performed.[45, 46]

The majority of patients with bone marrow involve-

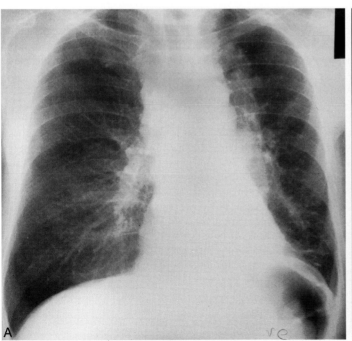
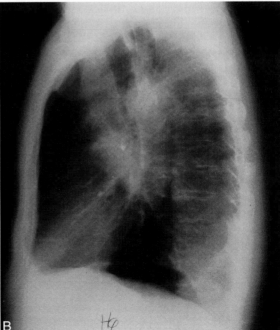

FIGURE 12–1. Lung cancer appearing as a mediastinal mass. PA chest radiograph *(A)* and lateral view *(B)* demonstrate bilateral mediastinal enlargement and minor central infiltration in the left lung. Bronchoscopy revealed small cell carcinoma.

TABLE 12–3. Major Presenting Symptoms and Signs in 1129 Patients with Small Cell Carcinoma

	CHUTE ET AL[30] (N = 326) (%)	GREEN ET AL[28] (N = 260) (%)	HUHTI ET AL[29] (N = 113) (%)	KATO ET AL[27] (N = 138) (%)	MARTINI ET AL[39] (N = 292) (%)
Cough	51	56	50	84	43
Dyspnea	41	29	38	45	21
Hemoptysis	24	26	26	49	24
Chest pain	36	28	40	54	31
Anorexia	30	12	—	—	20
Fatigue	37	17	12	59	12
Weight loss	48	31	37	57	24
Wheeze	—	—	—	31	2
Hoarseness	12	8	—	16	10
Dysphagia	—	3	—	3	—
Pneumonia	—	13	—	30	—
Atelectasis	35	11	—	—	3
Pleural effusion	—	13	—	—	2
Fever	14	18	27	—	6
Asymptomatic	2*	4	8	1	—

— = Not stated.
*Including 1529 patients with all histologic subtypes of lung cancer.

ment have normal peripheral blood findings, but thrombocytopenia is observed in 6% to 17% of patients with bone marrow involvement.[43, 44, 47] A leukoerythroblastic picture, defined as the presence of immature myeloid and erythroid precursors in the peripheral blood, is present in 10% to 37% of patients with bone marrow involvement.[43, 44, 47] In contrast, a leukoerythroblastic picture with a normal bone marrow examination is observed in less than 1% of the patients with SCLC. Circulating tumor cells in the peripheral blood (carcinocythemia) have been described.[48]

The occurrence of bone marrow metastases as the only site of extrathoracic disease is rare. In a review of 403 patients, only 1.7% had extensive disease based on isolated bone marrow involvement.[47]

Involvement of the bone is observed in 22% to 26% of SCLC patients at the time of diagnosis based on bone scans.[6]

Roentgenographic skeletal surveys are only infrequently positive at the time of diagnosis of SCLC. In a study by Hansen, two of 35 patients had radiographic evidence of osseous neoplastic involvement at the time of diagnosis, whereas a further 31% developed radiographic bone metastases subsequently during treatment.[49] Among the 15 patients with a positive bone marrow examination at diagnosis, only one had bone metastases on x-ray study. During therapy, however, bone radiographs occasionally revealed osteoblastic abnormalities.[50]

The symptoms caused by bone marrow metastases are vague and usually not painful, and pathologic fractures at the time of diagnosis of SCLC are rare.

Hepatic and Abdominal Metastases

Autopsy data show metastases to the liver in 74%, adrenals in 55%, abdominal lymph nodes in 55%, pancreas in 41%, and gastrointestinal tract in 14% of patients with SCLC.[5] Symptoms caused by metastases to

the gastrointestinal tract and abdominal lymph nodes are mostly vague and nonspecific, and antemortem diagnosis is unusual.[51]

During pretreatment staging, metastatic spread to the intra-abdominal organs is observed in 30% to 59% of patients with SCLC (see Table 12–2). Most frequently, the liver, adrenal glands, pancreas, and retroperitoneal and mesenteric lymph nodes are involved.[52-55] Although pathologic proof of these lesions usually is not available, they respond concordantly with lesions in other sites and almost certainly represent metastases.[56]

Pretreatment staging with a radionuclide liver scan, CT scan, peritoneoscopy, or ultrasound with liver biopsy suggests or documents liver metastases in approximately 25% of all patients with SCLC.[6, 57, 58] Hepatic seeding most often occurs in patients with evidence of metastatic disease elsewhere, and in some series, it is statistically associated with bone marrow involvement and with distant metastases in several other organs.[6, 57]

SCLC has a predilection for metastases to the pancreas and constitutes a high percentage of all lung cancer metastases to that organ. The symptoms include jaundice[59] and acute pancreatitis.[60, 61] In one study including 125 patients, 12 had jaundice at diagnosis.[59] In five of these patients, jaundice was due to pancreatic metastases resulting in extrahepatic biliary obstruction, and in seven patients, jaundice was due to diffuse hepatic metastases without extrahepatic obstruction. The frequency of pancreatitis due to metastatic spread is unknown, but in one study, three cases of acute pancreatitis occurred among 40 patients with SCLC at diagnosis or during the course of the disease.[62]

Central Nervous System Metastases

CNS metastases can be categorized as intracranial, leptomeningeal, and spinal.[63]

CNS metastases occur more frequently in SCLC, both at initial presentation and as an area for tumor progression or recurrence compared with the other histologic cell types of lung cancer.[64]

At autopsy, the frequency of CNS metastases is about 50%.[65–67] The brain is the most common site of intracranial metastases, and multiple metastases are more common than solitary types. Once one site of CNS metastatic disease is discovered, the probability of demonstrating metastases at other CNS sites increases greatly.[65, 67] In a compilation by Bunn, 41% of patients had brain metastases, 44% had cerebellar metastases, 16% had pituitary metastases, 19% had leptomeningeal metastases, and 13% had spinal or epidural metastases.[67]

Intracranial Metastases

At the time of diagnosis, the frequency of brain metastases in patients with SCLC varies from 0% to 23%.[66] This wide range reflects variations in the selection of patients, variations in diagnostic scrutiny, and whether or not only symptomatic patients have been evaluated. In a compilation of 11 studies including more than 1600 patients, about 10% of all patients with SCLC had brain metastases at diagnosis, and another 18% (range 6% to 30%) developed clinical signs of brain metastases during therapy.[66]

The risk of brain metastases and the frequency with which they are diagnosed are also influenced by survival time. The probability of developing brain metastases reaches 80% in patients surviving 2 years.[65] Similar results have subsequently been observed by others.[68] In a series from Copenhagen, the cumulative risk reached 50% after survival of 2 years.[66]

The prognostic implications of the presence of brain metastases are disputed. In the study by Hazel and associates,[69] 21 patients were found to have brain metastases as the only site of extensive disease. No deleterious effect on survival was found in this group of patients compared to 100 patients with limited disease, although none of the CNS-limited patients experienced long-term remissions. Others have found CNS metastases to have a poor prognostic influence, with median survival rates ranging from 2 to 6 months despite the use of radiotherapy.[70, 71] A possible explanation is the inclusion of only symptomatic patients in some of the studies.[71] However, in the study by Crane and colleagues no difference in survival was observed between 14 symptomatic and 8 asymptomatic patients presenting with brain metastases.[70]

A longer survival time has been observed in some studies among patients presenting with brain metastases compared with patients who develop this complication during therapy.[69, 71] Two possible explanations are (1) that brain metastases at presentation are effectively treated by chemotherapy[72] or (2) that brain metastases observed at the time of diagnosis are less resistant to radiotherapy than metastases arising during treatment.

In a recent study by Giannone and colleagues[73] including 429 patients, 10% presented with brain metas-

tases. In 18 patients, the brain was the only site of metastatic disease, whereas the remaining 25 patients had at least one additional metastatic site. Median survival of patients with only one site of metastatic disease was 11 months, whereas patients with metastases to additional sites lived for only 5 months. Furthermore, the survival time in patients with brain metastases as the only metastatic site was similar to that in patients with limited disease (13 months).

Leptomeningeal Metastases

Leptomeningeal metastases, or meningeal carcinomatosis, rarely appear at the time of presentation. In a compilation of more than 1500 patients with SCLC, 0.5% had meningeal carcinomatosis at the time of diagnosis, whereas another 5% to 18% of the patients developed this complication during therapy.[66] As with brain metastases the frequency appears to have increased with prolonged patient survival.[65, 74] In two studies, the actuarial probability of developing meningeal carcinomatosis increased rapidly over the first 2 to 3 years to 20% to 25%.[66, 67] As with brain metastases, meningeal carcinomatosis is diagnosed at the time of progressive systemic disease in the majority of patients,[66, 67] and a review of autopsy series revealed that meningeal carcinomatosis was found in 19% of 344 patients with SCLC.[67]

Spinal Metastases

Spinal metastases consist of epidural metastases, vertebral body metastases with collapse, compression and leptomeningeal involvement, and intramedullary metastases.[63]

Lung cancer is the most common primary tumor in patients with spinal metastases, accounting for 19% to 33% of cases.[75, 76] In a consecutive series of 102 patients with lung cancer and metastatic spinal cord compression, 40% of the patients had SCLC, 26% had adenocarcinoma, 18% had squamous cell carcinoma, and 9% had large cell carcinoma.[77] The anatomic level of spinal cord metastases is the thoracic region in more than two-thirds of the patients.[77]

In patients with SCLC, the frequency of spinal cord compression at diagnosis varies from 1% to 3%.[65, 78, 79] Only between 25% and 50% of patients with spinal metastases are diagnosed at the time of initial presentation of the lung cancer.[78, 79] In total, 4% to 9% of SCLC patients develop spinal cord compression during treatment, and an increase in frequency to 18% 2 years after the start of treatment has been described.[65, 67]

Differences in presentation and pathogenesis have been proposed for spinal cord compression arising either early or late in the natural history of SCLC. Eighty-three to one hundred percent of the patients presenting with cord compression have pain in the back, and 93% to 100% have radiographic or scintigraphic evidence of bone destruction.[78, 79] In contrast, patients developing cord compression while on therapy are characterized by a high frequency of prior or simultaneous CNS metastases, back pain in 44% to 47%, and radiographic or scintigraphic signs of bone destruction in only 19% to 28%.[78, 79]

Intramedullary spinal cord metastases are rare both at presentation and during treatment of SCLC, and the prevalence is difficult to determine.[65, 80, 81] In one study, four of 57 patients with SCLC developed intramedullary metastases during therapy,[80] but in many cases, leptomeningeal metastases and intramedullary metastases are present simultaneously.[81]

PARANEOPLASTIC SYNDROMES

The term paraneoplastic syndrome is used to identify a constellation of signs and symptoms secondary to cancer that occurs at a site distant from the tumor or its metastases. Paraneoplastic syndromes can be due to the production of systemic factors such as polypeptides, hormones, growth factors, cytokines, and autoimmunity or immune complex production. Paraneoplastic syndromes are present only in a minority of patients with lung cancer but affect several organs including the hematologic, renal, neurologic, endocrinologic, dermatologic, and gastrointestinal systems.

If a paraneoplastic syndrome occurs in conjunction with SCLC, it is usually present at the time of diagnosis. However, some patients first develop a paraneoplastic syndrome during the course of their disease. It has been estimated that approximately 20% of the patients with SCLC will develop some type of paraneoplastic syndrome during the course of their disease.[82] If one considers the anorexia and the cachexia that usually accompany SCLC as a paraneoplastic syndrome, this percentage probably approaches 100%.[82]

Paraneoplastic Endocrine Syndromes

This review focuses on two major groups of paraneoplastic syndromes: (1) those resulting in endocrinologic and metabolic disturbances and (2) those resulting in neurologic paraneoplastic disturbances.

In patients with SCLC or carcinoids, many peptides producing proven or potential paraneoplastic syndromes are known, as shown in Table 12–4.[83] At present, the function of many of these hormones such as bombesin and physalamin are not known.

Table 12–5 lists the frequency of peptide hormone elevations in the blood of patients with SCLC.[83] The observed frequencies are much higher than those of the clinically recognized paraneoplastic syndromes, because fragments, subunits, or precursors secreted by tumor cells are often biologically inactive.

The most frequent paraneoplastic endocrine syndromes in patients with SCLC include the syndrome of inappropriate antidiuretic hormone production (SIADH), Cushing's syndrome, and nonmetastatic hypercalcemia, which are discussed in more detail in the following.

TABLE 12–4. Mammalian Brain Peptides Producing Proven or Potential Paraneoplastic Syndromes in Small Cell Lung Cancer or Carcinoid Tumors

Neurohypophyseal hormones
  Vasopressin
  Neurophysins
Pituitary peptides
  Adrenocorticotrophic hormone
  β-endorphin
  Melanocyte-stimulating hormone
  Growth hormone
Nonbrain Hormones
  Parathormone
  β-hCG
Gastrointestinal peptides
  Vasoactive intestinal peptide
  Neurotensin
  Glucagon
  Bombesin
  Gastrin-releasing peptide
  Somatostatin
Others
  Calcitonin
  Physalaemin
  Neuron-specific enolase

Modified from Bunn PA, Ridgway ER: Paraneoplastic syndromes. In DeVita VT, Hellmann S, Rosenberg SA (eds): Cancer: Principles and Practice of Oncology. Philadelphia, J.B. Lippincott, 1993, pp 2026–2071.

Syndrome of Inappropriate Antidiuresis

The paraneoplastic endocrine syndrome most frequently associated with SCLC is SIADH. Tumor production of arginine vasopressin (AVP) and antidiuretic hormone (ADH) can result in this syndrome, which consists of hyponatremia, urine inappropriately higher in osmolarity than the plasma, and high urinary sodium concentrations in the face of serum hyponatremia.[83]

The usual presentation of SIADH is hyponatremia. The major clinical symptoms are caused by the water intoxication (i.e., hypo-osmolarity and hyponatremia). These symptoms include altered mental status, confusion, psychotic behavior, lethargy, seizures, and coma.[83] Measurements of blood ADH or urinary ADH excretion have shown significant elevations in 30% to 40% of all patients with SCLC at diagnosis.[84–87] The

TABLE 12–5. Peptide Hormone Elevations in the Blood of Patients with Small Cell Lung Cancer

HORMONE	PATIENTS WITH SIGNIFICANTLY ELEVATED LEVELS (%)
ACTH	30–69
Calcitonin	48–64
ADH	30–40
Parathormone	27
β-hCG	1–32
Growth hormone	0
Gastrin-releasing peptide	74
Neuron-specific enolase	69
Neurophysins	65

Modified from Bunn PA, Ridgway ER: Paraneoplastic syndromes. In DeVita VT, Hellmann S, Rosenberg SA (eds): Cancer: Principles and Practice of Oncology. Philadelphia, J.B. Lippincott, 1993, pp 2026–2071.

frequency of SIADH depends on the methods used for identification of the syndrome.[84, 87] Although the levels of AVP are elevated, clinical manifestations of SIADH are relatively uncommon. Collected series have shown that 4% to 5% of SCLC patients have clinically evident SIADH with hyponatremia at diagnosis, but the frequency of SIADH at presentation varies according to the definition in the different series.[84, 85, 88–91] In one large series, SIADH was present in 11% of the cases with SCLC at diagnosis, but only 27% of patients who fulfilled the diagnostic criteria for SIADH had clinical signs of their hyponatremia with water intoxication.[91] Furthermore, the clinical syndrome does not seem to correlate with the stage of the disease or the metastatic pattern. SIADH is reported to occur in more than 80% of the patients at the time of diagnosis, but it can be seen for the first time also at relapse.[91]

Evidence of SIADH by abnormal water-loading test in SCLC patients indicates that up to 60% of patients have subclinical SIADH.[84–86]

Atrial natriuretic peptide (ANP) has also a potent natriuretic activity, and elevated plasma levels have been demonstrated in patients with SIADH.[92] Kamoi and associates described a patient with SCLC and hyponatremia who had sustained high plasma levels of ANP with normal levels of ADH, suggesting that ANP produced the hyponatremia.[93] Examination of the tumor tissue showed no tumor secretion of ANP or ADH, indicating an increased secretion of ANP by atrial tissue.

Bliss and colleagues have evaluated tumor and tumor cell lines from hyponatremic patients with SCLC, where no detectable AVP messenger RNA was present.[94] They found that the tumors produced ANP messenger RNA and immunoreactive ANP.

Recently, significantly elevated levels of ANP and AVP in tumor tissue have also been demonstrated at autopsy in a patient with SCLC.[95]

Cushing's Syndrome

SCLC is the most common tumor associated with ectopic adrenocorticotropic hormone (ACTH) production and approximately 50% of the patients with ectopic ACTH production will have a diagnosis of SCLC.[83, 96]

Clinically, ectopic ACTH syndrome in SCLC includes hypokalemia, hyperglycemia, edema, muscle weakness or atrophy, hypertension, and weight loss.[83] The ectopic Cushing's syndrome in SCLC differs from the classic Cushing's syndrome due to its rapid development and lack of the classic cushingoid features in most cases.[82, 83]

The incidence of ectopic production of ACTH in patients with SCLC varies widely. Like SIADH, the diagnosis depends on the definition.[82, 83] The frequency of significant elevated levels of immunoreactive ACTH in sera of patients with SCLC varies from 24% to 30% depending on the radioimmunoassay used.[83, 86, 88, 97, 98] A much lower percentage of patients have a subclinical form of Cushing's syndrome, and

clinical Cushing's syndrome is only found in 0.4% to 2% of patients with lung cancer of all histologic types.[83] In SCLC, 1% to 5% of the patients have symptoms from ectopic ACTH production at diagnosis or during the course of disease.[88, 90, 99–101] In two recent studies, ectopic Cushing's syndrome with clinical signs of hypercortisolism was observed in 0.8% and 2.4% of 840 and 545 patients, respectively, at the time of diagnosis.[99, 100]

A poor survival time has been previously reported in patients with SCLC and ectopic Cushing's syndrome, but the observations were anecdotal.[88, 90, 101] In the studies by Shepherd and colleagues and Delisle and associates, median survival times were 3.6 and 4.0 months, respectively, for patients with ectopic ACTH production at initial presentation.[99, 100] Furthermore, Dimopoulos and colleagues reported a median survival of only 12 days from commencement of treatment in a series of 11 patients.[102] The reason for the short survival time of patients with SCLC and ectopic Cushing's syndrome is not clear, but infectious complications occurred in all three studies[99, 100, 102] and have also been reported by others.[103]

Two paraneoplastic endocrine syndromes with simultaneously elevated levels of ectopic AVP and ectopic ACTH have been described in a few patients with SCLC.[104]

Hypercalcemia

Hypercalcemia, a common syndrome complicating lung cancer, was observed during the clinical course in 12.5% of patients with mainly squamous cell histology in one large series.[105] In contrast, hypercalcemia is rare in patients with SCLC and, in most series, is reported to occur in less than 3% of patients.[106, 107]

In patients with SCLC, hypercalcemia is nearly always associated with bone or bone marrow metastases.[106–108]

Because hypercalcemia is rare both at the time of diagnosis and during the course of the disease in patients with SCLC, one should raise the question of a non–small cell histology, a combined histology, or concomitant hyperparathyroidism, in case hypercalcemia is present.

Paraneoplastic Neurologic Syndromes

In patients with established cancer, true paraneoplastic syndromes account for only a minority of neurologic problems, and they are diagnosed by exclusion. Most frequent neurologic complications are caused directly by the tumor or its metastases, by endocrine and electrolyte abnormalities, or by spinal or cerebral vascular diseases.[109]

Elrington and colleagues[110] studied the neurologic status of 150 patients presenting with SCLC. Neuromuscular or autonomic deficits, including muscular weakness, and abnormal cardiovascular reflexes, were common and occurred in up to 44% of cases. Furthermore, two patients had myasthenic syndrome, and one had subacute sensory neuropathy, while four patients presented with symptoms from cerebral metastases demonstrated on CT scan of the brain.[110]

In about 50% of patients, the paraneoplastic neurologic symptoms precede the discovery of the cancer. Furthermore, the course of the neurologic paraneoplastic abnormalities is frequently independent of the clinical course of the tumor in contrast to most other paraneoplastic syndromes, even though it has been described that the symptoms disappear if successful antineoplastic treatment is instituted. According to current knowledge, autoimmune mechanisms are involved in these syndromes.[111] The most likely explanation is that the tumor and nerve tissue share common antigens, and the immune response against tumor cell antigens may evoke production of antibodies that cross-react with neuronal antigens.[112]

Numerous neurologic syndromes, or "remote effects," have been described.[83] Table 12–6 shows some of the different syndromes observed in patients with SCLC categorized by area within the nervous system.[109]

Subacute Cerebellar Degeneration

Subacute cerebellar degeneration is characterized by subacute progressive cerebellar failure with ataxia, dysarthria, and hypotonia.[109, 113, 114] Furthermore, dementia is frequent. Anticerebellar antibodies in serum and cerebrospinal fluid have been observed in a patient with SCLC, and remission of the cerebellar dysfunction has been described[113] following pneumonectomy in a patient with SCLC.[114]

Dementia

Dementia is the most common encephalopathy to accompany SCLC.[82] The onset can be acute or chronic and can occur prior to, during, or following treatment. Dementia is often associated with other neurologic abnormalities or pre-existent diseases.

The dementia usually presents as forgetfulness, loss of memory, or confusion. There is little relationship between the prognosis of the dementia and tumor burden, and antineoplastic treatment does not necessarily result in improvement.

Limbic Encephalitis

Limbic encephalitis is characterized by progressive dementia and degenerative changes in the hippocampus and amygdaloid nuclei with uncharacteristic neurologic symptoms.[115, 116] Improvement in symptoms has been described following chemotherapy in a patient with SCLC.[116]

Optic Neuritis and Retinopathy

Optic neuritis is characterized by decreased vision and scotomas, and it is closely related to the visual paraneoplastic syndrome presenting with binocular loss of the vision in patients with SCLC.[117, 118] In patients with retinopathy, there is a specific loss of retinal cells owing to the immune deposits of antibodies shared by the retinal cells and SCLC tumor cells.[118]

Peripheral Nerves

Peripheral neuropathies can be categorized as symmetric sensory peripheral neuropathy that develops late in the course of the disease or acute or subacute severe combined sensorimotor neuropathy with progressive symptoms that often appears before other sign of the neoplasm.[119]

The sensory neuropathy in patients with SCLC is characterized by subacute distal sensory loss and loss of deep tendon reflexes with normal muscle strength. An immunologic mechanism has also been postulated as the cause of this paraneoplastic neurologic syndrome.[120, 121]

Autonomic and Visceral Neuropathy

Autonomic and visceral neuropathy has been especially associated with SCLC.[122, 123] The symptoms include intestinal pseudo-obstruction, gastroparesis, neurogenic bladder, and autonomic insufficiency, especially orthostatic hypotension.

TABLE 12–6. Paraneoplastic Syndromes of the Nervous System in Patients with Small Cell Carcinoma

SYNDROME	CLINICAL FEATURES	REFERENCES
Central Nervous System		
Subacute cerebellar degeneration	Subacute progresssive cerebellar failure	109, 113, 114
Dementia	Acute to slow progressive, but variable presentation	82
Limbic encephalitis	Dementia	115, 116
Optic neuritis/retinopathy	Decreased vision unilaterally or bilaterally	117, 118
Peripheral Nerves		
Sensory neuropathy	Sensory loss including deep tendon reflexes with normal muscle strength	120, 121
Visceral neuropathy	Intestinal pseudo-obstruction, gastroparesis, neurogenic bladder, autonomic insufficiency	122, 123
Muscle and Neuromuscular Function		
Myasthenic syndrome (Eaton-Lambert syndrome)	Muscle weakness of proximal muscles, dysarthria, ptosis, blurred vision, autonomic dysfunction	124, 125

Myasthenic Syndrome (Eaton-Lambert Syndrome)

The myasthenic syndrome is a rare, paraneoplastic neurologic syndrome, which is strongly associated with lung cancer, especially SCLC.[124] In a study of 50 patients with myasthenic syndrome, carcinoma was detected in 25, of whom 21 had SCLC. SCLC was evident within 2 years of onset of symptoms of the myasthenic syndrome in 20 out of 21 cases, and at 3.8 years, it also appeared in the remaining patient.[124] Muscle weakness and fatigue of proximal muscles, especially the pelvic girdle and thigh, are typical. Other symptoms include dysarthria, blurred vision, ptosis, and autonomic dysfunction.[124] Compared with patients with true myasthenia gravis in whom muscle strength diminishes with exercise, muscle strength improves with exercise, and the response to edrophonium chloride is poor in patients with the myasthenic syndrome.

Lambert reported in his original paper that 6% of all patients with SCLC develop this syndrome.[125] In more recent studies, about 1% of patients with SCLC present with the myasthenic syndrome.[110]

Different studies now indicate that autoimmune mechanisms are involved in the myasthenic syndrome in patients with SCLC.[126, 127] The relationship between response to antitumor therapy; pharmacologic or immunologic treatment, or both; and the activity of the myasthenic syndrome in subjects with SCLC is variable.[55, 128, 129] In the experience of Chalk and associates, 7 of 11 patients with SCLC and myasthenic syndrome who survived for more than 2 months after tumor therapy and treatment for the myasthenic syndrome (plasma exchange, prednisolone) demonstrated substantial neurologic improvement.[129]

SELECTED REFERENCES

Bunn PA, Ridgway ER: Paraneoplastic syndromes. *In* DeVita VT, Hellmann S, Rosenberg SA (eds): Cancer: Principles and Practice of Oncology. 4th Ed. Philadelphia, J.B. Lippincott, 1993, pp 2026–2071.
   An excellent review of all types of paraneoplastic syndromes, especially focusing on lung cancer.
Stahel RA, Ginsberg R, Havemann K, et al: Staging and prognostic factors in small cell lung cancer: A consensus report. *In* Hansen HH, Kristjansen PEG (eds): Management of Small Cell Lung Cancer: Third IASLC Workshop on Small Cell Lung Cancer. Amsterdam, Elsevier, 1989, pp 1–8.
   An international consensus report describing the present staging system of SCLC, including recommendations for staging procedures in clinical practice and clinical trials. In addition, the impact of histologic subclassification is given together with a summary of prognostic factors in SCLC.

REFERENCES

1. Ledermann JA: Extrapulmonary small cell carcinoma. Postgrad Med J 68:79, 1992.
2. Levenson RM, Ihde DC, Matthews MJ, et al: Small cell carcinoma presenting as an extrapulmonary neoplasm: Sites of origin and response to chemotherapy. J Natl Cancer Inst 67:607, 1981.
3. Remick SC, Ruckdeschel JC: Extrapulmonary and pulmonary small-cell carcinoma: Tumor biology, therapy, and outcome. Med Pediatr Oncol 20:89, 1992.
4. Matthews MJ, Kanhouwa S, Pickren J, et al: Frequency of residual and metastatic tumor in patients undergoing curative surgical resection for lung cancer. Cancer Chemother Rep 4:63, 1973.
5. Matthews MJ: Problems in morphology and behavior of bronchopulmonary malignant disease. *In* Israel L, Chahinian AP (eds): Lung Cancer: Natural History, Prognosis, and Therapy. New York, Academic Press, 1976, pp 23–62.
6. Ihde DC: Staging evaluation and prognostic factors in small-cell lung cancer. *In* Aisner J (ed): Contemporary Issues in Clinical Oncology: Lung Cancer. New York, Churchill Livingstone, 1985, pp 241–268.
7. Stahel RA, Ginsberg R, Havemann K, et al: Staging and prognostic factors in small cell lung cancer: A consensus report. *In* Hansen HH, Kristjansen PEG (eds): Management of Small Cell Lung Cancer: Third IASLC Workshop on Small Cell Lung Cancer. Amsterdam, Elsevier, 1989, pp 1–8.
8. Feinstein AR, Sosin DM, Wells CK: The Will Rogers phenomenon: Stage migration and new diagnostic techniques as a source of misleading statistics for survival in cancer. N Engl J Med 312:1604, 1985.
9. Ihde DC, Hansen HH: Staging procedures and prognostic factors in small cell lung cancer. *In* Greco FA, Oldham RK, Bunn PA (eds): Small Cell Lung Cancer. New York, Grune & Stratton, 1981, pp 261–283.
10. Lassen U, Østerlind K, Hansen M, et al: Long term survival in small-cell lung cancer: Posttreatment characteristics in patients surviving five to 18 + years. Proc Am Soc Clin Oncol 12:326, 1993.
11. Ihde DC, Makuch RW, Carney DN, et al: Prognostic implications of stage of disease and sites of metastases in patients with small cell carcinoma of the lung treated with intensive combination chemotherapy. Am Rev Respir Dis 123:500, 1981.
12. Livingston RB, Trauth LJ, Greenstreet RL: Small cell carcinoma: Clinical manifestations and behavior with treatment. *In* Greco FA, Oldham RK, Bunn PA (eds): Small Cell Lung Cancer. New York, Grune & Stratton, 1981, pp 285–300.
13. Mountain CF, Carr DT, Anderson WAD: A system for the clinical staging of lung cancer. AJR Am J Roentgenol 120:130, 1974.
14. Zelen M: Keynote address on biostatistics and data retrieval. Cancer Chemother Rep 4:31, 1973.
15. Fox W, Scadding JG: Medical research council comparative trial of surgery and radiotherapy for primary treatment of small-celled or oat-celled carcinoma of bronchus. Lancet ii:63, 1973.
16. Hainau B, Dombernowsky P, Hansen HH, et al: Cell proliferation and histologic classification of bronchogenic carcinoma. J Natl Cancer Inst 59:1113, 1977.
17. Shackney SE, Straus MJ, Bunn PA: The growth characteristics of small cell carcinoma of the lung. *In* Greco AF, Oldham RK, Bunn PA (eds): Small Cell Lung Cancer. New York, Grune & Stratton, 1981, pp 225–234.
18. Brigham BA, Bunn PA, Minna JD, et al: Growth rates of small cell bronchogenic carcinomas. Cancer 42:2880, 1978.
19. Handelsman H: The treatment of lung cancer: Perspectives and critique. J Surg Oncol 9:443, 1977.
20. Garland LH, Coulson W, Wollin E: The rate of growth and apparent duration of untreated primary bronchial carcinoma. Cancer 16:694, 1963.
21. Hyde L, Yee J, Wilson R, et al: Cell type and the natural history of lung cancer. JAMA 5:140, 1965.
22. Elmendorff HV: Die lebenserwartung von patienten mit inoperablem carcinom. Zeitschrift für Krebsforschung 71:289, 1968.
23. Roswit B, Patno ME, Rapp R, et al: The survival of patients with inoperable lung cancer: a large-scale randomized study of radiation therapy versus placebo. Radiology 90:688, 1968.
24. Wolf J, Patno ME, Roswit B, et al: Controlled study of survival of patients with clinically inoperable lung cancer treated with radiation therapy. Am J Med 40:360, 1966.

25. Green RA, Humphrey E, Close H, et al: Alkylating agents in bronchogenic carcinoma. Am J Med 46:516, 1969.
26. Hyde L, Wolf J, McCracken S, et al: Natural course of inoperable lung cancer. Chest 64:309, 1973.
27. Kato Y, Ferguson TB, Bennett DE, et al: Oat cell carcinoma of the lung. Cancer 23:517, 1969.
28. Green N, Kurohara SS, George FW III, et al: The biologic behavior of lung cancer according to histologic type. Radiol Clin Biol 41:160, 1972.
29. Huhti E, Sutinen S, Reinilä A, et al: Lung cancer in a defined geograhical area: History and histological types. Thorax 35:660, 1980.
30. Chute CG, Greenberg ER, Baron J, et al: Presenting conditions of 1539 population-based lung cancer patients by cell type and stage in New Hampshire and Vermont. Cancer 56:2107, 1985.
31. Cohen MH, Matthews MJ: Small cell bronchogenic carcinoma: A distinct clinicopathologic entity. Semin Oncol 5:234, 1978.
32. Byrd RB, Carr DT, Miller WE, et al: Radiographic abnormalities in carcinoma of the lung as related to histological cell type. Thorax 24:573, 1969.
33. Miller WE: Roentgenographic manifestations of lung cancer. In Strauss MJ (ed): Lung Cancer: Clinical Diagnosis and Treatment. New York, Grune & Stratton, 1977, pp 129–136.
34. Kreisman H, Wolkove N, Quoix E: Small cell lung cancer presenting as a solitary pulmonary nodule. Chest 101:225, 1992.
35. Quoix E, Fraser R, Wolkove N, et al: Small cell lung cancer presenting as a solitary pulmonary nodule. Cancer 66:577, 1990.
36. Hansen SW, Aabo K, Østerlind K: Lung abscess in small cell carcinoma of the lung during chemotherapy and corticosteroids: An analysis of 276 consecutive patients. Eur J Respir Dis 68:7, 1986.
37. Chaudhuri MR: Primary pulmonary cavitating carcinomas. Thorax 28:354, 1973.
38. Cohen MH: Signs and symptoms of bronchogenic carcinoma. In Strauss MJ (ed): Lung Cancer: Clinical Diagnosis and Treatment. New York, Grune & Stratton, 1977, pp 85–94.
39. Martini N, Wittes RE, Hilaris BS, et al: Oat cell carcinoma of the lung. Clin Bull 5:144, 1975.
40. Tandon RK: The significance of pleural effusions associated with bronchial carcinoma. Br J Dis Chest 60:49, 1966.
41. Pearlberg JL, Sandler MA, Lewis JW, et al: Small-cell bronchogenic carcinoma: CT evaluation. AJR Am J Roentgenol 150:265, 1988.
42. Livingston RB, McCracken JD, Trauth CJ, et al: Isolated pleural effusion in small cell lung carcinoma: Favorable prognosis. Chest 81:208, 1982.
43. Bezwoda WR, Lewis D, Livini N: Bone marrow involvement in anaplastic small cell lung cancer: Diagnosis, hematologic features, and prognostic implications. Cancer 58:1762, 1986.
44. Hirsch F, Hansen HH, Dombernowsky P, et al: Bone-marrow examination in the staging of small-cell anaplastic carcinoma of the lung with special reference to subtyping. Cancer 39:2563, 1977.
45. Hirsch FR, Hansen HH, Hainau B: Bilateral bone-marrow examinations in small-cell anaplastic carcinoma of the lung. Acta Pathol Microbiol Scand Sect A 87:59, 1979.
46. Østerlind K, Andersen PK: Prognostic factors in small cell lung cancer: Multivariate model based on 778 patients treated with chemotherapy with or without irradiation. Cancer Res 46:4189, 1986.
47. Campling B, Quirt I, DeBoer G, et al: Is bone marrow examination in small-cell lung cancer really necessary? Ann Intern Med 105:508, 1986.
48. Ejeckam GC, Sogbein SK, McLeish WA: Carcinocythemia due to metastatic oat-cell carcinoma of the lung. Can Med Assoc J 120:336, 1979.
49. Hansen HH: Bone metastases in lung cancer: A clinical study in 200 consecutive patients with bronchogenic carcinoma and its therapeutic implications for small cell carcinoma. Copenhagen, Munksgaard, 1974, pp 1–225.
50. Napoli LD, Hansen HH, Muggia FM, et al: The incidence of osseous involvment in lung cancer with special reference to the development of osteoblastic changes. Radiology 108:17, 1973.
51. Doyle LA, Aisner J: Clinical presentation of lung cancer. In Roth JA, Ruckdeschel JC, Weisenburger TH (eds): Thoracic Oncology. Philadelphia, W.B. Saunders, 1989, pp 52–76.
52. Harper PG, Houang M, Spiro SG, et al: Computerized axial tomography in the pretreatment assessment of small-cell carcinoma of the bronchus. Cancer 47:1775, 1981.
53. Mirvis SE, Whitley NO, Aisner J, et al: Abdominal CT in the staging of small-cell carcinoma of the lung: Incidence of metastases and effect on prognosis. AJR Am J Roentgenol 148:845, 1987.
54. Abrams J, Doyle LA, Aisner J: Staging, prognostic factors, and special considerations in small cell lung cancer. Semin Oncol 15:261, 1988.
55. Jenkyn LR, Brooks PL, Forcier RJ, et al: Remission of the Lambert-Eaton syndrome and small cell anaplastic carcinoma of the lung induced by chemotherapy and radiotherapy. Cancer 46:1123, 1980.
56. Ihde DC, Dunnick NR, Johnston-Early A, et al: Abdominal computed tomography in small cell lung cancer: Assessment of extent of disease and response to therapy. Cancer 49:1485, 1982.
57. Dombernowsky P, Hirsch F, Hansen HH, et al: Peritoneoscopy in the staging of 190 patients with small-cell anaplastic carcinoma of the lung with special reference to subtyping. Cancer 41:2008, 1978.
58. Hansen SW, Jensen F, Pedersen NT, et al: Detection of liver metastases in small-cell lung cancer: A comparison of peritoneoscopy with liver biopsy and ultrasonography with fine-needle aspiration. J Clin Oncol 5:255, 1987.
59. Johnson DH, Hainsworth JD, Greco FA: Extrahepatic biliary obstruction caused by small-cell lung cancer. Ann Intern Med 102:487, 1985.
60. Stewart KC, Dickout WJ, Urschel JD: Metastasis-induced acute pancreatitis as the initial manifestation of bronchogenic carcinoma. Chest 104:98, 1993.
61. Chowhan NM, Madajewicz S: Management of metastases-induced acute pancreatitis in small cell carcinoma of the lung. Cancer 65:1445, 1990.
62. Yeung K, Haidak DJ, Brown JA, et al: Metastasis-induced acute pancreatitis in small cell bronchogenic carcinoma. Arch Intern Med 139:552, 1979.
63. Posner JB: Management of central nervous system metastases. Semin Oncol 4:81, 1977.
64. Newman SJ, Hansen HH: Frequency, diagnosis, and treatment of brain metastases in 247 consecutive patients with bronchogenic carcinoma. Cancer 33:492, 1974.
65. Nugent JL, Bunn PA, Matthews MJ, et al: CNS metastases in small cell bronchogenic carcinoma. Cancer 44:1885, 1979.
66. Pedersen AG: Diagnostic procedures in the detection of CNS metastases from small cell lung cancer. In Hansen HH (ed): Lung Cancer: Basic and Clinical Aspects. Boston, Martinus Nijhoff, 1986, pp 153–183.
67. Bunn PA, Rosen ST: Central nervous system manifestations of small cell lung cancer. In Aisner J (ed): Contemporary Issues in Clinical Oncology: Lung Cancer. New York, Churchill Livingstone, 1985, pp 287–305.
68. Maurer LH, Tulloh M, Weiss RB, et al: A randomized combined modality trial in small cell carcinoma of the lung: Comparison of combination chemotherapy-radiation therapy versus cyclophosphamide-radiation therapy effects of maintenance chemotherapy and prophylactic whole brain irradiation. Cancer 45:30, 1980.
69. Hazel GA, Scott M, Eagan RT: The effect of CNS metastases on the survival of patients with small cell cancer of the lung. Cancer 51:933, 1983.
70. Crane JM, Nelson MJ, Ihde DC, et al: A comparison of computed tomography and radionuclide scanning for detection of brain metastases in small cell lung cancer. J Clin Oncol 2:1017, 1984.
71. Hirsch FR, Paulson OB, Hansen HH, et al: Intracranial metastases in small cell carcinoma of the lung: Prognostic aspects. Cancer 51:529, 1983.
72. Kristensen CA, Kristjansen PEG, Hansen HH: Systemic chemotherapy of brain metastases from small-cell lung cancer: A review. J Clin Oncol 10:1498–1502, 1992.
73. Giannone L, Johnson DH, Hande KR, et al: Favorable prognosis of brain metastases in small cell lung cancer. Ann Intern Med 106:386, 1987.

74. Rosen ST, Aisner J, Makuch RW, et al: Carcinomatous lepto-meningitis in small cell lung cancer: A clinicopathologic review of the National Cancer Institute experience. Medicine 61:45, 1982.

75. Sørensen PS, Børgesen SE, Rohde K, et al: Metastatic epidural spinal cord compression: Results of treatment and survival. Cancer 65:1502, 1990.

76. Stark RJ, Henson RA, Evans SJW: Spinal metastases: A retrospective survey from a general hospital. Brain 105:189, 1982.

77. Bach F, Agerlin N, Sørensen JB, et al: Metastatic spinal cord compression secondary to lung cancer. J Clin Oncol 10:1781, 1992.

78. Pedersen AG, Bach F, Melgaard B: Frequency, diagnosis, and prognosis of spinal cord compression in small cell bronchogenic carcinoma. Cancer 55:1818, 1985.

79. Goldman JM, Ash CM, Souhami RL, et al: Spinal cord compression in small cell lung cancer: A retrospective study of 610 patients. Br J Cancer 59:591, 1989.

80. Murphy KC, Feld R, Evans WK, et al: Intramedullary spinal cord metastases from small cell carcinoma of the lung. J Clin Oncol 1:99, 1983.

81. Weissman DE, Grossman SA: Simultaneous leptomeningeal and intramedullary spinal metastases in small cell lung carcinoma. Med Pediatr Oncol 14:54, 1986.

82. Goodman GE, Livingston RB: Small cell lung cancer. Curr Probl Cancer 13:1–54, 1989.

83. Bunn PA, Ridgway ER: Paraneoplastic syndromes. In DeVita VT, Hellmann S, Rosenberg SA (eds): Cancer: Principles and Practice of Oncology. 4th. Ed. Philadelphia, J.B. Lippincott, 1993, pp 2026–2071.

84. von Rohr A, Cerny T, Joss RA, et al: Das syndrom der inadäquaten ADH-sekretion (SIADH) beim kleinzelligen bronchuskarzinom. Schweiz Med Wochenschr 121:1271, 1991.

85. Comis RL, Miller M, Ginsberg SJ: Abnormalities in water homeostasis in small cell anaplastic lung cancer. Cancer 45:2414, 1980.

86. Hansen M, Hansen HH, Hirsch FR, et al: Hormonal polypeptides and amine metabolites in small cell carcinoma of the lung, with special reference to stage and subtypes. Cancer 45:1432, 1980.

87. Hansen M: Clinical implications of ectopic hormone production in small cell carcinoma of the lung. Dan Med Bull 28:221, 1981.

88. Bondy PK, Gilby ED: Endocrine function in small cell undifferentiated carcinoma of the lung. Cancer 50:2147, 1982.

89. Hainsworth JD, Workman R, Greco FA: Management of the syndrome of inappropriate antidiuretic hormone secretion in small cell lung cancer. Cancer 51:161, 1983.

90. Lokich JJ: The frequency and clinical biology of the ectopic hormone syndromes of small cell carcinoma. Cancer 50:2111, 1982.

91. List AF, Hainsworth JD, Davis BW, et al: The syndrome of inappropriate secretion of antidiuretic hormone (SIADH) in small-cell lung cancer. J Clin Oncol 4:1191, 1986.

92. Cogan E, DeGiève MF, Philpart I, et al: High plasma levels of atrial natriuretic factor in SIADH. N Engl J Med 314:1258, 1986.

93. Kamoi K, Ebe T, Hasegawa A, et al: Hyponatremia in small cell lung cancer: Mechanisms not involving inappropriate ADH secretion. Cancer 60:1089, 1987.

94. Bliss DP, Battey JF, Linnoila RI, et al: Expression of the atrial natriuretic factor gene in small cell lung cancer tumors and tumor cell lines. J Natl Cancer Inst 82:305, 1990.

95. Shimizu K, Nakano S, Nakano Y, et al: Ectopic atrial natriuretic peptide production in small cell lung cancer with the syndrome of inappropriate antidiuretic hormone secretion. Cancer 68:2284, 1991.

96. White A, Clark AJL, Stewart MF: The synthesis of ACTH and related peptides by tumors. Bailleres Clin Endocrinol Metab 4:1, 1990.

97. Hansen M, Pedersen AG: Tumor markers in patients with lung cancer. Chest 89:219S, 1986.

98. Gropp C, Havemann K, Scheuer A: Ectopic hormones in lung cancer patients at diagnosis and during therapy. Cancer 46:347, 1980.

99. Delisle L, Boyer MJ, Warr D, et al: Ectopic corticotropin syndrome and small-cell carcinoma of the lung: Clinical features, outcome and complications. Arch Intern Med 153:746, 1993.

100. Shepherd FA, Laskey J, Evans WK: Cushing's syndrome associated with ectopic corticotropin production and small-cell lung cancer. J Clin Oncol 10:21, 1992.

101. Abeloff MD, Trump DL, Baylin SB: Ectopic adrenocorticotrophic (ACTH) syndrome and small cell carcinoma of the lung—assessment of clinical implications in patients on combination chemotherapy. Cancer 48:1082, 1981.

102. Dimopoulos MA, Fernandez JF, Samaan NA, et al: Paraneoplastic Cushing's syndrome as an adverse prognostic factor in patients who die early with small cell lung cancer. Cancer 69:66, 1992.

103. Sieber SC, Dandurand R, Gelfman N, et al: Three opportunistic infections associated with ectopic corticotropin syndrome. Arch Intern Med 149:2589, 1989.

104. Pierce ST, Metcalfe M, Banks ER, et al.: Small cell carcinoma with two paraendocrine syndromes. Cancer 69:2258, 1992.

105. Bender RA, Hansen H: Hypercalcemia in bronchogenic carcinoma: A prospective study of 200 patients. Ann Intern Med 80:205, 1974.

106. Hayward ML, Howell DA, O'Donnell JF, et al: Hypercalcemia complicating small-cell carcinoma. Cancer 48:1643, 1981.

107. Stuart-Harris R, Ahern V, Danks JA, et al: Hypercalcaemia in small cell lung cancer: Report of a case associated with parathyroid hormone–related protein (PTHrP). Eur J Cancer 29A:1601, 1993.

108. Yoshimoto K, Yamasaki R, Sakai H, et al: Ectopic production of parathyroid hormone by small cell lung cancer in a patient with hypercalcemia. J Clin Endocrinol Metab 68:976, 1989.

109. Patchell RA, Posner JB: Neurologic complications of systemic cancer. Neurol Clin 3:729, 1985.

110. Elrington GM, Murray NMF, Spiro SG, et al: Neurological paraneoplastic syndromes in patients with small cell lung cancer: A prospective survey of 150 patients. J Neurol Neurosurg Psychiatry 54:764, 1991.

111. Kornguth SE: Neuronal proteins and paraneoplastic syndromes. N Engl J Med 321:1607, 1989.

112. Anderson NE: Anti-neuronal antibodies and neurological antineoplastic syndromes. Aust N Z J Med 19:379, 1989.

113. Greenlee JE, Lipton HL: Anticerebellar antibodies in serum and cerebrospinal fluid of a patient with oat cell carcinoma of the lung and paraneoplastic cerebellar degeneration. Ann Neurol 19:82, 1986.

114. Paone JF, Jeyasingham K: Remission of cerebellar dysfunction after pneumonectomy for bronchogenic carcinoma. N Engl J Med 17:156, 1980.

115. Case records of the Massachusetts general hospital. N Engl J Med 319:849, 1988.

116. Brennan LV, Craddock PR: Limbic encephalopathy as a non-metastatic complication of oat cell lung cancer. Am J Med 75:518, 1983.

117. Grunwald GB, Kornguth SE, Towfighi J, et al: Autoimmune basis for visual paraneoplastic syndrome in patients with small cell lung carcinoma: Retinal immune deposits and ablation of retinal ganglion cells. Cancer 60:780, 1987.

118. Thirkill CE, Fitzgerald P, Sergott RC, et al: Cancer-associated retinopathy (CAR syndrome) with antibodies reacting with retinal, optic-nerve, and cancer cells. N Engl J Med 321:1589, 1989.

119. Croft PB, Wilkinson M: The incidence of carcinomatous neuromyopathy in patients with various types of carcinoma. Brain 88:427, 1965.

120. Graus F, Elkon KB, Cordon-Cardo C, et al: Sensory neuronopathy and small cell lung cancer: Antineuronal antibody that also reacts with the tumor. Am J Med 80:45, 1986.

121. Kimmel DW, O'Neill BP, Lennon VA: Subacute sensory neuronopathy associated with small cell lung carcinoma: Diagnosis aided by autoimmune serology. Mayo Clin Proc 63:29, 1988.

122. Chinn JS, Schuffler MD: Paraneoplastic visceral neuropathy as a cause of severe gastrointestinal motor dysfunction. Gastroenterology 95:1279, 1988.

123. Schuffler MD, Baird HW, Fleming CR, et al: Intestinal pseudo-obstruction as the presenting manifestation of small-cell carcinoma of the lung. Ann Intern Med 98:129, 1983.

124. O'Neill JH, Murray NMF, Newsom-Davis J: The Lambert-Eaton myasthenic syndrome. Brain 111:577, 1988.

125. Lambert EH, Rooke ED: Myasthenic state and lung cancer. In

Brain WR, Norris FH (eds): The remote effects of cancer on the nervous system. New York, Grune & Stratton, 1965, pp 67–80.

126. Vincent A, Lang B, Newsom-Davis J: Autoimmunity to the voltage-gated calcium channel underlies the Lambert-Eaton myastenic syndrome, a paraneoplastic disorder. Trends Neurosci 12:496, 1989.

127. Morris CS, Esiri MM, Marx A, et al: Immunocytochemical characteristics of small cell lung carcinoma associated with the Lambert-Eaton myasthenic syndrome. Am J Pathol 140:839, 1992.

128. Clamon GH, Evans WK, Shepherd FA, et al: Myasthenic syndrome and small cell cancer of the lung. Arch Intern Med 144:999, 1984.

129. Chalk CH, Murray NMF, Newsom-Davis J, et al: Response of the Lambert-Eaton myasthenic syndrome to treatment of associated small-cell lung carcinoma. Neurology 40:1552, 1990.

13 TREATMENT OF SMALL CELL LUNG CANCER

David H. Johnson and Donald R. Eisert

Small cell lung cancer (SCLC) is a common malignancy seen almost exclusively in smokers.[1–5] Unlike non–small cell lung cancer, SCLC is usually disseminated at diagnosis and is therefore not amenable to cure with surgery or thoracic radiotherapy (TRT) alone.[1–3, 6] Indeed, if left untreated, SCLC is a rapidly fatal process, with few patients surviving beyond 4 to 6 months. With the recognition that this malignancy is chemoresponsive, considerable improvement in survival has been achieved during the past three decades. At present, virtually all patients are treated with some form of chemotherapy with or without TRT depending on the extent of disease at the time of diagnosis. Surgical resection largely has been abandoned but still may play a role in the management of this malignancy in rare circumstances.[7, 8] This chapter reviews current concepts in the management of SCLC.

CHEMOTHERAPY

Single Agents

The beneficial effect of chemotherapy in SCLC was firmly established in a Veterans' Administration trial in which single agent cyclophosphamide was demonstrated to significantly prolong survival.[9] Subsequently, numerous antineoplastic agents were shown to possess activity against SCLC. Effective single agents are defined by their ability to effect an objective response rate of ≥30% in previously untreated patients.[10] Active agents include nitrogen mustard, doxorubicin, methotrexate, ifosfamide, etoposide, teniposide, vincristine, vindesine, nitrosureas, cisplatin, and its analogue carboplatin.[4, 11, 12] Several new agents with unique mechanisms of action recently have been shown to possess activity against SCLC, including paclitaxel (Taxol)[13] and docetaxel (Taxotere), as well as the camptothecin derivatives topotecan and CPT-11.[14, 15] Despite the large number of active agents, SCLC is rarely treated with single agents.

Combination Chemotherapy

Combination chemotherapy is capable of effecting high objective response rates in SCLC and is associated with substantial survival benefit.[6] The superiority of combination therapy over single agents is well established.[16–18] Furthermore, the simultaneous administration of multiple agents is superior to the sequential administration of the same drugs.[17] Although there are many different drug combinations that yield excellent response rates and survival results against SCLC, direct comparisons of so-called standard regimens are rare, and no specific regimen has been found to be ideal for all patients. Consequently, the choice of induction regimen is usually dictated by the medical condition of the patient and, to some degree, by whether or not thoracic radiotherapy is to be used.[19]

With virtually any standard combination chemotherapy regimen, objective response rates range from 75% to 85% irrespective of initial stage, with complete responses occurring more frequently in patients with limited disease compared with those with extensive disease.[1–3, 6] Tumor regression typically occurs rapidly after one or two courses of treatment yielding effective palliation of most tumor-related symptoms.[6] Median survival ranges from 8 to 14 months depending on initial stage, while survival beyond 2 years is unusual except in limited disease. In most series, survival at 2 years from diagnosis is approximately 20% to 25% among patients with stage disease and ≤5% in extensive disease.[1–3] The best long-term survival is achieved in patients with limited-stage receiving concurrent TRT.[20, 21]

Although combination chemotherapy is necessary for optimal management of SCLC, there is no consensus as to what constitutes the best regimen or the optimal duration of therapy. Among the regimens listed in Table 13–1, cisplatin plus etoposide has become one of the more commonly used regimens for many reasons. Regimens containing etoposide appear to yield slightly better survival results than nonetoposide regimens, although the survival differences are of modest clinical significance.[22] In the setting of relapsed SCLC, the combination of cisplatin and etoposide is capable of producing objective response rates of equal to or more than 50% in patients who have experienced a recurrence after cyclophosphamide-based therapy.[23, 24] No other drug combination has yielded response rates of this magnitude in a similar setting.[25] Furthermore, in previously untreated patients, cisplatin plus etoposide yields excellent overall response rates and survival results that are equivalent

TABLE 13–1. Standard Chemotherapy Regimens for Small Cell Lung Cancer

CAV:	
Cyclophosphamide	1000 mg/m² IV Day 1
Doxorubicin (Adriamycin)	45–50 mg/m² IV Day 1
Vincristine	1.4 mg/m² IV Day 1 (maximum, 2 mg) Repeat every 3 weeks
CAE:	
Cyclophosphamide	1000 mg/m² IV Day 1
Doxorubicin (Adriamycin)	45 mg/m² IV Day 1
Etoposide	50 mg/m²/day IV Days 1–5 Repeat every 3 weeks
PE:	
Cisplatin	60–80 mg/m² IV Day 1
Etoposide	80–120 mg/m²/day IV, Days 1–3 Repeat every 3 weeks
CAV alternating with PE:	
CAV as above with	
Cisplatin	25 mg/m² IV, Days 1–3
Etoposide	100 mg/m²/day IV, Days 1–3 Repeat every 3 weeks
CBDCA-E:	
Carboplatin	100 mg/m²/day IV Days 1–3
Etoposide	120 mg/m²/day IV Days 1–3 Repeat every 4 weeks

Modified from DeVore RF, Johnson DH: Lung cancer: Chemotherapy. *In* Brain MC, Carbone PP (eds): Current Therapy in Hematology—Oncology. 4th Ed. Philadelphia, B.C. Dekker, Inc., 1992, pp 245–249.

to cyclophosphamide- or doxorubicin-based regimens, albeit with less host-related toxicity.[26–30] Cisplatin and etoposide is particularly well suited for the simultaneous administration of radiotherapy, given its lower incidence of toxicity and the putative radiation-sensitizing effect of both drugs.[31, 32] Thus, for many clinicians, cisplatin plus etoposide has become the de facto standard induction regimen for patients with SCLC.[6, 19]

The optimal duration of induction chemotherapy for SCLC is unknown. In recent clinical trials, treatment duration has ranged from a few weeks to several months.[29, 30] Randomized studies have not established a survival advantage for longer durations of therapy.[33] Furthermore, maintenance chemotherapy does not prolong survival in SCLC (Table 13–2).[34–36] Of note, in a trial conducted by the Southeastern Cancer Study Group (SECSG), patients who achieved an objective response to induction chemotherapy were randomized to no further therapy or two courses of a different non–cross resistant chemotherapy regimen as consolidation treatment.[37] Patients given consolidation

treatment experienced superior median and long-term survival. These data suggest that brief consolidation treatment after maximum response to induction chemotherapy may warrant further study. At present, routine treatment beyond four to six cycles of induction chemotherapy should be avoided because it may result in increased toxicity and can have an adverse impact on the patient's quality of life.[35]

Patients with SCLC often have concomitant cardiac or pulmonary diseases that may preclude the use of certain agents such as cisplatin or ifosfamide, which normally require aggressive hydration for safe administration.[38] In the patient with underlying cardiac disease, carboplatin can be substituted for cisplatin without loss of treatment efficacy in patients with extensive-stage disease.[39–41] Cyclophosphamide-based therapy may be preferred in patients with renal insufficiency given the potential nephrotoxicity of cisplatin and the renal excretion of carboplatin and etoposide.[42, 43]

Complications of standard chemotherapy regimens include myelosuppression in approximately 30% of patients, with documented infections developing in fewer than 5%.[44] Febrile neutropenic episodes occur rarely or frequently depending on the intensity of induction therapy. With standard doses of cisplatin plus etoposide, life-threatening neutropenia develops in no more than 2% to 5% of patients.[28] Cyclophosphamide-based therapy, on the other hand, is associated with a higher incidence of neutropenia.[1, 45] Treatment-related mortality, usually due to sepsis, occurs in fewer than 5% of patients. The incidence of gastrointestinal side effects varies but nausea, emesis, and mucositis are common, especially in combined modality regimens. New supportive care measures such as 5-HT₃ antiemetics and hematopoietic growth factors are available to help minimize or ameliorate many of these complications.[46, 47] The availability of hematopoietic growth factors has influenced the way in which patients and physicians view chemotherapy-induced myelosuppression. However, these agents must be used judiciously because, in some circumstances, they have proved detrimental.[48] Of note, prophylactic antibiotics may be just as efficacious for the prevention of fever during neutropenia as the more expensive hematopoietic growth factors.[49]

Late-developing complications related to chemotherapy also occur and include pulmonary fibrosis, cardiac toxicity, and second malignancies.[44, 50–52] In ad-

TABLE 13–2. Maintenance Chemotherapy

REFERENCE	NUMBER OF PATIENTS	NUMBER OF TREATMENT CYCLES	MAINTENANCE THERAPY	NO MAINTENANCE THERAPY
Bleehen et al[35]	265/497*	6 versus 12	35 week	29 week
Spiro et al[33]	610	4 versus 8	44 week (LD)	44 week (LD)
			40 week (ED)	34 week (ED)
Clarke et al[34]	202	4 versus 14	54 week	52 week
Giaccone et al[121]	434/687*	5 versus 12	39 week	41 week

*Number of patients randomized to maintenance versus no maintenance chemotherapy out of total number entered.
LD = Limited disease; ED = extensive disease.

TABLE 13–3. Alternating Non–Cross Resistant Chemotherapy Trials

		MEDIAN SURVIVAL (MONTHS)			
REFERENCE	**NUMBER OF PATIENTS**	**CAV (%)**	**PE (%)**	**CAV/PE (%)**	**P VALUE**
Evans et al[58]	289	8.0	—	9.6	.03
Fukuoka et al[29]	142	8.7	8.3	9.0	.898
Roth et al[30]	437	8.6	8.3	8.1	.425

CAV = cyclophosphamide, doxorubicin (Adriamycin), vincristine; PE = cisplatin, etoposide; CAV/PE = CAV alternating with PE.

dition, there is a disturbing incidence of neurotoxicities exhibited as mild dementia, ataxia, and other neurologic abnormalities primarily in patients who received prophylactic cranial irradiation that may be related to the interaction of certain agents and irradiation.[53, 54] The relationship of neurotoxicity to cranial irradiation is discussed later.

Alternating Non–Cross Resistant Chemotherapy

The development of drug resistance is the principal reason for the failure of existing chemotherapy regimens to effectively eradicate chemoresponsive neoplasms such as SCLC.[55] One strategy employed to prevent or delay the emergence of drug-resistant cells is to simultaneously administer multiple active agents, each at its individual optimal dose.[56, 57] However, owing to an overlap in toxicity profiles, it is often impossible to use combinations of active agents at their individual optimum dose level without incurring unacceptable host toxicity. Using mathematical modeling, Goldie and Coldman have suggested that alternation of two chemotherapy regimens of relatively comparable efficacy could potentially lessen host toxicity while minimizing the development of drug resistance.[56, 57] The strategy of administering non–cross resistant regimens on an alternating schedule has received extensive clinical testing during the past decade with disappointing results (Table 13–3).[29, 30, 58–60]

Canadian investigators observed an improved median survival using a regimen of cyclophosphamide, doxorubicin (Adriamycin), and vincristine (CAV) alternating with cisplatin and etoposide compared with CAV alone in extensive-stage SCLC.[58] However, these results were not confirmed in two subsequent randomized trials.[29, 30] In the latter trials, cisplatin plus etoposide alone was as effective as the alternating regimen in patients with extensive stage disease. In

one study, alternating non–cross-resistant chemotherapy yielded a statistically superior survival in patients with limited disease.[29] However, the latter data are at variance with other cooperative group trials, leaving the merit of this strategy in limited disease SCLC in doubt.[59, 60]

The failure of these efforts to substantiate the superiority of the alternating non–cross resistant chemotherapy strategy is most likely due to the lack of true non–cross resistance for the regimens employed.[29, 30] To be effective, it is necessary for the regimens to be of relatively comparable efficacy, and each must be capable of salvaging a reasonable percentage of patients who fail the alternative regimen.[55, 57] This is clearly not the case with CAV and cisplatin plus etoposide (Table 13–4). Thus, an adequate test of the Goldie-Coldman hypothesis awaits the development of regimens that are more nearly non–cross resistant.

Dose Escalation

Yet another means of overcoming drug resistance is to escalate the dose of an antineoplastic drug. Both in preclinical trials and in clinical studies, dose escalation has proved to be an effective method of increasing the rates of complete remission and cures in patients with selected chemoresponsive neoplasms.[61, 62] An early trial comparing standard doses of cyclophosphamide, methotrexate, and lomustine with higher doses of these agents seemed to validate this approach in SCLC.[63] Subsequent randomized trials, however, failed to substantiate the utility of further dose escalation, at least to the level possible in an outpatient setting.[28, 45] For example, the SECSG compared high dose CAV induction therapy with standard dose CAV, and while a superior complete response (CR) rate was observed, there was no improvement in median survival (Table 13–5).[45] Furthermore, life-threatening toxicities were more common with high-dose CAV. Similar results were reported by a Canadian group.[64] More recently, standard-dose cisplatin plus etoposide has been prospectively compared with high-dose cisplatin plus etoposide.[28] As expected, myelosuppression was greater with the more intensive regimen, but there was no difference in overall response rates or median or 1-year survival rates.

Even greater dose escalation has been attempted in nonrandomized trials without substantial improvement in survival despite impressive complete and

TABLE 13–4. Response to Crossover Chemotherapy in Alternating Non–Cross Resistant Chemotherapy Trials

REFERENCE	CAV TO PE	PE TO CAV	P VALUE
Fukuoka et al[29]	9/39 (23%)	1/13 (8%)	.21
Roth et al[30]	13/59 (22%)	5/41 (12%)	.15

CAV = cyclophosphamide, doxorubicin (Adriamycin), vincristine; PE = cisplatin, etoposide; CAV/PE = CAV alternating with PE.

TABLE 13–5. Randomized Dose Escalation Trials

REFERENCE	CHEMOTHERAPY	COMPLETE RESPONSE (%)	OVERALL RESPONSE (%)	MEDIAN SURVIVAL	P VALUE
Johnson et al[45]	HD-CAV	22	63	29.3 week	>.05
	SD-CAV	12	53	34.7 week	
Figueredo et al[64]	HD-CAV	21	71	ns	.968
	SD-CAV	22	61	ns	
Ihde et al[28]	HD-PE	23	86	11.4 month	.68
	SD-PE	22	83	10.7 month	

HD = High-dose; SD = standard-dose; CAV = cyclophosphamide, doxorubicin (Adriamycin), vincristine; PE = cisplatin, etoposide.

overall response rates.[65–70] Some of these trials have employed autologous bone marrow transplantation to facilitate restoration of hematopoiesis.[65, 67] Because widespread dissemination is commonplace, tumor contamination of bone marrow is a distinct possibility that limits the usefulness of autologous marrow rescue. Newer methods of marrow protection may permit future studies of dose escalation, but available data do not suggest that this will be a productive strategy to pursue.

Collectively, the available data indicate that dose escalation beyond that which produces modest hematologic toxicity is *not* beneficial to the patient with SCLC. Accordingly, the most effective regimen with the least amount of myelosuppression should be used in patients treated in a nonstudy setting.

Weekly Chemotherapy

Although dose escalation per se has not proved beneficial in the management of SCLC, the concept of dose intensity remains appealing.[71] One method of increasing the exposure of malignant cells to an increased amount of antineoplastic agent is to shorten the interval between cycles of treatment.[72] Maintenance of dose intensity—the amount of drug delivered per unit time—is thought to be a crucial aspect of successful management of chemoresponsive neoplasms[71] and may be important in SCLC.

Drug resistance in SCLC is either inherently present or develops rapidly during the course of treatment, possibly even as a consequence of therapy.[55] Clinically, drug resistance is exhibited by the rapid regrowth of SCLC in virtually every case shortly after discontinu-

ing treatment or, in some cases, during therapy.[1] During planned breaks in chemotherapy administration, which is needed to allow recovery from toxicity by normal tissues, tumor cells can regrow and mutation to drug resistance can occur. Frequent administration of chemotherapy without breaks for toxicity may minimize the development of chemoresistance by limiting tumor regrowth between cycles of therapy. To overcome this potential cause of treatment failure, a strategy of rapid chemotherapy administration has undergone extensive testing in recent years.[73–79]

Typical of these dose-intensity trials is a Southwest Oncology Group (SWOG) study in which SCLC patients were treated with doxorubicin (40 mg/m^2) and cyclophosphamide (400 mg/m^2) in week 1, methotrexate (200 mg/m^2) and vincristine (1.4 mg/m^2) in week 2, etoposide (75 mg/m^2/day $\times$ 3 days) and cisplatin (60 mg/m^2) in week 3 followed by vincristine alone in week 4.[74] Median survival of patients with limited disease was approximately 17 months, whereas patients with extensive disease survived a median of 11.4 months (Table 13–6). Although life-threatening toxicities were common, the majority of patients received at least 80% of the planned drug dosages. In a similar trial, Miles and coworkers alternated cisplatin (50 mg/m^2) and etoposide (75 mg/m^2/day $\times$ 2 days) with ifosfamide (2 g/m^2) and doxorubicin (25 mg/m^2) on a weekly basis for 12 consecutive weeks in patients with SCLC.[75] The overall response rate exceeded 90% and median survivals were 58 and 42 weeks in patients with limited-stage and extensive disease, respectively (Table 13–6).

Impressive results also have been reported by Canadian investigators who administered cisplatin (25 mg/m^2) for 9 consecutive weeks along with vincris-

TABLE 13–6. Weekly Chemotherapy Trials

REFERENCE	CHEMOTHERAPY	DURATION	PATIENT NUMBER	OVERALL RESPONSE (%)	MEDIAN SURVIVAL
Taylor et al[74]	CAVEPM	16 weeks	34 LD	82	16.6 months
			42 ED	81	11.4 months
Miles et al[75]	PEIA	12 weeks	45 LD	91	58 weeks
			25 ED	92	42 weeks
Murray et al[122]	CODE	9–12 weeks	—	—	—
			48 ED	94	61 weeks

CAVEPM = cyclophosphamide, doxorubicin (Adriamycin), vincristine, etoposide, cisplatin, methotrexate; PEIA = cisplatin, etoposide, ifosfamide, doxorubicin; CODE = cisplatin, vincristine (Oncovin), doxorubicin, etoposide; LD = limited disease; ED = extensive disease.

TABLE 13–7. Randomized Trials of Weekly Chemotherapy

REFERENCE	CHEMOTHERAPY	NUMBER OF PATIENTS	OVERALL RESPONSE	MEDIAN SURVIVAL	P VALUE
Miles et al[80]	PE/CAV every 3 weeks	311	78%	44 weeks	NS
	PEIA weekly		81%	46 weeks	
Sculier et al[81]	CAE every 3 weeks	101	62%	43 weeks	.34
	AECPVnVM weekly	98	69%	49 weeks	

PE/CAV = cisplatin plus etoposide alternating with cyclophosphamide, doxorubicin (Adriamycin), vincristine; PEIA = cisplatin, etoposide, ifosfamide, doxorubicin; CAE = cyclophosphamide, doxorubicin, etoposide; AECPVnVM = doxorubicin, etoposide, cyclophosphamide, cisplatin, vindesine, vincristine, methotrexate.

tine (1 mg/m² weeks 1, 2, 4, 6, and 8) plus doxorubicin (25 mg/m²) and etoposide (80 mg/m²/day × 3 days) during weeks 1, 3, 5, 7, and 9 to a select group of patients with extensive SCLC.[76] Chest (20 Gy/5 fractions) and prophylactic cranial irradiation (20 Gy/ 5 to 7 fractions) were administered to patients with no residual disease outside the thorax on completion of chemotherapy. The overall response rate was 94%, which included a 40% complete response rate. With chest radiotherapy, the complete response improved to 56%. Median survival was 61 weeks, and the 2-year survival rate was 30%; both figures represent marked improvements over the usual results in extensive disease (Table 13–6). Although life-threatening granulocytopenia occurred in 56% of patients, there were only four episodes of fever during granulocytopenia requiring hospitalization and one patient died of sepsis. Similar results have been reported by Japanese investigators.[77]

Although the aforementioned pilot studies all provide encouraging results, two recently completed randomized trials comparing standard chemotherapy to weekly chemotherapy have failed to demonstrate any survival benefit with weekly therapy (Table 13–7).[80, 81] British investigators prospectively compared a weekly chemotherapy regimen to a standard regimen of CAV alternating with cisplatin and etoposide.[80] The trial accrued 311 SCLC patients with good prognostic features (limited or extensive disease with Eastern Cooperative Oncology Group [ECOG] performance status ≤1 and alkaline phosphatase ≤1.5 the upper limit of normal).[82] Overall response rates (78% versus 81%), complete response rates (33% versus 30%), and median survivals (44 weeks versus 46 weeks) were not significantly different. Furthermore, hematologic toxicity was greater in the weekly chemotherapy regimen. Probably as a result of the greater hematologic

toxicity, patients treated weekly failed to receive the intended dose of chemotherapy. Whether or not the availability of hematopoietic growth factors have an impact on the ability to deliver more drug safely and what impact increased drug delivery may have on survival remains to be determined.

Late Intensification

Virtually all SCLC patients who achieve a remission eventually relapse and die of their malignancy.[1, 3] This observation has lead many investigators to administer additional high-dose treatment following initial tumor regression (i.e., late-intensification chemotherapy) based on the tenets of the Norton-Simon hypothesis, which states [that] as a tumor regresses, its growth fraction increases. Consequently, chemotherapy dose should not be compromised.[83] For example, Humblet and associates treated 101 SCLC patients with a standard chemotherapy regimen every 3 weeks for three courses.[84] On restaging, patients with limited disease in partial or complete response and patients with extensive disease in complete response were randomized to receive further conventional-dose chemotherapy or high-dose chemotherapy consisting of cyclophosphamide (6 g/m²), etoposide (500 mg/m²) and BCNU (300 mg/m²), followed by autologous bone marrow transplantation. Only 45 patients (39 with limited disease, 6 with extensive disease) were actually randomized out of 101 patients entered into the trial (22 received conventional chemotherapy, and 23 were given late-intensification chemotherapy). The median relapse-free survival time after randomization was 28 weeks with late-intensification chemotherapy compared with 10 weeks with conventional therapy (p = .002). Median overall survival times, however, were not statistically different (68 weeks and 55 weeks, respectively; p = .13) (Table 13–8). Although patients with

TABLE 13–8. Late-Intensification Chemotherapy

REFERENCE	NUMBER OF PATIENTS	STAGE	LI CHEMOTHERAPY	PER CENT RECEIVING LI	MEDIAN SURVIVAL
Humblet et al[84]	101	LD + ED	CEB	45	68 weeks (+LI) 55 weeks (LI)
Ihde et al[85]	29	ED	CE	28	5.5 months
Spitzer et al[86]	32	LD	CEV	37	14.0 months
Goodman et al[87]	58	LD	C	36	11.1 months
Smith et al[88]	36	LD + ED	C	38	10.0 months

LD = limited disease; ED = extensive disease; C = cyclophosphamide; E = etoposide; V = vincristine; B = BCNU; LI = late-intensification.

limited-stage disease receiving late-intensification therapy had a median survival of 84 weeks, this was not significantly different from the conventional-dose therapy group (60 weeks; p = .06). Similar disappointing results have been reported by other investigators (Table 13–8).[84–88]

With the availability of better supportive care measures such as hematopoietic growth factors and peripheral blood stem cell infusions, further investigation of late-intensification therapy may be warranted. However, few SCLC patients are candidates for this type of therapy and it has been recommended that future studies be confined to patients with limited-stage disease in complete response and possibly complete responding patients with extensive-stage disease who have a relatively low tumor burden at diagnosis.[89] In addition, adequate attention must be given to control of the intrathoracic tumor in these trials. For example, Humblet and colleagues noted that 15 of 16 patients with limited-stage disease receiving late-intensification therapy relapsed at the site of the primary tumor, confirming the inability of high-dose therapy to completely eradicate local disease.[84] Recently, Elias and colleagues have attempted to address this shortcoming by administering late-intensification chemotherapy to SCLC patients achieving a complete or near complete response followed through chest (50 to 56 Gy) and brain irradiation.[90] In a small, highly select group of patients, these investigators reported a 2-year actuarial disease-free survival rate of 57%. Nine of 11 patients (82%) remain disease free at 2 years or more of follow-up. Although promising, these data obviously require confirmation in a prospective, randomized trial. Whether such a trial can ever be successfully mounted is questionable because a large number of patients would be required. Even when patients are selected, fewer than 40% have proved sufficiently healthy to proceed with late-intensification chemotherapy (Table 13–8).[84–87]

Salvage Chemotherapy

On relapse, some SCLC patients may still be in good physical condition and desirous of further treatment. Unfortunately, few drugs or drug combinations are capable of effecting tumor regression in this setting.[25] The success of salvage chemotherapy depends on multiple factors, including

- The interval between cessation of initial therapy and the detection of recurrence,
- the nature of the response to initial therapy, and
- the composition of the initial chemotherapy.[25, 91–93]

The longer the interval between completion of induction therapy and recognition of relapse, the greater is the possibility of a favorable response to second-line treatment.[92] A favorable response to second-line therapy also is more likely if the patient experienced an objective tumor regression with the initial drug regimen.[92, 94] In circumstances in which more than 12 months have elapsed, retreatment with the original drug regimen may produce a second tumor regression.[91] A short interval between completion of induc-

tion therapy and recurrence usually portends a poor outcome, especially if the interval is 3 months or less.

Second-line chemotherapy with cisplatin plus etoposide following a cyclophosphamide-based induction regimen is capable of effecting a second response in up to 50% of patients.[23, 24] Unfortunately, the reverse sequence is considerably less successful.[25, 95] In patients failing initial treatment with cisplatin plus etoposide, it may be possible to obtain a second response using oral etoposide administered for several consecutive days.[94, 96] Oral etoposide has been combined with cisplatin and ifosfamide to obtain an impressive response rate in heavily pretreated SCLC patients including individuals who had relapsed from cisplatin plus etoposide therapy.[97] This regimen, however, is associated with considerable toxicity, potentially negating its palliative benefits.

Treatment of Elderly and Medically Unfit Patients

SCLC usually develops in the sixth or seventh decade of life. Consequently, additional medical problems are likely to be present, including cardiac disease, chronic obstructive pulmonary disease, hypertension, diabetes, peripheral vascular disease, and other malignancies.[98] As a result, older patients frequently take medications for their concomitant illnesses, and these agents can sometimes interfere with the effectiveness or metabolism of certain antineoplastic agents. Furthermore, older patients may be less tolerant of aggressive chemotherapy for a variety of physiologic and pharmacologic reasons, making their management more challenging.[99–101]

Despite the obvious difficulties encountered in managing SCLC in older patients, age per se has not been shown to be an independent prognostic factor in this disease.[102–104] Advancing age, however, can lessen the ability of an individual to tolerate standard doses of induction therapy.[98, 102] In a retrospective review of 122 elderly SCLC patients (i.e., ≥70 years) treated at the University of Toronto, Shepherd and colleagues reported that fewer than 50% were able to receive the planned course of chemotherapy and only two patients completed chemotherapy without a dose reduction.[102] Survival directly correlated with the amount of treatment received. Older patients able to tolerate 4 cycles or more of chemotherapy had a median survival of 10.7 months compared with 3.9 months for patients limited to three cycles or less of treatment. Median survival for patients receiving no therapy was only 1.1 months. The most common reason for failing to receive full course chemotherapy was myelosuppression.

Other investigators also have questioned the wisdom of aggressively treating older patients with SCLC.[98] In another retrospective analysis, an Australian group observed a high rate of toxicity in a group of elderly SCLC patients (70 to 80 years) treated with intensive chemotherapy.[98] Although response rates were higher with intensive combination chemotherapy regimens (84% versus 54%; p = .006), survival was not significantly improved over that achieved with so-called gentle therapy (i.e., single agent etoposide or radiotherapy). Only two of 72 patients survived more than 2 years. Half of all patients failed to complete the planned course of intensive therapy usually because of major toxicity, patient refusal, or the development of an intercurrent illness. Collectively, these data indicate that standard combination chemotherapy may not be appropriate for all older patients with SCLC.[103]

Although the best regimen for treating older or medically unfit patients is not well established, some investigators have employed single agent etoposide in this population with impressive results.[105–109] For example, in one trial confined to patients older than 70 years of age, five consecutive days of oral etoposide (160 mg/m[2]/day) yielded a median survival of 16 months in patients with limited disease and 9 months in patients with extensive disease.[107] A variety of doses and schedules of oral etoposide have been used, all of which are capable of producing excellent results, albeit with differing levels of myelosuppression (Table 13–9).[107–109] Oral etoposide is well absorbed and well tolerated, producing only modest hematologic toxicity when administered in relatively low doses of 50 mg once or twice daily.[108, 110] Still to be determined, however, is the optimal dose and schedule of oral etoposide. Additional treatment choices for older patients include cisplatin and etoposide; carboplatin and etoposide; or cyclophosphamide, doxorubicin, and etoposide. Each of these regimens has advantages in selected patients. The specific regimen employed should be dictated by the underlying status of the patient.

Drug Development

The optimal method by which new agents should be evaluated in patients with SCLC is the subject of considerable controversy.[111–114] Traditionally, phase II agents have been employed in patients with SCLC only after standard chemotherapy has been used, an approach still preferred by some experts.[114, 115] This approach ensures that no patient is denied the potential benefits of standard chemotherapy. However, testing new agents in previously treated patients may lead to an unacceptably high-false negative response rate.[116] To avoid this dilemma, new agents can be tested in chemotherapy-naive patients. The latter approach is considered ethically objectionable by some clinicians because patients can be subjected to the toxic effects of an inactive drug.

The ECOG and the National Cancer Institute of Canada (NCIC) have employed Phase II agents as initial therapy in carefully selected, previously untreated SCLC patients.[117–119] For these trials, the following criteria are used: patients must have extensive disease, a good performance status (ECOG ≤2), and no severe organ impairment that might require a rapid tumor response. Furthermore, patients must have adequate hepatic and renal function and cannot have an underlying illness that would prevent the administration of salvage chemotherapy consisting of cisplatin and etoposide. In addition to these criteria, any patient who progresses after one cycle of therapy or who fails to achieve a partial response after two courses of investigational agent is switched to cisplatin plus etoposide. All patients are closely monitored throughout the time the new agent is being given. ECOG and NCIC have tested several Phase II agents using this approach without observing an adverse affect on survival, even when the agent under study proved to be inactive.[118, 119]

An equally cogent argument can be made for continuing the practice of testing new agents only in patients who have failed standard induction therapy. Virtually all active agents in SCLC have yielded an objective response rate of 10% or more in previously treated patients.[114, 115] If a 10% response rate in previously treated patients is accepted as indicative of activity, then a two-stage sequential design for Phase II trials in SCLC can be developed.[115] A target enrollment of 20 patients in the initial phase of the study would allow for early termination of the trial if four or more patients respond because the agent under investigation would have at least a 10% activity level. If none of the initial 20 patients responds, the agent

TABLE 13–9. Use of Etoposide in Elderly Patients

REFERENCE	DOSE AND SCHEDULE	NUMBER OF PATIENTS	OVERALL RESPONSE (%)	MEDIAN SURVIVAL
Smit et al[107]	160 mg/m[2] p.o. × 5 days; repeat every 4 weeks	35	71	16.0 months (LD) 9.0 months (ED)
Clark et al[108]	50 mg p.o. BID × 14 days; repeat every 3 weeks	25	76	7.0 months (ED)
	50 mg p.o. daily × 21 days; repeat every 4 weeks	27	52	5.0 months (ED)
	50 mg p.o. BID × 10 days; repeat every 3 weeks	26	70	6.5 months (ED)
Gatzemeier et al[109]	167 mg/m[2] p.o. × 3 days; repeat every 8–10 days	55	56	7.5 months (LD) 6.5 months (ED)

LD = limited disease; ED = extensive disease.

under investigation would not be subjected to further analysis because the study design allows one to exclude a true response rate of more than 10.9% at the 90% confidence level. A 90% confidence level increases the power to identify truly active agents and only slightly increases the possibility of mislabeling an inactive agent as active. If 1 to 3 patients respond, an additional 15 patients are required to complete the evaluation of the investigational agent. With this study design, a maximum of 35 patients are needed to adequately assess the activity of a Phase II agent.

RADIATION THERAPY

Since the Medical Research Council's (MRC) prospective trial comparing surgery and radiotherapy in SCLC[123, 124] and improved median survival with the addition of single agent cyclophosphamide to thoracic irradiation,[125] the role of chemotherapy has expanded and combination chemotherapy has become the cornerstone of all treatment for SCLC.[126] However, because of high failure rates at the site of the primary disease and in the central nervous system, the role of radiation therapy continues to be explored and defined.

The major contribution of thoracic irradiation is local tumor control,[127] and local control of the intrathoracic tumor is a sine qua non for cure.[128] The addition of TRT can decrease chest failures from 72% to 43%.[129] Although chemotherapy combinations can achieve complete response rates of ~50% and overall response rates of more than 80%, local recurrence rates vary between 30% and 80%, and the rate of 2-year disease-free survival rarely surpasses 15% to 20%.[130]

In a consensus meeting on the management of small cell cancer in 1988, it was concluded that "a definitive recommendation for TRT in combined modality regimens cannot yet be made."[20] SCLC shares many of the features of tumors curable by combination chemotherapy: rapid progression, short doubling time, high growth fraction, sensitivity to multiple chemotherapeutic agents and radiation therapy, and a high incidence of complete remissions,[131] but from the many reported trials, it is difficult to state with certainty that thoracic radiotherapy is of benefit in SCLC. In an effort to answer this question, two meta-analyses have been performed.[20, 21] In looking at 16 randomized trials over the past 15 years, inconsistent results have been reported. Pignon and coworkers[21] performed a meta-analysis on 2140 patients with limited disease enrolled in 13 randomized trials. Sufficient information was available in 2103 patients, 1862 (88%) of whom have died. A study conducted by Osterlind[132] found a negative effect of thoracic irradiation. The meta-analysis demonstrated that the addition of radiotherapy corresponded to a 14% decrease in the risk of death, 18% if the Osterlind trial is excluded. Warde and colleagues[20] found the rate difference for treatment benefit was 25% but also noted that the addition of TRT increased the risk of treatment-related death. Both studies found an increase in overall survival of 5.4%.

Pignon's study did not find a significant difference for treatment by using alternating, concurrent, or sequential administration of radiotherapy, nor was the relative risk of early radiotherapy (<60 days) significant.[21] Based on these analyses, TRT does reduce the risk of dying of SCLC, but as often noted earlier, at the price of increased toxicity.

Treatment Considerations

Prospective randomized trials have failed to define the optimal volume to be irradiated, the preferred dose and fractionation scheme, the integration and timing with chemotherapy, and the treatment technique.

Volume

Because chemotherapy is highly cytotoxic to SCLC, it is unclear whether every cell must be irradiated to produce a cure. However, it is likely that the sites of bulk disease may harbor the most resistant cells.[133] Generally the primary tumor with 1- to 2-cm margins is included in the treatment volume. SWOG based the volume on the tumor before the administration of chemotherapy,[60] whereas no difference in local control was seen when the postchemotherapy volume was irradiated.[134] Not all chest failures represent a failure of TRT. In a retrospective review, Mira and Livingston[135] found only 28% of patients had definite tumor growth in the irradiated field and 72% had initial chest recurrence outside the irradiated volume. Other reports have found 80% failures at the site of initial tumor in patients with limited disease who attained a CR.[136] The supraclavicular nodes do not have to be treated routinely; however, they should be included when the primary is an upper lobe lesion, when there is clinical or evidence on computed tomography (CT) of enlarged (≥1 cm) supraclavicular nodes, or mediastinal nodes above the level of the carina.[137] The contralateral hilum does not need to be included in the treatment port.[138]

White and colleagues[139] performed a retrospective quality control review of SWOG protocol 7628 and clearly demonstrated the importance of careful treatment planning. Of 298 patients treated, 140 patients were evaluable for major violations, which were defined as (1) 5% to 10% underdose of any involved area, (2) 10% or more underdose of any area, (3) 10% or more overdose of a critical structure, (4) wrong fractionation (wrong daily dose of treatment or only 1 field per day), or (5) wrong area (missed the brain or supraclavicular fossa or both). One hundred and two major violations were identified in 44 patients. The most frequent errors involved the treatment volume and shielding. The violations led to a significant increase in chest failures and a decrease in survival. The findings and significance levels are presented in Table 13–10. Three-dimensional treatment planning is in its infancy but holds the promise of allowing delivery of doses to the tumor while limiting doses to normal tissues.[140]

TABLE 13–10. Impact of Radiotherapy Treatment Planning on Failure Patterns

FACTOR	NO PROTOCOL VIOLATION	PROTOCOL VIOLATION	P
Median survival (all patients)	60 weeks	40 weeks	.002
Median survival (CR/PR after induction)	65 weeks	39 weeks	.014
Improvement in response after induction	48%	27%	.05
Chest failure	55%	77%	.047
Chest failure in patients who achieved CR	34%	69%	.042

CR = Complete response; PR = partial response.

From White JE, Chen T, McCracken J, et al: The influence of radiation therapy quality control on survival, response rates, and sites of relapse in oat cell carcinoma of the lung. Preliminary report of a Southwest Oncology Group study. Cancer 50:1084–1090, 1982.

Dose

Rapid tumor regression with radiotherapy led to the belief that SCLC was a radiosensitive tumor and required a relatively low radiation dose, in the range of 30 to 45 Gy.[130] However, SCLC has a high growth fraction compared with other tumors,[141] and the rapid regression seen may be more related to tumor kinetics than to radiosensitivity.[142] However, it may be possible that doses that are ineffective when thoracic radiotherapy is used alone could be effective when combined with chemotherapy.[143] Choi and Carey[144] demonstrated increasing local control with increasing dose, with 60% local control at 30 Gy, 79% at 40 Gy, and 88% at 48 Gy; unfortunately, local control was measured over an interval of only 4 months.[144]

Eaton and associates, reporting for the CALGB, found 37.5% in-field recurrences with doses less than 42 Gy, 13% with doses above 42 Gy, and none when the dose was greater than 45 Gy.[145] SWOG found that 30 Gy versus 45 Gy did not influence the survival rate, but the CR rate was significantly higher (p = 0.02) with the higher dose.[139] However, the higher dose resulted in a higher level of toxicity.[142] Arriagada and coworkers have escalated the radiotherapy dose from 45 Gy to 55 Gy to 65 Gy in consecutive trials without an increase in long-term local control, and a dose of 55 Gy is recommended.[146] A subsequent protocol using TID fractionation for the first series and administering up to 61 Gy did not show significant improvement in CR, and 37% of patients had isolated local failures.[147] Increasing doses of radiotherapy appear to delay the time to local recurrence.[136, 146, 148] Even administering a single fraction of 12.5 Gy by a 360-degree arc has been tried; the majority of patients developed transient esophagitis, but no unusual toxicities were observed.[149] It is recommended that dose schema of 50 Gy or more or altered fractionation be used.[148]

Sequence of Combined Modality Therapy

Chemotherapy and radiotherapy can be combined in basically three ways: sequential, concurrent or alternating, as shown diagrammatically in Figures 13–1 to 13–4. Each has, or has had, its proponents. In early combined modality trials, treatment was generally sequential with either initial chemotherapy or initial radiotherapy.

Tubiana and coworkers[150] have developed the rationale for combining alternating radiotherapy and chemotherapy. The combination has two aims: (1) potentiation of one of the two modalities by the other or an additive effect on tumor without an increase in toxicity, and (2) the use of radiotherapy to control the primary tumor or sanctuary site and chemotherapy to control disseminated disease, which is referred to as spatial cooperation. Neither treatment should interfere with the other, and both modalities should be given in full doses to be effective. If one delays chemotherapy for radiotherapy, occult metastases would be allowed to proliferate; conversely, delay of radiotherapy for chemotherapy is detrimental because drugs often are not effective on bulky tumors. These arguments led to the initiation of a series of consecutive French trials of alternating chemotherapy and radiotherapy protocols in the treatment of SCLC. The Looney model proposes the use of alternating chemotherapy and radiotherapy to decrease the side effects while remaining therapeutically active.[151]

As an option to alternating chemotherapy and radiotherapy, concurrent treatment can be used and may possess an advantage. According to the Goldie-Coldman model, combination chemotherapy, using non–cross resistant drugs, is a way to achieve an increased therapeutic effect,[151] and sequential rather than simultaneous administration of two agents may increase the probability of development of a resistant tumor cell line.[152] Multiple drug resistance tends to appear before a curative effect is achieved, and radiotherapy can be used as a non–cross resistant treatment and is better delivered early before resistant cells appear and metastases occur.[151] However, drug-resistant SCLC is not completely cross resistant to ionizing radiation.[153] A consistent trend toward improved response and overall survival rates has been demonstrated when chemotherapy was administered concomitantly with TRT.[130] Approaches that do not delay chemotherapy for the administration of radiotherapy appear to possess superior antitumor effectiveness.[2]

In early studies, patients were frequently treated in a sequential manner, as shown in Figure 13–1. An improvement in long-term survival may be seen when TRT is used.[154] In a trial of cyclophosphamide, doxorubicin, and vincristine (CAV) and methotrexate, patients were randomized to receive 40 Gy in 20 fractions at week 10. The disease-free 4-year survival rate

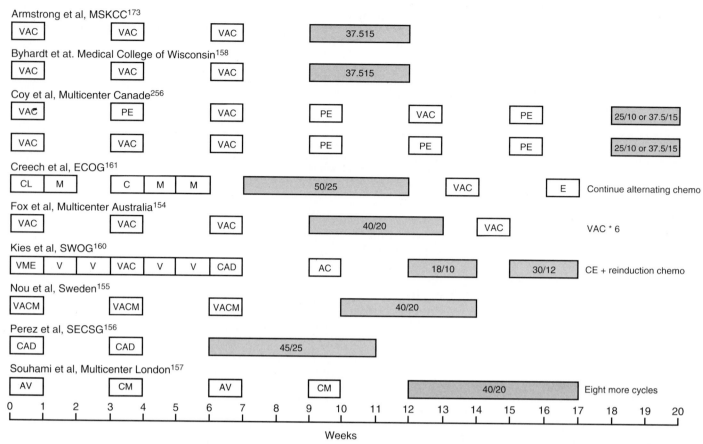

FIGURE 13–1. Sequential chemotherapy and radiotherapy. V = Vincristine; A = doxorubicin (Adriamycin); C = cyclophosphamide; P = cisplatin; E = etoposide; L = lomustine; M = methotrexate; D = dacarbazine; Pr = procarbazine.

was 12% with thoracic irradiation; there were no 4-year survivors without thoracic irradiation (p = .025).[155] When patients fail single modality TRT, the response to salvage chemotherapy may be disappointing. In a randomized Southeastern Cancer Study Group (SECSG) trial of concomitant versus delayed chemotherapy, disease free survival (DFS) was im-

proved with the combination. In the delayed arm, chemotherapy was given at relapse following TRT (43%), and none responded.[156]

Combination sequential chemoradiotherapy does not always lead to improved results. In a randomized trial, Souhami and associates[157] concluded that for patients with limited-stage and extensive-stage disease,

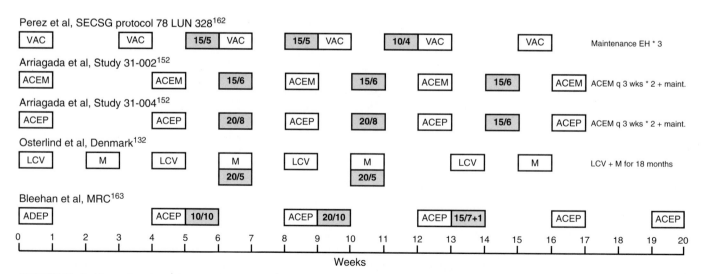

FIGURE 13–2. Alternating chemotherapy and radiotherapy. V = Vincristine; A = doxorubicin (Adriamycin); C = cyclophosphamide; P = cisplatin; E = etoposide; L = lomustine; M = methotrexate; D = dacarbazine; Pr = procarbazine.

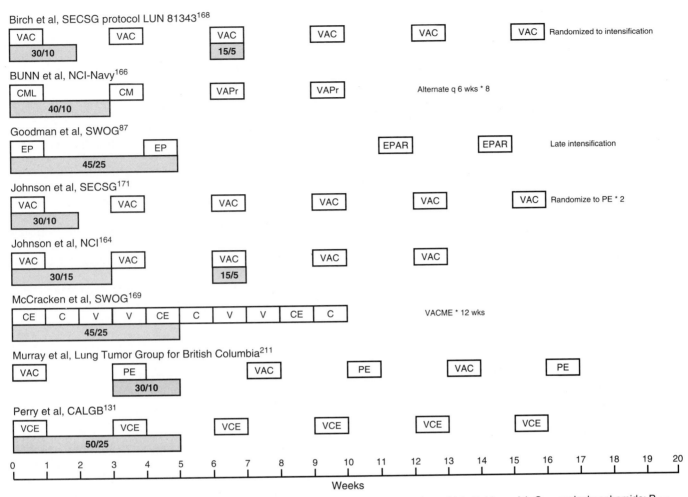

FIGURE 13–3. Concurrent chemotherapy and early radiotherapy. V = Vincristine; A = doxorubicin (Adriamycin); C = cyclophosphamide; P = cisplatin; E = etoposide; L = lomustine; M = methotrexate; D = dacarbazine; Pr = procarbazine.

the response to chemotherapy was the major determinant of prognosis. In a comparison of two consecutive trials, it was believed that survival was improved by the addition of TRT (p < .01).[158] In a

different scheme of chemotherapy and split course radiotherapy consisting of 60 Gy in 20 fractions with weekly etoposide, only 1 of the 26 patients (4%) failed locally.[159] SWOG conducted a trial of chemotherapy

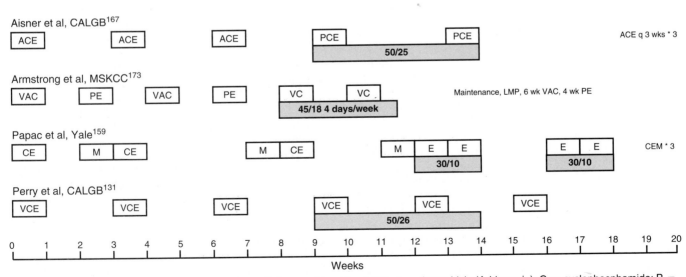

FIGURE 13–4. Concurrent chemotherapy and late radiotherapy. V = Vincristine; A = doxorubicin (Adriamycin); C = cyclophosphamide; P = cisplatin; E = etoposide; L = lomustine; M = methotrexate; D = dacarbazine.

and randomization to split course radiotherapy to 48 Gy in 22 fractions. After radiotherapy, CRs increased from 33% to 47%. TRT did not affect median or long-term survival but did decrease the number of chest relapses from 72% to 50%; interruption of the chemotherapy for radiotherapy had no adverse effect on overall tumor control, toxicity, or quality of life.[160] A statistically significant survival advantage was seen in patients receiving TRT[161] despite significant toxicity.

Various methods of alternating chemotherapy and radiotherapy are diagrammatically shown in Figure 13–2. The SECSG tested the concept of alternating chemotherapy and radiotherapy in limited SCLC by randomizing patients to receive TRT with the third, fourth, and fifth cycles of chemotherapy. The addition of TRT resulted in a significant improvement in CR (48% versus 62%), median survival (49 weeks versus 60 weeks), and 2-year survival (23% versus 40%). A significant reduction in chest failures (52% versus 36%) was also seen. Life-threatening toxicities were seen in only 1%.[162]

In a randomized trial, Osterlind and coworkers[132] found split course radiotherapy, consisting of two courses of 20 Gy in five fractions, significantly decreased chest relapses from 85% to 61% (p = 0.005), 72%, and 44% (p = 0.013), respectively, among autopsied patients. Although irradiated patients had a longer response duration, median survival was decreased; the differences were not significant.

Toxicity of alternating regimens may be significant. In two nonrandomized consecutive studies, Arriagada and associates[152] employed doxorubicin, etoposide, cyclophosphamide, and methotrexate with alternating TRT. Because of excessive toxicity, the methotrexate was replaced by cis-platinum, and 45 Gy were increased to 55 Gy. Isolated local recurrences were reduced from 25% to 9.5%, and median survival time was increased from 14 months to 20 months with the higher dose. This improvement, however, was largely the result of decreased treatment-related lethal toxicity.

Bleehen and colleagues[163] gave chemotherapy alternating with TRT. Because of the cis-platin, only 1 of 12 patients (8%) received six cycles of chemotherapy and all three courses of radiotherapy; 25% of patients received no radiotherapy. When the cis-platin dose was lowered, the treatment schema was substantially more tolerable. Based on this experience, it was believed that a large multicenter MRC randomized trial of alternating versus conventional scheduling was not feasible.[163]

Various methods of combining concurrent chemotherapy and radiotherapy are shown in Figures 13–3 and 13–4. In 1976, Johnson and colleagues[164] reported on the results of concurrent CAV chemotherapy with TRT, 20 to 30 Gy, in 21 consecutive patients with limited and extensive disease. Twenty of 21 patients (95%) attained a complete response with considerable toxicity, including 62% of patients who required nutritional support and three patients (14%) who developed esophageal stricture. Although no patient developed pneumonitis, all developed pulmonary

fibrosis,[164] and the ability to attain a CR in 95% was independently confirmed.[165] Toxicity is increased with concurrent chemoradiotherapy and modifications in the radiotherapy technique may be necessary. Doses of 40 Gy in 15 fractions concurrent with the first cycle of chemotherapy resulted in CR in 81%, but 67% of patients experienced moderate or severe esophageal toxicity requiring modifications in radiotherapy to shield the esophagus; severe late pulmonary toxicity was seen in 14 of 96 patients (15%); 10% lethal toxicity was observed with the majority in the combined modality arm; and five patients died in CR. The risk of dying from SCLC was significantly reduced (p = .003).[166] A trial of intense chemotherapy consisting of doxorubicin, cyclophosphamide, and etoposide with concurrent TRT, 40 Gy in 20 fractions with a 10 Gy boost at the fourth cycle with the doxorubicin replaced by cis-platin during radiotherapy, was conducted by the Cancer and Leukemia Group B (CALGB). Severe or life-threatening leukopenia was seen in 90% of patients. Severe or life-threatening pneumonitis was seen in 7% of patients who required mechanical ventilatory support. Although the 2 year survival rate was only 41%, 25% of patients survived for more than 4 years.

Not all toxicities require modification of the radiotherapy but may require modifications in the chemotherapy. The SECSG conducted a trial of alternating chemotherapy (78 LUN 328, Fig. 13–2)[162] and concurrent treatment (LUN 81343, Fig. 13–3).[168] When the TRT was delivered in weeks 1, 2, and 7, accrual to induction randomization was stopped when an interim analysis showed a significant difference in toxicity, and the induction chemotherapy schema was modified. The concomitant chemoradiotherapy significantly decreased local recurrences, whether alone or with other failure, whereas the alternating scheme resulted in a significant decrease in failures confined to the thorax only. Concurrent chemoradiotherapy resulted in 5% toxic deaths compared with 2% for the alternating scheme. Grade 3 to 4 esophagitis was reduced from 15% to 9% with the alternating schedule.[168] The combination of cis-platin, etoposide, and vincristine with concurrent TRT followed by consolidation chemotherapy is difficult to administer. Only two-thirds of 156 eligible patients completed the entire program. Overall, the toxicity was believed to be generally acceptable and reversible with better survival than in previous SWOG studies.[169] SWOG conducted a trial of concurrent TRT with cis-platin and etoposide followed by consolidation with etoposide, cis-platin, doxorubicin, and vincristine and subsequent cyclophosphamide intensification led to a 12% fatal toxicity rate (19% for patients going on to intensification) and was poorly tolerated, with only 36% completing all treatment.[87] In a randomized trial employing concurrent chemotherapy, radiotherapy given concurrently with the fourth, versus the first cycle, is advantageous, resulting in improved failure-free survival and a trend toward improved survival (p = .078). Patients given TRT concurrent with the first cycle demonstrated a failure to thrive and 14% of patients lost more than 10% of their body weight even though they received reduced doses of chemotherapy.[131] Not all toxicities are severe. The combination of CAV, alternating with cisplatin and etoposide (PE) and TRT, 45 Gy with 2.5-Gy fractions 4 days per week, resulted in 59% of patients developing esophagitis; however, in the majority, this problem was mild. Thirty-five per cent attained a CR after chemotherapy, and 65% achieved a complete response after TRT. No patient failed locally only. The median survival was 21 months. The 1-, 2-, and 3-year survival rates were 83%, 46% and 33%, respectively.[170] Johnson and associates[171] delivered 30 Gy in 10 fractions concurrently with induction VAC chemotherapy. A boost of 15 Gy in five fractions was given to residual tumor or the site of previous gross disease concomitantly with the third chemotherapy cycle. No significant difference in CR, overall response rate, median survival, or 2- or 5-year survival was found among 297 assessable patients. However, a significant increase in progression-free survival and response duration was attained by the addition of TRT. The price was significantly increased severe toxicity. The various response criteria, toxicities, and sites of failure are presented, along with p values, in Table 13–11 and are representative of concurrent schema. It is clear that TRT may require modification of subsequent chemotherapy.

Fractionation

Because SCLC possesses a high growth fraction, short cell cycle times and absence of a shoulder on cell survival curves, it is an ideal tumor for treatment by hyperfractionation. Small fraction size, as used in hyperfractionated schema, causes less normal tissue damage, but the time between fractions must be adequate to allow for normal tissue repair. Also, with no shoulder, tumor kill is exponential,[172] and with greater

cell kill each day, there is less chance for repopulation in a rapidly cycling tumor.[130] Because SCLC is so prolific, it is possible that cells could move from a relatively radioresistant phase of the cell cycle (the S phase) into a more radioresponsive phase (the G_2-M border).[133]

These factors make the combination of cisplatin and etoposide and hyperfractionated radiotherapy attractive. Armstrong and coworkers[173] conducted a trial comparing concurrent 2.5 Gy fractions 4 days per week to sequential 1.5 Gy BID; each arm received 45 Gy total. Although thoracic control was better with the daily fractionation (p < .05), the 2-year survival was better in the BID arm (p = .07),[173, 174] but no patient on the BID arm survived without disease. Chronic pulmonary complications were more common in the BID arm but were more severe in the once-daily arm.[174] It appears that the use of chemotherapy with hyperfractionated radiotherapy is important. Using thoracic radiotherapy to 48 Gy, delivered by split course twice-daily fractionation, a complete response was seen in 36% of patients and an overall response was seen in 100% of patients.[175] With additional follow-up, local control was attained in 97%.[77]

Hyperfractionated TRT can be combined with chemotherapy in an alternating fashion. This has the major theoretical advantage of avoiding the toxic effects resulting from the concurrent administration of chemotherapy and radiotherapy and may allow full-dose chemotherapy and radiotherapy without an undue delay of either modality.[172]

However, toxicity may not be significantly decreased by alternating chemotherapy and hyperfractionated radiotherapy.[172, 177] In 1988, Turrisi and associates[178] reported on a trial of cis-platin and etoposide delivered concurrently with BID TRT initiated within 24 hours of each other. A time period of 4 to 6 hours was mandated between two daily fractions of 1.5 Gy

TABLE 13–11. Toxicities Associated with Chemotherapy ± Radiotherapy

FACTOR	CAV + TRT	CAV	P
CR	46%	38%	.14
Overall response	67%	64%	.58
Median survival	14.4 mos	12.8 mos	.92
2-year survival	33%	23.5%	.077
5-year survival	16%	12%	.36
2-year progression-free survival	39%	15%	.002
Response duration	14.6 mos	7.8 mos	.0005
1 or more Grade-4 toxicities	73%	56%	.002
Life-threatening myelosuppression	60%	39%	.001
Fever and neutropenia requiring parenteral antibiotics	27%	16%	.007
Stomatitis and esophagitis preventing eating	13%	1%	<.001
Severe weight loss (>10%)	41%	23%	<.001
Per cent of patients receiving 80% or more of prescribed chemotherapy	57%	75%	.006
Doxorubicin	58%	78%	.003
Total failures	52%	74%	<.001
Thoracic failures only	22%	47%	<.001
Thoracic and distant failures	6%	15%	.007
Distant failures only	24%	12%	.003

From Johnson DH, Bass D, Einhorn LH, et al: Combination chemotherapy with or without thoracic radiotherapy in limited-stage small-cell cancer: A randomized trial of the Southeastern Cancer Study Group. J Clin Oncol 11:1223–1229, 1993.

to allow for repair of normal tissues. The principal toxicity was esophagitis, which was severe in only 13% of patients; three patients developed strictures, and no pulmonary toxicity was observed. All 21 patients with pure SCLC responded, whereas neither patient with variant histology responded. No in-field failures were reported. With a median follow-up of 22 months, the 2-year survival rate was 57%.[178] The treatment fields were generally considered conservative. Supraclavicular lymph nodes were treated for upper lobe lesions, and the contralateral hilum was never treated.[138] In a follow-up report of 32 patients, a CR was obtained in 93% but 39% of patients progressed from a CR. Only two of four patients with variant histology responded. Local control was achieved in 84%, and only two patients (6%) failed in the supraclavicular fossa. The 4-year survival rate was 46%.[138] Forty-five per cent of patients relapsed, five had the thorax as the first site of failure; all four variant histologies were in this group. A 13% treatment-related mortality rate was seen.[179] The variant histology appears to be important when considering hyperfractionation. Hyperfractionation is attractive because SCLC has a rather small shoulder on the cell survival curve while the variant histology has cell survival characteristics similar to large cell lung cancer with a substantial capacity to accumulate sublethal damage.[180, 181] The broader shoulder of the variant histology may account for the failures, and this argument is true for mixed histologies as well. Johnson and associates[182] gave concurrent PE and BID TRT at doses up to 45 Gy. A CR was achieved in 89%, and an overall response was seen in 100% of patients. The actuarial survival rate at 1 year was 95%, and at 2 years it was 83%. Only 1 of 18 patients (6%) experienced a chest failure. Although two patients developed esophageal stricture, no patient was hospitalized for pneumonitis. With additional follow-up, a CR was achieved in 81%, with overall response seen in 100%; the actuarial 1- and 2-year survival rate was >90% and 65%, respectively.[183] In an ECOG pilot study of 40 patients using the same schema, the 1- and 2-year survival rates were 67% and 36%, respectively. Of 14 failures, only three (8%) were local.[184, 185]

Other Considerations for the Use of Radiotherapy

Although there is controversy when using TRT in patients with a CR, even greater controversy exists in patients who have attained only a partial response (PR) after chemotherapy. The addition of TRT can control the thoracic disease, may prevent complications of progression, and may provide the prospect for long-term survival for some patients. Among 65 patients enrolled in two studies conducted at Memorial Sloan Kettering Cancer Center (MSKCC), 24 patients (37%) attained a CR after induction chemotherapy, whereas 24 patients (37%) who achieved a PR went on to achieve a CR following TRT. At 1 year, the actuarial thoracic control was 87% in chemotherapy-induced CRs and 72% in CR after TRT. The corresponding 5-year figures were 59% and 21% (not significant). However, actuarial freedom from distant failure was significantly less in patients who failed to attain a CR after induction chemotherapy.[173]

Because of the concept that SCLC is a systemic disease at diagnosis, use of extended radiotherapy fields has been tried in an effort to control likely sites of extrathoracic metastases. Treatment of the neuroaxis,[158] upper abdomen,[144] or entire ipsilateral lung[169, 172, 186] adds little therapeutically and is often poorly tolerated.[144, 158] In the mid-1970s, 10 to 15 Gy following chemotherapy was delivered to regions of extrathoracic spread identified at diagnosis; this process was termed radiotherapy consolidation.[164]

Total body irradiation (TBI) has been attempted with no significant improvements in results.[187–190] Hemi-body irradiation (HBI) has also failed to influence results significantly,[191–196] and if careful attention is not given to technique and dose, nearly 70% of patients suffer lethal pneumonitis.[197]

Complications of Combined Modality Therapy

The use of chemoradiotherapy is associated with a significant incidence of pulmonary complications. Because many chemotherapy schema consisted of CAV, pulmonary fibrosis has been a complication in many cases.[45] Many chemotherapeutic agents, including bleomycin, cyclophosphamide, methotrexate, mitomycin, procarbazine, busulphan, and doxorubicin, can damage lung tissue.[198–200] Doxorubicin is particularly damaging because it can stimulate a so-called recall phenomenon.[201, 202] In one study, 11 of 80 patients (28%) developed life-threatening pulmonary toxicity, and 10% died of pulmonary complications. Pulmonary toxicity has not proved to be a major limiting factor in nonconcurrent chemotherapy regimens.[203]

Pulmonary toxicity generally has an acute phase (pneumonitis), occurring 6 to 12 weeks after radiotherapy, and a late phase (fibrosis), occurring 6 months following treatment.[198, 204, 205] The area irradiated on the initial port film does not correlate with developing pneumonitis.[203] It is possible that some type of hypersensitivity phenomenon is responsible.[205, 206] Although radiation pneumonitis is often clinically silent, a fulminant course leading to death may be seen.[205] In a CALGB trial of doxorubicin, cyclophosphamide, and etoposide (ACE) followed by TRT, fatal ARDS occurred in 8% of patients and grade 3 or 4 pneumonitis was seen in 18% of patients. When ACE following TRT was discontinued, no additional cases of ARDS were seen.[207] Generally, the symptoms of pneumonitis subside spontaneously over several weeks.[205]

After 3 to 6 months, patients may develop radiation fibrosis, which is often asymptomatic. Fibrosis may occur without antecedent pneumonitis.[205] Unlike pulmonary pneumonitis, which is a bilateral process, pulmonary fibrosis demonstrates dense infiltrates that are strictly confined to the radiation therapy field.[203] A

TABLE 13–12. Failure Patterns with and without Elective Brain Irradiation

BRAIN FAILURES	WITH EBI (%)	WITHOUT EBI (%)	P
All Patients			
Brain only failure	8	27	.04
Brain as first failure	14	46	.004
All brain failures	20	58	.001
CR in chest			
CR in thorax	61	85	
Brain only failure	9	27	.1
Brain as first failure	18	45	.04
All brain failures	23	50	.04
Durable local control (never fail)	73	45	.05
Brain failure	25	70	.03

CR = Complete response; EBI = elective brain irradiation.

From Rosenstein M, Armstrong J, Kris M, et al: A reappraisal of the role of prophylactic cranial irradiation in limited small cell lung cancer. Int J Radiat Oncol Biol Phys 24:43–48, 1992.

50% incidence of visible increase in lung density on a CT scan is predicted with doses equivalent to 32.9 Gy in 15 fractions.[208] A significantly lower vital capacity and FEV_1 is found and is worse than expected with radiotherapy alone. These values may improve over months when patients have been treated with chemotherapy alone but do not improve in irradiated patients. Lung fibrosis progresses between 6 and 12 months and stabilizes.[298] By using quantitative lung perfusion scans and the radiotherapy planning film, it may be possible to predict which patients are at particularly high risk of pulmonary toxicity and in whom an alteration of treatment technique is necessary.[209, 210]

Doxorubicin can also contribute to damage of the esophagus, and as many as 25% of patients may experience severe esophagitis,[202] but not all have found this to be a problem.[211] The development of esophagitis is dose related; it is seen in 12% of patients receiving more than 40 Gy and less than 55 Gy.[212] Strictures may develop.[213]

Elective Brain Irradiation

The literature discusses the use of prophylactic cranial irradiation (PCI) as a method of decreasing the morbidity of brain metastases; no evidence exists that metastases to the brain are prevented by irradiating the brain. A better term is elective brain irradiation (EBI). The presumption is that patients already harbor micrometastases in a sanctuary site, and the use of irradiation in an elective fashion can prevent the clinical appearance of disease. The incidence of brain metastases depends on how patients are evaluated, with the highest incidence in autopsy series. Hansen and colleagues noted that with increased survival, increased brain metastases were seen and the researchers proposed the use of EBI.[214] Patients surviving 2 years have an 80% cumulative actuarial probability of developing a central nervous system (CNS) metastasis,[215] but the CNS is identified as the site of relapse in fewer than 5% of patients.[127, 169] Approximately one-half of patients have clinically silent metastases.[217]

The role of EBI continues to be investigated and remains controversial; it is generally accepted that EBI decreases the appearance of brain metastasis but does not increase survival. When patients do fail in the brain, this may be the greatest cause of patient morbidity and the direct cause of death in more than 40%.[218] As the stage of disease increases, the risk of developing brain metastases in patients attaining a CR increases from 15% for Stage I to 80% for Stage IIIB.[219] The use of EBI in patients who have attained a CR decreases brain relapses from a range of 20% to 58% to a range of 2% to 18%.[129, 144, 146, 220, 221, 222] Selected patients who have failed after previous CNS irradiation may benefit from retreatment; patients generally improve at least one level in neurologic function status.[223]

In a review of randomized trials of EBI, a significant reduction in the rate of CNS relapses is seen without a significant survival advantage,[224, 225] but individual nonrandomized studies may demonstrate a significant survival advantage with the use of EBI.[221, 226, 227] In a study of non–SCLC, the Radiation Therapy Oncology Group (RTOG) found that EBI does not significantly decrease the cumulative probability of brain metastases but appears to delay their onset.[228] EBI is recommended in all patients with limited disease who attain a CR,[2, 221, 224, 229] and it appears to be ineffective in patients who do not attain a CR.[230, 231] Table 13–12 presents the experience of MSKCC with the use of EBI.[221] The arguments for EBI focus on improvements in the quality of life rather than its duration.[232–234] Serial CT scans are not effective as a surveillance tool.[235]

The question of when EBI should be given remains ill defined, but with increasing experience, it appears that a window exists that defines when EBI is effective. Delaying EBI leaves more patients at risk for brain metastases for a longer period of time.[234] A study was conducted in which EBI was delivered at Day 1 or at Week 12 or 24, or no EBI was given. No significant differences between Day 1 and Week 12 or 24 were identified; it was concluded that EBI is not necessary during induction.[230] EBI should be separated from chemotherapy,[2, 218, 236, 229] but when EBI is given after two to three courses of chemotherapy, 7% of patients develop brain metastases versus 26% when given after five to six courses.

Hansen and coworkers[237] did not find a significant alteration in the occurrence of brain metastases when EBI was delayed until Week 12. If EBI is delayed longer, nearly 20% of patients develop brain metastasis.[211, 232, 238] It has been proposed that EBI will result in the treatment of 77 extra patients in order to benefit 3; it was concluded that cranial irradiation should be withheld for patients who develop metastases.[239]

Doses for EBI are gradually becoming better defined; the choice of the dose-fractionation scheme is a balance between controlling intracranial disease versus the subsequent development of neurologic toxicity. When 40 Gy in 20 fractions are given, a response is seen in 86%; when 30 Gy in 10 fractions or 20 Gy in 5 fractions are used, the response rate falls to 37.5%. One has to treat this data with caution because a selection process, rather than dose, could be responsible.[232] The dose per fraction should be between 2 and 3 Gy per fraction.[229] Treatment with less than 2 Gy per fraction is likely to cause excessive normal tissue damage; therefore, the use of a more conventional fractionation scheme is strongly recommended.[240] It appears that there is no difference between 25 and 30 Gy in 10 fractions, and no clinically detectable late sequelae were seen. With these two schema, the cumulative risk of developing brain relapse is 10% at 1 year.[241] ECOG has adopted 25 Gy in 10 fractions as its standard for EBI, and there are no reports of serious late effects with this regimen.[133] The delivery of 20 Gy in five fractions is poorly tolerated[229, 242] and should not be used. EBI contributes to myelosuppression even though less than 10% of the bone marrow volume is in the irradiated volume.[242, 243]

Although neurotoxicity has been recognized for over 15 years,[244] the recognition of significant neurologic sequelae in seven of 10 patients surviving 30 months or more stimulated careful investigation of the consequences in the CNS of EBI.[245]

A myriad of symptoms have been associated with the neurotoxicity of EBI. Recent memory loss, poor attention span, dementia, apathy, abulia, difficulty with walking and balance, difficulty writing, paresthesias, weakness, optic atrophy, psychomotor retardation, organic brain syndrome, confusion, speech impairment, inability to concentrate, symptoms of a combination of corticospinal and cerebellar tract signs or tonic-clonic seizures may be seen.[164, 229, 246–248] Eighty-seven per cent of patients report an abnormal neurologic symptom; memory loss (73%) or difficulty with walking or balance (67%) are the most frequent (53). Signs include gait abnormalities, muscle weakness, intention tremor, and peripheral neuropathy.[229] Seventy-one per cent of patients have an abnormal neurologic examination, 64% of patients have a gait abnormality, and 20% will have muscle weakness or tremors.[53] Older patients seem more susceptible to toxic effects.[246] Symptoms develop 14 to 54 months after EBI; the median onset is 24 to 35 months.[236, 249]

Based on serial pre-therapy and post-therapy CT scans, 23% of patients demonstrate cerebral atrophy on the pretreatment scan, although all patients may have this finding after EBI and all changes are likely to be progressive.[250] CT scans also demonstrate cerebral atrophy, ventricular dilatation, and diffuse low attenuation changes in the periventricular white matter.[236, 246, 247, 249, 251] MRI scans demonstrate subcortical white matter changes.[246, 249] Although periventricular hyperintensity may be normal in this age group, all patients who received EBI demonstrated this finding on MRI.[53] Despite these radiologic changes, most of the studies reporting on the clinical neurotoxicity associated with EBI given after chemotherapy find fewer than 20% of patients experience this complication. Laukkanen and colleagues[218] have recommended delaying EBI until completion of all chemotherapy.

If EBI is not a part of the treatment protocol, a number of patients will fail in the brain and will undergo therapeutic cranial irradiation, but irradiation of the brain after the clinical appearance of metastases from SCLC does not rival the benefits of EBI.[252] Thirty-nine of 225 patients (17%) developed brain metastases after initiation of chemotherapy, and 13 of 24 patients with limited-disease with brain metastases had no evidence of other metastases before death. This is a group of patients who had much to gain from EBI.[232] Clinically apparent metastases to more than one area of the neuroaxis is seen in 20% of patients.[215] After confirming the presence of metastases, patients should be started on steroids preceding the initiation of whole brain irradiation.[253] When patients are irradiated to 30 Gy in 15 fractions, 92% will attain a CR or PR, but 89% will have residual disease at autopsy.[215] Using 40 Gy in 20 fractions results in major symptomatic improvement in 46% of patients, unfortunately 45% of patients will show no improvement or progress.[216] A similar dose schedule may result in CR in 32% and a PR in 30%, but 65% will develop recurrent or progressive brain disease. Actuarial median response duration may be dose related, doses 40 Gy or more result in a survival time of 10 months, but patient selection is likely an important factor.[254] Median survival from the start of cranial irradiation is only 1 to 4 months, and patients die of progressive disease.[215, 255]

SURGERY

Because of the poor results obtained with surgery alone in early series of patients with small cell lung cancer, surgical resection has rarely been employed.[7, 8] However, a number of retrospective studies of selected patients (limited-stage disease and no or early node involvement) who have had surgical resection and systemic chemotherapy have shown improved survival and local control when compared with historical controls who were not resected.[7, 257–259] Shepherd and associates reported on 119 patients treated with combined modality therapy, including surgical resection.[7] Seventy-nine patients had surgery initially, and 40 patients had chemotherapy first with no difference between these groups. The median survival for the entire group was 26 months, with a projected 5-year survival rate of 39%. The 35 pathologic Stage I

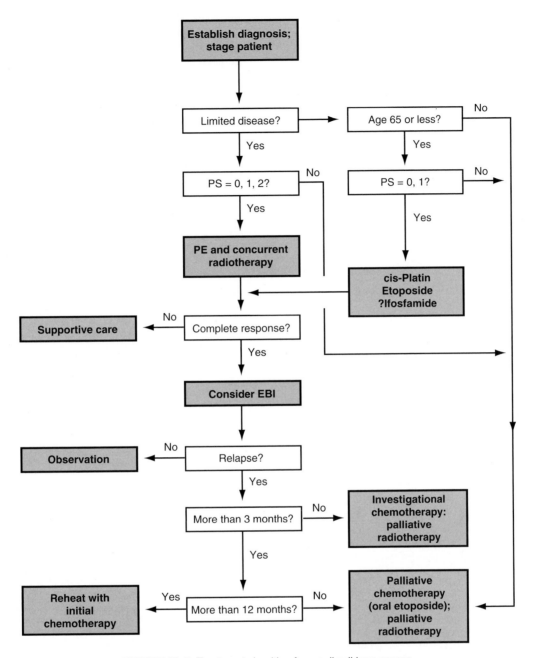

FIGURE 13–5. Treatment algorithm for small cell lung cancer.

patients (of the 69 who had clinical Stage I disease) had a projected 5-year survival rate of 51%, whereas for pathologic Stage II and III patients, it was 28% and 19%, respectively. Osterlind and associates, however, reported that there was no difference in survival in a retrospective study of patients who were clinically deemed operable who either did or did not undergo resection.[260]

Lad and colleagues[261] reported a randomized, prospective trial of surgical resection in 340 patients with limited-stage disease. Sixty five per cent (223 patients) achieved an objective response to chemotherapy, of which 144 were randomized (68 to surgery and 76 to no surgery). The resection rate was 83%, with an 18%

pathologic complete remission rate. There was no difference in survival between the two arms, however, with a 2-year survival rate of 20%.

However, the chemotherapy used in this study is not as effective as current regimens. Surgery should not be considered part of the standard treatment for Dnadvanced small cell lung cancer. The question of surgery most often arises following removal of a solitary lung nodule that is diagnosed as small cell lung cancer. Surgical resection of peripheral tumors with a standard lobectomy, provided there are no extensive lymph node metastases, does provide adequate local control of the tumor and significant long-term survival when combined with chemotherapy.

Atypical Bronchial Carcinoid

Bronchial carcinoids make up 1% to 2% of lung neoplasms.[262, 263] Of this group, approximately 10% to 34% are atypical carcinoids (AC),[262, 264] as defined by cellular atypia, necrosis, architectural disorder, or increased mitotic rate in the presence of a recognizable carcinoid pattern.[265] These tumors demonstrate a more aggressive behavior than well-differentiated typical carcinoids (TC)[264, 266] and are believed by many pathologists to be an intermediate tumor between typical carcinoid and small cell lung cancer.[266] The prognosis of bronchial carcinoids is related to the histology (AC versus TC) and stage.[264] Surgical resection is the treatment of choice,[264] with consideration of chemotherapy following resection for AC.[263]

SUMMARY

Chemotherapy represents the cornerstone of SCLC management (Fig. 13–5). Although no one chemotherapy regimen is optimal for all patients, cisplatin and etoposide is a reasonable initial choice for most patients irrespective of stage. The therapeutic advantage of this regimen is most apparent in patients with limited-stage disease in whom concurrent thoracic radiotherapy is now routinely used. In extensive-stage SCLC, individual patient factors and physician preference play a larger role in determining the choice of initial therapy. For example, the presence of renal dysfunction or cardiac disease may preclude the use of therapy requiring hydration. Drug substitutions such as carboplatin for cisplatin are unlikely to substantially alter outcome and can be used even in the absence of randomized trials demonstrating therapeutic comparability. Furthermore, given the relatively modest improvement in median survival achieved with combination chemotherapy and the general lack of curability of extensive-stage disease, single agent therapy may be an acceptable alternative for selected patients, particularly those who are elderly and may not be good candidates for more intensive therapy.

A better understanding of the basic biology of SCLC will undoubtedly lead to better treatment options. For the present, continued empiric clinical investigations are our best hope of advancing our knowledge of the treatment of this largely preventable malignancy.

Although the role of radiotherapy continues to be defined, some recommendations can be made. Thoracic irradiation should be reserved for patients with limited-stage disease who attain a CR to combination chemotherapy. Our bias is to deliver chemoradiotherapy in a concurrent fashion. Doses of 50 Gy or more at 1.8 to 2 Gy per fraction should be used. The prechemotherapy volume should be used for the initial volume. The spinal cord dose must not exceed 40 Gy. After the administration of 45 Gy, the field size can be reduced and an alternate field arrangement planned. Our preference is to use opposed oblique fields. The supraclavicular nodes should be included in selected cases and routine inclusion does not seem warranted. The treatment volume does not need to include the contralateral hilum. EBI continues to be recommended in patients who would benefit from TRT. The radiation therapy should be separated from chemotherapy, and 2-Gy fractions are recommended. The total dose should be between 25 and 30 Gy. With these guidelines, patients should tolerate treatment without excessive toxicity or morbidity.

SELECTED REFERENCES

Arriagada R, Le Chevalier T, Baldeyrou P, et al: Alternating radiotherapy and chemotherapy schedules in small cell lung cancer, limited disease. Int J Radiat Oncol Biol Phys 11:1461–1467, 1985.
This is one of a series of reports on consecutive French protocols employing alternating radiotherapy and chemotherapy. Based on the results of escalating doses of thoracic irradiation, a total dose of 55 Gy is recommended.

Johnson BE, Ihde DC, Bunn PA, et al. Patients with small cell lung cancer treated with combination chemotherapy with or without irradiation. Ann Intern Med 103:430–438, 1985.
Reports on the long term follow-up of patients treated at the NCI using concurrent radiotherapy and chemotherapy.

Johnson BE, Patronas N, Hayes W, et al. Neurologic, computed cranial tomographic, and magnetic resonance imaging abnormalities in patients with small cell lung cancer: Further follow-up of 6- to 13-year survivors. J Clin Oncol 8:48–56, 1990.
This is a report on the long-term neurologic toxicities, as well as the results of imaging studies, of elective brain irradiation. It also documents that some patients experience a slow decline in neuropsychologic function long after completion of treatment.

Pignon JP, Arriagada R, Ihde DC, et al. A meta-analysis of thoracic radiotherapy for small cell lung cancer. N Engl J Med 327:1618–1624, 1992.
The authors report on a meta-analysis of randomized trials investigating the role of radiotherapy in patients with limited-stage SCLC. Based on this analysis, thoracic irradiation results in an improved overall survival of approximately 5%. It was not possible to identify a preferred method of combining chemotherapy and radiotherapy.

Turrisi AT, Glover DJ, Mason BA. A preliminary report: Concurrent twice-daily radiotherapy plus platinum-etoposide chemotherapy for limited small cell lung cancer. Int J Radiat Oncol Biol Phys 15:183–187, 1988.
This is the initial report employing concurrent platinum and etoposide chemotherapy and twice-daily thoracic irradiation. For patients with limited disease, this is a promising combination and has been repeated in a prospective randomized ECOG trial. The study employed limited radiation fields; the supraclavicular lymph nodes were not routinely irradiated, and the contralateral hilum was not included in the irradiated volume.

REFERENCES

1. Johnson DH, Greco FA: Small cell carcinoma of the lung. Crit Rev Oncol Hematol 4:303–336, 1986.
2. Seifter EJ, Ihde DC: Therapy of small cell lung cancer: A perspective on two decades of clinical research. Semin Oncol 15:278–299, 1988.
3. Viallet J, Ihde DC: Small cell carcinoma of the lung: Clinical and biological aspects. Crit Rev Oncol Hematol 11:109–135, 1991.
4. Minna JD, Pass H, Glatstein E, Ihde DC: Cancer of the lung. *In* DeVita VT, Hellman S, Rosenberg SA (eds): Cancer, Principles and Practice of Oncology. 3rd Ed. Philadelphia: J.B. Lippincott, 1989.
5. Boring CC, Squires TS, Tong T: Cancer statistics. CA Cancer J Clin 42:19–38, 1992.

6. Ihde DC: Chemotherapy of lung cancer. N Engl J Med 327:1434–1441, 1992.
7. Shepherd FA, Ginsberg RJ, Feld R, et al: Surgical treatment for limited small cell lung cancer. The University of Toronto Lung Oncology Group experience. J Thorac Cardiovasc Surg 101:385–393, 1991.
8. Shepherd FA, Ginsberg R, Patterson GA, et al: Is there ever a role for salvage operations in limited small cell lung cancer? J Thorac Cardiovasc Surg 101:196–200, 1991.
9. Green RA, Humphrey E, Close H, Patno ME: Alkylating agents in bronchogenic carcinoma. Am J Med 46:516–525, 1969.
10. Joss RA, Cavalli F, Goldhirsch A, et al: New drugs in small cell lung cancer. Cancer Treat Rev 13:157–176, 1986.
11. Johnson DH: New drugs in the management of small cell lung cancer. Lung Cancer 5:221–231, 1989.
12. Ettinger D, Finkelstein D, Ritch P, et al: Randomized trial of single agents vs combination chemotherapy in extensive stage small cell lung cancer. Proc Am Soc Clin Oncol 11:295, 1992.
13. Ettinger DS, Finkelstein DM, Sarma R, Johnson DH: Phase II study of taxol in patients with extensive-stage small cell lung cancer: An Eastern Cooperative Oncology Group study. Proc Am Soc Clin Oncol 12:329, 1993.
14. Masuda N, Fukuoka M, Kununoki Y, et al: CPT-11: A new derivative of camptothecin for the treatment of refractory or relapsed small cell lung cancer. J Clin Oncol 10:1225–1229, 1992.
15. Slichenmyer WJ, Rowinsky EK, Donehower RC, Kaufmann SH: The current status of camptothecin analogues as antitumor agents. J Natl Cancer Inst 85:271–291, 1993.
16. Bleehen NM, Fayers PM, Girling DJ, Stephens RJ: Survival, adverse reactions and quality of life during combination chemotherapy compared with selective palliative treatment for small cell lung cancer. Report to the Medical Research Council by its Lung Cancer Working Party. Resp Med 83:51–58, 1989.
17. Lowenbraun S, Bartolucci A, Smalley RV, Lynn M, Krauss S, Durant J: The superiority of combination chemotherapy over single agent chemotherapy in small cell lung carcinoma. Cancer 44:406–413, 1979.
18. Alberto P, Brunner KW, Martz G, et al: Treatment of bronchogenic carcinoma with simultaneous or sequential combination chemotherapy, including methotrexate, cyclophosphamide, procarbazine and vincristine. Cancer 38:2208–2216, 1976.
19. Johnson DH: Treatment of limited-stage small cell lung cancer: Recent progress and future directions. Lung Cancer 9(Suppl 1):S1–S19, 1993.
20. Warde P, Payne D: Does thoracic irradiation improve survival and local control in limited-stage small cell lung carcinoma of the lung? A meta-analysis. J Clin Oncol 10:890–895, 1992.
21. Pignon JP, Arriagada R, Ihde DC, et al: A meta-analysis of thoracic radiotherapy for small cell lung cancer. N Engl J Med 327:1618–1624, 1992.
22. Johnson DH, Hainsworth JD, Hande KR, Greco FA: Current status of etoposide in the management of small cell lung cancer. Cancer 67:231–244, 1991.
23. Evans WK, Feld R, Osoba D, et al: VP-16 alone and in combination with cisplatin in previously treated patients with small cell lung cancer. Cancer 53:1461–1466, 1984.
24. Porter LL, Johnson DH, Hainsworth JD, Hande KR, Greco FA: Cisplatinum and VP-16-213 combination chemotherapy for refractory small cell carcinoma of the lung. Cancer Treat Rep 69:479–481, 1985.
25. Andersen M, Kristjansen PEG, Hansen HH: Second-line chemotherapy in small cell lung cancer. Cancer Treat Rev 17:427–436, 1990.
26. Sierocki JS, Hilaris BS, Hopfan S, et al: cis-Dichlorodiammineplatinum(II) and VP-16-213: An active induction regimen for small cell carcinoma of the lung. Cancer Treat Rep 63:1593–1597, 1979.
27. Evans WK, Shepherd FA, Feld R, et al: VP-16 and cisplatin as first-line therapy for small cell lung cancer. J Clin Oncol 3:1471–1477, 1985.
28. Ihde DC, Mulshine JL, Kramer BS, et al: Randomized trial of high vs. standard dose etoposide (VP16) and cisplatin in extensive stage small cell lung cancer. Proc Am Soc Clin Oncol 10:240, 1991.
29. Fukuoka M, Furuse K, Saijo N, et al: Randomized trial of cyclophosphamide, doxorubicin, and vincristine versus cisplatin and etoposide versus alternation of these regimens in small cell lung cancer. J Natl Cancer Inst 83:855–861, 1991.
30. Roth BJ, Johnson DH, Einhorn LH, et al: Randomized study of cyclophosphamide, doxorubicin, and vincristine versus etoposide and cisplatin versus alternation of these two regimens in extensive stage small cell lung cancer: A phase III trial of the Southeastern Cancer Study Group. J Clin Oncol 10:282–291, 1992.
31. Double EB: Keynote address: Platinum-radiation interactions. NCI Monogr 6:315–319, 1988.
32. Chang AYC, Gu Z, Keng P, Sobel S: Radiation sensitizing effects of topoisomerase I and II inhibitors. Proc Am Assoc Cancer Res 32:389, 1991.
33. Spiro SG, Souhami RL, Geddes DM, et al: Duration of chemotherapy in small cell lung cancer: A Cancer Research Campaign trial. Br J Cancer 59:578–585, 1989.
34. Clarke SJ, Bell DR, Woods RL, Levi JA: Maintenance chemotherapy for small cell carcinoma of the lung: Long term follow-up. Proc Am Soc Clin Oncol 8:248, 1989.
35. Bleehen NM, Fayers PM, Girling DJ, Stephens RJ: Controlled trial of twelve versus six courses of chemotherapy in the treatment of small cell lung cancer. Br J Cancer 59:584–590, 1989.
36. Feld R, Evans WK, DeBoer G, et al: Combined modality induction therapy without maintenance chemotherapy for small cell carcinoma of the lung. J Clin Oncol 4:294–304, 1984.
37. Einhorn LH, Greco FA, Crawford J, et al: Cisplatin plus etoposide consolidation following cyclophosphamide, doxorubicin, and vincristine in limited small cell lung cancer. J Clin Oncol 6:451–456, 1988.
38. Aisner J, Abrams J: Cisplatin for small cell lung cancer. Semin Oncol 16:2–9, 1989.
39. Smith IE, Evans BD, Gore ME, et al: Carboplatin (Paraplatin; JM8) and etoposide (VP-16) as first-line combination therapy for small cell lung cancer. J Clin Oncol 5:185–189, 1987.
40. Bishop JF, Raghaven D, Stuart-Harris R, et al: Carboplatin (CBDCA, JM-8) and VP-16-213 in previously untreated patients with small cell lung cancer. J Clin Oncol 5:1574–1578, 1987.
41. Evans WK, Eisenhauer E, Hughes P, et al: VP-16 and carboplatin in previously untreated patients with extensive small cell lung cancer: A study of the National Cancer Institute of Canada Clinical Trials Group. Br J Cancer 58:464–468, 1988.
42. Johnson DH: Recent developments in chemotherapy treatment of small cell lung cancer. Semin Oncol 20:315–325, 1993.
43. D'Incalci M, Rossi C, Zucchetti M, et al: Pharmacokinetics of etoposide in patients with abnormal renal and hepatic function. Cancer Res 46:2566–2571, 1986.
44. Abeloff MD, Klastersky J, Drings PD, et al: Complications of treatment of small cell carcinoma of the lung. Cancer Treat Rep 67:21–26, 1983.
45. Johnson DH, Einhorn LH, Birch R, et al: A randomized comparison of high-dose versus conventional-dose cyclophosphamide, doxorubicin, and vincristine for extensive-stage small cell lung cancer: A phase III trial of the Southeastern Cancer Study Group. J Clin Oncol 5:1731–1738, 1987.
46. Einhorn LH, Nagy C, Werner K, Finn AL: Ondansetron: A new antiemetic for patients receiving cisplatin chemotherapy. J Clin Oncol 8:731–735, 1990.
47. Crawford J, Ozer H, Stoller R, et al: Reduction by granulocyte colony-stimulating factor of fever and neutropenia induced by chemotherapy in patients with small cell lung cancer. N Engl J Med 325:164–170, 1991.
48. Bunn PA, Crowley J, Hazuka M, et al: The role of GM-CSF in limited stage SCLC: A randomized phase III study of the Southwest Oncology Group (SWOG). Proc Am Soc Clin Oncol 11:292, 1992.
49. de Jongh CA, Wade JC, Finley R, et al: Trimethoprim/sulfamethoxazole versus placebo: A double-blind comparison of infection prophylaxis in patients with small cell carcinoma of the lung. J Clin Oncol 1:302–307, 1983.
50. Johnson DH, Porter LL, List AF, et al: Acute non-lymphocytic leukemia following treatment of small cell lung cancer. Am J Med 81:962–968, 1986.
51. Heyne KH, Lippman SM, Lee JJ, et al: The incidence of second

primary tumors in long-term survivors of small cell lung cancer. J Clin Oncol 10:1519–1524, 1992.

52. Sagmen U, Lishner M, Maki E, et al: Second primary malignancies following diagnosis of small cell lung cancer. J Clin Oncol 10:1525–1533, 1992.

53. Johnson BE, Patronas N, Hayes W, et al: Neurologic, computed cranial tomographic, and magnetic resonance imaging abnormalities in patients with small cell lung cancer: Further follow-up of 6- to 13-year survivors. J Clin Oncol 8:48–56, 1990.

54. Turrisi AT: Brain irradiation and systemic chemotherapy for small cell lung cancer: Dangerous liaisons? J Clin Oncol 8:196–199, 1990.

55. Goldie JH, Coldman AJ: The genetic origin of drug resistance in neoplasms: Implications for systemic therapy. Cancer Res 44:3643–3653, 1984.

56. Goldie JH, Coldman AJ: A mathematic model for relating drug sensitivity of tumors to their spontaneous mutation rate. Cancer Treat Rep 63:1727–1733, 1979.

57. Goldie JH, Coldman AJ, Gudauskas GA: Rationale for the use of alternating non-cross-resistant chemotherapy. Cancer Treat Rep 66:439–449, 1982.

58. Evans WK, Feld R, Murray N, et al: Superiority of alternating non-cross-resistant chemotherapy in extensive small cell lung cancer. Ann Intern Med 107:451–458, 1987.

59. Feld R, Evans WK, Coy P, et al: Canadian multicenter randomized trial comparing sequential and alternating administration of two non-cross-resistant chemotherapy combinations in patients with limited small cell carcinoma of the lung. J Clin Oncol 5:1401–1409, 1987.

60. Goodman GE, Crowley JJ, Blasko JC, et al: Treatment of limited small cell lung cancer with etoposide and cisplatin alternating with vincristine, doxorubicin, and cyclophosphamide versus concurrent etoposide, vincristine, doxorubicin, and cyclophosphamide and chest radiotherapy: A Southwest Oncology Group study. J Clin Oncol 8:39–47, 1990.

61. Frei E, Canellos G: Dose: A critical factor in cancer chemotherapy. Am J Med 69:585–594, 1980.

62. Schabel FM, Griswold DP, Corbett TH, et al: Testing therapeutic hypotheses in mice and man: Observations on the therapeutic activity against advanced solid tumors of mice treated with anticancer drugs that have demonstrated or potential clinical utility for treatment of advanced solid tumors in man. In DeVita VT, Busch H (eds): Methods in Cancer Research. Cancer Drug Development Part B. New York, Academic Press, Inc., 1979, pp 4–52.

63. Cohen MH, Creaven PJ, Fossieck BE, et al: Intensive chemotherapy of small cell bronchogenic carcinoma. Cancer Treat Rep 61:349–354, 1977.

64. Figueredo AT, Hryniuk WM, Strautmanis I, et al: Co-trimoxazole prophylaxis during high-dose chemotherapy of small cell lung cancer. J Clin Oncol 3:54–64, 1985.

65. Harper PG, Souhami RL: Intensive chemotherapy with autologous bone marrow transplantation in small cell carcinoma of the lung. Rec Adv Cancer Res 97:146–156, 1985.

66. Johnson DH, Wolff SN, Hainsworth JD, et al: Extensive-stage small cell bronchogenic carcinoma: Intensive induction chemotherapy with high-dose cyclophosphamide plus high-dose etoposide. J Clin Oncol 3:170–175, 1985.

67. Farha P, Spitzer G, Valdivieso M, et al: High-dose chemotherapy and autologous bone marrow transplantation for the treatment of small cell lung carcinoma. Cancer 52:1351–1355, 1983.

68. Johnson DH, DeLeo MJ, Hande KR, et al: High-dose induction chemotherapy with cyclophosphamide, etoposide, and cisplatin for extensive-stage small cell lung cancer. J Clin Oncol 5:703–709, 1987.

69. Wolff SN, Johnson DH, Hande KR, et al: High-dose etoposide as single agent chemotherapy for small cell carcinoma of the lung. Cancer Treat Rep 67:957–958, 1983.

70. Souhami RL, Harper PG, Linch D, et al: High-dose cyclophosphamide with autologous marrow transplantation as initial treatment of small cell carcinoma of the bronchus. Cancer Chemother Pharmacol 8:31–34, 1982.

71. Hryniuk WM: The importance of dose intensity in the outcome of chemotherapy. In DeVita VT, Hellman S, Rosenberg SA (eds): Important Advances in Oncology 1988. Philadelphia: J.B. Lippincott, 1988, pp 121–141.

72. Murray N: The importance of dose and dose intensity in lung cancer chemotherapy. Semin Oncol 14(Suppl 4):20–28, 1987.

73. Tabbara IA, Quesenberry PJ, Hahn SS, Stewart M: Treatment of small cell carcinoma with weekly combination chemotherapy. A pilot study. Anticancer Res 9:189–192, 1989.

74. Taylor CW, Crowley J, Williamson SK, et al: Treatment of small cell lung cancer with an alternating chemotherapy regimen given at weekly intervals: A Southwest Oncology Group pilot study. J Clin Oncol 8:1811–1817, 1990.

75. Miles DW, Earl HM, Souhami RL, et al: Intensive weekly chemotherapy for good-prognosis patients with small cell lung cancer. J Clin Oncol 9:280–285, 1991.

76. Murray N, Shah A, Osoba D, et al: Intensive weekly chemotherapy for the treatment of extensive-stage small cell lung cancer. J Clin Oncol 9:1632–1638, 1991.

77. Fukuoka M, Takada M, Masuda N, et al: Dose intensive weekly chemotherapy with or without recombinant granulocyte colony-stimulating factor in extensive-stage small cell lung cancer. Proc Am Soc Clin Oncol 11:290, 1992.

78. Wampler GL, Ahlgren JD, Schulof RS: A pilot study of intensive weekly chemotherapy for extensive disease small cell lung carcinoma. Cancer Invest 10:97–102, 1992.

79. Kudoh S, Fukuoka M, Negoro S, et al: Weekly dose-intensive chemotherapy in patients with small cell lung cancer: A pilot study. Am J Clin Oncol 15:29–34, 1992.

80. Miles DW, Souhami RL, Spiro SG, et al: A randomized trial comparing "standard" 3 weekly with weekly chemotherapy in patients with small cell lung cancer. Proc Am Soc Clin Oncol 11:289, 1992.

81. Sculier JP, Paesmans M, Bureau G, et al: Multiple drug weekly chemotherapy versus combination regimen in small cell lung cancer: A phase III randomized study conducted by the European Lung Cancer Working Party. J Clin Oncol 11:1858–1865, 1993.

82. Souhami RL, Bradbury I, Geddes DM, et al: Prognostic significance of laboratory parameters measured at diagnosis in small cell carcinoma of the lung. Cancer Res 45:2878–2882, 1985.

83. Norton L, Simon R: Tumor size, sensitivity to therapy, and design of treatment schedules. Cancer Treat Rep 61:1307–1317, 1977.

84. Humblet Y, Symann M, Bosly A, et al: Late intensification chemotherapy with autologous bone marrow transplantation in selected small cell carcinoma of the lung: A randomized study. J Clin Oncol 5:1864–1873, 1987.

85. Ihde DC, Deisseroth AB, Lichter AS, et al: Late intensive combined modality therapy followed by autologous bone marrow infusion in extensive-stage small cell lung cancer. J Clin Oncol 4:1443–1454, 1986.

86. Spitzer G, Farha P, Valdivieso M, et al: High-dose intensification therapy with autologous bone marrow support for limited small cell bronchogenic carcinoma. J Clin Oncol 4:4–13, 1986.

87. Goodman GE, Crowley J, Livingston RB, et al: Treatment of limited small cell lung cancer with concurrent etoposide/cisplatin and radiotherapy followed by intensification with high-dose cyclophosphamide: A Southwest Oncology Group study. J Clin Oncol 9:453–457, 1991.

88. Smith IE, Evans BD, Harland SJ, et al: High-dose cyclophosphamide with autologous bone marrow rescue after conventional chemotherapy in the treatment of small cell lung carcinoma. Cancer Chemother Pharmacol 14:120–124, 1985.

89. Livingston RB: Small cell lung cancer—whither late intensification? J Clin Oncol 4:1437–1438, 1986.

90. Elias AD, Ayash L, Frei E, et al: Intensive combined modality therapy for limited-stage small cell lung cancer. J Natl Cancer Inst 85:559–566, 1993.

91. Batist G, Ihde DC, Zabell A, et al: Small cell carcinoma of the lung: Reinduction therapy after late relapse. Ann Intern Med 98:472–474, 1983.

92. Giaccone G, Ferrati P, Donadio M, et al: Reinduction chemotherapy in small cell lung cancer. Eur J Cancer 23:1697–1699, 1987.

93. Vincent M, Evans B, Smith I: First-line chemotherapy rechallenge after relapse in small cell lung cancer. Cancer Chemother Pharmacol 21:45–48, 1988.

94. Johnson DH, Greco FA, Strupp J, et al: Prolonged administra-

tion of oral etoposide in patients with relapsed or refractory small cell lung cancer: A phase II trial. J Clin Oncol 8:1613–1617, 1990.

95. Shepherd FA, Evans WK, MacCormick R, et al: Cyclophosphamide, doxorubicin and vincristine in etoposide- and cisplatin-resistant small cell lung cancer. Cancer Treat Rep 71:941–944, 1987.

96. Einhorn LH, Bond WH, Hornback N, Joe BT: Phase II trial of oral VP-16 in refractory small cell lung cancer: A Hoosier Oncology Group study. Semin Oncol 17:32–35, 1990.

97. Faylona E, Loehrer P, Einhorn L, et al: A phase II study of daily oral VP-16 + ifosfamide + cisplatin for previously treated small cell lung cancer: A Hoosier Oncology Group trial. Proc Am Soc Clin Oncol 11:307, 1992.

98. Findley MPN, Griffin AM, Raghavan D, et al: Retrospective review of chemotherapy for small cell lung cancer in the elderly: Does the end justify the means? Eur J Cancer 27:1597–1601, 1991.

99. Balducci L, Parker M, Sexton W, Tantranond P: Pharmacology of antineoplastic agents in the elderly patient. Semin Oncol 16:76–84, 1989.

100. Walsh SJ, Begg CB, Carbone PP: Cancer chemotherapy in the elderly. Semin Oncol 16:66–75, 1989.

101. Egorin MJ: Cancer pharmacology in the elderly. Semin Oncol 20:43–49, 1993.

102. Shepherd FA, Goss P, Evans W, et al: Treatment of small cell lung cancer in the elderly. Proc Am Soc Clin Oncol 10:241, 1991.

103. Goss GD, Logan D, Maroun J, Stewart D, Yau J, Evans WK: Chemotherapy in elderly patients with small cell lung cancer. Proc Am Soc Clin Oncol 11:290, 1992.

104. Poplin E, Thompson B, Whitacre M, Aisner J: Small cell carcinoma of the lung: Influence of age on treatment outcome. Cancer Treat Rep 71:291–296, 1987.

105. Johnson PWM, Seymour MT, Waines A, et al: Etoposide as a single agent in small cell lung cancer: As good as combination chemotherapy? Proc Am Soc Clin Oncol 11:291, 1992.

106. Johnson DH: Treatment of the elderly patient with small cell lung cancer. Chest 103:72S–74S, 1993.

107. Smit EF, Carney DN, Harford P, et al: A phase II study of oral etoposide in elderly patients with extensive small cell lung cancer. Thorax 44:631–633, 1989.

108. Clark PI, Cottier B: The activity of 10-, 14-, and 21-day schedules of single-agent etoposide in previously untreated patients with extensive small cell lung cancer. Semin Oncol 19(Suppl 14):36–39, 1992.

109. Gatzemeier U, Neuhauss R, Heckmayr M: Single agent oral etoposide in advanced NSCLC (chronic daily) and in elderly patients with SCLC. Lung Cancer 7(Suppl):102, 1991.

110. Hande KR, Krozely MG, Greco FA, et al: Bioavailability of low-dose oral etoposide. J Clin Oncol 11:374–377, 1993.

111. Aisner J: Identification of new drugs in small cell lung cancer: Phase II agents first? Cancer Treat Rep 71:1131–1133, 1987.

112. Cullen M: Evaluating new drugs in patients with chemosensitive tumours: Ethical dilemmas in extensive small cell lung cancer. Lung Cancer 5:1–7, 1989.

113. Ettinger DS: Evaluation of new drugs in untreated patients with small cell lung cancer: Its time has come. J Clin Oncol 8:374–377, 1990.

114. Grant SC, Gralla RJ, Kris MG, et al: Single-agent chemotherapy trials in small cell lung cancer, 1970 to 1990: The case for studies in previously treated patients. J Clin Oncol 10:484–498, 1992.

115. Grant SC, Kris MG: Phase II trials in small cell lung cancer: Shouldn't we be doing better? J Natl Cancer Inst 84:1058–1059, 1992.

116. Simon RM: Design and conduct of clinical trials. In DeVita VT, Hellman S, Rosenberg SA (eds): Cancer, Principles and Practice of Oncology. 3rd Ed. Philadelphia, J.B. Lippincott, 1989, pp 396–420.

117. Blackstein M, Eisenhauer EA, Wierzbicki R, Yoshida S: Epirubicin in extensive small cell lung cancer: A phase II study in previously untreated patients: A National Cancer Institute of Canada Clinical Trials Group study. J Clin Oncol 8:385–389, 1990.

118. Evans WK, Eisenhauer EA, Cormier Y, et al: Phase II study of

amonafide: Results of treatment and lessons learned from the study of an investigational agent in previously untreated patients with extensive small cell lung cancer. J Clin Oncol 8:390–395, 1990.

119. Ettinger DS, Finkelstein DM, Abeloff MD, et al: Justification for evaluating new anticancer agents in selected untreated patients with extensive-stage small cell lung cancer: An Eastern Cooperative Oncology Group randomized study. J Natl Cancer Inst 84:1077–1084, 1992.

120. DeVore RF, Johnson DH: Lung cancer: Chemotherapy. In Brain MC, Carbone PP (eds): Current Therapy in Hematology—Oncology. 4th Ed. Philadelphia, B.C. Dekker, Inc., 1992, pp 245–249.

121. Giaccone G, Dalesio O, McVie G, et al: Maintenance chemotherapy in small cell lung cancer: Long-term results of a randomized trial. J Clin Oncol 11:1230–1240, 1993.

122. Murray N, Osoba D, Shah A, et al: Brief intensive chemotherapy for metastatic non-small cell lung cancer: A phase II study of weekly CODE regimen. J Natl Cancer Inst 83:190–194, 1991.

123. Fox W, Scadding JG: Medical Research Council comparative trial of surgery and radiotherapy for primary treatment of small-celled or oat-celled carcinoma of bronchus. Lancet 2:63–65, 1973.

124. Miller AB, Fox W, Tall R: Five-year follow-up of the Medical Research Council Comparative trial of surgery and radiotherapy for the primary treatment of small or oat-celled carcinoma of the bronchus. Lancet 2:501–505, 1969.

125. Bergsagel DE, Jenkin RDT, White DM, et al: Lung cancer: Clinical trial of radiotherapy alone versus radiotherapy plus cyclophosphamide. Cancer 30:621–627, 1972.

126. Aisner J, Alberto P, Comis R, et al: Role of chemotherapy in small cell lung cancer: A consensus report of the International Association for the Study of Lung Cancer Workshop. Cancer Treat Rep 67:37–43, 1983.

127. Salazar OM, Creech RH: "The state of the art" toward defining the role of radiation therapy in the management of small cell bronchogenic carcinoma. Int J Radiat Oncol Biol Phys 6:1103–1117, 1980.

128. Cox JD, Byhardt R, Komaki R, et al: Interaction of thoracic irradiation and chemotherapy on local control and survival in small cell carcinoma of the lung. Cancer Treat Rep 63:1251–1255, 1979.

129. Cox JD, Holoye PY, Byhardt RW, et al: The role of thoracic and cranial irradiation for small cell carcinoma of the lung. Int J Radiat Oncol Biol Phys 8:191–196, 1982.

130. Haraf DJ, Devine S, Ihde DC, Vokes EE: The evolving role of systemic therapy in carcinoma of the lung. Semin Oncol 19:72–87, 1992.

131. Perry MC, Eaton WL, Propert KJ, et al: Chemotherapy with or without radiation therapy in limited small-cell carcinoma of the lung. N Engl J Med 316:912–918, 1897.

132. Osterlind K, Hansen HH, Hansen HS, et al: Chemotherapy versus chemotherapy plus irradiation in limited small cell lung cancer. Results of a controlled trial with five years follow-up. Br J Cancer 54:7–17, 1986.

133. Turrisi AT: Innovations in multimodality therapy for lung cancer—combined modality management of limited small-cell lung cancer. Chest 103:56S–59S, 1993.

134. Wilson HE, Stanley K, Vincent RG: Comparison of chemotherapy alone versus chemotherapy and radiation therapy of extensive small cell carcinoma of the lung. J Surg Oncol 23:181–184, 1983.

135. Mira JG, Livingston RB: Evaluation and radiotherapy implications of chest relapse patterns in small cell lung carcinoma treated with radiotherapy-chemotherapy. Cancer 46:2557–2565, 1980.

136. McMahon LJ, Herman TS, Manning MR: Patterns of relapse in patients with small cell carcinoma of the lung treated with Adriamycin-cyclophosphamide chemotherapy and radiation therapy. Cancer Treat Rep 63:359–362, 1979.

137. Johnson DH, Turrisi AT, Chang AY, et al: Alternating chemotherapy and twice-daily thoracic radiotherapy in limited-stage small-cell lung cancer: A pilot study of the Eastern Cooperative Oncology Group. J Clin Oncol 11:879–884, 1993.

138. Turrisi AT: Local failure (LF) and local control (LC) in limited small cell lung cancer (LSCLC): Influence of thoracic radiother-

apy factors and variant histology. (Abstract.) Int J Radiat Oncol Biol Phys 17(Suppl 1):201, 1989.

139. White JE, Chen T, McCracken J, et al: The influence of radiation therapy quality control on survival, response, and sites of relapse in oat cell carcinoma of the lung. Preliminary report of a Southwest Oncology Group study. Cancer 50:1084–1090, 1982.

140. Emami B, Manolis J, Barest G, et al: Three-dimensional treatment planning for lung cancer. Int J Radiat Oncol Biol Phys 21:217–227, 1991.

141. Vogelsang GB, Abeloff MD, Ettinger DS, Booker SV: Long-term survivors of small cell carcinoma of the lung. Am J Med 79:49–56, 1985.

142. Catane R, Lichter A, Lee YJ, et al: Small cell lung cancer: Analysis of treatment factors contributing to prolonged survival. Cancer 48:1936–1943, 1981.

143. Cox JD, Byhardt RW, Wilson JF, et al: Dose-time relationships and the local control of small cell carcinoma of the lung. Radiology 128:205–208, 1978.

144. Choi CH, Carey RW: Small cell anaplastic carcinoma of lung. Reappraisal of current management. Cancer 37:2651–2657, 1976.

145. Eaton WL, Maurer H, Glicksman A, et al: The relationship of infield recurrences to prescribed tumor dose in small cell carcinoma of the lung. Int J Radiat Oncol Biol Phys 7:1223, 1981.

146. Arriagada R, Le Chevalier T, Ruffie P: Alternating radiotherapy and chemotherapy in 173 consecutive patients with limited small cell lung carcinoma. Int J Radiat Oncol Biol Phys 19:1135–1138, 1990.

147. Arriagada R, Kramar A, LeChevalier T, et al: Competing events determining relapse-free survival in limited small-cell lung carcinoma. J Clin Oncol 10:447–451, 1992.

148. Choi NC, Carey RW: Importance of radiation dose in achieving improved loco-regional tumor control in limited stage small-cell lung carcinoma: An update. Int J Radiat Oncol Biol Phys 17:307–310, 1989.

149. Thatcher N, Lind M, Stout R, et al: Carboplatin, ifosfamide and etoposide with mid-course vincristine and thoracic radiotherapy for 'limited' stage small cell carcinoma of the bronchus. Br J Cancer 60:98–101, 1989.

150. Tubiana M, Arriagada R, Cosset JM: Sequencing of drugs and radiation. Cancer 55:2131–2139, 1985.

151. Saijo N: Combined modality therapy for small cell lung cancer. Oncology 49(Suppl 1):2–10, 1992.

152. Arriagada R, Le Chevalier T, Baldeyrou P, et al: Alternating radiotherapy and chemotherapy schedules in small cell lung cancer, limited disease. Int J Radiat Oncol Biol Phys 11:1461–1467, 1985.

153. Ochs JJ, Tester WJ, Cohen MH, et al: "Salvage" radiation therapy for intrathoracic small cell carcinoma of the lung progressing on combination chemotherapy. Cancer Treat Rep 67:1123–1126, 1983.

154. Fox RM, Woods RL, Brodie GN, Tattersall M: A randomized study: Small cell anaplastic lung cancer treated by combination chemotherapy and adjuvant radiotherapy. Int J Radiat Oncol Biol Phys 6:1083–1085, 1980.

155. Nou E, Brodin O, Bergh J: A randomized study of radiation treatment in small cell bronchial carcinoma treated with two types of four-drug chemotherapy regimens. Cancer 62:1079–1090, 1988.

156. Perez CA, Krauss S, Bartolucci AA, et al: Thoracic and elective brain irradiation with concomitant or delayed multiagent chemotherapy in the treatment of localized small cell carcinoma of the lung: A randomized prospective study by the Southeastern Cancer Study Group. Cancer 47:2407–2413, 1981.

157. Souhami RL, Geddes DM, Spiro SG, et al: Radiotherapy in small cell cancer of the lung treated with combination chemotherapy: A controlled trial. Br Med J 288:1643–1646, 1984.

158. Byhardt RW, Cox JD, Libnoch JA, et al: Multiagent chemotherapy, prophylactic neuroaxis irradiation and consolidative irradiation for small cell carcinoma of the lung. Am J Clin Oncol 8:504–511, 1985.

159. Papac R, Yung S, Bien R, et al: Improved local control of thoracic disease in small cell lung cancer with higher dose thoracic irradiation and cyclic chemotherapy. Int J Radiat Oncol Biol Phys 13:993–998, 1987.

160. Kies MS, Mira JG, Crowley JJ, et al: Multimodal therapy for limited small-cell lung cancer: A randomized study of induction chemotherapy with or without thoracic radiation in complete responders; and with wide-field versus reduced-field radiation in partial responders: A Southwest Oncology Group study. J Clin Oncol 5:592–600, 1987.

161. Creech R, Richter M, Finkelstein D: Combination chemotherapy with or without consolidation radiation therapy for regional small cell carcinoma of the lung. (Abstract.) Proc Am Soc Clin Oncol 7:196, 1988.

162. Perez CA, Einhorn L, Oldham RK, et al: Randomized trial of radiotherapy to the thorax in limited small-cell carcinoma of the lung treated with multi-agent chemotherapy and elective brain irradiation: A preliminary report. J Clin Oncol 2:1200–1208, 1984.

163. Bleehen NM, Girling DJ, Gregor A, et al: A Medical Research Council phase II trial of alternating chemotherapy and radiotherapy in small-cell lung cancer. The Medical Research Council Lung Cancer Working Party. Br J Cancer 64:775–779, 1991.

164. Johnson RE, Brereton HD, Kent CH: Small-cell carcinoma of the lung: Attempt to remedy causes of past therapeutic failure. Lancet 2:289–291, 1976.

165. Greco FA, Einhorn LH, Richardson RL, Oldham RK: Small cell lung cancer: Progress and perspectives. Semin Oncol 5:323–335, 1978.

166. Bunn PA, Lichter A, Makuch R, et al: Chemotherapy alone or chemotherapy with chest radiation therapy in limited stage small cell lung cancer. Ann Intern Med 106:655–662, 1987.

167. Aisner J, Goutsou M, Mauer LH, et al: Intensive combination chemotherapy, concurrent chest irradiation, and warfarin for the treatment of limited-disease small cell lung cancer: A cancer and leukemia B pilot study. J Clin Oncol 10:1230–1236, 1992.

168. Birch R, Omura GA, Greco FA, et al: Patterns of failure in combined chemotherapy and radiotherapy for limited small cell lung cancer: Southeastern Cancer Study Group experience. NCI Monogr 6:265–270, 1988.

169. McCraken JD, Janaki LM, Crowley JJ, et al: Concurrent chemotherapy/radiotherapy for limited small-cell lung carcinoma: A Southwest Oncology Group Study. J Clin Oncol 8:892–898, 1990.

170. Shank B, Scher H, Hilaris BS, et al: Increased survival with high-dose multifield radiotherapy and intensive chemotherapy in limited small cell carcinoma of the lung. Cancer 56:2771–2778, 1985.

171. Johnson DH, Bass D, Einhorn LH, et al: Combination chemotherapy with or without thoracic radiotherapy in limited-stage small-cell lung cancer: A randomized trial of the Southeastern Cancer Study Group. J Clin Oncol 11:1223–1229, 1993.

172. Mornex F, Trillet V, Chauvin F, et al: Hyperfractionated radiotherapy alternating with multidrug chemotherapy in the treatment of limited small cell lung cancer (SCLC). Int J Radiat Oncol Biol Phys 19:23–30, 1990.

173. Armstrong JG, Rosenstein MM, Scher HI, et al: Limited small cell lung cancer: Prognostic significance of a complete response to the induction phase of chemotherapy followed by thoracic irradiation. Radiology 178:875–878, 1991.

174. Armstrong JG, Rosenstein MM, Kris MG, et al: Twice daily thoracic irradiation for limited small cell lung cancer. Int J Radiat Oncol Biol Phys 21:1269–1274, 1991.

175. Frytak S, Shaw EG, Eagan RT, et al: Hyperfractionated thoracic radiotherapy (HTRT) and infusion cisplatin based chemotherapy (CT) for small cell lung cancer (SCLC)—A preliminary report. (Abstract.) Proc Am Soc Clin Oncol 8:239, 1989.

176. Frytak S, Shaw R, Eagan E, et al: Accelerated hyperfractionated split-course thoracic radiotherapy (AHSCTRT) and infusion cisplatin based chemotherapy for small cell lung cancer. Proc Am Soc Clin Oncol 9:234, 1990.

177. Hoskin PJ, Parton D, Yarnold JR, et al: Intercalated radiochemotherapy in small cell lung cancer: Toxicity and implications for future regimens. Radiother Oncol 20:177–180, 1991.

178. Turrisi AT, Glover DJ, Mason BA: A preliminary report: Concurrent twice-daily radiotherapy plus platinum-etoposide chemotherapy for limited small cell lung cancer. Int J Radiat Oncol Biol Phys 15:183–187, 1988.

179. Turrisi AT, Glover DJ: Thoracic radiotherapy variables: Influ-

ence on local control in small cell lung cancer limited disease. Int J Radiat Oncol Biol Phys 19:1473–1479, 1990.

180. Mitchell JB, Morstyn G, Russo A, Carney DN: In vitro radiobiology of human lung cancer. Cancer Treat Symp 2:3–10, 1985.

181. Carney D, Mitchell J, Kinsella T: In vitro radiation and chemotherapy sensitivity of established cell lines of human small cell lung cancer and its large cell morphological variants. Cancer Res 43:2806–2811, 1983.

182. Johnson BE, Grayson J, Woods E, et al: Limited (LTD) stage small cell lung cancer (SCLC) treated with concurrent etoposide/cisplatin (VP/PLAT) plus BID chest radiotherapy (RT). (Abstract.) Proc Am Soc Clin Oncol 8:228, 1989.

183. Johnson BE, Salem C, Nesbitt J, et al: Limited (LTD) stage small cell lung cancer (SCLC) treated with concurrent BID chest radiotherapy and etoposide/cisplatin (VP/PT) followed by chemotherapy (CT) selected by in vitro drug sensitivity testing (DST). (Abstract.) Proc Am Soc Clin Oncol 10:240, 1991.

184. Turrisi AT, Wagner H, Glover D, et al: Limited small cell lung cancer (LSCLC): Concurrent BID thoracic radiotherapy (TRT) with platinum-etoposide (PE): An ECOG study. (Abstract.) Proc Am Soc Clin Oncol 9:230, 1990.

185. Johnson DH, Turrisi AT, Chang AY, et al: Alternating chemotherapy (CT) and thoracic radiotherapy (TRT) in limited small-cell lung cancer (LSCLC): A test of the Looney hypothesis. (Abstract.) Proc Am Soc Clin Oncol 10:243, 1991.

186. Tourani JM, Levy R, Even P, Andrieu JM: Short intensive five-drug chemotherapy (CT) followed by extensive irradiation for limited small-cell lung cancer (LSCLC). Improved response rate and survival. A pilot study. (Abstract.) Proc Am Soc Clin Oncol 10:245, 1991.

187. Qasim MM: Total-body irradiation in oat cell carcinoma of the bronchus. Clin Radiol 32:37–39, 1981.

188. Byhardt RW, Cox JD, Wilson JF, et al: Total body irradiation vs. chemotherapy as a systemic adjuvant for small cell carcinoma of the lung. Int J Radiat Oncol Biol Phys 5:2043–2048, 1979.

189. Elias AD, Ayash L, Skarin AT, et al: High-dose combined alkylating agent therapy with autologous stem cell support and chest radiotherapy for limited small-cell lung cancer. Chest 103:433S–435S, 1993.

190. Das S, Scott JS, Clark RA, et al: Total body irradiation as an alternative to systemic chemotherapy in small-cell anaplastic lung cancer. Br J Clin Pract 44:571–573, 1990.

191. Urtasun RC, Belch A, Bodnar RN: Hemibody radiation, an active therapeutic modality for the management of patients with small cell lung cancer. Int J Radiat Oncol Biol Phys 9:1575–1578, 1983.

192. Brincker H, Hindberg J, Hansen PV: Cyclic alternating polychemotherapy with or without upper and lower half-body irradiation in small cell anaplastic lung cancer. A randomized study. Eur J Cancer Clin Oncol 23:205–211, 1987.

193. Mason BA, Richter MP, Catalano RB, Creech RB: Upper hemibody and local chest irradiation as consolidation following response to high-dose induction chemotherapy for small cell bronchogenic carcinoma—A pilot study. Cancer Treat Rep 66:1609–1612, 1982.

194. Salazar OM, Creech RH, Rubin P, et al: Half-body and local chest irradiation as consolidation following response to standard induction chemotherapy for disseminated small cell lung cancer. Int J Radiat Oncol Biol Phys 6:1093–1102, 1980.

195. Huttner J, Wiener N, Quadt C, et al: A randomized clinical trial comparing systemic radiotherapy versus chemotherapy versus local radiotherapy in small cell lung cancer. Eur J Cancer Clin Oncol 25:933–937, 1989.

196. Belch AR, Urtasun RC, Bodnar D, Kinney B: Use of hemibody irradiation as a non-cross-resistant agent in combination with systematic chemotherapy in small cell lung cancer. NCI Monogr 6:271–274, 1988.

197. Eichorn HJ, Huttner J, Dalluge KH: Preliminary report on "one-time" and high dose irradiation of the upper and lower half-body in patients with small cell lung cancer. Int J Radiat Oncol Biol Phys 9:1459–1465, 1983.

198. Arriagada R, Cueto Ladron de Guevara J, Hanzen C, et al: Limited small cell lung cancer treated by combined radiotherapy and chemotherapy: Evaluation of a grading system of lung fibrosis. Radiother Oncol 14:1–8, 1989.

199. Trask CWL, Joannides T, Harper PG, et al: Radiation-induced lung fibrosis after treatment of small cell carcinoma of the lung with very high-dose cyclophosphamide. Cancer 55:57–60, 1988.

200. Ginsberg SJ, Comis RL: The pulmonary toxicity of antineoplastic agents. Semin Oncol 9:34–51, 1982.

201. McInerney DP, Bullimore J: Reactivation of radiation pneumonitis by Adriamycin. Br J Radiol 50:224–227, 1977.

202. Verschoore J, Lagrange JL, Boublil JL, et al: Pulmonary toxicity of a combination of low-dose doxorubicin and irradiation for inoperable lung cancer. Radiother Oncol 9:281–288, 1987.

203. Brooks BJ Jr, Seifter EJ, Walsh TE, et al: Pulmonary toxicity with combined modality therapy for limited stage small-cell lung cancer. J Clin Oncol 4:200–209, 1986.

204. Gross NJ: Pulmonary effects of radiation therapy. Ann Intern Med 86:81–92, 1977.

205. Davis SD, Yankelevitz DF, Henschke CI: Radiation effects on the lung: Clinical features, pathology, and imaging findings. Am J Roentgen 159:1157–1164, 1992.

206. Roberts CM, Foulcher E, Zaunders JJ, et al: Radiation pneumonitis: A possible lymphocyte-mediated hypersensitivity reaction. Ann Intern Med 118:696–700, 1993.

207. Maurer H, Modeas C, Goutsou M, et al: Adult respiratory distress syndrome (ARDS) after combined modality chemotherapy (CT) and radiation therapy (RT) in limited disease (LD) small cell lung cancer (SCLC). (Abstract.) Proc Am Soc Clin Oncol 9:229, 1990.

208. Mah K, Van Dyk J, Keane T, Poon PY: Acute radiation induced pulmonary damage: A clinical study on the response to fractionated radiation therapy. Int J Radiat Oncol Biol Phys 13:179–188, 1987.

209. Curran WJ, Moldofsky PJ, Solin LJ: Observations on the predictive value of perfusion lung scans on post-irradiation pulmonary function among 210 patients with bronchogenic carcinoma. Int J Radiat Oncol Biol Phys 24:31–36, 1992.

210. Rubenstein JH, Richter MP, Moldofsky PJ, Solin LJ: Prospective prediction of post-radiation therapy lung function using quantitative lung scans and pulmonary function testing. Int J Radiat Oncol Biol Phys 15:83–87, 1988.

211. Murray N, Shah A, Brown E, et al: Alternating chemotherapy and thoracic radiotherapy with concurrent cisplatin-etoposide for limited stage small cell carcinoma of the lung. Semin Oncol 13(Suppl 3):24–30, 1986.

212. Hellman S, Kligerman MM, Von Essen CF, Scibetta MP: Sequelae of radical radiotherapy of carcinoma of the lung. Radiology 82:1055–1061, 1964.

213. Greco FA, Brereton HD, Kent H, et al: Adriamycin and enhanced radiation reaction in normal esophagus and skin. Ann Intern Med 85:294–298, 1976.

214. Hansen HH: Should initial treatment of small cell carcinoma include systemic chemotherapy and brain irradiation? Cancer Chemother Rep 4:239–241, 1973.

215. Nugent JL, Bunn PAJ, Matthews M, et al: CNS metastases in small cell bronchogenic carcinoma. Increasing frequency and changing pattern with lengthening of survival. Cancer 44:1885–1893, 1979.

216. Hirsch FR, Paulson OB, Hansen HH, Larsen HO: Intracranial metastases in small cell carcinoma of the lung: Prognostic aspects. Cancer 51:529–533, 1983.

217. Hirsch FR, Paulson OB, Hansen HH, Vraa-Jensen J: Intracranial metastases in small cell carcinoma of the lung: Correlation of clinical and autopsy findings. Cancer 50:2433–2437, 1982.

218. Laukkanen E, Klonoff H, Allan B, et al: The role of prophylactic brain irradiation in limited stage small cell lung cancer: clinical, neuropsychologic, and CT sequelae. Int J Radiat Oncol Biol Phys 14:1109–1117, 1988.

219. Ichinose Y, Hara N, Ohta M, et al: Brain metastases in patients with limited small cell lung cancer achieving complete remission. Correlation with TNM staging. Chest 96:1332–1335, 1989.

220. Jacobs RH, Greenberg A, Bitran JD, et al: A 10-year experience with combined modality therapy for stage III small cell lung carcinoma. Cancer 58:2177–2184, 1986.

221. Rosenstein M, Armstrong J, Kris M, et al: A reappraisal of the role of prophylactic cranial irradiation in limited small cell lung cancer. Int J Radiat Oncol Biol Phys 24:43–48, 1992.

222. Komaki R, Cox JD, Whitson W: Risk of brain metastasis from

small cell carcinoma of the lung related to length of survival and prophylactic irradiation. Cancer Treat Rep 65:811–814, 1981.

223. Crane J, Lichter A, Ihde D, et al: Therapeutic cranial radiotherapy (RT) for brain metastases in small cell lung cancer (SCLC). (Abstract.) Proc Annu Meet Am Assoc Cancer Res 24:145, 1983.

224. Pedersen AG, Kristjansen PEG, Hansen HH: Prophylactic cranial irradiation and small cell lung cancer. Cancer Treat Rev 15:85–103, 1988.

225. Abner A: Prophylactic cranial irradiation in the treatment of small-cell carcinoma of the lung. Chest 103:445S–448S, 1993.

226. Liu X, Li X, Pang YB, Li Q, et al: The results of treatment in 100 patients with limited-stage small cell lung cancer. Cancer 71:326–331, 1993.

227. Komaki R, Byhardt RW, Anderson T, et al: What is the lowest effective biologic dose for prophylactic cranial irradiation? Am J Clin Oncol 8:523–527, 1985.

228. Russell AH, Pajak TE, Selim HM, et al: Prophylactic cranial irradiation for lung cancer patients at high risk for development of cerebral metastasis: Results of a prospective randomized trial conducted by the Radiation Therapy Oncology Group. Int J Radiat Oncol Biol Phys 21:637–643, 1991.

229. Johnson BE, Becker B, Goff WB, et al: Neurologic, neuropsychologic, and computed cranial tomography scan abnormalities in 2- to 10-year survivors of small-cell lung cancer. J Clin Oncol 3:1659–1667, 1985.

230. Rosen ST, Makuch RW, Lichter AS, et al: Role of prophylactic cranial irradiation in prevention of central nervous system metastases in small cell lung cancer: Potential benefit restricted to patients in complete response. Am J Med 74:615–624, 1983.

231. Levitt M, Meikle A, Murray N, Weinerman B: Oat cell carcinoma of the lung: CNS metastasis in spite of prophylactic brain irradiation. Cancer Treat Rep 62:131–133, 1978.

232. Lucas CF, Robinson B, Hoskin PJ, et al: Morbidity of cranial relapse in small cell lung cancer and the impact of radiation therapy. Cancer Treat Rep 70:565–570, 1986.

233. Rosenman J, Choi NC: Improved quality of life of patients with small-cell carcinoma of the lung by elective irradiation of the brain. Int J Radiat Oncol Biol Phys 8:1041–1043, 1982.

234. Lee JS, Umsawasdi T, Barkley HT, et al: Timing of elective brain irradiation: A critical factor for brain metastasis-free survival in small cell lung cancer. Int J Radiat Oncol Biol Phys 13:697–704, 1987.

235. Hardy J, Smith I, Cherryman G, et al: The value of computed tomographic (CT) scan surveillance in the detection and management of brain metastases in patients with small cell lung cancer. Br J Cancer 62:684–686, 1990.

236. Fleck JF, Einhorn LH, Lauer RC, et al: Is prophylactic cranial irradiation indicated in small-cell lung cancer? J Clin Oncol 8:209–214, 1990.

237. Hansen HH, Dombernowsky P, Hansen M, Rygard J: Prophylactic irradiation in bronchogenic small cell anaplastic carcinoma: A comparative trial of localized versus extensive radiotherapy including prophylactic brain irradiation in patients receiving combination chemotherapy. Cancer 46:279–284, 1980.

238. Zatopek NK, Holoye PY, Ellerbroek NA, et al: Resectability of small-cell lung cancer following induction chemotherapy in patients with limited disease (Stage II-IIIb). Am J Clin Oncol 14:427–432, 1991.

239. Baglan RJ, Marks JE: Comparison of symptomatic and prophylactic irradiation of brain metastases from oat cell carcinoma of the lung. Cancer 47:41–45, 1981.

240. Herskovic AM, Orton CG: Elective brain irradiation for small cell anaplastic lung cancer. Int J Radiat Oncol Biol Phys 12:427–429, 1986.

241. Stockdale AD, Rostom AY: Upper-half body irradiation for oat cell carcinoma of the bronchus. Br J Radiol 62:563–564, 1989.

242. Feld R, Clamon GH, Blum R, et al: Short course prophylactic cranial irradiation for small cell lung cancer. Am J Clin Oncol 8:371–376, 1985.

243. Lee JS, Umsawasdi T, Dhingra HM, Barkley HT: Effects of brain irradiation and chemotherapy on myelosuppression in small cell lung cancer. J Clin Oncol 4:1615–1619, 1986.

244. Bunn PAJ, Nugent JL, Matthews MJ: Central nervous system metastases in small cell bronchogenic carcinoma. Semin Oncol 5:314–322, 1978.

245. Lauer RC, Fleck JF, Antony A, Einhorn L: Is prophylactic cranial irradiation indicated in small cell lung cancer? (Abstract.) Proc Am Soc Clin Oncol 7:209, 1988.

246. Lishner M, Feld R, Payne DG, et al: Late neurological complications after prophylactic cranial irradiation in patients with small-cell lung cancer: The Toronto Experience. J Clin Oncol 8:215–221, 1990.

247. Frytak S, Shaw JN, O'Neill BP, et al: Leukoencephalopathy in small cell lung cancer patients receiving prophylactic cranial irradiation. Am J Clin Oncol 12:27–33, 1989.

248. Looper JD, Einhorn LH, Garcia SA, et al: Severe neurologic problems following successful therapy for small cell lung cancer (SCLC). (Abstract.) Proc Am Soc Clin Oncol 3:231, 1984.

249. So NK, O'Neill BP, Frytak S, et al: Delayed leukoencephalopathy in survivors with small cell lung cancer. Neurology 37:1198–1201, 1987.

250. Craig JB, Moody D, Cruz JM, et al: Prospective evaluation of changes in computed cranial tomography in patients with small cell lung carcinoma treated with chemotherapy and prophylactic cranial irradiation. J Clin Oncol 2:1151–1156, 1984.

251. Lee JS, Umsawasdi T, Lee YY, et al: Neurotoxicity in long-term survivors of small cell lung cancer. Int J Radiat Oncol Biol Phys 12:313–321, 1986.

252. Cox JD, Komaki R, Byhardt RW, Kun LE: Results of whole brain irradiation for metastases from small cell carcinoma of the lung. Cancer Treat Rep 64:957–966, 1980.

253. Posner J: Management of central nervous system metastasis. Semin Oncol 4:81–91, 1977.

254. Carmichael J, Crane JM, Bunn PA, et al: Results of therapeutic cranial irradiation in small cell lung cancer. Int J Radiat Oncol Biol Phys 14:455–459, 1988.

255. Van Hazel GA, Scott M, Eagan RT: The effect of CNS metastases on the survival of patients with small cell cancer of the lung. Cancer 51:933–937, 1983.

256. Coy P, Hodson I, Payne DG, et al: The effect of dose of thoracic irradiation on recurrence in patients with limited stage small cell lung cancer. Initial results of a Canadian multicenter randomized trial. Int J Radiat Oncol Biol Phys 14:219–226, 1988.

257. Prasad US, Naylor AR, Walker WS, et al: Long-term survival after pulmonary resection for small cell carcinoma of the lung. Thorax, 44:784, 1989.

258. Friess GG, McCracken JD, Troxell ML, et al: Effect of initial resection of small-cell carcinoma of the lung: a review of Southwest Oncology Group Study 7628. J Clin Oncol 3:964, 1985.

259. Macchiarini P, Hardin M, Basolo F, et al: Surgery plus adjuvant chemotherapy for T1-3N0M0 small-cell lung cancer: Rationale for current approach. Am J Clin Oncol 14:218, 1991.

260. Osterlind K, Hansen M, Hansen H, et al: Treatment policy of surgery in small cell carcinoma of the lung: Retrospective analysis of a series of 874 consecutive patients. Thorax 40:272, 1985.

261. Lad T, Thomas P, Piantadosi S: Surgical resection of small-cell lung cancer—a prospective randomized evaluation. (Abstract.) Proc Annu Meet Am Soc Clin Oncol 10:A835, 1991.

262. Harpole D Jr, Feldman JM, Buchanan S, et al: Bronchial carcinoid tumors: A retrospective analysis of 126 patients. Ann Thorac Surg 54(1):50–54, 1992.

263. Arishita GI, Ostrow LB, Kline AL: Atypical carcinoid tumor of the lung: A case report and discussion of the literature. (Review). Milit Med 154(8):421–424, 1989.

264. Davila DG, Dunn WF, Tazelaar HD, et al: Bronchial carcinoid tumors. [Review]. Mayo Clin Proceed 68(8):795–803, 1993.

265. Grote TH, Macon WR, Davis B, et al: Atypical carcinoid of the lung. A distinct clinicopathologic entity. Chest 93(2):370–375, 1988.

266. DeCaro LF, Paladugu R, Benfield JR, et al: Typical and atypical carcinoids within the pulmonary APUD tumor spectrum. J Thorac Cardiovasc Surg 86:528–536, 1983.

SPECIAL CONSIDERATIONS

14 SUPERIOR SULCUS TUMORS

Frederick L. Grover and Ritsuko Komaki

HISTORY

The first description of a superior sulcus tumor is attributed to Edwin Hare,[1] a house surgeon at Stafford County General Infirmary, who, in a letter in 1838 to the London Medical Gazette, described a patient who presented with a history of pain, tingling, and numbness in the distribution of the left ulnar nerve. The patient had Horner's syndrome and a palpable tumor in the "inferior triangular space" on the left side of the neck, and as the tumor grew, the patient developed paraplegia and urinary retention and eventually succumbed. At postmortem examination, Hare noted a hard tumor that extended superiorly toward the origin of the brachial plexus with involvement of the carotid artery, the cervical sympathetic nerves, and the vagus and phrenic nerves. In addition, the tumor was attached to the spine and intervertebral foramina.

In 1932, Tobias[2] described an apical-costovertebral syndrome caused by an apical tumor. He described the pain, the anatomy, and other clinical aspects of this syndrome, noting that it could be caused by bronchogenic carcinoma. Pancoast first reported four cases of "apical chest tumors" in 1924,[3] and in 1932,[4] he gave his well-known Chairman's Address to the Section of Radiology at the 83rd Annual Session of the American Medical Association entitled "Superior Pulmonary Sulcus Tumor—Tumor Characterized by Pain, Horner's Syndrome, Destruction of Bone, and Atrophy of Hand Muscles." In this report, he presented seven cases, including those previously reported. He emphasized that the x-ray observations were "a sharply defined shadow in the apex of the thorax, destruction of one, two or all three of the upper ribs in their posterior aspects and the adjacent transverse processes, and sometimes slight vertebral body erosion." He noted the characteristic clinical signs of pain

in the distribution of the eighth cervical nerve and first and second thoracic nerves, with wasting of the muscles of the hand, and Horner's syndrome. Pancoast, however, believed that the tumor was epithelial in its histopathology and thought it might arise from an embryonal rest. He did not realize, as Tobias did, that bronchogenic carcinoma was the likely cause of the syndrome. The belief that the superior sulcus tumor was extrapulmonary persisted through the middle 1930s.[5] By the middle 1940s, it became apparent that the primary etiology of superior sulcus tumors was bronchogenic carcinoma.[6, 7]

Initially, only radiation treatment was attempted because these tumors were thought to be unresectable. The first successful removal of Pancoast's tumor due to bronchogenic carcinoma was performed in 1950 by Chardack and MacCallum.[8] This resection was accomplished by upper lobectomy with en bloc resection of the first and second ribs and removal of roots C7, C8, and T1. The patient was given postoperative radiotherapy in case any microscopic foci of tumor remained. Chardack and MacCallum[9] reported his follow-up in 1956, noting that this patient died 5 years and 10 months after the postoperative radiotherapy, but a postmortem examination revealed no evidence of recurrence or of metastasis. In 1957, Dontas[10] reported eight patients who had operative treatment of superior sulcus tumors. Initially, this author divided only the attachments of the tumor to the thoracic outlet area as a palliative procedure. In his latter four patients, however, upper lobectomy with removal of the adjacent ribs was performed. The first four patients died of tumor recurrence. The exact survival periods of the latter four were not reported, although no patients had local recurrence.

Shaw and colleagues[11] made a very important contribution to the care of superior sulcus tumors by reporting their experience in treating 18 patients with preoperative radiation therapy followed by en bloc surgical resection in 4 to 6 weeks. These authors thus demonstrated a high resectability rate, minimal complication rate, good palliation, and the possibility for cure in patients with superior sulcus tumors treated with preoperative radiation followed by en bloc surgical resection. The first such patient was treated in 1956 and was reported to be alive 27 years later.[12]

DEFINITION

The superior sulcus tumor was described by Pancoast in 1932, as noted earlier.[4] Paulson[13] noted that these tumors are "bronchogenic carcinomas developing peripherally in the apex of the lungs and invading the superior pulmonary sulcus." They are, he stated, ". . . frequently low grade epidermoid carcinomas that grow slowly and metastasize late." Situated in the narrow confines of the thoracic inlet, they invade the lymphatics of the endothoracic fascia and involve, by direct extension, the lower roots of the brachial plexus, the intercostal nerves, the stellate ganglion, the sympathetic chain, and adjacent ribs and vertebrae, producing the severe pain and Horner's syndrome (pupillary constriction, ptosis of upper eyelid, slight elevation of lower lid, sinking in of eyeball, narrowing of palpebral fissure, and anhidrosis and flushing of the affected side of face) that characterize Pancoast's syndrome.

DIAGNOSIS

Symptoms

Paulson[14] noted that initially patients experience localized pain in the shoulder and along the vertebral border of the scapula. This pain later extends down the ulnar nerve distribution of the arm to the elbow, indicating involvement of T1, and finally to the ulnar surface of the forearm and to the fourth and fifth fingers of the hand due to C8 nerve involvement. He reported that as the tumor enlarges and extends farther into the thoracic inlet, the sympathetic chain and stellate ganglion will be involved, producing Horner's syndrome and anhidrosis of the ipsilateral face and upper extremity. He further stated that either the first or second ribs or the vertebral bodies may be involved, which increases the pain, and if the spinal canal or cord is involved, the symptoms of a spinal cord tumor are present. He noted that pulmonary symptoms are usually not the presenting complaints. Paulson[15] also reported that with further involvement of the brachial plexus "weakness and atrophy of the muscles of the hand occur, accompanied by loss of the triceps reflex."

In one series,[16] 34 of 37 patients were treated for cervical osteoarthritis or bursitis of the shoulder before they were diagnosed as having a superior sulcus tumor. The incorrect diagnosis had been carried for an average of 5 to 7 months, and for one patient, 4 years passed without a correct diagnosis. In a report of 26 patients with superior sulcus tumors, Miller and colleagues[17] found that 25 patients had shoulder girdle or arm pain, eight had Horner's syndrome, and 21 had some degree of either cough, hemoptysis, or shortness of breath. Attar and associates[18] noted that 44% of 73 patients in a group with fairly advanced superior sulcus tumors had pain around the shoulder and that it radiated along the ulnar distribution of the arm in 22 patients. Pulmonary symptoms were present in 14% of patients, 25% had palpable supraclavicular nodes, 23% had significant weight loss, and 5% had superior vena cava syndromes. Horner's syndrome was present in 34% of patients, sensory disturbance and muscle weakness in 8%, spinal cord involvement with paraplegia in 5%, recurrent nerve paralysis in 10%, and phrenic nerve paralysis in 4%. It should be noted, however, that many of these are signs and symptoms of late-stage disease and are not typical of a well-localized superior sulcus tumor (Table 14–1).

Physical Examination

The physical examination of these patients may reveal increased pain with abduction of the arm, muscle weakness, atrophy of the muscles of the hand, loss of the triceps reflex, and Horner's syndrome.[14, 15] Patients frequently support the elbow of the involved extremity to decrease their pain. Depending on the stage of the disease process, the supraclavicular nodes may be enlarged and evidence of spinal tract involvement such as paraplegia may also be present. If the recurrent laryngeal nerve is involved, the patient is hoarse, and if compression of the vena cava is present, neck vein and upper body venous distention is observed.

Radiologic Evaluation

Chest Radiographs

There are two main problems in making the radiographic diagnosis of superior sulcus tumors,[19] both resulting in failure to make an early diagnosis of the lesion. First, a soft tissue mass without bony destruction might be missed or may often be misinterpreted as pleural thickening on regular chest radiographs. A

TABLE 14–1. Superior Sulcus Tumors: Signs and Symptoms

SIGN OR SYMPTOM	INCIDENCE* (%)
Shoulder pain	44 to 96
Arm and/or head pain	30 to 75
Numbness of arm	22
Weakness or atrophy of arm or head	8 to 13
Horner's syndrome	14 to 34
Pulmonary symptoms	14 to 81
Weight loss	23 to 35
Superior vena cava syndrome	5
Cord symptoms	5

*Range of signs and symptoms in literature.

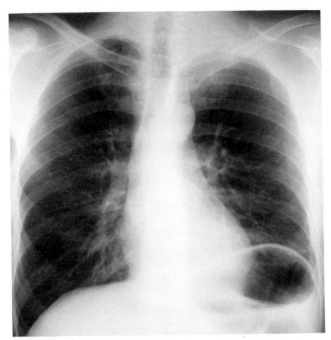

FIGURE 14–1. A homogeneous shadow extends medially from the apical pleural thickening toward the suprahilar region. The percutaneous biopsy of the lesion showed poorly differentiated adenocarcinoma.

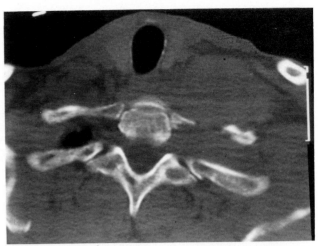

FIGURE 14–3. The CT scan shows a left apical mass destroying the left first rib and extending close to the foramen.

shadow extending medially from the pleural thickening toward the hilus is more suggestive of a malignant tumor (Fig. 14–1). These cases are better shown with apical lordotic or slightly oblique views (Fig. 14–2). The second problem may occur because the ordinary chest radiograph or apical lordotic film does not show bony destruction. Additional anteroposterior views of the lower cervical–upper dorsal spine or a tomogram may demonstrate bony destruction.[19]

Computed Tomography

Computed tomography (CT) can better demonstrate the relationship of the superior sulcus tumor to ante-

rior structures (subclavian artery and vein, trachea, and esophagus) and posterior structures (chest wall and vertebral bodies) than conventional radiography, and it provides information that helps determine operability (Figs. 14–3 and 14–4).[20] CT scanning of the lower cervical region and upper thorax is useful for identifying the following contraindications for an adequate resection:

1. Involvement of the great vessels at the thoracic inlet, primarily the subclavian artery and vein.
2. Involvement of the trachea or esophagus.
3. Extensive brachial plexus invasion.
4. Extensive chest wall invasion, particularly invasion of the vertebral bodies and spinal cord.

If CT of the thorax shows mediastinal nodal enlargement or evidence of direct mediastinal invasion, surgical resection of the tumor may be contraindicated. However, mediastinoscopy must be performed in the case of enlarged mediastinal nodes in order to be absolutely certain whether or not they are involved with tumor.

The diagnosis of a superior sulcus bronchogenic carcinoma based on the history, physical examination,

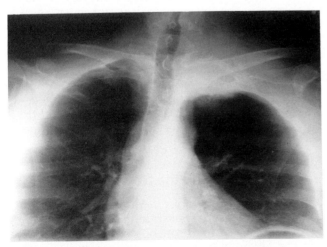

FIGURE 14–2. This apical lordotic roentgenogram shows the destruction of the left posterior first rib.

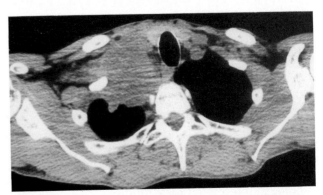

FIGURE 14–4. The CT scan shows the apical mass invading the left subclavian artery and vein as well as the left anterior chest wall. This lesion was considered to be unresectable because of the advanced local extension.

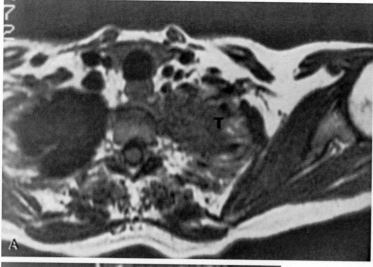

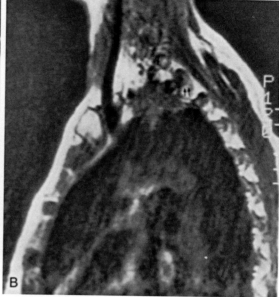

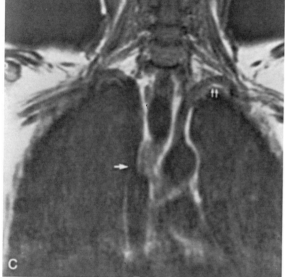

FIGURE 14–5. Magnetic resonance imaging findings. *A*, Superior sulcus tumor. The extent of this left apical carcinoma (T) is difficult to assess in the axial plane. *B*, Sagittal scan demonstrates that the tumor extends beyond the apex of the lung but does not involve the brachial plexus. It abuts the posterior wall of the subclavian artery (*single arrow*) and involves the first rib (*double arrows*). *C*, Coronal scan demonstrates the left paratracheal and the contralateral mediastinal nodal involvement (*arrow*). The subclavian artery is patent (*double arrows*).

and radiologic findings is accurate more than 95% of the time according to Paulson.[13] There are, however, numerous other entities that may masquerade as superior sulcus carcinoma.[21–24] It is therefore necessary to obtain a definitive diagnosis before planning treatment for these patients.

Magnetic Resonance Imaging

Display of the anatomy of the superior sulcus on thin-section coronal and sagittal images showed significant accuracy compared with CT scans (0.94 accuracy with MRI, 0.63 with CT scans) correlated to the surgical specimen (15 patients) and the patients' clinical symptoms (17 patients), according to Heelan and his colleagues.[25] This comparison was conducted prospectively, independently, and blindly when the diagnostic radiologist interpreted these studies.

Sagittal and coronal T1-weighted magnetic resonance imaging (MRI) through the superior sulcus offers improved diagnostic accuracy compared with CT

scanning, especially in evaluating invasion of the superior sulcus tumor into the lower neck (Fig. 14–5). MRI should be performed before surgery to detect invasion into the lower neck. It is not meaningful to perform complete MRI of the whole thorax and upper abdomen in the patients with superior sulcus tumor and no symptoms of abdominal metastasis. Using MRI to improve accuracy in staging lung cancer in the other areas, such as the upper abdomen, is not warranted. Therefore, in patients with superior sulcus tumor, focused coronal and sagittal T1-weighted MRI is a useful adjunct to routine, dynamic CT scanning of the chest (Fig. 14–5).

Bronchoscopy and Fine-Needle Aspiration

Bronchoscopic examination frequently is not diagnostic. Hepper and colleagues[26] initially reported only a 16% positive yield by bronchoscopic examination before the advent of fiberoptic bronchoscopy. With fiberoptic bronchoscopy and intrabronchial brushing, this yield should be somewhat higher. Attar and coworkers[18] noted that bronchoscopy yielded positive cytologic findings in 13 of 43 patients (30%) in whom it was used. Miller and colleagues[17] found that sputum cytology and bronchoscopy were diagnostic in 31% of patients. Because of the low diagnostic yield with bronchoscopy in the face of a need for preoperative diagnosis, attention has been directed to other diagnostic methods. McGoon,[27] in 1964, described a transcervical technique, using a supraclavicular approach lateral to the sternal head of the sternocleidomastoid muscle passing through the scalene fat pad. This approach allows identification of the tumor and its relationship to the subclavian artery, brachial plexus, and sympathetic nerves so that it can be safely wedged or needle biopsy can be performed. Siderys and Pittman[28] reported on the use of the Vim-Silverman needle directed into the chest posteriorly via the second or third intercostal space with the patient in the prone position. In 1974, Walls and colleagues[29] noted that 26 of 27 patients with superior sulcus tumors were diagnosed cytologically by fine-needle aspiration via a posterior approach. In addition to identifying the extent of the tumor, CT can be used to direct the position of needles to diagnose superior sulcus tumors.[30] In 1985, Paulson and colleagues[31] reported on 24 patients in whom percutaneous fine-needle biopsies were performed by a radiologist using a cervical approach with image-intensified fluoroscopy with television monitoring and CT. The diagnostic yield was noted to be greater than 95%. The advantage of CT is its ability to display clearly the exact location of the needle within the lesion. The disadvantages of CT-guided biopsies are the high unit cost, relatively high radiation dose, and the length of time needed to perform the procedure compared with fluoroscopic- and ultrasonographic-guided biopsies.[30] It would appear, therefore, that if the diagnosis is not obtained with flexible bronchoscopy and brushing, fine-needle aspiration of the tumor using the above-mentioned techniques should be performed expeditiously so that treatment can be undertaken.

STAGING

Paulson[13–15, 32] has consistently stressed the importance of proper preoperative staging of patients with superior sulcus lesions. In a report of his experience through 1983, he noted that only 3 of 17 patients with hilar or mediastinal nodal involvement survived 1 year, and none survived for 2 years. Of those patients without nodal involvement at operation, 44% lived for 5 years or longer. The overall survival rate was 31% at 5 years. This experience involved 78 patients treated with preoperative radiation therapy and surgical resection. Paulson thus advocates performance of mediastinoscopy, or scalene node biopsy if scalene nodes are palpable, in all patients prior to initiation of therapy.

Stanford and colleagues,[33] in 1980, noted that a group of patients who had negative preoperative staging and were treated by preoperative radiation followed by en bloc resection had a 5-year survival of 49.7%. The survival rate was only 13.1% in a second group of patients who either had localized nodal involvement or were not staged preoperatively. A third group, who were considered inoperable and were given palliative radiation, had a 4-year survival of 5.5%. This review again emphasizes the importance of adequate staging and the importance of nodal involvement to survival. Attar and associates[18] noted that all his patients with mediastinal nodal involvement died shortly after operation and emphasized in his closing remarks after presentation of his paper that "adequate preoperative assessment is extremely important if we hope to obtain good results in patients with Pancoast tumors." Ginsberg[34] reported the Toronto experience, noting that "stringent preoperative assessment of these patients is done to rule out distant metastasis resulting in resection in only 10 of 72 patients." Paulson[13] listed the contraindications to operation of superior sulcus tumors, including "extensive invasion of the brachial plexus, subclavian artery, and either the bodies of lamina of their vertebrae, mediastinal involvement (particularly perinodal), venous obstruction, and distant metastases. In some instances, ipsilaterally involved mediastinal or scalene nodes have been resected for palliation of severe pain. However, the survival rate of these patients has been low."

If the superior sulcus tumor is located more anteriorly, the subclavian artery might be involved, which is one of the contraindications for resection of the tumor. If the brachial plexus is involved by a tumor that is extending more superiorly, surgery might be contraindicated or sacrifice of the brachial plexus is necessary. When the tumor is located more posteriorly at the superior sulcus (typical Pancoast's tumor), the patient may have Horner's syndrome due to the involvement of the sella ganglion or vertebral body with or without extension of the tumor into the foramen. Depending on the extent of disease, surgery may be feasible with combined effort by a thoracic surgeon and a neurosurgeon. The superior sulcus tumor has to be specified as anteriorly located or more posteriorly located, which will influence the resectability or the dose arrangement of the radiotherapy boost.

TREATMENT AND RESULTS

Preoperative Radiation Therapy and Surgical Resection

Preoperative radiation therapy and surgical resection were first reported by Shaw and coworkers in 1961.[11] This original series has been continued by Paulson[13–15] and updated on several occasions. The treatment consists of delivering 3000 cGy using megavoltage equipment in 10 fractions over 12 elapsed days to the area of the tumor in the superior pulmonary sulcus, the chest wall, and the superior mediastinum beyond the midline. Three weeks after the completion of the radiotherapy, the patients undergo surgical resection. The surgical resection consists of an extended en bloc resection of the primary tumor and chest wall, including the entire first rib and the posterior portions of the second and third ribs (Fig. 14–6). In addition, the resection may include part of the first three thoracic vertebrae, encompassing the transverse processes, the intercostal nerve roots, the eighth cervical nerve root, the lower trunk of the brachial plexus, part of the stellate ganglion, and the dorsal sympathetic chain. The involved lung is resected by either a lobectomy or a segmental resection, and the entire procedure is accompanied by a radical dissection of the regional, hilar, and mediastinal lymph nodes.

As of 1983, Paulson's series[15] totaled 131 patients who started treatment with combined preoperative radiation and en bloc surgical resection. Of the 79 patients operated on after the preoperative radiation, only one was judged to have an unresectable tumor. Therefore, 78 of these patients (60%) completed the combined treatment. The operative mortality rate was 2.6%. The survival rate for those completing combined treatment was 31% at 5 years, 26% at 10 years, and 22% at 15 years (Fig. 14–7 and Table 14–2). Only 3 of 17 patients who had either hilar or mediastinal nodal involvement survived 1 year, and none survived 2 years. Forty-four per cent of those who did not have nodal involvement at operation survived 5 years or more, 33% for 10 years, and 30% for 15 years.

Other surgical series have reported on combined preoperative radiation and surgical resection using the Paulson technique. In the report by Miller and colleagues,[17] the preoperative radiation dose varied from 2000 to 4000 cGy over a time span of 4 days to 4 weeks, but the most common regimen was that of Paulson.[15] Attar and colleagues[18] initially gave 5500 to 6000 cGy preoperatively over a 4-week period, but they noted a high rate of morbidity and mortality in the group that received this level of radiation and therefore decreased the dose of radiation to that used by Paulson and colleagues. Ginsberg[34] also uses a dose of 3000 cGy preoperatively. Beyer and Weisenburger[35] noted that those patients who received at least 5500 cGy showed a better response and appeared to have increased survival. The preoperative radiation dosage employed by Devine and associates[36] was 3000 to 3500 cGy over 2 weeks in 25 of their patients and 4500 to 5000 cGy over 5 to 5.5 weeks in 15 of their patients. They noted no difference in resectability or survival between the groups receiving the two dosages.

Attar and associates[18] reported on 19 patients who underwent preoperative radiation followed by en bloc resection and noted a 23% 3-year survival rate. Miller and colleagues[17] reported on 26 patients who underwent combined radiation treatment and en bloc resection. There was one early postoperative death, and 32% survived for 5 years. Stanford and colleagues[33] noted a 5-year survival rate of 49.7% in patients undergoing preoperative radiation followed by en bloc resection if their preoperative staging was positive or if they were not preoperatively staged. Beyer

and Weisenburger[35] treated 28 patients who had localized disease with megavoltage radiation with or without surgical resection and had an actuarial survival rate of 22% at 5 years. They noted, however, that the 15 patients who received combined radiation and surgery had a 45% 5-year survival rate. Ginsberg[34] reported that 72 patients with Pancoast's tumors were seen between 1966 and 1976 at the University of Toronto. Fifty were deemed inoperable after screening and staging procedures. Ten underwent preoperative radiation and resection with a 40% 2-year survival rate. Twelve patients also had limited disease with no evidence of metastasis and, although thought to be surgical candidates, were never referred for surgery and received only radiation therapy. Only two of those patients (17%) survived 24 months.

Martini[37] discussed 145 patients treated at Memorial Hospital in New York City over a 36-year period, 29 of whom were treated by external radiation alone, 68 by operation without preoperative radiation, and 48 by preoperative radiation followed by resection. He noted that only 9% treated by operation alone had resectable tumors as compared with 23% who received preoperative radiation. He did note, however, that at their institution, a large group of patients did not have resectable tumors at exploration, with or without preoperative radiation therapy. This is perhaps because many patients were explored without preoperative mediastinoscopy and more sophisticated imaging evaluation, such as CT or MRI. He noted a mean survival time of 6 months with external radiation alone, 30 months with preoperative radiation followed by resection, and 10 months with operation alone. His group also found that if the tumor was not resectable at exploration, the combination of implantation of radon seeds and external radiation (4000 cGy in 4 weeks) provided a better survival rate than external radiation therapy alone (12 months versus 6 months), although patients treated with postoperative radiation alone had more extensive tumor. Devine and colleagues[36] reported a 2-year survival of 29% and a 5-year survival of 14% in patients who completed preoperative radiation and surgery. They noted, however, that 30% of patients for whom preoperative radiation therapy followed by surgical therapy was planned did not undergo surgical resection.

Over the past several years, there have been several other reports of sizable series of patients treated with a combination of preoperative radiation and surgical resection. Anderson, Moy, and Holmes[38] reported the UCLA experience in which 21 patients received preoperative radiation followed by resection, resulting in a 5-year survival rate of 34%. They also advocated radiation by iridium implants postoperatively to 3000 cGy if the tumor was close to the vertebral bodies and nerve roots at the time of operation. Mathisen's[39] group reported on 21 patients who underwent combined therapy at the Massachusetts General Hospital and noted three operative deaths with a median survival time of 24 months and an actuarial survival rate of 55% in 3 years and 27% at 5 years. Long-term palliation of pain was achieved in 72% of the patients.

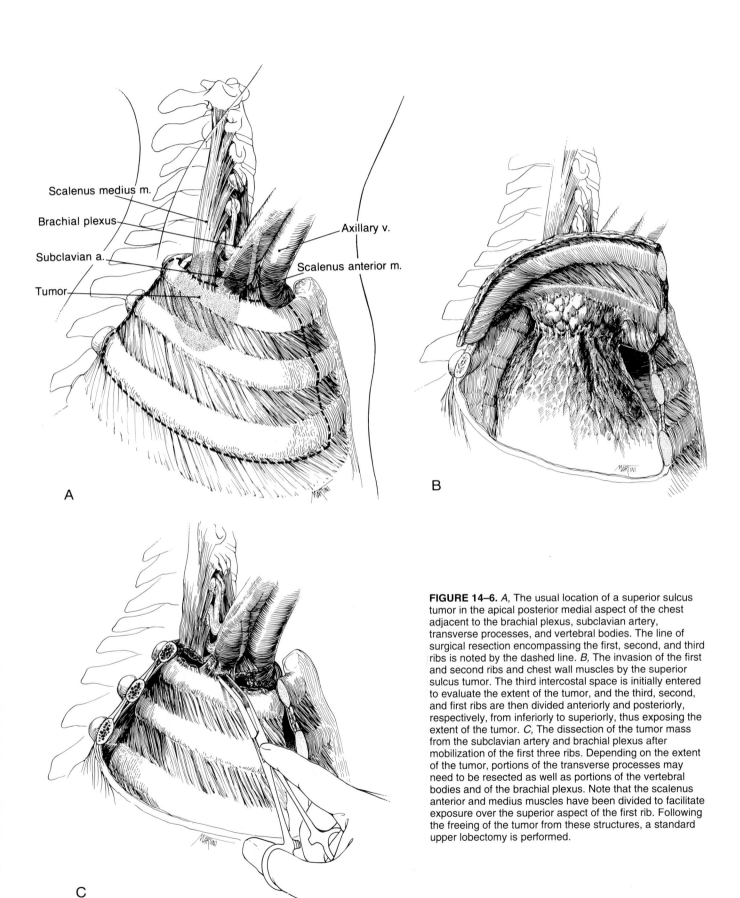

Scalenus medius m.

Brachial plexus

Subclavian a.

Tumor

Axillary v.

Scalenus anterior m.

A

B

C

FIGURE 14–6. *A,* The usual location of a superior sulcus tumor in the apical posterior medial aspect of the chest adjacent to the brachial plexus, subclavian artery, transverse processes, and vertebral bodies. The line of surgical resection encompassing the first, second, and third ribs is noted by the dashed line. *B,* The invasion of the first and second ribs and chest wall muscles by the superior sulcus tumor. The third intercostal space is initially entered to evaluate the extent of the tumor, and the third, second, and first ribs are then divided anteriorly and posteriorly, respectively, from inferiorly to superiorly, thus exposing the extent of the tumor. *C,* The dissection of the tumor mass from the subclavian artery and brachial plexus after mobilization of the first three ribs. Depending on the extent of the tumor, portions of the transverse processes may need to be resected as well as portions of the vertebral bodies and of the brachial plexus. Note that the scalenus anterior and medius muscles have been divided to facilitate exposure over the superior aspect of the first rib. Following the freeing of the tumor from these structures, a standard upper lobectomy is performed.

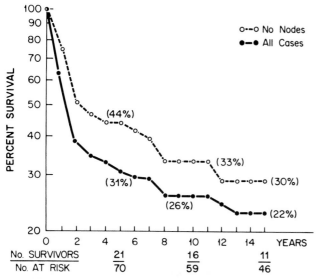

FIGURE 14–7. Graph showing 5-, 10-, and 15-year actuarial survival curves of 78 patients after combined preoperative radiation, followed by en bloc surgical resection (1956–1983) in patients with no lymph nodes involved and including those with nodal involvement. (From Paulson DL: Technical considerations in stage III disease: The "superior sulcus" lesion. *In* Delarue NC, Eschapasse H [eds]: International Trends in General Thoracic Surgery, Vol I. Philadelphia, W.B. Saunders, 1985.)

Shahian, Neptune, and Ellis[40] reported on 18 patients treated with preoperative radiation and resection, 14 of whom underwent supplemental postoperative radiotherapy because of positive lymph nodes, tumor at the resection margins, or both. There were no hospital deaths and the overall 5-year observed survival rate for the entire series was 56%. These authors believed that the addition of postoperative radiotherapy for those with unfavorable operative findings resulted in long-term survivals in the groups with positive margins or nodes that were comparable to those with negative nodes and margins. Ricci and his colleagues[41] from Rome reported on 56 patients with superior sulcus tumors, 32 of whom received preoperative radiation and 4 of whom also received postoperative radiotherapy. This group used Paulson's approach in 30 cases and Dartevelle's in 11, and the 5-year survival rate was 34%, with four patients undergoing preoperative radiation and radical resection. Sartori and his colleagues[42] from Padua, Italy, reported on 42 patients with superior sulcus tumors who received preoperative radiation followed by en bloc resection of the

tumor, chest wall, and adjacent structures with one perioperative death and a median survival time of 14 months and a 5-year actuarial survival rate of 25%. They confirmed poor results in patients with vertebral invasion, subclavian artery invasion, or N2 disease.

Surgical Resection Only

Surgical resection without radiotherapy is not the usual course of treatment for patients with superior sulcus tumors. One of the reasons for this is the low resectability rate in patients who have not had the benefit of preoperative radiation. As noted, Martini[37] and Hilaris and colleagues[43] found that only 9% of 68 patients had resectable tumors as compared with 23% of 48 patients who had preoperative radiation. However, some patients with well-localized disease and very small tumors do well with extended resection only. Attar and colleagues[18] reported a 60% survival rate at 3 years in five such patients. The paucity of other articles reporting experience with surgery alone indicates that this treatment modality is seldom used.

Dartevelle and his colleagues[44] from France have recently reported another surgical approach for radical resection of superior sulcus tumors that have extensive involvement of the adjacent structures above the thoracic inlet, in particular the subclavian artery and vein and the brachial plexus. They offer this approach in lieu of or in combination with the classic posterior approach described by Paulson in these patients who have extensive involvement above the thoracic inlet because of more complete exposure of the inlet structures that have been invaded. This approach involves a large L-shaped anterior cervical incision, removal of the medial half of the clavicle, dissection or resection of the subclavian vein, division of the anterior scaleneus muscle and resection of the cervical portion of the phrenic nerve if it is invaded, exposure of the subclavian and vertebral arteries, dissection of the brachial plexus up to the spinal foramen, resection of invaded ribs, and en bloc removal of the chest wall and lung tumor either directly or by an extension of the cervical incision into the deltopectoral groove. As noted, this can be complemented by adding a posterior thoracotomy, if needed (Figs. 14–8 to 14–11).

Surgical Resection with Postoperative Radiation Therapy

There is no established role for postoperative radiation therapy to improve survival in patients with car-

TABLE 14–2. Results of Treatment of Superior Sulcus Tumors*

TREATMENT	LOCAL CONTROL (%)	SURVIVAL (%)			
		2-year	3-year	5-year	10-year
Preoperative XRT† and surgical resection	31 to 70	29 to 40	23	13 to 50	26
Surgical resection only	53	—	—	15 to 60	—
Surgical resection with postoperative XRT	0 to 56	—	7	15	—
XRT only	33 to 55	17	7 to 28	3.5 to 23	—

*Large range of results reflects varying stages of carcinoma among institutions.
†XRT = X-ray treatment.

external irradiation alone, or implant and external irradiation). Twelve patients survived longer than 5 years after the treatment, and ten (83%) had resection of the tumor, implantation, and external irradiation (4000 cGy in 4 weeks). Nine patients developed nonfatal complications after incomplete resection and interstitial implants. Complications were related either to surgery or to radiation therapy. Surgical complications were atelectasis, bronchopneumonia, subcutaneous emphysema, and wound infection. Those related to radiation therapy included esophagitis and a lung abscess secondary to tumor necrosis.

A more recent report on 85 patients with superior sulcus tumors by Komaki and colleagues[47] at The University of Texas M.D. Anderson Cancer Center revealed that surgery and radiotherapy was more effective in controlling the superior sulcus tumor and improving survival compared with the results with the use of either modality alone. There were 43 pa-

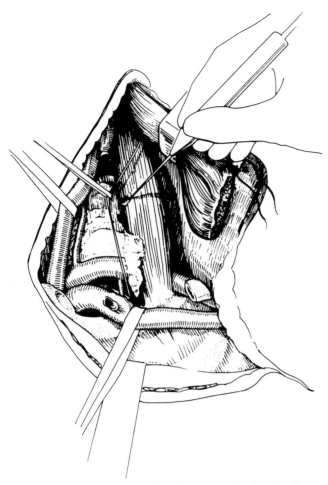

FIGURE 14–8. Exposure of subclavian artery after division of insertion of anterior scalenus muscle on first rib. (From Dartevelle PG, Chapelier AR, Macchiarini P, et al: Anterior transcervical-thoracic approach for radical resection of lung tumors invading the thoracic inlet. J Thorac Cardiovasc Surg 105:1025–1034, 1993.)

cinoma of the lung who have had complete surgical resection without gross or microscopic residual tumor, nor has its role been established for patients showing no metastasis to the regional lymph nodes, including peribronchial, hilar, or mediastinal lymph nodes. This applies to any site of cancer of the lung, although superior sulcus tumors have less tendency to involve hilar lymph node metastasis.

Martini and McCormack[45] reported on 170 patients with superior sulcus tumors who were treated at Memorial Hospital in New York City from 1938 to 1978. A group of 127 patients underwent surgery, and their 5-year survival rate was 17% compared with 3.4% for the inoperable patients, although the staging work-up was not complete and inoperable patients were treated palliatively. Among the 127 patients who underwent operation, 20 patients had curative surgery and their 5-year survival rate was 28.9%. The remaining patients received postoperative brachytherapy and achieved survival rates of 14.0% to 14.7%. Hilaris and associates[46] reported on 116 patients with superior sulcus tumors treated by irradiation alone or combined surgical resection and irradiation (implant,

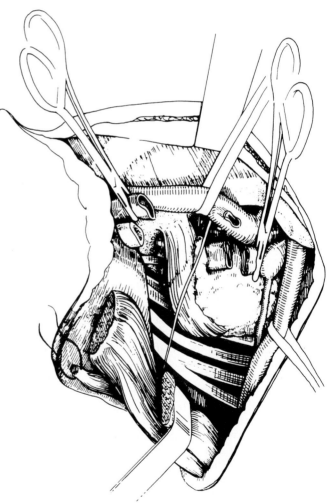

FIGURE 14–9. The subclavian artery can be freed from tumor by dividing all collateral branches (vertebral artery is generally preserved if not invaded), and if it is involved, it can be divided proximally and distally. (From Dartevelle PG, Chapelier AR, Macchiarini P, et al: Anterior transcervical-thoracic approach for radical resection of lung tumors invading the thoracic inlet. J Thorac Cardiovasc Surg 105:1025–1034, 1993.)

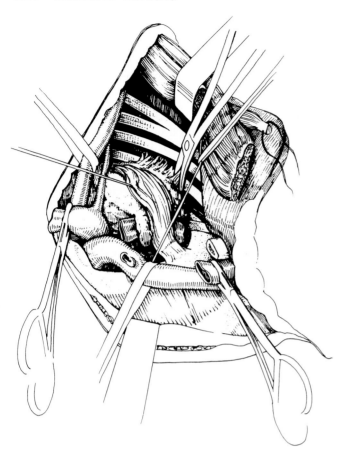

FIGURE 14–10. The spread of tumor to brachial plexus requires an out-in side neurolysis if upper nerve roots are involved or a resection of T1 if lower trunk or nerve roots are involved. (From Dartevelle PG, Chapelier AR, Macchiarini P, et al: Anterior transcervical-thoracic approach for radical resection of lung tumors invading the thoracic inlet. J Thorac Cardiovasc Surg 105:1025–1034, 1993.)

tients with superior sulcus tumor categorized as Stage IIIA and 42 patients as Stage IIIB. Surgery was a component of treatment more frequently in patients with Stage IIIA than in Stage IIIB disease (p <.05), and chemotherapy was used significantly more often in patients with Stage IIIB disease (p <.01). Stage IIIA patients had a 46.5% 1-year survival rate compared with 21% for Stage IIIB (p = .0042). When surgery was a component of treatment, 52% (13/25) lived longer than 2 years compared with 22% (13/60) when the lesion was unresectable. Fifty-two patients (61%) had local control, and their survival was significantly better than those who did not achieve local control (p <.01). High performance status, less than 5% weight loss, and lack of direct extension into vertebral bodies were highly significant factors for better survival. Surgical resection should be used whenever possible for superior sulcus tumors. Patients with unresectable lesions should receive high-dose photon or neutron radiation therapy.

Dartevelle and his colleagues[44] reported 2- and 5-year actuarial survival rates of 50% and 31%, respectively, with a median follow-up time of 2.5 years. None of their patients received preoperative radiation, 14% had surgery alone, and 86% had surgery followed by postoperative irradiation. Therefore, this is a group of patients who had extensive invasion of the superior sulcus area and who were able to be resected in spite of not receiving preoperative radiation, probably largely due to the added exposure that the anterior transcervical thoracic approach provides, as well as more adequate evaluation by modern imaging studies.

Patients with Inoperable Disease

Whenever patients with superior sulcus tumors are considered to be inoperable for medical reasons or the lesions are surgically unresectable, they can receive radiation therapy or combined modality therapy, depending on the histologic findings.

Morris and Abadir[48] recommended radiotherapy alone for superior sulcus tumors. They reported 26 cases and showed that high-dose radiation therapy (nominal single dose [NSD] 1900 rets [equivalent to 7000 cGy in 7 weeks] or higher) controlled direct bony

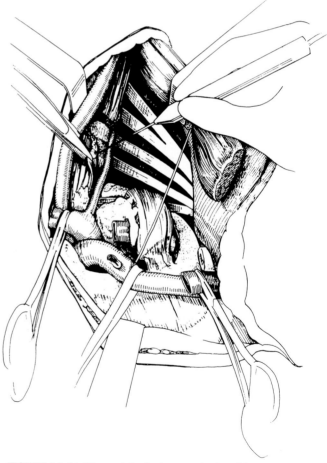

FIGURE 14–11. The vertebral artery can be freed from tumor, the prevertebral muscles detached from vertebral bodies, and both the stellate ganglion and the sympathetic chain isolated and eventually resected. (From Dartevelle PG, Chapelier AR, Macchiarini P, et al: Anterior transcervical-thoracic approach for radical resection of lung tumors invading the thoracic inlet. J Thorac Cardiovasc Surg 105:1025–1034, 1993.)

invasion better than lower doses (less than 1900 rets). Ahmad and colleagues[49] treated 48 patients by irradiation alone using either cobalt-60 or cesium-137 teletherapy to give between 5000 cGy and 6000 cGy in 5 to 6 weeks. Their actuarial survival rate was 28% at 3 years and 21% at 5 years. They encountered no severe complications among the patients who received radiation therapy alone, except some fibrosis observed in the radiographs that produced no symptoms. Other experiences with treating superior sulcus tumors by external radiation therapy were reported by Van Houtte and colleagues.[50] This group reported 31 patients with superior sulcus tumors treated with external radiation therapy in doses ranging from 2000 cGy to 7000 cGy, and the overall 5-year survival rate was 18%. They found that doses below 5000 cGy and bone invasion were each associated with a higher rate of local recurrence.

At the Medical College of Wisconsin,[51] 36 patients with superior sulcus tumors were treated by external irradiation only between 1963 and 1977. Local control correlated positively with the field size and the median survival. The patients who failed locally did not survive beyond 2 years. Between 1978 and 1983, an additional 32 patients with inoperable superior sulcus tumors were studied.

Relief of pain was achieved in 91% of all patients presenting with pain. The reversal of hoarseness was achieved in only 6 of 10 patients. Three-fourths of the patients with Horner's syndrome responded to the irradiation. The disease-free survival rates were 65%, 38%, 25%, and 15% at 12 months, 24 months, 36 months, and 48 months, respectively (Fig. 14–12). No patients survived beyond 24 months if the primary tumor was not controlled in the chest. The pattern of failure showed the brain to be the most common site of distant metastases after the completion of chest irradiation (23 of 68 patients, 34%). No fatal complications occurred as a result of external radiation therapy alone.

In the series studied by Anderson, Moy, and Holmes,[38] 27 patients received radiation only and this group had no 5-year survivors. The majority of these patients received between 4000 to 6000 cGy because they were either unresectable, refused surgery, were medically too ill for resection, or had distant metastasis. Ricci and his colleagues[41] reported on 15 inoperable patients who were treated by radiation therapy with a 2-year survival rate of 6%. These patients received 6000 cGy.

High-energy external radiotherapy is therefore recommended for patients proved to have superior sulcus tumors by means of CT-guided aspiration cytologic techniques or biopsy who are unable to have surgical resection because of the extent of the disease or are inoperable for medical reasons. The field must be generous enough to encompass the upper mediastinum and the vertebral bodies as well as the supraclavicular region. The total minimum tumor dose should be 6000 cGy administered in 6 to 6½ weeks. CT planning dosimetry is very helpful in determining the adequate dose to the tumor, adjacent structures, and regional lymph nodes and in sparing critical organs such as the spinal cord, esophagus, and excessive volume of the lung. As with other sites of inoperable non–small cell lung cancer, chemotherapy may add to results of radiation but clinical trials focused on superior sulcus tumors are lacking.

SUMMARY

In conclusion, it has been demonstrated that superior sulcus bronchogenic carcinomas, if presenting without distant metastasis or regional nodal involvement, can be treated with success comparable to that found with other non–small cell bronchogenic carcinomas. In patients who have no evidence of distant metastasis, who have a negative mediastinoscopy, and whose CT scan implies a relatively well-localized superior sulcus tumor, it appears that the treatment offering the greatest degree of success is preoperative radiation followed by en bloc surgical resection of the primary tumor, the upper three ribs, portions of the brachial plexus, and the transverse processes and sympathetic chain as necessary based on the extent of involvement. If a patient with negative findings on mediastinoscopy undergoes an operation and nodal

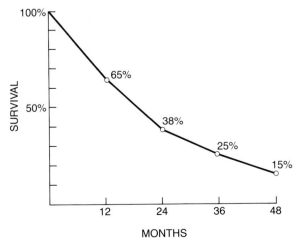

FIGURE 14–12. Disease-free survival in patients with superior sulcus tumor treated by external irradiation alone.

DIAGNOSTIC AND STAGING WORK-UP OF SUPERIOR SULCUS TUMOR

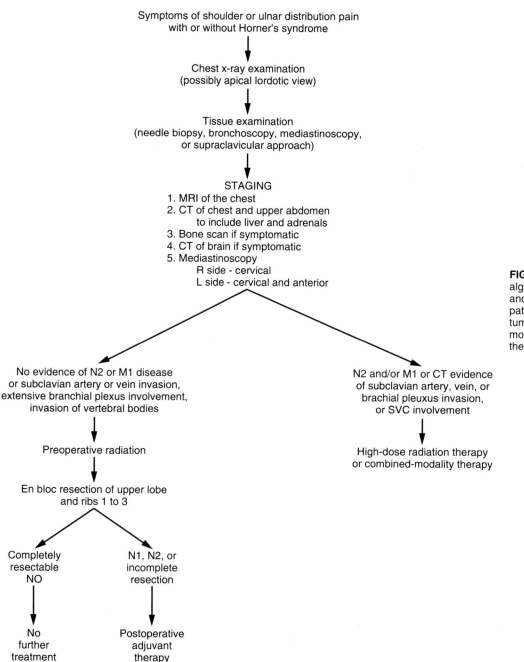

FIGURE 14–13. This treatment algorithm illustrates the diagnostic and staging work-up of the patient with a superior sulcus tumor with the therapy deemed most appropriate, depending on the stage of disease.

involvement is found in the hilum or mediastinum at the time of resection, it would seem prudent to offer that patient postoperative adjuvant therapy. If residual tumor from the primary site is left in the thoracic apex at the time of surgery, brachytherapy with postoperative radiation treatment may be advisable. Those patients who have extensive involvement of structures above the thoracic inlet, including the subclavian artery, vein, and the brachial plexus, may benefit from Dartevelle's cervical approach, sometimes used in combination with the classic posterior thoracotomy approach. For the patient who has a large apical mass with involvement of the superior vena cava, or evidence of very extensive involvement of the vertebral bodies and brachial plexus, or evidence of mediastinal nodal metastases at mediastinoscopy, it seems that the treatment of choice would be high-dose radiotherapy or combined modality therapy (Fig. 14–13).

SELECTED REFERENCES

Komaki R, Mountain CF, Holbert JM et al: Superior sulcus tumors: Treatment selection and results for 85 patients without metastasis (M0) at presentation. Int J Radiat Oncol Biol Phys 19:31–36, 1990. *Between January 1977 and December 1987, 85 patients with superior sulcus tumor were treated definitively at The University of Texas M.*

D. Anderson Cancer Center. All patients had CT scans of the chest and other adequate metastatic workup. Forty-three were classified as clinical Stage IIIA and 42 Stage IIIB. Stage IIIA patients had a 46.5% 2-year survival rate compared to 20.6% for Stage IIIB (p = .0042). When surgery was a component of treatment, 52% (13/25) lived 2 years or longer, compared with 22% (13/60) when surgery was not a part of treatment. Overall, 52 patients (61%) had local control which was the most important factor for the long-term survival. In patients with unresectable tumors, total dose of radiation therapy was important in achieving local control. Ten of 11 patients treated with neutrons had local control. This report recommends that if the tumor is resectable, surgical resection should be considered. Postoperative radiation therapy was preferred because split course radiation therapy was disadvantageous. The patients with unresectable superior sulcus tumors should receive high-dose photon (higher than 65 Gy in 6½ weeks) or neutron radiation therapy.

Komaki R, Roh J, Cox JD, et al: Superior sulcus tumors: Results of irradiation of 36 patients. Cancer 48:1563–1568, 1981.
Results of 36 patients with superior sulcus tumors who were treated primarily with radiation are described. Eighty-six percent of patients had relief of symptoms for a median of 12 months after radiation. Forty-seven percent achieved local control, and a 5-year actuarial survival rate of 23% was reported. Therefore, it is demonstrated that radiation therapy is also an effective mode of therapy for superior sulcus tumors, particularly those that have surgical contraindications.

Neal CR, Amdur RJ, Mendenhall WM et al: Pancoast tumor: Radiation therapy alone versus preoperative radiation therapy and surgery. Int J Radiat Oncol Biol Phys 21:651–660, 1991.
The authors reported 73 patients with Pancoast tumor. Forty-one patients were treated by preoperative radiation therapy (usually 30 Gy in 2 weeks or 45 Gy in 5 weeks) and 32 patients were treated by radiation therapy alone (usually 65 Gy to 70 Gy in 6½ to 8 weeks). Although 41 patients initially scheduled to received preoperative radiation therapy followed by surgery, surgery was not performed in 29% for various reasons. There was no significant difference in the absolute or cause-specific survival rates between treatment groups, but severe complications were significantly common in patients receiving combined therapy. They emphasized selection bias of patients by reviewing two dozen articles dealing with radiation therapy alone versus radiation therapy plus surgery for treatment of Pancoast tumors.

Pancoast HK: Superior pulmonary sulcus tumor. JAMA 99:1391–1396, 1932.
This paper was delivered by Pancoast as the Chairman's Address to the Section of Radiology in 1932. In the report he presented seven cases, describing the x-ray findings and clinical signs and symptoms of superior sulcus tumors. It was largely because of this paper that superior sulcus tumors have also been called "Pancoast's syndrome," and this paper is therefore historically important.

Paulson DL: Technical considerations in stage III disease: The "superior sulcus" lesion. In Delarue NC, Eschapasse H (eds): International Trends in General Thoracic Surgery, Vol I. Philadelphia, W.B. Saunders, 1985, pp 121–133.
The Dallas experience of Paulson and Shaw is updated. This involves preoperative radiation followed by en bloc resection of the upper lobe and first three ribs originally reported in 1960. In this series of 78 patients, 31%, 26%, and 22% survived 5, 10, and 15 years, respectively.

Shaw RR, Paulson DL, Kee JL: Treatment of the superior sulcus tumor by irradiation followed by resection. Ann Surg 154:29–40, 1961.
This important paper reports 18 patients treated with preoperative radiation therapy followed by en bloc surgical resection in 4 to 6 weeks. Therefore, it introduces the concept of preoperative shrinkage of these tumors followed by radical resection of the tumor and adjacent chest wall. This therapy has continued to be the treatment of choice for well-localized N0 and N1 superior sulcus tumors.

REFERENCES

1. Hare ES: Tumor involving certain nerves. London Med Gas 1:16–18, 1838.
2. Tobias JW: Sindrome apico-costo-vertebral dolorosa por tumor, apexiano. Su valor diagnostico en el cancer primitivo pulmonar. Rev Med Lat Am 19:1522–1556, 1932.
3. Pancoast HK: Importance of careful roentgenray investigation of apical chest tumors. JAMA 83:1407–1411, 1924.
4. Pancoast HK: Superior pulmonary sulcus tumor. JAMA 99:1391–1396, 1932.
5. Graef I, Steinberg I: Superior pulmonary sulcus tumor: A case exhibiting a malignant epithelial neoplasm of unknown origin with Pancoast's syndrome. AJR Am J Roentgenol 36:293–300, 1936.
6. James I, Page W: Miniature scar-carcinoma of the lung and the "upper sulcus tumor" of Pancoast. Br J Surg 32:85–90, 1944.
7. Herbut PA, Watson JS: Tumor of the thoracic inlet producing Pancoast syndrome. Arch Pathol 42:88–103, 1946.
8. Chardack WM, MacCallum JD: Pancoast syndrome due to bronchogenic carcinoma: Successful surgical removal and postoperative irradiation. J Thorac Surg 25:402–412, 1953.
9. Chardack WM, MacCallum JD: Pancoast tumor: Five-year survival without recurrence or metastases following radical resection and postoperative irradiation. J Thorac Surg 31:535–542, 1956.
10. Dontas NS: The Pancoast syndrome. Br J Tuberc 51:246–250, 1957.
11. Shaw RR, Paulson DL, Kee JL: Treatment of the superior sulcus tumor by irradiation followed by resection. Ann Surg 154:29–40, 1961.
12. Shaw RR: Pancoast's tumor. Ann Thorac Surg 37:343–344, 1984.
13. Paulson DL: III. Superior sulcus carcinomas. In Sabiston D, Spencer F (eds): Gibbons Surgery of the Chest, Vol I. Philadelphia, W.B. Saunders, 1983, pp 506–515.
14. Paulson DL: Carcinomas in the superior pulmonary sulcus. J Thorac Cardiovasc Surg 70:1095–1104, 1975.
15. Paulson DL: Technical considerations in stage III disease: The "superior sulcus" lesion. In Delarue NC, Eschapasse H (eds): International Trends in General Thoracic Surgery, Vol I. Philadelphia, W.B. Saunders, 1985, pp 121–133.
16. Ziporyn T: Upper body pain: Possible tipoff to Pancoast tumor. JAMA 246:1759–1763, 1981.
17. Miller JI, Mansour KA, Hatcher CR: Carcinoma of the superior pulmonary sulcus. Ann Thorac Surg 28:44–47, 1979.
18. Attar S, Miller JE, Satterfield J, et al: Pancoast's tumor: Irradiation or surgery? Ann Thorac Surg 28:578–586, 1979.
19. Simon H, Moon AC: Pitfalls in the diagnosis of pancoast tumor. Radiology 82:235–239, 1982.
20. Webb WR, Jeffrey RB, Godwin JD: Thoracic computed tomography in superior sulcus tumors. J Comput Assist Tomogr 5:361–365, 1981.
21. Johnson DH, Hainsworth JD, Greco FA: Pancoast's syndrome and small cell lung cancer. Chest 82:602–606, 1982.
22. Aletras H, Papaconstantinou C: Pancoast's syndrome following an intrapleural rupture of a hepatic echinococcus cyst. Scand J Thorac Cardiovasc Surg 16:283–287, 1982.
23. Chen KTK, Padmanabhan A: Pancoast syndrome caused by extramedullary plasmacytoma. J Surg Oncol 24:117–118, 1983.
24. Eiben C, Indihan FJ, Hunter SW: Thoracic actinomycosis mimicking the Pancoast syndrome. Minn Med 66:541–544, 1983.
25. Heelan RT, Demas BE, Caravelli JF, et al: Superior sulcus tumor: CT and MR imaging. Radiology 170:637–641, 1989.
26. Hepper NGG, Herskovic T, Witten DM, et al: Thoracic inlet tumors. Ann Intern Med 54:979–989, 1966.
27. McGoon DC: Transcervical technique for removal of specimen from superior sulcus tumor for pathologic study. Ann Surg 159:407–410, 1964.
28. Siderys H, Pittman JN: Percutaneous needle biopsy of the lung in cases of superior sulcus tumors. J Thorac Cardiovasc Surg 53:716–720, 1967.
29. Walls WJ, Thornbury JR, Naylor B: Pulmonary needle aspiration biopsy in the diagnosis of Pancoast tumors. Radiology 111:99–102, 1974.
30. Wallace S, Carrasco CH, Charnsangavej C, et al: Contributions of interventional radiology to diagnosis and management of the cancer patient. In Bragg DG, Rubin P, Youker JE (eds): Oncologic Imaging. Elmsford, New York, Pergamon Press, 1984, pp 587–593.
31. Paulson DL, Weed TE, Rian RL: Cervical approach for percutaneous needle biopsy of Pancoast tumors. Ann Thorac Surg 39:586–587, 1985.

32. Paulson DL: The importance of defining location and staging of superior pulmonary sulcus tumors. (Editorial.) Ann Thorac Surg 15:549–551, 1973.

33. Stanford W, Barnes RP, Tucker AR: Influence of staging in superior sulcus (Pancoast) tumors of the lung. Ann Thorac Surg 29:406–409, 1980.

34. Ginsberg RJ: Discussion of Attar S, Miller JE, Satterfield J, et al: Pancoast's tumor: Irradiation or surgery? Ann Thorac Surg 28:578–586, 1979.

35. Beyer DC, Weisenburger T: Superior sulcus tumors. Am J Clin Oncol 8:24–25, 1985.

36. Devine JW, Mendenhall WM, Million RR, et al: Carcinoma of the superior pulmonary sulcus treated with surgery and/or radiation therapy. Cancer 5:941–943, 1986.

37. Martini N: Discussion of Attar S, Miller JE, Satterfield J, et al: Pancoast's tumor: Irradiation or surgery? Ann Thorac Surg 28:578–586, 1979.

38. Anderson TM, Moy PM, Holmes EC: Factors affecting survival in superior sulcus tumors. J Clin Oncol 4(11):1598–1603, 1986.

39. Mathisen DJ, Grillo HC, Wright CD, et al: Superior sulcus tumors: Results of combined treatment (irradiation and radical resection). J Thorac Cardiovasc Surg 94:69–74, 1987.

40. Shahian DM, Neptune WB, Ellis FH: Pancoast tumors: Improved survival with preoperative and postoperative radiotherapy. Ann Thorac Surg 43:32–38, 1987.

41. Ricci C, Rendina EA, Venuta F, et al: Superior pulmonary sulcus tumors: Radical resection and palliative treatment. Int Surg 74:175–179, 1989.

42. Sartori F, Rea F, Calabro F, et al: Carcinoma of the superior pulmonary sulcus: Results of irradiation and radical resection. J Thorac Cardiovasc Surg 104(3):679–683, 1992.

43. Hilaris BS, Luomanen RK, Beattie EJ: Integrated irradiation and surgery in the treatment of apical lung cancer. Cancer 27:1369–1378, 1971.

44. Dartevelle PG, Chapelier AR, Macchiarini P, et al: Anterior transcervical-thoracic approach for radical resection of lung tumors invading the thoracic inlet. J Thorac Cardiovasc Surg 105(6):1025–1034, 1993.

45. Martini N, McCormack P: Therapy of Stage III (non-metastatic disease). Semin Oncol 10:95–110, 1983.

46. Hilaris BS, Martini N, Luomanen RKJ, et al: The value of preoperative radiation therapy in apical cancer of the lung. Surg Clin North Am 54:831, 1974.

47. Komaki R, Mountain CF, Holbert JM et al: Superior sulcus tumors: Treatment selection and results for 85 patients without metastasis (M0) at presentation. Int J Radiat Oncol Biol Phys 19:31–36, 1990.

48. Morris RW, Abadir R: Pancoast tumors: The value of high-dose radiotherapy. Radiology 132:717–719, 1979.

49. Ahmad K, Fayos JV, Kirsch MM: Apical lung carcinoma. Cancer 54:913–917, 1984.

50. Van Houtte P, MacLennan I, Poulter C, et al: External radiation in management of superior sulcus tumors. Cancer 54:223–227, 1984.

51. Komaki R, Roh J, Cox JD, et al: Superior sulcus tumors: Results of irradiation of 36 patients. Cancer 48:1563–1568, 1981.

15 SUPERIOR VENA CAVA SYNDROME

Minesh P. Mehta and Timothy J. Kinsella

INTRODUCTION

The constellation of clinical and radiographic findings resulting from compromised blood flow through the superior vena cava (SVC) is encountered relatively frequently, especially in association with a variety of thoracic neoplasms, and is referred to as the SVC syndrome (SVCS). A thorough understanding of this entity requires an appreciation of the intricate venous anatomy and physiology of the thorax and abdomen. The etiologic factors are numerous and varied, resulting in a wide spectrum of clinical findings and severity. In most instances, a proper diagnostic work-up is necessary for appropriate therapeutic intervention. The prognosis, in terms of palliation, is usually excellent, but long-term survivorship is achieved only in a minority of patients, usually those with benign lesions as the causative factor.

ANATOMIC AND PHYSIOLOGIC CORRELATES

Venous Drainage of the Thorax

Superior Vena Cava

The union of the right and left brachiocephalic veins results in the formation of the SVC, which is the final common vessel draining the bulk of venous blood from the upper thorax, both upper extremities, and the head and neck region.[1] The average length of the SVC is 7 cm, with the final 1.5 cm embedded within the reflection of the pericardial sac around the right atrium. The SVC is located in the superior and middle mediastinum. It originates behind the first right costal cartilage, traverses posterior to the first and second intercostal spaces, and terminates in the right atrium at the level of the third intercostal space. Because it is large (average diameter of 2 cm) and thin walled and lacks valves, it maintains blood at a low pressure and therefore is easily compressible. The SVC is completely encircled by numerous lymph nodes, and its complicated anatomic relationships are best understood by reviewing its cross-sectional anatomy, as illustrated in the computed tomography (CT) scan in Figure 15–1.

Azygos Venous System

The azygos venous system,[1] which consists of several interconnected veins, provides the major auxiliary pathway for venous drainage when the SVC is compromised. It is a low-pressure system with incomplete valves, permitting reversal of blood flow direction and thus enabling shunting of venous return from side to side—from the SVC to the inferior vena cava (IVC) and from interconnecting veins that allow bypass of SVC obstruction. Figure 15–2 is a schematic of the interconnections within this system.

The segmental lumbar veins on the right are typically interconnected by one or two longitudinally placed ascending lumbar veins, which connect inferiorly with either the common iliac vein or the IVC. Under normal physiologic conditions, the negative intrathoracic pressure induces blood flow in a cephalad direction into the azygos vein, which is the thoracic continuation of the right ascending lumbar vein. On the right, the azygos also collects blood from the posterior intercostal veins; several esophageal, mediastinal, and pericardial veins; and the bronchial veins

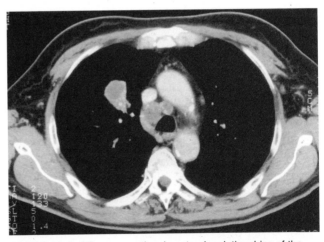

FIGURE 15–1. CT cross-sectional anatomic relationships of the superior vena cava (SVC). *Anterior,* The anterior margins of the right lung and pleura, as well as the pericardium inferiorly separate the cava from the internal thoracic artery, superior internal mammary nodes, and the first three intercostal spaces, costal cartilages, and sternum. *Posterior,* The trachea, the paratracheal lymph nodes, and the right vagus nerve are located posteromedially, while the posterolateral relations include the right lung and pleura. The esophagus is a distant left posterior relation. *Right,* The right phrenic nerve and right pleura are located to the right of the cava. *Left,* The ascending aorta and the commencement of the brachiocephalic artery form the left-sided relations of the SVC. Note the enlarged lymph nodes abutting the posterior wall of the SVC, as well as a primary neoplasm in the right upper lobe of the lung.

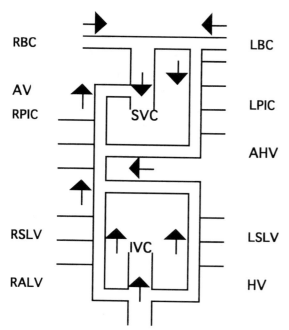

FIGURE 15–2. The azygos system. Schematic illustration of the azygos venous system. The right and left segmental lumbar veins (RSLV, LSLV) empty into the right ascending lumbar vein (RALV) and the hemiazygos vein (HV). These veins continue into the azygos vein (AV) and connect with the inferior vena cava (IVC). The right and left posterior intercostals (RPIC, LPIC) empty into the azygos vein and the accessory hemiazygos vein (AHV), the latter draining into the AV inferiorly and left brachiocephalic (LBC) vein superiorly. The LBC vein and right brachiocephalic (RBC) vein form the superior vena cava (SVC), which receives the AV posteriorly as it enters the right atrium.

just before its termination into the posterior aspect of the SVC immediately above the level of the pericardial reflection.

On the left, the segmental lumbar as well as the lower posterior intercostal veins drain into the longitudinally traversing hemiazygos vein, which empties into the azygos by crossing over and fusing with it at approximately the eighth thoracic vertebral level. In addition, the azygos receives the accessory hemiazygos vein through a variable communicating vein, approximately at the level of the seventh thoracic vertebra. The accessory hemiazygos drains the left upper posterior intercostals and the left bronchial veins and communicates with the left brachiocephalic vein superiorly.

Veins of the Vertebral Column

The vertebral venous system represents another low-pressure, intercommunicating network capable of altering the direction of blood flow and permitting communication between the SVC and IVC.[1] At any given transverse level, an almost bicircumferential system exists, consisting of an internal plexus within the canal and an external plexus outside the vertebral bodies. Each of these plexuses has anterior and posterior venous arches. An extensive net of interconnecting, valveless, thin-walled tributaries connects the plexuses. These transverse plexuses communicate with a

series of longitudinal veins that also do not contain valves and therefore can support directional change. Inferiorly, these veins are in continuity with the common iliacs and the lumbar veins, which empty into the IVC and the azygos system, respectively. Superiorly, communication is maintained into both the azygos and the SVC through the intercostal veins.

Lateral Thoracic Veins

The lateral thoracic veins are longitudinally oriented vessels that can also provide alternative circulatory pathways in the event of SVC obstruction. They can shunt blood into the azygos system through the posterior intercostals or into the IVC through the superior epigastric, which empties into the femoral vein.

Internal Mammary Veins

These vessels provide another detour, either into the IVC through the inferior epigastric emptying into the iliac vein or into the azygos through the intercostal veins.

An Animal Model for SVCS

In an elegant series of experiments in dogs, Carlson[2] documented the effects of ligating the SVC. When the SVC was ligated below the level of the azygos, none of the animals was able to survive, suggesting that other compensatory pathways are unable to acutely compensate for sudden, complete SVC occlusion below the azygos. Ligation above the level of the azygos in seven dogs resulted in significant acute symptoms, including listlessness and cyanosis, but within approximately 1 week, collateral blood flow developed, permitting survival and recovery. These experiments suggest that the azygos system represents the most important collateral pathway and is able to compensate for even acute and complete SVC occlusion. Interestingly, in further experiments, Carlson was able to document that staged ligation of the SVC and the azygos were compatible with life, suggesting that nonazygos collaterals can also support life, although not in an acute setting.

Collateral Circulatory Pathways

Collateral venous pathways in humans have been extensively described by McIntire and Sykes[3] and Klassen et al.[4] More recently, Stanford et al[5] demonstrated the development of multiple collateral pathways in SVCS using venography. The technique of radionuclide venography has resulted in a substantial improvement in our understanding of the development of these collateral channels.[6, 7] In a radionuclide analysis of the SVC in 70 patients with SVCS, Muramatsu et al[7] identified several major and minor collateral pathways, depending on whether the obstruction was above or at the azygos. These include several of the pathways described earlier, but they also demonstrated an important collateral pathway by which blood is transported to the contralateral brachiocephalic vein through the jugular venous arch (Fig. 15–3). A tabular listing of the major pathways is provided in Table 15–1. In supra-azygos obstruction, shunting of blood to the nonoccluded contralateral brachiocephalic vein via the jugular venous arch appears to be the most important pathway. Other major pathways include the lateral thoracic, which shunts blood into the azygos via the posterior intercostals; the vertebral venous plexus; and the internal mammary pathway. In obstructions involving the azygos orifice, all of the major pathways shunt blood into the IVC (Fig. 15–4) through the lateral thoracic-superior epigastric route, the internal mammary-inferior epigastric route, the cervical vertebral network-azygos route, and the lateral thoracic-posterior intercostal-azygos route.

Other unusual and collateral pathways include systemic-to-pulmonary venous shunting[8]; direct shunting between the right subclavian vein and the left ventricle[9]; collateral channels connecting the upper extremity veins and the portal vein via the paraumbilical veins, resulting in a scintigraphic "hot spot" in the liver,[10] and, interestingly, via the cerebral sinuses.[7] In

TABLE 15–1. Collateral Pathways in SVCS Identified by Radionuclide Superior Cavography

MAJOR PATHWAYS				
Shunt	Intermediary	System	n	%*
A. SUPRA-AZYGOS OCCLUSION (n = 73)				
Jugular arch	Brachiocephalic	SVC	29	40
Lateral thoracic	Intercostal/azygos	SVC	18	25
Cervical net	Vertebral/azygos	SVC	18	25
Lateral thoracic	Internal thoracic	SVC	18	25
B. PARA-AZYGOS OCCLUSION (n = 12)				
Lateral thoracic	Superior epigastric	IVC	7	58
Internal thoracic	Inferior epigastric	IVC	5	42
Cervical net	Azygos	IVC	4	33
Lateral thoracic	Intercostal/azygos	IVC	3	25

SVCS = superior vena cava syndrome, SVC = superior vena cava, IVC = inferior vena cava.

*Percentages do not add up to 100 because of multiple collaterals in some cases.

Modified from Muramatsu T, Miyame T, Dohi Y: Collateral pathways observed by radionuclide superior cavography in 70 patients with superior vena caval obstruction. Clin Nucl Med 16:332–336, 1991.

addition, left-sided as well as bilateral SVCs have been reported,[11] and these have very unusual drainage patterns, including the coronary sinus, pulmonary venous atrium, and so on. Obviously, the presence of

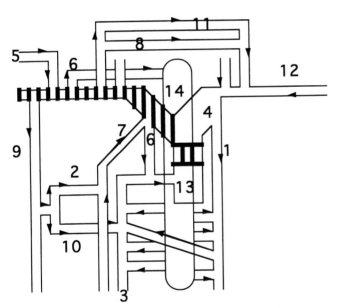

FIGURE 15–3. Collateral pathways in supra-azygos caval occlusion. The hashed areas represent occlusion of the SVC (13) affecting the right side, but not affecting the azygos (3). The pathways include

1. The jugular venous arch (8) to the left subclavian (12), left brachiocephalic (4) and accessory hemiazygos (1).
2. The lateral thoracic (9) to the posterior intercostals (10) into the azygos.
3. The cervical venous network (6) into the vertebral venous plexus (14) which communicates with the azygos as well as the SVC.
4. The lateral thoracic-anterior intercostal (2)-internal mammary (7) pathway.
5. Via the cephalic vein (5) into the subclavian (12).
6. The cerebral sinus route (11).

(Modified from Muramatsu T, Miyame T, Dohi Y: Collateral pathways observed by radionuclide superior cavography in 70 patients with superior vena caval obstruction. Clin Nucl Med 16:332–336, 1991.)

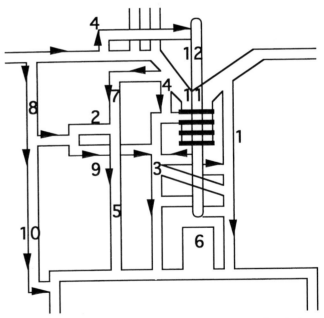

FIGURE 15–4. Collateral pathways in para-azygos caval occlusion. When the occlusion involves the orifice of the azygos (3, shaded area), the major collaterals drain into the IVC (6) or its branches, as follows:

1. Lateral thoracic (8) to superior epigastric (10) to IVC.
2. Internal mammary (7), to inferior epigastric (5) to IVC.
3. Cervical venous network (4), to azygos system (3), to IVC.
4. Lateral thoracic to posterior intercostal (9), to azygos to IVC.

(Modified from Muramatsu T, Miyame T, Dohi Y: Collateral pathways observed by radionuclide superior cavography in 70 patients with superior vena caval obstruction. Clin Nucl Med 16:332–336, 1991.)

TABLE 15–2. Mechanistic Model for the Causes of Superior Vena Cava Syndrome

	EXTRINSIC	INTRAVASCULAR	LUMINAL
Benign	Retrosternal goiter	Catheter thrombus	Endothelial hyperplasia
Malignant	Lymphoma	Tumor thrombus	Angiosarcoma

SVC occlusion in these situations results in rather dramatic and unusual collateralization.

ETIOLOGY

Mechanistic Considerations

The vascular flow within the SVC can be impeded by significant extrinsic compression, intraluminal thrombosis, direct invasion or infiltration of the vessel wall, or a combination of any of these mechanisms. The etiologic considerations in any of these scenarios could include benign as well as malignant conditions. This relatively simple mechanistic model allows for easy categorization of the enormous number of possible causes of SVCS. A working example of this concept is illustrated in Table 15–2.

Although it is unclear which mechanism predominates, Roswitt and coworkers[12] have suggested that even when extrinsic compression is highly suspected, as in lung cancer, thrombotic events may be present in 40% to 50% of patients. The therapeutic implications of this situation as it pertains to the use of thrombolytic therapy are discussed later. Interestingly, thrombotic occlusion in these cases can also occur as a result of tumor thrombi,[13] which poses a different set of management issues.

The Changing Spectrum

The first published and recorded instance of SVCS is generally credited to William Hunter,[14] who in 1757 described the syndrome as a consequence of a syphilitic aneurysm. In fact, for the most part, SVCS was regarded as a relatively rare entity before the latter half of this century. McIntire and Sykes[3] provided an extensive review of all literature published up to 1949 and found only 502 cases. In this series, 63% of cases were associated with benign causes such as aortic aneurysm (30%); chronic mediastinitis, usually tuberculous, syphilitic or fungal (16%); idiopathic mediastinal fibrosis (12%); and other miscellaneous benign causes (5%). One-third of cases (34%) were associated with a primary malignant thoracic tumor, and metastatic disease accounted for only 3%. In 1954, Schechter[15] reported that 40% of 274 cases of SVCS were due to syphilitic aneurysms or tuberculous mediastinitis, and the remainder had a malignant etiology.

With improved antibiotic management of syphilis and tuberculosis, these diseases have become extremely rare causes of SVCS. Paralleling the dramatic increase in lung cancer,[16] this neoplasm has become the leading cause of SVCS. In 1962, Effler and Groves[17]

reported on a series of 64 patients from the Cleveland Clinic and noted that 16 patients had a benign etiology, including granuloma, goiter, fibrosing mediastinitis, and idiopathic causes. Lung cancer was the most common diagnosis.

In a 1967 literature review by Banker and Maddison[18] of 438 cases, only 15% had a benign etiology; again, lung cancer was the most common cause (65%). Kamiya et al[19] reviewed the Japanese experience in 734 patients from 1949 to 1965 and found that almost three-fourths of the patients had an intrathoracic malignancy as a causative factor for SVCS. In 1979, Lochridge and associates[20] found that the proportion of SVCS with malignancy as the etiology had escalated to 97%. In other more recent studies,[21–26] the proportion of patients with underlying malignancy as the cause of SVCS ranged from 78% to 97%, with an average of 88%. This is illustrated clearly in Figure 15–5, and Table 15–3.

Common Malignant Causes

Thoracic malignancies account for the overwhelming majority of patients with SVCS encountered in routine practice. Extrinsic compression by a rapidly proliferating tumor is often the primary etiologic factor. In descending order, the most common malignancies re-

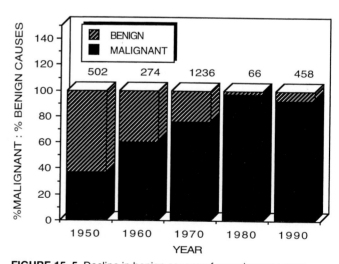

FIGURE 15–5. Decline in benign causes of superior vena cava syndrome (SVCS) since 1950. The graph is a composite depiction of the declining proportionate contribution of benign diseases as a cause of SVCS. The data are extracted from references 3, 15, and 17 to 26, and represent the proportions for the preceding decade. The solid bars represent the percentage contribution from malignant causes, and the striped bars represent benign causes. The numbers above the bars represent total patient numbers used to calculate the breakdown.

TABLE 15–3. Changing Spectrum of Superior Vena Cava Syndrome Etiology

YEAR	STUDY	NO. OF PATIENTS	ETIOLOGY Benign %	ETIOLOGY Malignant %
1948	McIntire and Sykes[3]	502	63	37
1954	Schechter[15]	274	40	60
1962	Effler and Groves[17]	64	25	75
1965	Kamiya et al[19]	734	26	74
1967	Banker and Maddison[18]	438	20	80
1979	Lochridge et al[20]	66	3	97
1981	Schraufnagel et al[21]	107	3	97
1981	Parish et al[22]	86	22	78
1986	Bell et al[23]	138	1	99
1987	Fincher[24]	39	13	87
1990	Chen et al[25]	45	7	93
1990	Yellin et al[26]	43	16	84
	Total	2536	30	70

sponsible for SVCS are small cell lung cancer (SCLC), squamous cell lung cancer, adenocarcinoma and large cell lung cancer, lymphoma, metastases, germ cell tumors, and thymic neoplasms. Lung cancer has been reported to account for 67% to 82% of cases of SVCS[27]; lymphomas, 5% to 15%; and metastases, 3% to 20%. In a composite analysis of 267 cases of SVCS reported in three different series[23, 25, 26] within the past 7 yr, the distribution was as follows: lung, 69%; miscellaneous (including benign), 16%; lymphoma, 7%; metastases, 4%; and germ cell tumors and thymic neoplasms, 2% each. This distribution is illustrated in Figure 15–6.

Lung Cancer

As early as 1953, Roswitt and colleagues[12] recognized that the rapidly increasing and significant number of patients with inoperable bronchogenic carcinoma implied that this disease would become the leading cause of SVCS. In a retrospective review of 4100 patients with lung cancer treated between 1965 and 1984, Armstrong and associates[28] identified 99 patients, or roughly 2.5%, with SVCS. Salsali and Clifton[29] noted the occurrence of SVCS in 4% of 4960 patients. The exact incidence of SVCS is unknown, but

assuming that of the 150,000 annual cases of lung cancer seen in the United States, 120,000 are inoperable, and using an average rate of 3%, it can be deduced that there should be approximately 3600 cases of SVCS resulting from lung cancer annually; furthermore, because lung cancer causes approximately 60% of all cases of SVCS, an estimated annualized incidence of 6000 is projected.

In a comprehensive literature review, Ahmann[30] evaluated a total of 1986 patients with SVCS reported in the literature through 1984 and provided a histologic breakdown of the 1086 patients (55% of all patients with SVCS) who had SVCS as a consequence of lung cancer. In his analysis, SCLC was the most frequent histologic diagnosis, accounting for 32% of patients, followed by squamous cell (15%), undifferentiated carcinoma (8%), adenocarcinoma (5%), and large cell (4%). Ahmann further analyzed 720 cases from 18 series in which detailed histologic assessment was available after the 1967 recommendations by the World Health Organization (WHO) to subdivide lung cancer into the four broad categories of epidermoid carcinoma, adenocarcinoma, large cell carcinoma, and small cell carcinoma. In this second limited analysis, Ahmann found that SCLC accounted for 40% of SVCS

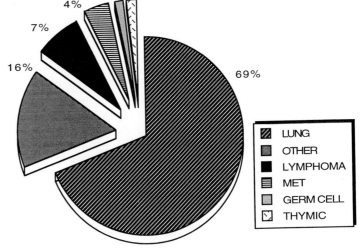

FIGURE 15–6. Distribution of various malignancies causing SVCS. (Data from Chen,[25] Yellin,[26] and Bell.[23])

TABLE 15–4. Histologic Types of Lung Cancer Causing Superior Vena Cava Syndrome

STUDY	YEAR	Small Cell	Squamous	Adenocarcinoma	Large Cell	Other
Rosenbloom[31]	1949	3	3	0	0	3
Szur and Bromley[32]	1956	13	3	7	1	6
Geller[33]	1963	1	0	0	0	2
Skinner et al[34]	1965	5	5	2	0	7
Salsali and Cliffton[35]	1965	85	6	11	0	23
Urschel and Paulson[36]	1966	8	13	2	6	24
Salsali and Cliffton[37]	1968	24	0	11	0	37
Ghosh and Cliffton[38]	1973	27	12	0	0	30
Armstrong et al[39]	1975	1	0	0	0	1
Kane et al[40]	1976	8	0	0	0	0
Avasthi and Moghissi[41]	1977	1	2	0	1	0
Davenport et al[42]	1978	20	5	1	0	0
Lochridge[20]	1979	8	12	4	4	26
Scarantino et al[43]	1979	13	7	3	13	12
Parish et al[22]	1981	12	12	11	8	2
Shimm et al[44]	1981	8	6	3	4	0
Schraufnagel et al[21]	1981	19	24	6	1	17
Bell et al[23]	1986	77	41	23	31	2
Armstrong et al[45]	1987	42	26	17	11	3
Chen et al[25]	1990	3	11	5	0	7
Yellin et al[26]	1990	4	6	6	2	12
Total		382	194	112	82	214

caused by lung cancer. The squamous, adeno, and large cell types accounted for 18%, 9%, and 7%, respectively, and other variants made up the remaining 26%. This analysis has been expanded to include more recent series, and the data are presented in Table 15–4. Of a total of 984 patients with SVCS resulting from lung cancer reported in 21 series, the percentage contribution from the various histologies was 39% for small cell, 22% for other histologic subtypes, 20% for squamous, 11% for adenocarcinoma, and 8% for large cell (Fig. 15–7).

Given the fact that SCLC is responsible for only 25%[46] of all lung cancer, its inordinate contribution to the development of SVCS (almost 40%) can be explained only on the basis of its typically central location, a very high incidence of nodal metastases, and a significantly faster tumor-doubling time than most other histologic types of lung cancer. Although SVCS develops approximately 3% of the time with non–small cell histologies, it occurs in approximately 10% to 12% of patients with SCLC.[47–49]

Lymphoma

Lymphomas usually account for about 7% to 10% of all causes of SVCS[23, 25, 26, 50] and, as a group, constitute the second most common etiologic factor in the development of SVCS. Analogous to the rationale for the inordinate contribution of SCLC to the causation of SVCS, these neoplasms are also rapidly proliferating and frequently produce bulky mediastinal adenopathy leading to a high incidence of SVCS. Conversely, although Hodgkin's disease can produce large mediastinal masses, the relatively slow rate of growth prevents a high rate of SVCS. Lymphoblastic lymphoma and diffuse large cell lymphoma are the two most frequently encountered histologies.[50] The incidence of SVCS in lymphoblastic lymphoma approaches 21%. Miller and colleagues[51] have reported a significant association between the extent of sclerosis in a lymphoma and the development of SVCS. About 7% of patients with non-Hodgkin's lymphoma develop a diffuse large cell variant with significant sclerosis, and this entity is associated with SVCS almost 100% of the time.

Germ Cell Neoplasms

Primary mediastinal germ cell tumors are an extremely rare entity; yet these neoplasms account for almost 2% of malignant causes of SVCS.[23, 25, 26] The

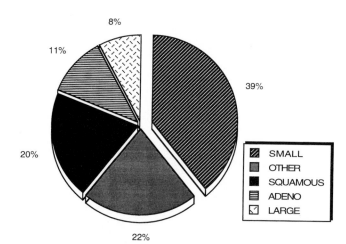

FIGURE 15–7. Percentage distribution of lung cancer–associated cases of SVCS by histologic type. (Data relating to 984 patients in 21 series; see references 20 to 23, 25, 26, and 31 to 45.

explanation for this also is their rapid growth, which is noted in all germ cell tumors except the mature teratoma. Almost 20% of patients with primary mediastinal germ cell tumors develop SVCS.[52]

Thymic Neoplasms

Thymoma, the most common tumor of the anterior mediastinum, expresses malignant behavior about one-third to one-half of the time, but invasion of the great vessels is rare.[53, 54] This fact, together with its rather slow growth rate, is responsible for only about 2% SVCS from thymoma.[55] When it does occur, SVCS is more from extrinsic compression than from vascular invasion. Rarely, direct invasion into the right atrium leads to the development of SVCS.[56] Airan and colleagues[57] recently reviewed the association of malignant thymoma with SVCS.

Metastases

Metastatic disease to the lungs or mediastinum, or both, accounts for 4% of SVCS caused by malignancies.[23, 25, 26] Breast cancer is the most frequent diagnosis, possibly related to metastases to the internal mammary chain of nodes. With increasing survival of patients with metastatic disease, this cause is likely to also increase in frequency and must always be borne in mind when addressing the differential diagnoses for SVCS.

Uncommon Malignant Causes of SVCS

A number of case reports[58-70] have documented the large variety of tumors that are known to have caused SVCS, most reporting tumors of hematogenous origin such as leukemic infiltrates, granulocytic sarcomas, plasmacytomas, and so on. These are presented as a summary in Table 15–5.

TABLE 15–5. Uncommon Malignancies Causing Superior Vena Cava Syndrome

CAUSE	STUDY
Granulocytic sarcoma (AML)	Varma et al[58]
Chronic lymphocytic leukemia	de Mayolo et al[59]
Cardiac lymphoma	Hwang et al[60]
Cardiac rhabdomyosarcoma	Bishop et al[61]
Plasmacytoma	Davis et al[62]
Thyroid carcinoma	Thomas et al[63]
Intracaval paraganglioma	Rutegard et al[64]
Right atrial metastases	Nishida et al[65]
Intracaval metastases	Korobkin and Gasano[66]
Mediastinal carcinoid	Aggarwal et al[67]
Angiosarcoma	Sunderrajan et al[68]
Leiomyosarcoma	Sunderrajan et al[68]
Liposarcoma	Sunderrajan et al[68]
Fibrosarcoma	Sunderrajan et al[68]
Malignant mesothelioma	Martin et al[69]
Histiocytosis X	Kuten et al[70]

Etiologic Associations in the Pediatric Age Group

In the pediatric population, SVCS is extremely rare. In a review of the world literature published in 1983,[71] a total of 175 pediatric cases of SVCS were identified, most associated with benign iatrogenic causes such as caval catheters, ventriculoatrial shunts, and cardiovascular surgery, but lymphoproliferative diseases also contributed to the development of the syndrome. Small infants are especially susceptible to catheter-associated vascular thrombosis. In infants weighing less than 10 kg, thrombotic complications are noted in 15% to 20% compared with only 4% in those weighing more than 10 kg.[72] Grisoni and colleagues[73] noted that premature and low-birth-weight infants were at highest risk, with an overall 21% thrombosis rate in a neonatal intensive care unit. The factors that increase this risk include placement outside the SVC (15% outside the SVC versus 0% in the SVC),[74] catheter material (polyvinyl more than Silastic),[75] and increased solution osmolality and viscosity.[76]

In adolescence, mediastinal tumors are the main cause of SVCS. Despite the fact that mediastinal masses are not altogether rare in this population, the occurrence of SVCS is distinctly unusual. In a study of 607 such patients, D'Angio and associates[77] reported only nine patients (1.5%) with SVCS. Lymphomas are by far the most common malignant cause of SVCS in the pediatric population,[78] and as in adults, non-Hodgkin's lymphoma, particularly the diffuse large cell and the lymphoblastic types, predominates. Neurogenic tumors such as neuroblastoma and ganglioneuroma, thymoma, sarcoma, and teratoma have also been reported to cause SVCS. Ingram and coworkers[79] have analyzed the proportion of various mediastinal masses that lead to SVCS in a cohort reported from St. Jude's Children's Hospital (Fig. 15–8). Germ cell tumors, with a 20% rate, have the highest

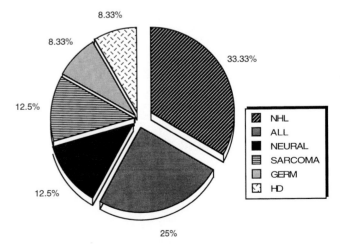

FIGURE 15–8. Malignancies causing SVCS in children. NHL = Non-Hodgkin's lymphoma; ALL = Acute lymphoblastic leukemia; HD = Hodgkin's disease. (Data from Ingram L, Rivera GK, Shapiro DN: Superior vena cava syndrome associated with childhood malignancy: Analysis of 24 cases. Med Pediatr Oncol 18:476–481, 1990.)

incidence of SVCS. Of a total of 114 children with germ cell neoplasms, 10 presented with mediastinal masses, of whom 2 (20%) developed SVCS.

Nonmalignant Causes of SVCS

Nonmalignant etiologies of SVCS, although significantly less frequent[3] than in the first half of the decade, continue to remain an important causative factor for SVCS. An analysis of published literature suggests that benign causes may be responsible for approximately 12%[23, 25, 26] of cases of SVCS. Although an extremely large number of conditions fall in this category, the most common include mediastinal fibrosis and central venous devices. The latter group is becoming increasingly common owing to the widespread use of these devices and is a particularly common cause in the pediatric population.[72] Mahajan and colleagues[73] reviewed the benign causes of SVCS in a series of 16 patients in 1975 and found that mediastinal fibrosis from histoplasmosis was the most frequent cause, accounting for 12 of 16 cases. Other causes included retrosternal thyroid, aortic aneurysm, and congestive heart failure. A listing of several nonmalignant causes of SVCS is presented in Table 15–6.[73, 80–111]

CLINICAL FEATURES

Is This a Medical Emergency?

Older medical literature[35, 42, 112] has suggested that SVCS is a medical emergency, requiring the institution

TABLE 15–6. Nonmalignant Causes of Superior Vena Cava Syndrome

CAUSE	STUDY
Bronchogenic cysts	80
Aortic pseudoaneurysm	81
	82
Subclavian aneurysm	83
Superior vena cava stenosis	84
Pericardial hematoma	85
Entomophthoromycosis	86
Histoplasmosis	87
	88
Nocardia infection	89
Blastomycosis	90
Filarial adenopathy	91
Septic thrombii	92
Tuberculous mediastinitis	93
Pacemaker leads	94
	95
Central venous catheter	96–102
Peritoneovenous shunt	103
Transvenous electrode	104
Substernal goiter	80
	105
Intravascular papillary endothelial hyperplasia	106
Angioimmunoblastic lymphadenopathy	107
Systemic lupus erythematosus	108
Sarcoidosis	109
Behçet's disease (vasculitis)	110
Radiation fibrosis	73
Idiopathic thrombosis	111

of emergency radiotherapy. This belief was based on the assumption that sudden, dramatic occlusion of the SVC and the azygos system would result in the so-called wet brain syndrome,[17] i.e., the development of cerebral edema secondary to venous obstruction. Such acute cerebral edema has been implicated as the causative factor in the development of seizures, drowsiness, stupor, and other serious neurologic sequelae. Hussey and colleagues[112] have stated that in more than 10% of their patients, SVCS was the cause of rapid death. Lokich and Goodman[113] suggested that in addition to irreversible central nervous system damage, significant pulmonary symptoms, possibly as a consequence of pulmonary edema, are likely to occur unless emergency radiation is instituted.

Roswitt et al[12] eloquently described, "The superior vena cava obstruction syndrome in bronchial cancer is a grave symptom-complex which grows in severity as the venous pressure mounts in the great vein and its tributaries. The patient experiences progressive dyspnea, cough and orthopnea, aggravated greatly in the prone position. He is soon able to breathe only in the erect posture and dares not lie down. There is progressive edema of the head, neck and upper extremities and a peculiar reddish cyanosis of the skin which grows more intensely on recumbency. As the cerebral venopressure rises, the patient suffers headaches, vertigo, drowsiness, stupor and unconsciousness. Unless decompression therapy with x-ray irradiation and/or nitrogen mustard is effective, death comes finally as a result of cerebral anoxemia, failure of the respiratory center or strangulation/edema of the glottis and respiratory passages."

Although this description is very colorful and graphic, it is probably far from the truth in the vast majority of cases. In several recent publications,[21, 30] this picture of SVCS has been challenged. In a review of 1986 cases, Ahmann[30] was able to find only one case where death was directly attributable to SVC obstruction. Many examples of long-term survival with unrelieved SVCS were reported by Ahmann. The widely described central nervous system symptoms are, in most instances, secondary to brain metastases.[26] Thomas and colleagues[63] reviewed the possibility of sudden death in patients with SVCS resulting from massive angioinvasion by tumor. To date, there have been only eight well-documented such cases, all as a consequence of anaplastic or follicular carcinoma of the thyroid. Other than these exceptional situations, there are no reasonable grounds to believe that unrelieved SVCS is fatal in and of itself.

Presenting Features

A review of 426 patients in five recent publications[21, 22, 25, 26, 28] reveals that there is clearly a male preponderance (252 men and 174 women, ratio 1.4:1). The mean age was 53.6 years. In most patients, the syndrome is of insidious onset with slow development of symptoms, and a short interval to presentation is highly correlated with either an underlying malignancy or catheter-induced thrombotic occlusion, whereas nonmalignant etiologies other than catheters are associated with long-standing symptoms. In this group of patients, the median time from onset of first symptom to actual presentation ranged from 3.2 to 6.5 wk for patients with malignant disease and 60 to 168 wk for patients with nonmalignant conditions, once again clearly underscoring the fact that occlusion of the SVC is a relatively slow process. The time span reported here is sufficient for the development of collateral circulation, which minimizes the acute impact of the syndrome.

Further review of the data from 319 patients from the above series[22, 25, 26, 28] shows that the most common symptoms (Fig. 15–9) (in descending order) were dyspnea (54%), suffusion (54%), cough (29%), and arm or facial swelling (23%). Less common symptoms include chest pain, dysphagia, syncope, obtundation, hemoptysis, and headache. Particularly notable is the extremely low rate of obtundation (1.6%), again belying the noxious reputation of SVCS.

In a similar analysis of presenting signs in a series of 256 patients from three studies,[22, 25, 28] the most common signs (Fig. 15–10) (in descending order) were facial and extremity edema (66%), engorged neck (60%) and chest (58%) veins, cyanosis (21%), and plethora (17%). Among the earliest and most prominent signs of SVCS are numerous, dilated, vertically oriented, tortuous cutaneous veins above the inferior rib cage margin.[114] By occluding a venule with two fingers, stripping the blood along the vessel, and then releasing one of the fingers, one can determine the direction of blood flow. For veins above the umbilicus, instead of the normal cephalad course, the drainage is commonly caudad. Less common signs include Horner's syndrome, vocal cord paralysis, and abnormal cardiac murmurs. Rare presentations described in the literature range from an unusual case of bilateral chylothorax[115] associated with SVCS to the development

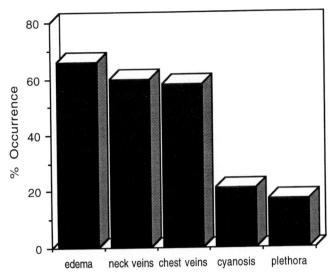

FIGURE 15–10. Common signs in SVCS. (Data from Parish,[22] Chen,[25] and Armstrong.[28])

of acute macular neuroretinopathy[116] as a consequence of hypoperfusion from SVCS. In an analysis of 724 biopsy-proven cases of SCLC being evaluated for the presence of SVCS, Urban and associates[49] found 87 cases of SVCS, and in this subgroup, there was a considerably higher risk of concurrent brain metastases (22% versus 11%). Such findings may in part explain the neurologic symptoms that have been ascribed to SVCS in the past.

Clinical Features in the Pediatric Population

Unlike the adult with SVCS, the child with SVCS truly constitutes a medical emergency[71] because in the child, the SVC is tightly locked in a tiny thoracic compartment in close proximity to the tracheobronchial tree, and airway compromise is a frequent accompaniment when an underlying malignancy is suspected. D'Angio and coworkers[77] have described a so-called superior mediastinal syndrome that differs from SVCS in that severe tracheal and venous compression go hand in hand. In addition, these children face potentially life-threatening risks from anesthesia as tracheal compression is observed in more than one-half of the cases.[117] Therefore, although judicious minimally invasive procedures are justifiable, more aggressive and invasive procedures should be undertaken only in a major tertiary care center with personnel who have expertise in this special situation. In the clinically very serious case, the overzealousness to establish a histologic diagnosis should be superseded by an empiric pretherapy debulking option using radiotherapy.[79]

DIAGNOSTIC WORK-UP

Lokich and Goodman[113] suggested that "the pitfalls in the management of SVCS relate to overzealous efforts

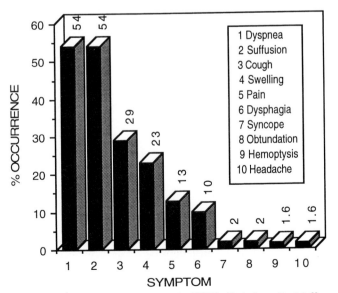

FIGURE 15–9. Common symptoms in SVCS. (Data from Parish,[22] Chen,[25] Yellin,[26] and Armstrong.[28])

to establish the site of obstruction and to determine a specific histopathologic diagnosis." This statement reflected three assumptions:

1. That diagnostic studies, particularly invasive ones, are associated with undue risk of life-threatening complications, such as respiratory obstruction, aspiration, and hemorrhage.

2. That SVCS is a medical emergency, and extensive diagnostic work-up may imply a delay in emergency therapy, leading to a poorer outcome.

3. That the most common causes of SVCS are malignant neoplasms, predominantly those expected to respond rapidly and dramatically to a course of radiotherapy, and therefore the exact histopathologic definition is moot in most cases.

This traditional view has recently been challenged on several grounds.[13, 21, 26, 30] Ahmann[30] challenged these concepts and emphasized the need for a thorough but expeditious diagnostic work-up based on the following conclusions:

1. That diagnostic studies, even invasive ones, are not associated with undue morbidity. In an analysis of 843 diagnostic procedures, including 217 bronchoscopies, 197 contrast venographic studies, 120 lymph node biopsies, 119 thoracotomies, 96 nuclear venographies, 53 mediastinoscopies, and 41 other miscellaneous studies, he found only 10 reported complications (1.2%), suggesting that in most patients with SVCS, even invasive procedures can be performed relatively safely.

2. That SVCS may be an acute condition in some patients, but it is hardly ever a medical emergency, and there is almost always time to pursue a definitive diagnosis.

3. That the spectrum of etiologic factors that can lead to SVCS is so varied that a policy of instituting emergency radiotherapy without a diagnosis may result in some patients with benign diseases receiving unnecessary radiation and some malignant tumors such as SCLC could potentially be better treated by other approaches such as chemotherapy.

A large variety of diagnostic tests are available for the assessment of SVCS, and the actual work-up has to be individualized to the particular clinical situation. Chen and colleagues[25] proposed an algorithm for evaluation of SVCS, starting with a chest CT and working up toward more invasive procedures (Fig. 15–11). Minimally invasive studies such as CT, magnetic resonance imaging (MRI), ultrasound, scintigraphy, and venography are helpful in determining the location and extent of obstruction, whereas more invasive tests such as sputum cytology, bronchial washings/biopsy, thoracentesis, pleural biopsy, thoracoscopy, CT-guided needle biopsy, lymph node biopsy, and mediastinoscopy assist in establishing a histologic diagnosis, a process that should be required in most cases of SVCS.

Chest Radiograph

A chest radiograph often is one of the earliest studies obtained, and although it is not diagnostic of SVCS, it

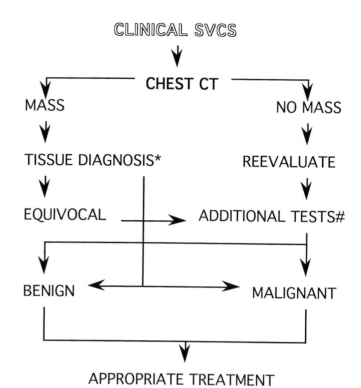

FIGURE 15–11. Chen's algorithm for diagnostic work-up of SVCS. *Includes sputum cytology, thoracentesis, needle aspirate, bronchoscopy. #Includes superior venacavography, mediastinoscopy, thoracotomy. (Modified from Chen JC, Bongard F, Klein SK: A contemporary perspective on superior vena cava syndrome. Am J Surg 160:207–211, 1990.)

often establishes the presence of a mediastinal mass as noted by a widened mediastinum. Approximately four of five patients are reported to have significant findings on chest radiography.[22] Right-sided lesions typically outnumber those on the left by a ratio of more than 4:1.[12] The presence of a so-called aortic nipple, i.e., a dilated left superior intercostal vein that produces a shadow overlying the aorta, has been reported to be predictive of SVCS.[118] Other findings include pleural effusion, hilar mass, pulmonary infiltrates, cardiomegaly, and enlarged or calcified nodes, or both[22, 28] (Fig. 15–12).

Computed Chest Tomography

Chest CT probably is one of the most frequently used imaging techniques for SVCS. Chen and associates[25] reported a diagnostic accuracy of 100% for chest CT. CT is particularly useful in evaluating extrinsic compression and may also provide some detail regarding collateral circulation. Schwartz and coworkers[119] used CT with contrast in 18 patients with SVCS and found only one false negative. Engel and associates[120] stated that a CT diagnosis of SVCS may be made based on the presence of both the so-called direct sign, i.e., nonopacification of central venous structures such as the SVC or brachiocephalic vein, and the indirect sign, i.e., opacification of collateral venous channels. In an analysis of 36 patients with SVCS, Trigaux and Van Beers[121] reported that opacification of the subcuta-

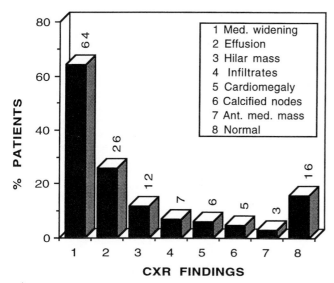

FIGURE 15–12. Chest x-ray findings in patients with SVCS. (From Parish JM, Marschke RF Jr, Dines DE, Lee RE: Etiologic conditions in superior vena cava syndrome. Mayo Clin Proc 56:407–413, 1981.)

neous anterior channel was highly diagnostic and specific (96%) for SVCS. CT also may be able to predict the subsequent evolution of the syndrome in asymptomatic patients.[122] Moncada and coworkers[123] suggested that the addition of CT phlebography to standard CT provides accurate delineation of the location and extent of SVC obstruction. In addition, this procedure may allow for better definition of radiotherapy portals, permit accurate localization for biopsy, and document collateral circulation. The main limitation of CT is the necessity for intravenous contrast with the possibility of attendant contrast reactions, which can theoretically be of major consequence in a patient with compromised cardiorespiratory status, and the possibility of adverse effects on renal function.

Magnetic Resonance Imaging

MRI provides multiplanar anatomic detail that allows for easy visualization of the extrinsic mass in transverse, sagittal, and coronal planes. Coronal MRI offers the earliest indication of an impending obstruction because it is exquisitely sensitive in detecting the aortic nipple.[124] The fact that flowing blood generates a signal void and therefore appears black on T1-weighted images provides a natural contrast to examine vascular structures such as the SVC. However, MRI has several disadvantages, including cost; lack of availability in some locations; lack of adequate pulmonary visualization; inability to resolve calcific patterns; significantly greater artifacts from clips, respiratory, and cardiac motion; and the lack of general availability of MRI-compatible equipment that often accompanies a patient with SVCS to an imaging unit.[125] In a comparison of three cross-sectional imaging modalities—CT, MRI, and ultrasound—Khimji and Zeiss[126] suggested that MRI has potential and ap-

parent advantages in the evaluation of a patient with SVC.

Sonography

Sonographic techniques for the evaluation of SVCS, although not frequently used, have been described, and in the pregnant patient they may represent a useful alternative to other potentially more hazardous approaches. The normal subclavian vein shows rhythmic motion with respiration, collapsing with inspiration. In SVCS, this transient collapse is not evident.[127] A recently described sonographic technique, transesophageal echocardiography (TEE), is a safe bedside procedure that is excellent for evaluating the SVC and its surrounding structures, particularly in the acutely ill patient.[128] TEE allows visualization of the SVC at several levels up to the right atrium, thereby permitting evaluation of the location of the obstruction, and therefore is far more accurate than transthoracic echocardiography. In three patients described by Ayala and associates,[128] transthoracic echocardiography failed to visualize the SVC adequately, but TEE was able to provide accurate diagnostic information.

Single-Photon Emission Tomography

With advances in single-photon emission tomography (SPECT) technology and the use of high doses of the radionuclide gallium-67, there has been a recent resurgence of interest in using gallium-67 SPECT in the evaluation of intrathoracic malignancies. Compared with planar images, SPECT provides increased contrast resolution and three-dimensional localization. In addition, current technology permits the creation of composite SPECT-CT images, which are particularly useful for establishing the physiologic status of ambiguous CT objects and for identifying pathologic areas not clearly delineated by CT. Swayne and Kaplan[129] have summarized the role of gallium-67 SPECT in the evaluation of SVCS and have described an unusual case of poorly differentiated adenocarcinoma causing SVCS that was not detected by CT because of its intravascular location but was identified by gallium-67 SPECT-CT image correlation.

Venography

Contrast venography (phlebography, angiocardiography) was applied in the evaluation of SVCS as early as the 1940s[130] and allowed the first true assessment of the site and nature of the obstruction as well as the pattern of collateral development. When combined with pressure measurements, it permits additional physiologic assessment and has been described as affording "unequaled precision for localization of venous obstruction in bronchogenic carcinoma and for determining the extent and efficiency of the collateral circulation."[12] In more recent studies, Dyet and Moghisi[131] and Stanford et al[5] demonstrated that venography is capable of providing accurate information regarding vessel patency and the level of obstruction, and the latter information is particularly useful if surgery is being contemplated. These studies have clearly documented that obstruction of the SVC at the junction of the azygos is the most common presentation, occurring 72% of the time. Lokich and Goodman[113] suggested that venography should be avoided because interruption of the integrity of the vessel wall in the face of considerably elevated vascular pressure could result in excessive hemorrhage. In the Mayo Clinic study,[22] superior venacavography was not found to be a useful procedure in making the diagnosis, and the authors reported that elevated venous pressures of 200 mm Hg made the procedure hazardous because of the difficulty in stopping bleeding. However, in the literature review of Ahmann,[30] the author was able to document, of 197 patients, only one case (0.5%) of relatively minor and transient toxicity resulting from contrast venography, thus challenging the notion that venography is an excessively morbid procedure in the setting of SVCS. From a practical standpoint, venography may find application in only a small number of patients, i.e., those being considered for surgery[131] and those patients in whom there is lack of an adequate response from radiotherapy, suggesting the possibility of obstruction extending beyond the treatment fields.[13]

Radionuclide Venography

Radionuclide venography (RNV), also referred to as scintigraphy, is a minimally invasive alternative to contrast venography and is performed using technetium-99m. Although this technique provides information analogous to venography,[6, 7] it does not allow adequate assessment of vessel caliber and potential graft sites—information that is crucial if surgery is contemplated. In view of this, scintigraphy cannot be considered a routine diagnostic study for the evaluation of SVCS. In an analysis of 220 RNV studies of the upper extremity in patients with indwelling central venous catheters, Podoloff and Kim[132] found obstruction in 123 patients, 26 of whom also underwent contrast venography. Significant agreement was noted in 19 cases (73%), but there were seven false-positive cases (27%) with RNV. Further analysis of these cases revealed that if the RNV diagnosis is based solely on the slow-flow pattern, there is a high likelihood of false positivity. In a report on 20 patients with SVCS secondary to lung cancer, Maxfield and Meckstroth[133] reported that RNV provided prognostic information for radiotherapy. The safety of RNV has been documented by the complete lack of morbid events in 96 studies documented by Ahmann.[30]

Establishing a Histologic Diagnosis

Once considered almost dangerous,[113] modern studies[13, 21–26, 30] all call for a thorough effort at establishing a tissue diagnosis. Commonly used procedures include bronchoscopy, lymph node biopsy, sputum cytology, thoracotomy, mediastinoscopy, bone marrow

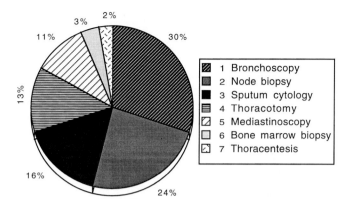

FIGURE 15–13. Commonly employed diagnostic procedures in SVCS. (Data from Schraufnagel,[21] Armstrong,[28] and Painter.[134])

biopsy, and thoracentesis. Figure 15–13 is a summary of the more commonly used procedures. Bronchoscopy is the most frequently used procedure and is positive approximately 50% of the time. Sputum cytology is also useful in 50% of cases, particularly with SCLC. Thoracotomy as a procedure has the highest diagnostic yield (98%),[134] followed by mediastinoscopy (77%) and thoracentesis (73%). Other procedures have lower yields, as illustrated in Figure 15–14. Painter and Karpf[134] reported complications in five of nine patients (56%) when performing mediastinoscopy. In a more recent report, Callejas et al[135] attempted diagnostic mediastinoscopy on eight patients with SVCS and reported two complications (25%). These complication rates are higher than expected, and in the series of 53 mediastinoscopies compiled by Ahmann,[30] the morbidity rate was much lower (three of 53, or 6%). Although the exact reasons for these highly variable morbidity rates are unclear, it is possible that the

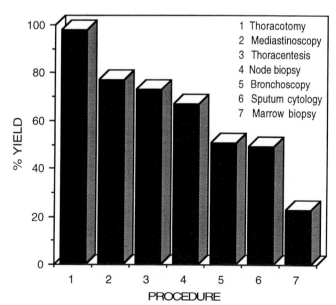

FIGURE 15–14. The diagnostic yield of various procedures in the evaluation of patients with SVCS. (Data from Schraufnagel,[21] Armstrong,[28] and Painter.[134])

lower rates may be a reflection of under-reporting or selection bias.

More recently, CT-guided needle biopsy, ultrasound-guided needle aspiration biopsy,[136] percutaneous atherectomy,[137] and thoracoscopic biopsy have also been used. To a lesser extent, significantly elevated serum human chorionic gonadotropin-beta subunit and/or alpha-fetoprotein may constitute sufficient evidence for germ cell histology if a definitive tissue diagnosis is not feasible.

THERAPEUTIC CONSIDERATIONS

Goals of Therapy

The major therapeutic goals in the management of SVCS include palliation of symptoms in the noncurable situation, aggressive management of potentially curable malignancies with both palliation and possible cure as major objectives, cure of SVCS when the underlying etiology is nonmalignant, and minimal treatment-related morbidity in all patients. Because approximately 80% of SVCS is caused by lung cancer, lymphoma, thymic tumors, germ cell neoplasms, and metastases, the most commonly used therapeutic options include radiation and chemotherapy either alone or in combination. However, other measures, such as surgical reconstruction, vascular stents, angioplasty, thrombolytic therapy, anticoagulation, steroids, diuretics, and other medical and supportive measures, have been used in the management of SVCS. In all instances in which an underlying neoplasm is suspected, therapy directed at the neoplasm as soon as possible is likely to achieve reversal of the symptoms.

Radiation Therapy

Radiotherapy probably is the most frequently used definitive therapeutic modality in the management of SVCS. In a composite of analysis of 381 patients with SVCS reported in four different studies[21, 22, 26, 28] (Fig. 15–15), radiotherapy was found to be the most frequently used therapeutic modality. As stand-alone therapy, it was used in 53% of cases, and overall, it was used in 68% of patients. The reason for the frequent application of radiation therapy is its efficacy in managing bronchogenic carcinoma, both small and non–small cell; non-Hodgkin's lymphoma; germ cell tumors; thymic malignancies; and metastatic tumors. It also is relatively easy to apply, even in very sick patients.

There are three major issues that need to be addressed in the radiotherapeutic management of SVCS: fractionation schema, total dose, and field size. Because of the paucity of well-controlled, prospective, randomized trials, these issues often are a matter of institutional practice.

Fractionation

Whether the initial fractions of radiation should be large or not is a matter of considerable debate. Oppo-

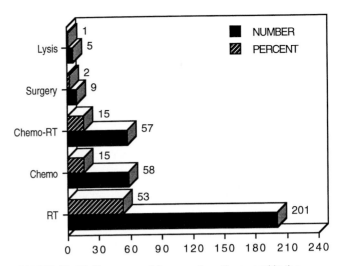

FIGURE 15–15. Frequency of therapeutic options used in the treatment of SVCS. RT = Radiotherapy; Chemo = chemotherapy; Chemo-RT = combined chemotherapy and radiotherapy; lysis = thrombolytic therapy. (Data from Schraufnagel,[21] Parish,[22] Yellin,[26] and Armstrong.[28])

nents of this concept have suggested the lack of any prospective, randomized trials supporting the use of large fractions, the possibility of enhanced late tissue toxicity, the theoretical possibility of radiation-induced edema that could cause clinical deterioration, and the fact that most tumors in this location are relatively sensitive even to conventional fraction sizes of 1.8 to 2.0 Gy.

Proponents of large fraction radiation during the early phase have recommended using approximately three fractions of 3 to 4 Gy, each followed by conventional fractions, to a total dose of 30 to 60 Gy.[28, 42, 113] In a series of animal experiments and clinical trials, Rubin and associates[43, 138] suggested that the use of initial large fraction radiation is most efficacious in SVCS. In a few small studies in which large versus small fractions have been evaluated, large fraction radiation appeared to produce faster relief. For example, Armstrong and colleagues[28] reported that improvement occurred in less than 2 wk in 70% of patients who received initial high-dose fractions compared with 56% of patients who received conventional radiation, although this difference was not statistically significant. Fisherman and Bradfield[139] and Scarantino and associates[43] both reported on nonrandomized groups of patients treated with conventional versus high-dose fractions and suggested that there was faster symptomatic resolution in the latter group.

Dose

The total dose is a function of the tumor type and the underlying host characteristics. A prospective, randomized, dose-seeking trial has not been performed, but Armstrong and coworkers[28] reported on their institutional experience using varying dose levels to treat non–SCLC causing SVCS. A dose of less than 20 Gy resulted in a 50% response rate, whereas higher doses produced response rates of 86%, 93%, and 100%

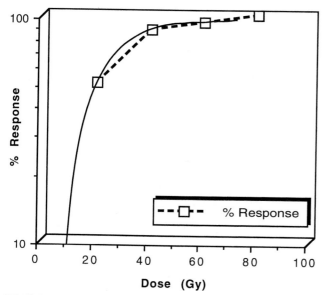

FIGURE 15–16. Dose-response relationship. The data points are extracted from Armstrong,[28] and a third order polynomial is fitted.

at dose levels up to 40, 60, and more than 60 Gy, respectively. When these data are plotted on a semilog graph, as in Figure 15–16, and a polynomial curve is fitted, there is a strong suggestion for a dose-response relationship mimicking the classic sigmoid radiation-response curves. It appears that there is a very steep dose-response curve from 20 to 40 Gy and a plateauing effect thereafter. Based on such retrospective data, a minimum dose of 40 Gy would be considered necessary for SVCS caused by non–SCLC.

The actual total dose for non–SCLC treated definitively with conventional fractionation is 60 Gy,[140] although recent data suggest that superior results may be achieved with hyperfractionated[141] or even accelerated[142] regimens. Patients with limited-stage SCLC also very clearly benefit when thoracic radiation is incorporated into the chemotherapeutic regimen,[143] and some recent studies suggest that upfront rather than delayed[144] and possibly hyperfractionated radiation[145] may be beneficial. In this instance, the total dose is usually 45 Gy, administered as 1.5 Gy twice daily. For the treatment of lymphoma, the addition of thoracic radiation provides a more durable response than chemotherapy only.[50]

Field Size

The third crucial issue in radiotherapy for SVCS is field shaping. Obviously, every effort needs to be made to encompass the full extent of the tumor in every case. Attention also needs to be directed to regional lymph nodes in specific situations. More important, cases of radiation failure have been described where the reason for failure is a thrombus extending beyond the radiation portal, and when this is included in the field, prompt response is achieved.[13]

Chemotherapy

Some of the earliest clinical experience with chemotherapy was with combined-modality therapy using

radiation and nitrogen mustard in patients with non–SCLC and SVCS.[12] Armstrong and coworkers[28] reported that in patients with non–SCLC and SVCS, the addition of chemotherapy does not produce a survival advantage. Since that time, the focus of chemotherapy in the treatment of SVCS has shifted primarily to SCLC and lymphoma. These malignancies are generally systemic and chemosensitive. With the use of chemotherapy only for SVCS caused by SCLC, Urban and associates[49] described a response rate of 81% in 87 patients. In a smaller series of 22 patients with SCLC causing SVCS, Dombernowsky and Hansen[48] reported symptomatic resolution in all patients with a median response time of 7 days. In a nonrandomized series of 56 patients with SVCS resulting from SCLC, Maddox and colleagues[146] noted reversal of SVCS in 64% with radiation, 83% with combined therapy, and 100% with chemotherapy. Figure 15–17 illustrates the high resolution rates of SVCS from SCLC achieved with chemotherapy only in four separate series. Although a higher incidence of brain metastases has been reported in association with SVCS in SCLC,[49] SVCS per se is not an adverse prognostic factor. In view of a recent meta-analysis[143] demonstrating a survival advantage with the addition of thoracic radiation, it should be strongly considered in this group of patients provided they have limited-stage disease. Also, in view of the recent NCI-Canada study[144] as well as previous studies by Turrisi and Glover,[145] thoracic radiation should be considered earlier rather than later. To expedite such an approach, a platinum-based chemotherapy approach rather than an adriamycin-based approach is recommended.

Chemotherapy has also been advocated in SVCS caused by non-Hodgkin's lymphoma.[50] In the study from M. D. Anderson Hospital, 28 patients were treated with radiation, chemotherapy, or a combination. All patients achieved an excellent response within 2 wk of therapy, but no survival advantage was apparent for any modality. In the study from

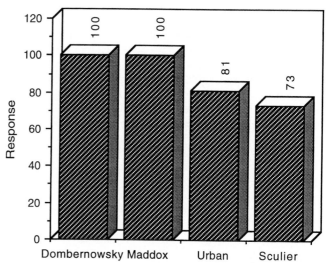

FIGURE 15–17. SVCS reversal rates in small cell lung cancer with chemotherapy. (From Dombernowsky,[48] Maddox,[146] Urban,[49] and Sculier.[47])

Washington University Mallinckrodt Institute,[28] 11 patients with lymphoma were treated with radiation only, and six were treated with chemoradiotherapy. Actuarial survival at 5 yr was 41%, and no difference by therapy was apparent.

Anticoagulation

Because more than half of the patients with SVCS actually have a thrombotic occlusion as part of their syndrome, it is appealing to consider the use of anticoagulants in these patients. They have often been used in conjunction with other measures for the treatment of SVCS, but proper documentation of their effectiveness in a controlled fashion is not forthcoming. It is in fact quite possible that anticoagulation may interfere with invasive diagnostic testing and therefore cannot be routinely recommended. Adelstein and colleagues[147] documented an increased risk of thromboembolic events after initiation of chemotherapy and therefore recommend beginning anticoagulation together with cytostatic agents. Urban and coworkers[49] proposed that a possible explanation of a lack of survival disadvantage in his group of 87 patients with SCLC and SVCS (who also had a higher incidence of brain metastases) compared with the larger group of patients with SCLC and no SVCS is the use of anticoagulation in the former group. This explanation is based on data, including a randomized trial,[148] suggesting that both heparin[149] and warfarin improve the outcome in SCLC.

Pacemaker-induced SVCS is a rare condition[102] that has been managed by anticoagulation. Thrombosis as well as fibrotic occlusion and infectious vegetations can cause SVC occlusion from any indwelling system. Of the approximately 30 cases reported, only one was not anticoagulated, and this patient died of pulmonary emboli. Of the 19 patients who were treated initially with anticoagulation, 14 (74%) improved clinically but did not develop recanalization. Whether this represents successful therapy from anticoagulation or simply the development of compensatory collaterals is unclear. Parenthetically, if thrombolytic therapy is not contemplated, indwelling systems that cause SVCS should, in general, be removed, particularly if any infection is suspected. Catheter removal should be accompanied by anticoagulation to avoid embolization.

Thrombolytic Therapy

Gray and colleagues[150] summarized the literature pertaining to thrombolytic therapy of SVCS. In their series of 16 patients, they were able to achieve complete clot lysis in nine (56%). Eleven of these patients had a central venous line that was present in the face of thrombotic SVCS, and of this group, eight (73%) recanalized. They concluded that urokinase is probably superior to streptokinase and that a short duration of symptoms (less than 5 days) is predictive of a good response. In all patients in whom the lysis was successful, catheter function was preserved and there

was no need to remove these devices. Recombinant tissue-type plasminogen activator has also recently been reported[151] as being useful in catheter-associated thrombotic SVCS.

Angioplasty

Percutaneous transluminal angioplasty has recently been used in a small number of patients with pacemaker-related thrombotic or fibrotic occlusion.[102, 103, 152] The technique appears to be promising and may either delay or avoid the need for reconstructive surgery in some patients.

Intravascular Stents

Advances in percutaneous interventional vascular techniques have allowed the development of intravascular stents, which are beginning to find application in the management of both benign and malignant SVCS. In a series of six patients with malignant SVCS, Solomon and associates[153] were able to achieve complete resolution in five. Rosch and colleagues[154] described complete symptom relief in 22 of 22 patients using the Gianturco-Rosch self-expandable Z-stents. Twenty of 22 patients had a malignant etiology for their SVCS, with advanced symptomatology, and 13 of these patients had received radiation therapy. Additional successful cases have been reported by Irving and coworkers[155] (16 of 17 successful in recurrent malignant SVCS) and Oudkerk and associates[156] (19 of 22 successful in recurrent malignant SVCS). Therefore, with a cumulative success rate of approximately 92%, intravascular stents are a promising new modality for patients with recurrent or progressive cancer. In addition, these intravascular techniques can also be combined with endovascular thrombectomy.[157]

Surgical Reconstruction

Because of the relatively short life expectancy of many patients with malignant SVCS, surgical reconstruction and bypass techniques have primarily been reserved for patients with nonmalignant SVCS. However, with improvements in the management of malignant SVCS, more patients are becoming longer-term survivors, and a cohort of patients with recurrent SVCS is emerging. A number of surgical interventions have been described for this group of patients. Such methods can be categorized as either autografts (most often, the saphenous vein), venous homografts, or artificial grafts (e.g., Gore-Tex or Dacron).

Venous autografts produce the best results but are not always feasible because of the lack of availability of adequate lengths of spare vein. Commonly used veins include the saphenous, left innominate, internal jugular, femoral, azygos, and umbilical. Other autologous alternatives include the use of a pedicle created from the right atrium or the pericardium. Venous homografts, although more readily available, have a late patency rate of only 10% to 37%. Their inherent antigenicity elicits an inflammatory reaction characterized by intimal thickening and perivascular fibrosis. Synthetic grafts do not have an antigenicity problem but are susceptible to intraluminal thrombosis because of their surface properties. In humans, the patency rate of polytetrafluoroethylene (Gore-Tex) grafts is 62%.[54]

Chiou and associates[54] described the successful use of such grafts in the management of patients with malignant thymoma with venous invasion. Such tumors would previously have been considered inoperable. The technique has also been successfully used in children.[158] Using spiral vein grafts constructed from the saphenous vein, Doty and colleagues[159] demonstrated long-term patency in seven of nine grafts for as long as 15 years when used in a patient without a malignancy. Piccione et al[160] were able to achieve patency in six of six patients with malignant SVCS using autologous pericardial graft. Larsson and Lepore[161] and Gloviczki and coworkers,[162] in two independent reports, have described the use of various graft techniques in a total of 28 patients, 12 with underlying malignancy. Therefore, surgical reconstruction remains a viable option in patients with an underlying benign etiology and may even prove beneficial in selected patients with malignancies.

Medical Management

Nonspecific medical measures that are likely to provide comfort and stabilize the patient include bed rest with elevation of the head and oxygen, both of which reduce venous pressure and cardiac output. Diuretics with salt restriction have been empirically used to reduce edema but could lead to dehydration and thrombosis. Steroids have been routinely used by some to "block the inflammatory reaction resulting from radiotherapy," but in an experimental model, Green and associates[163] debunked this fallacy, and the use of steroids must be considered of unproven benefit except in patients with concomitant brain metastases or laryngeal edema.

OUTCOME

Symptomatic Relief

Although it is expected that almost all patients with SVCS resulting from nonmalignant causes will achieve symptomatic relief with appropriate therapy, only 50% to 70% of patients with underlying malignancy achieve such relief. In an analysis of 367 such patients in five series[21, 22, 25, 26, 28] (Table 15–7), clinical response was noted in 248 patients (68%). Of 166 patients treated with radiation only, the response rate was 69%, whereas in the 45 patients treated with chemotherapy only, the response rate was 84%. In general, response is achieved within 2 wk but may be a function of the initial radiation fraction size as reported by Armstrong and coworkers.[28] When larger fraction size is used, 70% respond within 2 wk compared with 56% when the fraction size is smaller.

TABLE 15–7. Response Rates for Malignant Superior Vena Cava Syndrome

THERAPY	SERIES	NO. OF PATIENTS	%
Overall relief rate	Schraufnagel et al[21]	248/367	68
Radiation	Parish et al[22]	115/166	69
Chemotherapy	Chen et al[25]	38/45	84
Chemoradiotherapy	Yellin et al[26]	25/36	69
Surgery	Armstrong et al[28]	8/11	73

Venographic Response

In an effort to document the objective venographic response to therapy, Ahmann[30] evaluated the literature for serial venographic as well as autopsy evidence of recanalization. Of 35 cases with serial venograms, clinical response was noted in 30 (86%). Although 19 patients (54%) were noted to have improved flow on follow-up venograms, 16 (46%) demonstrated no response. Similarly, in 99 cases with autopsy results, persistent obstruction was noted in 75 (76%). The discordance between verifiable restoration of flow dynamics and clinical response can probably be explained by the development of collateral circulation.

Survival

The survival of a patient with SVCS is in large measure dependent on the underlying condition. The presence of SVCS itself does not specifically impact survival in most instances. In a review of five series,[21, 22, 25, 26, 28] the mean survival for patients with malignancy ranged from 12 to 40.2 wk. In the series of Armstrong and colleagues,[28] the median survival of all patients was 22 wk. A significant effect of histology was noted, with the 5-yr survival rate dropping from 41% for lymphoma to 5% for SCLC to 2% for non–SCLC. Figure 15–18 is a composite plot of survival information

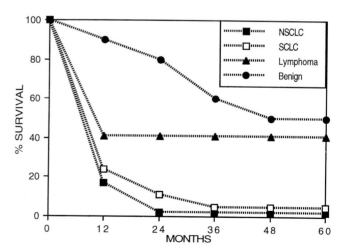

FIGURE 15–18. Survival of patients with SVCS. (Data from Armstrong[28] and Cancer Consult: Review of the Current Concepts in the Management of Superior Vena Cava Syndrome, 1990.)

for various causes of SVCS compiled from the literature.

SUMMARY

The SVCS refers to a combination of clinical and radiographic findings resulting from compromised blood flow through the SVC, a clinical situation that is frequently seen in association with a variety of thoracic neoplasms. This compromise of vascular flow can result from extrinsic compression, intraluminal thrombosis, direct invasion, or infiltration of the vessel wall. When initially described in the eighteenth century, syphilitic aneurysms accounted for most cases of this syndrome, but almost 90% of the cases are now accounted for by an underlying malignancy, the most common being lung cancer, followed by lymphoma, metastases, germ cell tumors, and thymic neoplasms.

Because of the dramatic clinical presentation, the syndrome was previously thought of as a medical emergency and emergency radiotherapeutic management was considered standard. Recent data suggest that sudden death from SVC obstruction is extremely rare, and there are no reasonable grounds to suggest that unrelieved compression of the SVC is fatal in and of itself. The modern approach to this syndrome therefore centers around obtaining an adequate radiographic and tissue diagnosis. The major therapeutic goals include palliation of symptoms in the noncurable situation, aggressive management of potentially curable malignancies with both palliation and possible cure as major objectives, cure of the syndrome when the underlying etiology is nonmalignant, and minimization of treatment-related morbidity in all patients. Radiotherapy remains the most frequently used definitive therapeutic modality, being used in more than one-half to two-thirds of all cases. Based on retrospective data, it appears that a minimum dose of 40 Gy is necessary to alleviate symptoms. Other therapeutic modalities that have been used in the management of the syndrome and are finding increasing application include chemotherapy, particularly for SCLC and lymphoma; anticoagulation; thrombolytic therapy; angioplasty; intravascular stents; and surgical reconstruction. In addition to these approaches, nonspecific medical measures to provide comfort and stabilize the patient are frequently used.

With adequate management, approximately two-thirds of the patients can be palliated. The survival is a function of the underlying etiology, and for the vast majority of whose obstruction is a consequence of an underlying malignancy, the mean survival ranges from 12 to 40 wk. The overall survival outlook for SVCS therefore continues to remain very poor.

SELECTED REFERENCES

1. Lokich JJ, Goodman R: Superior vena cava syndrome: Clinical management. JAMA 231:58–61, 1975.
   This reference has considerable historical interest in that it contributed in large measure to the widespread misconception that SVCS is a dire medical emergency where the primary aim is immediate radiotherapeutic intervention in the absence of a serious attempt at making a diagnosis. In this regard, this article has shaped past medical practice in several centers and continues to exert a significant influence on practice patterns.
2. Carlson HA: Obstruction of the superior vena: An experimental study. Arch Surg 29:669–677, 1934.
   If you can retrieve this article from your local library, a copy should go into your "classic papers" folder. In a truly elegant series of experiments, Carlson uncovered the major physiologic concepts that underlie this syndrome and provides an elegant anatomic understanding of collateral circulation. The significance of time in allowing the development of collaterals, a concept crucial to the understanding of SVCS, is explained.
3. Armstrong BA, Perez CA, Simpson JR, et al: Role of irradiation in the management of superior vena cava syndrome. Int J Radiat Oncol Biol Phys 13:531–539, 1987.
   This article, which was written by a medical student, may be the most comprehensive clinical single institution review of SVCS. The records of 125 cases of SVCS were culled. The etiologic factors, clinical characteristics, response patterns, and role of initial large fraction radiation in attaining rapid response are well described. The influence of histology on outcome is clarified.
4. Ahmann FR: A reassessment of the clinical implications of the superior vena caval syndrome. J Clin Oncol 2:961–969, 1984.
   This review article is the most comprehensive, combining data from more than 90 publications and 1986 patients. Four major conclusions are arrived at: (1) unrelieved SVCS is not life threatening; (2) diagnostic procedures, even invasive ones, can safely be performed in SVCS; (3) successful palliation does not always require re-establishment of SVC patency; and (4) SCLC is the most common cause of SVCS. This article has in large measure attempted to challenge and reverse the concepts proffered by Lokich and Goodman.
5. Ingram L, Rivera GK, Shapiro DN: Superior vena cava syndrome associated with childhood malignancy: Analysis of 24 cases. Med Pediatr Oncol 18:476–481, 1990.
   This is a comprehensive, single-institution review of pediatric SVCS, suggesting that in children, SVCS often results in an acute clinical presentation, requiring urgent intervention. The occurrence of the superior mediastinal syndrome in which airway compromise frequently accompanies SVCS and may lead to significant anesthetic risk is noted. Hematologic malignancies dominate as the causative factor.

REFERENCES

1. Warwick R, Williams PL: Angiology. In Warwick R, Williams PL (eds): Gray's Anatomy. 35th Ed. Edinburgh, Longman, 1973, pp 700–704.
2. Carlson HA: Obstruction of the superior vena: An experimental study. Arch Surg 29:669–677, 1934.
3. McIntire TT, Sykes EM: Obstruction of the superior vena cava: A review of the literature and report of two personal cases. Ann Intern Med 30:925–960, 1948.
4. Klassen KP, Andrews NC, Curtis GM: Diagnosis and treatment of superior vena caval obstruction. AMA Arch Surg 63:311–326, 1951.
5. Stanford W, Jolles H, Ell S, et al: Superior vena cava obstruction: A venographic classification. Am J Roentgenol 148:62–69, 1987.
6. Maxfield WS, Meckstroth GR: Technetium-99m superior vena cavography. Radiology 92:913–917, 1969.
7. Muramatsu T, Miyamae T, Dohi Y: Collateral pathways observed by radionuclide superior cavography in 70 patients with superior vena caval obstruction. Clin Nucl Med 16:332–336, 1991.
8. Gale B, Chen C, Chun KJ, et al: Systemic to pulmonary venous shunting in superior vena cava obstruction: Unusual myocardial and thyroid visualization. Clin Nucl Med 15:246–250, 1990.
9. Taki J, Bunko H, Tonami N, et al: Shunt between right subcla-

vian vein and the left heart in superior vena cava obstruction due to lung cancer. Clin Nucl Med 15:251–253, 1990.

10. Suneja SK, Teal JS: Discrepant sulfur colloid and radioparticle liver uptake in superior vena cava obstruction: Case report. J Nucl Med 30:113–116, 1989.

11. Zellers TM, Hagler DJ, Julsrud PR: Accuracy of two-dimensional echocardiography in diagnosing left superior vena cava. J Am Soc Echo 2:132–138, 1989.

12. Roswitt B, Kaplan G, Jacobson HG: The superior vena cava obstruction syndrome in bronchogenic carcinoma. Radiology 61:722–737, 1953.

13. Kumar PP, Good RR: Need for invasive diagnostic procedures in the management of superior vena cava syndrome. J Natl Med Assoc 81:41–47, 1989.

14. Hunter W: The history of an aneurysm of the aorta with some remarks on aneurysms in general. Med Observ Inq 1:323–357, 1757.

15. Schechter MM: The superior vena cava syndrome. Am J Med Sci 227:46–56, 1954.

16. Boring CC, Squires TS, Tong T: Cancer statistics, 1993. CA Cancer J Clin 43:7–26, 1993.

17. Effler DB, Groves LK: Superior vena caval obstruction. J Thorac Cardiovasc Surg 43:574–584, 1962.

18. Banker VP, Maddison FE: Superior vena cava syndrome secondary to aortic disease: Report of two cases and review of the literature. Dis Chest 51:656–662, 1967.

19. Kamiya K, Nakata Y, Naiki K, et al: Superior vena cava syndrome. J Vasc Dis 4:59–65, 1967.

20. Lochridge SK, Knibble WP, Doty DB: Obstruction of the superior vena cava. Surgery 85:14–24, 1979.

21. Schraufnagel DE, Hill R, Leech JA, et al: Superior vena caval obstruction: Is it a medical emergency? Am J Med 70:1169–1174, 1981.

22. Parish JM, Marschke RF, Dines DE, et al: Etiologic considerations in superior vena cava syndrome. Mayo Clin Proc 36:407–413, 1981.

23. Bell DR, Woods RL, Levi JA: Superior vena caval obstruction: A 10-year experience. Med J Aust 145:566–568, 1986.

24. Fincher RE: Superior vena cava syndrome: Experience in a teaching hospital. South Med J 80:1243–1245, 1987.

25. Chen JC, Bongard F, Klein SR: A contemporary perspective on superior vena cava syndrome. Am J Surg 160:207–211, 1990.

26. Yellin A, Rosen A, Reichert N, et al: Superior vena cava syndrome: The myth—the facts. Am Rev Resp Dis 141:1114–1118, 1990.

27. Nieto AF, Doty DB: Superior vena cava obstruction, clinical syndrome, etiology, and treatment. Curr Probl Cancer 10:442–484, 1986.

28. Armstrong BA, Perez CA, Simpson JR, et al: Role of irradiation in the management of superior vena cava syndrome. Int J Radiat Oncol Biol Phys 13:531–539, 1987.

29. Salsali M, Cliffton EE: Superior vena caval obstruction in carcinoma of the lung. NY State J Med 69:2875–2880, 1969.

30. Ahmann FR: A reassessment of the clinical implications of the superior vena caval syndrome. J Clin Oncol 2:961–969, 1984.

31. Rosenbloom SE: Superior vena obstruction in primary cancer of the lung. Ann Intern Med 31:470–478, 1949.

32. Szur L, Bromley LL II: Obstruction of the superior vena cava in carcinoma of bronchus. Br Med J 2:1273–1276, 1956.

33. Geller W: The mandate for chemotherapeutic decompression in superior vena caval obstruction. Radiology 81:385–387, 1963.

34. Skinner DB, Salzman EV, Scannell JG: The challenge of superior vena caval obstruction. J Thorac Cardiovasc Surg 49:824–833, 1965.

35. Salsali M, Cliffton EE: Superior vena caval obstruction with carcinoma of the lung. Surg Gynecol Obstet 121:783–788, 1965.

36. Urschel HC, Paulson DL: Superior vena caval obstruction. Dis Chest 49:155–165, 1966.

37. Salsali M, Cliffton EE: Superior vena caval obstruction with lung cancer. Ann Thorac Surg 6:437–442, 1968.

38. Ghosh BV, Cliffton EE: Malignant tumors with superior vena cava obstruction. NY State J Med 73:283–289, 1973.

39. Armstrong P, Hayes DF, Richardson PH: Transvenous biopsy of carcinoma of bronchus causing superior vena caval obstruction. Br Med J 1:662–663, 1975.

40. Kane RC, Cohen MH, Broder LE, et al: Superior vena caval obstruction due to small cell anaplastic lung carcinoma. JAMA 235:1717–1718, 1976.

41. Avasthi RB, Moghissi K: Malignant obstruction of the superior vena cava and its palliation: A report of four cases. J Thorac Cardiovasc Surg 74:244–248, 1977.

42. Davenport D, Ferree C, Blake D, et al: Treatment of malignant superior vena caval obstruction. Cancer 42:2600–2603, 1978.

43. Scarantino C, Salazar OM, Rubin P, et al: The optimum radiation schedule in treatment of superior vena caval obstruction: Importance of ^{99m}Tc scintiangiograms. Int J Radiat Oncol Biol Phys 5:1987–1995, 1979.

44. Shimm DS, Lugue GL, Tigsby LC: Evaluating the superior vena cava syndrome. JAMA 245:951–953, 1981.

45. Armstrong BA, Perez CA, Simpson JR, et al: Role of irradiation in the management of superior vena cava syndrome. Int J Radiat Oncol Biol Phys 13:531–539, 1987.

46. Johnson DH, Greco FA: Small cell lung cancer: Current perspectives. Am J Med Sci 293:377–389, 1987.

47. Sculier JP, Evans WK, Feld R, et al: Superior vena caval obstruction syndrome in small cell lung cancer. Cancer 57:847–851, 1986.

48. Dombernowsky P, Hansen HH: Combination chemotherapy in the management of superior vena caval obstruction in small cell anaplastic carcinoma of the lung. Acta Med Scand 204:513–516, 1978.

49. Urban T, Lebeau B, Chastang C, et al: Superior vena cava syndrome in small-cell lung cancer. Arch Intern Med 153:384–387, 1993.

50. Perez-Soler R, McLaughlin P, Velasquez WS, et al: Clinical features and results of management of superior vena cava syndrome secondary to lymphoma. J Clin Oncol 2:260–266, 1984.

51. Miller JB, Variakojis D, Bitran J, et al: Diffuse histiocytic lymphoma with sclerosis: A clinicopathologic entity frequently causing superior vena caval obstruction. Cancer 47:748–756, 1981.

52. Holbert BL, Libshitz HI: Superior vena caval syndrome in primary germ cell tumors. Can Assoc Radiol J 37:182–184, 1986.

53. Cohen DJ, Ronnigen LD, Graeber GM, et al: Management of patients with malignant thymoma. J Thor Cardiovasc Surg 87:301–307, 1984.

54. Chiou GT, Chen CL, Wei J, et al: Reconstruction of superior vena cava in invasive thymoma. Chest 97:502–503, 1990.

55. Large SR, Shneerson JM, Stovin PG, et al: Surgical pathology of thymomas: 20 Year experience. Thorax 41:51–54, 1986.

56. Fujio A, Kitano M, Asakura S, et al: Intracaval and intraatrial growth of thymoma: Report of a long surviving case. Nippon Kyobu Shikkan Gakkai Zasshi 23:934–939, 1985.

57. Airan B, Sharma R, Iyer KS, et al: Malignant thymoma presenting as intracardiac tumor and superior vena caval obstruction. Ann Thorac Surg 50:989–991, 1990.

58. Varma S, Varma N, Dhar S, et al: Cytodiagnosis of granulocytic sarcoma presenting as superior vena cava syndrome in acute myeloblastic leukemia: A case report. Acta Cytol 36:371–372, 1992.

59. de Mayolo JA, Sridhar KS, Kunhardt B, et al: Superior vena cava obstruction in a patient with chronic lymphocytic leukemia and lung cancer. Am J Clin Oncol 15:352–355, 1992.

60. Hwang MH, Brown A, Piao ZE, et al: Cardiac lymphoma associates with superior vena caval syndrome and cardiac tamponade: Case history. Angiology 41:328–332, 1990.

61. Bishop WT, Chan NH, MacDonald IL, et al: Malignant primary cardiac tumour presenting as superior vena cava obstruction syndrome. Can J Cardiol 6:259–261, 1990.

62. Davis SR, King HS, Le Roux J, et al: Superior vena cava syndrome caused by an intrathoracic plasmacytoma. Cancer 68:1376–1379, 1991.

63. Thomas S, Sawhney S, Kapur BM: Case report: Bilateral massive internal jugular vein thrombosis in carcinoma of the thyroid: CT evaluation. Clin Radiol 43:433–434, 1991.

64. Rutegard J, Granstrand M, Aberg T: Intracaval paraganglioma causing superior vena cava syndrome. Eur J Cardio-Thorac Surg 6:337–338, 1992.

65. Nishida H, Grooters RK, Coster D, et al: Metastatic right atrial

tumor in colon cancer with superior vena cava syndrome and tricuspid obstruction. Heart Vessels 6:125–127, 1991.

66. Korobkin M, Gasano VA: Intracaval and intracardiac extension of malignant thymoma: CT diagnosis. J Comput Assist Tomogr 13:348–350, 1989.

67. Aggarwal P, Sharma SK, Chattopadhyay TK, et al: Mediastinal carcinoid tumor with unusual manifestations. Postgrad Med J 65:327–328, 1989.

68. Sunderrajan EV, Luger AM, Rosenholtz MJ, et al: Leiomyosarcoma in the mediastinum presenting as superior vena cava syndrome. Cancer 53:2553–2556, 1984.

69. Martin AA, Sitton JE, Daroca PJ, et al: Superior vena cava syndrome associated with malignant mesothelioma. J Louis State Med Soc 149:33–35, 1991.

70. Kuten A, Jose B, O'Shea PA: Superior vena cava syndrome secondary to histiocytosis-X in a child: Case report. Med Pediatr Oncol 7:225–228, 1979.

71. Issa PY, Brihi ER, Janin Y, et al: Superior vena cava syndrome in childhood: Report of ten cases and review of the literature. Pediatrics 71:337–341, 1983.

72. Moore RA, McNicholas KW, Naidech H: Clinically silent venous thrombosis following internal and external jugular central venous cannulation in pediatric cardiac patients. Anesthesiology 62:640–643, 1985.

73. Grisoni ER, Mehta SK, Connors AF: Thrombosis and infection complicating central venous catheterization in neonates. J Pediatr Surg 21:772–776, 1986.

74. Effman EL, Ablow RC, Touloukian RJ, et al: Radiographic aspects of total parenteral nutrition during infancy. Radiology 127:195–201, 1978.

75. Ladefoged K, Efsen F, Krogh CJ, et al: Long-term parenteral nutrition. II. Catheter-related complications. Scand J Gastroenterol 16:913–919, 1981.

76. Raszka WV, Smith FR, Pratt SR: Superior vena cava syndrome in infants. Clin Pediatr 28:195–198, 1989.

77. D'Angio GJ, Mitus A, Evans AE: The superior mediastinal syndrome in children with cancer. Am J Roentgenol Radiol Ther Nucl Med 93:537–544, 1965.

78. Yellin A, Mandel M, Rechavi G, et al: Superior vena cava syndrome associated with lymphoma. Am J Dis Child 146:1060–1063, 1992.

79. Ingram L, Rivera GK, Shapiro DN: Superior vena cava syndrome associated with childhood malignancy: Analysis of 24 cases. Med Pediatr Oncol 18:476–481, 1990.

80. Gomes MN, Hufnagel CA: Superior vena cava obstruction: A review of the literature and report of two cases due to benign intrathoracic tumors. Ann Thorac Surg 20:344–359, 1975.

81. McFalls EO, Palac R, Gately H, et al: Pseudoaneurysm formation with superior vena caval syndrome 7 years after aortic composite graft placement. Ann Thorac Surg 48:704–705, 1989.

82. Rosin MD, Ridley PD, Maxwell PH: Rupture of a pseudoaneurysm of a saphenous vein coronary arterial bypass graft presenting with superior caval venous obstruction. Int J Cardiol 25:121–123, 1989.

83. Yavuzer S, Cobanli B, Kavukcu S, et al: Aneurysms of an aberrant right subclavian artery: A rare cause of the superior vena cava syndrome. Vasa 18:69–73, 1989.

84. Weber HS, Markowitz RI, Hellenbrand WE, et al: Pulmonary venous collaterals secondary to superior vena cava stenosis: A rare cause of right to left shunting following repair of a sinus venosus atrial septal defect. Pediatr Cardiol 10:49–51, 1989.

85. Maggiano HJ, Higgins TL, Lobo W, et al: Superior vena cava syndrome after open heart surgery. Cleve Clin J Med 59:93–95, 1992.

86. Coelho Filho JC, Pereira J, Rabello A Jr: Mediastinal and pulmonary entomophthoromycosis with superior vena cava syndrome: Case report. Rev Inst Med Trop Sao Paulo 31:430–433, 1989.

87. Urschel HC Jr, Razzuk MA, Netto GJ, et al: Sclerosing mediastinitis: Improved management with histoplasmosis titer and ketoconazole. Ann Thorac Surg 50:215–221, 1990.

88. Zufferey P, Chapuis L, Monti M: Superior vena cava syndrome due to chronic granulomatous mediastinitis. Vasa 19:341–344, 1990.

89. Pitchenik AE, Zaunbrecher F: Superior vena cava syndrome caused by *Nocardia asteroides*. Am Rev Respir Dis 117:795–797, 1978.

90. Lagerstorm CF, Mitchell HG, Graham BS, et al: Chronic fibrosing mediastinitis and superior vena caval obstruction from blastomycosis. Ann Thorac Surg 54:764–765, 1992.

91. Seetharaman M, Bahadur P, Shrinivas V, et al: Filarial mediastinal lymphadenitis: Another cause of superior vena cava syndrome. Chest 94:871–872, 1988.

92. Sola JE, Stone MM, Wise B, et al: Atypical thrombotic and septic complications of totally implantable venous access devices in patients with cystic fibrosis. Pediatr Pulm 14:239–242, 1992.

93. Kulpati DD, Gupta R, Saha MM, et al: Fibrosing mediastinitis: A rare cause of superior vena caval obstruction. Ind J Chest Dis Allied Sci 31:291–294, 1989.

94. Mazzetti H, Dussaut A, Tentori C, et al: Superior vena cava occlusion and/or syndrome related to pacemaker leads. Am Heart J 125:831–837, 1993.

95. Murakami Y, Matsuno Y, Izumi S, et al: Superior vena cava syndrome as a complication of DDD pacemaker implantation. Clin Cardiol 13:298–300, 1990.

96. Preston CI, Poynton CH, Williams LB: Intermittent superior vena cava syndrome caused by a Hickman catheter. Clin Oncol 4:60–61, 1992.

97. Raska WV Jr, Smith FR, Pratt SR: Superior vena cava syndrome in infants. Clin Pediatr 28:195–198, 1989.

98. Caglar MK, Tolboom J: Successful treatment of superior vena cava syndrome with urokinase in an infant with a central venous catheter. Helv Paediatr Acta 43:483–486, 1989.

99. Belcastro S, Susa A, Pavanelli L, et al: Thrombosis of the superior vena cava due to a central catheter for total parenteral nutrition. JPEN 14:31–33, 1990.

100. Beers TR, Burnes J, Fleming CR: Superior vena caval obstruction in patients with gut failure receiving home parenteral nutrition. JPEN 14:474–479, 1990.

101. Aujla N, McCauley J, Sorkin M: Superior vena cava syndrome due to subclavian hemodialysis catheters. Milit Med 155:274–277, 1990.

102. Goudevenos JA, Reid PG, Adams PC, et al: Pacemaker-induced superior vena cava syndrome: Report of four cases and review of the literature. Pacing Clin Electrophysiol 12:1890–1895, 1989.

103. Meinertz T, Kasper W, Lohr-Schwaab S, et al: Percutaneous recanalization and dilation of a thrombotically occluded superior vena cava in a patient with a peritoneovenous shunt. J Hepatol 9:91–94, 1989.

104. Antonelli D, Rosenfeld T, Kaveh Z: Intermittent superior caval venous syndrome due to permanent transvenous electrode. Int J Cardiol 23:125–127, 1989.

105. Cengiz K, Aykin A, Demirci A, et al: Intrathoracic goiter with hyperthyroidism, tracheal compression, superior vena cava syndrome, and Horner's syndrome. Chest 97:1005–1006, 1990.

106. Park JY, Chung-Park M, Snow M: Intravascular papillary endothelial hyperplasia of superior vena cava: A rare cause of the superior vena cava syndrome. Thorax 46:272–273, 1991.

107. Sanghvi S, Kothari AS, Hathi BC, et al: Angioimmunoblastic lymphadenopathy presenting as superior vena caval obstruction. Chest 100:1721–1722, 1991.

108. Van der Brink H, Vroom TM, van der Laar MA, et al: Superior vena cava syndrome caused by systemic lupus erythematosus in a patient with long-standing rheumatoid arthritis. J Rheumatol 17:240–243, 1990.

109. Fincher RM, Sherman EB: Superior vena caval obstruction due to sarcoidosis. South Med J 79:1306–1308, 1986.

110. Thomas I, Helmold ME, Nychay S: Behçet's disease presenting as superior vena cava syndrome. J Am Acad Dermatol 26:863–865, 1992.

111. Walsh GC, Norton GI, Baird MM, et al: Idiopathic thrombosis of the superior vena cava. Can Med Assoc J 76:292–295, 1957.

112. Hussey HH, Katz S, Yater WM: The superior vena caval syndrome: Report of thirty-five cases. Am Heart J 31:1–26, 1946.

113. Lokich JJ, Goodman R: Superior vena cava syndrome: Clinical management. JAMA 231:58–61, 1975.

114. Hirschmann JV, Raugi GJ: Dermatologic features of the superior vena cava syndrome. Arch Dermatol 128:953–956, 1992.

115. Warren WH, Altman JS, Gregory SA: Chylothorax secondary to obstruction of the superior vena cava: A complication of the LeVeen shunt. Thorax 45:978–979, 1990.

116. Leys M, Van Slycken S, Koller J, et al: Acute macular neuroretinopathy after shock. Bull Soc Belge D Ophtalmol 241:95–104, 1991.
117. Neuman GC, Weingarten AE, Abramowitz RM, et al: The anesthetic management of the patient with an anterior mediastinal mass. Anesthesiology 60:144–147, 1984.
118. Carter MM, Tarr RW, Mazer MJ, et al: The "aortic nipple" as a sign of impending superior vena caval obstruction. Chest 87:775–777, 1985.
119. Schwartz EE, Goodman LR, Haskin ME: Role of CT scanning in superior vena cava syndrome. Am J Clin Oncol 9:71–78, 1986.
120. Engel IA, Auh YH, Rubenstein WA, et al: CT diagnosis of mediastinal and thoracic inlet venous obstruction. Am J Roentgenol 141:521–526, 1983.
121. Trigaux JP, Van Beers B: Thoracic collateral venous channels: Normal and pathologic CT findings. J Comput Assist Tomogr 14:769–773, 1990.
122. Bechtold RE, Wolfman NT, Karstaedt N, et al: Superior vena caval obstruction: Detection using CT. Radiology 157:485–487, 1985.
123. Moncada R, Cardella R, Demos TC, et al: Evaluation of the superior vena cava syndrome by axial CT and CT phlebography. Am J Roentgenol 143:731–736, 1984.
124. Medera M, Meydam K, Schmitt WG: MRI visualization of the aortic nipple. Cardiovasc Intervent Radiol 11:29–35, 1988.
125. Loehr SP, Baker DM, Link KM, et al: MRI evaluation of the mediastinum part 1: Anterior mediastinum. MRI Decisions 24–32, May/June 1993.
126. Khimji T, Zeiss J: MRI versus CT and US in the evaluation of a patient presenting with superior vena cava syndrome: Case report. Clin Imag 16:269–271, 1992.
127. Gooding GA, Hightower DR, Moore EH, et al: Obstruction of the superior vena cava or subclavian veins: Sonographic diagnosis. Radiology 159:663–667, 1986.
128. Ayala K, Chandrasekaran K, Karalis DG, et al: Diagnosis of superior vena caval obstruction by transesophageal echocardiography. Chest 101:874–876, 1992.
129. Swayne LC, Kaplan IL: Gallium SPECT detection of neoplastic intravascular obstruction of the superior vena cava. Clin Nucl Med 14:823–826, 1989.
130. Neuhoff H, Sussman ML, Nabatoff RA: Angiocardiography in the differential diagnosis of pulmonary neoplasms. Surgery 25:178–183, 1949.
131. Dyet JF, Moghisi K: Role of venography in assessing patients with superior vena obstruction caused by bronchial carcinoma for bypass operations. Thorax 35:628–630, 1980.
132. Podoloff DA, Kim EE: Evaluation of sensitivity and specificity of upper extremity radionuclide venography in cancer patients with indwelling central venous catheters. Clin Nucl Med 17:457–462, 1992.
133. Maxfield WS, Meckstroth GR: Tc-99m superior vena cavography. Radiology 92:913–918, 1969.
134. Painter TD, Karpf M: Superior vena cava syndrome: Diagnostic procedures. Am J Med Sci 285:2–6, 1983.
135. Callejas MA, Rami R, Catalan M, et al: Mediastinoscopy as an emergency diagnostic procedure in superior vena cava syndrome. Scand J Thorac Cardiovasc Surg 25:137–139, 1991.
136. Chen CH, Kuo ML, Shih JF, et al: Ultrasonically guided needle aspiration biopsy in the diagnosis of advanced superior vena cava syndrome. Chung Huai Hsueh Rsa Chih-Chinese Med J 50:119–124, 1992.
137. Dake MD, Zemel G, Dolmatch BL, et al: The cause of superior vena cava syndrome: Diagnosis with percutaneous atherectomy. Radiology 174:957–959, 1990.
138. Rubin P, Green J, Holzwasser G, et al: Superior vena caval syndrome: Slow low dose versus rapid high dose schedules. Radiology 81:388–401, 1963.
139. Fisherman WH, Bradfield JS: Superior vena caval syndrome: Response with initially high daily dose irradiation. South Med J 66:677–680, 1973.
140. Perez CA, Stanley K, Grundy G, et al: Impact of irradiation technique and tumor extent in tumor control and survival of patients with unresectable non-oat cell carcinoma of the lung: Report by the Radiation Therapy Oncology Group. Cancer 50:1091–1099, 1982.
141. Cox JD, Azarnia N, Byhardt RW, et al: A randomized phase I/II trial of hyperfractionated radiation therapy with total doses of 60.0 Gy to 79.2 Gy: Possible survival benefit with >69.6 Gy in favorable patients with Radiation Therapy Oncology Group stage III non-small cell lung carcinoma: Report of Radiation Therapy Oncology Group 83-11. J Clin Oncol 8:1543–1555, 1990.
142. Saunders MI, Dische S: Continuous, hyperfractionated, accelerated radiotherapy (CHART) in non-small cell carcinoma of the bronchus. Int J Radiat Oncol Biol Phys 19:1211–1215, 1990.
143. Pignon JP, Arriagada R, Ihde DC, et al: A meta-analysis of thoracic radiotherapy for small-cell lung cancer. N Engl J Med 327:1618–1624, 1992.
144. Murray N, Coy P, Pater J, et al: Importance of timing for thoracic irradiation in the combined modality treatment of limited stage small cell lung cancer. J Clin Oncol 11:336–344, 1993.
145. Turrisi AT, Glover DJ: Thoracic radiotherapy variables: Influence on local control in small cell lung cancer limited disease. Int J Radiat Oncol Biol Phys 19:1473–1479, 1990.
146. Maddox AM, Valdivieso M, Lukeman J, et al: Superior vena cava obstruction in small cell bronchogenic carcinoma. Cancer 52:2165–2172, 1983.
147. Adelstein DJ, Hines JD, Carter SG, et al: Thromboembolic events in patients with malignant superior vena cava thrombosis and obstruction. Arch Intern Med 149:1209–1213, 1985.
148. Chahinian AP, Propert KJ, Ware JH, et al: A randomized trial of anticoagulation with warfarin and of alternating chemotherapy in extensive small cell lung cancer by the Cancer and Leukemia Group. J Clin Oncol 53:2046–2052, 1984.
149. Lebeau B, Chastang CI, Brechot JM: Subcutaneous heparin treatment increases complete response rate and overall survival in small cell lung cancer. Lung Cancer 7(suppl):129, 1991.
150. Gray BH, Olin JW, Graor RA, et al: Safety and efficacy of thrombolytic therapy for superior vena cava syndrome. Chest 99:54–59, 1991.
151. Greenberg S, Kosinski R, Daniels J: Treatment of superior vena cava thrombosis with recombinant tissue type plasminogen activator. Chest 99:1298–1301, 1991.
152. Grace AA, Sutters M, Schofield PM: Balloon dilatation of pacemaker induced stenosis of the superior vena cava. Br Heart J 65:225–226, 1991.
153. Solomon N, Wholey MH, Jarmolowski CR: Intravascular stents in the management of superior vena cava syndrome. Catheter Cardiovasc Diag 23:245–252, 1991.
154. Rosch J, Uchida BT, Hall LD, et al: Gianturco-Rosch expandable Z-stents in the treatment of superior vena cava syndrome. Cardiovasc Intervent Radiol 15:319–327, 1992.
155. Irving JD, Dondelinger RF, Reidy JF, et al: Gianturco self-expanding stents: Clinical experience in the vena cava and large veins. Cardiovasc Intervent Radiol 15:328–333, 1992.
156. Oudkerk M, Heystraten FM, Stoter G: Stenting in malignant vena caval obstruction. Cancer 71:142–146, 1993.
157. Yedlicka JW Jr, Carlson JE, Hunter DW, et al: Thrombectomy with the transluminal endarterectomy catheter (TEC) system: Experimental study and case report. J Vasc Intervent Radiol 2:343–347, 1991.
158. Lemmer JH Jr, Behrendt DM, Beekman RH, et al: Pedicled right atrial-pericardial tissue conduit for bypass of the obstructed superior vena cava in children. J Thorac Cardiovasc Surg 98:417–420, 1989.
159. Doty DB, Doty JR, Jones KW: Bypass of superior vena cava: Fifteen years' experience with spiral vein graft for obstruction of superior vena cava caused by benign disease. J Thorac Cardiovasc Surg 99:889–896, 1990.
160. Piccione W Jr, Faber LP, Warren WH: Superior vena caval reconstruction using autologous pericardium. Ann Thorac Surg 50:417–419, 1990.
161. Larsson S, Lepore V: Technical options in reconstruction of large mediastinal veins. Surgery 111:311–317, 1992.
162. Gloviczki P, Pairolero PC, Cherry KJ, et al: Reconstruction of the vena cava and of its primary tributaries: A preliminary report. J Vasc Surg 11:373–381, 1990.
163. Green J, Rubin P, Holzwasser G: The experimental production of superior vena caval obstruction. Radiology 81:406–414, 1963.

16 CHEMOPREVENTION OF LUNG CANCER

Jin S. Lee, Scott M. Lippman, and Waun K. Hong

Lung cancer is the most rapidly increasing type of cancer in the world and has been a leading cause of cancer death in the United States and many other western countries.[1] Continuing efforts at primary prevention of lung cancer by smoking cessation have led to a modest decrease in the number of smokers in the United States.[2] However, given the trend of worldwide increase in consumption of tobacco products and nicotine's addictive effects,[3] cigarette smoking will continue to be a major public health problem worldwide. More disturbing is that even after successful smoking cessation, the risk of developing lung cancer stays high for more than a decade.[4] Once cancer develops, the overall treatment outcome remains suboptimal, as reflected by a 5-year survival rate of approximately 10%, which has been only minimally improved over the past three decades.[5] In addition, earlier hopes to reduce the lung cancer mortality by detecting the lung cancer in an earlier stage with regular chest radiographs or sputum cytology, or both, have not been fulfilled.[6] Clearly, alternative approaches are needed as a means of reducing lung cancer mortality.

One approach is chemoprevention, which received renewed interest in the last 5 years after clinical demonstration of the chemical inhibition of cancer development in patients with head and neck cancers[7] and those with xeroderma pigmentosum.[8] The study of head and neck cancer is particularly relevant to lung chemoprevention. Lung and head and neck cancers are related regionally by their location in the aerodigestive tract and biologically by their causative links to tobacco.[9] Head and neck clinical chemoprevention study is currently more mature than the lung. Head and neck chemoprevention has served as a clinical model for design and interpretation strategies of lung chemoprevention. Therefore, this chapter reviews studies relevant to carcinogenesis and chemoprevention in the lung and head and neck.

HISTOLOGIC CHANGES IN THE AERODIGESTIVE TRACTS OF SMOKERS

Lung cancer, like other epithelial cancers, is viewed as an end-product of the multistep carcinogenic process.[10] The driving force behind this process is thought to be genetic damage caused by continuous exposure to carcinogens, such as those contained in cigarette smoke. Genetic damage is evidenced by the linear relationship between the DNA adduct formation in human lung and cigarette smoking,[11–13] and the increased frequency of micronuclei in high-risk tissue and premalignant lesions.[14] Hypothetically, the greater the degree of genetic damage, the greater the risk of cancer development.

Although the causal association between cigarette smoking and lung cancer was initially entertained in the late 1920s and 1930s,[15] it was not until 1950 that the causal relationship was demonstrated by well-designed clinical studies, one from the United States[16] and one from Great Britain.[17] Subsequently, in the 1950s and early 1960s, many investigators reported histologic changes in the bronchial epithelium that were associated with chronic smoking and lung cancer,[18] including basal cell hyperplasia, stratification, squamous cell metaplasia, and carcinoma in situ. Most notable is the work of Auerbach and associates,[19] who carefully examined serial sections of the entire tracheobronchial trees of chronic smokers and patients who died of lung cancer. They recorded three major types of epithelial changes: (1) an increase in the number of cell rows, (2) loss of cilia, and (3) the presence of atypical cells. They analyzed those findings singly and in combination with other variables. There was a consistent direct correlation between the frequency of these epithelial changes and the amount of cigarette smoking, as shown in Table 16–1. The most striking finding was the frequency of carcinoma in situ, a lesion composed entirely of atypical cells without cilia in an average thickness of five or more cell rows, which was observed in 15.0% of the sections from those who died of lung cancer. No such lesion was found among men who never smoked regularly, and very few were found among light smokers, but they were found in 4.3% of sections from men who smoked one to two packages of cigarettes a day and 11.4% of sections from those who smoked two or more packages of cigarettes a day. Similar findings were reported even in passive smokers.[20] These findings are consistent with the concept of field cancerization, which was initially introduced by Slaughter and colleagues in 1953 to describe the diffuse mucosal changes observed in patients with head and neck can-

TABLE 16–1. Histologic Changes in Bronchial Epithelium According to Smoking History Compared with Lung Cancer Patients. Percentage of Sections with Histologic Changes

HISTOLOGIC CHANGES	Never Smoked (n = 3324)	SMOKERS				LUNG CANCER (n = 2784)
		< 0.5 PPD (n = 1834)	0.5–1.0 PPD (n = 3016)	1–2 PPD (n = 7062)	≥ 2 PPD (n = 1787)	
Lesions with cilia						
Hyperplasia (≥ 3 rows)	9.4	35.5	40.3	63.8	76.2	78.6
≥ 70% atypical cells	0.1	0.4	1.0	4.8	30.0	67.9
≥ 90% atypical cells	0.0	0.1	0.1	0.1	0.6	11.2
Lesions without cilia						
Overall	6.0	10.2	12.6	19.7	28.3	27.4
100% atypical cells	0.0	0.3	0.8	4.3	11.4	15.0

PPD = packs per day.

Modified from Auerbach O, Stout AP, Hammond EC, et al: Changes in bronchial epithelium in relation to cigarette smoking and in relation to lung cancer. N Engl J Med 265:253–267, 1961.

cers.[21] Slaughter studied resected tissue specimens from patients with squamous cell cancer of the oral cavity. Three primary histologic abnormalities were described in the tissue surrounding the resected tumors: hyperplasia (an increase in the number of rows in the epithelium), hyperkeratinization, and dyskaryosis (atypia). Furthermore, when serial sections of the entire surgical specimen were examined, separate foci of in situ and invasive carcinoma were frequent findings. It is conceivable, therefore, that the entire aerodigestive tract epithelium is exposed to and preconditioned by carcinogenic agents, such as those included in the cigarette smoke, and is at increased risk of developing cancer.

GENETIC EVIDENCE OF FIELD CANCERIZATION

Genetic alterations in lung cancer involve both activation of the dominantly acting cellular oncogenes and the inactivation or chromosomal deletion of the recessive or tumor-suppressor genes.[22, 23] Because the inactivation of tumor-suppressor genes requires at least two genetic changes, lung cancer cells must have suffered many separate genetic changes. A conservative estimate based on the cytogenetic and molecular changes places the number of genetic mutations between 10 and 20.[23] The genetic events specific for the multistep carcinogenic process at each organ site have not yet been fully identified. Nevertheless, complex cytogenetic abnormalities are consistently found not only in tumor cells[24–26] but also in normal and nonmalignant lung tissue samples from patients with lung cancer.[24, 26] Unfortunately, the majority of conventional cytogenetic studies have been performed after short-term culture or on tumor-derived cell lines; therefore, the possibility of in vitro culture artifacts could not be completely excluded. Using the premature chromosome condensation (PCC) technique, which allows cytogenetic analysis of slowly proliferating or nonproliferating cell populations and thereby overcomes the problems associated with cell culture,

investigators were able to demonstrate cytogenetic abnormalities present in the normal and premalignant lung tissue samples obtained from patients with lung cancer and compared the results with those found from the tumor specimens.[27–29] Of most interest was that the distribution of chromosome numbers per cell in the normal lung samples was similar to that in the corresponding tumor specimen.[28, 29] In addition, even though an exact concordance in cytogenetic abnormalities did not exist, the tumor cells and normal cells shared some cytogenetic abnormalities. These results strongly support the notion that chromosomal changes accumulate *during* a multistep carcinogenic process rather than occurring subsequent to malignant transformation. Further supporting evidence for field cancerization comes from the studies of genetic alterations in paraffin-embedded tissue sections using a chromosome in situ hybridization technique[30–32] and DNA content analysis after Feulgen staining.[33] Using biotinylated chromosome 7- and 17-specific centromeric DNA probes (Oncor Inc., Gaithersburg, MD), chromosomal polysomies were found not only in tumor cells[30] but also in the chronic smokers' bronchial mucosa and in the histologically defined premalignant lesions such as bronchial metaplasia and oral leukoplakia.[31, 32] Because not all smokers develop lung cancer, careful examination of bronchial tissue samples for genetic alterations might allow us to identify individuals at high risk for malignant transformation.

Recent molecular studies provide more support for the concept of field carcinogenesis. Chung and co-workers[34] reported a high rate of discordance in the presence or locus (within the gene) of p53 mutation in primary or second primary tumor within individual patients. These data suggest an independent genetic origin of cancers within the epithelial field at risk.

SECOND PRIMARY TUMORS

As predicted by the concepts of field cancerization and multistep carcinogenic process, there is a high risk of developing second primary tumors among patients with lung cancer[35] and head and neck cancer who have been successfully treated for their first primary tumor. In one series, 26% of patients with primary laryngeal carcinomas developed a second primary tumor in the lung.[36] The risk of second primary tumors is increased in patients with resected non–small cell lung cancer and exceeds 10% in a selected series of patients with Stage I non–small cell lung cancer (Table 16–2).[37–42] More strikingly, the risk of developing second primary tumors is very high in long-term survivors of small cell lung cancer.[43–48] Heyne and associates[47] reported that the 8-year cumulative risk of developing second primary tumors in long-term survivors of small cell lung cancer was 50%. Of particular interest, non–small cell lung cancer is the major cause of late mortality in long-term survivors of small cell lung cancer.[44, 48]

CHEMOPREVENTIVE AGENTS

Chemoprevention study grew in large part out of the epidemiologic data demonstrating the existence of dietary inhibitors of carcinogenesis.[49, 50] It is difficult to sort out from epidemiologic studies what specific compounds within complex foods provide anticarcinogenic (or carcinogenic) effects.[51] The cancer-preventive data from epidemiology, however, led to in vitro and in vivo (animal) laboratory studies of specific components of complex foods.[52, 53] These studies discovered many agents with laboratory anticarcinogenic activity and began to suggest toxicity profiles of these agents. But carcinogenesis and toxicity studies in animals do not necessarily translate closely to effects in humans. Carefully controlled clinical chemoprevention trials are required to establish definitively the role (activity and toxicity) of specific natural or synthetic agents in cancer prevention.[54] Several agents currently undergoing clinical study are described here.

Retinol (Vitamin A)

Vitamin A and its synthetic analogues are collectively referred to as retinoids. The retinoids appear to act by binding to a specific set of retinoic acid receptors (RAR) and retinoid-X-receptors (RXR).[55] The binding of retinoids to these receptors results in binding to specific nuclear sites and regulation of multiple genes. Current studies are attempting to elucidate the specific transcriptional changes that occur as a result of this binding. Overall, it is hypothesized that retinoids induce differentiation in cells that have lost normal regulatory mechanisms. Retinol and the synthetic retinoids are noted to produce significant toxic effects if given in high doses. Many synthetic retinoids have now been developed, and several of these have undergone extensive clinical testing.

Isotretinoin (13-*cis*-retinoic acid)

One of the most actively studied retinoids in chemoprevention trials is 13-*cis*-retinoic acid.[56] Its mechanism of action is unknown, although it most likely functions by inducing differentiation in cells. One problem with 13-*cis*-retinoic acid has been its toxicity in early clinical trials. Because any toxicity can be a problem when treating for long periods of time individuals who do not have cancer, attention has been given to identifying agents that produce few and mild toxic effects. A recent study has confirmed that 13-*cis*-retinoic acid has biologic activity in humans when given at a relatively low dose of 0.5 mg/kg/day.[57] At this dose level, side effects are minimal and rarely require cessation of therapy.

Etretinate

Etretinate is a vitamin A derivative that has been found to inhibit or prevent papillomas and carcinomas in mice.[58] Etretinate may not only induce differentiation but also may act by altering the immune system.[59] Its toxicity is similar to that seen with other synthetic retinoids, and it has been used in several clinical studies.

Retinyl Palmitate

Retinyl palmitate is a synthetic retinoid being used in a large lung cancer chemoprevention trial in Europe. The mechanism of action is probably similar to that of the other retinoids. Early studies indicated that toxicity may be a problem with this agent, but it has been given in doses as high as 300,000 IU daily without significant toxic effects.[60]

TABLE 16–2. Selected Studies on the Incidence of Second Primary Tumors in Patients with Non–Small Cell Lung Cancer

INVESTIGATORS	STUDY GROUP	NO. OF PATIENTS	RESULTS
Shields[37]	Resected patients who survived > 10 years	257	51 Patients with SPT (25 patients with SPT of the lung)
Van Bodegon[38]	All patients with 1° carcinoma of the lung	1,540	153 Patients with SPT of lung (89 metachronous)
Thomas[39, 40]	T_1N_0 patients after resection	907	0.9 SPT of lung/100 patients/year
Smith[41]	All resected patients	1,400	55 Patients with SPT of lung (49 metachronous)
Pairolero[42]	Postsurgical Stage I patients in long-term follow-up study	346	35 Patients with SPT of lung (2.2 SPT/100 patients/year)

SPT = Second primary tumor.

Other Retinoids

Although the above-mentioned agents have been used in several clinical trials, other synthetic retinoids are also being studied. 4-Hydroxy-phenylretinamide (4-HPR) is among the most active synthetic retinoids in preclinical models and appears to cause fewer toxic effects than other retinoids; therefore, 4-HPR is a high priority in National Cancer Institute (NCI)–sponsored clinical studies.[52] All-*trans*-retinoic acid is being used in the management of acute promyelocytic leukemia in several clinical trials; however, its toxicity would appear to limit its usefulness in chemoprevention.[61]

Beta-Carotene

A naturally occurring agent, beta-carotene is found in yellow and green leafy vegetables and is a precursor to vitamin A. Beta-carotene is a prototype for the class of compounds known as carotenoids. Several prospective studies have identified an inverse correlation between dietary beta-carotene intake and lung cancer.[51, 62] Interestingly, three of four of these studies that evaluated dietary retinol intake as well did not find the same correlation for vitamin A intake.[63–65] Furthermore, selected studies that correlated increased serum levels of beta-carotene with a decreased risk of lung cancer did not identify a similar correlation for vitamin A.[66, 67] The mechanism of action for beta-carotene remains unknown, although it is believed to act by inducing differentiation in proliferating epithelium following its metabolism to retinol. However, beta-carotene and other carotenoids may have an additional mechanism not found in synthetic retinoids—the ability to scavenge free radicals.[68] A major advantage of beta-carotene and other carotenoids is that they are generally well tolerated and produce few side effects, but long-term use of beta-carotene may result in decreased levels of vitamin E, which may compromise its activity.[69]

Vitamin E

Lower-than-normal levels of vitamin E have been found to correlate with an increased risk of lung cancer in epidemiologic studies.[66] The function of vitamin E, a fat-soluble vitamin, appears to be the neutralization of free radicals in the lipid membrane. The chemopreventive efficacy of this agent is being evaluated in randomized clinical trials.

Vitamin B$_{12}$ and Folate

Preclinical data indicates that cigarette smoking may lead to a reduction in serum folate levels, which in at least one study correlated with an increased incidence of bronchial metaplasia.[70] The mechanism of action is not known, but data from one clinical trial indicate that this combination has biologic activity in the respiratory epithelium.[71]

Selenium

Epidemiologic data suggest that lower-than-normal levels of selenium may correlate with an increased risk of lung cancer, and animal models have shown that this agent has chemopreventive activity.[52] Selenium appears to act as an antioxidant. Unfortunately, the therapeutic ratio between active levels of selenium and toxic levels may be quite narrow; therefore, various selenium compounds are being investigated.

N-Acetylcysteine

N-Acetylcysteine is a synthetic precursor of intracellular cysteine that reduces intracellular glutathione levels.[52] It has significant activity in lung cancer preclinical models and has no significant toxicity in humans. At present, a large randomized trial is evaluating the efficacy of this agent in preventing second primary tumors in patients with a history of resected lung cancers.

CLINICAL TRIALS

Chemoprevention trials present unique problems in study design because, by definition, study individuals do not have cancer and the development of cancer remains the ultimate primary endpoint for the evaluation of chemoprevention agents. Because the participants are usually healthy subjects without cancer and are required to take the experimental agent over a long period of time, toxicity and compliance are of major importance for the success of a study.[72] On the other hand, the occurrence of lung cancer is not a frequent event in most populations, and even in high-risk groups, it may take many years to develop; large samples and prolonged follow-up, therefore, are necessary to achieve statistical significance. As such, only a few chemoprevention trials have been designed for the general population. The Physicians' Health Study[73] used a 2 × 2 factorial design to evaluate the benefits of aspirin and beta-carotene for primary prevention of cardiovascular disease and cancer. Accrual of 22,071 United States male physicians has been completed, and data analysis is awaited. The study was designed to have a greater than 90% probability of detecting a 20% reduction in cancer incidence in the beta-carotene group at an average of 7.5 years follow-up. A newly funded Women's Health study is conducting a trial of beta-carotene, vitamin E, and aspirin for the primary prevention of cancer and cardiovascular disease among over 40,000 United States female nurses aged 50 or older.[74] Unfortunately, this type of trial requiring thousands of participants and many years of follow-up entails tremendous expense. Methods that decrease the number of subjects or shorten the duration of follow-up are imperative for practical evaluation of multiple chemoprevention strategies.

One approach to decrease the sample size is to focus on high-risk groups, such as those with personal (e.g., smoking) or occupational risk factors (e.g., asbestos exposure, mining). Ongoing primary chemoprevention trials in these high-risk groups are listed in Table 16–3. The trials have generally used naturally occurring nutrients as the chemoprevention agents. Results from these primary cancer chemoprevention trials are not yet available. Another approach is to identify biomarkers that might be associated with specific stages of the carcinogenic process that can be used to select high-risk individuals and also be used as an intermediate endpoint to assess the effect of chemopreventive agents on the tissue at risk.[75] Short-term chemoprevention trials on subjects selected by presence of bronchial metaplasia or sputum atypia also are examples of this approach. A third approach is to focus on those who had been cured of a primary tumor, which is reviewed here in more detail.

PHASE III CHEMOPREVENTION TRIALS

Cigarette Smokers and Asbestos-Exposed Individuals

In an attempt to decrease the sizes of the samples necessary to define the effectiveness of chemoprevention strategies, investigators are evaluating the efficacy of several agents in individuals who smoke cigarettes. Cigarette smoking remains the single most important risk factor for the development of lung cancer; heavy smokers have a relative risk of 13.3.[76] Because smokers are at a relatively high risk of developing lung cancer, the number of subjects needed to show the effectiveness of chemoprevention is much lower. Several randomized trials are evaluating the role of retinoids in preventing the development of lung cancer in smokers.

A pilot trial from the University of Pittsburgh randomized 400 male and female smokers to receive either 15 mg or 30 mg of beta-carotene or placebo.[77] Beta-carotene levels were increased in the group receiving beta-carotene, confirming compliance, and toxicity was minimal, demonstrating the feasibility of a large randomized trial of beta-carotene in smokers.

The University of Washington in Seattle has completed the vanguard portion of a large randomized trial comparing the efficacy of 25,000 IU of retinol, 30 mg of beta-carotene, a combination of both agents, or placebo in a 2 × 2 factorial trial in individuals with a smoking history of 20 pack-years or more.[78, 79] The advantage of a vanguard format is that the first cohort of subjects confirms the feasibility of performing a randomized trial. In addition to collecting compliance and short-term toxicity data, this group will continue with the study and provide data on potential long-term complications before extended follow-up on the majority of subjects. The vanguard portion has completed accrual of 1029 individuals, and compliance in this group exceeds 90%, as determined by self-reporting and periodic pill counts. The only toxic effect reported is mild yellowing of the skin in individuals receiving beta-carotene.

These investigators are also studying the effectiveness of 25,000 IU of retinol plus 30 mg of beta-carotene versus placebo in 816 male smokers with a history of occupational asbestos exposure. Individuals exposed to asbestos have an increased risk of lung cancer, with a relative risk of 1.4 to 2.6 over that of the general population.[80] Furthermore, asbestos exposure and cigarette smoking in combination increases the relative risk of lung cancer over that of the general population to 28.8.[81] Occupational asbestos exposure for this trial was defined as at least 15 years since the first exposure to asbestos in a job title consistent with high asbestos exposure or changes on chest radiography consistent with asbestos-induced pleural or parenchymal pulmonary disease, or both. As in the trial in smokers, compliance was high and toxicity was minimal.

Based on these pilot studies, a large-scale randomized trial, the Carotene and Retinol Efficacy Trial (CARET), is under way to evaluate the efficacy of 30 mg of beta-carotene plus 25,000 IU of retinol versus placebo in 13,000 smokers and 4000 asbestos-exposed smokers. As of July 1990, more than 4600 patients had been randomized, and accrual is anticipated to be completed in 1998.[78] The primary endpoint is the development of lung cancer or mesothelioma, and secondary endpoints include other malignancies and deaths from all causes.

The largest randomized trial evaluating the efficacy

TABLE 16–3. Selected Chemoprevention Trials of Lung and Upper Aerodigestive Tract Cancers in High Risk Groups

TRIAL	AGENT	STUDY POPULATION	CANCER SITES
Finland	Beta-carotene, Alpha-tocopherol	Smokers	Lung
Univ. Texas-Tyler	Beta-carotene, retinol	Asbestos exposure	Lung
Univ. Texas-Tyler	Etretinate	Asbestos exposure	Lung
CARET Study, Seattle	Beta-carotene, retinol	Smokers, asbestos exposure	Lung
Univ. Pittsburgh	Beta-carotene	Smokers	Lung
Univ. Alabama	Folic acid, B_{12}	Smokers	Lung
China (Yunnan)	Beta-carotene, retinol, Alpha-tocopherol, selenium	Tin miners	Lung
NCI/Huixian Study	Selenium, zinc, riboflavin	Huixian, China	Esophagus

CARET = Carotene and Retinol Efficacy Trial; NCI = National Cancer Institute.
Modified from Boone CW, Delloff GJ, Malone WE: Identification of candidate cancer chemopreventive agents and their evaluation in animal models and human clinical trials: A review. Cancer Res 50:2–9, 1990.

of chemoprevention of lung cancer in smokers was begun in Finland in 1984 by the National Public Health Institute of Finland in collaboration with the United States National Cancer Institute.[82, 83] Five hundred and ninety smoking males were invited to participate in the study; a 1-year pilot trial evaluated the feasibility of a large-scale trial.[82] Forty per cent were randomized; one-third of the invited individuals were not randomized because their current smoking habits had decreased to smoking fewer than five commercially manufactured cigarettes daily. After a 3-month run-in period on placebo, subjects were randomized using a 2 × 2 factorial design to receive either 20 mg of synthetic beta-carotene, 50 mg of alpha-tocopherol (vitamin E), a combination of both agents, or placebo daily. Compliance was excellent and toxicity was minimal. Based on these preliminary results, a large randomized trial was begun in 1985.[83] A total of 29,133 Finnish male smokers 50 to 69 years of age were randomly assigned to one of the four regimens. After a median follow-up of 6.1 years (range, 5 to 8), 876 new cases of lung cancer were diagnosed. Unexpectedly, those who received beta carotene had 18% higher incidence of lung cancer (95% confidence interval, 3 to 36%) than those who did not. Total mortality was also higher among those who received beta-carotene by 8% (95% confidence interval, 1 to 16%), primarily because there were more deaths from lung cancer and ischemic heart disease. There was no significant reduction in the incidence of lung cancer among those who received alpha-tocopherol. These results raise the possibility that these substances may have harmful as well as beneficial effects. However, longer follow-up of the participants in this trial and data from other large ongoing trials are required to determine the full spectrum of the effects of these agents.

Tin Miners

Another randomized trial is evaluating chemopreventive agents in miners. Tin miners in the Yunnan Province in Southern China with more than 10 years of mining experience have been found to develop lung cancer at the rate of 1% per year.[84] A pilot study investigated the feasibility of using beta-carotene, retinol, vitamin E, and selenium to prevent lung cancer in this high-risk group. As part of the pilot portion of the trial, 358 individuals were randomized to receive either 25,000 IU vitamin A, 50 mg of beta-carotene, 800 IU of vitamin E, 400 mg of selenium, or placebo in a 2 × 4 factorial design. Compliance approximated 90%, as determined by pill counts and serum levels of all four agents tested, and toxicity was not a significant problem; therefore, a full-scale trial is now being planned.

TRIALS USING INTERMEDIATE MARKERS

General Considerations

Many different biologic phenomena, such as histologic changes in bronchial epithelium, cytogenetic ab-

normalities, and increases in proliferative cells, are being investigated as potential intermediate markers of carcinogenesis.[75] The study of these markers will improve our understanding of the development of lung cancer. Researchers hypothesize that if a molecular abnormality was known to be associated with the development of a specific malignancy, reversal of the molecular abnormality would reverse the probability of developing cancer. Unfortunately, because the specific steps in lung carcinogenesis remain unknown, studies involving intermediate endpoints still require validation by the primary endpoint, the development of lung cancer. Nevertheless, intermediate markers are being used in two ways.[85] First, intermediate markers allow identification of individuals at increased risk of developing lung cancer. The identification by a specific marker of an increased risk of lung cancer allows selection of a subset of patients in which the projected number of cancers is high enough to allow completion of a trial with a relatively limited number of subjects. Second, trials evaluating the efficacy of chemopreventive agents use intermediate markers to determine whether or not an agent is having a biologic effect and allow detection of an agent's activity without waiting for the development of invasive cancer, thereby greatly decreasing the study sample size and duration of follow-up.

Clinical-Histologic Premalignancy Studies

Head and Neck Carcinogenesis Trials

Chemoprevention study in the oral cavity has served as a model system for the design of trials in the lung. Chemoprevention studies of the premalignant oral lesion leukoplakia, an intermediate marker for carcinogenesis throughout the aerodigestive tract, are particularly relevant to lung chemoprevention. This lesion is a white patch found anywhere on the mucosa of the oral cavity or oropharynx that cannot be scraped off or classified as any other disorder. Oral leukoplakia is tobacco related, a precursor of squamous cell carcinoma, easily monitored by physical examination and biopsy, has excellent preclinical models, and is related to carcinogenesis in the lung through its etiology and biology and through field carcinogenesis. These features make oral leukoplakia an excellent model system for preliminary clinical study of chemoprevention agents with potential activity throughout the upper aerodigestive tract and lung.[86, 87]

Many agents under study in the lung, including retinoids, beta-carotene, vitamin E, and selenium, have been tested in chemoprevention trials in oral leukoplakia.[88–92] Of these agents only the retinoids have undergone the rigor of randomized trials, which are briefly reviewed below.

Non-randomized studies of retinoids in oral leukoplakia were first reported in the 1950s. To date, a total of five randomized trials have been published. The first was a 3-month, placebo-controlled, double-blind trial of high-dose 13-cis-retinoic acid that was reported by Hong and associates in 1986.[93] Forty-four

TABLE 16–4. Completed Phase II Trials Using Intermediate Endpoints

INVESTIGATORS	STUDY ENDPOINT	TREATMENT	EVALUABLE SUBJECTS	RESULT
Saccomanno[99]	Degree of atypia on sputum cytology	13-cRA 1–2.5 mg/kg/day	26	No improvement
Heimburger[71]	Squamous metaplasia on sputum cytology	Folate 10 mg/day; vitamin B_{12} 500 μg; Placebo	36 37	Improvement in treatment group (p = .03)
Arnold[100]	Degree of atypia on sputum cytology	Etretinate 25 mg/day Placebo	71 67	No improvement compared with placebo group
Misset[108]	Metaplasia index using biopsy samples	Etretinate 25 mg/day	40	Reduction in metaplasia index in 29 subjects
Lee[109]	Metaplasia index using biopsy samples	13-cRA 1 mg/kg/day Placebo	33 34	No improvement compared with placebo group

patients were enrolled. The clinical response was 67% in the retinoid group and 10% in the placebo group (p = .0002). Reversal of dysplasia (histologic response) was observed in 54% of the retinoid group and 10% of the placebo group (p = .01). Although significantly active, high-dose 13-*cis*-retinoic acid mucocutaneous toxicity was not acceptable for widespread usage and over half of the retinoid clinical responders relapsed within 3 months of discontinuing therapy.

A second trial, sponsored by the NCI, was designed to address these problems of toxicity and relapse.[94] Seventy patients were enrolled. The design included a 3-month high-dose induction, followed by a 9-month maintenance phase, in which responding patients were randomized to low-dose 13-*cis*-retinoic acid or beta-carotene. Clinical maintenance-phase progression rates were 8% in the low-dose retinoid group and 55% in the beta-carotene group (p < .001). Maintenance-phase toxicity was generally mild though significantly greater in the low-dose 13-*cis*-retinoic acid group than in the beta-carotene group.

The favorable activity and toxicity profiles of low-dose 13-*cis*-retinoic acid in oral leukoplakia studies was the basis for the dosage used in the design of the large-scale NCI Phase III trials to prevent second primary tumors in early stage head and neck and lung cancer patients (discussed later).

Three other randomized oral leukoplakia studies have been reported. Natural vitamin A has produced a 57% clinical complete response rate in betel nut chewers from Asia.[95] These results were significantly better than the 3% complete regression rate in the placebo group. The histologic response rate was also greater in the vitamin A than the placebo group. A randomized, placebo-controlled trial from China reported significant activity of a synthetic retinamide in oral leukoplakia.[96] The most recent randomized trial was designed to prevent relapse in patients whose oral lesions were resected.[97] The most recent report of this Italian trial indicates a significantly lower relapse rate in the fenretinide group (7.7%) than that in the nontreatment control group (29%). The relapse rate in the retinoid group closely approximates the progression rate of 8% in the earlier low-dose 13cRA maintenance study.[94]

Lung Carcinogenesis Trials

Several chemoprevention trials are using reversal of histologic and cytologic abnormalities as an endpoint (Table 16–4). These trials are, in large part, based on the observation of Saccomanno and coworkers,[98] who after sequential cytologic examinations of exfoliated bronchial cells in the sputum of uranium miners, concluded that human lung cancers develop through a series of identifiable stages, namely squamous cell metaplasia, squamous cell metaplasia with atypia (mild, moderate, or severe), carcinoma in situ, and invasive carcinoma.

Saccomanno and colleagues[99] treated 26 subjects in a nonrandomized trial; all subjects had documented abnormalities in sputum samples subjected to cytologic analysis ranging from moderate atypical metaplasia to overt carcinoma. The subjects received 1 to 2.5 mg/kg/day of 13-*cis*-retinoic acid. No improvement was found in the degree of atypia after this treatment, but alterations in cellular morphology were noted, including increased intracytoplasmic and intranuclear vacuolation, bizarre nuclear shapes, nuclear membrane rupture, and pyknotic nuclei.

Three randomized placebo-controlled trials have incorporated sputum cytology studies of bronchial squamous metaplasia and atypia as a potential intermediate endpoint marker for lung chemoprevention trials. The first trial by Heimburger and associates[71] evaluated the effects of folate and vitamin B_{12} on squamous metaplasia in smokers, which was based on the hypothesis that a folate deficiency secondary to cigarette smoking was a contributing factor in the development of bronchial metaplasia. Several investigators had previously reported that smokers with bronchial squamous metaplasia had lower plasma folate levels than smokers without bronchial squamous metaplasia. Three hundred and eleven males with a smoking history of at least 20 pack-years were evaluated for the presence of bronchial squamous metaplasia by cytologic measures. One hundred and eight male smokers who showed squamous metaplasia on at least one of the initial three samples were invited to return for entry into the study. Of these, 80 individuals were randomized to receive either placebo or folate (10 mg) and vitamin B_{12} (500 μ) orally for 4 months, and 73 were evaluable. Plasma folate and red blood cell folate were found to markedly increase in the group that received folate and vitamin B_{12}, whereas no change was noted in the placebo group. At both study entry and termination, sputum was resampled five times during a 10- to 14-day period, and the worst cytologic score of the five samples from each subject was used in analysis. The number of subjects in whom the worst sputum cytology score improved after 4 months of intervention was significantly higher in the 36 subjects who received folate and vitamin B_{12} than in the 37 subjects who received placebo (38.9% versus 16.2%; p = .03). However, the significance of this finding is tempered by substantial spontaneous variation in sputum cytologies. Despite the fact that all the study subjects had squamous metaplasia on at least one of the initial three sputum samples on screening, repeat examination of five subsequent sputum samples obtained on study termination failed to show squamous metaplasia in 24 (32.9%) of the 73 evaluable subjects.

In the second randomized trial, Arnold and colleagues[100] screened 298 subjects with minimum of a 15 pack-year history of cigarette smoking for the presence of atypia on sputum cytology; of those 298 subjects, 229 demonstrated sufficient atypia to be eligible for the study. One hundred and fifty individuals who showed mild atypia on at least two of three specimens or moderate or severe atypia on at least one of three specimens were randomized to receive either placebo or etretinate 25 mg orally/day. Compliance was high, as documented by pill counts and serum etretinate levels: There were detectable levels of etretinate in 92.8% of subjects in the etretinate group but in only 2.3% of subjects in the placebo group.[101] Of the 138 evaluable subjects who completed 6 months of treatment, 23 (32.4%) of 71 subjects on etretinate and 20 (29.9%) of 67 subjects on placebo showed improvement in the degree of atypia (p = .45). In a subset of smokers who had moderate or severe atypia, 16 (32%) of 50 individuals improved on etretinate and 16 (30.2%) of 53 improved on placebo (p = .51). Again, this study demonstrated that the observed improvement was in most part due to substantial variation in sputum cytology results. But the lack of a difference in the rate of improvement in sputum atypia between the two groups led to the conclusion that etretinate at the dose used in that study had no impact on sputum atypia as detected by sputum cytology.

The third trial[102] evaluating the effects of beta-carotene and retinol on sputum atypia in workers exposed to asbestos is ongoing. The study is based on two observations: First, the presence of marked atypia in the sputum of asbestos-exposed workers is a risk factor for the development of lung cancer, whereas low levels of atypia or normal sputum cytology are predictive of not developing cancer.[103] Second, serum beta-carotene levels in this group of patients are very low, and increasing them may be beneficial.[104] Individuals with a significant history of asbestos exposure were screened for dysplasia by sputum cytologic analysis. Individuals who successfully completed a 6-week run-in period were randomized to receive either 50 mg of beta-carotene per day and 25,000 IU retinol every other day or placebo. Initial sputum cytologic examinations found normal sputum in 8.2%, squamous metaplasia in 39.4%, mild atypia in 41.2%, moderate atypia in 10.1%, and severe atypia in 1.1%. Cancer was not identified in any of the initial specimens. The primary endpoint of this trial is change in the sputum cytology. At last report, 1073 patients had been screened and 705 had been randomized. Compliance is estimated at approximately 93%, and only 14.4% of patients on the treatment arm have serum beta-carotene levels below the 75th percentile level of the placebo group, which indicates that supplementation is being achieved.

The advantage of sputum atypia as an intermediate endpoint marker lies in its wide use and noninvasiveness. However, this marker's disadvantage is in its high variability on repeat sampling and its high rate of spontaneous improvement,[105] as exemplified by the randomized trial of Arnold and colleagues,[100] in which improvement in sputum atypia was noted not only in 32.4% of 71 etretinate-treated subjects but also in 29.9% of 67 subjects in the placebo-treated group. Using squamous metaplasia documented by histologic evaluation of standard bronchoscopic biopsy specimens as a study endpoint, French investigators[106–108] evaluated the effects of etretinate on the bronchial metaplasia index in 70 smokers with a smoking history of 15 pack-years or more. In that nonrandomized trial, the investigators obtained bronchial biopsies from 10 standardized regions during fiberoptic bronchoscopy. A metaplasia index was calculated for each patient indicating the number of sections exhibiting squamous cell metaplasia compared with the total number of sections counted. The patients who had a metaplasia index greater than 15% were treated daily for 6 months with etretinate 25 mg orally. At the time of the first report, 12 patients had completed the prescribed therapy, and the metaplasia index had decreased in 10 of the 11 subjects evaluated.[106] The follow-up report showed that out of the 40 evaluable participants, 29 (72.5%) had reductions in metaplasia index. The mean metaplasia index decreased from 34.6% before treatment to 27% following treatment (p < .001) despite continued smoking.[108] Four patients who ceased smoking were not included in this analysis; their metaplasia indices were reported to have decreased to 0%.

Encouraged by these promising results, investigators at the M.D. Anderson Cancer Center conducted a randomized placebo-controlled trial using 13-*cis*-retinoic acid as a chemopreventive agent.[109] Eligible subjects had a history of smoking for more than 15 pack-years; all underwent bronchoscopy, with biopsies obtained at six designated sites. Individuals with either dysplasia or a metaplasia index greater than 15% were randomized to receive either 13-*cis*-retinoic acid (1 mg/kg/day) or placebo for 6 months. As of the most recent report, 69 patients had undergone follow-up bronchoscopy. Nineteen of 35 subjects on 13-*cis*-retinoic acid and 20 of 34 subjects on placebo had a decrease in 8% or more. Furthermore, nine subjects in each group had complete reversal of metaplasia index. When the results were analyzed according to smoking status, statistically significant reductions in metaplasia index were noted among subjects in both groups who had stopped smoking before the repeat bronchoscopy was performed.

This trial and that by Arnold and colleagues[100] failed to demonstrate a significant reversal of squamous metaplasia by two widely studied retinoids, 13-cis-retinoic acid and etretinate. Nevertheless, these studies demonstrate several issues that need to be addressed. First, as mentioned earlier, a high degree of variability exists in studies using cytologic or histologic changes as intermediate endpoints. Because the control groups of all of the randomized trials reported significant changes in the measured marker, these changes probably represent the degree of random change inherent in the intermediate markers used. Second, the grading of atypia by sputum cytologic analysis is very subjective, requiring confirmation by multiple investigators. Third, despite the known variability of squamous metaplasia, it was possible to quantitate the global effects of smoking cessation by the sizable changes in the metaplasia index. This point has a very important clinical implication. In future trials, if a biomarker is to be used as a surrogate endpoint, the confounding effects of smoking cessation should be taken into consideration. Finally, although histologic changes in the bronchial epithelium have been considered to correlate with the risk of lung cancer, they have not been proved to relate directly to the development of lung cancer, nor has reversal of these lesions been proved to reverse cancer risk. Therefore, the beneficial effects seen in some studies using changes in the bronchial epithelium detected by either bronchoscopy or sputum cytologic analysis will require confirmation in chemoprevention trials in which the primary endpoint is the development of cancer. Conversely, a lack of significant improvement in these intermediate biomarkers does not rule out the possibility that an agent will have activity in preventing lung cancer. Therefore, the lack of benefit should not dampen the enthusiasm for designing new chemoprevention trials, nor should it be used to justify discontinuation of ongoing trials. Rather, there is a need to continue to develop biomarkers that may be more predictive of clinical outcome.

A recent placebo-controlled trial in 114 smokers studied the effects of beta-carotene on micronuclei frequency in sputum cytology specimens.[110] Micronuclei frequency is a short-term marker of clastogenic exposure to DNA. During the 14-week intervention, a 47% decrease in micronuclei counts was observed in the beta-carotene group compared with a 16% decrease in the placebo group. Although this finding is interesting, micronuclei frequency is a nonspecific and highly variable endpoint that creates many difficulties of interpretation. Micronuclei frequency has been extensively studied in the context of oral leukoplakia intervention trials and has been found to show no correlation with histopathology or with clinical or histologic

response to many chemopreventive agents, including retinoids, beta-carotene, and vitamin E.

PATIENTS AT RISK FOR SECOND PRIMARY TUMORS

As mentioned earlier, patients with a history of aerodigestive tract tumors have a markedly increased risk of developing lung and head and neck cancer[35, 36]; several chemoprevention trials have, therefore, used this group of patients to evaluate the efficacy of chemopreventive agents.

Head and Neck Trials

In a recently reported Phase III study, adjuvant 13-cis-retinoic acid has been found to decrease the rate of second primary tumor development.[7, 9] Patients with Stage I to IV squamous cell carcinoma of the head and neck who were rendered disease-free after local therapy (surgery and/or radiotherapy) were randomized to receive 13-cis-retinoic acid (50 to 100 mg/m^2/day) or placebo for 12 months. Adjuvant 13-cis-retinoic acid had no effect on the patterns of primary disease recurrence—local, regional, or distant. There was a statistically significant difference (p = .0046), however, between the two study arms in the rate of second primary tumor development (Fig. 16–1). In the most recent report (median follow-up of 55 months), seven patients (14%) in the 13-cis-retinoic acid group developed second primaries compared with 16 patients (31%) in the placebo group. This reduction in second primary tumors associated with 13-cis-retinoic acid treatment remains statistically significant (p = .04). The average annual second primary tumor rate in the retinoid group was 3.1% compared with a placebo rate of 6.8%, representing a rate reduction of 54%. The high dose of 13-cis-retinoic acid used in this study produced frequent moderate-to-severe toxicities, including cheilitis, dry skin, and conjunctivitis.

As expected with relatively short-term retinoid intervention, the difference in overall second primary tumor rates between the 13-cis-retinoic acid and placebo arms has diminished over time with long-term follow-up.[111] The greatest difference between the study arms occurred within the first 2 years (odds ratio, 6.9), dropping significantly with extended follow-up (odds ratio, approximately 2).

In a subset analysis, 13-cis-retinoic acid had a greater effect on second primaries occurring within the tobacco-exposed field of the head and neck, esophagus, and lungs than on the overall analysis of second primaries occurring at any site. Four patients (8%) in the 13-cis-retinoic acid arm and 14 patients (27%) in the placebo arm have developed tobacco-related second primary tumors (p = .008). Furthermore, the retinoid effect on second primary tumor development within the target epithelial field at risk (head and neck, lung and esophagus) has persisted. The odds ratio (13-cis-retinoic acid versus placebo second primary tumor rates) between the study arms

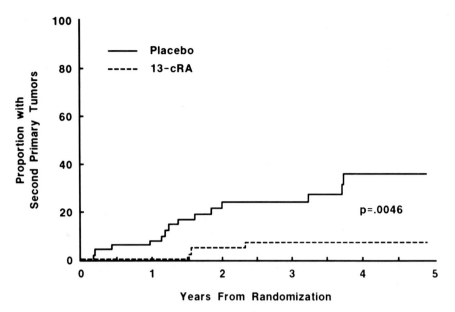

FIGURE 16–1. Cumulative risk of developing second primary tumors after 13-*cis*-retinoic acid treatment in head and neck cancer patients. (From Lippman SM, Hong WK: Retinoid chemoprevention of upper aerodigestive tract carcinogenesis. *In* DeVita VT, Hellman S, Rosenberg SA [eds]: Important Advances in Oncology 1992. Philadelphia, J.B. Lippincott, 1992, pp 93–109.)

has remained at approximately 5 throughout the study follow-up. This finding is unprecedented. Previous studies from preclinical in vivo models and clinical trials have found that the chemopreventive activity of retinoids declines after stopping the intervention.

Because of the substantial toxicity observed with high-dose 13-*cis*-retinoic acid and the need for long-term intervention, current head and neck and lung second primary tumor chemoprevention trials are studying lower 13-*cis*-retinoic acid doses, which have their bases in oral leukoplakia intervention studies.

Notwithstanding its reduced second primary tumor rates, the 13-*cis*-retinoic acid group did not have a statistically significant improvement in survival over the placebo group. Survival figures at the median follow-up of 55 months are 62% in the 13-*cis*-retinoic acid group and 53% in the placebo group (p = .37). Several factors contributed to the lack of a significant retinoid impact on overall survival: (1) identical rates of primary disease recurrence (not second primary tumors) in both arms, (2) a high drop-out rate in the 13-*cis*-retinoic acid arm due in large part to significant toxicity of the retinoid at high doses, and (3) improved second primary tumor survival in the placebo group due to early detection and therapy.

This 13-*cis*-retinoic acid adjuvant head and neck trial led directly to two large-scale NCI trials developed at M.D. Anderson Cancer Center and activated through the multicenter cooperative group network in the United States. These Phase III trials are testing the efficacy of low-dose (30 mg/kg/day) 13-*cis*-retinoic acid to prevent second primary tumors associated with head and neck and lung cancer in stage T1–N0 patients.[112] The head and neck study was activated through the Radiation Therapy Oncology Group (RTOG) in February 1992 and, as of July 1994, has accrued over 500 of 1080 planned patients. The number of person-years of follow-up for the trial is relatively low at the present time. Early information from

this study suggests that the treatment is well tolerated. The lung trial is discussed in detail later.

Four other large-scale trials in chemoprevention for head and neck second primary tumors are being conducted, two in the United States and two in Europe.[112] The United States trials are testing beta-carotene (50 mg/day) and very low dose 13-*cis*-retinoic acid (5 to 10 mg/day). One of the European trials is a multicenter effort called EUROSCAN and involves 13 countries and 40 cancer centers.[113] This trial employs a 2 × 2 factorial design to test retinyl palmitate (300,000 IU/day in year 1; 150,000 IU/day in year 2) and N-acetyl-cysteine (600 mg/day for 2 years) in patients previously treated for early-stage squamous cancer of the larynx or oral cavity or early stage non–small cell lung cancer (non–SCLC). The other European trial is a French cooperative trial of low-dose etretinate (25 mg/day for 2 years) in patients with T1–2, N0–1 squamous cell cancer of the oral cavity and oropharynx.

Lung Trials

Because cancers of the head and neck and lung share the common etiologic and biologic features of field and multistep carcinogenesis, strategies for chemoprevention of second primary tumors in patients with head and neck cancers might be expanded to those with lung cancers. As discussed earlier, individuals with stage I non–SCLC cancer have an increased risk of developing a second primary tumor of the lung (see Table 16–2).

In a recently reported randomized trial, Pastorino and associates[60, 114] studied 307 patients who had complete resection of a stage I non–SCLC of the lung. Patients were eligible if they had microscopic residual disease, as long as they received consolidation with adjuvant radiotherapy. Patients were randomized to receive either 300,000 IU of retinyl palmitate daily (150 patients) or no treatment (157 patients) for 12 months. The primary endpoints for this adjuvant trial were tumor recurrence and second primary tumor (SPT). Compliance was estimated to be over 80%, that is, over 80% of doses were taken correctly during this period, and toxicity was minimal; three patients withdrew because of symptoms that may have been related to the drug. With a median follow-up of 46 months, 37% of the patients in the retinyl group had developed either recurrence or a second primary tumor, compared with 48% of the patients in the placebo group. Overall, second primary tumors occurred in 29 of the control patients and in 18 of the patients on retinyl palmitate. Multiple second primary tumors developed only in the control group. The average annual second primary tumor rate was 4.8% in the control group and 3.1% in the 13-*cis*-retinoic acid group, reflecting a 35% reduction in the average annual second primary rate in the retinoid arm. The majority of second primary tumors (more than 70%) were tobacco related, such as those located in the head and neck, lung, and bladder. Tobacco-related second primaries developed in 13 patients in the retinoid group and 25 in the control group. In a subset analysis, the time to development of a tobacco-related second primary tumor (based on patient count rather than SPT count) was significantly longer in the retinoid group than in the placebo group (p = .045) (Fig. 16–2). The 5-year disease-free survival rate was 64% for the treated group and 51% for the control group (p = .054). The overall survival rate was better in the group that received retinoid treatment (66%) than in the placebo group (57%), but the difference was not statistically significant (p = .3).

The mechanism of retinoid chemoprevention in the lung and head and neck carcinogenesis is under intensive study. Nuclear RARs, members of the steroid receptor family, have been shown to mediate retinoid effects. Recent preclinical and clinical data suggest that reduced RAR-beta expression is associated both with the progression of head and neck carcinogenesis and possibly with retinoid activity.[112] Recent in vitro and in vivo work also suggest a critical role of RAR-beta in lung cancer.[115-118] Taken together, these data suggest the intriguing possibility that retinoid suppression of second primary tumor development throughout the aerodigestive tract may result from regulation of RAR-beta.

The EORTC trial,[113] as indicated above, is completing a large prospective randomized trial testing the efficacy of retinyl palmitate or N-acetylcysteine, or both, versus placebo in the prevention of relapse and second primary tumors in patients who have had either head and neck and lung cancer. Patients treated for squamous cell carcinoma of the larynx (T1–3, N1–0), squamous cell carcinoma of the oropharynx (T1–2, N0–1), or non–SCLC of the lung (T1–2, N0–1, and T3N0) are eligible and are randomized to receive retinyl palmitate, N-acetylcysteine, a combination of both agents, or placebo. Accrual of the target 2000 patients should now be complete.

Finally, a randomized Intergroup trial (NCI I91-0001) has been activated to test the efficacy of 13-*cis*-retinoic acid in preventing the occurrence of second primary tumors following the resection of Stage I non–SCLC.[119] Patients who have had a non–SCLC resected whose tumor is either T1 or T2 and N0M0 and who are 6 weeks to 36 months into the postresection period are eligible. Following an 8-week placebo run-in period, during which patients must consume at least 75% of their capsules, patients are randomized to receive either 13-*cis*-retinoic acid (30 mg/day) or placebo for 3 years. The lower dose of 13-*cis*-retinoic acid was chosen because a significant number of patients in the previous head and neck trial[7] discontinued therapy because of toxic effects when 13-*cis*-retinoic acid was given at 50 mg/m²/day. Furthermore, recent evidence indicates that 13-*cis*-retinoic acid at the lower dose has significant biologic activity in aerodigestive tract carcinogenesis: It was effective in maintaining remissions of oral leukoplakia.[94] The accrual goal for this study is 1260 patients, a number that will allow detection of a 50% reduction in the incidence of second primary tumors with an 80% power assuming an incidence of second primary tumors of 2% to 3% per year. As of September 1994, approximately 600 patients had been entered on the study, and accrual is increasing as the study opens throughout all major cooperative oncology groups with more than 100 institutions now registered.

The high rate of second primary tumors in patients with aerodigestive tract malignancies allows smaller sample sizes than would be possible with other high-risk groups. Research in this group has several disadvantages, however. Distinction of a second primary tumor from relapse of a primary can be difficult, because the two tumors may be of similar histologic types and the lung is a frequent site of metastasis for both head and neck cancer and non–SCLC of the lung. Also, the time to the development of a cancer may be long, necessitating several years of follow-up to detect an advantage for a given chemoprevention strategy.

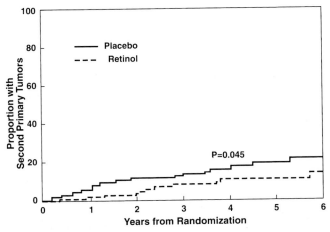

FIGURE 16–2. Cumulative risk of developing second primary tumors in the chemoprevention field (lung, head and neck, or bladder) after treatment with retinyl palmitate in non–small cell lung cancer patients. (Redrawn from Pastorino U, Infante M, Maioli M, et al: Adjuvant treatment of stage I lung cancer with high-dose vitamin A. J Clin Oncol 11:1216–1222, 1993.)

In addition, the need for chemoprevention study to complement established smoking cessation measures in SCLC is pressing because cured SCLC patients have one of the highest rates of second primary tumor development.[35]

SCREENING AND EARLY DETECTION

Prevention of lung cancer deaths by detecting the cancer at an earlier, more treatable stage via screening remains an attractive option.[6] In the 1970s, three large NCI-sponsored randomized studies assessed the efficacy of lung cancer screening with chest x-ray study and sputum cytology in approximately 30,000 male smokers. Two studies, the Memorial-Sloan Kettering Lung Project (MSKLP) and the Johns Hopkins Lung Project (JHLP) compared annual chest x-ray screening with chest x-ray study plus every 4-month sputum cytology assessments.[120, 121] Both studies found that the addition of standard sputum cytology assessments to chest x-ray study did not improve resectability, survival, or mortality rates. These two studies did not assess the impact of chest x-ray screening because all subjects in both studies underwent annual chest x-ray studies.

The third study, the Mayo Lung Project, compared a group in which dual screening (chest x-ray study plus 4-month cytology) was obtained to a control group in which screening was recommended but compliance was not enforced.[122] Approximately half of the control group had annual chest x-ray studies. Therefore, the study actually compared an intensively screened group to a less consistently and less intensively screened group. The studies all showed no improvement in mortality rate (the number of cancer deaths per number of subjects screened) in the more intensively screened group (122 lung cancer deaths or a mortality rate of 3.2 per 1000 patients per year) than in the control group (115 deaths or 3.0 per 1000).

However, because the screened group had a higher resectability rate (46% versus 32%) and 5-year survival rate (33% versus 15%), the fatality rate (number of cancer deaths per number of cancer cases) was significantly lower in the screened group (59% versus 72%, p = .016). The still unexplained problem, which accounted for the equivalent overall lung mortality rates in the two study groups (despite improved survival and fatality rates in the screened group), was that the absolute number of lung cancer cases detected in the screened group was greater than the number in the control group (122 versus 115). The explanation for the difference of 46 lung cancer cases between the screened and control groups is unknown and has been the subject of continuing discussion and debate.[123, 124] Proposed explanations for the increased lung cancer incidence in this and the one other randomized study that evaluated the role of chest x-ray screening (from Czechoslovakia) include screening bias (overdiagnosis, selection, lead-time and length bias) and chance imbalance (statistical chance alone or a chance imbalance of cancer risk factors). The fa-

vored explanation, that of overdiagnosis (i.e., diagnosis of clinically unimportant [benign] lung cancer),[123] is not supported by findings of large autopsy series or by the survival rates of screen-detected but not resected lung cancers from the large screening studies.[124]

Despite these unresolved issues, a consistent finding in all study groups that included chest x-ray screening (both study groups from the MSKLP and JHLP studies and the screened group from the Mayo study) was that the 5- to 10-year lung cancer survival rates were roughly threefold higher than the lung cancer survival rates in the Mayo control group and the general population (i.e., NCI SEER figures). These findings suggest that chest x-ray screening may be beneficial.

Based on the many issues discussed earlier, the potential role of standard chest x-ray screening of high-risk subjects is still incompletely resolved. However, newer biochemical and molecular markers of malignancy may allow detection of very early lung lesions before they are detectable with standard sputum cytology or chest x-ray study techniques. Tockman and associates[125] screened the first available stored sputum cytology samples from 69 patients previously entered in the Johns Hopkins Lung Project (discussed earlier) using two monoclonal antibodies developed against antigens found on SCLC and non–SCLC cell lines. As a control, 40 samples were randomly selected from the 537 subjects with less than marked atypia who did not go on to develop lung cancer. Also included in the analysis were all three subjects with marked atypia who did not develop lung cancer. A total of 26 patients who did develop lung cancer were randomly selected: 15 from the 40 patients with less than marked atypia, and 11 from the 46 individuals with marked atypia. Of these 26 patients, 22 first-collected sputum samples were satisfactory for analysis after immunostaining and 14 of these were positive for antibody staining, achieving a sensitivity of 64%. The average interval from the first specimen to the diagnosis of lung cancer in the false-negative population was 57 months, whereas the interval in the true-positive population averaged approximately 24 months. Re-evaluation of later sputum samples from the false-negative patients revealed several additional positive specimens, increasing the sensitivity to 91%.

A large prospective trial is under way to assess the efficacy of these monoclonal antibodies in identifying second primary cancer lung cancer in patients who have completed treatment for stage I non–SCLC. Second primary lung tumors, for the purpose of this study, are defined as (1) lung cancer of different histology than the index cancer or (2) cancer of the same histology with features of primary lung cancer occurring more than 2 years after the index tumor and developing in a different lobe. Overall, second primary tumors in non–SCLC develop at a rate of 4% to 5% per year in prospective studies.[114] Data from the Lung Cancer Study Group indicate that the annual rate of second primary lung cancer development in this patient population is approximately 3%. The results from this *second primary* tumor early detection may have important implications for subsequent *primary* lung cancer early detection studies.

The early detection protocol has been modified to include essentially identical eligibility criteria as in the lung cancer second primary tumor chemoprevention trial testing low-dose 13-*cis*-retinoic acid (INT NCI I91-0001). Therefore, patients with T1–2,N0 non–SCLC after definitive resection who have nonmalignant sputum cytology are eligible to enter two related studies (one of early detection and one of retinoid chemoprevention). This novel strategy includes optimal usage of NCI or health care resources to help coordinate and enhance patient accrual in both large-scale trials. Furthermore, these studies illustrate, in part, the close relationship of the two evolving cancer control modalities of early detection and chemoprevention.

CONCLUSION AND FUTURE DIRECTIONS

Despite many significant advances in recent decades, treatment and primary prevention efforts have not made a significant impact on morbidity and mortality resulting from major cancers, such as those of the lung, head and neck, and colon. Primary prevention is difficult to institute not only because it requires changing behavioral patterns (e.g., getting smokers to quit) but it also does not help many people already exposed to potentially lethal carcinogens. Chemoprevention, a new cancer control modality, is a multidisciplinary approach involving clinicians, epidemiologists, statisticians, basic scientists, and behavioral scientists. The two fundamental theories of multistep carcinogenesis and field carcinogenesis have provided the conceptional framework on which chemoprevention study is constructed. Early clinical trials have suggested that chemoprevention has great potential, and the results of several ongoing, large randomized trials will clarify the effectiveness of current chemoprevention strategies. Although it is designed to work as an adjunct to, rather than as a replacement for, established cancer treatment and control modalities, development of effective chemopreventive strategies will decrease the cancer-related morbidity and mortality, not only from those arising in the upper aerodigestive tract but also in many other sites. Further efforts to identify new chemopreventive agents and optimization of the use of available agents, combined with identification of useful intermediate biomarkers, are expected to generate exciting results.

SELECTED REFERENCES

Chung KY, Mukhopadhyay T, Kim J, et al: Discordant p53 gene mutations in primary head and neck cancers and corresponding second primary cancers of the upper aerodigestive tract. Cancer Res 53:1676–1683, 1993.
This study of primary head and neck tumors and second primary tumors provided molecular support for the concept of field carcinogenesis. The study found a high rate of discordance of p53 mutations in the primary and related second primary tumors strongly suggesting an independent genetic origin of these tumors.

Hong WK, Lippman SM, Itri LM, et al: Prevention of second primary tumors in squamous cell carcinoma of the head and neck. N Engl J Med 323:795–801, 1990.
This was a Phase III placebo-controlled adjuvant trial of high-dose isotretinoin in head and neck cancer. The study observed a significantly lower rate of second primary tumors in the retinoid arm. There was no difference between the arms in the rate of primary tumor recurrence (local, regional, distant) or survival.

Lee JS, Lippman SM, Benner SE, et al: Randomized placebo-controlled trial of isotretinoin in chemoprevention of bronchial squamous metaplasia. J Clin Oncol 12:937–945, 1994.
This was a randomized placebo-controlled trial of isotretinoin in chronic smokers with bronchial metaplasia and dysplasia determined by bronchoscopic biopsies. The study found no effect of the retinoid on the reversal of metaplasia. Smoking cessation was the only factor that significantly correlated with reversal of metaplasia.

Lippman SM, Benner SE, Hong WK: Cancer chemoprevention. J Clin Oncol 12:851–873, 1994.
An extensive review of the most important advances in biologic studies and clinical trials in the field of cancer chemoprevention.

Pastorino U, Infante M, Maioli M, et al: Adjuvant treatment of stage I lung cancer with high-dose vitamin A. J Clin Oncol 11:1216–1222, 1993.
This was a Phase III adjuvant trial of high-dose retinyl palmitate versus no treatment in Stage I non–small cell lung cancer. The trial reported a significant increase in the time to development of a tobacco-related second primary tumor. Nonsignificant improvements in disease-free survival and overall survival were observed in the retinoid arm.

Tockman MS, Gupta PK, Myers JD, et al: Sensitive and specific monoclonal antibody recognition of human lung cancer antigen on preserved sputum cells: A new approach to early lung cancer detection. J Clin Oncol 6:1685–1693, 1988.
This study provided evidence that lung cancer screening with more sensitive biologic markers could lead to earlier cancer detection. The study employed monoclonal antibodies (known to react with lung cancer surface antigens) on stored sputum cytology samples from the Johns Hopkins Lung Project, a large screening study from the 1970s.

REFERENCES

1. Parkin DM, Laara E, Muir CS. Estimates of the worldwide frequency of 16 major cancers in 1980. Int J Cancer 41:184–197, 1988.
2. Centers for Disease Control: Cigarette smoking among adults—United States, 1991. MMWR 42:230–233, 1993.
3. The health consequences of smoking. Nicotine addiction: A report of the surgeon general. U.S. Dept of Health and Human Services, 1988.
4. Garfinkel L, Stellman SD: Smoking and lung cancer in women: Findings in a prospective study. Cancer Res 48:6951–6955, 1988.
5. Boring CC, Squires TS, Tong T, Montgomery S: Cancer Statistics. CA Cancer J Clin 44:7–26, 1994.
6. Frost JK, Fontana RS, McClamed MR, et al: Early lung cancer detection: Summary and conclusions. Am Rev Respir Dis 130:565–570, 1984.
7. Hong WK, Lippman SM, Itri LM, et al: Prevention of second primary tumors with isotretinoin in squamous cell carcinoma of the head and neck. N Engl J Med 323:795–801, 1990.
8. Kraemer KH, DiGiovanna JJ, Moshell AN, et al: Prevention of skin cancer in xeroderma pigmentosum with the use of isotretinoin. N Engl J Med 318:1633–1637, 1988.
9. Lippman SM, Hong WK: Retinoid chemoprevention of upper aerodigestive tract carcinogenesis. In DeVita VT, Hellman S, Rosenberg SA (eds): Important Advances in Oncology 1992. Philadelphia, J.B. Lippincott Company, 1992, pp. 93–109.
10. Sporn MB: Carcinogenesis and cancer: Different perspectives on the same disease. Cancer Res 51:6215–6218, 1991.
11. Garner RC, Cuzick J, Jenkins D, et al: Linear relationship between DNA adducts in human lung and cigarette smoking. IARC Sci Publ 104:421–426, 1990.

12. Phillips DH, Schoket B, Hewer A, et al: Influence of cigarette smoking on the levels of DNA adducts in human bronchial epithelium and white blood cells. Int J Cancer 46:569–575, 1990.

13. Phillips DH, Hewer A, Martin CN, et al: Correlation of DNA adduct levels in human lung with cigarette smoking. Nature 336:790–792, 1988.

14. Stich HF: Micronucleated exfoliated cells as indicator for genotoxic damage and as markers in chemoprevention trials. J Nutr Growth Cancer 4:9–18, 1987.

15. Oschsner A, DeBakey M: Carcinoma of the lung. Arch Surg 42:209–258, 1941.

16. Wynder EL, Graham EA: Tobacco smoking as a possible etiologic factor in bronchogenic carcinoma: A study of six hundred and eighty-four proved cases. JAMA 143:329–336, 1950.

17. Doll R, Hill AB: Smoking and carcinoma of the lung: Preliminary report. Br Med J 2:739–748, 1950.

18. Lee JS, Hong WK. Biology of preneoplastic lesions. In Roth JA, Cox JD, Hong WK (eds): Lung Cancer. Cambridge, Mass., Blackwell Scientific Publications, 1993, pp 34–56.

19. Auerbach O, Stout AP, Hammond EC, et al: Changes in bronchial epithelium in relation to cigarette smoking and in relation to lung cancer. N Engl J Med 265:253–267, 1961.

20. Trichopoulus D, Mollo F, Tomatis L, et al: Active and passive smoking and pathological indicators of lung cancer risk in an autopsy series. JAMA 268:1697–1701, 1992.

21. Slaughter DP, Southwick HW, Smejkal W: "Field cancerization" in oral stratified squamous epithelium: Clinical implications of multicentric origin. Cancer 6:963–968, 1953.

22. Inman DS, Harris CC: Oncogenes and tumor suppressor genes in human lung carcinogenesis. Crit Rev Oncog 2:161–171, 1991.

23. Ihde DC, Minna JD. Non-small cell lung cancer. Part I. Biology, diagnosis, and staging. Curr Probl Cancer 15:61–104, 1991.

24. Lee JS, Pathak S, Hopwood V, et al: Involvement of chromosome 7 in primary lung tumor and nonmalignant normal lung tissue. Cancer Res 47:6349–6352, 1987.

25. Miura I, Siegfried JM, Resau J, et al: Chromosome alterations in 21 non-small cell lung carcinomas. Genes, Chromosomes and Cancer 2:328–338, 1990.

26. Sozzi G, Miozzo M, Tagliabue E, et al: Cytogenetic abnormalities and overexpression of receptors for growth factors in normal bronchial epithelium and tumor samples of lung cancer patients. Cancer Res 51:400–404, 1991.

27. Hittelman WN, Wang ZW, Cheong N, et al: Premature chromosome condensation and cytogenetics of human solid tumors. Cancer Bulletin 41:298–305, 1989.

28. Sohn HY, Cheong N, Wang ZW, Hong WK, et al: Detection of aneuploidy in normal lung tissue adjacent to lung tumor by premature chromosome condensation. Cancer Genet Cytogenet 41:250, 1989.

29. Hittelman WN, Cheong N, Sohn HY, et al: Tumorigenesis and tumor response: View from the (prematurely condensed) chromosome. In Obe G, Natarajan AT (eds). Chromosomal Aberrations: Basic and Applied Aspects (Advances in Mutagenesis Research). Berlin, Springer-Verlag, 1990, pp. 101–112.

30. Kim SY, Lee JS, Ro JY, et al: Interphase cytogenetics in paraffin sections of lung tumors by non-isotopic in-situ hybridization: Mapping genotype/phenotype heterogenicity. Am J Pathol 142:307–317, 1993.

31. Voravud N, Shin DM, Ro JY, et al: Increased polysomies of chromosome 7 and 17 during head and neck cancer multistage tumorigenesis. Cancer Res 53:2874–2883, 1993.

32. Lee JS, Kim SY, Hong WK, et al: Detection of chromosomal polysomy in oral leukoplakia, a premalignant lesion. J Natl Cancer Inst 85:1951–1954, 1993.

33. Gazdar AF, Hung J, Walker L, et al: Extensive areas of dysplasia and aneuploidy of the entire bronchial mucosal tract accompanies non-small cell lung cancers (NSCLC) and provides evidence for the field cancerization theory. Proc Am Soc Clin Oncol 12:334, 1993.

34. Chung KY, Mukhopadhyay T, Kim J, et al: Discordant p53 gene mutations in primary head and neck cancers and corresponding second primary cancers of the upper aerodigestive tract. Cancer Res 53:1676–1683, 1993.

35. Ihde DC, Tucker MA: Secondary primary malignancies in small cell lung cancer: A major consequence of modest success. J Clin Oncol 10:1511–1513, 1992.

36. Christensen P, Joergensen K, Munk J, et al: Hyperfrequency of pulmonary cancer in a population of 415 patients treated for laryngeal cancer. Laryngoscope 97:612–614, 1987.

37. Shields TW, Humphrey EW, Higgins GA, et al: Long term survivors after resection of lung carcinoma. J Thorac Cardiovasc Surg 76:439–442, 1978.

38. Van Bodegon PC, Wagenaar SS, Corrin B, et al: Second primary lung cancer: Importance of long term follow-up. Thorax 44:788–793, 1989.

39. Thomas P, Rubinstein L: The Lung Cancer Study Group: Cancer recurrence after resection: T1N0 non-small cell lung cancer. Ann Thorac Surg 49:242–247, 1990.

40. Thomas PA, Rubinstein L: The Lung Cancer Study Group: Late appearance of malignancies after surgery for T1N0 non-small cell lung cancer. Lung Cancer 7 (Suppl):82, 1991.

41. Smith RA, Nigan BK, Thompson JM. Second primary lung carcinoma. Thorax 31:507–516, 1976.

42. Pairolero PC, Williams DE, Bergstrahl EJ, et al: Postsurgical stage I bronchogenic carcinoma: Morbid implications of recurrent disease. Ann Thorac Surg 38:331–338, 1984.

43. Craig J, Powell B, Muss HB, Kawamoto E, et al: Second primary bronchogenic carcinomas after small cell carcinoma: Report of two cases and review of the literature. Am J Med 176:1013–1020, 1984.

44. Johnson BE, Ihde DC, Matthews MJ, et al: Non-small cell lung cancer: Major cause of late mortality in patients with small cell lung cancer. Am J Med 80:1103–1110, 1986.

45. Osterlind K, Hansen HH, Hansen M, et al: Mortality and morbidity in long-term surviving patients treated with chemotherapy with or without irradiation for small cell lung cancer. J Clin Oncol 4:1044–1052, 1986.

46. Sagman U, Lishner M, Maki E, et al: Second primary malignancies following diagnosis of small cell lung cancer. J Clin Oncol 10:1525–1533, 1992.

47. Heyne KH, Lippman SM, Lee JJ, et al: The incidence of second primary tumors in long-term survivors of small cell lung cancer. J Clin Oncol 10:1519–1524, 1992.

48. Richardson GE, Vernon DJ, Phelps R, et al: Second tumors are the major cause of late mortality in long term survivors of small cell lung cancer. Lung Cancer 7(Suppl):175, 1991.

49. Hirayama T: Diet and Cancer. Nutr Cancer 1:67–81, 1979.

50. Willett WM, McMahon B: Diet and cancer: An overview. N Engl J Med 310:633–638, 1984.

51. Ziegler RG, Sund AF, Craft NE, et al: Does β-carotene explain why reduced cancer risk is associated with vegetable and fruit intake? Cancer Res 52 (Suppl):2060s–2066s, 1992.

52. Boone CW, Kelloff GJ, Malone WE: Identification of candidate cancer chemopreventive agents and their evaluation in animal models and human clinical trials: A review. Cancer Res 50:2–9, 1990.

53. Kelloff GJ, Boone CW, Malone WI: Recent results in preclinical and clinical drug development of chemopreventive agents at the National Cancer Institute. In Wattenberg L, Lipkin M, Boone CW, Kelloff GJ (eds): Cancer Chemoprevention. Boca Raton, Florida, CRC Press, 1992, pp 41–56.

54. Lippman SM, Benner SE, Hong WK. Cancer chemoprevention. J Clin Oncol 12:851–873, 1994.

55. Lehmann JM, Dawson MI, Hobbs PD, et al: Identification of retinoids with nuclear receptor subtype-selective activities. Cancer Res 51:4804–4809, 1991.

56. Lippman SM, Hong WK: 13-cis-retinoic acid and cancer chemoprevention. Natl Cancer Inst Monogr 13:111–115, 1992.

57. Lippman SM, Benner SE, Hong WK: Retinoids in chemoprevention of head and neck carcinogenesis. Prev Med 22:693–700, 1993.

58. Bollag W: Therapeutic effect of aromatic retinoid acid analog on chemically induced skin papillomas and carcinomas in mice. Eur J Cancer 10:731–737, 1974.

59. Bruley-Rosset M, Hercent T, Martinez J, et al: Prevention of spontaneous tumors of aged mice by immunopharmacological manipulation: Study of immune anti-tumor mechanisms. J Natl Cancer Inst 66:1113–1119, 1981.

60. Pastorino U, Soresi E, Clerici M, et al: Lung cancer chemoprevention with retinol palmitate. Acta Oncol 27:773–782, 1988.

61. Smith MA, Parkinson DR, Cheson BD, et al: Retinoids in cancer therapy. J Clin Oncol 10:839–864, 1992.

62. Kvale G, Bjelke E, Gart JJ: Dietary habits and lung cancer risk. Int J Cancer 31:397–405, 1983.

63. Shekelle RB, Lepper M, Liu S, Maliza C, et al: Dietary vitamin A and risk of cancer in the Western Electric Study. Lancet 2:1185–1190, 1981.

64. Paganini-Hill A, Chao A, Ross RK, et al: Vitamin A, β-carotene, and the risk of cancer: A prospective study. J Natl Cancer Inst 79:443–448, 1987.

65. Krombout D: Essential micronutrients in relation to carcinogenesis. Am J Clin Nutr 45:1361–1367, 1987.

66. Menkes MS, Constock GW, Vuilleumier JP, et al: Serum β-carotene, vitamins A and E, selenium and the risk of lung cancer. N Engl J Med 315:1250–1254, 1986.

67. Willett WC, Polk BP, Underwood BA, et al: Relation of serum vitamins A and E and carotenoids to the risk of cancer. N Engl J Med 310:430–434, 1989.

68. Peto R, Doll R, Buckley JD, Sporn MB. Can dietary β-carotene materially reduce human cancer rates? Nature 290:201–208, 1981.

69. Xu MJ, Plezia PM, Alberts DS, et al: Reduction in plasma or skin α-tocopherol concentration with long-term administration of β-carotene in humans and mice. J Natl Cancer Inst 84:1559–1565, 1992.

70. Heimburger DC, Krumdieck CL, Alexander CB, et al. Localized folic acid deficiency and bronchial metaplasia in smokers: Hypothesis and preliminary report. Nutr Int 3:54–60, 1987.

71. Heimburger DC, Alexander CB, Birch R, et al: Improvement in bronchial squamous metaplasia in smokers treated with folate and vitamin B$_{12}$. Report of a preliminary randomized, double-blind intervention trial. JAMA 259:1525–1530, 1988.

72. Chemoprevention Clinical Trials: U.S. Department of Health and Human Services, Washington, D.C., U.S. Government Printing Office, 1984.

73. Hennekens CH: Issues in the design and conduct of clinical trials. J Natl Cancer Inst 73:1473–1476, 1984.

74. Buring JE, Hennekens CH: The Women's Health Study: Summary of the study design. J Myocard Ischemia 4:27–29, 1993.

75. Lee JS, Hong WK, Ro JY, et al: Determination of biomarkers for intermediate end points in chemoprevention trials. Cancer Res 52 (Suppl):2707S–2710S, 1992.

76. Stampfer MJ, Willet WE, Hennekens CH: Choice of populations for cancer prevention trials. In Moon TE, Micozzi MS (eds): Nutrition and cancer prevention: Investigation of the role of micronutrients. New York: Marcel Dekker, 1989, pp 473–482.

77. Greenwald P, Cullen JW, Kelloff G, Pierson HF: Chemoprevention of lung cancer. Chest 96:14S–17S, 1989.

78. Grizzle J, Omenn G, Goodman G, et al: Design of the β-carotene and retinol efficacy trial (CARET) for chemoprevention of cancer in populations at high risk: Heavy smokers and asbestos-exposed workers. In Pastorino U, Hong WK (eds): Chemoimmuno Prevention of Cancer. New York, Thieme Medical Publishers 1991, pp 167–176.

79. Omenn GS: A double-blind randomized trial with beta-carotene and retinol in persons at high risk for lung cancer due to occupational asbestos exposure and/or cigarette smoking. Public Health Rev 16:99–125, 1988.

80. Hodgson JT, Jones RD: Mortality of asbestos workers in England and Wales 1971–1981. Br J Indust Med 43:1158–1164, 1986.

81. Kjuus H, Skjaerven R, Langard S, et al: A case-reference study of lung cancer, occupational exposure and smoking. II. Role of asbestos exposure. Scand J Work Environ Health 12:203–209, 1986.

82. Albanes D, Virtamo J, Rautalahta M, et al: Pilot study: The US-Finland lung cancer prevention trial. J Nutr Growth Cancer 3:207–214, 1986.

83. The Alpha-Tocopherol Beta Carotene Cancer Prevention Study Group: The effects of vitamin E and beta carotene on the incidence of lung cancer and other cancers in male smokers. N Engl J Med 330:1029–1035, 1994.

84. Xuan XZ, Schatzakin A, Mao BL, et al: Feasibility of conducting a lung cancer chemoprevention trial among tin miners in Yunnan, PR China. Cancer Causes and Control 2:175–182, 1991.

85. Lippman SM, Lee JS, Lotan R, et al: Biomarkers as intermediate end points in chemoprevention trials. J Natl Cancer Inst 82:555–560, 1990.

86. Rosin MP, Dunn BP, Stich HF: Use of intermediate end points in quantitating the response of precancerous lesions to chemopreventive agents. Canadian J Physiol Pharmacol 65:483–487, 1987.

87. Silverman S, Gorsky M, Lozada F: Oral leukoplakia and malignant transformation: A follow-up study of 257 patients. Cancer 53:563–568, 1984.

88. Wolf K: Zur vitamin A behandlung der leukoplakien. Arch Klin Exp Derm 206:495–498, 1957.

89. Silverman S, Renstrup G, Pindborg JJ: Studies in oral leukoplakias: III. Effects of vitamin A comparing clinical, histopathologic, cytologic and hematologic responses. Acta Odont Scand 21:271–292, 1963.

90. Stich HF, Rosin MP, Hornby AP, et al: Remission of oral leukoplakia and micronuclei in tobacco/betel quid chewers treated with beta carotene and with beta carotene plus vitamin A. Int J Cancer 42:195–199, 1988.

91. Garewal HS, Meyskens FL, Killen D, et al: Response of oral leukoplakia to beta-carotene. J Clin Oncol 8:1715–1720, 1990.

92. Benner SE, Winn RJ, Lippman SM, et al: Regression of oral leukoplakia with α-tocopherol: A community clinical oncology program chemoprevention study. J Natl Cancer Inst 85:44–47, 1993.

93. Hong WK, Endicott J, Itri LM, et al: 13-cis-retinoic acid in the treatment of oral leukoplakia. N Engl J Med 315:1501–1505, 1986.

94. Lippman SM, Batsakis JG, Toth BB, et al: Comparison of low-dose isotretinoin with beta carotene to prevent oral carcinogenesis. N Engl J Med 328:15–20, 1993.

95. Stich HF, Hornby AP, Matthew B, et al: Response of oral leukoplakias to the administration of vitamin A. Cancer Lett 40:93–101, 1988.

96. Han J, Lu Y, Sun Z, et al: Evaluation of N-4-(hydroxycarbophenyl) retinamide as a cancer prevention agent and as a cancer chemotherapeutic agent. In Vivo 4:153–160, 1990.

97. Chiesa F, Tradati N, Marazza M, et al: Prevention of local relapses and new localizations of oral leukoplakias with the synthetic retinoid fenretinide (4-HPR): Preliminary results. Eur J Cancer 28:97–102, 1992.

98. Saccomanno G, Archer VE, Auerbach O, et al: Development of carcinoma of the lung as reflected in exfoliated cells. Cancer 33:256–270, 1974.

99. Saccomanno G, Moran PG, Schmidt RD, et al: Effect of 13-cis-retinoids on premalignant and malignant cells of lung origin. Acta Cytol 26:78–85, 1982.

100. Arnold AM, Browman GP, Levin MN, et al: The effect of synthetic retinoid etretinate on sputum cytology: Results from a randomized trial. Br J Cancer 65:737–743, 1992.

101. Browman G, Arnold A, Booker I, Johnstone B, et al: Etretinate blood levels in monitoring of compliance and contamination in a chemoprevention trial. J Natl Cancer Inst 81:795–798, 1989.

102. McLarty J, Yanagihara R, Girard W, et al: β-carotene, retinol and lung cancer chemoprevention: Study design and present status. In Pastorino U, Hong WK (eds): Chemoimmuno prevention of cancer. New York, Thieme Medical Publishers, 1991, pp 161–165.

103. Yanagihara R, McLarty J, Heiger L, et al: The predictive value of sputum bronchial dysplasia in subjects at risk for lung cancer. Proc Am Soc Clin Oncol 6:166, 1987.

104. McLarty J, Yanagihara R, Riley L: Characteristics of subjects with high and low serum β-carotene: Implications for lung cancer risk. Proc Am Soc Clin Oncol 6:228, 1987.

105. Band PR, Feldstein M, Saccomanno G: Reversibility of bronchial marked atypia: Implications for chemoprevention. Cancer Detect Prev 9:157–160, 1986.

106. Gouveia J, Mathe G, Hercend T, et al: Degree of bronchial metaplasia in heavy smokers and its regression after treatment with a retinoid. Lancet 1:710–712, 1982.

107. Mathe G, Gouveia J, Hercent T, et al: Correlation between precancerous bronchial metaplasia and cigarette consumption, and preliminary results of retinoid treatment. Cancer Detect Prev 5:461–466, 1982.

108. Misset JC, Mathe G, Santelli G, et al: Regression of bronchial epidermoid metaplasia in heavy smokers with etretinate treatment. Cancer Detect Prev 9:167–170, 1986.

109. Lee JS, Lippman SM, Benner SE, et al: Randomized placebo-controlled trial of isotretinoin in chemoprevention of bronchial squamous metaplasia. J Clin Oncol 12:937–945, 1994.

110. van Poppel G, Kok FJ, Hermus RJ: Beta-carotene supplementation in smokers reduces the frequency of micronuclei in sputum. Br J Cancer 66:1164–1168, 1992.

111. Benner SE, Pajak TF, Lippman SM, et al: Prevention of second primary tumors with isotretinoin in squamous cell carcinoma of the head and neck: Long term follow-up. J Natl Cancer Inst 86:140–141, 1994.

112. Lippman SM, Hong WK: Not Yet Standard: Retinoids versus second primary tumors. J Clin Oncol 11:1204–1207, 1993.

113. Pastorino U, Zandwijk NV, DeVries N, et al: European chemoprevention trials in patients with lung cancer or head and neck cancer, using high dose retinol palmitate and N-acetyl-cystein (NAC). (Abstract.) Biomed Pharmacother 46:331, 1992.

114. Pastorino U, Infante M, Maioli M, et al: Adjuvant treatment of stage I lung cancer with high-dose vitamin A. J Clin Oncol 11:1216–1222, 1993.

115. Xu X-C, Ro JY, Lee JS, et al: Differential expression of nuclear retinoic acid receptors in surgical specimens from head and neck "normal," hyperplastic, premalignant and malignant tissues. (Abstract.) Proc Am Assoc Cancer Res 34:551, 1993.

116. Gebert JF, Moghal N, Frangioni JV, et al: High frequency of retinoic acid receptor beta abnormalities in human lung cancer. Oncogene 6:1859–1868, 1991.

117. Houle B, Leduc F, Bradley WEC: Implication of RARβ in epidermoid (squamous) lung cancer. Genes Chromosome Cancer 3:358–366, 1991.

118. Houle B, Rochette-Egly C, Bradley WEC: Tumor-suppressive effect of the retinoic acid receptor β in human epidermoid lung cancer cells. Proc Natl Acad Sci USA 90:985–989, 1993.

119. Huber MH, Lee JS, Hong WK: Chemoprevention of lung cancer. Semin Oncol 20:128–141, 1993.

120. Melamed MR, Flehinger BJ, Zaman MB, et al. Screening for early lung cancer: Results of the Memorial-Sloan Kettering study in New York. Chest 86:44–53, 1984.

121. Tochman MS. Survival and mortality from lung cancer in a screened population: The Johns Hopkins study. Chest 89:325S–326S, 1986.

122. Fontana RS, Sanderson DR, Taylor WF, et al. Early lung cancer detection: Results of the initial (prevalence) radiologic and cytologic screening in the Mayo Clinic study. Am Rev Respir Dis 130:561–565, 1984.

123. Eddy D: Screening for lung cancer. Ann Intern Med 111:232–237, 1989.

124. Strauss GM, Gleason RE, Sugarbaker DJ: Screening for lung cancer re-examined: A reinterpretation of the Mayo Lung Project randomized trial on lung cancer screening. Chest 103:337S–341S, 1993.

125. Tockman MS, Gupta PK, Myers JD, et al: Sensitive and specific monoclonal antibody recognition of human lung cancer antigen on preserved sputum cells: A new approach to early lung cancer detection. J Clin Oncol 6:1685–1693, 1988.

Part II

CANCER OF THE ESOPHAGUS

17 ESOPHAGEAL CANCER—OVERVIEW

Jack A. Roth

Several promising developments have occurred related to the prevention and therapy of esophageal cancer since the first edition of *Thoracic Oncology*. One of the most significant observations is the rapid increase in adenocarcinomas in white males, which now account for almost half of esophageal cancers in the United States (see Chapter 18). Esophageal cancer remains one of the most variable forms of cancer with respect to racial, ethnic, and geographic incidence. There are several regions where the incidence exceeds 100 per 100,000. Thus, cancer of the esophagus is a global health problem.[1, 2]

Progress has been made in identifying premalignant lesions in the esophagus that are associated with a markedly increased risk of developing invasive esophageal cancer (see Chapters 18 and 19). The presence of Barrett's epithelium (columnar-lined esophagus) increases the risk of developing adenocarcinoma at least 30-fold. Dysplastic squamous epithelium also increases the risk of developing squamous cancers. A recent randomized vitamin supplement protocol lowered the incidence of esophageal cancer in Chinese receiving a combination of beta-carotene, vitamin E, and selenium (see Chapter 19). This suggests that prevention strategies may be an effective way of reducing the incidence of esophageal cancer in high-risk individuals. Prevention is the preferred course because the success rate of treating invasive cancer is low.

Unfortunately, patients with esophageal cancer frequently do not seek medical attention until the tumor is advanced. The clinical presentation and natural history of esophageal cancer are discussed in Chapter 20. Palliation of symptoms with minimal morbidity is a major objective in the treatment of these patients because many patients present with locally advanced unresectable tumors. Surgical bypass no longer has a role in palliating patients because of its high morbidity rate. Intubation is a useful modality. Combination chemotherapy and radiation therapy combined with endoscopic laser resection can offer durable palliation.[3, 4]

The histologic distinctions between the various degrees of preneoplasia are described in detail in Chapter 21. A variety of less common esophageal neoplasms are also discussed. Once malignancy is diagnosed, accurate staging and determination of resectability is necessary. Noninvasive staging studies are still unable to reliably predict resectability. However, these studies are useful for preoperative planning and detection of distant metastases. The indications for diagnostic imaging for esophageal cancer and the outcome of these studies is described in Chapter 22. Preoperative and intraoperative staging of esophageal cancer is still not standardized. Chapter 23 provides a detailed analysis of the staging classification and staging procedures.

Refinements in surgical technique and preoperative and postoperative care have reduced the mortality and morbidity rates resulting from esophagectomy. Some controversy still exists as to the optimal procedure for resection of esophageal cancer. The most frequently used techniques are described in Chapter 24. Little difference in outcome can be shown for the most commonly used procedures.[5] However, knowledge of these techniques is useful because the extent and location of the tumor may dictate the optimal operative approach.

Radiation therapy remains a mainstay of palliative therapy and is an important component of combined modality treatment protocols. As discussed in Chapters 25 and 26, the combination of radiation therapy with chemotherapy has improved survival over radiation therapy alone.[3] Induction chemotherapy prior to surgery has also resulted in apparent increases in survival in several studies.[6, 7] These clinical trials and ongoing intergroup randomized trials are discussed in Chapter 26.

REFERENCES

1. Day NE, Munoz N: Esophagus. In Schottenfeld D, Fraumeni JF Jr (eds): Cancer Epidemiology and Prevention. Philadelphia, W.B. Saunders, 1982, pp 569–623.
2. Li JY: Epidemiology of esophageal cancer in China. Monogr Natl Cancer Inst 62:113–120, 1982.
3. Herskovic A, Martz K, Al-Sarraf M, et al: Combined chemotherapy and radiotherapy compared with radiotherapy alone in patients with cancer of the esophagus. N Engl J Med 326:1593–1598, 1992.
4. McCaughan JS, Williams TE, Bethel BH: Palliation of esophageal malignancy with photodynamic therapy. Ann Thorac Surg 40:113–120, 1985.
5. Putnam JB Jr, Suell DA, Natarajan G, et al: A comparison of three techniques of esophagectomy for carcinoma of the esophagus from one institution with a residency training program. Ann Thorac Surg 57(2):319–325, 1994.
6. Roth JA, Pass HI, Flanagan MM, et al: Randomized clinical trial of preoperative and postoperative adjuvant chemotherapy with cisplatin, vindesine and bleomycin for carcinoma of the esophagus. J Thorac Cardiovasc Surg 96:242–248, 1988.
7. Forastiere AA, Orringer MB, Perez T, et al: Concurrent chemotherapy and radiation therapy followed by transhiatal esophagectomy for local-regional cancer of the esophagus. J Clin Oncol 8:119–127, 1990.

BIOLOGY OF ESOPHAGEAL CANCER

18 EPIDEMIOLOGY AND GENESIS OF ESOPHAGEAL CANCER

William J. Blot

OVERVIEW

This chapter reviews and updates the epidemiology of esophageal cancer. Worldwide mortality statistics indicate that this cancer varies substantially both within and between countries. In parts of China and Iran and several other areas of the world, it is by far the most common cancer. In the United States, overall esophageal cancer rates have been rising steadily among blacks but not among whites, and the tumor now ranks as the second leading cause of cancer death among black men under age 55. There are remarkable differences in demographic patterns by cell type, however. In the United States and western Europe, incidence rates of esophageal adenocarcinomas are rapidly rising, and among white males, these rates now surpass those for squamous cell carcinomas. Cigarette smoking and alcoholic beverage drinking are the major causes of esophageal cancer in western countries, and account for the fourfold excess in males compared with females. Smoking and drinking are strongly linked to squamous cell tumors, whereas their role in adenocarcinomas is yet to be adequately characterized. Nutritional deficiencies may also contribute to the etiology of this cancer. Epidemiologic studies implicate diets low in fruits and vegetables, and although the reasons for the clustering of esophageal cancer in high-risk areas around the world are unknown, the local diets are often characterized by a low intake of several vitamins and minerals. Further research may help clarify the role of nutrition and other factors and their interaction with tobacco and alcohol intake, and may provide new information useful toward the prevention of these cancers.

THE EPIDEMIOLOGY OF ESOPHAGEAL CANCER

Esophageal cancer exhibits unusual epidemiologic features that distinguish it from all other cancers. In this chapter, the epidemiology of this neoplasm is updated from a prior review,[1] summarizing what is known about the causes of esophageal cancer in this country and various parts of the world. The chapter highlights the changing patterns of this cancer, including the emergence of esophageal adenocarcinoma as a principal cell type in the United States.

Descriptive Statistics

Geographic Variation. Esophageal cancer varies more worldwide than any other cancer.[2-4] Table 18-1 provides some indication of the international variation, noting that annual age-adjusted incidence rates of esophageal cancer range from less than 5 cases per 100,000 population among whites in the United States and in several other countries to over 100 per 100,000 in high-risk locales in China and Iran.

Differences in rates of esophageal cancer within countries are often substantial. The geographic distribution of death rates from esophageal cancer within China, for example, is marked. Some of the highest rates in the world occur in Linxian, a rural county of 800,000 persons, where esophageal cancer is the leading cause of death. The area is characterized by a dry climate, relatively infertile soil (until recently), and a population with chronic mild (subclinical) deficiencies of multiple nutrients.[5] Table 18-2 lists mortality rates from the tumor among Linxian adults aged 40 to 69. Rates in the county are nearly 10 times the Chinese

TABLE 18–1. Esophageal Cancer Incidence Among Males Around the World

GEOGRAPHIC AREA	INCIDENCE RATE (*)
Linxian, China; Caspian region of Iran, USSR	100 +
Transkei, South Africa; Parts of Kazakhstan, USSR;	50–99
Northern France	20–49
Hong Kong; Singapore (Chinese): Most areas of China; Miyagi, Japan; India; Caribbean Islands; Brazil; France; United States (blacks)	10–19
Most areas of Japan; United Kingdom; New Zealand; Southern Europe	5–9
Canada; United States (white); Australia; Israel; Colombia; Western Africa; Scandinavia; Central and Eastern Europe	<5

*Annual rates per 100,000 adjusted to the world standard population. Data from references 1 to 4, generally applicable to the period around the mid 1980s.

national level, which, in turn, is nearly 10 times the rate among similarly aged whites in the United States. Even within Linxian, there is variation, with the excess being most severe in its northern communes.

The situation in China is similar to the situation in Iran and Uzbekistan. In certain areas bordering the Caspian Sea, esophageal cancer mortality rates exceeding 100 per 100,000 are found.[3] The areas tend to be marked by dry climates and impoverished (compared to the United States) conditions. Notable are the steep gradients in the death rates as one moves away from the cluster centers.[6] Nevertheless, substantially elevated rates can be considered to exist in a broad belt stretching from Iran in the west across the southern former Soviet republics into China. Although incidence rates are not as high to the south of this region, esophageal cancer is one of the most common tumors in India and neighboring countries.[2]

Areas of elevated mortality from esophageal cancer are not limited to Asia. Clusters of high incidence have been reported among black men in the Transkei and other regions of South Africa and in Kenya and bordering areas of East Africa.[3] Esophageal cancer is also one of the more common tumors in certain islands of the Caribbean and in parts of Europe. In some regions in Brittany in northern France, for example, esophageal cancer occurs over three times more frequently than the national average.[3, 7]

Within the United States, esophageal cancer also varies geographically, with the diversity greatest for blacks.[8] Among urban areas, rates in Washington, D.C. exceed those in the other urban areas by a fairly wide margin. Some clustering of elevated mortality from esophageal cancer has also been observed among blacks in coastal counties in the southeast, particularly the low country in South Carolina. The geographic variation among blacks is greater for esophageal cancer than for any other tumor, with rates in high-risk regions exceeding those in low-risk regions by nearly fivefold, in contrast to 2.4-fold for lung can-

cer and 1.3-fold for prostate cancer, the two leading cancers among blacks.[9] Although differences are not as great for whites, esophageal cancer exhibits greater variation in mortality among men than any cancer except rectal cancer.[9]

One of the distinctive patterns of esophageal cancer among both whites and blacks in the United States is the consistently higher rates in urban than in rural areas. The urban excess among white males is higher for esophageal cancer than for any other type except oral cancer.[9] For males of both racial groups, mortality rates are nearly twice as high in highly populated counties compared with lightly populated counties throughout the country.

The observation of substantial geographic variation suggests that potent environmental agents capable of inducing esophageal cancer also vary geographically. Just what these agents may be in the United States and elsewhere is discussed later in this review. In the following section, further characterization of the incidence of esophageal cancer according to the demographic indices of age, sex, and race is described. Variation in rates across these factors provides additional clues to the etiology of this cancer.

Occurrence Rates by Age, Sex, and Race. Throughout the world, esophageal cancer is a disease of mid- to late adulthood, rarely occurring in persons below age 25. Rates tend to rise steadily with age, as shown in Figure 18–1, where the age curves for esophageal cancer mortality over the 5-year period from 1985 to 1989 among white American men and women are displayed. The median age at death is 66 for males and 67 for females.[10] Throughout the world, most of the tumors occur among persons in the 50- to 70-year age range.[2, 7] The age patterns are similar for squamous cell carcinomas and adenocarcinomas.[11]

In the United States and other western nations, esophageal cancer occurs much more frequently among males than among females, with the preponderance among males even more pronounced for adenocarcinomas than for squamous cell carcinomas of the esophagus.[11, 12] Table 18–3 shows a sex ratio among whites of 6.5 for adenocarcinoma and 2.5 for squamous cell cancers. In high-risk areas of China, Iran, and the former Soviet Union, however, esophageal cancers (predominantly squamous cell cancers) appear almost as often in women as in men.[3, 4] In only a

TABLE 18–2. Esophageal Cancer Mortality Rates Among Linxian Adults Age 40–69

AREA	MORTALITY RATE
Linxian county	470
Linxian's northern communes	760
China	56
United States (blacks)	19
United States (whites)	5

Annual rates per 100,000 population adjusted in 5-year age groups to the Linxian population. Data from Blot and Li.[75]

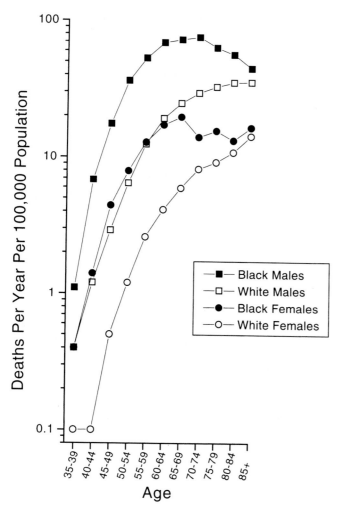

FIGURE 18–1. Age-specific esophageal cancer mortality rates in the United States from 1985 to 1989 by sex and race.

than among whites in the United States, but adenocarcinomas occur more often among whites (Table 18–3).[11] The excess in blacks of squamous cell carcinoma is even greater among young persons, exceeding sixfold for those below 55 years of age.[12] Such a high black-to-white ratio is seen for no other cancer. The difference is such that squamous cell esophageal cancer is one of the most common malignancies among black men under age 55 (second only to lung cancer), while still being a relatively rare cancer among similarly aged whites.

Time Trends. Available national mortality data from Europe and North America show relatively stable total esophageal cancer rates in most countries.[7] There are some exceptions, such as the more than 50% decline in rates in Finland and Switzerland since the 1950s, whereas slight increases have been reported in Scotland. There is some evidence to suggest that esophageal cancer has been a problem in Linxian China for hundreds of years. Data available for the past 25 years indicate that rates are generally stable, although some decline has been detected among younger persons in the 1980s.[13] In the South African Transkei, esophageal cancer was apparently uncommon until this century, with the elevated incidence arising only within the past 30 to 59 years.[14]

Within the United States, rates of overall esophageal cancer mortality among white men and women have been fairly steady since the 1950s.[8] For American blacks, on the other hand, esophageal cancer death rates rose steadily from the 1950s to 1980s.[12] Mortality has nearly doubled among blacks over the 4 decades. For nonwhites there are strong cohort effects, with higher age-specific rates for successively later born cohorts. The generational increase is slowing, however, with blacks born after 1930 not experiencing a continuing rise in esophageal cancer death. The increasing mortality among blacks is not simply due to detection of esophageal cancer that in the past would have gone undiagnosed, since esophageal cancer is, at least when compared with other tumors, easily identified. Furthermore, as noted below, the tumors are usually fatal regardless of race, so that the escalating trend among blacks is not attributable to poorer medical care.

Whereas the increasing rates of esophageal cancer (mainly squamous cell tumors) among blacks appear

few areas of the world (Sri Lanka, Singapore [non-Chinese], and some of the localities in Iran) is esophageal cancer reported more often in females.[2, 3]

Striking differences according to racial or ethnic background have been observed in several parts of the world. The differences raise the possibility of differences in genetic susceptibility, but as noted later, differences in environmental exposures may be more important in most situations. Squamous cell esophageal cancer occurs much more often among blacks

TABLE 18–3. Annual Age-Adjusted Incidence Rates of Esophageal Cancer from 1976 to 1987 by Histologic Type, Sex, and Race*

Cell Type	MEN		WOMEN	
	White	Black	White	Black
Squamous cell carcinoma	3.0 (3040)	16.8 (1475)	1.2 (1641)	4.6 (506)
Adenocarcinoma	1.3 (1311)	0.4 (37)	0.2 (242)	0.0 (4)
Other/NOS†	0.6 (628)	1.6 (133)	0.2 (327)	0.6 (61)

*Rates are per 100,000 population and are age-adjusted to the United States standard population. Numbers of cases in SEER registries (covering approximately 10% of the United States population) are given in parentheses.
†NOS indicates type of cancer not otherwise specified.
Data from Blot et al.[11]

to be abating, the incidence of adenocarcinoma is rising among whites and blacks (Fig. 18–2). In the United States, the increases in rates of esophageal adenocarcinoma through the 1980s have been on the order of 5% to 10% per year, a faster pace than virtually any other cancer.[11] As shown in Figure 18–2, by 1988 to 1990, among white men adenocarcinomas accounted for nearly half of all esophageal cancers.[15] If these trends have persisted, rates of adenocarcinoma as of this writing (1994) will be over 50% greater than rates of squamous cell carcinomas. The percentages of adenocarcinomas among blacks and white females, although increasing, remain much lower (Table 18–3).

Survival Rates. The chances of surviving esophageal cancer are low.[16] Relative 5-year survival rates in the United States have improved slightly over time, but still remain poor. In the latest reporting period, only 8% of patients survived 5 or more years. The survival rates are low in both men and women and in whites and blacks, although they are slightly better for women and whites. The median survival time during the 1980s was 9 months. The high fatality results in rates of esophageal cancer incidence and mortality being nearly equal, and thus the two terms are often used interchangeably in this report. Survival patterns for squamous cell carcinomas and adenocarcinomas appear to be generally similar.

The unusual demographic patterns of esophageal cancer provide a series of clues to the environmental and host determinants of this fatal disease. In the next section, analytic evidence relevant to the identification and characterization of the causes of esophageal cancer is summarized.

Risk Factors

Tobacco. The major causes of esophageal cancer in the United States and other western countries are cigarette smoking and alcoholic beverage consumption. Epidemiologic investigations, both cohort (prospective) and case-control (retrospective) studies, have consistently shown increased risks of esophageal cancer among smokers. Table 18–4 presents estimates of the relative risk of esophageal cancer among cigarette smokers derived from three large follow-up surveys (the American Cancer Society's cohort mortality study of nearly 1,000,000 American men and women,[17] a 16-year follow-up of 250,000 United States veterans,[18] and a survey ascertaining deaths over a 20-year period among 34,000 British doctors[19]). Smokers experienced about a fivefold increased death rate of esophageal cancer compared with nonsmokers. In the two surveys in which dose-response trends were evaluated, the excess rose to about tenfold among heavy cigarette smokers.[18, 19] The elevated risks held not only for cigarette smokers, because 4-fold increases were found for users of cigars or pipes exclusively.[17, 19] Risks were elevated among users of mentholated and non-mentholated cigarettes, and the higher prevalence of use of menthol brands by blacks does not account for their higher rates of esophageal cancer.[20] As noted in reports by the United States Surgeon General[21] and the International Agency for Research on Cancer,[22] the findings from these and other cohort and case-control investigations leave little doubt that smoking is a cause of esophageal cancer.

Most of the investigations of smoking's effects pertain to squamous cell carcinomas. Evidence regarding risk factors for esophageal adenocarcinomas is scanty, in part because of the rarity of these cell types in the

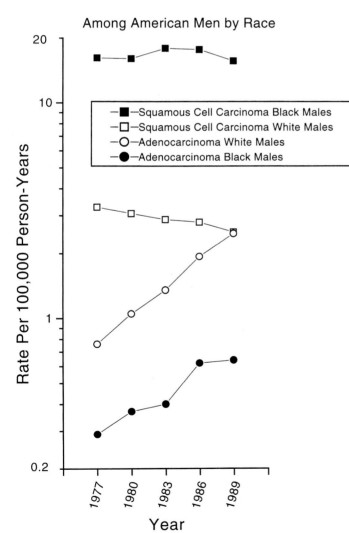

FIGURE 18–2. Trends in age-adjusted incidence rates of squamous cell carcinomas and adenocarcinomas of the esophagus among American men by race.

TABLE 18–4. Relative Risks of Esophageal Cancer Among Cigarette Smokers in Three Large Prospective Studies

STUDY COHORT	RELATIVE RISK
American Cancer Society volunteers	4.2
United States veterans	6.4
British doctors	4.7

Shown are ratios of esophageal cancer mortality rates in cigarette smokers compared to nonsmokers.
Data from Hammond,[17] Rogot and Murray,[18] and Doll and Peto.[19]

past. Available comparisons of traits of patients with adenocarcinomas of the esophagus (often combined with patients with gastric cardia adenocarcinomas), however, tend to show that smoking is a risk factor, although the association is not as strong as for squamous cell cancers.[23-26]

Smoking, along with alcohol drinking, is a major contributor to the male excess of esophageal cancer (particularly squamous cancers), and accounts for some part of the higher rates among blacks in the United States because the prevalence of smoking is now higher among black men than white men.[27] Smoking also plays a role in the high rates of esophageal cancer among blacks in South Africa, although pipes more than cigarettes have been implicated among persons from the Transkei.[28]

In parts of India, esophageal cancer has been reported in higher frequency not only among smokers but also among chewers of quids containing tobacco, betel, and other ingredients.[29] In Sri Lanka, habitual quid chewing is thought to account for the unusual observation of higher esophageal cancer rates among females, who usually practice the habit, than males.[30] Effects of tobacco, as opposed to betel or other constituents of the chews, cannot be distinguished in this part of the world. Surveys in Bombay[31, 32] found that excess risks were not as great when tobacco was included in the quid, suggesting that other constituents may be responsible for the association with esophageal cancer, but a stronger effect for tobacco-containing chews was noted in southern India.[33] Although some increase in risk was noted in case-control studies in New York[34, 35] and Puerto Rico,[36] little information is available to evaluate American chewing tobacco or snuff as risk factors for esophageal cancer.

In the areas of the world with the very highest rates of esophageal cancer, tobacco does not appear to play a major role. Some increase in risk was linked to cigarette smoking in Iran,[37] with a twofold excess of the malignancy among female smokers, and in China,[38] but smoking was not particularly common in either area. There also was no association with the chewing of nass, a mixture containing, tobacco, lime, ash and other ingredients. The chewing of residues from opium pipes has been implicated, however.[39] The habit is practiced more in the high-risk Caspian areas and more often among patients with the tumor. Biochemical evidence of exposure comes from the detection of urinary metabolites of morphine more often in members of households where the cancer patients lived.[39] The likelihood that this exposure may contribute to the elevated cancer risk is increased by the identification of mutagenic substances in the opium residues. Mutagenic activity has also been described for pipe tobacco residues of the type often chewed by residents of the Transkei.[40]

Alcohol. A history of heavy consumption of alcohol is often a characteristic of patients with esophageal cancer in the United States and other western countries. This clinical impression is borne out by epidemiologic investigations, which clearly demonstrate

TABLE 18–5. Areas with Alcohol-Associated Elevated Esophageal Cancer Rates

AREA	TYPE OF BEVERAGE IMPLICATED
Northern France	Apple brandy
Transkei, South Africa	Maize beer
Puerto Rico	Home-brewed and other rum
Brazil	Cachaca (distilled from sugar cane)
Coastal South Carolina	Moonshine whiskey
Washington, D.C.	Hard liquor

Data from Blot.[42]

that high consumption of alcohol, particularly when combined with cigarette smoking, may greatly increase esophageal cancer risk.[41, 42] Several cohort studies of heavy alcohol consumers have examined esophageal cancer risk. In Finland, a 70% excess of esophageal cancer was found among 250,000 registered "alcohol misusers," whereas three- to fourfold excesses were reported among male alcoholics there and in Canada.[43, 44] In Japan, esophageal cancer mortality was significantly higher among smokers who drank alcoholic beverages than among smokers who did not.[45] Case-control studies have been more numerous, and these consistently show higher relative risks among heavy drinkers.[41]

Drinking of alcoholic beverages has been associated in several clusters of elevated esophageal cancer mortality rates around the world (Table 18–5).[42] In each case, a particular beverage has been implicated, including apple brandies in France, maize beer in the South African Transkei, sugar cane distilled beverages in Puerto Rico and South America, and moonshine whiskeys in South Carolina. The common ingredient is ethanol, but the variation in risks of esophageal cancer with the alcoholic beverages suggests some contribution from other ingredients in the specific beverages.

Increases in risk from drinking can be substantial. Table 18–6 shows risk estimates from an investigation into the high mortality rates from esophageal cancer in Brittany.[3, 46] Risks increased strikingly with increasing amount of alcoholic beverages drunk within each smoking category, with differences between high and low alcohol consumption ranging from about 20- to 50-fold. Smoking exhibited an independent but

TABLE 18–6. Relative Risks of Esophageal Cancer According to Amount of Alcohol and Tobacco Consumed, Brittany, France

| ALCOHOL (gm/day) | TOBACCO (gm/day) | | | |
	0–9	10–19	20–29	30 +
0–40	1.0*	3.4	3.2	7.8
41–80	7.3	8.4	8.8	35.0
81–120	11.8	13.6	12.6	83.0
121 +	49.6	65.9	137.6	155.6

*Reference category.

Data from Parkin et al,[2] adapted from a case-control study of esophageal cancer (predominantly squamous cell carcinomas) among men in Brittany.[46]

smaller effect; however, it combined with drinking in a multiplicative fashion in enhancing esophageal cancer risk: Among those who were both heavy drinkers and heavy smokers, the relative excess exceeded 100-fold. The effects of alcohol are evident among non-smokers, however, and conversely, the effects of smoking are found among nondrinkers.[47] Rising risks of esophageal cancer among nonsmokers according to amount of alcohol consumed have also been reported elsewhere.[48]

Results qualitatively similar to those in France have been found in the United States. In a case-control study in New York, heavy drinkers who were moderate smokers were found to have 25 times the risk of esophageal cancer of smokers who did not drink.[34] Alcohol consumption was also found to be the major risk factor and to be responsible for the high esophageal cancer rates among black men in Washington, D.C.[48, 49] A sixfold excess was found among heavy drinkers. The excess persisted after controlling for smoking, and a significant alcohol-associated increase was noted even among those who did not smoke. This study revealed increases in risk among both hard liquor and beer or wine drinkers, although the association was stronger for spirits consumption. In coastal South Carolina, regular drinking of moonshine whiskeys was reported by nearly 90% of black male patients with esophageal cancer.[50] The significant excess risks associated with this habit appear to account for much of the excess mortality among area blacks. Similar observations of exceptionally high risks among heavy drinkers have been made elsewhere in the United States,[51, 52] Puerto Rico,[36] South America,[53] and Japan.[45] Studies of two cohorts of brewery workers with presumed high intake of beer have yielded differing results: No excess of esophageal cancer was noted among Guiness employees in Dublin,[54] but an increase was detected among Carlsburg brewers in Denmark.[55] Nearly all of these studies focused on males, but the patterns appear likely to hold for females as well.

The large majority of studies examining the role of alcohol drinking on esophageal cancer pertains primarily to squamous cell carcinomas. Limited data suggest that adenocarcinomas may also be related to drinking but to a considerably lesser extent.[24–26]

Despite the strong associations between alcohol and tobacco consumption and the risk of esophageal cancer, trends in the intake of these products tend not to correlate with trends in esophageal cancer mortality in several western countries,[56, 57] suggesting that other factors are also involved.

Diet and Nutritional Deficiency. The worldwide patterns of esophageal cancer incidence exhibit some correlation with patterns of nutrition and diet.[58] Populations in areas with the highest cancer rates tend to have low nutritional status. Marginally low levels of beta-carotene, retinol, vitamins A and C, several B vitamins, magnesium, zinc, and certain minerals have been noted in China, Iran, and South Africa. Wheat and corn are often the staple foods. Case-control stud-

ies in Iran[31] and South Africa[59, 60] have documented the lower intake of fruits and vegetables and higher consumption of wheat or maize, or both, among the cancer patients. Consumption of maize has been linked to elevated risk also in northern Italy, where rates of esophageal cancer are only moderately high.[61] Pickled vegetable intake has been associated with an increased risk of esophageal cancer in Hong Kong,[62] but case-control studies have not confirmed the initial suspicions that pickled vegetables were responsible for the high rates in Linxian.[38, 63] Frank clinical nutritional deficiencies are rare, but biochemical studies have shown low urinary or blood concentrations of several substances, particularly riboflavin.[59, 64–65] In Linxian, for example, nearly 90% of the population exhibits depressed riboflavin levels, measured by erythrocyte glutathione reductase coefficients corresponding to those signaling deficiency in the United States.[65] There is some suspicion that such low nutritional status may enhance the risk of esophageal cancer induced by carcinogens (possibly including nitrosamines, mycotoxins, and physical irritants ingested via the consumption of some foods[66] in the local environments. Similar promotion of cancer risk has been demonstrated in laboratory animals maintained on diets deficient in vitamin A and other micronutrients.[67, 68] In rats, zinc deficiencies have enhanced nitrosamine-induced esophageal carcinogenesis.[69] Riboflavin deficiency, which can induce esophageal hyperplasia in baboons, has promoted skin carcinogenesis in mice.[70] Conversely, supplementation with several nutrients has been found to block chemically induced cancer in a number of animal studies.[67, 68] Thus, there is experimental evidence to suggest that nutrition may be involved in the late stages of the process leading to cancer, particularly esophageal cancer.

There is also compelling epidemiologic evidence. One of the earliest suggestions that nutritional deficiency may increase the risk of cancer came from the observation of hypopharyngeal and upper esophageal cancer among women in northern Sweden with Plummer-Vinson syndrome.[71] The condition is characterized not only by iron deficiency but also by low levels of several nutrients including riboflavin. Esophageal cancer has also been linked to celiac disease,[72] a familial malabsorption disorder of the small intestine that may lead to deficiencies of various nutrients. Case-control studies in the United States also suggest that nutritional factors contribute to esophageal cancer risk. In the survey among black men in Washington, D.C., significantly more of the cancer patients were reported to have had lower intake of fruits and vegetables, fresh meat and fish, and dairy products throughout their adult life than the controls.[73] The risk of esophageal cancer associated with low intake of these food groups was about twofold, after adjusting for alcoholic beverage intake. In a hospital-based study in western New York, a twofold excess of esophageal cancer was reported among men in the lowest compared with the highest categories of estimated intake of vitamins A and C and fruits and vegetables.[51] Lower vegetable intake was also noted in case-control studies in New York City,[34] Los Angeles,[52] and South Carolina,[50] and poorer nutritional status was described among esophageal cancer patients in Puerto Rico.[36] In studies that have attempted to discriminate between effects of beta-carotene and retinol, the evidence has clearly favored a protective role for beta-carotene but not retinol.[50, 74] The disease itself affects dietary habits, but these investigations attempted to ascertain nutritional habits prior to onset during most of adulthood. In a prospective survey of 250,000 adults in Japan, lower esophageal cancer mortality from 1965 to 1975 was found among those who reported daily fruit and meat intake in 1965.[45]

To evaluate the hypothesis that vitamins and minerals may influence esophageal cancer risk, two randomized human trials were launched in Linxian.[75] In the first, approximately 3400 persons with cytologically diagnosed severe dysplasia of the esophagus were randomly allocated into one of two treatment groups. One group received a daily supplement of a multiple vitamin and mineral preparation, the other a placebo. For most of the nutrients, the doses in the supplements were about two to three times the United States Recommended Daily Allowances (RDA). In the second trial, about 30,000 villagers were randomly allocated into treatment groups according to the specifications of a fractional factorial statistical design assessing four combinations of nutrients: retinol and zinc; riboflavin and niacin; vitamin C and molybdenum; and beta-carotene, vitamin E, and selenium. The daily doses received in this general population trial were one to two times the United States RDAs for most of the nutrients, so that the marginal deficiencies were corrected and the population levels of the supplemented nutrients approximated those of the upper quartile of the United States population. After 5 years of supplementation, death rates from cancer were significantly lower (RR = 0.87) among those who received a combination of beta-carotene, vitamin E, and selenium.[76] No significant benefits were seen for the other combinations, although some lowering of esophageal cancer incidence was noted among those receiving riboflavin and niacin. The reduction offers a hopeful sign that supplementation with these antioxidants may prove to be of benefit in cancer prevention, at least in certain high-risk areas. No significant reduction in cancer rates was seen in the smaller dysplasia trial, although a greater proportion of those receiving multiple vitamins and minerals rather than placebo showed regression of the dysplasia.[77] In a 13-month randomized trial in a neighboring Chinese county involving weekly administration of retinol, zinc, and riboflavin, the prevalence of esophagitis and dysplasia was similar in the treated and untreated groups.[78] However, a nonsignificant reduction in esophagitis was found in Uzebekistan among persons treated for 20 months with beta-carotene, retinol, and vitamin E.[79] The exportability of these findings to the United States population is not clear, but it does appear likely that improved nutrition helps lower the incidence of esophageal cancer among individuals at high risk.

Other Factors. Existing evidence indicates that smoking, alcohol, and dietary and nutritional factors account for the bulk of esophageal tumors in western societies. Esophageal cancers have been reported following exposure to other environmental agents, however. Esophageal cancer deaths were found 2.5 times more frequently than expected in a follow-up of 17,600 asbestos insulation workers in the United States and Canada, although other surveys of asbestos-exposed workers generally have not found risks as high.[80] Cohort studies in Sweden found nearly 10 times the expected numbers of esophageal cancers among vulcanization workers,[81] and a nearly three-fold excess among workers in several jobs involving exposure to combustion products,[82] but clues to occupational factors such as this have been sparse. Ionizing radiation may also increase the risk of esophageal cancer. About twice as many esophageal cancers have thus far occurred among Hiroshima and Nagasaki atomic bomb survivors exposed to 200 or more compared with less than 10 cGy from the 1945 explosions.[83] A twofold excess of esophageal cancer has also been observed among patients given x-ray therapy for ankylosing spondylitis.[84] Other physical irritants of the esophagus may predispose individuals to increased risk. The drinking of exceptionally hot beverages has been associated with elevated risk of esophageal cancer in studies in Japan and Singapore.[45, 85] In Singapore, a threefold excess was found among persons who consumed burning hot teas.[63] Heavy consumption of mate, a tea drunk at high temperatures, has recently been associated with a large increase in risk of esophageal cancer in Uruguay[53] and smaller increases in Brazil.[86] Thermal irritation from drinking teas at exceptionally hot temperatures in these areas as well as in high-risk areas of Iran[87] may be responsible. The drinking of tea per se, and the accompanying ingestion of tannins, had been postulated as contributing to the high rates of esophageal cancer in Curaçao and among blacks in coastal South Carolina,[88] but indigenous teas now appear to be exonerated.[50] Indeed green tea contains flavonoids, isothiocyanates, phenols, and other compounds that have been postulated to play a protective role,[89] and a significantly lowered risk of esophageal cancer has been reported among drinkers of green tea in Shanghai.[90]

Little is known about the role of viral agents in the etiology of esophageal cancer, but papillomaviruses have been identified in several patients.[91] The virus is convincingly associated with cancers of the uterine cervix and may play a more general role in human carcinogenesis. Although the clustering of elevated rates in relatively confined geographic areas in several parts of the world raises the possibility of familial susceptibility to esophageal cancer, there is little evidence to indicate that genetic predisposition to the malignancy is common. A genetically determined association between tylosis and esophageal cancer has been reported[92] but appears to be rare and not involved in high-risk areas such as Iran.[3] In China, however, familial clustering has been reported, with risks of esophageal cancer elevated among those with a parent or sibling with the cancer.[93, 94]

For adenocarcinomas, clinical reports indicate that most tend to arise from columnar-lined (metaplastic) epithelium, commonly known as Barrett's esophagus.[95] Barrett's esophagus shares the race and sex predilections of esophageal adenocarcinoma, also being much more common among white males than other groups. Barrett's esophagus is related to duodenal-gastrointestinal reflux disease, with damage resulting from both abnormal (for the esophagus) acid and alkaline exposures, but its causes also are largely unknown. Clinical reports suggest that patients with esophageal adenocarcinoma often have a prior history of hiatal hernia or duodenal ulcer.[23, 26]

CONCLUSIONS AND SUMMARY

The epidemiologic features of esophageal cancer distinguish this tumor from all other malignancies. It is the most common cancer in certain parts of the world, occurring more frequently in Linxian and near the Caspian Sea, for example, than all cancers combined in the United States. The marked geographic variation seems due largely to environmental factors, but their clear identification has eluded detection. Nutritional factors seem involved and may enhance risk resulting from the interaction of several esophageal insults. Current laboratory and epidemiologic research offers some promise of clarifying the causes of the clustering, although past experience indicates that the task is not an easy one. Within the United States ample evidence is available to take preventive action to reduce the incidence of squamous cell carcinomas of the esophagus, because its major causes—tobacco and alcohol—have been determined. Death rates can be reliably predicted to fall following the reduction of smoking and heavy alcohol consumption. Smoking and drinking contribute to the epidemic of the tumor among black Americans, but the excess among blacks compared with that of whites (which reaches over sixfold among those under age 55) may be influenced by other determinants, including nutrition. The causes of the rapidly rising rates of adenocarcinomas of the esophagus, and reasons for its occurrence primarily among white men, are enigmatic. Additional research on the etiology of this emerging cell type is warranted and may provide information crucial to the development of readily implementable preventive strategies.

SELECTED REFERENCES

Blot WJ, Devesa SS, Kneller RW, Fraumeni JF Jr: Rising incidence of adenocarcinoma of the esophagus and gastric cardia. JAMA 265:1287–1289, 1991; and 270:1320, 1993.
This study using national cancer incidence data documents the changing patterns of esophageal cancer in the United States. Rates of adenocarcinoma of the esophagus among white males were shown to have tripled from the mid 1970s to late 1980s, with concomitant but less steep rises for gastric cardia cancers. Increases also were observed among women and black males. By 1990, adenocarcinoma was the most common histologic type of esophageal cancer among white men.
Brown LM, Blot WJ, Schuman S, et al: Environmental factors and

high risk of esophageal cancer among men in coastal South Carolina. J Natl Cancer Inst 80:1620–1628, 1988.
This case-control study assessed many of the potential risk factors for squamous cell carcinomas of the esophagus in an area of the United States with an unusually high mortality rate from this cancer. Consumption of alcohol, particularly moonshine whiskies, was shown to account for much of the clustering of elevated rates, whereas risk was significantly reduced among those with high fruit intake.
International Agency for Research on Cancer: Tobacco smoking. IARC Monogr Eval Carcinog Risks Hum 38:1–396, 1986.
This monograph presents data from around the world showing that tobacco smoking is a cause of esophageal cancer, with risk rising in proportion to amount smoked.
Kabat G, Ng S, Wynder EL: Tobacco, alcohol intake, and diet in relation to adenocarcinoma of the esophagus and gastric cardia. Cancer Causes Control 4:123–132, 1993.
In one of the few epidemiologic studies of esophageal adenocarcinoma, risk factors were examined for the combined category of adenocarcinomas of the esophagus and gastric cardia. The risks of these cancers were found to be doubled among smokers and heavy drinkers, and risk decreased with increasing dietary fiber intake.

REFERENCES

1. Blot WJ: The epidemiology of esophageal cancer. In Roth J, Rukdeschel J, Weisenburger T (eds): Thoracic Oncology. Philadelphia, W.B. Saunders, 1989, pp 295–304.
2. Parkin M, Muir C, Whelan S, et al: Cancer Incidence in Five Continents, Vol VI. Lyon, International Agency for Research on Cancer, 1992.
3. Day NE, Munoz N: Esophagus. In Schottenfeld D, Fraumeni J (eds): Cancer Epidemiology and Prevention. Philadelphia, W.B. Saunders, 1982, pp 569–623.
4. Li JY: Epidemiology of esophageal cancer in China. Monogr Natl Cancer Inst 62:113–120, 1982.
5. Yang OS: Research on esophageal cancer in China: A review. Cancer Res 40:2633–2644, 1980.
6. Mahboubi E, Kmet J, Cook P, et al: Oesophageal cancer studies in the Caspian littoral of Iran: The Caspian cancer registry. Br J Cancer 28:197–214, 1973.
7. Kurihara M, Aoki K, Hisamachi S: Cancer Mortality Statistics in the World 1950–1985. Nagoya, Japan, Univ Nagoya Press, 1989.
8. Fraumeni JF, Blot WJ: Geographic variation in esophageal cancer mortality in the United States. J Chron Dis 30:759–767, 1977.
9. Blot WJ, Fraumeni JF: Geographic epidemiology of cancer in the United States. In Schottenfeld D, Fraumeni J (eds): Cancer Epidemiology and Prevention. Philadelphia, W.B. Saunders, 1982, pp. 179–193.
10. Young JL, Percy CL, Asire AJ: Surveillance, Epidemiology, and End Results: Incidence and Mortality Data 1973–77. NIH Pub No 81-2330, Washington, 1981.
11. Blot WJ, Devesa SS, Kneller RW, Fraumeni JF Jr: Rising incidence of adenocarcinoma of the esophagus and gastric cardia. JAMA 265:1287–1289, 1991.
12. Blot WJ, Fraumeni JF Jr: Trends in esophageal cancer mortality among U.S. blacks and whites. Am J Public Health 77:296–298, 1987.
13. Lu JB, Yang WX, Liu JM, et al: Trends in morbidity and mortality for esophageal cancer in Linxian county 1959–1983. Int J Cancer 36:643–645, 1985.
14. Rose EF, McGlashan ND: The spatial distribution of esophageal cancer in the Transkei, South Africa. Br J Cancer 31:197–206, 1979.
15. Blot WJ, Devesa SS, Fraumeni JF Jr: Continuing climb in rates of esophageal adenocarcinoma: An update. JAMA 270:1320, 1993.
16. Miller BA, Ries L, Hankey B, et al: Cancer Statistics Review 1973–1989. DHHS, NIH Pub No 92-2789, Bethesda, 1992.
17. Hammond EC: Smoking in relation to death rates of one million men and women. Monogr Natl Cancer Inst 19:127–204, 1966.
18. Rogot E, Murray JL: Smoking and causes of death among U.S. veterans: 16 years of observation. Public Health Rep 95:1525–1536, 1976.

19. Doll R, Peto R: Mortality in relation to smoking: 20 years' observation on male British doctors. BMJ 2:1525–1536, 1976.

20. Hebert J, Kabat G: Menthol cigarette smoking and oesophageal cancer. Int J Epidemiol 18:37–44, 1989.

21. Surgeon General: The Health Consequences of Smoking: Cancer. DHHS, Washington, 1982.

22. International Agency for Research on Cancer: Tobacco smoking. IARC Monogr Eval Carcinog Risks Hum 38:1–396, 1986.

23. MacDonald WC, MacDonald JB: Adenocarcinoma of the esophagus and/or gastric cardia. Cancer 60:1094–1098, 1987.

24. Gray JR, Goldman AJ, MacDonald WC: Cigarette and alcohol use in patients with adenocarcinoma of the gastric cardia or lower esophagus. Cancer 69:2227–2231, 1992.

25. Kabat G, Ng S, Wynder EL: Tobacco, alcohol intake, and diet in relation to adenocarcinoma of the esophagus and gastric cardia. Cancer Causes Control 4:123–132, 1993.

26. Brown LM, Silverman DT, Pottern LM, et al: Adenocarcinoma of the esophagus and esophagogastric junction in white men in the United States: Alcohol, tobacco, and socioeconomic factors. Cancer Causes Control 5:333–340, 1994.

27. Fiore MC, Novotny TE, Pierce JP, et al: Trends in cigarette smoking in the United States, the changing influence of gender and race. JAMA 261:49–55, 1989.

28. Bradshaw E, Schonland M: Smoking, drinking, and esophageal cancer in African males in Johannesburg, South Africa. Br J Cancer 30:157–163, 1974.

29. Gupta P, Pindborg J, Mehta FS: Comparison of carcinogenicity of betel quid with and without tobacco: an epidemiologic review. Ecol Dis 4:213–219, 1992.

30. Stephen SJ, Uragoda CG: Some observations on esophageal cancer in Ceylon, including its relation to betel chewing. Br J Cancer 24:11–15, 1970.

31. Jussawalla DJ: Esophageal cancer in India. J Cancer Res Clin Oncol 99:29–33, 1981.

32. Jussawalla DJ, Desphands VA: Evaluation of cancer risk in tobacco chewers and smokers: An epidemiologic assessment. Cancer 28:244–252, 1971.

33. Shanta V, Krishnamurthi S: Further study in aetiology of carcinomas of the upper alimentary tract. Br J Cancer 17:8–23, 1963.

34. Wynder EL, Bross IJ: A study of etiological factors in cancer of the esophagus. Cancer 14:389–413, 1961.

35. Wynder EL, Stellman SD: Comparative epidemiology of tobacco-related cancers. Cancer Res 37:4608–4622, 1977.

36. Martinez I: Factors associated with cancer of the esophagus, mouth, and pharynx in Puerto Rico. J Natl Cancer Inst 42:1069–1094, 1969.

37. Cook-Mozaffari PJ, Azordkegan F, Day NE, et al: Esophageal cancer studies in the Caspian littoral of Iran: Results of a case-control study. Br J Cancer 39:293–309, 1979.

38. Li JY, Ershow AG, Chen J, et al: A case-control study of cancer of the esophagus and gastric cardia in Linxian. Int J Cancer 43:755–761, 1989.

39. Ghadirian P, Stein GF, Gorodetzky C, et al: Oesophageal cancer studies in the Caspian littoral of Iran: some residual results, including opium use as a risk factor. Int J Cancer 35:593–597, 1985.

40. Hewer T, Rose E, Ghadirian P, et al: Ingested mutagens from opium and tobacco pyrolysis products and cancer of the esophagus. Lancet ii:494–496, 1978.

41. International Agency for Research on Cancer: Alcohol Drinking. IARC Monogr Eval Carcinog Risks Hum 44:1–378, 1988.

42. Blot WJ: Alcohol and cancer. Cancer Res 52:2119s–2123s, 1992.

43. Hakulinen T, Lehtimaki L, Lehtonen M, Teppo L: Cancer morbidity among two males cohorts with increased alcohol consumption. J Natl Cancer Inst 52:1711–1714, 1974.

44. Schmidt W, Popham RE: The role of drinking and smoking in mortality from cancer and other causes in male alcoholics. Cancer 47:1031–1041, 1981.

45. Hirayama T: Diet and cancer. Nutr Cancer 1:67–81, 1979.

46. Tuyns AJ, Pequiqnot G, Jensen OM: Le cancer de esophageal en Ille et Vilaine en function des niveaux de consomation d'alcool et de tabac: Des risques qui se multiplient. Bull Cancer (Paris) 64:63–65, 1977.

47. Tuyns AJ: Esophageal cancer in non-smoking drinkers and non-drinking smokers. Int J Cancer 32:443–444, 1983.

48. LaVecchia C, Negri E: The role of alcohol in oesophageal cancer in nonsmokers and of tobacco in nondrinkers. Int J Cancer 43:784–785, 1989.

49. Pottern LM, Morris LE, Blot WJ, et al: Esophageal cancer among black men in Washington, D.C. I: alcohol, tobacco, and other risk factors. J Natl Cancer Inst 67:777–783, 1981.

50. Brown LM, Blot WJ, Schuman S, et al: Environmental factors and high risk of esophageal cancer among men in coastal South Carolina. J Natl Cancer Inst 80:1620–1625, 1988.

51. Mettlin C, Graham S, Priore S, et al: Diet and cancer of the esophagus. Nutr Cancer 2:143–147, 1981.

52. Yu MC, Garabrandt DA, Peters J, Mack T: Tobacco, alcohol, diet, occupation and carcinoma of the esophagus. Cancer Res 48:3843–3848, 1988.

53. DeStefani E, Munoz N, Esteve J, et al: Mate drinking, alcohol, tobacco, diet and esophageal cancer in Uruguay. Cancer Res 50:426–431, 1990.

54. Dean G, MacLennan R, McLaughlin H, Shelley E: Causes of death of blue-collar workers at a Dublin brewery 1954–1973. Br J Cancer 40:581–589, 1979.

55. Jensen OM: Cancer morbidity and causes of death among Danish brewery workers. Int J Cancer 23:454–463, 1979.

56. Moller H, Boyle P, Maisonneuve P, et al: Changing mortality from esophageal cancer in males in Denmark and other European countries in relation to changing levels of alcohol consumption. Cancer Causes Control 1:181–188, 1990.

57. Cheng KK, Day NE, Davies TW: Oesophageal cancer mortality in Europe: Paradoxical time trend in relation to smoking and drinking. Br J Cancer 65:613–617, 1992.

58. VanRensburg SJ: Epidemiologic and dietary evidence for a specific nutritional predisposition to esophageal cancer. J Natl Cancer Inst 67:243–251, 1981.

59. VanRensburg SJ, Bradshaw ES, Bradshaw D, Rose EF: Esophageal cancer in Zulu men, South Africa: A case-control study. Br J Cancer 51:399–405, 1985.

60. VanRensburg SJ, Benade AS, Rose EF, DuPleiss JP: Nutritional status of African populations predisposed to esophageal cancer. Nutr Cancer 4:206–216, 1983.

61. Franceschi S, Bidoli E, Baron A, LaVecchia C: Maise and risk of cancers of the oral cavity, pharynx, and esophagus in northeastern Italy. J Natl Cancer Inst 82:1407–1411, 1990.

62. Cheng KK, Day NE, Duffy SW, et al: Pickled vegetables in the aetiology of oesophageal cancer in Hong Kong Chinese. Lancet 334:1314–1318, 1992.

63. Yu Y, Taylor PR, Li JY, et al: Retrospective cohort study of risk factors for esophageal cancer in Linxian, People's Republic of China. Cancer Causes Control 4:195–202, 1993.

64. Munoz N, Crespi M, Grassi A, et al: Precursor lesions of esophageal cancer in high risk populations in Iran and China. Lancet 1:876–879, 1982.

65. Yang CS, Sun Y, Yang Q, et al: Vitamin A and other deficiencies in Linxian, a high esophageal cancer incidence area in north China. J Natl Cancer Inst 73:1449–1453, 1984.

66. Yang CS: Nitrosamines and other etiological factors in the esophageal cancer in north China. Banbury Rpt 12:487–501, 1982.

67. National Research Council: Diet and Health. Washington, National Academy of Science, 1989.

68. Birt DF: Update on effects of vitamins A, C, and E and selenium on carcinogenesis. Proc Soc Exp Biol Med 183:311–320, 1986.

69. Gabriel GN, Schrazer TF, Newberne PM: Zinc deficiency, alcohol, and a retinoid: Association with esophageal cancer in rats. J Natl Cancer Inst 68:785–789, 1982.

70. Foy H, Kondi A: The vulnerable esophagus: Riboflavin deficiency and squamous cell dysplasia of the skin and the esophagus. J Natl Cancer Inst 72:941–948, 1984.

71. Larson LG, Sandstorm A, Westling P: Relationship of Plummer Vinson disease to cancer of upper alimentary tract in Sweden. Cancer Res 35:3308–3316, 1975.

72. Holmes GK, Stokes PL, Sorahan TM, et al: Coeliac disease, gluten-free diet, and malignancy. Gut 17:612–619, 1976.

73. Ziegler RG, Morris LE, Blot WJ, et al: Esophageal cancer among black men in Washington, D.C. II: Role of nutrition. J Natl Cancer Inst 67:1199–1202, 1981.

74. Decarli A, Liati P, Negri E, et al: Vitamin A and other dietary factors in the etiology of esophageal cancer. Nutr Cancer 10:29–37, 1987.

75. Blot WJ, Li JY: Some considerations in the design of a nutrition intervention trial in Linxian. Monogr Natl Cancer Inst 69:29–34, 1985.

76. Blot WJ, Li JY, Taylor PR, et al: Nutrition intervention trials in Linxian, China: Supplementation with specific vitamin/mineral combinations, cancer incidence, and disease-specific mortality in the general population. J Natl Cancer Inst 85:1483–1492, 1993.

77. Li JY, Taylor PR, Li B, et al: Nutrition intervention trials in Linxian, China: Multiple vitamin/mineral supplementation, cancer incidence and disease-specific mortality among adults with esophageal dysplasia. J Natl Cancer Inst 85:1492–1498, 1993.

78. Munoz N, Wahrendorf J, Bang LJ, et al: No effect of riboflavin, retinol, and zinc on prevalence of precancerous lesions of esophagus. Lancet ii:111–114, 1985.

79. Zardize D, Evstifeeva P, Boyle P: Chemoprevention of oral leukoplakia and chronic esophagitis in an area of high incidence of oral and esophageal cancer. Ann Epidemiol 3:225–234, 1993.

80. Selikoff IJ, Hammond EC, Seidman H: Mortality experience of insulation workers in the United States and Canada, 1943–1976. Ann N Y Acad Sci 330:91–116, 1979.

81. Norell S, Ahblom A, Lipping H, Osterblom L: Esophageal cancer and vulcanization work. Lancet i:462–463, 1983.

82. Gustavisson P, Hogstedt C, Evanoff B: Increased risk of esophageal cancer among workers exposed to combustion products. Arch Environ Health 48:243–245, 1993.

83. Radiation Effects Research Foundation: Life Span Study Report 9, 1950–1978. Supplementary Tables. Radiation Effects Research Foundation, Hiroshima, 1981.

84. Smith PG: Late effects of x-ray treatment of ankylosing spondylitis. In Boice J, Fraumeni J (eds): Radiation Carcinogenesis. New York, Raven Press, 1984, pp 107–118.

85. DeJong UW, Breslow N, Hong JG, et al: Etiological factors in esophageal cancer in Singapore Chinese. Int J Cancer 13:291–303, 1974.

86. Victora C, Munoz N, Day NE, et al: Hot beverages and oesophageal cancer in southern Brazil: A case-control study. Int J Cancer 39:710–716, 1987.

87. Ghadirian P: Thermal irritation and esophageal cancer in northern Iran. Cancer 60:1909–1914, 1987.

88. Morton JF: Tentative correlations of plant usage and esophageal cancer zones. Economic Botany 24:217–226, 1970.

89. Yang CS, Wang ZY: Tea and cancer. J Natl Cancer Inst 85:1038–1049, 1993.

90. Gao YT, McLaughlin JK, Blot WJ, et al: Reduced risk of esophageal cancer associated with green tea consumption. J Natl Cancer Inst 86:855–858, 1994.

91. Hille JJ, Markowitz S, Margolius KA, Isaacson C: Human papillomavirus and carcinoma of the esophagus. N Eng J Med 312:1707, 1985.

92. Shine J, Allison PR: Carcinoma of esophagus with tylosis. Lancet 1:951–953, 1966.

93. Hu N, Dawsey SM, Wu M, et al: Familial aggregation of esophageal cancer in Yangcheng county, Shanxi Province, China. Int J Epidemiol 21:877–882, 1992.

94. Carter CL, Hu N, Wu M, et al: Segregation analysis of esophageal cancer in 221 high risk Chinese families. J Natl Cancer Inst 84:771–776, 1992.

95. Rosenberg JC, Fromm D: Barrett's esophagus as a premalignant lesion. In Devita V, Hellman S, Rosenberg S (eds): Cancer Prevention. Philadelphia, J.B. Lippincott, 1992, pp 1–11.

19 THE PATHOBIOLOGY OF ESOPHAGEAL CANCER

Louis R. Bégin

EMBRYOLOGIC AND HISTOLOGIC ASPECTS AS RELATED TO NEOPLASIA

During week 4 of fetal life, the esophagus is a short, tubular, endodermal segment located between the pharynx and the caudal part of the foregut. It is originally lined by a thin layer of stratified columnar epithelium, which will proliferate to almost occlude the lumen and among which intraepithelial vacuoles begin to appear. Between weeks 4 and 7, this tubular segment lengthens considerably, with narrowing in its middle portion. Following extensive formation and coalescence of epithelial vacuoles, a lumen is reformed between weeks 6 and 7. Ciliated columnar cells first appear during week 8 in the middle third, and they will ultimately cover most of the stratified columnar epithelium by cephalad and caudal extension. At week 10, a single layer of columnar epithelium populates the proximal and distal ends of the esophagus.[1] Superficial (mucosal) cardiac-type glands are noted in the upper and lower ends of the esophagus after month 3. They originate from downward growth of this single layer of columnar epithelium into the lamina propria, with subsequent proliferation and differentiation. Stratified squamous epithelium appears at about month 5 in the middle third, progressively replacing the ciliated epithelium by cephalad and caudal extension. Because the most upper end of the esophagus is the last area to be replaced by squamous epithelium, ciliated columnar cells may temporarily persist within the first 2 to 3 days after birth. Deep (submucosal) glands start to develop around month 7, likely deriving from the squamous epithelium, and will mature mainly during the postnatal period. These glands are conceived as of minor salivary-type and embryologically linked to those of the oropharynx.[2] Development of the muscularis propria occurs during weeks 6 to 9 from the periendodermal mesoderm with subsequent formation of striated muscle in the most upper esophagus.

The mature esophagus has a mucosa that includes an epithelial lining, lamina propria, and muscularis mucosae. The epithelium consists of a nonkeratinizing, stratified squamous epithelium including a layer of basal and parabasal cells lacking glycogen (about 10% to 15% of the thickness), whereas overlying cells have a glycogen-rich clear cytoplasm (Fig. 19–1). Cells of esophageal intraepithelial neoplasia (EIN) and squamous cell carcinoma probably derive from the progenitor basal cell, parabasal cell, or both. Small cell carcinoma (at least some cases) might originate from a totipotential stem cell at that level. These cells have a high proliferative potential and express epidermal growth factor (EGF) receptors[3, 4] and have a high nucleolar organizer regions (NOR) mean number.[5] The lamina propria is the nonepithelial portion of the mucosa above the muscularis mucosae and consists of loose connective tissue, vessels, lymphatics, scattered inflammatory cells, and occasional superficial mucus-secreting (cardiac-type) glands. Superficial glands are diffusely scattered in the lamina propria, predominantly in the distal and proximal ends.[1] Found in 6% to 16% of esophagi, these glands have been variably considered as heterotopias, embryologic rests, or normal constituents.[1, 6] They have a tubuloalveolar configuration, open directly into the lumen, and are composed of mucinous cells secreting neutral mucin.[1] A genuine esophageal adenocarcinoma probably arising within these glands has been documented, according to Christensen and associates.[7] The mucosa and submucosa are delineated by a thin layer of smooth muscle, the muscularis mucosae.

The submucosa consists of loose collagenous tissue containing abundant vessels, lymphatics, and deep

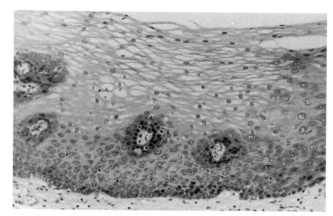

FIGURE 19–1. Normal esophageal mucosa characterized by a nonkeratinizing, stratified squamous epithelium. Nuclei are regular in size and shape, with evidence of normal surface maturation. The clear cytoplasm in superficial layers reflects a high cytoplasmic glycogen content. (Hematoxylin and eosin, 100 ×.)

mucus-secreting glands. These glands of tubuloalveolar configuration are unevenly distributed throughout the entire length of the esophagus but are more numerous in the upper and lower regions.[2] They consist mostly of mucinous cells, with or without a minor serous component, secreting acid mucin (Fig. 19–2).[1] Deep esophageal glands are conceived as of minor salivary-type and embryologically related to those of the oropharynx.[2] Adenoid cystic carcinoma of the esophagus presumably derives from these deep esophageal glands. The duct or glandular terminal portion of these glands may be involved with high-grade EIN (carcinoma in situ).[8, 9]

The muscularis propria is exclusively composed of smooth muscle in the distal esophageal half, whereas only about 5% of the proximal muscularis propria is composed of striated muscle.[10] The intervening segment consists of mixed muscle types, with a predominance of smooth muscle.[10] Esophageal leiomyosarcoma is native from the muscularis propria. On the other hand, primary rhabdomyosarcoma of the esophagus has been documented as arising in the distal third; therefore, striated muscle is not likely to be the native tissue of this neoplasm.

The adventitial layer is characterized by a serosa of pleuroperitoneal derivation lining only short segments of the esophagus,[2] whereas the esophagus is mostly surrounded by a fascia. Many lymphatics and nerve bundles are present at that level.[11] Therefore, the adventitial layer provides a fragile barrier to local tumor spread and is of significance in the high incidence of perineurial spreading when tumor reaches that level.[11]

The gastroesophageal (GE) junction is best defined as the distal-most end of the lower esophageal sphincter.[1] Recognizing that this is a relatively crude estimation, the GE junction is generally considered by the endoscopist to be about 40 cm from the incisors, with a range from 38 to 43 cm.[1] The mucosal squamocolumnar junction, which represents an abrupt interface between gray-white esophageal and pink-orange gastric epithelia, appears as a serrated but occasionally

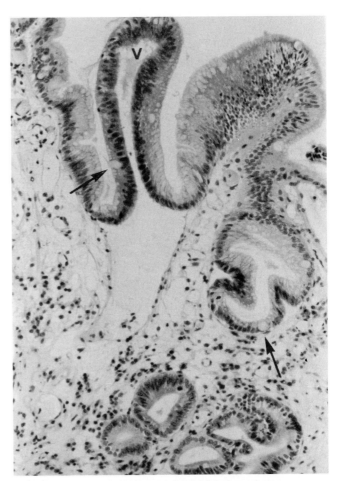

FIGURE 19–3. Barrett's mucosa, distal third of esophagus. Specialized type of glandular mucosa with surface villosities (V) and presence of goblet cells (*arrows*) resembling intestinal mucosa. There is no evidence of glandular epithelial dysplasia. (Hematoxylin and eosin, 100 ×.)

straight line of contrast (referred to as the Z line). It can be anatomically located within 2 cm (and even rarely 3 cm) above the GE junction. Therefore, endoscopic and histologic recognition of gastric-type mucosa within the most distal 2 to 3 cm esophageal segment above the GE junction should not be misinterpreted as Barrett's esophagus. On the other hand, involvement of at least 3 cm of the distal tubular esophagus by columnar epithelium-lined mucosa (Fig. 19–3) is a reflection of an acquired retrograde metaplastic process secondary to reflux esophagitis, referred to as Barrett's esophagus.[12] The large majority of genuine adenocarcinomas of the lower esophagus arise on this basis, whereas the proportion of esophageal adenocarcinomas arising from gastric-type heterotopias or esophageal mucinous glands is small.

Heterotopic (ectopic) gastric mucosa can occur anywhere in the esophagus, most often in the postcricoid (upper third) region, and has been found in 4.5% of infantile esophagi at autopsy. It is largely believed to be a congenital condition resulting from remaining rests of gastric precursor cells after incomplete replacement of the columnar epithelium by stratified

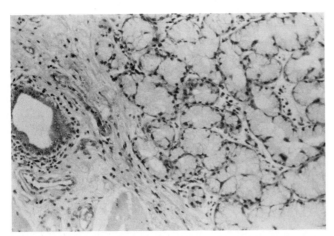

FIGURE 19–2. Normal deep mucus-secreting gland resembling a minor salivary gland. Note the abundant pale cytoplasmic mucinous content and basal positioning of nucleus. An intercalated duct is present on the left side. (Hematoxylin and eosin, 100 ×.)

squamous epithelium during embryogenesis.[7] Heterotopic gastric mucosa has been observed in 2% to 4% of patients undergoing endoscopy[13] and is sometimes designated as the inlet patch.[14] It appears as a sharply demarcated pink, velvety patch. As a result of frequently associated inflammation, ulceration, or both, glandular epithelial atypia can be present and should not be histologically misinterpreted as malignancy. On the other hand, recognizing the extremely low risk of malignant transformation in this setting, genuine cases of adenocarcinoma mostly of the upper esophagus and arising from heterotopic gastric mucosa have been reported.[7] By 1987, Christensen and colleagues[7] had found six acceptable cases in the literature, in addition to their own two cases. However, many more cases might have escaped documentation because the heterotopic focus was small or obliterated by tumor growth.

The lymphatic plexus is highly developed in the lamina propria and submucosa, and it is connected with lymphatics in the muscularis propria and adventitial layer as well.[1] The presence of a prominent longitudinal lymphatic system potentially allows significant intramucosal and/or submucosal neoplastic spreading beyond grossly visible tumor[1] and a variable or unpredictable pattern of lymphatogenous metastasis.

Argyrophilic cells have been found in 28% of esophagi examined by Tateishi and associates.[15] These cells are located in the basal region of the squamous epithelium but not in the glandular component. Argyrophilic cells were found to be more numerous as a result of certain factors in association with epithelial hyperplasia and chronic esophagitis.[16] The presence of these cells accounts for the rare occurrence of primary neuroendocrine esophageal neoplasia, namely carcinoid tumor and possibly small cell carcinoma.

Melanocytes have been found in the normal esophageal mucosa in 4% to 8% of esophagi at autopsy, either as scattered cells or as groups of cells in the basal region of the epithelium.[15–17] In a recent study, melanocytes were found in 30% of esophageal specimens with associated carcinoma.[16] The existence of this cell type, the occurrence of melanocytic hyperplasia (referred to as melanosis or melanocytosis) alone[16, 18] or in association with malignant melanoma,[19] and the presence of an associated junctional (in situ) melanocytic component in most cases of esophageal malignant melanoma[19, 20] support the concept of primary esophageal melanocytic neoplasia.

HANDLING OF CYTOLOGIC AND TISSUE MATERIAL FOR PATHOLOGIC ASSESSMENT

The use of the flexible fiberoptic endoscope allows good visual observation and direct biopsy of esophageal lesions. Although the biopsy specimens obtained with this technique are smaller than those obtained with the rigid endoscope, they are often multiple and can be taken at earlier stages and at more frequent intervals. Suction or aspiration biopsy is likely to provide a more substantial specimen that includes the submucosal stroma, whereas grasp biopsy may reveal only superficial epithelium, making histologic interpretation more difficult. The preferred site of biopsy should be the surface margin or surrounding mucosa of the lesion, avoiding as much as possible the necrotic areas and bleeding points. At least four to six fragments should be taken and immediately transferred to 10% buffered neutral formaldehyde, although the choice of fixative is not crucial. No precise orientation is required for embedding, but at least six levels of tissue should be histologically examined. However, there is some limitation in diagnostic interpretation. For instance, a mesodermal lesion or a carcinoma with mostly subepithelial invasion might be overlooked if only normal epithelium is sampled.[21] Ideally, biopsies should be coupled with brush cytology, which dislodges tumor cells by means of abrasion, especially when there is failure to pass the endoscope in a stenotic lesion.[21]

For endoscopic surveillance and biopsy monitoring of patients with Barrett's esophagus, the jumbo biopsy forceps, which acquires biopsy specimens that average 0.4 to 0.5 cm in diameter, is optimal. Use of these forceps requires passage of the therapeutic endoscope, which has a larger caliber than the more widely used screening instrument. Such large biopsy specimens increase the sample of tissue available for analysis and are not associated with an increased risk of complications.[22] Biopsy specimens should be taken at least every 2 cm in the four quadrants throughout the length of Barrett's mucosa.[23]

For exfoliative cytology, a lavage entails washing the mucosa with an isotonic saline solution. In order to provide optimal cytologic preservation, the fluid should be collected in an iced container and rapidly centrifuged, preferably in a refrigerated centrifuge. The sediment is spread evenly on frosted slides or on slides coated with albumin for adherence. Slides are then fixed immediately in 95% alcohol and stained according to Papanicolaou's method.

Brush specimens are collected under direct vision through the fiberoptic endoscope and should be obtained prior to biopsy. Cells must be retrieved from the nylon brush immediately to prevent drying the artifact. With the *direct method*, cells are removed from the brush directly onto the glass slide. Using a quick rotary movement, the brush is pressed firmly and evenly down the slide. This is repeated with a second slide. With the *indirect method*, the brush is immersed in a narrow-mouthed bottle that is filled with isotonic saline solution. Cells are dislodged by rigorous shaking of the brush and the entire fluid specimen is filtered through a millepore filter. For both direct and indirect methods, the glass slides are placed immediately in 95% alcohol and stained according to Papanicolaou's method.

An alternative method for collecting cytologic material has been proposed.[24] Following withdrawal of the forceps from the endoscope, the material from the tip of the biopsy forceps is gently smeared on a slide.

This imprint is immediately fixed in 95% alcohol and stained with Papanicolaou's method. Such a procedure combining cytologic smear and tissue material has shown 92% accuracy for diagnosis of gastroesophageal malignancy in a large survey.[24]

The following procedure is recommended for the handling of surgical specimens of esophagectomy or esophagogastrectomy. The specimen is dissected in a fresh state with a longitudinal opening opposite to the tumor, if feasible. If the gastric segment is included, it should be opened in continuity along the greater curvature. Periesophageal and perigastric lymph nodes should be dissected and identified according to their location as adjacent, proximal, and distal to the tumor. The specimen should then be pinned on a cork board, mucosal side up, and immersed in a large amount of formaldehyde for 12 to 24 hours. After photography, the following information should be recorded: length and size of specimen, size of tumor in regard to transverse and longitudinal axis, and degree of circumferential involvement. Gross configuration, depth of penetration, and relationship of tumor to margins and gastric segment should also be recorded. The peritumoral mucosa should be characterized, especially in appreciating EIN or Barrett's mucosa. Recommended sampling is as follows: four longitudinal sections of tumor at the deepest point of penetration, one including a portion of non-neoplastic mucosa proximal to the tumor and another a portion distal to the tumor (periesophageal soft tissue should be marked with India ink); at least two transverse sections of non-neoplastic mucosa, proximal and distal edge (if stomach is present, at least one section of the gastroesophageal junction); proximal and distal lines of resection; and one representative section of each lymph node.

PATHOLOGIC CONDITIONS ASSOCIATED WITH ESOPHAGEAL CARCINOMA

Long-standing achalasia,[25–31] corrosive or caustic injury,[32–36] sclerotherapy-related injury (likely a coincidental rather than causal association),[37–39] chronic radiation injury,[40–43] pharyngoesophageal (Zenker's) diverticulum,[44–47] epinephric esophageal diverticulum,[48] esophageal duplication cyst,[49] the Plummer-Vinson (Paterson-Kelly) syndrome,[50, 51] diffuse palmoplantar keratoderma (tylosis),[52, 53] celiac disease (nontropical sprue),[54, 55] the hiatal hernia or chronic esophagitis complex,[56] the acquired immunodeficiency syndrome (AIDS),[57, 58] human papillomavirus (HPV) infection,[59–62] and Barrett's esophagus[12, 21, 63–105] have all been associated with esophageal cancer. These conditions are discussed in Chapter 20.

Although most of the above-mentioned conditions have associated with an increased risk for the development of esophageal carcinoma, they account for only a small minority of cases. Except for Barrett's esophagus, these conditions have been associated mostly with squamous cell carcinoma. Esophageal adenocarcinoma is associated with Barrett's esophagus (Fig. 19–3) in most cases,[21, 63, 64] whereas the reported prevalence rate of adenocarcinoma in patients with newly diagnosed Barrett's esophagus is in the range of 8% to 27%.[12, 65–68] On the other hand, the incidence of esophageal adenocarcinoma developing in patients who present initially with Barrett's esophagus appears to be relatively low. The reported incidence has ranged from 1/52 to 1/141 patient-years, representing a $30\times$ to $125\times$ increased risk compared with that of the general population.[66, 68–72]

Risk Assessment in Barrett's Esophagus: Pathologic Correlates of Clinical Significance

Recognition of high-grade glandular epithelial dysplasia is considered to be the best marker indicative of a high risk for concurrent or subsequent development of adenocarcinoma in the setting of Barrett's esophagus. The cytoarchitectural criteria for diagnosing high-grade dysplasia are well defined,[23, 91] and there is a high degree of interobserver reproducibility in separating high-grade dysplasia from lesser degrees of abnormality.[91] The histologic appearance of glandular epithelial dysplasia is discussed in a subsequent section (see the section entitled Glandular Epithelial Dysplasia in Barrett's Mucosa).

The assessment of cellular DNA content by flow cytometry or image cytometry (using Feulgen-stained sections) has shown excellent correlation between an abnormal DNA content (aneuploidy) and the histologic diagnosis of dysplasia and adenocarcinoma.[93, 94] It has proved to be most useful in detecting a subset of patients whose biopsies were histologically indefinite or negative for dysplasia but who had DNA abnormalities similar to those otherwise seen only in dysplasia and adenocarcinoma.[93–95] Furthermore, in a recent study of 62 patients evaluated prospectively for a mean interval of 34 months, nine of 13 patients who showed aneuploid or increased G2/tetraploid cell populations (evidence of increased proliferative activity within cells) in their initial flow cytometric analysis developed high-grade dysplasia or adenocarcinoma during follow-up.[87] None of the 49 patients without these abnormalities progressed to high-grade dysplasia or adenocarcinoma. Neoplastic progression was characterized by progressive flow cytometric and histologic abnormalities.[87] Therefore, flow cytometry, in conjunction with histology, is most helpful in identifying a subset of patients with Barrett's esophagus who merit more frequent endoscopic surveillance for the early detection of high-grade dysplasia or adenocarcinoma.[87, 96] On the other hand, the clinical applicability of DNA flow cytometry and image cytometry in monitoring patients with Barrett's esophagus remains to be demonstrated.[96]

Alternative methods have been investigated in an attempt to identify a high-risk subset of patients with Barrett's mucosa.

Evaluation of the sulfomucin content of the nongoblet cell population of the specialized-type Barrett's mucosa has not proved to be useful as an indicator of neoplastic transformation. Sulfomucin in specialized-type Barrett's mucosa has been observed with equal frequency in cases with or without concurrent adenocarcinoma.[77] In another study, sulfomucin was present in biopsies of 73% of patients with a histologic diagnosis of dysplasia or adenocarcinoma, 78% of patients whose biopsies were indefinite for dysplasia, and 55% of patients whose biopsies were negative for dysplasia.[93]

The detection of epidermal growth factor (EGF) receptors in Barrett's mucosa is unlikely to be useful in segregating a high-risk subset of patients. EGF receptor expression and a heterogeneous pattern of staining have been observed in all six cases of nondysplastic, specialized-type Barrett's mucosa in the study of Poller and coworkers.[97] EGF receptor expression has also been observed in Barrett's mucosa by Jankowski and associates.[4] No significant difference of expression of EGF has been observed among the three different types of Barrett's mucosa, nor was it influenced by the absence or presence or the degree of dysplasia.[98]

The significance of immunocytochemically assessing the expression of transforming growth factor (TGF) alpha (a growth-promoting peptide) and proliferating cell nuclear antigen (PCNA) (an index of cellular proliferation) as a determinant of prognosis and clinical outcome in Barrett's mucosa is currently under investigation. Overexpression of TGF alpha and PCNA has been observed in the specialized type of Barrett's mucosa in contrast to the other types of Barrett's mucosa, including a relatively higher labeling index in the specialized-type Barrett's mucosa with high-grade dysplasia and adenocarcinoma as well.[81, 99]

The determination of the NOR mean number, using paraffin sections stained by the AgNOR reaction, has proved to be of limited value in distinguishing dysplasia from reactive changes.[100]

The pattern of p53 protein overexpression in Barrett's mucosa has been recently studied by multiparameter flow cytometric assay using biopsy material.[101] p53 protein overexpression within Barrett's mucosa was found in 5% of patients who were determined to be negative for dysplasia, 15% of patients with abnormalities in the indefinite or low-grade dysplasia range, 45% of patients with high-grade dysplasia, and 53% of patients with Barrett's-related adenocarcinoma. p53 protein overexpression was found in 9% of patients who had neither high-grade dysplasia nor adenocarcinoma.[101] Whether or not patients whose biopsy specimens show p53 protein overexpression are at increased risk for progression to adenocarcinoma remains to be determined by prospective studies.

Abdelatif and associates[102] studied the differential expression of c-myc and H-ras oncogenes in Barrett's mucosa using a nonradioactive in situ hybridization technique. Enhanced c-myc expression of approximately equal intensity was consistently observed in all grades of dysplasia and adenocarcinoma as well. H-ras was also consistently expressed in high-grade dysplasia and adenocarcinoma but not in low-grade dysplasia. Neither c-myc nor H-ras expression was detected in nondysplastic Barrett's mucosa. Whereas

overexpression of H-ras is a correlate of high-grade dysplasia, its value as a high-risk discriminant is not superior to high-grade dysplasia per se.

Garewal and colleagues[103] studied ornithine decarboxylase activity (known to be increased in certain premalignant conditions) in biopsy specimens of Barrett's mucosa from 15 patients. The enzyme activity was found to be significantly greater in four patients with dysplasia compared with 11 patients without dysplasia. However, it does not provide any discriminating value in recognizing high-risk patients.

In conclusion, recognition of high-grade dysplasia on histologic examination, possibly complemented by the identification of abnormal DNA ploidy, remains the most specific and sensitive marker in identifying patients at risk of developing adenocarcinoma. In such patients with a diagnosis of unequivocal high-grade dysplasia and without proven concurrent invasive adenocarcinoma, the question of management, namely prophylactic esophagectomy[67, 79, 88] versus enhanced endoscopy and biopsy surveillance,[23, 72, 78, 87] remains controversial. Such a decision must probably be made for each patient individually, because the possibility of detecting an occult superficial adenocarcinoma has to be weighed against the risk of operative mortality, whereas high-grade dysplasia may persist for years without clinical or histologic evidence of progression.[72, 84]

CLASSIFICATION OF ESOPHAGEAL CANCER

A classification scheme of esophageal cancer is included in Table 19–1. Although the classification frameworks proposed by both the World Health Organization[106] and Armed Forces Institute of Pathology[107] have served as guidelines for the present classification, some modification and expansion were believed to be necessary in order to reflect current concepts of pathobiology in esophageal neoplasia, as well as to fulfill the comprehensive requirements of this present text. Therefore, all types of documented tumors, regardless of rarity, are included in this classification scheme. As in most systems for classifying neoplasia, the histologic type of tumor is based principally on its cytoarchitectural differentiation, as determined by histologic examination, with the occasional use of ultrastructural or immunocytochemical techniques, or both. A term such as undifferentiated carcinoma, small cell variant, or NOS (not otherwise specified) refers to the lack of any cytoarchitectural differentiation and to the relative size of the tumor cells. Some tumors have been reported with a cumbersome terminology (e.g., squamous cell carcinoma with sarcomatoid features or small cell carcinoma), reflecting different concepts of histogenesis or stressing their cytoarchitecture. When many synonyms are used for one term, these are mentioned in the appropriate discussion. The qualitative term of NOS refers to the conventional profile of one tumor histologic type. Preinvasive neoplasia also has been included in the

TABLE 19–1. Classification of Esophageal Cancer

Preinvasive neoplasia
  Esophageal intraepithelial neoplasia
  Glandular epithelial dysplasia/adenocarcinoma in situ in
    Barrett's mucosa
Invasive malignant neoplasia
  Squamous cell carcinoma, NOS*
  Basaloid squamous cell carcinoma†
  Squamous cell carcinoma with sarcomatoid features†
  Verrucous squamous cell carcinoma†
  Adenocarcinoma, NOS
  Adenoid cystic carcinoma†
  Mucoepidermoid carcinoma†
  Adenosquamous carcinoma†
  Adenoacanthoma†
  Undifferentiated carcinoma, NOS
  Small cell carcinoma†
  Carcinoid tumor
  Malignant melanoma
  Sarcomas
    Leiomyosarcoma
    Fibrosarcoma
    Malignant fibrous histiocytoma
    Osteosarcoma
    Chondrosarcoma
    Synovial sarcoma
    Hemangiopericytoma
    Kaposi's sarcoma
    Rhabdomyosarcoma
    Liposarcoma
    Malignant schwannoma
    Malignant granular cell tumor
    Malignant mesenchymoma
  Choriocarcinoma
  Malignant lymphoma and Hodgkin's disease
  Extramedullary plasmacytoma
  Collision tumors
  Secondary and metastatic tumors
  Unclassified

*NOS = not otherwise specified.
†Special variants.

present classification scheme, although its natural history and rate of progression to invasive neoplasia remain unclear, particularly for EIN in the Western world.

ESOPHAGEAL INTRAEPITHELIAL NEOPLASIA

EIN is best defined as an abnormal squamous cell proliferative zone within the esophageal epithelium, without disruption of the basal lamina. This designation encompasses both dysplasia of variable degrees (mild, moderate, severe) and carcinoma in situ (also referred to as epithelial or intraepithelial carcinoma and even superficially spreading carcinomatous component when extensive).[108, 109] The concept of EIN is valid because it encompasses a spectrum of lesions that are frequently concurrent and confluent, and recognizes a cytoarchitectural continuum. The designation EIN is used for lesions of the aerodigestive and female genital tracts. EIN is further characterized as low-grade or high-grade, low-grade EIN corresponding to mild and moderate dysplasia, whereas high-grade EIN corresponds to severe dysplasia and carci-

noma in situ.[110] Delineation of EIN as low-grade versus high-grade probably offers a practical advantage because histologic discrimination between two sets rather than four sets of intraepithelial lesions is easier, more reproducible, and therefore allows comparative analysis among studies. For example, the significant lack of intraobserver and interobserver reproducibility for the distinction between mild and moderate dysplasia is well recognized.[111, 112]

Recognition of these two sets of intraepithelial lesions is justified from a pathobiologic perspective, particularly in recognizing high-grade EIN as a precursor lesion of invasive squamous cell carcinoma, whereas the role of low-grade EIN as a precursor lesion is unclear. In an autopsy study of 500 esophageal specimens without clinically overt esophageal carcinoma, both lesions of high-grade EIN referred to as severe dysplasia and carcinoma in situ were similarly found to be significantly associated with risk factors usually corresponding to those of clinical esophageal carcinoma, namely male gender, smoking, drinking, head and neck cancer, and multiple primary cancers.[113] However, such association was not found for lesions referred to as mild or moderate dysplasia, both of which are encompassed within the designation of low-grade EIN.[113]

Using an experimental rat model in which a full range of epithelial neoplastic lesions were induced by N-methyl-N-amylnitrosamine, Koga and coworkers[114] observed that the mean DNA content in severe dysplasia was similar to that of carcinoma in situ and superficial invasive carcinoma as well, whereas it was statistically higher than that of mild and moderate dysplasia (without any difference in the latter two lesions). The mean DNA content for mild and moderate dysplasia was nearly similar but statistically higher than that of normal esophageal mucosa. The DNA distribution patterns (according to the degree of dispersion and the peak modal value on the DNA histogram) were remarkably comparable for lesions of severe dysplasia, carcinoma in situ, and superficial invasive carcinoma as a group, including a similar proportion of type 3 pattern of high DNA ploidy. Conversely, types 1 and 2 patterns of low DNA ploidy were observed in 95% of lesions qualified as mild or moderate dysplasia.[114] In a study of human esophagi, Rubio and associates[112] also observed a similar pattern of DNA distribution (widely dispersed) in lesions of severe dysplasia and carcinoma in situ. On the other hand, low-grade EIN encompasses lesions whose role as a precursor of invasive carcinoma is far from being clarified.[112, 114, 115] A large proportion if not the majority of lesions of low-grade EIN (particularly mild dysplasia) remain stable or regress according to prospective cytology screening studies,[115] and many of these lesions might possibly be of reactive nature.[112, 116]

In practice, however, traditional terms such as dysplasia and carcinoma in situ are still widely used in reference to the esophagus since the designation of EIN has not yet gained wide acceptance. In terms of primary tumor site, high-grade EIN (carcinoma in situ) corresponds to Tis cancer in the TNM staging system adopted by the American Joint Committee on Cancer.[117]

The cytoarchitectural alterations of EIN are characterized by loss of cell polarity, cytoplasmic dedifferentiation, an increased nuclear and cytoplasmic ratio, variation in nuclear size and shape, and hyperchromasia with chromatin aberrations.[21, 110, 115] These nuclear changes are a reflection of alteration of the chromosomal contents. The presence of such cells up to one-third (mild dysplasia) or two-thirds (moderate dysplasia) of the epithelial thickness corresponds to low-grade EIN (Fig. 19–4). The presence of these cells in more than two-thirds of the epithelial thickness with some surface cytoplasmic maturation (severe dysplasia) or transepithelial involvement without maturation (carcinoma in situ) corresponds to high-grade EIN (Figs. 19–5 and 19–6). Mitotic figures, including atypical forms, are likely to be observed in high-grade EIN. Ductal and glandular involvement of deep esophageal glands by high-grade EIN (carcinoma in situ) in the setting of concurrent invasive carcinoma has been observed in nearly 20% of cases following a diligent search by Takubo and coworkers.[8] The epithelial-stromal interface is either straight or most often undulated, with epithelial buds bulging

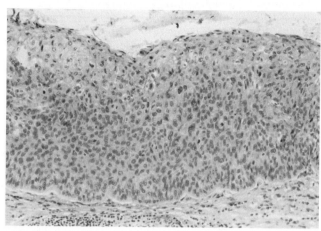

FIGURE 19–5. High-grade EIN. Nearly full-thickness neoplastic transformation of the esophageal epithelium is seen. Note loss of cell polarity and variation in nuclear size and shape. (Hematoxylin and eosin, 100 ×.)

into the lamina propria.[110] The overall grading of EIN in an intraepithelial lesion or overall assessment of a case is based on the most severe degree of histologic alteration observed.[110] Quantitative nuclear morphometric analysis might be of potential value in objectively discriminating EIN cells from normal or reac-

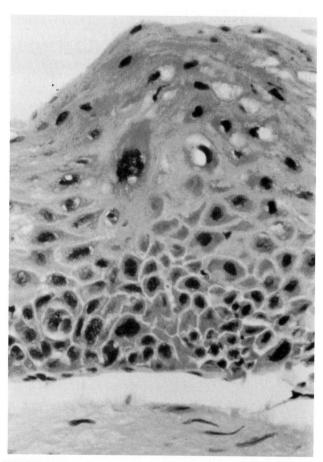

FIGURE 19–4. Low-grade esophageal intraepithelial neoplasia (EIN). There are loss of cell polarity, abnormal maturation, increased nuclear-cytoplasmic ratio, and nuclear hyperchromasia involving about one-half to two-thirds of the epithelium. (Hematoxylin and eosin, 250 ×.)

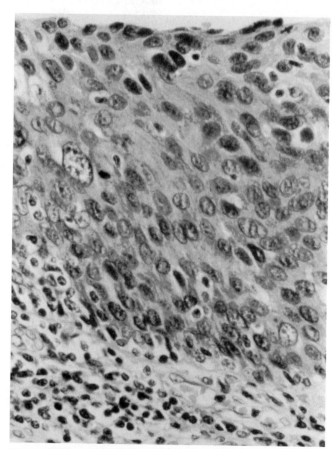

FIGURE 19–6. High-grade EIN. There is variation in nuclear size and shape, a high nuclear-cytoplasmic ratio, nuclear hyperchromasia with chromatin aberrations, and lack of surface maturation. (Hematoxylin and eosin, 250 ×.)

tive esophageal epithelial cells[118] but is unlikely to be used on a routine basis.

Hurlimann and associates[119] have recognized two main patterns of high-grade EIN (carcinoma in situ) with a distinct phenotype, one of which might represent the specific precursor of undifferentiated carcinoma, NOS. The usually encountered transepithelial pattern of high-grade EIN was composed of cells expressing keratins of high molecular weight and was often associated with keratinizing (well to moderately differentiated) squamous cell carcinoma. On the other hand, the infrequent pagetoid pattern of high-grade EIN, characterized by a discontinuous population of cells in the parabasal and basal regions, was composed of cells expressing keratins of low molecular weight. This pattern was highly associated with undifferentiated carcinoma, NOS, the latter expressing exclusively keratins of low molecular weight.[119]

Grossly, lesions of high-grade EIN are frequently inconspicuous, showing a subtle alteration of color or luster, or minimal change in the surface contour.[115] Lesions of EIN are likely to be enhanced and delineated by the application of Lugol's (iodine) solution or toluidine blue to the mucosal surface.[120, 121] A positive lesion is likely to appear as an unstained patch with Lugol's solution staining (the normal epithelium stains green-brown), and as a blue patch with toluidine blue staining. For the detection of high-grade EIN, the use of Lugol's solution offers greater sensitivity.[122] However, because the abnormal tinctorial character observed with these techniques is a reflection of hypercellularity and loss of cytoplasmic differentiation and maturation, a positive result can occur within reactive zones of repair or inflammation or within an atrophic epithelium.[122] Rarely, high-grade EIN (more precisely carcinoma in situ) may appear as a lesion with a slightly raised or depressed configuration and a smooth or irregular surface like the gross verrucous type or coarse type ascribed to superficial esophageal carcinoma (SEC).[123]

In areas in which there is a high incidence of invasive esophageal squamous cell carcinoma (particularly in parts of China), the overall prevalence of pure EIN on initial screening is within the range of 13% to 20%, whereas documentation of pure cases of high-grade EIN is sparse in Western countries.[124, 125] However, EIN (particularly high-grade EIN) is commonly observed in conjunction with superficial squamous cell carcinoma,[8, 9, 109–111, 126–128] as contiguous or separate mucosal lesions, and less often with advanced squamous cell carcinoma,* presumably because of obliteration of the residual intraepithelial neoplastic component by tumor in advanced disease. Following preoperative radiotherapy, the incidence of concurrent high-grade EIN is much lower (in the range of 10% to 15%), probably as a result of radiation-induced destruction.[9, 120, 122, 128, 130]

Substantial evidence supports the importance of high-grade EIN as a precursor of invasive squamous cell carcinoma. However, the progression rate and la-

tency period observed in high-risk populations of China, Iran, and South Africa is probably not applicable to high-risk populations of the Western world.[116] At any rate, the following observations support the concept of a sequence leading from EIN to squamous cell carcinoma.

In geographic areas known for a high incidence of esophageal carcinoma, such as China, the overall prevalence of EIN is estimated to be in the range of 13% to 20% and up to 38% in high-risk subsets of this population.[115] In a large Japanese study of 500 esophagi at autopsy, without clinically overt esophageal carcinoma, recognition of lesions of high-grade EIN was highly associated with risk factors corresponding to those of clinical esophageal carcinoma, such as male gender, smoking, drinking, head and neck cancer, and multiple primary cancers.[113]

Prospective studies examining the natural history of high-grade EIN are indicative of a significant risk for progression to invasive squamous cell carcinoma in high-risk populations of China. Lu and coworkers[131] in a prospective study of high-risk population in China, followed for 10 years, observed that high-grade EIN (severe dysplasia) was associated with about a threefold increased risk for developing invasive carcinoma compared with controls. In another large prospective follow-up study of high-risk population in China, invasive squamous cell carcinoma developed in about one-third of patients with biopsy proved dysplasia and chronic esophagitis, as opposed to 4% of patients with chronic esophagitis alone over a follow-up period of 30 to 78 months.[132] However, such progression rate has not been reproduced in a United States prospective study of a high-risk population in which dysplasia was diagnosed by cytology,[116] partly relating to the difficulty of distinguishing low-grade EIN from esophagitis-associated inflammatory epithelial atypia.

Concurrent and contiguous high-grade EIN is frequently observed in cases of superficial invasive squamous cell carcinoma[8, 9, 109–111, 126–128] and less often in cases of advanced squamous cell carcinoma.* The incidence of concurrent/contiguous high-grade EIN is proportionally lower as the associated invasive carcinoma shows a deeper level of invasion and higher tumor volume. The low incidence of concurrent high-grade EIN reported in preoperatively radiated esophagi is probably the result of radiation-induced destruction.[9, 120, 122, 128, 130] On the other hand, the discontinuous topography and multicentricity of high-grade EIN, observed in a significant proportion of cases of invasive squamous cell carcinoma, likely reflects field carcinomatous transformation. Concurrent and contiguous EIN has also been observed in three-quarters of cases of spontaneous squamous cell carcinoma in the chicken.[133]

A peculiar type of epithelial bud configuration in high-grade EIN is putatively considered to be the immediate precursor of microinvasion. In a thorough Chinese study of 64 esophageal specimens showing

---

*See references 8, 9, 107, 111, 120, 122, and 129.

*See references 8, 9, 107, 111, 120, 122, and 129.

high-grade EIN concurrent to superficial invasive squamous cell carcinoma, the presence of epithelial buds of varying length and width with irregular contours (referred to as Type 3) were observed in 88% of cases, mostly adjacent to the invasive carcinoma. Furthermore, microinvasion was seen to originate at the tips of these Type 3 epithelial buds in 21% of the specimens.[110] Similar observations have been reported using an experimental animal model[134] and in specimens of chicken esophagi with a spontaneous squamous cell carcinoma.[133]

In experimental carcinogenesis using a rat model to which nitrosamine compounds are administered, a full histopathologic continuum of EIN to superficial invasive squamous cell carcinoma to advanced invasive squamous cell carcinoma has been repeatedly induced, including similar abnormal DNA profiles for high-grade EIN and superficial invasive squamous cell carcinoma.[114]

Cytophotometric DNA analysis studies have shown similar patterns of DNA distribution and content between high-grade EIN and superficial invasive squamous cell carcinoma, both in human esophagi[112] and in the experimental rat model.[114]

The overexpression of nuclear protein p53 tumor suppressor gene product (as a reflection of a mutated form of p53) has been observed in EIN as well as in squamous cell carcinoma of the esophagus.[135]

On the other hand, there is evidence that lesions of EIN may remain stable or even regress. Prospective cytology screening studies in China have shown that the majority (80% to 85%) of lesions referred to as mild dysplasia remain stable or even regress, whereas 40% of lesions referred to as severe dysplasia regress over a 2- to 4-year period.[21, 115]

In the Western world, the diagnosis of EIN should be made with caution and by using stringent cytopathologic criteria, because epithelial changes related to chronic esophagitis or ulceration represent a potential source of misinterpretation. In *epithelial atypia of repair* or *inflammation,* enlarged nuclei can be observed in more than one-half of the epithelial thickness, in conjunction with increased mitotic activity. However, in contrast to EIN, there is no chromatin aberration or abnormal mitotic figure, whereas macronucleoli are often present. Following chemotherapy or regional radiotherapy, *esophageal epithelial atypia* is characterized by cells of increased size and abnormal shape, occasionally multinucleated, showing nuclear hyperchromasia and pleomorphism in conjunction with epithelial atrophy and lack of maturation[115, 122]; such changes should not to be misinterpreted as EIN. On the other hand, a white mucosal plaque interpreted as leukoplakia by the endoscopist is likely to represent *glycogenic acanthosis* or less often *hyperkeratosis* on histologic interpretation. Epithelial hyperplasia with large glycogen-rich cells without cytologic atypia is histologically characteristic of glycogenic acanthosis. Because they are multiple and occasionally confluent, lesions of glycogenic acanthosis have a predilection for the lower third of the esophagus[136] and are observed in 15% of all endoscopies.[136] The lesion is gray-white, has an ovoid nodular or plaquelike configuration, and measures up to 1.5 cm in diameter. This condition is not a precursor of carcinoma and may in fact represent a variant from normal.

Focal esophageal epithelial hyperplasia (some of these lesions are referred to as squamous cell papillomas), induced by HPV infection, has been recently documented.[59, 137] These lesions are similar to flat condylomata, as has been described in the epithelium of the lower female genital tract. Most patients had esophageal biopsy for non-neoplastic conditions, and their lesions were described as erythematous or white on endoscopic examination. They are histologically characterized by undulating squamous epithelial hyperplasia with koilocytosis, giant and multinucleated cells, hyperkeratosis, acanthosis, papillomatosis, and dyskeratosis. The presence of vacuolated cells with clear cytoplasm or perinuclear halos and nuclear pyknosis (koilocytosis) in superficial or middle epithelial layers is the most important criterion for recognizing the nature of this process.[59, 137] The significance of this lesion and HPV infection as a precursor of esophageal neoplasia is currently being investigated. In a recent study of 45 biopsy samples of esophageal squamous cell carcinoma, HPV DNA (including the most oncogenic types 16 and 18) has been detected by polymerase chain reaction in three cases.[61] In the study by Williamson and colleagues,[60] HPV DNA has been detected by in situ DNA hybridization in 71% of patients with esophageal squamous cell carcinoma, either in the tumor biopsy material (6 of 14 samplings) or in the adjacent mucosa (6 of 9 samplings). Furthermore, HPV DNA has been found by in situ DNA hybridization in 43% of patients with esophageal squamous cell carcinoma, mostly in the adjacent mucosa showing changes of EIN or epithelial hyperplasia.[59] In a separate study, Chang and coworkers[62] found HPV DNA by in situ DNA hybridization in 66% of specimens of low-grade to high-grade EIN.

INVASIVE ESOPHAGEAL CANCER

General Considerations

In collected series of patients with esophageal cancer, the overall topographic distribution without histologic stratification is as follows: 50% in the middle esophageal third, 30% to 40% in the lower third, and 10% to 20% in the upper third.[107, 138] However, overlapping is not infrequent,[129] and except in women afflicted with Plummer-Vinson (Paterson-Kelly) syndrome, the cervical (postcricoid) location is rare.[107] The major problem in regard to information about histologic stratification is the lack of stringent diagnostic pathologic criteria: (1) many series have included glandular neoplasms involving gastric cardia, most frequently of gastric derivation; (2) rare subtypes such as adenoid cystic carcinoma or adenosquamous carcinoma have been included in series of conventional adenocarcinoma or carcinoma at large; (3) adenocarcinoma superimposed on Barrett's esophagus, better understood lately, may involve gastric cardia and yet should be classified as of primary esophageal origin; (4) some series[122, 129] have classified as undifferentiated carcinoma any tumor displaying a significant undifferentiated component in spite of focal squamous cell differentiation (in fact, except for the small cell variant, undifferentiated carcinoma has been defined poorly).

The relative incidence of esophageal cancer in regard to major histologic types is as follows: squamous cell carcinoma, 87% to 90% (including superficial and advanced forms); primary adenocarcinoma, 5% to 10% (including tumors related to Barrett's esophagus); and undifferentiated carcinoma, 3% to 4%,[107] if defined as strict absence of squamous or glandular differentiation. All other tumors are rare and usually the object of case reports or retrospective surveys. Adenocarcinoma of the gastric cardia (of conventional type) is arbitrarily assigned to gastric origin in the absence of associated Barrett's esophagus, whereas squamous cell carcinoma of the gastroesophageal junction is assigned to the lower thoracic esophagus.

Superficial Squamous Cell Carcinoma

The concept of SEC (early esophageal carcinoma, superficially invasive carcinoma, microscopic carcinoma, microinvasive squamous cell carcinoma) has emerged in the late 1970s in the Chinese and Japanese literature. It reflects earlier detection and concomitant prognostic improvement mostly resulting from screening procedures (including cytologic surveillance) and periodic health examinations applied to high-risk populations in the Eastern world. Except for sporadic case reports, recognition of SEC in the Western world and reporting of small series has occurred in the last decade mostly as a result of the increased use of fiberoptic endoscopy, Lugol's (iodine) solution or toluidine blue application to the esophageal mucosa showing minimal alterations, and increased diagnostic awareness from the endoscopist.[127, 128, 139]

Although there is no consensus on the precise definition of SEC among authors, a currently accepted definition and the one used in this chapter is the following: invasive squamous cell carcinoma or undifferentiated carcinoma (NOS, non–small cell type) of the esophagus whose depth of invasion is not beyond the submucosa, regardless of the presence or absence of regional lymph node metastasis.[111, 115, 123, 126, 140, 141] Therefore, tumor invasion can be confined to the mucosa (within the lamina propria or muscularis mucosae) or submucosa. The designation SEC is considered valid when preoperative radiotherapy or chemotherapy, or both, and the presence of synchronous parenchymal and distant metastasis are excluded, and assuming that a thorough pathologic examination of the surgical specimen has been performed.[109–111, 142] On the other hand, some authors have restricted the use of the term SEC to cases without lymph node metastasis.[110, 127, 139] Some series have also included cases of high-grade EIN (carcinoma in situ, alternatively called intraepithelial or epithelial

carcinoma).* Furthermore, some authors have included tumors of a different histologic type such as adenocarcinoma, adenoid cystic carcinoma, adenosquamous carcinoma, squamous cell carcinoma with sarcomatoid features, sarcomas, and even malignant melanoma under the umbrella designation of SEC.[109, 123, 139, 142, 145]

In terms of primary tumor site, SEC coincides with T1 cancer in the TNM staging system adopted by the American Joint Committee on Cancer.[117]

Its occurrence rate among resected specimens of esophageal carcinoma at large is reported as 7% to 13% in the Western world,[126–128] whereas the occurrence rate among resected and nonresected esophageal carcinoma at large has been reported as 0.75% to 4%.[126, 139] In the Eastern world (large series from Japan), the occurrence rate among resected specimens of esophageal carcinoma has been reported as 9% to 11%[142, 146, 147] including lesions referred to as carcinoma in situ. Not surprisingly, the number of reported cases of SEC from Japan and China largely exceeds those reported in Europe and United States. It is largely diagnosed in males,[123, 126, 139, 148] with age ranging from the fourth to eight decade.[123, 148] In the Eastern world, a large proportion (more than half) of patients diagnosed with SEC are asymptomatic, their lesions being discovered through screening procedures or periodic health examination or being incidentally discovered during investigation for another problem. Otherwise, dysphagia is the most common symptom.[141–143, 146] On the other hand, in the Western world, dysphagia, retrosternal pain and heartburn are the most frequent symptoms encountered. A significant proportion of patients are also asymptomatic, SEC being fortuitously discovered during endoscopy for another reason.[123, 126–128, 139, 149] In a review of series of SEC cumulating a total number of 116 cases, the location was 53% in the middle esophageal third, 39% in the lower third, and 8% in the upper third,[126, 139, 143, 148] a distribution comparable to advanced squamous cell carcinoma of the esophagus.

The terminology used to describe the macroscopic (gross) appearance of SEC is most variable and cumbersome because Chinese, Japanese, and Western authors use different terminology. We find the descriptive scheme used by Bogomoletz and coworkers[123] most appropriate because it seems to reflect a greater diversity of tumor appearance for SEC encountered in the Western world.

In the macroscopic scheme used by Bogomoletz and associates[123] (and excluding their tumors not of a conventional squamous cell or undifferentiated cell, NOS, histologic type), five macroscopic types are recognized, either by endoscopy or inspection of the surgical specimen:

1. The *verrucous* type (38%), characterized by a single plateau-like lesion with an irregular surface or a convoluted lesion with alternating elevated nodules and narrow depressions. It probably encompasses the

---

*See references 109, 123, 126, 139, 141, 143, and 144.

appearance referred to as plaquelike or nodular by Schmidt and coworkers.[126]

2. The *coarse* type (33%), in which the mucosa has lost its normal glassy appearance, showing a more red coloration and a slightly raised or depressed configuration; alternating raised and depressed areas are often observed.

3. The *polypoid* type (13%), which exhibits a sessile or pedunculated configuration with a smooth or eroded surface.

4. The *normal* flat type (9%), in which the mucosa appears grossly normal but in which Lugol's (iodine) solution application discloses an unstained (iodine negative) zone.

5. The *ulcerating infiltrating* type (7%), whose appearance is most reminiscent of advanced squamous cell carcinoma, including a fungating appearance as well.

The verrucous and coarse types display some features ascribed to the plaque and erosive types in the Chinese scheme, but they also show other changes.[123] The polypoid type may partly correspond to the papillary type in the Chinese scheme. The normal flat type is the counterpart of the occult type in the Chinese scheme, whereas there is no Chinese counterpart for the ulcerating infiltrating type. Chinese investigators have recognized four basic macroscopic types for SEC,[144, 150] whose terminology is used as well in the Western literature:

1. The *plaque* type (the most common), characterized by a slightly elevated lesion with a granular mucosal aspect, loss of luster and subtle thickening; in most lesions of this type, invasion is confined to the mucosa.

2. The *erosive* type, showing a slightly depressed or eroded mucosal pattern with an irregular but sharply demarcated contour.

3. The *papillary* type, characterized by a papillary or polypoid protrusion, usually 1 to 3 cm in diameter with a well-demarcated contour.

4. The *occult* type (the least common), often showing an indistinct mucosal luster after fixation; in most cases, however, this appearance corresponds to high-grade EIN (carcinoma in situ).[144]

The plaque and erosive types account for more than 70% of the gross appearance observed for SEC in China, whereas no appearance resembling advanced squamous cell carcinoma is reported for SCE. Japanese authors use the same gross and endoscopic terminology as for early gastric carcinoma. It is complex, often including composite forms and not uniformly used among Japanese authors. The following basic macroscopic types are recognized: (1) *superficial*, (2) *protruding*, and (3) *excavated*. The superficial type is further qualified as *elevated*, *flat*, or *depressed*.[109, 140–143, 146, 148] The size of SEC with a conventional squamous cell histologic type ranges from 0.5 to 10 cm in major diameter, with about two-thirds of lesions measuring less than 3 cm.[123, 126–128, 139, 141] Even when invasion of the submucosa is observed, a significant proportion of

lesions measure less than 2 cm, as observed in 29% of the 89 cases reported by Ide and colleagues.[109] The presentation of SEC as multiple pedunculated polypoid lesions (without sarcomatoid features) is exceptional.[151]

In SEC, the histologic profile is similar to that of advanced carcinoma including a full range of squamous cell differentiation or an undifferentiated, NOS, histologic type.[123, 140, 143, 147, 148] The histologic grade has not been found to correlate with the depth of tumor invasion, the incidence of nodal metastasis, the survival, or the nuclear DNA ploidy index.[152, 153] Even at its earliest degree, invasion is usually recognized by the presence of a ragged stromal-epithelial interface, stromal fibrosis (desmoplasia), and associated chronic inflammation. In two Western series of SEC, including 68 patients, all esophageal specimens showed a chronic lymphoplasmacytoid cell infiltrate of variable intensity apposed to the invasive tumor component.[123, 126] In cases with marked inflammation, nodal enlargement secondary to reactive lymphoid hyperplasia was observed in about one-third of patients.[123] Perineurial invasion, considered to be one important route of tumor dissemination and frequently observed in advanced esophageal carcinoma, is not present in SEC.[11]

Mapping studies of whole surgical specimens of SEC have shown concurrent and multicentric high-grade (and to a lesser degree low-grade) EIN in the vast majority of specimens. In a study of 76 specimens from China,[110] the authors observed concurrent and adjacent areas of high-grade EIN (severe dysplasia/carcinoma in situ) in 66 cases (87%), including all specimens in which the depth of tumor invasion was confined within the lamina propria. In a Japanese study of 48 esophageal specimens with SEC (referred to as the main tumor), Kuwano and colleagues[9] observed concurrent and contiguous high-grade EIN (carcinoma in situ) in 33 patients (69%), more specifically in 88% of patients with tumor invasion confined to the mucosa and 65% of patients with tumor invasion within the submucosa. In one European series of 15 esophagectomy specimens with SEC, Anani and coworkers[111] observed concurrent and multicentric areas of EIN (both low-grade and high-grade) in all cases. These areas of EIN were either confluent or discontinuous and were always at least focally contiguous with carcinoma in situ and invasive carcinoma. Furthermore, extensive involvement of the esophageal specimen by high-grade EIN has been observed in about 20% to 35% of patients with SEC.[109, 111, 126] Concurrent areas of high-grade EIN (carcinoma in situ) at a distant location from the main tumor and within a separate segmental third of the esophagus were observed in all five cases of SEC studied by Kuwano and associates.[154] Furthermore, Rubio and colleagues[110] observed a relatively higher incidence of concurrent high-grade EIN (carcinoma in situ) with type III epithelial buds (buds of varying length and width with irregular contours; see the previous section on EIN) in cases of SEC in which invasion was beyond the lamina propria. This type of epithelial bud is currently believed to represent the most immediate morphologic precursor of microinvasion.[110] In conclusion, the above-mentioned observations in the setting of SEC would sustain:

1. The concept of a sequence in esophageal carcinogenesis leading from EIN to invasive squamous cell carcinoma, assuming that progressive obliteration and destruction of the contiguous intraepithelial neoplastic component occurs with deeper tumor invasion and increased tumor volume.

2. The concept of field effect in esophageal carcinogenesis, at least in a substantial number of esophageal squamous cell carcinomas.

In two series with a thorough evaluation of vascular (lymphatic or venular, or both) invasion in SEC, vascular invasion was observed in 33% to 40% of cases in which tumor invasion was confined to the mucosa and in 67% to 80% of cases in which tumor invasion was present in the submucosa.[11, 139] The presence of vascular invasion in SEC with tumor invasion in the submucosa has otherwise been reported in 43% to 60% of tumors.[8, 126, 143, 145, 148] In patients with SEC with tumor invasion confined to the mucosa, the reported incidence of regional lymph node metastasis has ranged from 0% to 8%,[8, 123, 126, 140–143] whereas the reported incidence has ranged from 11% to 75% (a range of 30% to 50% being probably most representative) with tumors invading the submucosa.* Therefore submucosal invasion in SEC is associated with a relatively high incidence of lymph node metastasis.

In a recent study of 16 cases of SEC with invasion of the submucosa, Ohno and associates[148] suggested that recognition of a prominent vertical tumor growth pattern rather than a horizontal tumor growth pattern might be a poor prognostic determinant. These authors reported that a tumor growth pattern referred to as the *massively penetrating (down growth) type*, defined as a ratio of submucosal tumor area to total (mucosal and submucosal) tumor area exceeding 0.2_3 was associated with a poor outcome. Indeed, this tumor growth pattern was observed in all four tumor-related deaths of their series, which occurred within 2 years of diagnosis. Furthermore, vascular invasion and lymph node metastasis were almost exclusively observed in conjunction with this tumor growth pattern.

Some retrospective studies, using surgical specimens with SEC, have examined nuclear characteristics for prognostic determination because it might be of value in predicting the extent of disease and in tailoring therapeutic strategies in a preoperative setting. Nuclear DNA ploidy (content) has been determined via cytophotometric analysis performed on paraffin-fixed sections stained by the Feulgen reaction and examined by the two-wavelength method.[145, 147, 153] Although it has been reported that lymph node metastasis was observed almost exclusively in cases with a high DNA ploidy index (Types 3 and 4: widely scattered DNA distribution histogram)[145, 153] or that the

nuclear DNA ploidy index was significantly higher in cases of SEC with nodal metastasis,[147] it has been observed that cases of SEC without nodal metastasis were distributed almost equally in the low and high nuclear DNA ploidy index groups as well.[145, 153] Therefore, determination of nuclear DNA ploidy has not been shown to have a high predictive value for nodal metastasis in SEC. In a comparative analysis, Inokuchi and coworkers[153] observed a high nuclear DNA ploidy index (Types 3 and 4: widely scattered DNA distribution histogram) in 69% of cases of SEC, compared with 82% of cases of advanced esophageal carcinoma, which does not represent a major difference. However, the Type 4 nuclear DNA ploidy (aneuploidy) was detected in 26% of cases of SEC as compared with 41% of cases of advanced esophageal carcinoma. In patients with SEC, recognition of Type 4 DNA ploidy (aneuploidy) has been associated with a 5-year survival of 10% in one study,[153] whereas more than one-half of the patients died of recurrent disease in another study.[145] These observations suggest that recognition of aneuploidy might be a poor prognostic determinant in SEC. Determination of the NOR mean number (which correlates with proliferative activity), using paraffin-embedded sections stained by the AgNOR reaction, has been studied in SEC. In a study of 39 cases, Maesawa and colleagues[147] reported that the NOR mean number was significantly higher in patients developing recurrence than in those surviving for more than 3 years without recurrence. On the other hand, the study of Miyasaki and coworkers[5] revealed that (1) determination of the NOR mean number was of little practical value in distinguishing between non-neoplastic epithelium, EIN, and invasive squamous cell carcinoma; (2) because significant intratumoral heterogeneity was present, this technique was of limited value in determining the aggressive potential of a tumor. Further studies are required to determine whether this technique has a significant role in the pathobiologic assessment of esophageal neoplasia. Maesawa and associates[142] reported that the *nuclear area* (NA) mean number, which is karyometrically estimated by using an image analysis system, was significantly higher in cases of SEC with lymph node metastasis and in patients developing recurrence within 3 years.

One Chinese study[155] has examined the natural history of untreated SEC, including 90 patients who for various reasons refused any form of therapy, with a follow-up of 19 to 78 months. Whereas a diagnosis of squamous cell carcinoma was histologically confirmed by endoscopic biopsy in all patients, it is unclear how the degree of mural invasion was ascertained and whether or not cases of high-grade EIN (carcinoma in situ) were included (although we suspect that cases of carcinoma in situ were included). Of these 90 patients with untreated SEC, 52 patients (58%) were found to have persistent superficial mucosal disease, 27 patients (30%) died of their disease with a mean survival of 53 months, eight patients progressed to advanced-stage disease, and three patients died of unrelated causes. From their study, these

---

*See references 8, 122, 123, 126, 140 to 143, and 148.

authors[155] estimated that the median survival of untreated SEC was 75 months and that the 5-year survival was 62%.

The overall crude 5-year survival rate for surgically treated SEC (recognizing that many series include carcinoma in situ and tumors other than of conventional squamous cell histologic type) is in the range of about 42% to 95%,[140, 143, 147, 156, 157] the highest figure reflecting the Chinese experience. The overall long-term 10-year survival rate is 36% in a large Japanese series.[156] This is remarkably better than the overall 5-year survival rate of less than 10% observed in the Western world for advanced esophageal carcinoma.[138, 158, 159] In SEC, a major difference in survival is observed when patients are stratified into those with tumor invasion confined to the mucosa or submucosa. In three large series of SEC (which were slightly contaminated by the inclusion of a few cases of carcinoma in situ in two of these series), patients with tumor invasion confined to the mucosa had a 5-year survival rate ranging from 66% to 88%, whereas patients with tumor invasion of the submucosa had a 5-year survival rate ranging from 48% to 55% (the lowest figure corresponding to a series excluding carcinoma in situ).[142, 145, 156] Conversely, the 10-year survival rate in patients with SEC with invasion confined to the mucosa and invasion within the submucosa was 59% and 36%, respectively, in a large series reported by the Japanese Committee for Registration of Esophageal Carcinoma Cases.[156] As a correlate, the presence of nodal metastasis in cases of SEC has mostly been observed in conjunction with tumor invasion of the submucosa and has been associated with a 5-year survival rate of 39%, as opposed to 72% in the absence of nodal metastasis.[142] Because SEC with invasion of the submucosa seems to represent a more aggressive subset of disease, some authors have suggested that the definition of SEC should be reconsidered and perhaps restricted to cases with tumor invasion confined to the mucosa, regardless of the nodal status.[140, 145, 156]

Advanced Squamous Cell Carcinoma

Advanced squamous cell carcinoma (epidermoid carcinoma) is by far the most frequent histologic type encountered among esophageal malignancy, and represents the one referred to in most epidemiologic and experimental studies on this topic. It accounts for 87% to 90% of esophageal malignancy, when defined with stringent histologic criteria (historically including a small proportion of superficial squamous cell carcinomas). Series with a reported incidence of 62% to 75% have excluded neoplasms with a significant undifferentiated component, in spite of focal squamous cell differentiation.[122, 127] Men are predominantly affected, with a male-to-female ratio of 4:1 to 6:1,[138, 156, 160, 161] and are mostly in their sixth and seventh decades.[162] However, postcricoid carcinoma usually afflicts females mostly in their fifth decade.

In two major autopsy series comprising 236 patients, squamous cell carcinoma had the following topographic distribution, based on the esophageal

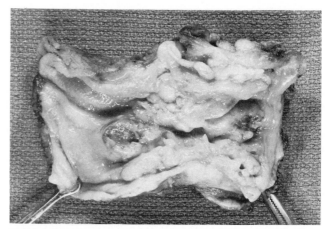

FIGURE 19–7. Distal third of esophagus displaying a squamous cell carcinoma (6 × 5 cm) of predominantly fungating type with superimposed ulceration.

level of predominant involvement: 9% to 10% in the upper third, 54% to 66% in the middle third, and 25% to 36% in the lower third.[138, 162] In about 20% of patients, there is regional overlapping, which is equally distributed between the upper and middle thirds, and the middle and lower thirds.[129] Using a different topographic scheme, the distribution is estimated to be about 5% in the cervical esophagus, 8% in the upper thoracic esophagus, 60% in the middle thoracic esophagus, and 27% in the lower thoracic esophagus, according to a Japanese series of nearly 5000 cases.[156] However, it is difficult to obtain comparative data with regard to site, because (1) two major systems of topographic mapping are used; (2) a substantial degree of submucosal, longitudinal spreading occurs, which obscures precise localization; and (3) postcricoid tumors may not have been included.

Three predominant macroscopic (gross) types are encountered in advanced squamous cell carcinoma,[107] although there is no consensus as to their relative incidence. The *fungating* type (Fig. 19–7) is characterized by a prominent, intraluminal growth with superimposed ulceration displaying a red-yellow surface. The intraluminal component may have a sessile, polypoid configuration or may be characterized by a plaquelike mass with a well-defined, sharp border.

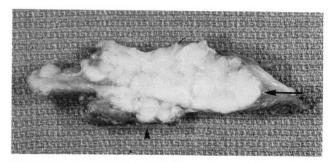

FIGURE 19–8. Cross-section of the tumor shown in Figure 19–7, showing a solid, gray-white, firm, neoplastic component. Note transmural penetration with periadventitial tumor nodules (*arrowhead*) and submucosal extension (*arrow*).

The degree of mural invasion is variable but is usually extensive (Fig. 19–8), and in most cases, only part of the circumference is involved. This type is variably reported in 11% to 60% of cases.[107, 138] The *ulcerating* type (Fig. 19–9) is a well-defined ulcer of variable depth, with a shaggy, yellow and dark red hemorrhagic surface. The border is slightly elevated, indurated, and irregular. Submucosal extension may give a somewhat nodular aspect to the surrounding mucosa. It is reported in 25% to 63% of patients,[107, 138] whereas it is the type most frequently encountered in our experience. The *infiltrating* type is reported in 15% to 26% of cases[107, 138] and is characterized by a predominantly mural pattern of growth. Circumferential involvement is frequent, with luminal stenosis, functional obstruction, and proximal dilatation. Superimposed shallow ulceration is usually present. The cut surface shows a prominent, intramural component with firm, gray-white, dry tumor tissue, with or without yellow foci of necrosis and a variable degree of transmural or longitudinal growth. Following radiotherapy, the tumor is likely to be of ulcerating type (in about two-thirds of patients) or infiltrating type (about one-fourth of cases).[122] The tumor size is variable, measuring between 2 and 5 cm in more than 50% of patients, and more than 5 cm in 40% of patients.[138, 162] The location, gross configuration (for the above-mentioned three types) and tumor size (particularly in the 3- to 10-cm range) are not significant prognostic determinants.[156, 163, 164] The occurrence of an occult second primary invasive carcinoma, most likely of the superficial form, has been observed in 7% of esophagectomy specimens in one study.[165]

A fourth macroscopic type referred to as a *polypoid* tumor has been recognized and found to be a good prognostic determinant.[166] Generally believed to be of rare occurrence, this type has been observed in 2% to 8% of cases of advanced squamous cell carcinoma in some series.[166] It is defined as an intraluminal polypoid tumor, measuring more than 3 cm, without mural constriction or ulceration, and with a conventional squamous cell histologic type.[166] It was traditionally

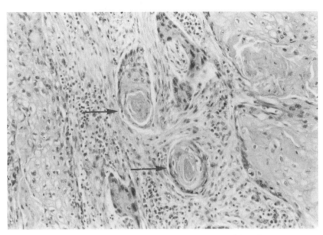

FIGURE 19–10. Well-differentiated squamous cell carcinoma. There are confluent sheets of cohesive, polygonal cells with keratin pearl formation (*arrows*). The epithelial-stromal interface is irregular with a desmoplastic fibrous response. (Hematoxylin and eosin, 100 ×.)

included in the fungating type.[166] In the study of Sasajima and associates,[166] the polypoid type was associated with a 5-year survival of 71%, as opposed to 11% with the other macroscopic types of squamous cell carcinoma as a control group, whereas the incidence of adventitial involvement was lower than in the latter control group.

Advanced squamous cell carcinoma, like the superficial form, is histologically characterized by invasive and confluent sheets of cohesive, polygonal, oval, or spindle-shaped cells with a sharp pushing or ragged stromal-epithelial interface. The associated stroma shows fibroblastic proliferation and collagen deposition (desmoplasia), with a variable degree of lymphoplasmacytoid cell inflammation. Well-differentiated tumors display prominent keratinization, including keratin pearls and cell dyskeratosis (Fig. 19–10). Cells have abundant, densely eosinophilic cytoplasm and hyperchromatic nuclei with coarse chromatin. Abnormal mitoses are often present. Poorly differentiated tumors display minimal evidence of keratinization, and are recognized as such in the presence of individual cell keratinization (large polygonal cells with densely eosinophilic cytoplasm and pyknotic nucleus) and intercellular bridges (reflecting artifactual membrane retraction between desmosomal attachments) (Figs. 19–11 and 19–12); otherwise cells show a high nuclear to cytoplasmic ratio, scanty amphophilic cytoplasm, and nuclear anaplasia. Moderately differentiated tumors have an intermediate character. Regional variation in the degree of differentiation is often seen, whereas necrosis is frequently encountered in less differentiated tumors. Loss of tumor cell cohesion may create a pseudoglandular pattern mimicking adenocarcinoma (Fig. 19–13); however, mucin stains are negative. In some cases, the tumor is characterized by the predominance of clear cells resulting from a glycogen-rich cytoplasm and hydropic cytoplasmic changes (in the absence of mucin) (Fig. 19–14). The histologic grade is moderately or poorly differentiated

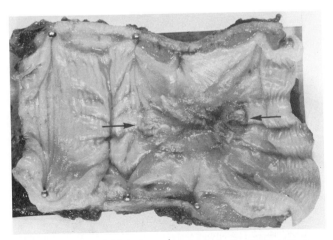

FIGURE 19–9. Distal third of esophagus displaying a squamous cell carcinoma (2.5 × 1.5 cm) of ulcerating type (*between arrows*). Note the irregularity of the ulcer bed and the raised nodular border.

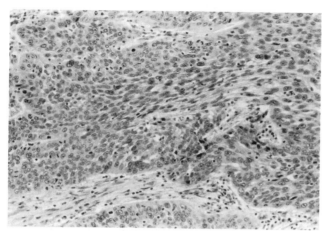

FIGURE 19–11. Poorly differentiated squamous cell carcinoma. There are sheets of cohesive polygonal cells with a focal spindle cell configuration on the right side. (Hematoxylin and eosin, 100 ×.)

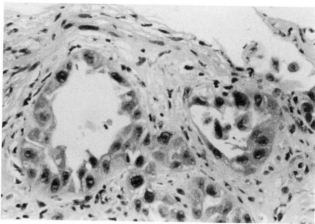

FIGURE 19–13. Squamous cell carcinoma with pseudoglandular features. Groups of cells with central loss of cohesiveness (acantholysis) mimicking glandular formations. Evidence of squamous cell differentiation elsewhere and the absence of mucin rule out adenocarcinoma. (Hematoxylin and eosin, 250 ×.)

in the majority of tumors.[106, 163] In the absence of any stigma of squamous differentiation and after exclusion of any other histologic type, a tumor is best classified as undifferentiated carcinoma, NOS.

It is generally believed that the histologic grade is not a prognostic determinant.[106, 164] However, in a recent study of 69 cases, Robey-Cafferty and coworkers[163] found that the histologic grade (degree of differentiation) was a significant independent prognostic indicator. In their study, the 5-year survival rate was 54% in patients with a well to moderately differentiated tumor, compared with about 6% with a poorly differentiated tumor (including undifferentiated carcinoma, NOS). No relationship has been established between the histologic grade and the degree of tumor radiosensitivity. In advanced carcinoma, a substantial degree of submucosal extension (longitudinal growth) away from the grossly visible tumor is likely to be present, whereas satellite submucosal metastases are occasionally seen.[138]

Mapping studies of whole esophagectomy specimens have revealed the presence of concurrent, contiguous high-grade EIN (carcinoma in situ) in 27% to 69% of cases of advanced carcinoma,[9, 87, 111, 120, 122] whereas noncontiguous and distant high-grade EIN, above or below the invasive tumor, has been observed in at least 13% of patients.[122] In a study of 179 patients, Soga and colleagues[108] found diffuse and extensive high-grade EIN (carcinoma in situ) up to a 20 mm distance from the main tumor in 6% of cases. However, in specimens exposed to preoperative radiotherapy, the incidence of concurrent high-grade EIN (carcinoma in situ) is much lower.[9, 122] The above-mentioned observations emphasize the need for thorough intraoperative evaluation of the esophageal resection margins, including mucosal staining with Lugol's (iodine) solution or toluidine blue in conjunction with frozen section assessment.[167, 168] However, the status of

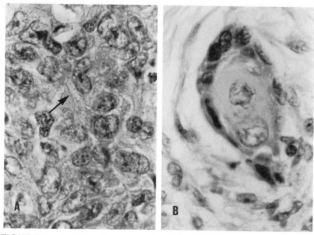

FIGURE 19–12. The diagnosis of poorly differentiated squamous cell carcinoma (the tumor in Figure 19–11) is confirmed by the presence of intercellular bridges (*arrow*) (*A*) and evidence of individual cell keratinization with abundant, dense eosinophilic cytoplasm (*B*). (Hematoxylin and eosin, 630 ×.)

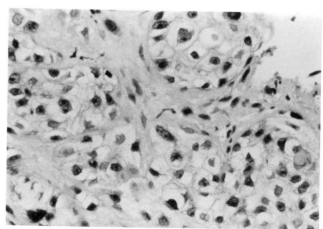

FIGURE 19–14. Squamous cell carcinoma with clear cell features. Groups of cells with clear cytoplasm due to hydropic changes or the presence of abundant glycogen in the cytoplasmic compartment. (Hematoxylin and eosin, 250 ×.)

resection margin is not statistically linked to survival.[163]

Vascular (venular or lymphatic) invasion is observed in 66% to 91% of cases,[8, 164] a higher incidence correlating with deeper tumor penetration.[8] Vascular invasion has not been found to be a prognostic determinant of significance in multivariate analysis.[163, 164] Transmural penetration up to the adventitia, with or without significant invasion of periesophageal tissues, is observed in the majority (over 75%) of cases following evaluation of esophagectomy specimens.[122, 156] The depth of tumor penetration in squamous cell carcinoma at large is a major prognostic determinant[157] and is the basic criterion for segregating the superficial form (SEC). It is also a prognostic determinant of significance in the advanced form regarding 5-year survival[156, 157, 164] and 10-year survival as well.[156] Whereas it is characteristically absent in SEC, perineurial invasion is observed in 32% of cases of advanced carcinoma in which invasion has reached the adventitia and in 50% of cases in which invasion of neighboring structures is present.[11, 169]

Tumor alteration associated with radiotherapy includes changes such as giant cell granulomata surrounding keratin material, increased cytoplasmic differentiation (larger volume of cytoplasm and dyskeratosis), and marked nuclear atypia (enlargement, hyperchromasia, pyknosis, and multinucleation). Vacuolar changes are frequently present.[122] Histopathologic changes attributable to preoperative chemotherapy can also be observed in esophageal squamous cell carcinoma following surgical resection. In a recent study by Darnton and coworkers,[170] using control cases, the following qualitative and quantitative changes were observed: (1) marked tumor regression in 5 of 12 cases, characterized by residual small foci of tumor cells in the submucosa or muscularis propria, frequently surrounded by a mixed cell inflammatory infiltrate (complete tumor regression was observed in one additional case); (2) a significant twofold reduction in the proportion of tumor epithelial component to stromal component; (3) localized fibrosis, chronic inflammation, and regeneration of a thin stratified surface epithelium over previously ulcerated tumor areas in all cases. However, no relationship was found between the degree of tumor response to chemotherapy and the histologic grade, based on comparison with biopsy material prior to chemotherapy.

The overall incidence of regional lymph node metastasis following surgical resection (series composed largely of advanced but also of a few cases of superficial carcinoma) has ranged from 48% to 77% and was found to correlate with the depth of tumor penetration.[8, 107, 122, 156] Lymph node status is a major prognostic determinant. Multivariate analysis has shown that regional lymph node metastasis is a poor prognostic determinant in regard to 5-year survival[164] and is associated with a high risk of recurrence within 2 years after surgery.[171] In a large Japanese series of nearly 4000 patients, the presence of regional nodal metastasis was found to be associated with a 5-year survival rate of 18% and a 10-year survival rate of 14%, as opposed to 41% and 32%, respectively, in the absence of nodal metastasis.[156] Using lymph node status as an independent predictor, Ellis and associates[157] found a 5-year survival rate of 32% in the absence of nodal metastasis, compared with less than 16% in the presence of nodal metastasis. With a positive nodal status, recognition of less than five positive versus five or more positive lymph nodes might be of prognostic significance in regard to 5-year survival[157] but needs to be further evaluated.

In two large series examining young adults with esophageal squamous cell carcinoma (defined as either less than age 49[172] or less than age 35[173]) as compared with older patients, no difference was found regarding tumor location, size, gross configuration, histologic grade, vascular invasion, or lymph node metastasis.[172, 173] Therefore, age is not influential on clinicopathologic parameters in esophageal squamous cell carcinoma.

Studies on tumor DNA ploidy (content) in advanced carcinoma have been variably performed by (1) cytophotometric analysis of paraffin-embedded sections stained with the Feulgen reaction and examined with the two-wavelength method[153, 171, 174–176]; (2) flow cytometry of paraffin-embedded tissue[163, 177–180]; and (3) flow cytometry of fresh tissue.[181] Furthermore, intratumoral heterogeneity has been recognized in esophageal carcinoma[177, 182] for which sampling is likely influential. Therefore, caution is warranted in making comparative analysis among different studies, whereas the reporting of conflicting results is not surprising. Whereas one study reported a correlation between DNA ploidy and the histologic grade,[179] other studies (including one with multivariate analysis) found that there was no such correlation.[175, 180] DNA ploidy has been correlated with the extent of mural tumor penetration in one study,[181] whereas no such association was found by other investigators.[176, 179] Alternatively, high DNA ploidy (Types 3 and 4, aneuploidy) has been[174, 178] or has not been[179] found to be associated with a higher incidence of lymph node metastasis. On the other hand, there are numerous studies that showed that the DNA ploidy of tumor cells reflects the aggressiveness of the tumor. Patients with a tumor characterized by a high DNA ploidy index (aneuploidy) were found to have a much higher incidence of early recurrence or hematogenous metastasis, or both, following surgical resection for advanced carcinoma[153, 171, 177–179, 181] and had a higher likelihood of dying within 2 years from their disease, independent of their nodal status.[174, 180] On the other hand, no correlation was observed between DNA ploidy and survival in one study.[163] Intratumoral heterogeneity in DNA ploidy (content) has been recently recognized in 37% to 43% of esophageal carcinomas that were of superficial or advanced form.[177, 182] Not surprisingly and as a correlate, variations in DNA ploidy indexes between the primary and metastatic tumors were found in about half of cases,[177] although the DNA ploidy index seen in a metastatic lesion was found to be similar to one of the indexes observed in the primary tumor in 88% to 100% of cases.[177, 182]

In advanced esophageal carcinoma, the presence of a high population density of Langerhans' cells (S-100 protein positive dendritic cells) admixed within the tumor cell population, has been statistically associated with a better 2-year survival rate.[183] This observation is likely a reflection of host defense against carcinoma. EGF has been implicated in mitogenesis and oncogenesis in the gastrointestinal tract. In an immunohistochemical study of 31 cases of esophageal squamous cell carcinoma, an elevated EGF receptor level within tumor cells was seen in 71% of cases.[3] However, no correlation was found between the EGF receptor level of the tumor and pathologic features such as lymph node metastasis, depth of tumor penetration, histologic grade, or vascular invasion.[3] Although loss of blood group antigen (antigens A, B, and H) expression within tumor cells (by immunocytochemical determination) has been found to correlate with advanced-stage disease, it has not been shown to be statistically linked to survival in a study of 69 cases by Robey-Cafferty and colleagues.[163] No correlation has been observed between the expression of the squamous cell carcinoma–related antigen within tumor cells (by immunocytochemical determination) and the prognosis of patients with esophageal carcinoma, although this antigen is an indicator of histologic differentiation.[183] Whether determination of the NOR mean number in esophageal carcinoma cells is of prognostic significance[5, 146] remains to be determined by further studies. It has been suggested that immunocytochemical staining of matrix metalloproteinases might be a useful technique for evaluating the malignant potential of esophageal carcinoma, particularly regarding invasiveness and metastatic capabilities. In a study of 29 cases of surgically resected esophageal carcinoma (including adjacent normal mucosa as a control), and using an immunocytochemical staining technique, Shima and coworkers[184] found that cytoplasmic expression of matrix metalloproteinases MMP-2 (Type IV collagenase/72-kilodalton gelatinase) and MMP-3 (stromelysin), which is mostly observed at the marginal or deeply invasive tumor component, was closely related to lymph node metastasis and vascular invasion. Immunocytochemical determination of the nuclear protein p53 tumor suppressor gene product (a proliferative cell nuclear antigen) in esophageal carcinoma cells has not proved to be useful in determining clinical outcome and prognosis of patients.[135] Whereas p53 expression was closely correlated with the malignant phenotype, including EIN, no significant correlation was observed between the percentage of tumor cells positive for p53 and the histologic grade, nuclear morphology, mitotic index, clinical stage, size of tumor, depth of tumor penetration or presence of vascular invasion.[135]

Postmortem examination has shown that in squamous cell carcinoma treated by different modalities, residual tumor is seen in 75% of cases, and transmural penetration with invasion of neighboring structures is observed in 60% of cases.[129] The trachea and bronchus are most often invaded (about half of the cases), followed by the aorta, pericardium, and pleura.[129] Fistula formation is observed in about one-third of patients, most often penetrating into the tracheobronchial tree.[129] Tumors of the upper esophageal third are particularly prone to be associated with perforation or fistula formation at the time of death.[129, 138] As expected, a preferential invasion of the trachea is observed for tumors of the upper esophageal third; the trachea, bronchus, and aorta for tumors of the middle third; and the bronchus, aorta, and pleuropericardium for tumors of the lower third.[129, 138] Postmortem examination has revealed the presence of nodal metastasis, including the mediastinal, abdominal, and cervical regions (in decreasing order of frequency), in about 75% of cases.[129] Nodal metastasis may be found at a significant distance from the primary esophageal tumor site, because 40% of tumors in the upper esophageal third had metastasized to abdominal lymph nodes and 38% of tumors in the lower third had metastasized to cervical lymph nodes in one postmortem study.[129] Concurrent nodal involvement both above and below the diaphragm has been observed in about one-third of cases.[129] Hematogenous metastases are observed in about 50% of cases and are likely to be associated with synchronous nodal involvement.[107, 129] Lung (31% to 52%) and liver (23% to 47%) are the sites of predilection, followed by pleura, bone, kidney, bronchus, nervous system, and stomach.[129, 162] The pattern of metastatic disease does not differ between treated and nontreated patients.[162] A synchronous or metachronous squamous cell carcinoma of the head and neck has been documented in 15% of cases of squamous cell carcinoma of the esophagus, as a reflection of exposure to common risk factors.[129] The most frequent cause of death is bronchopneumonia (in about one-third of cases), in association with the formation of a tracheoesophageal or bronchoesophageal fistula in about 40% of these patients.[129]

Basaloid Squamous Cell Carcinoma

Basaloid squamous cell carcinoma is a distinct variant of squamous cell carcinoma, which is well documented in the head and neck region and has recently been recognized in the esophagus as well.[185, 186] This neoplastic variant probably encompasses many tumors previously reported as adenoid cystic carcinoma (carcinoma with adenoid cystic differentiation) of the esophagus.[187] The clinical presentation, location, gross configuration, and aggressive biologic outcome appear similar to the advanced form of conventional squamous cell carcinoma.

The tumor is characterized by closely packed, moderately pleomorphic, basaloid cells forming variably sized lobules and trabeculae (Figs. 19–15 and 19–16). Larger lobules often show central, comedo-type necrosis (see Fig. 19–15), whereas cells at the periphery tend to exhibit nuclear palisading. Hyaline bands are often present around tumor lobules or in between anastomosing trabeculae (see Figs. 19–16 and 19–17). This hyaline material has been found to be periodic acid–Schiff (PAS) diastase-resistant positive[185, 186] and to contain laminin and Type 4 collagen.[186] Cytologi-

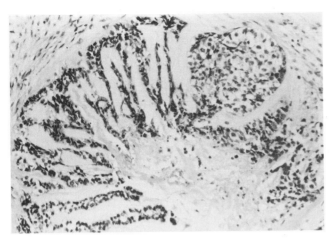

FIGURE 19–15. Basaloid squamous cell carcinoma. Large tumor lobule with central comedo-type necrosis and the presence of hyaline bands. (Hematoxylin and eosin, 100 ×.)

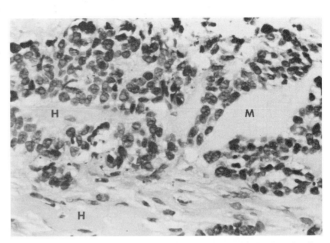

FIGURE 19–17. Basaloid squamous cell carcinoma. Basaloid cells with a high nuclear-cytoplasmic ratio, hyperchromatic vesicular nuclei, and individual cell necrosis. Note the presence of bandlike hyaline material (H) or microcystic space containing alcianophilic material (M). (Hematoxylin and eosin, 250 ×.)

cally, basaloid cells have a high nuclear to cytoplasmic ratio and dense hyperchromatic nuclei (see Fig. 19–17). Mitotic figures, including atypical forms, are often numerous. In most tumors, there is an associated major (30% to 50%) or minor component of conventional squamous cell carcinoma, whereas overlying high-grade EIN has been observed in half of the patients.[185, 186] Occasionally, microcystic or intertrabecular spaces containing alcianophilic basophilic material or true glandular spaces are observed.[185, 186] The basaloid component in this variant of squamous cell carcinoma generally shows poor and uneven staining for low molecular weight cytokeratin (e.g., AE1, CAM 5.2).[185]

This tumor rarely occurs, and was identified in 1.7% (three patients) of 178 consecutive cases of squamous cell carcinoma in one Japanese series.[188] On the other hand, Takubo and coworkers[188] observed a minor basaloid component in 9% of their 178 squamous cell carcinomas. The cell of origin is likely from the basal or parabasal region of esophageal epithelium.[189]

Squamous Cell Carcinoma with Sarcomatoid Features

Squamous cell carcinoma with sarcomatoid features (carcinosarcoma, pseudosarcoma, spindle cell carcinoma, carcinoma with spindle cell features, carcinoma with prominent spindle cells, polypoid carcinoma) is a variant of esophageal cancer with peculiar clinicopathologic features. The great variety of designations has reflected conflicting views on the histogenesis and biologic behavior of the sarcomatoid component. Whether this sarcomatoid component is epithelial or mesenchymal in origin and whether it is neoplastic or reactive in nature is still a controversial matter.

The term carcinosarcoma has been based on the assumption that this tumor was composed of distinctive carcinomatous and sarcomatous components, each one having its metastatic potential. The designation pseudosarcoma has implied that the sarcomatoid component was of metaplastic nature or non-neoplastic mesenchymal reactive nature, with potential metastases composed of carcinoma only. Terms such as spindle cell carcinoma or carcinoma with spindle cell features have stressed the concept of epithelial differentiation in the spindle cell component, based on ultrastructural or immunocytochemical observations. The designation polypoid carcinoma, in addition to stressing the epithelial nature of this tumor on ultrastructural[190] or immunocytochemical[191] grounds, has been proposed as a unifying term for this complex terminology, emphasizing gross configuration.[190] However, current evidence suggests that this plethora of terms has little practical use from a clinical standpoint[21, 190, 192, 193] and that this tumor is likely to represent a variant of squamous cell carcinoma with a distinct clinicopathologic presentation and biologic outcome. A retrospective comparative analysis of 16 reported cases of carcinosarcoma and 17 cases of pseudosarcoma showed no significant difference in regard to age, sex, tumor location, gross configura-

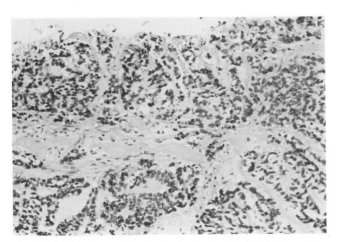

FIGURE 19–16. Basaloid squamous cell carcinoma. Solid grouping of basaloid cells with intervening microcystic spaces or hyaline bands. (Hematoxylin and eosin, 100 ×.)

tion, size, depth of penetration, histologic appearance, or prognosis.[192] Another study that compared 23 reported patients with carcinosarcoma and 19 patients with pseudosarcoma found no significant difference regarding the depth of tumor penetration, the histologic appearance of primary and metastatic tumors, and the clinical course.[190] In fact, overlapping histologic findings have been reported in studies of both primary and metastatic tumors, challenging the original concept and definition of this neoplasm.[190, 193]

This form of esophageal malignancy is very rare. The reported incidence has ranged from 0.5% to 2.7% among collected series.[160, 166, 194–196] By 1991, nearly 170 cases were reported according to Perch and colleagues.[197] The clinical presentation does not significantly differ from conventional squamous cell carcinoma.[160] Most patients are men in their sixth or seventh decade and present with dysphagia (two-thirds of patients), whereas the middle and lower esophageal thirds are the sites of predilection.[160, 194, 195]

Grossly, the majority of tumors have an intraluminal, polypoid, and pedunculated configuration (Fig. 19–18).[160, 194] However, occasional tumors have an ulcerating gross configuration similar to conventional squamous cell carcinoma, even in the absence of preoperative radiotherapy (up to 25% of cases in the large series by Iyomasa and colleagues).[160, 196] Whereas a wide range in size can be observed,[194] the mean tumor size was 7 cm (estimated to be significantly larger than for conventional squamous cell carcinoma) in a series of 20 cases reported by Iyomasa and coworkers.[160] The pedicle may be short and broad or long and narrow.[194, 196] Surface ulceration and tumor necrosis are frequently seen and the cut surface is yellow-white or gray-red (Fig. 19–18). In 80% to 85% of patients, tumor penetration is confined within the esophageal wall, regardless of the tumor size.[160, 190] Of these tumors, invasion is confined to the submucosa in about half of patients, and to the muscularis propria in the other patients.[160, 190] Tumors with transmu-

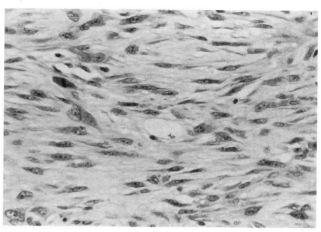

FIGURE 19–19. Squamous cell carcinoma with sarcomatoid features. Fibrosarcoma-like pattern with parallel alignment of malignant fibroblastic-like cells and intervening collagen deposition. (Hematoxylin and eosin, 250 ×.)

ral penetration (i.e., invasion of adventitia and periesophageal tissues) tend to have an ulcerating rather than polypoid configuration.[160] However, Gal and coworkers[196] observed transmural tumor penetration in four of eight polypoid tumors.

Histologically, the bulk of the tumor has a sarcomatoid appearance that is often reminiscent of a fibrosarcoma or malignant fibrous histiocytoma.[160, 193, 196, 198–200] It is characterized by a fascicular or storiform growth pattern of spindle cells with an eosinophilic or amphophilic cytoplasm, and hyperchromatic nuclei with or without macronucleoli (Fig. 19–19). A pleomorphic pattern of variably shaped cells with an abundant eosinophilic or foamy cytoplasm can be observed (Fig. 19–20). Admixed mononucleated or multinucleated giant cells with bizarre hyperchromatic nuclei and occasional pseudoinclusions are often present (Fig. 19–20). The number of mitoses, including

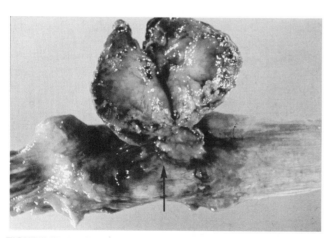

FIGURE 19–18. Squamous cell carcinoma with sarcomatoid features. A 2.5- × 2.0-cm tumor characterized by an intraluminal, polypoid configuration and a small base of mural implantation (*arrow*). Central section through the tumor reveals a gelatinous, white, and focally hemorrhagic appearance. (Courtesy of Dr. Réal Lagacé, Hôtel-Dieu de Québec, Québec, Canada.)

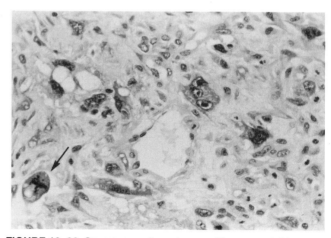

FIGURE 19–20. Squamous cell carcinoma with sarcomatoid features. Malignant fibrous histiocytoma-like pattern with a predominant population of malignant histiocytic-like cells and admixed mononucleated and multinucleated giant cells with an abundant, focally vacuolated cytoplasm. Note the presence of an atypical mitotic figure (*arrow*). (Hematoxylin and eosin, 250 ×.)

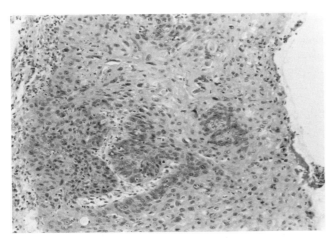

FIGURE 19–21. Squamous cell carcinoma with sarcomatoid features. High-grade EIN (carcinoma in situ) is present at the base and edge of the polypoid component. (Hematoxylin and eosin, 100 ×.)

atypical forms, is variable. The degree of cellularity and collagen deposition varies, whereas myxoid changes are occasionally encountered. Foci of chondroid, osseous, or myogenic (smooth muscle) differentiation are occasionally seen.[107, 198, 199, 201] In addition to the obviously malignant sarcomatoid elements, an apparently reactive fibroblastic and myofibroblastic proliferation (without nuclear atypia) is observed in most tumors of polypoid configuration.[198] Careful sampling and histologic examination are likely to reveal an EIN (Fig. 19–21), with or without an associated invasive carcinomatous component at the edge or base of pedicle.[196, 199, 200, 202] The invasive carcinomatous component is characterized by nests of cohesive polygonal cells with a full range of squamous differentiation (keratinization) (Fig. 19–22); it may occasionally be undifferentiated[196, 198] and rarely show focal glandular differentiation.[198] This component is intimately related to the sarcomatoid component, either sharply demarcated or blended with a transitional morphology, and is unlikely to be visible beyond the submucosal level (Fig. 19–22). On the other hand, the carcinomatous component can be very small, without significant admixture with the sarcomatoid component.[199] The entire spectrum of EIN (dysplasia and carcinoma in situ) has been observed in the adjacent mucosa.[192, 196, 199] On the other hand, the surface of the polypoid tumor may be extensively ulcerated (Fig. 19–23) or covered by atrophic squamous epithelium.[191, 200] Endoscopic biopsy is likely to show a carcinomatous or sarcomatoid spindle and pleomorphic cell component and should be performed away from necrotic or ulcerated areas.[200] Very rarely, adenocarcinoma has been the associated carcinomatous component,[194] and obviously such a lesion would best be referred to as an *adenocarcinoma with sarcomatoid features.*

Because of its frequent polypoid configuration in the esophagus, a benign polyp, malignant melanoma, or smooth muscle neoplasm should be distinguished from squamous cell carcinoma with sarcomatoid features. An *inflammatory pseudotumor (fibroid polyp)* may involve the esophagus as a polypoid lesion, usually associated with an area of ulceration. It is characterized by proliferating fibrovascular tissue with an ad-

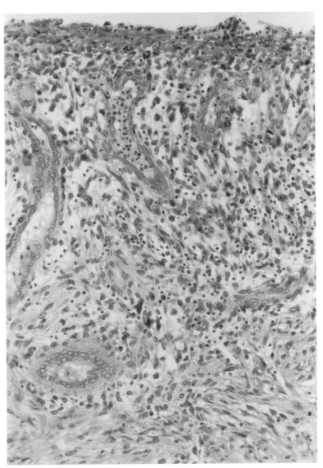

FIGURE 19–23. Squamous cell carcinoma with sarcomatoid features. A biopsy specimen obtained from an ulcerated area shows a granulation tissue-like appearance, precluding a confident diagnosis of malignancy. (Hematoxylin and eosin, 100 ×.)

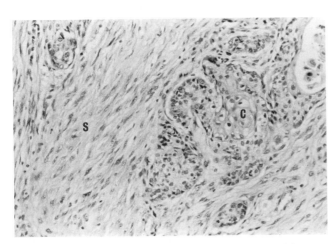

FIGURE 19–22. Squamous cell carcinoma with sarcomatoid features. Poorly differentiated carcinomatous component (C) admixed with sarcomatoid component (S). (Hematoxylin and eosin, 100 ×.)

mixed polymorphous inflammatory cell infiltrate, including eosinophils and lymphoid aggregates. Both the stroma and overlying epithelium are benign, although epithelial atypia of inflammation and repair may be present.[203] The lesion designated as *fibrovascular polyp* is closely related to the inflammatory pseudotumor but lacks significant inflammation.[107] *Malignant melanoma* may display sarcomatoid features. However, its melanocytic nature should be confirmed in the presence of intracytoplasmic melanin pigment, an associated radial junctional melanocytic component, and immunocytochemical reactivity for S-100 protein, vimentin, and HMB-45. A *smooth muscle neoplasm* shows features that are described under the heading of leiomyosarcoma.

Numerous studies have focused on phenotypic characterization of this tumor, in an attempt to understand the histogenesis of the sarcomatoid component. An immunocytochemical strong and diffuse expression of cytokeratin is observed in the carcinomatous component of all cases (Fig. 19–24),[196, 197, 199, 200] whereas vimentin is detected within the sarcomatoid component of most cases.[196, 198, 199] Focal immunoreactivity for cytokeratin within the sarcomatoid component has been observed in more than half of the cases reported by Gal and colleagues,[196] and has also been substantiated in other reports.[191, 196, 201, 204] On the other hand, many reports have stressed the absence of immunoreactivity for cytokeratin within the sarcomatoid component.[193, 197, 199, 202, 205] Immunoreactivity for cytokeratin has been observed within spindle cells of the transitional zone (interface between carcinomatous and sarcomatoid components) in almost half (9 of 20) of the cases studied by Wang and associates.[198] Furthermore, coexpression of keratin and vimentin has been observed in spindle cells of the transitional zone[198] and within cells of the carcinomatous component[196, 199] in a few cases. The expression of desmin or muscle-specific actin (HHF-35, Enzo), or both, has been detected within the sarcomatoid component in a few tumors,[198, 199] sustaining evidence of myogenic differentiation. In many cases, ultrastructural examination of the sarcomatoid spindle cells has shown, in

addition to abundant rough endoplasmic reticulum (putatively related to the synthesis of collagen), the presence of tonofilaments and desmosomes indicative of epithelial differentiation.[190, 192, 201, 206] On the other hand, some authors have exclusively observed features of fibroblastic, myofibroblastic, or fibrohistiocytic differentiation at the ultrastructural and immunocytochemical (positivity for alpha$_1$-antitrypsin and alpha$_1$-antichymotrypsin) levels.[199, 200] Recognizing the conflicting nature of this information, many observations would tend to support the assumption that the sarcomatoid component for its most part is of epithelial derivation and represents a metaplastic transformation[196] or a dedifferentiation[198] from the carcinomatous component, resulting in a mesenchymal phenotype. On the other hand, the possibility that a superimposed reactive fibroblastic and myofibroblastic proliferation is part of the sarcomatoid component in some tumors cannot be excluded.

The rarity of squamous cell carcinoma with sarcomatoid features and the lack of adequate follow-up documentation in many reports make the biologic assessment somewhat difficult. The prognosis has been traditionally viewed as better than that of conventional squamous cell carcinoma, including a quoted incidence of lymph node or hematogenous metastasis, of less than 20% to 30%[190, 192] and the reporting of many cases of long, disease-free survivals.[194] However, in two recent large series, nodal metastasis was documented in 50% to 65% of cases, an incidence not significantly different than that for conventional squamous cell carcinoma.[160, 196] In metastatic deposits, the tumor has most often a pure carcinomatous morphology, whereas a pure sarcomatoid or combined morphology is rarely observed.[160, 193, 199] In a series of 20 cases reported by Iyomasa and colleagues,[160] the 3-year survival for patients with squamous cell carcinoma with sarcomatoid features was 63%, as opposed to 28% for conventional squamous cell carcinoma as a control group. However, the 5-year survival was 27%, as compared with 22% for conventional squamous cell carcinoma as a control group, therefore without significant difference. This 5-year survival figure is less optimistic than the traditionally estimated crude survival rate of 50% for squamous cell carcinoma with sarcomatoid features.[190, 192, 203] The limited degree of tumor penetration in most cases is probably the reason for high surgical resectability and better 3-year survival. However, the significant potential for hematogenous metastasis in this tumor negatively affects the long-term survival.

Verrucous Squamous Cell Carcinoma

Although verrucous squamous cell carcinoma (verrucous acanthosis) is well documented in the oral cavity, its occurrence in the esophagus is extremely rare. By 1991, about 12 cases were reported in the English literature.[208] In half of patients, a history of heavy smoking and drinking has been documented, whereas in the other half, tumors have been associated with achalasia, corrosion injury–related stricture, or an esoph-

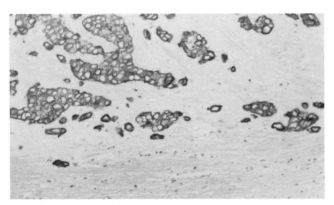

FIGURE 19–24. Squamous cell carcinoma with sarcomatoid features. Strong cytoplasmic immunoreactivity for cytokeratin AE1/AE3 within the poorly differentiated carcinomatous component. (Hematoxylin and eosin, 100 ×.)

ageal diverticulum.[209, 210] Verrucous squamous cell carcinoma should be distinguished from conventional squamous cell carcinoma of the esophagus in view of its much less aggressive course. Indeed, it is a slowly progressive, infiltrating tumor that rarely metastasizes to lymph nodes, although nodal enlargement may be present.[208, 210, 211] With early detection and adequate surgical treatment, the prognosis should be most favorable.[208, 210, 211]

The age has ranged from 36 to 76 years, with a mean of 61 years, whereas the ratio of men to women is 7:4. The most common symptoms are dysphagia, weight loss, and coughing. There is often a remarkably long delay between the first symptoms, the detection of a tumoral lesion, and the final diagnosis.[208]

The tumor occurs mainly in the upper third of the esophagus and is grossly characterized by a highly irregular shaggy, wartlike mucosal appearance including numerous white papillary projections, which may nearly fill the esophageal lumen. All tumors are large, involving at least 6 cm of esophageal length and the entire circumference. Transmural tumor penetration with or without invasion of surrounding structures has been reported in eight of 10 patients, whereas fistula formation has been observed in three patients.[208] Histologically, the luminal aspect is characterized by papillary projections of stratified squamous epithelium showing marked parakeratosis, hyperkeratosis, and some dyskeratosis. Nuclear atypia is usually minimal. There are intervening clefts containing keratin or cellular debris.[212] The deeper aspect is characterized by swollen, peglike infiltrating columns of squamous cells with marked keratinization. A pronounced degree of inflammation is present both within the papillae and at the basal aspect.[208, 210, 212] Volumetric expansion of these papillary structures by marked inflammation has been held partly responsible for luminal filling and obstructive symptoms.[208] Without correlation with clinical and radiologic findings, a diagnosis of malignancy may be impossible based on a surface biopsy only, in view of the well-differentiated cytoarchitectural character. However, a diagnosis can be made if deep, representative biopsy material is provided in conjunction with pertinent endoscopic and radiologic information.

This neoplasm should be distinguished from esophageal squamous cell papilloma[213, 214] or papillomatosis.[213, 215, 216] Squamous cell papilloma is an uncommon lesion of middle-aged men, usually solitary and with a predilection for the distal esophageal third. This lesion, particularly in the distal esophagus, is commonly associated with severe esophagitis or Barrett's esophagus.[213] It has a sessile and warty or semipedunculated and smooth configuration, ranging in size from 0.2 to 1.0 cm. Histologically, fibrovascular cores are covered by benign, commonly acanthotic, squamous epithelium with a prominent basal zone and complete surface maturation. Three architectural growth patterns are observed: an exophytic type (about half of cases); an endophytic type with inverted papillomatous proliferation; and an uncommon spiked type showing a prominent granular layer

and hyperkeratosis.[213] Koilocytosis, parakeratosis, and stromal inflammation are commonly present.[213] About half of these lesions were found to be positive for HPV, most commonly Type 16, in the study by Odze and colleagues.[213] Current evidence suggests that the synergistic action of mucosal irritation and HPV infection is involved in the pathogenesis of esophageal squamous cell papilloma. Further studies are required to determine the natural history of this lesion and its potential relationship, if any, to the development of esophageal intraepithelial neoplasia and carcinoma.

Hematogenous metastasis has not been reported in the setting of verrucous squamous cell carcinoma, whereas lymph node involvement has been observed in one case, possibly by contiguous tumor invasion.[208] Although the tumor has a low-grade malignant pathobiology, the prognosis is rather poor mostly because of local invasion and related complications. More than two-thirds of the patients have died of complications such as malnutrition, aspiration pneumonia, bronchoesophageal fistula formation, or dehiscence of anastomosis. Therefore, early detection and surgical resection are mandatory if the clinical condition of patient permits.[208]

Interestingly, although rare in humans, verrucous squamous cell carcinoma has a great resemblance to the malignant esophageal neoplasm induced in rats with methyl-alkyl-nitrosamines, in which case tumors are predominantly pedunculated and papillary.[217]

Glandular Epithelial Dysplasia in Barrett's Mucosa

Glandular epithelial dysplasia is, at present, the best defined premalignant lesion in Barrett's esophagus and is most often identified in the specialized-type mucosa. Contiguous glandular epithelial dysplasia, mostly high grade, has been observed in 50% to 100% of cases of adenocarcinoma related to Barrett's esophagus.[12, 63, 76, 79, 82–85] Furthermore, although the natural history of glandular epithelial dysplasia is unclear, many studies have confirmed the increased frequency and worsening of dysplasia and adenocarcinomatous transformation in a significant number of patients,[68, 72, 78, 87] tending to support the hypothesis of a sequence leading from glandular dysplasia to adenocarcinoma in situ to invasive adenocarcinoma. The pathobiologic significance of Barrett's mucosa and related dysplasia has been discussed previously (see the heading entitled Pathologic Conditions Associated with Esophageal Carcinoma).

Glandular dysplasia represents a combination of architectural and cytologic abnormalities that parallel one another in severity for each degree of dysplasia. However, one or the other parameter may predominate in a particular patient. Architectural changes include an exaggerated surface villiform configuration, whereas the glands may show papillary infoldings, irregular shapes, crowding, and cribriform patterns. Cytologic changes include nuclear enlargement, hyperchromasia, and pleomorphism; nuclear stratification; excessively large and abnormal nucleoli; abnor-

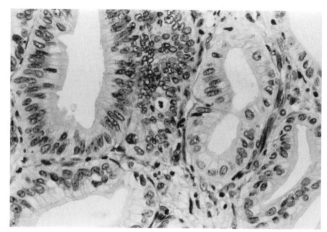

FIGURE 19–25. Transition between nondysplastic glands (*right half*) and low-grade glandular epithelial dysplasia (*left half*) in Barrett's mucosa. In dysplastic glands, nuclear stratification is confined to the lower half of glands, whereas nuclei are enlarged and hyperchromatic with distinctive nucleoli. (Hematoxylin and eosin, 250 ×.)

mal mitoses; cytoplasmic dedifferentiation (i.e., basophilia with decreased or absent mucin production); and increased nuclear/cytoplasmic ratio.[23, 91, 115] In low-grade dysplasia, architectural changes are modest, the cells retain the capacity for mucin production, and nuclear stratification is confined to the lower half of the cells (Fig. 19–25). High-grade dysplasia (encompassing adenocarcinoma in situ) is characterized by more profound architectural alterations, prominent nuclear abnormalities, markedly decreased or absent mucin production, and stratification of nuclei into the upper half of the cells (Fig. 19–26). A cribriform gland pattern is also indicative of high-grade dysplasia.[23, 91, 115] On the other hand, the designation *intramucosal adenocarcinoma* implies neoplastic invasion within the lamina propria but not beyond the muscularis mucosae and includes changes such as

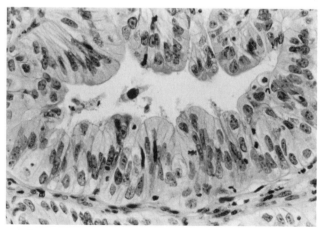

FIGURE 19–26. High-grade glandular epithelial dysplasia (adenocarcinoma in situ) in Barrett's mucosa. One neoplastic gland is characterized by nuclear stratification and nuclear features including enlargement, hyperchromasia with chromatin aberrations, large abnormal nucleoli, and mitotic figures. (Hematoxylin and eosin, 250 ×.)

angulation of glands, single cells or irregular clusters of cells in the lamina propria, sheets of cells, and a desmoplastic stromal response.[23, 115] Therefore, it represents a superficial form of adenocarcinoma.

In practice, we use this reporting scheme when a biopsy sampling of Barrett's mucosa is assessed: (1) negative for dysplasia; (2) indefinite for dysplasia or low-grade dysplasia; (3) high-grade dysplasia; (4) intramucosal invasive adenocarcinoma (notwithstanding that most biopsy specimens are not deep enough to rule out submucosal invasion). The grouping of indefinite for dysplasia and low-grade dysplasia is justified because there is a significant degree of interobserver variation in the distinction between both lesions.[91] On the other hand, there is a high degree of reproducibility in diagnosing high-grade dysplasia and intramucosal invasive adenocarcinoma as they can be separated from lesser degrees of abnormality with an interobserver agreement of 86%.[91]

Glandular dysplasia in Barrett's mucosa is usually not endoscopically (grossly) distinctive, the mucosa otherwise appearing red and velvety. In some cases, however, high-grade dysplasia may assume a polypoid configuration, measuring 0.5 to over 2.0 cm in diameter.[82, 84, 115, 218] Malignant transformation can occasionally occur in such polypoid lesions.[115]

Glandular dysplasia should be distinguished from *glandular epithelial atypia of inflammation or repair*. In the latter condition, the architecture is not significantly altered. Although nuclei are enlarged, they maintain their basal location, do not vary in size, lack chromatin aberrations, and typically contain prominent central nucleoli.[115] Furthermore, associated inflammation or fibrinopurulent exudate, or both, may be present.

Adenocarcinoma

Primary (genuine) adenocarcinoma of the esophagus is recognized as a distinct entity that is defined with stringent criteria,[64] although a current trend is to lump together tumors exclusively involving the esophagus with those involving the gastric cardia in view of the remarkable pathobiologic resemblance. The incidence reported has varied widely because of the paucity of genuine cases, unclear definition, and inclusion of lesions involving the gastric cardia. Such heterogeneity in reporting has made the pathobiologic assessment most difficult. Criteria for accepting a tumor as a genuine adenocarcinoma of the esophagus are presently defined as follows: (1) neoplastic involvement of the esophagus in the absence of a primary gastric tumor and without involvement of the gastroesophageal junction[64] or (2) neoplastic involvement of at least 75% of the esophagus in spite of invasion of the gastroesophageal junction, in conjunction with Barrett's esophagus.[63, 82] On the other hand, we prefer to classify adenoid cystic carcinoma and the adenosquamous-adenoacanthoma-mucoepidermoid carcinoma complex as specific subtypes, although many authors do not make such a distinction.[76, 219] The reported incidence of primary adenocarcinoma among esophageal malignancies has varied greatly, ranging from less than 1% to as high as 39% (a figure around 5% to 10% seems to be most representative).[64, 67, 85, 166, 220–225] On the other hand, there is evidence that the relative incidence of primary adenocarcinoma of the esophagus (and of the gastric cardia as well) is steadily rising in the United States, whereas the incidence of squamous cell carcinoma has remained relatively stable and the incidence of gastric adenocarcinoma is slightly declining.[22, 224, 226, 227] The rate of increase is about 4% to 10% per year among men, therefore exceeding those of any other type of cancer.[227] In a recent study comparing the 1935 to 1971 period with the 1974 to 1989 period, the incidence of esophageal adenocarcinoma was found to have increased of five- to sixfold.[226] Compared with squamous cell carcinoma, adenocarcinoma of the esophagus has been estimated to be six and a half times less frequently encountered.[161]

Patients affected by adenocarcinoma tend to be white males in their sixth to eighth decades, whether or not they also have Barrett's esophagus.[80, 222, 227, 228] The male-to-female ratio is in the range of 7 to 10, whereas the relative incidence rate in blacks is 30% that of whites.[161, 227] Dysphagia, pain, and weight loss are the usual symptoms on presentation. Adenocarcinoma of the esophagus arises in two basic clinicopathologic settings: (1) superimposed on Barrett's esophagus in the large majority (about 80% to 90%) of cases[21, 63, 64, 78, 80, 85]; and (2) without underlying Barrett's esophagus and of rare occurrence. The tumors without underlying Barrett's esophagus are assumed to be native from esophageal mucinous glands or heterotopic (ectopic) patches of gastric mucosa, as previously discussed.[7, 229, 230] However, the latter assumption may be difficult to verify because the destructive nature and size of the tumor may obscure any evidence of histogenesis. As a correlate, the site of predilection is the lower esophagus (about 80% to 90% of cases).[76, 82, 161, 223]

The gross configuration in *advanced adenocarcinoma of the esophagus* is not distinctive and has been described as fungating, polypoid, flat, ulcerating, annular or stenosing, or as a combination of patterns (Fig. 19–27).[76, 230] Superimposed ulceration is frequent,[76] but fistula formation is uncommon.[64] The tumor size ranges from 1 to 10 cm, usually between 3 cm and 6 cm.[64, 76, 82] In one study,[231] tumor size was found to be a prognostic determinant because tumors smaller than 6 cm were associated with a 5-year survival rate of 21%, whereas no 5-year survivor was found among patients with tumors larger than 6 cm. Barrett's esophagus–related adenocarcinoma is generally centered within few centimeters of the gastroesophageal junction (mean, 2 cm ± 0.3 cm).[80] Although rare, Barrett's esophagus–related adenocarcinoma has been documented in young adults and children.[232] The pathobiology does not differ from that of adult cases.

Histologically, the whole spectrum of glandular differentiation may be seen,[76, 223] and there is a strong resemblance to gastric adenocarcinoma.[63] Well-differentiated tumors have a distinct gland-forming pattern of small or large glands of simple or complex shape,

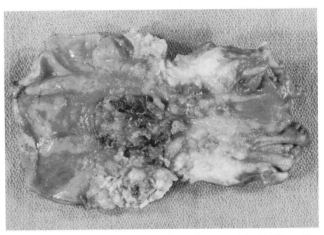

FIGURE 19–27. Adenocarcinoma of esophagus related to Barrett's mucosa. There is a sessile, shaggy, fungating, and ulcerating tumor with an ill-defined outline.

associated with a reactive stroma displaying a variable degree of inflammation and fibrosis (Fig. 19–28). Neoplastic glands have a haphazard arrangement, and individual cell infiltration may or may not be obvious. The glandular cell lining is simple or stratified with a variable degree of cytoplasmic differentiation. Cytologic stigmata of malignancy include loss of cell polarity, increased nuclear/cytoplasmic ratio, variation in nuclear size and shape, hyperchromasia, enlarged nucleoli, and an increased number of mitotic figures, including abnormal forms. Intracellular and extracellular mucin is present. With loss of tumoral differentiation, gland formation and mucin production are scanty (Fig. 19–29). Some tumors may be predominantly mucin producing with individual cells or cell clusters floating in abundant mucin.[63, 64] Other tumors may display a papillary pattern characterized by fibrovascular cores covered with a cuboidal or columnar neoplastic epithelium.[63, 64, 107] The latter pattern

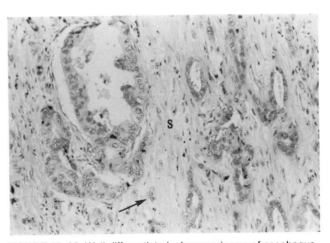

FIGURE 19–28. Well-differentiated adenocarcinoma of esophagus, arising within Barrett's mucosa. There is a disorganized pattern of infiltrative, neoplastic glands of variable size within a reactive desmoplastic stroma (S). Infiltrating individual neoplastic cells are present (*arrow*). (Hematoxylin and eosin, 100 ×.)

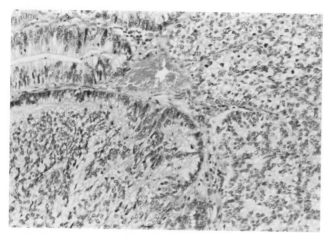

FIGURE 19–29. Poorly differentiated adenocarcinoma of the esophagus, arising within Barrett's mucosa. There is a predominant solid pattern of clear cells, whereas a small gland-forming component is seen in the upper left. (Hematoxylin and eosin, 100 ×.)

has been linked to a bulky, exophytic gross configuration.[63] Rarely, a signet-ring cell pattern, characterized by individual infiltrating cells with a large cytoplasmic mucin vacuole and eccentric positioning of the nucleus, may be seen.[64, 107, 221, 233] The presence of such a diffuse neoplastic pattern in the esophagus has been referred to as *linitis plastica*. According to Pazdur and colleagues,[234] three cases of esophageal linitis plastica were well documented in the literature by 1988 and showed the following characteristics: marked mural thickening with luminal stenosis, transmural tumor penetration, invasion of periesophageal tissues, and early metastatic dissemination. The proximal stomach and gastroesophageal junction should not be involved by neoplasia in order to accept such a case of primary esophageal derivation. Small gland and single cell patterns have been associated with an infiltrating tumor border, poor histologic differentiation, and positive resection margins.[76] Gössner[225] has suggested that an unusually large number of Barrett's esophagus–related adenocarcinomas would show focal squamous differentiation (referred to as "adenosquamous carcinoma") as a result of phenotypic instability of a single neoplastic cell line. However, such observation has not been corroborated by other authors nor in our own experience.

Three cases of *Paget's disease of the esophagus* have been reported.[235, 236, 237] Nonomura and associates[235] reported a unique case without associated invasive carcinoma and characterized by intraepithelial growth of individual or groups of cells within the lower part of the epithelium and with intraepithelial involvement of esophageal glands. Large, round cells with a pale cytoplasm and macronucleoli were characteristic, whereas mucin and expression of carcinoembryonic antigen (CEA) were detected within many pagetoid cells at the level of esophageal glands. The patient was a 60-year-old male with a 3-month history of dysphagia and pain whose endoscopy revealed an irregular and indurated mucosa. Conversely, mucin-nega-

tive pagetoid cells were contiguous to a poorly differentiated squamous cell carcinoma in one case,[237] whereas mucin-positive pagetoid cells were contiguous to an adenosquamous carcinoma in another case.[236]

By the time of diagnosis, esophageal adenocarcinoma is likely to show deep mural penetration, therefore representing an advanced form of disease. Transmural penetration and invasion of the adventitia has been reported in 76% to 88% of cases.[63, 76, 82, 83] A positive margin was present in 35% of cases in one study,[76] stressing the importance of intraoperative marginal assessment by frozen section. Multicentricity is occasionally observed.[76] The incidence of regional lymph node metastasis has ranged from 37% to 71%.[63, 76, 82, 83] The overall 2-year survival rate is 25% to 34%, whereas the 5-year survival rate is 14% to 24% (the former figure seems to be most representative).[67, 231, 238] The reported median survival time has ranged from 7 months to 23 months.[64, 76, 223, 239] At postmortem examination, lymphatogenous dissemination to mediastinal and abdominal lymph nodes, and hematogenous dissemination to lungs, liver, and vertebrae is the usual mode of metastatic involvement. Therefore, the overall outcome and prognosis of adenocarcinoma is comparable to squamous cell carcinoma.

The concept of *superficial (early) adenocarcinoma of the esophagus* has emerged,[78] by analogy with its squamous cell malignant counterpart. It is defined as invasive adenocarcinoma with a depth of penetration not beyond the submucosa, regardless of the nodal status. Whereas a few such cases have been included in series of adenocarcinoma at large,[63, 76, 82] superficial adenocarcinoma is likely to be detected during endoscopic surveillance of patients with high-grade dysplastic Barrett's mucosa.[78, 79, 88, 89] The prevalence rate of the superficial form in the setting of Barrett's esophagus–related adenocarcinoma has ranged from 24% to 67%.[78, 79, 88] In nearly half of these cases, there was no endoscopic or gross mucosal alteration suggestive of invasive neoplasia (the Barrett's mucosa otherwise looking red, velvety, or eroded).[78, 88, 90] In other cases, the endoscopic or gross appearance was clinically suspicious for invasive neoplasia and included mucosal changes such as a polypoid configuration (sessile and with a smooth surface), ulceration with a firm raised edge, a thickened and verrucous configuration, or a white plaque.[78, 88, 90] In one study, the tumor size ranged from 0.2 to 3.0 cm, whereas the mean length of associated Barrett's mucosa was 4.8 cm.[78] The histologic appearance is similar to advanced adenocarcinoma, most tumors showing a range of well to moderate glandular differentiation.[78] In one series of 12 patients, regional lymph node metastasis was present in one case only, whereas all patients (excluding two unrelated deaths) were alive without evidence of disease after a mean follow-up of 30 months.[78] The three patients reported by Altorki and coworkers[89] were node negative and alive without evidence of disease at 4 years, 4 years, and 8 years, respectively. An overall 5-year survival of 67% to 86% has been reported for superficial adenocarcinoma.[67, 88]

Therefore, the outcome and prognosis is somewhat comparable to superficial squamous cell carcinoma.

Some information has recently emerged regarding the effect of preoperative chemotherapy on the histologic and ultrastructural appearance of esophageal adenocarcinoma. In a study of 13 esophagectomy specimens in which patients had received preoperative chemotherapy, Darnton and associates[170] observed minor histologic changes in nine surgical specimens including a minor degree of fibrosis, chronic inflammation, and tumor cell regression. No significant alteration of the mean proportion of tumor epithelial to stromal component was observed. On the other hand, more obvious alterations have been observed at the ultrastructural level. Darnton and colleagues,[240] using 13 nontreated esophageal adenocarcinomas as controls, found ultrastructural evidence of cytotoxic damage in all 10 cases of esophageal adenocarcinoma in which patients had received preoperative chemotherapy. A variable proportion of neoplastic cells was found to show degenerative or regenerative changes, or both: rupture of nuclear or cytoplasmic membranes with discharge of cell content in the stroma; cytoplasmic vacuolar changes and increased number of secondary lysosomes; protrusion of cytoplasmic blebs into the lumen; and nuclear changes including karyopyknosis and karyorrhexis. Phagocytosing macrophages and admixed lymphocytes, eosinophils, and mast cells were present in the stroma.

The Pathobiologic Significance of Adenocarcinoma at the Gastric Cardia

Comparative analysis of genuine esophageal adenocarcinoma (most frequently in association with Barrett's esophagus) and adenocarcinoma of the gastric cardia and gastroesophageal junction has shown striking similarities from an epidemiologic, pathologic, and prognostic standpoint.[85, 218, 225–227, 241] The incidence of adenocarcinoma involving the gastric cardia has been steadily rising,[22, 226, 227] from 4% to 10% per year similarly to genuine esophageal adenocarcinoma.[227] In one study comparing the 1935 to 1971 period with the 1974 to 1989 period, a five- to sixfold increase in the incidence rate was observed, similarly to genuine esophageal adenocarcinoma.[226] Both tumors are characterized by a very high male-to-female ratio[218, 222, 227, 242] and occur with a much higher relative incidence among whites compared with blacks.[227] Both tumors are associated with an increased prevalence of duodenal ulcers and hiatal hernia.[85, 218] Many investigators have observed a similar pattern of alcohol and tobacco consumption among both groups of patients.[83, 85, 222, 243] In two pathologic studies comparing genuine adenocarcinoma of the esophagus with adenocarcinoma of the gastric cardia, no significant difference was observed regarding the pattern of tumor growth, degree of histologic differentiation, mucin production, stromal or inflammatory reaction, depth of invasion, likelihood of angioinvasion, and lymph node metastasis.[83, 85] The significant difference is the presence of high-grade glandular epithelial dysplasia in most cases of Barrett's esophagus–related adenocarcinoma (in about 90%), whereas dysplasia within the contiguous gastric mucosa is observed in no more than 20% of cases of adenocarcinoma of the gastric cardia. On the other hand, concurrent Barrett's mucosa has been recently reported to be present in a significant proportion (9% to 55%) of adenocarcinomas centered on the gastric cardia.[85, 222, 225, 226]

One study comparing 103 patients with adenocarcinoma of the gastric cardia and 28 patients with a genuine adenocarcinoma of the esophagus (half of which were associated with Barrett's esophagus) showed poor prognosis in both groups, with a median survival of 11 months and 7 months, respectively.[239] In both groups, the discrepancy between clinical and pathologic staging was striking, most patients having advanced disease at the time of surgical and pathologic evaluation.[239] In a recent study of 112 cases of surgically resected adenocarcinoma of the gastric cardia, Blomjous and associates[241] observed a cumulative 5-year metastatic rate of 64%, a locoregional recurrence rate of 36% (correlating with a positive surgical margin) and an overall 5-year survival rate of 24%.

Adenoid Cystic Carcinoma

First reported in 1950 as retrieved by Kabuto and coworkers[244] from the United States Naval Medical School Atlas of Pathology, adenoid cystic carcinoma (carcinoma with adenoid cystic differentiation) has been the object of an ongoing dispute in regard to its histogenesis and natural history, specifically in view of its resemblance to its salivary gland counterpart.[187, 245] This tumor is very rare. By 1991, only 55 cases were recorded in the English literature,[246–249] whereas an incidence of 0.75% to 1.2% has been reported among esophageal malignancies.[187, 246] On the other hand, Bogomoletz and colleagues[123] reported an incidence of 7% for adenoid cystic carcinoma in their series of 76 cases of superficial esophageal carcinoma. However, many such reported cases might be currently reclassified as basaloid squamous cell carcinomas. We use this designation for esophageal tumors showing a predominant pattern of adenoid cystic carcinoma, excluding tumors (most often squamous cell carcinoma) in which this pattern represents a minor or focal component.[250]

The tumor has a predilection for males (male-to-female ratio of about 3:1) in their sixth to eighth decades (range, 36 to 83 years; median age, 65 years).[251] Progressive dysphagia and obstruction are the common presenting symptoms, whereas the duration of symptoms before diagnosis is generally short (range, 2 weeks to 6 months).[251] However, most patients with a superficial tumor confined to the submucosa are asymptomatic, and the tumor is found incidentally.[123, 244, 246, 247] The tumor is most often located in the middle third (about two-thirds of cases), less often in the lower third, and rarely, in the upper third.[251] The gross configuration is either predominantly fungating (about one-third of cases), ulcerating, infiltrative, or less often, verrucous or polypoid.[123, 187, 246, 247, 249] The size is variable, while transmural penetration and invasion of periesophageal tissues is frequent.[187, 245, 246] Tumors confined to the submucosa have ranged from 1 to 5 cm in size.[123, 246, 247, 249] To our knowledge, no case of adenoid cystic carcinoma confined to the mucosa has been reported.

Adenoid cystic carcinoma of the esophagus is histologically characterized by a spectrum of solid, cribriform, or trabecular patterns. There is a population of monotonous, small, basaloid cells showing marked mitotic activity, possessing round-to-oval nuclei and scanty cytoplasm. The epithelial and stromal interface is smooth and sharp. Some eosinophilic, hyaline material, positive for PAS after diastase digestion, is seen most frequently within pseudocysts in cribriform areas or in between trabeculae. Ultrastructure has shown this material to be replicated basal lamina with admixed nondescript fibers, which is in contact with epithelial cells or myofibroblasts.[245] In addition, there are occasional glandular lumina with alcianophilic mucin and outlined by microvilli at the ultrastructural level.[245] The immunocytochemical phenotype resembles its salivary gland counterpart.[246, 247] However, some subtle morphologic differences have been noted in comparison with its salivary gland counterpart. Indeed, the following features have been noted to be most distinctive in the esophagus: the predominance of a solid pattern with focal necrosis, prominent nuclear overlapping and mitotic activity, and the continuity with the overlying mucosal surface in many tumors.[187, 245, 246] Furthermore, some tumors have been associated with high-grade EIN,[187, 245, 246] have shown foci of keratinizing squamous cell differentiation, or have rarely been associated with a synchronous separate squamous cell carcinoma.[123, 187, 246] Therefore, adenoid cystic carcinoma of the esophagus tends to be of intermediate to high histologic grade in reference to the conventional grading scheme of adenoid cystic carcinoma at large. A precise diagnosis by forceps biopsy is difficult in view of the limited architectural detail that is available, although cytologic malignancy should be obvious.[245]

The origin of adenoid cystic carcinoma of the esophagus is a matter of debate, two concepts of histogenesis being currently considered: (1) Small, superficial tumors confined to the submucosa have been documented with an intact overlying epithelium and without associated EIN,[244, 247–249] whereas in one case, the tumor was associated with and focally replacing submucosal glands.[248] These topographic observations and the ultrastructural resemblance to the intercalated duct cells of mucus-secreting glands[245] suggest an origin from the submucosal esophageal glands. (2) On the other hand, the following changes have been observed in a significant number of cases: direct continuity with overlying squamous cell epithelium, association with contiguous or noncontiguous EIN, and focal squamous cell differentiation.[187, 246] Such observations raise the assumption of a tumor arising from the surface squamous epithelium (perhaps best referred to as basaloid squamous cell carcinoma) or at

least associated surface epithelial neoplastic induction.[187]

Current evidence suggests that adenoid cystic carcinoma of the esophagus has a much more aggressive clinical behavior than its salivary gland counterpart, including a shorter duration of symptoms prior to diagnosis, a high tendency to metastasize, and a worse prognosis.[187, 246, 251] Petursson[251] in his review of 45 cases from the literature (including his own case) observed the development of metastasis in 76% of cases (including distant metastasis in a large percentage of patients), whereas the 1-year survival rate was 23%.[251] In their survey of the literature, Epstein and associates[187] reported a median survival of 9 months following diagnosis. This is in contrast to adenoid cystic carcinoma of the salivary glands, which has been associated with a 5-year survival of 60% to 70%.[252] On the other hand, tumors that were confined to the submucosa have proved to have a good prognosis including patients with long-term survival times, whereas nodal metastasis has been rarely encountered (2 of 10 cases).[123, 244, 246–249]

Mucoepidermoid Carcinoma

Mucoepidermoid carcinoma of the esophagus is defined as a tumor histologically resembling its salivary gland counterpart.[106] Unfortunately, many authors seem to use the designations of mucoepidermoid carcinoma and adenosquamous carcinoma synonymously. In our opinion, the term mucoepidermoid carcinoma should be restricted to a tumor showing a histologic type strictly similar to its salivary gland counterpart. We apply the term adenosquamous carcinoma to a tumor with a basic appearance of squamous cell carcinoma in which there are occasional and focal glandular elements. By 1990, about 36 cases were allegedly reported in the English literature.[253–256] Seven tumors referred to as having combined glandular and squamous elements[250] and some cases previously reported as adenoacanthoma might be added as well.[257] Patients described with this rare form of esophageal malignancy have been predominantly males (22 males/7 females) in their sixth or seventh decade (range, 46 to 81 years).[253, 255] The clinical presentation (dysphagia and weight loss of several months of duration), predilection for the lower (about half of cases) and middle esophageal thirds, the endoscopic and gross appearance, and radiologic features resemble squamous cell carcinoma.[255]

This tumor is characterized by an intimate mixture of squamous, mucus-secreting cells, and cells of intermediate type, the relative proportion of which may vary.[106] Mucous cells assume a cuboidal, columnar, or goblet shape with intracellular mucin, occasionally forming abortive glands. Signet-ring cells without mucin are rarely observed,[255, 258] ultrastructurally corresponding to intracytoplasmic spaces outlined by short microvilli.[255, 258] Squamous cells are usually present in the form of clumps or multilayered masses. Keratinization is uncommon, including intercellular bridges and occasional pearl formation. Intermediate

of 5 cm.[297] Satellite nodular lesions may be seen (about 12% of cases), sometimes at considerable distance from the primary tumor; because some of these are associated with multifocal junctional melanocytic cell proliferation, they might represent distinct primaries.[294, 297, 299] Mucosal macular pigmentation (so-called melanosis or melanocytosis) is observed in the surrounding mucosa in about one-quarter of cases, most often focal but occasionally diffuse.[297, 300] The cut surface is usually soft, gray-white or black, and dusty, depending on the relative degree of melanin content.

Histologically, the tumor is characterized by a solid pattern of noncohesive, round-to-polygonal cells or a fascicular or storiform pattern of spindle cells (with a sarcomatoid appearance) (Fig. 19–34). Most cells have abundant eosinophilic or dusty cytoplasm, vesicular nuclei, and prominent eosinophilic nucleoli (Fig. 19–35). Pleomorphic areas may be present, including bizarre cells and mononucleated or multinucleated giant cells.[19, 20] Mitoses are usually numerous, including atypical forms. Melanin deposition is seen in more than 90% of tumors.[20, 297] Histochemical staining with Fontana-Masson stain reveals intracytoplasmic, fine black granules of variable distribution, as a reflection

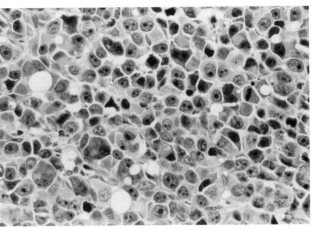

FIGURE 19–35. Primary malignant melanoma of esophagus. Population of noncohesive polygonal cells with abundant dusty and focally vacuolar cytoplasm. Nuclei are round to ovoid, with macronucleoli and frequent eccentric positioning. Cells were strongly immunoreactive for S-100 protein, HMB-45, and vimentin. (Hematoxylin and eosin, 250 ×.)

of melanogenesis within neoplastic melanocytes; the histochemical reactivity may be focal and found only after careful search. Some tumors are amelanotic (9% to 25% of cases in some series)[294, 298] and are likely to be misdiagnosed as undifferentiated carcinoma, sarcomatoid carcinoma, or even sarcoma. A small cell pattern in which cells have scanty cytoplasm and inconspicuous nucleoli, signet-ring cell features or balloon cell features have been occasionally observed[19] and could lead to a misdiagnosis of small cell carcinoma, poorly differentiated adenocarcinoma, or even malignant lymphoma. In such cases, immunocytochemical characterization is essential to confirm the melanocytic nature of the neoplasm. A full range of tumor penetration is observed, without any correlation with the metastatic potential.[294, 295] However, tumor invasion is often limited to the submucosa, and is characterized by a pushing rather than infiltrating border.[20, 293, 297, 301] Superimposed mild, chronic inflammation may be present.[297] A lateral lentiginous (in situ) component of atypical to frankly malignant melanocytes (resembling cutaneous lentigo maligna) is frequently present.[20, 297, 301–303] Furthermore, a diligent search often reveals a benign proliferation of hyperpigmented melanocytes in the overlying or adjacent mucosa (referred to as melanosis or melanocytosis when mucosal pigmentation is grossly seen).[19, 297, 298, 300, 304, 305]

The melanocytic phenotype of the tumor is best confirmed by immunocytochemical characterization, in which tumor cells are immunoreactive for S-100 protein, vimentin, and HMB-45 but are negative for cytokeratin or epithelial membrane antigen.[19, 20] On ultrastructural examination, tumor cells are united by junctional complexes and display intracytoplasmic Stages II to III melanosomes (so-called premelanosomes with a distinctive lattice-like arrangement) and dense bodies (Stage IV melanosomes).[20, 306] With a high index of suspicion in conjunction with immunocyto-

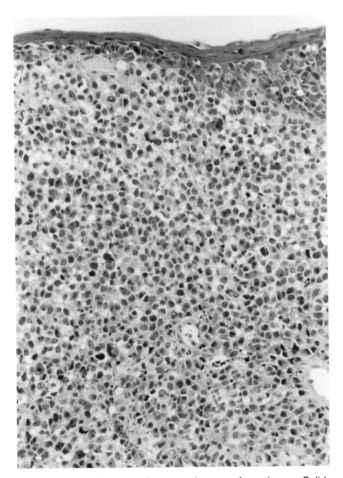

FIGURE 19–34. Primary malignant melanoma of esophagus. Solid pattern of noncohesive malignant cells. Note the overlying intact epithelium with a few intercalated malignant cells in the basal region. (Hematoxylin and eosin, 100 ×.) (Courtesy of Dr. Yvan Boivin, Hôtel-Dieu de Montréal, Montréal, Québec, Canada.)

chemical confirmation, a confident diagnosis of malignant melanoma is feasible on biopsy material.[294, 295]

The histogenesis of primary esophageal malignant melanoma is linked to the presence of esophageal melanocytes, presumably of ectodermal origin, which have been demonstrated in the basal region of the epithelium of 4% to 8% of normal esophagi.[15, 17] The presence of benign macular, black to brown lesions in the esophageal mucosa is referred to as melanosis or melanocytosis. It can occur alone[18] or in synchronous or asynchronous association with malignant melanoma.[19, 298, 300, 304, 305, 307] The pigmented character on endoscopic or gross examination is not only due to an increased number of benign melanocytes in the basal region of esophageal epithelium but also to an increase in the amount of melanin within these melanocytes and within keratinocytes (from passive transfer) and macrophages/fibroblasts in the lamina propria.[18] In one case of esophageal melanosis associated with malignant melanoma, a full range of cytologic atypia up to melanoma in situ was observed.[307] The above-mentioned observations leave no doubt in recognizing the existence of primary esophageal melanocytic neoplasia, whereas symptomatic metastatic malignant melanoma in the esophagus is exceedingly rare.[297]

The prognosis is poor, with an overall mean survival time of about 10 months and an overall 5-year survival rate not exceeding 2%.[297] About 40% of patients have nodal or hematogenous metastasis, or both, at the time of diagnosis.[294, 295, 297] About two-thirds of patients die within a year of the diagnosis, irrespective of therapeutic modalities, with disease-related death in 85% of cases.[297] At the time of diagnosis, about 70% of patients have a surgically resectable tumor.[293] Surgical resection, when feasible, is considered the treatment of choice, either for palliation or for cure, with an overall 5-year survival of 4% following radical surgery.[297] In an autopsy survey of 61 patients, metastases were seen in 84% of patients, most often in the liver (47% of cases with metastasis), mediastinum and mediastinal lymph nodes (41%), lung (29%), pleura (24%), supraclavicular lymph nodes (24%), followed by peritoneum and mesentery, brain, kidneys and adrenals, and other distant sites.[297] In another autopsy study of 29 patients, metastases were documented in 76% of cases with a similar topography of dissemination.[298]

Sarcomas

Leiomyosarcoma

Sarcomas of the esophagus are extremely rare, and represent no more than 5% of sarcomas of the gastrointestinal tract (nearly 50% of cases occurring in the stomach),[308] whereas an incidence of 0.5% (13 of 2526 cases) among esophageal malignancies has been reported in one study.[295] Leiomyosarcoma is the most frequently encountered type among them. Eighty-two cases were said to have been reported in the English literature (including a substantial proportion from Ja-

pan) by 1991.[197] On the other hand, using stringent criteria and including cases in which surgical resection was done (most of these being published after 1960), 39 cases were tabulated by Pélissier and co-workers[309] from the American and European literature, whereas 12 acceptable cases were subsequently published.[197, 295, 310] Otherwise, the genuine nature of many reported cases with poor pathologic documentation is doubtful, and therefore, the information provided on the pathobiology of this tumor should be assessed critically.

Most patients are in their sixth to eighth decades,[309, 311] and there is no significant difference in distribution between sexes (male-to-female ratio, 1:3).[295, 309, 311] The lower and middle esophageal thirds are most often involved.[295, 309, 311]

The gross configuration is variable. In more than half of cases, the tumor has an intraluminal and polypoid, lobulated, sessile, or pedunculated appearance.[295, 309] In about one-fourth of cases, the tumor is infiltrating, with a predominant extramural component invading periesophageal tissues.[295, 309] In a lesser proportion of cases, the tumor shows a combination of features as previously described, an intramural and circumscribed appearance (simulating a leiomyoma), or a diffuse infiltrating and stenosing configuration.[309] The cut surface appears gray-white, rubbery, and glistening. In contrast with leiomyoma, foci of softening, hemorrhage, or necrosis are likely to be present.[309, 311]

Histologically, the tumor is usually characterized by a fascicular pattern of spindle-shaped cells with an eosinophilic fibrillar cytoplasm and with a variable amount of intervening collagen (Fig. 19–36). Foci of palisading or hyalinization can be present, whereas some tumors may show epithelioid features. Poorly differentiated tumors may show marked pleomorphism, including multinucleated malignant cells. Mitotic figures, in conjunction with necrosis and/or hemorrhage, and large tumor size are likely to be the best indicators of metastatic potential for a smooth

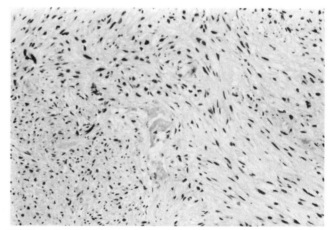

FIGURE 19–36. Well-differentiated leiomyosarcoma. There are interlacing bundles of spindle cells with nuclear hyperchromasia and anisonucleosis. This tumor was highly infiltrative and had mitotic activity (not illustrated here). (Hematoxylin and eosin, 100 ×.) (Courtesy of Dr. Yvan Boivin, Hôtel-Dieu de Montréal, Montréal, Québec, Canada.)

muscle neoplasm. However, although most leiomyomas are intramural and measure less than 5 cm in size, occasional tumors can reach a huge size.[312] Distinction between leiomyoma and leiomyosarcoma is unlikely to be achieved on biopsy material only or even on intraoperative frozen section assessment.[309, 312] Immunocytochemical reactivity for vimentin (best demonstrated on alcohol-fixed tissue) and negativity for melanocytic (S-100 protein, HMB-45) and epithelial (cytokeratin, epithelial membrane antigen) markers confirm the mesenchymal cell lineage. Immunoreactivity for desmin or muscle-specific actin, or both, further confirms the smooth muscle phenotype, although a negative result is often observed in borderline or malignant smooth muscle tumors of the gastrointestinal tract.

The natural history of esophageal leiomyosarcoma is unclear, since the follow-up is suboptimal for a majority of cases. Although it has been suggested that the disease is usually of slow growth in females with a polypoid tumor,[309, 311] some authors do not share this opinion.[295] The disease can be associated with local recurrence, particularly following tumoral excision (tumorectomy), and the mode of metastatic dissemination is characteristically hematogenous.[295, 309]

Fibrosarcoma

This type of sarcoma is defined as a malignant neoplasm composed of interlacing bundles of spindle-shaped fibroblasts and myofibroblasts with a characteristic herringbone pattern. For most reported cases of fibrosarcoma of esophageal origin, its actual existence is doubtful. The diagnosis was more popular in the 1950s and 1960s, and such cases would likely be reclassified now as either malignant fibrous histiocytoma or leiomyosarcoma. A neoplasm of extreme rarity, Goodner and colleagues[313] reported one case of fibrosarcoma among 1456 esophageal malignancies. Two acceptable cases were reported following radiotherapy to the neck after intervals of 29 years and 30 years, respectively, with prolonged survival in both cases.[313, 314]

Malignant Fibrous Histiocytoma

Three cases of malignant fibrous histiocytoma of the esophagus have been reported, including one in the Russian literature.[310, 315, 316] Samsonova and associates[316] reported a 12-cm exophytic tumor of the thoracic esophagus in a man in his sixth decade. Aagaard and coworkers[310] reported a 12-cm exophytic, obstructing tumor of the lower esophageal third in a 67-year-old male. The tumor invaded the left main bronchus, whereas metastases were observed in lymph nodes of the mesentery and in the liver. In their case, the tumor was originally misdiagnosed as an undifferentiated carcinoma, NOS. Sápi and colleagues[315] reported a 3.3-cm polypoid and pedunculated tumor in a 65-year-old man who presented with dysphagia. A polypectomy only was performed, whereas no follow-up was available.

Histologically, the tumor is characterized by a fascicular or storiform pattern of fibroblastic-like malignant cells, alternating with a pleomorphic pattern of histiocytic-like malignant cells. In addition, mononucleated or multinucleated giant cells with abundant amphophilic to eosinophilic cytoplasm, bizarre nuclei, and nuclear pseudoinclusions are often seen. Many cells contain hyaline globules, fat, or hemosiderin.[310, 315] On immunocytochemical characterization, tumor cells should be negative for epithelial, melanocytic, or myogenic markers, whereas immunoreactivity for vimentin and occasionally for alpha$_1$-antitrypsin is present.[315] Ultrastructure has revealed that most cells contain abundant rough endoplasmic reticulum, including dilated cisternae, which is indicative of fibroblastic differentiation. Lysosomes, myelin figures and pseudopodia have been observed in some cells, which are indicative of histiocytic differentiation.[315] The histogenesis of malignant fibrous histiocytoma is unclear, two views being currently considered: (1) the tumor would represent a sarcoma in which a primitive mesenchymal or fibroblastic-like cell shows both fibroblastic-like and histiocytic-like differentiation; and (2) the tumor would simply be a reflection of the end-stage of dedifferentiation of various sarcomas.

Osteosarcoma

Although osteosarcoma of the esophagus is found in dogs in association with *Spirocerca lupi*,[317] only one human case has been acceptably documented in the English literature.[318] A 70-year-old man underwent an esophagogastrectomy for a massive polypoid, 13-cm tumor of the lower esophagus. Histologically, a population of spindle- or stellate-shaped tumor cells with nuclear pleomorphism, mitoses, deposition of osteoid matrix, and admixed osteoclastic-like multinucleated cells was characteristic. The histogenesis has been ascribed to aberrant differentiation or metaplasia in neoplastic mesenchyme.[318]

Chondrosarcoma

One case of chondrosarcoma of the esophagus has been reported by Yaghmai and colleagues.[319] A 46-year-old man who presented with dysphagia of 6 months' duration, was found to have numerous firm, polypoid lesions covered with an intact mucosa in the middle and distal esophageal thirds. On imaging, the tumor was primarily in the esophageal wall with extramural expansion and was unrelated to the vertebral column. Four endoscopic biopsies revealed a well-differentiated chondrosarcoma characterized by a hyaline chondroid matrix, and features such as hypercellularity, multinucleated lacunae, variation in nuclear size and shape, and hyperchromasia. The patient refused surgery and died 8 months after diagnosis from local disease. Whether this is a pure chondrosarcoma or a component from a malignant mesenchymoma is unclear because the whole tumor was not available for pathologic examination. Malignant transformation of cartilaginous tracheobronchial remnants within the esophageal wall has been suggested to explain such an exceptional site for chondroid malignancy.[319]

Synovial Sarcoma

Four cases of synovial sarcoma have been reported in the English literature,[197, 295, 320, 321] including one case that has been reported twice.[197, 322] In three cases, the tumor occurred in patients younger than age 30, was located in the upper esophageal third, and had a polypoid or pedunculated configuration. These patients, following esophagectomy and postoperative radiotherapy, were alive without evidence of disease at 3 years, 6 years, and 16 years of follow-up, respectively.[197, 295, 321] In the fourth case, a 65-year-old female who presented with dysphagia and a palpable cervical mass was found to have an extensive, papilliferous tumor of the upper third of the esophagus. The patient expired 2 years after surgery and postoperative radiotherapy with recurrent disease but without distant metastasis.[320]

A biphasic pattern, including a cuboidal epithelial component forming clefts and glandlike spaces with eosinophilic secretions as well as a sarcomatous component of interlacing bundles of densely packed, short spindle cells, is histologically characteristic.[197, 295, 320–322] A dilated, capillary-type (hemangiopericytoid) vascular component may be present.[197] The epithelial component is immunoreactive for cytokeratin, whereas the mesenchymal component is positive for vimentin.[197]

Hemangiopericytoma

Two cases of hemangiopericytoma of the esophagus have been reported.[323, 324] Fisher[323] reported a case of an 81-year-old woman with a rapidly growing tumor that recurred and metastasized despite radiotherapy. Burke and Ranchod[324] reported, with optimal pathologic documentation, the case of a 23-year-old white man with a pedunculated, submucosal tumor who was alive 16 months after surgery. The tumor was characterized by a monophasic population of spindle-shaped cells forming a tuft woven pattern with branching thin-walled vessels of varying caliber. Ultrastructurally, cells were characterized by cytoplasmic processes with plasmalemmal plaques and pinocytic vesicles.

Kaposi's Sarcoma

A disease involving primarily homosexual and bisexual men and intravenous drug users, AIDS is etiologically linked to the retrovirus human immunodeficiency virus type 1 (HIV-1).[325–329] HIV-1 has a specific tropism for CD4-positive cells, which include lymphocytes, monocytes and macrophages.[330] Many of the immune defects noted in AIDS result from the depletion and functional defects in the CD4-positive helper or inducer subset of lymphocytes.[330] The mortality rate reaches 80% within a 2-year period, and 90% of

these patients are between 20 and 49 years of age.[331] As a consequence of this immune collapse, a myriad of opportunistic infections are encountered, as well as a significant incidence of Kaposi's sarcoma and malignant lymphoma. Both of these neoplasms may involve the gastrointestinal tract.[325, 329]

In postmortem studies (with a collective review of 105 patients), 50% to 77% of all patients had Kaposi's sarcoma and, of these, 50% to 70% had involvement of the gastrointestinal tract.[325–327] In fact, gastrointestinal involvement is one of the most frequent extracutaneous manifestations of Kaposi's sarcoma[325, 327] and characteristically reflects disseminated disease in other body sites, frequently in conjunction with at least cutaneous and/or nodal involvement.[325, 327, 329] In some cases, extensive involvement of the esophagus was documented.[325, 326] On the other hand, the clinical prevalence of Kaposi's sarcoma in AIDS patients has been decreasing in the last decade[332]; the cumulative percentage of patients with AIDS-related Kaposi's sarcoma has fallen to less than one-third of what it was in the early years of the epidemic.[332] This change in incidence possibly results from decreased infection with cytomegalovirus, which might possibly be a cofactor in the development of Kaposi's sarcoma.[332]

On endoscopic observation, the lesions appear as dark red mucosal macules or violaceous nodules measuring about 5 to 15 mm.[329] Endoscopic biopsies are positive in no more than 25% of cases, mostly because of the submucosal location of these lesions.[329] Numerous hemorrhagic mucosal and submucosal nodules separated by islands of preserved mucosa are characteristic on postmortem examination.[325] The tumor is histologically characterized by solid areas of spindle cells with entrapped red blood cells merging with primitive vascular channels and angiomatous areas containing well-formed vascular channels. Intracytoplasmic eosinophilic globules are characteristically present. Early small lesions can cause difficulty in recognition and may be confused with inflammatory lesions. Admixed lymphoplasmacytoid cells and siderophages are often present.[331, 333] Disseminated Kaposi's sarcoma has been documented as the immediate cause of death in 11% of patients (6 of 54 patients) with AIDS, usually as a result of fatal hemorrhage.[334] However, gastrointestinal involvement as such is unlikely to cause significant symptoms, although hemorrhage can be a serious complication with extensive disease.[326, 329]

Rhabdomyosarcoma

The existence of a genuine esophageal rhabdomyosarcoma is questionable in the absence of cytoplasmic cross striations or immunocytochemical or ultrastructural evidence of striated myogenic differentiation. Therefore, many reported cases might represent examples of poorly differentiated leiomyosarcoma or even malignant fibrous histiocytoma. At least one of these pathologic criteria should be fulfilled in order to accept a tumor as a genuine rhabdomyosarcoma: (1) presence of cells with unequivocal cross striations (best demonstrated with PTAH stain); (2) cytoplasmic immunoreactivity for myoglobin, in conjunction with desmin and/or muscle-specific actin; and (3) ultrastructural evidence of thin and thick myofilaments with Z-band material. Six reported cases fulfill indisputable criteria of acceptability.[335–340] The tumors were preferentially located in the middle and lower esophageal thirds. They were histologically characterized by a pleomorphic pattern, including plump or elongated cells with abundant eosinophilic cytoplasm, hyperchromatic nuclei, and macronucleoli. Myxoid changes or a small cell component were occasionally present. This appearance is characteristic of a pleomorphic type of rhabdomyosarcoma. Rhabdomyosarcoma is possibly arising from an undifferentiated mesenchymal progenitor cell, and is unlikely native from the esophageal striated muscle.[337, 339] This tumor has proved to have a dismal prognosis with rapid hematogenous or lymphatogenous metastatic dissemination.

Liposarcoma

Three cases of myxoid liposarcoma of the esophagus have been reported in the English literature.[341–343] Mansour and coworkers[341] reported the case of a 53-year-old male with a 4-cm pedunculated and polypoid tumor of the upper esophageal third. The patient was asymptomatic 1 year following local excision. Cooper and colleagues[342] reported the case of a 68-year-old man with a sessile, polypoid tumor of the lower third. The tumor was 7 cm in size with transmural tumor penetration. The patient had no evidence of disease 1 year following an esophagectomy. Baca and associates[343] reported the case of a 66-year-old woman who presented with a large polypoid, pedunculated tumor filling two-thirds of the dilated esophagus and arising from the upper third. A 12-cm tumor with focal necrosis was excised. No follow-up was available.

The overlying mucosa is intact, whereas the cut surface shows a soft gelatinous appearance. Histologically, the tumor is characterized by a myxoid population of bland spindle or stellate cells lying within a hyaluronic acid-rich matrix, a plexiform capillary vasculature, and admixed lipoblasts.[341, 342]

Malignant Schwannoma

Two cases of malignant schwannoma of the esophagus have been reported in the English literature,[197, 295] one of which was designated as *Triton tumor* because of the inclusion of rhabdomyoblasts. Caldwell and colleagues[295] reported the case of a polypoid tumor of the lower esophageal third in a 57-year-old woman. The patient died of postoperative complications. No significant histopathologic documentation was provided. Perch and coworkers[197] reported the case of a 22-year-old man who presented with a cauliflower-like, polypoid tumor of the upper third of the esophagus. The patient underwent an esophagectomy, followed by chemotherapy and radiotherapy, and was

alive without evidence of disease at 7-year follow-up. Pathologically, a multilobulated, 8-cm × 4-cm tumor was characterized by interlacing bundles of spindle-shaped cells with vacuolated areas and wavy nuclei. In some areas, there were large epithelioid cells with eosinophilic cytoplasm, which occasionally were multinucleated. The term Triton tumor refers to a malignant schwannoma with rhabdomyoblastic elements.

Malignant Granular Cell Tumor

Benign granular cell tumor is well known to occur in the esophagus, particularly the distal third, most commonly as a sessile or pedunculated polypoid, or nodular lesion with an intact mucosal surface.[344] About 190 cases have been so far reported.[344] A potential diagnostic pitfall on endoscopic biopsy is to misinterpret the surface pseudoepitheliomatous hyperplasia as a well-differentiated squamous cell carcinoma.

In our opinion, one indisputable case of *malignant* granular cell tumor of the esophagus has been reported in the German literature, based on the presence of associated lymph node metastasis.[345] On the other hand, seven other cases have been reported as malignant based on the large tumor size (ranging 4 to 10 cm), rapid recent growth, infiltrating pattern, and rapid recurrence following excision.[344] Among these eight cases, only two showed increased cellularity with nuclear atypia, pleomorphism, and a few mitoses.[346, 347] Granular cell tumor is otherwise histologically characterized by a solid pattern of polygonal cells, sometimes merging with fascicles of elongated cells. A granular and eosinophilic cytoplasm with PAS-diastase–resistant positive granules is characteristic. As tumor cells are immunoreactive for S-100 protein, the tumor is believed to be probably of Schwann cell derivation. Ultrastructurally, the cytoplasm is packed with lysosomes.

Malignant Mesenchymoma

A case of malignant mesenchymoma of the esophagus has been reported twice,[348, 349] originally by Haratake and colleagues.[348] A 50-year-old male presented with an acute episode of vomiting and was found to have a large intraluminal polypoid tumor in the middle esophageal third. An esophagectomy was performed following radiotherapy. The tumor was confined to the submucosa and measured 11 cm × 4 cm.

Choriocarcinoma

Three cases of primary esophageal choriocarcinoma have been reported, with no evidence of gonadal disease on postmortem examination.[350–352] Gynecomastia may be present and high levels of human chorionic gonadotropin can be demonstrated in serum or urine.[351, 352]

Hemorrhage and necrosis are prominent features on gross examination. The combination of cytotrophoblastic and syncytiotrophoblastic cellular components is histologically characteristic. Cytotrophoblastic cells are groups of more or less cohesive mononucleated cells with basophilic, focally vacuolated cytoplasm and round, pleomorphic hyperchromatic nuclei with prominent nucleoli. Syncytiotrophoblastic cells are multinucleated with abundant cytoplasm and clustering of hyperchromatic nuclei. These trophoblastic cellular elements may[350, 351] or may not[352] be associated with a carcinomatous-like component.

The histogenesis of extragonadal choriocarcinoma has been linked putatively to a displaced gonadal anlage, teratomatous transformation, or retrograde differentiation of tumor cells to the embryonal stage with the ability to form trophoblastic cells.[107] The course is aggressive, with rapid growth and hematogenous metastatic dissemination.

Malignant Lymphoma and Hodgkin's Disease

Clinical documentation of gastrointestinal tract involvement by malignant lymphoma is uncommon and has been observed in about 4% of cases,[353] whereas gastrointestinal involvement is found in about half of cases at autopsy.[353, 354] Clinical involvement of the esophagus by malignant lymphoma is observed in less than 2% of cases.[355] In most of these cases, it represents secondary invasion from the mediastinal lymph nodes or from the gastric fundus.[353-356] An exceptional case has also been documented in which esophageal involvement, accompanied by dysphagia and odynophagia, complicated longstanding cutaneous T-cell lymphoma of mycosis fungoides-type.[357] Genuine primary malignant lymphoma of the esophagus is very rare, about a dozen cases being documented.[357-365] Criteria of eligibility for a primary tumor include (1) predominant involvement of the esophagus, possibly with a few positive satellite lymph nodes; (2) absence of mediastinal and distant lymph node or splenic and hepatic involvement; and (3) a normal bone marrow.[363] However, malignant lymphoma of the esophagus in an immunocompromised host may become a more frequent neoplastic manifestation, especially in conjunction with AIDS. At least, four cases of high-grade malignant lymphoma, three of which were primary, have been reported in patients with AIDS.[357] Therefore, dysphagia in patients with AIDS requires proper investigation, including esophagoscopy and biopsy.

Dysphagia is the most common clinical manifestation of primary or secondary malignant lymphoma of the esophagus. On endoscopic or gross examination, a variety of patterns are encountered including a polypoid, nodular or ulcerative, or stenotic or stricture configuration.[356-359, 361-364, 366] The gross appearance is therefore often reminiscent of a conventional carcinoma. On the other hand, the presence of multiple submucosal nodules giving a varicoid appearance without ulceration[365] or a combination of many patterns could be suggestive of malignant lymphoma. Histologic documentation is suboptimal in most cases of non-Hodgkin's malignant lymphoma of the esophagus and such cases (either primary or secondary)

have been classified as small lymphocytic or plasmacytoid type (well-differentiated, low-grade),[362, 367] small cleaved cell type (poorly differentiated lymphocytic, intermediate-grade),[359, 368, 369] large cell type (histiocytic, intermediate-grade),[356, 358, 363] immunoblastic type (high-grade),[357, 366] T-cell type,[356, 357, 361] and Ki-1 (CD 30)–positive large cell type (high-grade).[360] The histologic features are similar to their nodal counterpart and are well described in standard monographs. Malignant lymphoma could be misinterpreted as an undifferentiated carcinoma on light microscopy; an immunocytochemical work-up is therefore essential for phenotypic characterization of a primitive-looking neoplasm. Lymphomatous cells are immunoreactive for leukocyte common antigen (CD 45), whereas they are negative for epithelial markers (cytokeratin, epithelial membrane antigen) and melanocytic markers (S-100 protein, HMB-45). Furthermore, immunoreactivity for L26 (CD 20) is indicative of a B-cell phenotype, whereas immunoreactivity for MT 1 (CD 43) is indicative of a T-cell phenotype. One case of Ki-1–positive large cell lymphoma, which shows a striking resemblance with undifferentiated carcinoma, NOS, has been reported as a primary tumor of the esophagus.[360] However, the primary nature is questionable because synchronous involvement of the liver and porta hepatis or pancreatic lymph nodes was present.[360] Exceptionally, this form of malignant lymphoma is nonimmunoreactive for leukocyte common antigen but is positive for Ki-1. Ultrastructurally, lymphomatous cells lack the presence of junctional complexes, melanosomes, mucin granules, or tonofilaments.

Lymphoid hyperplasia (pseudolymphoma) has been reported in the esophagus and should be considered in the differential diagnosis of malignant lymphoma.[370, 371] This lesion represents a florid follicular reaction of the B-cell lymphoid population and may include a significant number of large cells of follicular dendritic cell nature.[371] It has been associated with chronic stenosing ulcerating esophagitis and Barrett's mucosa.[370] It may have an exophytic appearance with associated mucosal ulceration. The lesion can be localized to the submucosa or may show extensive mural involvement.[370, 371] Distinction from malignant lymphoma is based on the presence of a follicular pattern with germinal centers, a polymorphic cell population (including lymphocytes at various stages of transformation, plasma cells, histiocytes, eosinophils, and dendritic cells), and the polytypic or polyclonal immunocytochemical character of the lymphoplasmacytoid cell population.[371] However, it is likely to be difficult to arrive at a definite diagnosis based on biopsy or cytologic material only.

Esophageal involvement with *Hodgkin's disease* is likely a secondary manifestation, associated with synchronous mediastinal contiguous disease.[354, 356, 372] Two cases with primary presentation have been reported.[373, 374] Stein and colleagues[374] reported a 30-year-old man with progressive dysphagia who underwent surgical resection by sharp dissection and subsequent radiotherapy. Histology revealed a nodular sclerosing variant characterized by fibrosis with an admixture of lymphocytes, plasma cells, eosinophils, histiocytes, and Reed-Sternberg cells. The patient developed recurrent mediastinal disease 3 years later. Chiolero[373] reported a case with a midesophageal stricture without any mediastinal or distal nodal involvement at autopsy.

Extramedullary Plasmacytoma (Myeloma)

Primary esophageal involvement with extramedullary plasmacytoma is extremely rare, with only two cases being documented.[375, 376] For acceptance of an extramedullary plasmacytoma, the following criteria should be fulfilled: (1) absence of Bence Jones proteinuria; (2) normal serum electrophoresis; (3) normal bone marrow; and (4) absence of hepatic and splenic involvement.[376] This neoplasm is characterized by round or ovoid cells with an amphophilic cytoplasm and a large, frequently eccentric nucleus displaying a "cartwheel" chromatin. A few binucleated cells may be present. Surgical resection followed by radiotherapy has been recommended.[376]

Secondary and Metastatic Tumors

Direct invasion of the esophagus may occur with a malignancy from the stomach, hypopharynx, larynx, thyroid, or tracheobronchial tract.[377] Metastatic involvement of the esophagus is well documented following breast carcinoma and is likely a reflection of lymphatogenous dissemination, in conjunction with involvement of mediastinal or periesophageal lymph nodes.[378] The mean interval between mastectomy and esophageal symptoms, most commonly progressive dysphagia, is 8 years. The middle esophageal third is preferentially affected, with concentric stricture and overlying intact mucosa.[378]

Metastatic malignant melanoma to the esophagus has been observed as nodular lesions mostly at the mucosal and submucosal level in 4% of patients with disseminated malignant melanoma,[379] and is unlikely to be symptomatic.[297] In fact, only 11 cases of symptomatic metastatic melanoma were reported by 1993.[380] In these cases, the tumor was most often polypoid and submucosal, without any mucosal junctional or lentiginous component or associated melanosis.[380] All patients died within 11 months, with a median survival of 5 months following esophageal manifestations.[380]

Metastasis to the esophagus has also occurred with primary tumors of lung, pancreas, testis, eye, prostate, bone, liver, bladder, rectum, kidney, cervix, and endometrium[377] and may produce clinical and radiologic findings suggestive of primary benign or malignant esophageal disease.[381, 382]

CYTOPATHOLOGY OF ESOPHAGEAL MALIGNANCY

Endoscopic brush cytology and biopsy are well-established complementary techniques for obtaining a diagnosis of esophageal malignancy.[383–386] Furthermore, meticulous care in the handling of the cytologic material is required to achieve an optimal rate of detection. An unsatisfactory specimen with insufficient numbers of poorly preserved cells should be repeated and not interpreted as benign.

In a prospective European study of symptomatic patients in which 100 verified esophagogastric tumors were collected, the cumulative diagnostic accuracy of combined biopsy and brush cytology was significantly better (96%) than with biopsy (83%) or cytology alone (85%).[383] In a Japanese survey of patients suspected of having upper gastrointestinal malignancy, including 116 cases of verified esophageal cancer, Kasugai and associates[385] demonstrated a high diagnostic accuracy with endoscopically directed biopsy and brush cytology: 90% for biopsy, 97% for brush cytology, and 99% for combined modalities. In the diagnosis of carcinoma of the lower esophagus and gastric cardia, biopsy touch smear cytology has been shown to be highly accurate. Indeed, in a 4-year prospective study of 64 patients suspected of having a malignant lesion in this location, Young and colleagues[387] observed a sensitivity of 100% for biopsy touch smear cytology compared with 82% for brush cytology and 89% for biopsy. Brush cytology also appears much more reliable than biopsy for stenosing tumors and may be the only means of obtaining diagnostic tumor cells in such instances.[21, 383] Following irradiation, brushing is likely to be superior to lavage because abrasion frees cells that are entrapped within cicatricial tissue. On the other hand, multiple biopsies are preferable to cytology for diagnosing a polypoid lesion.[383]

In China, for the screening of a high-risk population and the detection of superficial esophageal carcinoma or high-grade EIN, the *abrasive balloon-mesh technique* is widely used.[386, 388] It offers a diagnostic accuracy of about 90% and appears as a simple, painless, and accurate method of early detection.[386, 388] A single- or double-lumen tube made of rubber or plastic with an inflatable balloon, the latter being covered by a cotton mesh net, is used. Smears are prepared from collected material as previously discussed. An alternative method is to use a *suction-abrasive tube* with which the entire length of the esophagus is sampled.[389] The end of the tube with abraded material is immersed and shaken in normal saline. The fluid is then centrifugated and the sediment smeared on a ground-glass slide with subsequent fixation and staining. In South Africa, the *abrasive brush capsule* has been used for the screening of a high-risk population.[390, 391] It consists of a sponge within a capsule, attached to a long thread, which is swallowed with water. The capsular covering of the sponge dissolves and the sponge expands to be then withdrawn through the esophagus. This technique has been shown to have a high sensitivity (90%) and specificity (100%) in detecting carcinoma.[390] In China, as a result of improvements in early diagnosis and surgical intervention, the 5-year survival has risen from 10% in the 1960s to 30% for patients with advanced carcinoma and 90% for those with superficial carcinoma in the 1970s.[386, 388] The role of cytology in screening a high-risk population (in countries such as China, Iran or South Africa) is obvious, considering that about 20% to 40% of cases of superficial carcinoma are not detected by esophagoscopy or radiography alone.[386] However, this approach is probably not justified or even applicable in the Western world, where the detection of superficial carcinoma is likely to be achieved by endoscopy and biopsy.[123] Furthermore, in a prospective study among asymptomatic high-risk Veterans in the United States, the abrasive balloon-mesh cytology technique was not found to have a significant value in screening for superficial carcinoma.[116] In the study by Jacob and associates[116] including 28 patients diagnosed with esophageal EIN by abrasive balloon-mesh cytology, only one patient progressed to invasive carcinoma, whereas cytologic changes were reassessed later as normal or inflammatory atypia in 86% of cases or persistent EIN in 7% of cases.[116] These authors believed that this technique was of limited use as a screening method for early detection of esophageal carcinoma, probably because of the low incidence of this disease in United States, the coexistence of peptic esophagitis in this high-risk population, the difficulty of cytologically distinguishing inflammatory atypia from EIN, and the far less predictable EIN-to-carcinoma sequence in the high-risk population in the United States.[116]

A most comprehensive cytopathologic description of esophageal premalignant and malignant lesions has been provided by Shu.[386, 388] The cytologic smear from the *normal esophagus* is characterized by a majority of cells from the intermediate layers and about 10% from the superficial layers. Parabasal cells are very rare. Admixed columnar-gastric or respiratory cells may be seen. *Atypical* (inflammation-related) *esophageal cells* are often admixed with inflammatory cells, originating from the intermediate or superficial layers. Enlargement of the nuclei is slight, with a round nuclear contour and a finely dispersed chromatin. *Dysplastic esophageal cells* (EIN) retrieved in low-grade dysplasia have enlarged and hyperchromatic nuclei measuring less than three times the normal size of cells from the intermediate or superficial layers. In high-grade dysplasia, the nuclei are more than three times larger, with marked hyperchromasia and there is an increased number of dysplastic parabasal cells. *Squamous carcinoma cells* are usually found singly, are polygonal and comparatively uniform in shape, and have malignant nuclear characteristics, including fiber and spindle forms (Fig. 19–37). In *superficial carcinoma*, malignant cells are few and mostly round or oval. Well-differentiated cancer cells predominate, and large numbers of dysplastic cells are present in the background. In *advanced carcinoma*, malignant cells are often numerous, including sheets of pleomorphic cells. Dysplastic cells are few, and the background is dirty.

The *tumor grade* may be estimated on cytologic grounds according to Shu.[386, 388] Well-differentiated squamous carcinoma cells are mostly polygonal or bizarrely shaped, with abundant red or orange cyto-

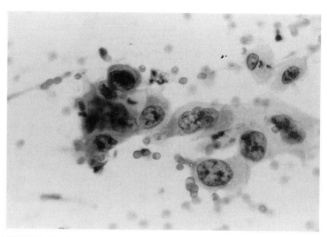

FIGURE 19–37. Invasive squamous cell carcinoma, brush cytology. Groups of polygonal and elongated cells with abundant, dense blue cytoplasm. Nuclei are hyperchromatic with an irregular nuclear membrane and clumps of dense chromatin. (Papanicolaou, 400 ×.)

plasm (Fig. 19–37). The nuclear-cytoplasmic ratio is slightly increased with frequent spindle, fiber, tadpole, or polygonal cell shapes. Nuclei are large and hyperchromatic. Moderately differentiated squamous carcinoma cells are mostly round to oval and look like parabasal cells with blue cytoplasm. The nuclear-cytoplasmic ratio is moderately increased with one or several visible nucleoli. These cells are most common in smears that represent a superficial carcinoma. Poorly differentiated squamous carcinoma cells are usually small and much more uneven in size, are often round or oval with scanty cytoplasm, and have well-defined cell and nuclear borders. The nuclear-cytoplasmic ratio is high, and nucleoli are prominent. Often, cells assume an irregular form, and only so-called naked hyperchromatic nuclei are apparent.

Esophageal squamous and gastric cardia glandular tumors were differentiated cytologically with an accuracy of 97% in a study by Shu.[386] The most common cause of error is in the distinction between poorly differentiated squamous cell carcinoma and adenocarcinoma. Otherwise, the cytologic profile of esophageal adenocarcinoma is similar to gastric adenocarcinoma, both consisting of clumps of cells with nuclear overlapping, common peripheral border, columnar or cuboidal cell shape, eccentric positioning of nucleus, prominent nucleolus, and cytoplasmic vacuolation (Fig. 19–38).

Brush cytology could theoretically play an important role as a complementary technique in the evaluation of patients with Barrett's esophagus.[392, 393] However, although cytologic interpretation is highly accurate in identifying Barrett's esophagus–related dysplastic or adenocarcinoma cells, it is not reliable in distinguishing low-grade from high-grade glandular epithelial dysplasia.[394] Furthermore, its value has not been explored in a prospective study comparing its efficacy with that of endoscopic biopsy.

On cytologic preparation, small cell carcinoma is characterized by isolated cells two to three times the size of a lymphocyte, with minimal or absent cyto-

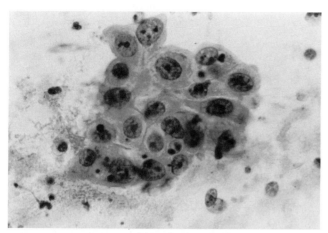

FIGURE 19–38. Adenocarcinoma of lower esophagus and gastric cardia, brush cytology. Cluster of cohesive polygonal cells with a common peripheral border. The cytoplasm is focally vacuolated. Nuclei are round with finely dispersed chromatin, with the presence of one to three prominent nucleoli. (Papanicolaou, 400 ×.)

plasm, and sometimes forming cell clusters with nuclear molding.[271, 280] Nuclei are round to oval, with an evenly distributed finely to coarsely granular chromatin, and with small or inconspicuous nucleoli.[271, 280] The crushed artifact (smeared nuclear material and nuclear streaking) often observed on forceps biopsy is not present on cytologic preparation.[280]

Cytologic brushing may be useful in the diagnosis of malignant melanoma.[303, 304] The background is often dirty. Round or spindle-shaped tumor cells, isolated or in clusters, with one or multiple prominent nucleoli, are observed. The presence of occasional intranuclear vacuoles (so-called pseudoinclusions) is characteristic, and the cytoplasm may contain granules of brown melanin pigment.

In sarcomatoid squamous cell carcinoma, the cytologic smear may reveal sheets or single malignant squamous cells, both keratinizing and nonkeratinizing, variably shaped (often spindle) cells with wispy cytoplasm, and scattered multinucleated cells.[199, 395]

In one case of malignant fibrous histiocytoma, the diagnosis was cytologically suggested in the presence of abundant and bizarre giant cells, in addition to a few osteoclastic-like multinucleated cells.[315]

Radiation-induced changes, most striking in the first 3 months (but sometimes persisting up to 6 months), should not be misinterpreted as malignancy or EIN. In this setting, changes such as abnormal cell shape, increased cell size with abundant cytoplasm, multinucleation and vacuolation are suggestive of radiation effect.

SELECTED REFERENCES

Mandard AM, Chasle J, Marnay J, et al: Autopsy findings in 111 cases of esophageal cancer. Cancer 48:329–335, 1981.
An excellent clinicopathologic study based on autopsy material, focusing predominantly on cases of squamous cell carcinoma. It includes a thorough mapping of locoregional disease, as well as the pattern of metastatic dissemination. Correlation is established between

clinical staging and postmortem findings, and the natural history is well delineated. Some emphasis is given to major associated diseases, including associated malignancies and cause of death.

Mandard AM, Marnay J, Gignoux M, et al: Cancer of the esophagus and associated lesions: Detailed pathologic study of 100 esophagectomy specimens. Hum Pathol 15:660–669, 1984.
A detailed pathologic analysis of 100 surgical esophagectomy specimens with systematic examination of the entire resected specimen by subserial sectioning in order to characterize the invasive carcinoma and associated mucosal anomalies. Most of the information relates to squamous cell carcinoma with or without an undifferentiated component. The association and definition of esophageal intraepithelial neoplasia is discussed. The degree of mural tumor penetration in correlation with lymph node metastasis or vascular invasion is discussed. The effect of preoperative radiotherapy is studied.

Shu Y-J: Cytopathology of the esophagus. An overview of esophageal cytopathology in China. Acta Cytol 27:7–16, 1983.
A most complete and comprehensive paper on the significance and diagnostic criteria of the cytopathology of the esophagus. A comparative description of normal, atypical, dysplastic (intraepithelial neoplasia) and cancer cells is described in detail and well illustrated for both squamous cell carcinoma and adenocarcinoma. The accuracy of this procedure and its value for early detection of carcinoma is emphasized.

Smith RRL, Hamilton SR, Boitnott JK, et al: The spectrum of carcinoma arising in Barrett's esophagus. A clinicopathologic study of 26 patients. Am J Surg Pathol 8:563–573, 1984.
A detailed clinicopathologic study of esophageal adenocarcinoma, arising in conjunction with Barrett's esophagus. Optimal characterization of the invasive tumor as well as adjacent Barrett's mucosa (with emphasis on glandular epithelial dysplasia) is provided. The natural history is well defined.

Sons HU, Borchard F: Esophageal cancer. Autopsy findings in 171 cases. Arch Pathol Lab Med 108:983–988, 1984.
A study of esophageal cancer on autopsy material, with more than 90% of cases being squamous cell carcinomas. There is emphasis on the pattern of locoregional and distant metastatic disease and major complications. The literature is thoroughly reviewed and well presented.

REFERENCES

1. DeNardi FG, Riddell RH: Esophagus. *In* Sternberg SS (ed): Histology for Pathologists. New York, Raven Press, 1992, pp 515–532.
2. Enterline H, Thompson J: Pathology of the Esophagus. New York, Springer-Verlag, 1984.
3. Ozawa S, Ueda M, Ando N, et al: High incidence of EGF receptor hyperproduction in esophageal squamous cell carcinomas. Int J Cancer 39:333–337, 1987.
4. Jankowski J, Murphy S, Coghill G, et al: Epidermal growth factor receptors in the eosophagus. Gut 33:439–443, 1992.
5. Miyazaki S, Sasano H, Suzuki T, et al: Nucleolar organizer regions in human esophageal disorders: Comparison with proliferating cell nuclear antigen by immunostaining. Mod Pathol 5:396–401, 1992.
6. De La Pava S, Pickren JW, Adler RH: Ectopic gastric mucosa of the esophagus. A study on histogenesis. NY State J Med 64:1831–1835, 1964.
7. Christensen WN, Sternberg SS: Adenocarcinoma of the upper esophagus arising in ectopic gastric mucosa. Am J Surg Pathol 11:397–402, 1987.
8. Takubo K, Takai A, Takayama S, et al: Intraductal spread of esophageal squamous cell carcinoma. Cancer 59:1751–1757, 1987.
9. Kuwano H, Matsuda H, Matsuoka H, et al: Intra-epithelial carcinoma concomitant with esophageal squamous cell carcinoma. Cancer 59:783–787, 1987.
10. Meyer GW, Austin RM, Brady CE III, et al: Muscle anatomy of the human esophagus. J Clin Gastroenterol 8:131–134, 1986.
11. Takubo K, Takai A, Sasajima K, et al: Perineural spread of esophageal carcinoma. *In* Siewert JR, Hölscher AH (eds): Diseases of the Esophagus. New York, Springer-Verlag, 1988, pp 89–92.

12. Spechler SJ, Goyal RK: Barrett's esophagus. N Engl J Med 315:362–371, 1986.
13. Feller SC, Weaver GA: Heterotopic gastric mucosa in the upper esophagus. (Correspondence.) Gastroenterology 90:257–258, 1986.
14. Jabbari M, Goresky CA, Lough J, et al: The inlet patch: Heterotopic gastric mucosa in the upper esophagus. Gastroenterology 89:352–356, 1985.
15. Tateishi R, Taniguchi H, Wada A, et al: Argyrophil cells and melanocytes in esophageal mucosa. Arch Pathol 98:87–89, 1974.
16. Ohashi K, Kato Y, Kanno J, et al: Melanocytes and melanosis of the oesophagus in Japanese subjects—analysis of factors effecting their increase. Virchows Arch [A] 417:137–143, 1990.
17. De La Pava S, Nigogosyan G, Pickren JW, et al: Melanosis of the esophagus. Cancer 16:48–50, 1963.
18. Yamazaki K, Ohmori T, Kumagai Y, et al: Ultrastructure of oesophageal melanocytosis. Virchows Arch [A] 418:515–522, 1991.
19. Symmans WF, Grimes MM: Malignant melanoma of the esophagus: Histologic variants and immunohistochemical findings in four cases. Surg Pathol 4:222–234, 1991.
20. DiCostanzo DP, Urmacher C: Primary malignant melanoma of the esophagus. Am J Surg Pathol 11:46–52, 1987.
21. Ming SC: Tumors of the Esophagus and Stomach. Atlas of Tumor Pathology, fascicle 7, 2nd series. Washington, DC, Armed Forces Institute of Pathology, 1985 (Suppl).
22. Haggitt RC: Adenocarcinoma in Barrett's esophagus: A new epidemic? (Editorial.) Hum Path 23:475–476, 1992.
23. Reid BJ, Weinstein WM, Lewin KJ, et al: Endoscopic biopsy can detect high-grade dysplasia or early adenocarcinoma in Barrett's esophagus without grossly recognizable neoplastic lesions. Gastroenterology 94:81–90, 1988.
24. Gupta RK, Rogers KE: Endoscopic cytology and biopsy in the diagnosis of gastroesophageal malignancy. Acta Cytol 27:17–22, 1983.
25. Peracchia A, Segalin A, Bardini R, et al: Esophageal carcinoma and achalasia: Prevalence, incidence and results of treatment. Hepatogastroenterology 38:514–516, 1991.
26. Meijssen MAC, Tilanus HW, van Blankenstein M, et al: Achalasia complicated by oesophageal squamous cell carcinoma: A prospective study in 195 patients. Gut 33:155–158, 1992.
27. Csendes A, Braghetto I, Mascaro J, et al: Late subjective and objective evaluation of the results of esophagomyotomy in 100 patients with achalasia of the esophagus. Surgery 104:469–475, 1988.
28. Chuong JJH, DuBovik S, McCallum RW: Achalasia as a risk factor for esophageal carcinoma. A reappraisal. Dig Dis Sci 29:1105–1108, 1984.
29. Agha FP, Keren DF: Barrett's esophagus complicating achalasia after esophagomyotomy. A clinical, radiologic, and pathologic study of 70 patients with achalasia and related motor disorders. J Clin Gastroenterol 9:232–237, 1987.
30. Goodman P, Scott LD, Verani RR, et al: Esophageal adenocarcinoma in a patient with surgically treated achalasia. Dig Dis Sci 35:1549–1552, 1990.
31. Proctor DD, Fraser JL, Mangano MM, et al: Small cell carcinoma of the esophagus in a patient with longstanding primary achalasia. Am J Gastroenterol 87:664–667, 1992.
32. Appelqvist P, Salmo M: Lye corrosion carcinoma of the esophagus. A review of 63 cases. Cancer 45:2655–2658, 1980.
33. Isolauri J, Markkula H: Lye ingestion and carcinoma of the esophagus. Acta Chir Scand 155:269–271, 1989.
34. Hoplins RA, Postlethwait RW: Caustic burns and carcinoma of the esophagus. Ann Surg 194:146–148, 1981.
35. Gerzić Z, Kneźević J, Milićević M, et al: Postcorrosive stricture and carcinoma of the esophagus. In Siewert JR, Hölscher AH (eds): Diseases of the Esophagus. New York, Springer-Verlag, 1988, pp 113–117.
36. Giudicelli R, Fuentes P, Garbe L, et al: Malignant transformation after caustic esophageal injury: Report of five cases. In Siewert JR, Hölscher AH (eds): Diseases of the Esophagus. New York, Springer-Verlag, 1988, pp 52–54.
37. Kokudo N, Sanjo K, Umekita N, et al: Squamous cell carcinoma after endoscopic injection sclerotherapy for esophageal varices. Am J Gastroenterol 85:861–864, 1990.
38. McCormick PA, Sawyer A, McIntyre N, et al: Carcinoma of the esophagus and long-term sclerotherapy. Endoscopy 21:152, 1989.
39. Guillemot F, Bonniere P, Bretagne JF, et al: Esophageal cancer and endoscopic sclerosis of esophageal varices: A fortuitous association? Gastroenterol Clin Biol 12:858–861, 1988.
40. Marin ML, Marin RH, Geller SA, et al: Carcinoma of the esophagus arising in patients with prior exposure to radiotherapy. In Siewert JR, Hölscher AH (eds): Diseases of the Esophagus. New York, Springer-Verlag, 1988, pp 122–125.
41. Ogino T, Kato H, Tsukiyama I, et al: Radiation-induced carcinoma of the esophagus. (Letter.) Acta Oncol 31:475–477, 1992.
42. O'Connell EW, Seaman WB, Ghahremani GG: Radiation-induced esophageal carcinoma. Gastrointest Radiol 9:287–291, 1984.
43. Goffman TE, McKeen EA, Curtis RE, et al: Esophageal carcinoma following irradiation for breast cancer. Cancer 52:1808–1809, 1983.
44. Møller Jensen B, Kruse-Andersen S, Andersen K: Carcinoma in a pharyngeal diverticulum. (Letter.) J Clin Gastroenterol 11:119, 1989.
45. Bowdler DA, Stell PM: Carcinoma arising in posterior pharyngeal pulsion diverticulum (Zenker's diverticulum). Br J Surg 74:561–563, 1987.
46. Wychulis AR, Gunnlaugsson GH, Clagett OT: Carcinoma occurring in pharyngoesophageal diverticulum: Report of three cases. Surgery 66:976–979, 1969.
47. Huang B-s, Unni KK, Payne WS: Long-term survival following diverticulectomy for cancer in pharyngoesophageal (Zenker's) diverticulum. Ann Thorac Surg 38:201–210, 1984.
48. Saldana JA, Cone RO, Hopens TA, et al: Carcinoma arising in an epiphrenic esophageal diverticulum. Gastrointest Radiol 7:15–18, 1982.
49. Tapia RH, White VA: Squamous cell carcinoma arising in a duplication cyst of the esophagus. Am J Gastroenterol 80:325–329, 1985.
50. Entwhistle CC, Jacobs A: Histological findings in the Paterson-Kelly syndrome. J Clin Pathol 18:408–413, 1965.
51. Wynder EL, Hultberg S, Jacobsson F, et al: Environmental factors in cancer of the upper alimentary tract: A Swedish study with special reference to Plummer-Vinson (Paterson-Kelly) syndrome. Cancer 10:470–487, 1957.
52. Harper PS, Harper RMJ, Howel-Evans AW: Carcinoma of the esophagus with tylosis. Q J Med 39:317–333, 1970.
53. Howel-Evans W, McConnell RB, Clarke CA, et al: Carcinoma of the esophagus with keratosis palmaris et plantaris (tylosis): A study of two families. Q J Med 27:413–429, 1958.
54. Selby WS, Gallagher ND: Malignancy in a 19-year experience of adult celiac disease. Dig Dis Sci 24:684–688, 1979.
55. Holmes GKT, Stokes PL, Sorahan TM, et al: Coeliac disease, gluten-free diet, and malignancy. Gut 17:612–619, 1976.
56. Kuylenstierna R, Munck-Wikland E: Esophagitis and cancer of the esophagus. Cancer 56:837–839, 1985.
57. Bernal A, del Junco GW: Endoscopic and pathologic features of esophageal lymphoma: A report of four cases in patients with acquired immune deficiency syndrome. Gastrointest Endosc 32:96–99, 1986.
58. Frager DH, Wolf EL, Competiello LS, et al: Squamous cell carcinoma of the esophagus in patients with acquired immunodeficiency syndrome. Gastrointest Radiol 13:358–360, 1988.
59. Chang F, Syrjanen S, Shen Q, et al: Human papillomavirus (HPV) DNA in esophageal precancer lesions and squamous cell carcinomas from China. Int J Cancer 45:21–25, 1990.
60. Williamson AL, Jaskiesicz K, Gunning A: The detection of human papillomavirus in oesophageal lesions. Anticancer Res 11:263–265, 1991.
61. Toh Y, Kuwano H, Tanaka S, et al: Detection of human papillomavirus DNA in esophageal carcinoma in Japan by polymerase chain reaction. Cancer 70:2234–2238, 1992.
62. Chang F, Shen Q, Zhou J, et al: Detection of human papillomavirus DNA in cytologic specimens derived from esophageal precancer lesions and cancer. Scand J Gastroenterol 25:383–388, 1990.
63. Haggitt RC, Tryzelaar J, Ellis FH, et al: Adenocarcinoma complicating columnar epithelium-lined (Barrett's) esophagus. Am J Clin Pathol 70:1–5, 1978.

64. Reyes CV, Wang T: Primary adenocarcinoma of the esophagus: A review of 12 cases. J Surg Oncol 18:153–158, 1981.
65. Naef AP, Savary M, Ozzello L: Columnar-lined esophagus: An acquired lesion with malignant predisposition. Report on 140 cases of Barrett's esophagus with 12 adenocarcinomas. J Thorac Cardiovasc Surg 70:826–835, 1975.
66. Cameron AJ, Ott BJ, Payne WS: The incidence of adenocarcinoma in columnar-lined (Barrett's) esophagus. N Engl J Med 313:857–859, 1985.
67. Streitz JM, Ellis FH, Gibb SP, et al: Adenocarcinoma in Barrett's esophagus. A clinicopathologic study of 65 cases. Ann Surg 213:122–125, 1991.
68. Williamson WA, Ellis FH, Gibb SP, et al: Barrett's esophagus. Prevalence and incidence of adenocarcinoma. Arch Intern Med 151:2212–2216, 1991.
69. Spechler SJ, Robbins AH, Rubins HB, et al: Adenocarcinoma and Barrett's esophagus. An overrated risk? Gastroenterology 87:927–933, 1984.
70. van der Veen AH, Dees J, Blankensteijn JD, et al: Adenocarcinoma in Barrett's oesophagus: An overrated risk. Gut 30:14–18, 1989.
71. Iftikhar SY, James PD, Steele RJC, et al: Length of Barrett's oesophagus: An important factor in the development of dysplasia and adenocarcinoma. Gut 33:1155–1158, 1992.
72. Hameeteman W, Tytgat GNJ, Houthoff HJ, et al: Barrett's esophagus: Development of dysplasia and adenocarcinoma. Gastroenterology 96:1249–1256, 1989.
73. Cameron AJ, Lomboy CT: Barrett's esophagus: Age, prevalence, and extent of columnar epithelium. Gastroenterology 103:1241–1245, 1992.
74. Qualman SJ, Murray RD, McClung HJ, et al: Intestinal metaplasia is age related in Barrett's esophagus. Arch Pathol Lab Med 114:1236–1240, 1990.
75. Paull A, Trier JS, Dalton MD, et al: The histologic spectrum of Barrett's esophagus. N Engl J Med 295:476–480, 1976.
76. Smith RRL, Hamilton SR, Boitnott JK, et al: The spectrum of carcinoma arising in Barrett's esophagus. A clinicopathologic study of 26 patients. Am J Surg Pathol 8:563–573, 1984.
77. Jauregui HO, Davessar K, Hale JH, et al: Mucin histochemistry of intestinal metaplasia in Barrett's esophagus. Mod Pathol 1:188–192, 1988.
78. De Baecque C, Potet F, Molas G, et al: Superficial adenocarcinoma of the oesophagus arising in Barrett's mucosa with dysplasia: A clinico-pathological study of 12 patients. Histopathology 16:213–220, 1990.
79. Hamilton SR, Smith RRL: The relationship between columnar epithelial dysplasia and invasive adenocarcinoma arising in Barrett's esophagus. Am J Clin Pathol 87:301–312, 1987.
80. Hamilton SR, Smith RRL, Cameron JL: Prevalence and characteristics of Barrett esophagus in patients with adenocarcinoma of the esophagus or esophagogastric junction. Hum Pathol 19:942–948, 1988.
81. Gray MR, Hall PA, Nash J, et al: Epithelial proliferation in Barrett's esophagus by proliferating cell nuclear antigen immunolocalization. Gastroenterology 103:1769–1776, 1992.
82. Thompson JJ, Zinsser KR, Enterline HT: Barrett's metaplasia and adenocarcinoma of the esophagus and gastroesophageal junction. Hum Pathol 14:42–61, 1983.
83. Kalish RJ, Clancy PE, Orringer MB, et al: Clinical epidemiologic and morphologic comparison between adenocarcinomas arising in Barrett's esophageal mucosa and in the gastric cardia. Gastroenterology 86:461–467, 1984.
84. Lee RG: Dysplasia in Barrett's esophagus: A clinicopathologic study of six patients. Am J Surg Pathol 9:845–852, 1985.
85. Wang HH, Antonioli DA, Goldman H: Comparative features of esophageal and gastric adenocarcinomas: Recent changes in type and frequency. Hum Pathol 17:482–487, 1986.
86. Rubio CA, Åberg B: Barrett's mucosa in conjunction with squamous carcinoma of the esophagus. Cancer 68:583–586, 1991.
87. Reid BJ, Blount PL, Rubin CE, et al: Flow-cytometric and histological progression to malignancy in Barrett's esophagus: Prospective endoscopic surveillance of a cohort. Gastroenterology 102:1212–1219, 1992.
88. Pera M, Trastek VF, Herschel A: Barrett's esophagus with high-grade dysplasia: An indication for esophagectomy? Ann Thorac Surg 54:199–204, 1992.
89. Altorki NK, Sunagawa M, Little AG, et al: High-grade dysplasia in the columnar-lined esophagus. Am J Surg 161:97–99, 1991.
90. McArdle JE, Lewin KJ, Randall G, et al: Distribution of dysplasias and early invasive carcinoma in Barrett's esophagus. Hum Pathol 23:479–482, 1992.
91. Reid BJ, Haggitt RC, Rubin CE, et al: Observer variation in the diagnosis of dysplasia in Barrett's esophagus. Hum Pathol 19:166–178, 1988.
92. Rosenberg JC, Budev H, Edwards RC, et al: Analysis of adenocarcinoma in Barrett's esophagus utilizing a staging system. Cancer 55:1353–1360, 1985.
93. Haggitt RC, Reid BJ, Rabinovitch PS, et al: Barrett's esophagus. Correlation between mucin histochemistry, flow cytometry, and histologic diagnosis for predicting increased cancer risk. Am J Pathol 131:53–61, 1988.
94. James PD, Atkinson M: Value of DNA image cytometry in the prediction of malignant change in Barrett's oesophagus. Gut 30:899–905, 1989.
95. McKinley MJ, Budman DR, Grueneberg D, et al: DNA content in Barrett's esophagus and esophageal malignancy. Am J Gastroenterol 82:1012–1015, 1987.
96. Garewal HS, Sampliner RE, Fennerty MD: Flow cytometry in Barrett's esophagus. (Editorial.) What have we learned so far? Dig Dis Sci 36:548–551, 1991.
97. Poller DN, Steele RJC, Morrell K: Epidermal growth factor receptor expression in Barrett's esophagus. Arch Pathol Lab Med 116:1226–1227, 1992.
98. Jankowski J, Coghill G, Tregaskis B, et al: Epidermal growth factor in the oesophagus. Gut 33:1448–1453, 1992.
99. Jankowski J, McMenemin R, Hopwood D, et al: Proliferating cell nuclear antigen in oesophageal diseases; correlation with transforming growth factor alpha expression. Gut 33:587–591, 1992.
100. Burke AP, Sobin LH, Shekitka KM, et al: Correlation of nucleolar organizer regions and glandular dysplasia of the stomach and esophagus. Mod Pathol 3:357–360, 1990.
101. Ramel S, Reid BJ, Sanchez CA, et al: Evaluation of p53 protein expression in Barrett's esophagus by two-parameter flow cytometry. Gastroenterology 102:1220–1228, 1992.
102. Abdelatif OMA, Chandler FW, Mills LR, et al: Differential expression of c-myc and H-ras oncogenes in Barrett's epithelium. A study using colorimetric in situ hybridization. Arch Pathol Lab Med 115:880–885, 1991.
103. Garewal HS, Sampliner R, Gerner E, et al: Ornithine decarboxylase activity in Barrett's esophagus: A potential marker for dysplasia. Gastroenterology 94:819–821, 1988.
104. Rosengard AM, Hamilton SR: Squamous carcinoma of the esophagus in patients with Barrett esophagus. Mod Pathol 2:2–7, 1989.
105. Paraf F, Fléjou J-F, Potet F, et al: Esophageal squamous carcinoma in five patients with Barrett's esophagus. Am J Gastroenterol 87:746–750, 1992.
106. Watanabe H, Jass JR, Sobin LH: Histological Typing of Oesophageal and Gastric Tumors. (2nd Ed.) New York, Springer-Verlag, 1990.
107. Ming SC: Tumors of the Esophagus and Stomach. Atlas of Tumor Pathology, fascicle 7, 2nd series. Washington, DC, Armed Forces Institute of Pathology, 1973.
108. Soga J, Tanaka O, Sasaki K, et al: Superficial spreading carcinoma of the esophagus. Cancer 50:1641–1645, 1982.
109. Ide H, Murata Y, Okushima N, et al: Clinicopathological study of the development of early esophageal carcinoma. In Siewert JR, Hölscher AH (eds): Diseases of the Esophagus. New York, Springer-Verlag, 1988, pp 45–51.
110. Rubio CA, Liu F-s, Zhao H-Z: Histological classification of intraepithelial neoplasias and microinvasive squamous carcinoma of the esophagus. Am J Surg Pathol 13:685–690, 1989.
111. Anani PA, Gardiol D, Savary M, et al: An extensive morphological and comparative study of clinically early and obvious squamous cell carcinoma of the esophagus. Pathol Res Pract 187:214–219, 1991.
112. Rubio CA, Auer GU, Kato Y, et al: DNA profiles in dysplasia and carcinoma of the human esophagus. Anal Quant Cytol Histol 10:207–210, 1988.
113. Takiyama W, Moriwaki S, Mandai K, et al: Dysplasia in the

human esophagus: Clinicopathological study on 500 esophagi at autopsy. Jpn J Clin Oncol 22:250–255, 1992.

114. Koga Y, Sugimachi K, Kuwano H, et al: Cytophotometric DNA analysis of esophageal dysplasia and carcinoma induced in rats by N-methyl-N-amylnitrosamine. Eur J Cancer Clin Oncol 24:643–651, 1988.

115. Antonioli DA: Esophagus. *In* Henson DE, Albores-Saavedra J (eds): Pathology of Incipient Neoplasia. (2nd Ed.) Philadelphia, W.B. Saunders, 1993, pp 64–84.

116. Jacob P, Kahrilas PJ, Desai T, et al: Natural history and significance of esophageal squamous cell dysplasia. Cancer 65:2731–2739, 1990.

117. Beahrs OH, Henson DE, Hutter RVP, Kennedy BJ: Manual for Staging of Cancer. (4th Ed.) Philadelphia, J.B. Lippincott, 1992, pp 57–59.

118. Lindholm J, Rubio CA, Kato Y, et al: A morphometric method to discriminate normal from dysplastic carcinoma in situ squamous epithelium in the human esophagus. Pathol Res Pract 184:297–305, 1989.

119. Hurlimann O, Galdiol D: Immunohistochemistry of dysplasias and carcinomas of the esophageal epithelium. Pathol Res Pract 184:567–576, 1989.

120. Mandard AM, Tourneux J, Gignoux M, et al: *In situ* carcinoma of the esophagus: Macroscopic study with particular reference to the Lugol test. Endoscopy 12:51–57, 1980.

121. Hix WR, Wilson WR: Detection of occult carcinoma of the esophagus by toluidine blue staining in high-risk patients. *In* Siewert JR, Hölscher AH (eds): Diseases of the Esophagus. New York, Springer-Verlag, 1988, pp 118–120.

122. Mandard AM, Marnay J, Gignoux M, et al: Cancer of the esophagus and associated lesions: Detailed pathologic study of 100 esophagectomy specimens. Hum Pathol 15:660–669, 1984.

123. Bogomoletz WV, Molas G, Potet F: Superficial squamous cell carcinoma of the esophagus. A report of 76 cases and review of the literature. Am J Surg Pathol 13:535–546, 1989.

124. Ushigome S, Spjut HJ, Noon GP: Extensive dysplasia and carcinoma in situ of esophageal epithelium. Cancer 20:1023–1029, 1967.

125. Sotus PC, Majmudar B, Symbas PN: Carcinoma in situ of the esophagus. JAMA 239:335–336, 1978.

126. Schmidt LW, Dean PJ, Wilson RT: Superficially invasive squamous cell carcinoma of the esophagus. A study of seven cases in Memphis, Tennessee. Gastroenterology 91:1456–1461, 1986.

127. Barge J, Molas G, Maillard JN, et al: Superficial oesophageal carcinoma: An oesophageal counterpart of early gastric cancer. Histopathology 5:499–510, 1981.

128. Benasco C, Combalia N, Pou JM, et al: Superficial esophageal carcinoma: A report of 12 cases. Gastrointest Endosc 31:64–67, 1985.

129. Mandard AM, Chasle J, Marnay J, et al: Autopsy findings in 111 cases of esophageal cancer. Cancer 48:329–335, 1981.

130. Ohta H, Nakazawa S, Segawa K, et al: Distribution of epithelial dysplasia in the cancerous esophagus. Scand J Gastroenterol 21:392–398, 1986.

131. Lu J-B, Wang W-X, Dong W-Z, et al: A prospective study of esophageal cytological atypia in Linxian county. Int J Cancer 41:805–808, 1988.

132. Qiu S, Yang G: Precursor lesions of esophageal cancer in high-risk populations in Henan province, China. Cancer 62:551–557, 1988.

133. Rubio CA, Liu F-S: Spontaneous squamous carcinoma of the esophagus in chickens. Cancer 64:2511–2514, 1989.

134. Rubio CA: Epithelial lesions antedating oesophageal carcinoma. I. Histologic study in mice. Pathol Res Pract 176:269–275, 1983.

135. Sasano H, Miyazaki S, Gooukon Y, et al: Expression of p53 in human esophageal carcinoma: An immunohistochemical study with correlation to proliferating cell nuclear antigen expression. Hum Pathol 23:1238–1243, 1992.

136. Stern Z, Sharon P, Ligumsky M, et al: Glycogenic acanthosis of the esophagus. Am J Gastroenterol 74:261–263, 1980.

137. Winkler B, Capo V, Reumann W, et al: Human papillomavirus infection of the esophagus. A clinicopathologic study with demonstration of papillomavirus antigen by the immunoperoxidase technique. Cancer 55:149–155, 1985.

138. Sons HU, Borchard F: Esophageal cancer. Autopsy findings in 171 cases. Arch Pathol Lab Med 108:983–988, 1984.

139. Froelicher P, Miller G: The European experience with esophageal cancer limited to the mucosa and submucosa. Gastrointest Endosc 32:88–90, 1986.

140. Goseki N, Koike M, Yoshida M: Histopathologic characteristics of early stage esophageal carcinoma. A comparative study with gastric carcinoma. Cancer 69:1088–1093, 1992.

141. Sato T, Sakai Y, Kajita A, et al: Radiographic microstructures of early esophageal carcinoma: Correlation of specimen radiography with pathologic findings and clinical radiography. Gastrointest Radiol 11:12–19, 1986.

142. Kato H, Tachimori Y, Watanabe H, et al: Superficial esophageal carcinoma. Surgical treatment and the results. Cancer 66:2319–2323, 1990.

143. Sugimachi K, Ohno S, Matsuda H, et al: Clinicopathologic study of early stage esophageal carcinoma. Br J Surg 76:759–763, 1989.

144. Liu FS, Li L, Qu SL: Clinical and pathological characteristics of early oesophageal cancer. Clin Oncol 1:539–557, 1982.

145. Sugimachi K, Kitamura K, Matsuda H, et al: Proposed new criteria for early carcinoma of the esophagus. Surg Gynecol Obstet 173:303–308, 1991.

146. Shimazu H, Kobori O, Shoji M, et al: Superficial carcinoma of the esophagus. Gastroenterol Jpn 18:409–416, 1983.

147. Maesawa C, Masuda T, Tamura G, et al: Prognostic assessment of superficial squamous cell carcinoma of the esophagus using karyometric analysis and nucleolar organizer regions. J Surg Oncol 51:164–168, 1992.

148. Ohno S, Mori M, Tsutsui S, et al: Growth patterns and prognosis of submucosal carcinoma of the esophagus. A pathologic study. Cancer 68:335–340, 1991.

149. Burke EL, Sturm J, Williamson D: The diagnosis of microscopic carcinoma of the esophagus. Am J Dig Dis 23:148–151, 1978.

150. Li M, Li P, Li B: Recent progress in research on esophageal cancer in China. Adv Cancer Res 33:173–250, 1980.

151. Tekeste H, Latour F: Squamous cell carcinoma of esophagus presenting as multiple pedunculated polyps. Dig Dis Sci 31:433–437, 1986.

152. Sugimachi K, Ide H, Okamura T, et al: Cytophotometric DNA analysis of mucosal and submucosal carcinoma of the esophagus. Cancer 53:2683–2687, 1984.

153. Inokuchi K, Kuwano H, Sugimachi K, et al: Cytophotometric DNA analysis of superficial and advanced carcinoma of the esophagus. *In* Siewert JR, Hölscher AH (eds): Diseases of the Esophagus. New York, Springer-Verlag, 1988, pp 31–34.

154. Kuwano H, Morita M, Matsuda H, et al: Histopathologic findings of minute foci of squamous cell carcinoma in the human esophagus. Cancer 68:2617–2620, 1991.

155. Guanrei Y, Songliang Q, He H, et al: Natural history of early esophageal squamous carcinoma and early adenocarcinoma of the gastric cardia in the People's Republic of China. Endoscopy 20:95–98, 1988.

156. Iizuka T, Isono K, Kakegawa T, et al: Parameters linked to ten-year survival in Japan of resected esophageal carcinoma. Japanese Committee for Registration of Esophageal Carcinoma Cases. Chest 96:1005–1011, 1989.

157. Ellis FH Jr, Watkins E Jr, Krasna MJ, et al: Staging of carcinoma of the esophagus and cardia: A comparison of different staging criteria. J Surg Oncol 52:231–235, 1993.

158. Earlam R, Cunha-Melo JR: Oesophageal squamous cell carcinoma. I. A critical review of surgery. Br J Surg 67:381–390, 1980.

159. Earlam R, Cunha-Melo JR: Oesophageal squamous cell carcinoma. II. A critical review of radiotherapy. Br J Surg 67:457–461, 1980.

160. Iyomasa S, Kato H, Tachimori Y, et al: Carcinosarcoma of the esophagus: A twenty-case study. Jpn J Clin Oncol 20:99–106, 1990.

161. Yang PC, Davis S: Incidence of cancer of the esophagus in the US by histologic type. Cancer 61:612–617, 1988.

162. Anderson LL, Lad TE: Autopsy findings in squamous-cell carcinoma of the esophagus. Cancer 50:1587–1590, 1982.

163. Robey-Cafferty SS, El-Naggar AK, Sahin AA, et al: Prognostic factors in esophageal squamous carcinoma. A study of histologic features, blood group expression, and DNA ploidy. Am J Clin Pathol 95:844–849, 1991.

164. Sugimachi K, Matsuura H, Kai H, et al: Prognostic factors of esophageal carcinoma: Univariate and multivariate analyses. J Surg Oncol 31:108–112, 1986.

165. Kuwano H, Ohno S, Matsuda H, et al: Serial histologic evaluation of multiple primary squamous cell carcinomas of the esophagus. Cancer 61:1635–1638, 1988.

166. Sasajima K, Takai A, Taniguchi Y, et al: Polypoid squamous cell carcinoma of the esophagus. Cancer 64:94–97, 1989.

167. Kuwano H, Kitamura K, Baba K, et al: Determination of the resection line in early esophageal cancer using intraoperative endoscopic examination with Lugol staining. J Surg Oncol 50:149–152, 1992.

168. Sugimachi K, Tsutsui S, Kitamura K, et al: Lugol stain for intraoperative determination of the proximal surgical margin of the esophagus. J Surg Oncol 46:226–229, 1991.

169. Takubo KT, Takai A, Yamashita K, et al: Light and electron microscopic studies of perineurial invasion by esophageal carcinoma. JNCI 74:987–993, 1985.

170. Darnton SJ, Allen SM, Edwards CW, et al: Histopathological findings in oesophageal carcinoma with and without preoperative chemotherapy. J Clin Pathol 46:51–55, 1993.

171. Matsuura H, Kuwano H, Morita M, et al: Predicting recurrence time of esophageal carcinoma through assessment of histologic factors and DNA ploidy. Cancer 67:1406–1411, 1991.

172. Mori M, Ohno S, Tsutsui S, et al: Esophageal carcinoma in young patients. Ann Thorac Surg 49:284–286, 1990.

173. Patil PK, Patel SG, Mistry RC, et al: Cancer of the esophagus in young adults. J Surg Oncol 50:179–182, 1992.

174. Matsuura H, Sugimachi K, Ueo H, et al: Malignant potentiality of squamous cell carcinoma of the esophagus predictable by DNA analysis. Cancer 57:1810–1814, 1986.

175. Sugimachi K, Koga Y, Mori M, et al: Comparative data on cytophotometric DNA in malignant lesions of the esophagus in the Chinese and Japanese. Cancer 59:1947–1950, 1987.

176. Stephens JK, Bibbo M, Dytch H, et al: Correlation between automated karyometric measurements of squamous cell carcinoma of the esophagus and histopathologic and clinical features. Cancer 64:83–87, 1989.

177. Tsutsui S, Kuwano H, Mori M, et al: A flow cytometric analysis of DNA content in primary and metastatic lesions of esophageal squamous cell carcinoma. Cancer 70:2586–2591, 1992.

178. Kaketani K, Saito T, Kobayashi M: Flow cytometric analysis of nuclear DNA content in esophageal cancer. Aneuploidy as an index for highly malignant potential. Cancer 64:887–891, 1989.

179. Ruol A, Segalin A, Panozzo M, et al: Flow cytometric DNA analysis of squamous cell carcinoma of the esophagus. Cancer 65:1185–1188, 1990.

180. Böttger T, Störkel S, Stöckle M, et al: DNA image cytometry. A prognostic tool in squamous cell carcinoma of the esophagus? Cancer 67:2290–2294, 1991.

181. Sanekata K, Nishihira T, Kasai M: The prognostic value of flow cytometric DNA analysis in human esophageal carcinomas. In Siewert JR, Hölscher AH (eds): Diseases of the Esophagus. New York, Springer-Verlag, 1988, pp 81–84.

182. Sasaki K, Murakami T, Murakami T, et al: Intratumoral heterogeneity in DNA ploidy of esophageal squamous cell carcinomas. Cancer 68:2403–2406, 1991.

183. Matsuda H, Mori M, Tsujitani S, et al: Immunohistochemical evaluation of squamous cell carcinoma antigen and S-100 protein-positive cells in human malignant esophageal tissues. Cancer 65:2261–2265, 1990.

184. Shima I, Sasaguri Y, Kusukawa J, et al: Production of matrix metalloproteinase-2 and metalloproteinase-3 related to malignant behavior of esophageal carcinoma. Cancer 70:2747–2753, 1992.

185. Tsang WYW, Chan JKC, Lee KC, et al: Basaloid-squamous carcinoma of the upper aerodigestive tract and so-called adenoid cystic carcinoma of the oesophagus: The same tumour type? Histopathology 19:35–46, 1991.

186. Takubo K, Mafune K, Tanaka Y, et al: Basaloid-squamous carcinoma of the esophagus with marked deposition of basement membrane substance. Acta Pathol Jpn 41:59–64, 1991.

187. Epstein JI, Sears DL, Tucker RS, et al: Carcinoma of the esophagus with adenoid cystic differentiation. Cancer 53:1131–1136, 1984.

188. Takubo K, Sasajima K, Yamashita K, et al: Morphological heterogeneity of esophageal carcinoma. Acta Pathol Jpn 38:180–189, 1989.

189. Rubio CA, Liu FS: The histogenesis of the microinvasive basal cell carcinoma of the esophagus. Pathol Res Pract 186:223–227, 1990.

190. Osamura RY, Shimamura K, Hata J, et al: Polypoid carcinoma of the esophagus. A unifying term for "carcinosarcoma" and "pseudosarcoma." Am J Surg Pathol 2:201–208, 1978.

191. Kuhajda FP, Sun TT, Mendelsohn G: Polypoid squamous carcinoma of the esophagus. A case report with immunostaining for keratin. Am J Surg Pathol 7:495–499, 1983.

192. Matsusaka T, Watanabe H, Enjoji M: Pseudosarcoma and carcinosarcoma of the esophagus. Cancer 37:1546–1555, 1976.

193. Martin MR, Kahn LB: So-called pseudosarcoma of the esophagus. Nodal metastases of the spindle cell element. Arch Pathol Lab Med 101:604–609, 1977.

194. Xu L, Sun C, Wu LH, et al: Clinical and pathological characteristics of carcinosarcoma of the esophagus: Report of four cases. Ann Thorac Surg 37:197–203, 1984.

195. Turnbull AD, Rosen P, Goodner JT, et al: Primary malignant tumors of the esophagus other than typical epidermoid carcinoma. Ann Thorac Surg 15:463–473, 1973.

196. Gal AA, Martin SE, Kernen JA, et al: Esophageal carcinoma with prominent spindle cells. Cancer 60:2244–2250, 1987.

197. Perch SJ, Soffen EM, Whittington R, et al: Esophageal sarcomas. J Surg Oncol 48:194–198, 1991.

198. Wang Z-Y, Itabashi M, Hirota T, et al: Immunohistochemical study of the histogenesis of esophageal carcinosarcoma. Jpn J Clin Oncol 22:377–386, 1992.

199. Kimura N, Tezuka F, Ono I, et al: Myogenic expression in esophageal polypoid tumors. Arch Pathol Lab Med 113:1159–1165, 1989.

200. Linder J, Stein RB, Roggli VL, et al: Polypoid tumor of the esophagus. Hum Pathol 18:692–700, 1987.

201. Hanada M, Nakano K, Ii Y, et al: Carcinosarcoma of the esophagus with osseous and cartilagenous production: A combined study of keratin immunohistochemistry and electron microscopy. Acta Pathol Jpn 34:669–678, 1984.

202. Ooi A, Kawahara E, Okada Y, et al: Carcinosarcoma of the esophagus. An immunohistochemical and electron micrscopic study. Acta Pathol Jpn 36:151–159, 1986.

203. LiVolsi VA, Perzin KH: Inflammatory pseudotumors (inflammatory fibrous polyps) of the esophagus. A clinicopathologic study. Am J Dig Dis 20:475–481, 1975.

204. Agha FP, Keren DF: Spindle-cell squamous carcinoma of the esophagus. AJR Am J Roentgenol 145:541–545, 1985.

205. Mauro M, Cristina L, Giorgio S, et al: Carcinosarcoma vs. pseudosarcoma. (Letter.) Am J Surg Pathol 9:388, 1985.

206. Du Boulay CEH, Isaacson P: Carcinoma of the oesophagus with spindle cell features. Histopathology 5:403–414, 1981.

207. Nichols T, Yokoo H, Craig RM, et al: Pseudosarcoma of the esophagus. Three new cases and review of the literature. Am J Gastroenterol 72:615–622, 1979.

208. Biemond P, ten Kate FJW, van Blankenstein M: Esophageal verrucous carcinoma: Histologically a low-grade malignancy but clinically a fatal disease. J Clin Gastroenterol 13:102–107, 1991.

209. Agha FP, Weatherbee L, Sams JS: Verrucous carcinoma of the esophagus. Am J Gastroenterol 79:844–849, 1984.

210. Minielly JA, Harrison EG Jr, Fontana RS, et al: Verrucous squamous cell carcinoma of the esophagus. Cancer 20:2078–2087, 1967.

211. Meyerowitz BR, Shea LT: The natural history of squamous verrucose carcinoma of the esophagus. J Thorac Cardiovasc Surg 61:646–649, 1972.

212. Koerfgen HP, Husemann B, Giedl J, et al: Verrucous carcinoma of the esophagus. Endoscopy 20:326–329, 1988.

213. Odze R, Antonioli D, Shocket D, et al: Esophageal squamous papillomas. A clinicopathologic study of 38 lesions and analysis for human papillomavirus by the polymerase chain reaction. Am J Surg Pathol 17:803–812, 1993.

214. Quitadamo M, Benson J: Squamous papilloma of the esophagus: A case report and review of the literature. Am J Gastroenterol 83:194–201, 1988.

215. Waterfall WE, Somers S, Desa DJ: Benign oesophageal papillomatosis. A case report with a review of the literature. J Clin Pathol 33:111–115, 1978.

216. Fekete F, Chazouillères O, Ganthier V, et al: Un cas de papillomatose oesophagienne de l'adulte. Gastroenterol Clin Biol 12:66–70, 1988.

217. Stinson SF: Animal model: Esophageal carcinoma in the rat induced with Methyl-alkyl-nitrosamines. Am J Pathol 96:871–874, 1979.

218. MacDonald WC, MacDonald JB: Adenocarcinoma of the esophagus and/or gastric cardia. Cancer 60:1094–1098, 1987.

219. Raphael HA, Ellis FH Jr, Dockerty MB: Primary adenocarcinoma of the esophagus: 18-year review and review of literature. Ann Surg 164:785–796, 1966.

220. Bosch A, Frias Z, Caldwell WL: Adenocarcinoma of the esophagus. Cancer 43:1557–1561, 1979.

221. Cederqvist C, Nielsen J, Berthelsen A, et al: Adenocarcinoma of the oesophagus. Acta Chir Scand 146:411–415, 1980.

222. Rogers EL, Goldkind SF, Iseri OA, et al: Adenocarcinoma of the lower esophagus. A disease primarily of white men with Barrett's esophagus. J Clin Gastroenterol 8:613–618, 1986.

223. Steiger Z, Wilson RF, Leichman L, et al: Primary adenocarcinoma of the esophagus. J Surg Oncol 36:68–70, 1987.

224. Alpern HD, Buell C, Olson J: Increasing percentage of adenocarcinoma in primary carcinoma of the esophagus. (Letter.) Am J Gastroenterol 84:574, 1989.

225. Gössner W: Pathology of adenocarcinoma of the esophagus and the gastroesophageal junction. *In* Siewert JR, Hölscher AH (eds): Diseases of the Esophagus. New York, Springer-Verlag, 1988, pp 39–44.

226. Pera M, Cameron AJ, Trastek VF, et al: Increasing incidence of adenocarcinoma of the esophagus and esophagogastric junction. Gastroenterology 104:510–513, 1993.

227. Blot WJ, Devesa SS, Kneller RW, et al: Rising incidence of adenocarcinoma of the esophagus and gastric cardia. JAMA 265:1287–1289, 1991.

228. Harvey JC, Kagan AR, Hause D, et al: Adenocarcinoma arising in Barrett's esophagus. J Surg Oncol 45:162–163, 1990.

229. Dawson JL: Adenocarcinoma of the middle oesophagus arising in an oesophagus lined by gastric (parietal) epithelium. Br J Surg 51:940–942, 1964.

230. Carrie A: Adenocarcinoma of upper end of the oesophagus arising from ectopic gastric epithelium. Br J Surg 37:474, 1950.

231. Li H, Walsh TN, Hennessy TPJ: Carcinoma arising in Barrett's esophagus. Surg Gynecol Obstet 175:167–172, 1992.

232. Hassall E, Dimmick JE, Magee JF: Adenocarcinoma in childhood Barrett's esophagus: Case documentation and the need for surveillance in children. Am J Gastroenterol 88:282–288, 1993.

233. Chejfec G, Jablokow VR, Gould VE: Linitis plastica carcinoma of the esophagus. Cancer 51:2139–2143, 1983.

234. Pazdur R, Olencki T, Herman GE: Linitis plastica of the esophagus. Am J Gastroenterol 83:1395–1397, 1988.

235. Nonomura A, Kimura A, Mizukami Y, et al: Paget's disease of the esophagus. J Clin Gastroenterol 16:130–135, 1993.

236. Norihisa Y, Kakudo K, Tsutsumi Y, et al: Paget's extension of esophageal carcinoma. Immunohistochemical and mucin histochemical evidence of Paget's cells in the esophageal mucosa. Acta Pathol Jpn 38:651–658, 1988.

237. Yates DR, Koss LG: Paget's disease of the esophageal epithelium. Arch Pathol 86:447–452, 1968.

238. Sanfey H, Hamilton SE, Smith RRL, et al: Carcinoma arising in Barrett's esophagus. Surg Gynecol Obstet 161:570–574, 1985.

239. Fein R, Kelsen DP, Geller N, et al: Adenocarcinoma of the esophagus and gastroesophageal junction. Prognostic factors and results of therapy. Cancer 56:2512–2518, 1985.

240. Darnton SJ, Antonakopoulos GN, Newman J, et al: Effects of chemotherapy on ultrastructure of oesophageal adenocarcinoma. J Clin Pathol 45:979–983, 1992.

241. Blomjous JGAM, Hop WCJ, Langenhorst BLAM, et al: Adenocarcinoma of the gastric cardia. Recurrence and survival after resection. Cancer 70:569–574, 1992.

242. Mori M, Kitagawa S, Iida M, et al: Early carcinoma of the gastric cardia. A clinicopathologic study of 21 cases. Cancer 59:1758–1766, 1987.

243. Gray JR, Coldman AJ, MacDonald WC: Cigarette and alcohol use in patients with adenocarcinoma of the gastric cardia or lower esophagus. Cancer 69:2227–2231, 1992.

244. Kabuto T, Taniguchi K, Iwanaga T, et al: Primary adenoid cystic carcinoma of the esophagus. Report of a case. Cancer 43:2452–2456, 1979.

245. Sweeney EC, Cooney T: Adenoid cystic carcinoma of the esophagus. A light and electron microscopic study. Cancer 45:1516–1525, 1980.

246. Cerar A, Juteršek A, Vidmar S: Adenoid cystic carcinoma of the esophagus. A clinicopathologic study of three cases. Cancer 67:2159–2164, 1991.

247. Blaauwgeers JLG, Allema JH, Bosma A, et al: Early adenoid cystic carcinoma of the upper oesophagus. Eur J Surg Oncol 16:77–81, 1990.

248. Akamatsu T, Honda T, Nakayama J, et al: Primary adenoid cystic carcinoma. Report of a case and its histochemical characterization. Acta Pathol Jpn 36:1707–1717, 1986.

249. Kim JH, Lee MS, Cho SW, et al: Primary adenoid cystic carcinoma of the esophagus: A case report. Endoscopy 23:38–41, 1991.

250. Kuwano H, Ueo H, Sugimachi K, et al: Glandular or mucus-secreting components in squamous cell carcinoma of the esophagus. Cancer 56:514–518, 1985.

251. Petursson SR: Adenoid cystic carcinoma of the esophagus. Complete response to combination chemotherapy. Cancer 57:1464–1467, 1986.

252. Spiro RH, Huvos AG, Strong EW: Adenoid cystic carcinoma of salivary origin: A clinicopathologic study of 242 cases. Am J Surg 128:512–520, 1974.

253. Bombi JA, Riverola A, Bordas JM, et al: Adenosquamous carcinoma of the esophagus. A case report. Pathol Res Pract 187:514–519, 1991.

254. Karaki Y, Katoh H, Shimazaki K, et al: Histogenesis of adenosquamous carcinoma of the esophagus. *In* Siewert JR, Hölscher AH (eds): Diseases of the Esophagus. New York, Springer-Verlag, 1988, pp 60–63.

255. Sasajima K, Watanabe M, Takubo K, et al: Mucoepidermoid carcinoma of the esophagus: Report of two cases and review of the literature. Endoscopy 22:140–143, 1990.

256. Ozawa S, Ando N, Shinozawa Y, et al: Two cases of resected esophageal mucoepidermoid carcinoma. Jpn J Surg 19:86–92, 1989.

257. McPeak E, Arens WL: Adenoacanthoma of esophagus. Report of one case with consideration of tumor's resemblance to so-called salivary gland tumor. Arch Pathol Lab Med 44:385–390, 1947.

258. Takubo K, Takai A, Yamashita K, et al: Carcinoma with signet ring cells of the esophagus. Acta Pathol Jpn 37:989–995, 1987.

259. Bell-Thomson J, Haggitt RC, Ellis FH Jr: Mucoepidermoid and adenoid cystic carcinomas of the esophagus. J Thorac Cardiovasc Surg 79:438–446, 1980.

260. Woodard BH, Shelburne JD, Vollmer RT, et al: Mucoepidermoid carcinoma of the esophagus: A case report. Hum Pathol 9:352–354, 1978.

261. Majmudar B, Dillard R, Susann PW: Collision carcinoma of the gastric cardia. Hum Pathol 9:471–473, 1978.

262. Dodge OG: Gastro-oesophageal carcinoma of mixed histological type. J Pathol 81:459–471, 1961.

263. Wanke M: Collision tumour of the cardia. Virchows Arch [A] 357:81–86, 1972.

264. McKeown F: Oat-cell carcinoma of the oesophagus. J Pathol 64:889–891, 1952.

265. Beyer KL, Marshall JB, Diaz-Arias AA, et al: Primary small-cell carcinoma of the esophagus. Report of 11 cases and review of the literature. J Clin Gastroenterol 13:135–141, 1991.

266. Reyes CV, Chejfec G, Jao W, et al: Neuroendocrine carcinomas of the esophagus. Ultrastruct Pathol 1:367–376, 1980.

267. Briggs JC, Ibrahim NBN: Oat cell carcinoma of the oesophagus: A clinico-pathological study of 23 cases. Histopathology 7:261–277, 1983.

268. Tennvall J, Johansson L, Albertsson M: Small cell carcinoma of the esophagus: A clinical and immunohistopathologic review. Eur J Surg Oncol 16:109–115, 1990.

269. Isolauri J, Mattila J, Kallioniemi O-P: Primary undifferentiated small cell carcinoma of the esophagus: Clinicopathological and flow cytometric evaluation of eight cases. J Surg Oncol 46:174–177, 1991.

270. Nichols GL, Kelsen DP: Small cell carcinoma of the esophagus.

The Memorial Hospital experience 1970 to 1987. Cancer 64:1531–1533, 1989.

271. Horai T, Kobayashi A, Tateishi R, et al: A cytologic study on small cell carcinoma of the esophagus. Cancer 41:1890–1896, 1978.

272. Rosenthal SN, Lemkin JA: Multiple small cell carcinomas of the esophagus. Cancer 51:1944–1946, 1983.

273. Sarma DP: Oat cell carcinoma of the esophagus. J Surg Oncol 19:145–150, 1982.

274. Imai T, Sannohe Y, Okano H: Oat cell carcinoma (apudoma) of the esophagus. A case report. Cancer 41:358–364, 1978.

275. Mori M, Matsukuma A, Adachi Y, et al: Small cell carcinoma of the esophagus. Cancer 63:564–573, 1989.

276. Tateishi R, Taniguchi K, Horai T, et al: Argyrophil cell carcinoma (apudoma) of the esophagus. A histopathologic entity. Virchows Arch [A] 371:283–294, 1976.

277. Tanoue S, Shimoda T, Suzuki M, et al: Anaplastic carcinoma of the esophagus. Acta Pathol Jpn 33:831–841, 1983.

278. Sato T, Mukai M, Ando N, et al: Small cell carcinoma (non-oat cell type) of the esophagus concomitant with invasive squamous cell carcinoma and carcinoma in situ. A case report. Cancer 57:328–332, 1986.

279. Matsusaka T, Watanabe H, Enjoji M: Anaplastic carcinoma of the esophagus. Report of three cases and their histogenetic consideration. Cancer 37:1352–1358, 1976.

280. Hoda SA, Hajdu SI: Small cell carcinoma of the esophagus. Cytology and immunohistology in four cases. Acta Cytol 36:113–120, 1992.

281. Attar BM, Levendoglu H, Rhee H: Small cell carcinoma of the esophagus. Report of three cases and review of the literature. Dig Dis Sci 35:145–152, 1990.

282. Rivera F, Matilla A, Fernandez-Sanz J, et al: Oat cell carcinoma of the esophagus. Case description and review of the literature. Virchows Arch [A] 391:337–344, 1981.

283. Watson KJR, Shulkes A, Smallwood RA, et al: Watery diarrhea-hypokalemia achlorhydria syndrome and carcinoma of the esophagus. Gastroenterology 88:798–803, 1985.

284. Bosman FT, Louwerens JWK: APUD cells in teratomas. Am J Pathol 104:174–180, 1981.

285. Ho KJ, Herrera GA, Jones JM, et al: Small cell carcinoma of the esophagus: Evidence for a unified histogenesis. Hum Pathol 15:460–468, 1984.

286. Brenner S, Heimlich H, Widman M: Carcinoid of esophagus. NY State J Med 69:1337–1339, 1969.

287. Dutt AK, Kutty MK, Balasegaram M, et al: Carcinoid tumour: A report of 4 cases with unusual sites of origin. Med J Malaysia 23:216–219, 1969.

288. Rankin R, Nirodi NS, Browne MK: Carcinoid tumour of the oesophagus: Report of a case. Scott Med J 25:245–249, 1980.

289. Younghusband JD, Aluwihare APR: Carcinoma of the oesophagus: Factors influencing survival. Br J Surg 57:422–430, 1970.

290. Chong FK, Graham JH, Madoff IM: Mucin-producing carcinoid ("composite tumor") of upper third of esophagus. A variant of carcinoid tumor. Cancer 44:1853–1859, 1979.

291. Imura H, Matsukura S, Yamamoto H, et al: Studies on ectopic ACTH producing tumors. II. Clinical and biochemical features of 30 cases. Cancer 35:1337–1339, 1975.

292. Brodman HR, Pai BN: Malignant carcinoid of the stomach and distal esophagus. Am J Dig Dis 13:677–681, 1968.

293. Chalkiadakis G, Wihlm JM, Morand G, et al: Primary malignant melanoma of the esophagus. Ann Thorac Surg 39:472–475, 1985.

294. Kato H, Watanabe H, Tachimori Y, et al: Primary malignant melanoma of the esophagus: Report of four cases. Jpn J Clin Oncol 21:306–313, 1991.

295. Caldwell CB, Bains MS, Burt M: Unusual malignant neoplasms of the esophagus. Oat cell carcinoma, melanoma, and sarcoma. J Thorac Cardiovasc Surg 101:100–107, 1991.

296. Garfinkle JM, Cahan WG: Primary melanocarcinoma of the esophagus: First histologically proved case. Cancer 5:921–926, 1952.

297. Sabanathan S, Eng J, Pradhan GN: Primary malignant melanoma of the esophagus. Am J Gastroenterol 84:1475–1481, 1989.

298. Taniyama K, Suzuki H, Sakuramachi S, et al: Amelanotic malignant melanoma of the esophagus: Case report and review of the literature. Jpn J Clin Oncol 20:286–295, 1990.

299. Yamashita Y, Hirai T, Mukaida H, et al: Primary malignant melanoma of the esophagus—a case report. Jpn J Surg 19:498–501, 1989.

300. Piccone VA, Klopstock R, LeVeen HH, et al: Primary malignant melanoma of the esophagus associated with melanosis of the entire esophagus. First case report. J Thorac Cardiovasc Surg 59:865–870, 1970.

301. Boulafendis D, Damiani M, Sie E, et al: Primary malignant melanoma of the esophagus in a young adult. Am J Gastroenterol 80:417–420, 1985.

302. Takubo K, Kanda Y, Ishii M, et al: Primary malignant melanoma of the esophagus. Hum Pathol 14:727–730, 1983.

303. Ludwig ME, Shaw R, de Suto-Nagy G: Primary malignant melanoma of the esophagus. Cancer 48:2528–2534, 1981.

304. Aldovini D, Detassis C, Piscioli F: Primary malignant melanoma of the esophagus. Brush cytology and histogenesis. Acta Cytol 27:65–68, 1983.

305. Kreuser ED: Primary malignant melanoma of the esophagus. Virchows Arch [A] 385:49–59, 1979.

306. Frable WJ, Kay S, Schatzki P: Primary malignant melanoma of the esophagus: An electron microscopic study. Am J Clin Pathol 58:659–667, 1972.

307. Guzman RP, Wightman R, Ravinsky E, et al: Primary malignant melanoma of the esophagus with diffuse melanocytic atypia and melanoma in situ. Am J Clin Pathol 92:802–804, 1989.

308. Dougherty MJ, Compton C, Talbert M, et al: Sarcomas of the gastrointestinal tract. Separation into favorable and unfavorable prognosic groups by mitotic count. Ann Surg 214:569–574, 1991.

309. Pélissier E, Bachour A, Angonin R, et al: Léiomyosarcome de l'oesophage. A propos d'un cas avec revue de la littérature. Chirurgie 115:467–475, 1989.

310. Aagaard MT, Kristensen IB, Lund O, et al: Primary malignant non-epithelial tumours of the thoracic oesophagus and cardia in a 25-year surgical material. Scand J Gastroenterol 25:876–882, 1990.

311. Choh JH, Khazei AH, Ihm HJ: Leiomyosarcoma of the esophagus: Report of a case and review of the literature. J Surg Oncol 32:223–226, 1986.

312. Rubin RA, Lichtenstein GR, Morris JB: Acute esophageal obstruction: A unique presentation of a giant intramural esophageal leiomyoma. Am J Gastroenterol 87:1669–1671, 1992.

313. Goodner JT, Miller TR, Watson WL: Sarcoma of the esophagus. AJR Am J Roentgenol 89:132–139, 1963.

314. Goolden AWG: Radiation cancer of the pharynx. Brit Med J 2:1110–1112, 1951.

315. Sápi Z, Papp I, Bodó M: Malignant fibrous histiocytoma of the esophagus. Report of a case with cytologic, immunohistologic and ultrastructural studies. Acta Cytol 36:121–125, 1992.

316. Samsonova VA, Minkovieh LD: Malignant fibrous histiocytoma of the esophagus. Arkh Patol 50:65–67, 1988.

317. Ribelin WE, Bailey WS: Esophageal sarcomas associated with *Spirocerca lupi* infection in the dog. Cancer 11:1241–1246, 1958.

318. McIntyre M, Webb JN, Browning GCP: Osteosarcoma of the esophagus. Hum Pathol 13:680–682, 1982.

319. Yaghmai I, Ghahremani GG: Chondrosarcoma of the esophagus. AJR Am J Roentgenol 126:1175–1177, 1976.

320. Palmer BV, Levene A, Shaw HJ: Synovial sarcoma of the pharynx and oesophagus. J Laryngol Otol 97:1173–1176, 1983.

321. Amr SS, Shihabi NK, Hajj HA: Synovial sarcoma of the esophagus. Am J Otolaryngol 5:266–269, 1984.

322. Bloch MJ, Iozzo RV, Edmunds LH, et al: Polypoid synovial sarcoma of the esophagus. Gastroenterology 92:229–233, 1987.

323. Fisher JH: Hemangiopericytoma: A review of twenty cases. Can Med Assoc J 83:1136–1139, 1960.

324. Burke JS, Ranchod M: Hemangiopericytoma of the esophagus. Hum Pathol 12:96–100, 1981.

325. Guarda LA, Luna MA, Smith JL Jr, et al: Acquired immune deficiency syndrome: Postmortem findings. Am J Clin Pathol 81:549–557, 1984.

326. Welch K, Finkbeiner W, Alpers CE, et al: Autopsy findings in the acquired immune deficiency syndrome. JAMA 252:1152–1159, 1984.

327. Niedt GW, Schinella RA: Acquired immunodeficiency syndrome. Clinicopathologic study of 56 autopsies. Arch Pathol Lab Med 109:727–734, 1985.

328. Amberson JB, DiCarlo EF, Metroka CE, et al: Diagnostic pathology in the acquired immunodeficiency syndrome. Surgical pathology and cytology experience with 67 patients. Arch Pathol Lab Med 109:345–351, 1985.

329. Gelb A, Miller S: AIDS and gastroenterology. Am J Gastroenterol 81:619–622, 1986.

330. Said JW: Pathogenesis of HIV infection. *In* Nash G, Said JW (eds): Pathology of AIDS and HIV Infection. Montreal, Canada, W.B. Saunders, 1992, pp 15–18.

331. Millard PR: AIDS: Histopathological aspects. J Pathol 143:223–239, 1984.

332. Nash G: Epidemiology of HIV infection. *In* Nash G, Said JW (eds): Pathology of AIDS and HIV Infection. Montreal, Canada, W.B. Saunders, 1992, pp 3–7.

333. Francis ND, Parkin JM, Weber J, et al: Kaposi's sarcoma in acquired immune deficiency syndrome (AIDS). J Clin Pathol 39:469–474, 1986.

334. Moskowitz L, Hensley GT, Chan JC, et al: Immediate causes of death in acquired immunodeficiency syndrome. Arch Pathol Lab Med 109:735–738, 1985.

335. Wolfensberger R: Ueber ein Rhabdomyom der Speiserohre. Beitr Pathol Anat 15:490–526, 1894.

336. Stout AP, Lattes R: Tumors of the Esophagus. Atlas of Tumor Pathology, fascicle 20. Washington, DC, Armed Forces Institute of Pathology, 1957.

337. Sumiyoshi A, Sannoe Y, Tanaka K: Rhabdomyosarcoma of the esophagus: A case report with sarcoid-like lesions in its draining lymph nodes and the spleen. Acta Pathol Jpn 22:581–589, 1972.

338. Wobbes T, Rinsma SG, Holla AT, et al: Rhabdomyosarcoma of the esophagus. Arch Chir Neerl 27:69–75, 1975.

339. Vartio T, Nickels J, Hockerstedt K, et al: Rhabdomyosarcoma of the oesophagus. Light and electron microscopic study of a rare tumour. Virchows Arch [A] 386:357–361, 1980.

340. Chetty R, Learmonth GM, Price SK, et al: Primary oesophageal rhabdomyosarcoma. Cytopathology 2:103–108, 1991.

341. Mansour KA, Fritz RC, Jacobs DM, et al: Pedunculated liposarcoma of the esophagus: A first case report. J Thorac Cardiovasc Surg 86:447–450, 1983.

342. Cooper GJ, Boucher NR, Smith JHF, et al: Liposarcoma of the esophagus. Ann Thorac Surg 51:1012–1013, 1991.

343. Baca I, Klempa I, Weber JT: Liposarcoma of the esophagus. Eur J Surg Oncol 17:313–315, 1991.

344. Orlowska J, Pachlewski J, Gugulski A, et al: A conservative approach to granular cell tumors of the esophagus: Four case reports and literature review. Am J Gastroenterol 88:311–315, 1993.

345. Obiditsch-Mayer I, Salzer-Kuntschik M: Malignes, "gekorntzelliges neurom," sogenanntes "myoblastenmyom," des oesophagus. Beitr Pathol Anat 125:357–373, 1961.

346. Ohmori T, Arita N, Uraga N, et al: Malignant granular cell tumor of the esophagus. A case report with light and electron microscopic, histochemical, and immunohistochemical study. Acta Pathol Jpn 37:775–783, 1987.

347. O'Connell DJ, Mahon H, Meester TR: Multicentric tracheobronchial and oesophageal granular cell myoblastoma. Thorax 33:596–602, 1978.

348. Haratake J, Jimi A, Horie A, et al: Malignant mesenchymoma of the esophagus. Acta Pathol Jpn 34:925–933, 1984.

349. Onomura K, Ohno M, Uchino A, et al: CT of malignant mesenchymoma of the esophagus. Gastrointest Radiol 14:202–204, 1989.

350. McKechnie JC, Fechner RE: Choriocarcinoma and adenocarcinoma of the esophagus with gonadotropin secretion. Cancer 27:694–701, 1971.

351. Sasano N, Abe S, Satake O, et al: Choriocarcinoma mimicry of an esophageal carcinoma with urinary gonadotropic activities. Tohoku J Exp Clin Med 100:153–163, 1970.

352. Trillo AA, Accettullo LM, Yeiter TL: Choriocarcinoma of the esophagus: Histologic and cytologic findings. A case report. Acta Cytol 23:69–74, 1979.

353. Herrmann R, Panahon AM, Barcos M, et al: Gastrointestinal involvement in non-Hodgkin's lymphomas. Cancer 46:215–222, 1980.

354. Ehrlich AN, Stalder G, Geller W, et al: Gastrointestinal manifestations of malignant lymphoma. Gastroenterology 54:1115–1121, 1968.

355. Rosenberg SA, Diamond HD, Jaslowitz B, et al: Lymphosarcoma: A review of 1269 cases. Medicine 40:31–84, 1961.

356. Agha FP, Schnitzer B: Esophageal involvement in lymphoma. Am J Gastroenterol 80:412–416, 1985.

357. Kim OD, Cantave I, Schlesinger PK: Esophageal involvement by cutaneous T-cell lymphoma, mycosis fungoides type: Diagnosis by endoscopic biopsy. J Clin Gastroenterol 12:178–182, 1990.

358. Berman MD, Falchuk KR, Trey C, et al: Primary histiocytic lymphoma of the esophagus. Dig Dis Sci 24:883–886, 1979.

359. Matsuura H, Saito R, Nakajima S, et al: Non-Hodgkin's lymphoma of the esophagus. Am J Gastroenterol 80:941–946, 1985.

360. Pearson JM, Borg-Grech A: Primary Ki-1 (CD 30)-positive, large cell, anaplastic lymphoma of the esophagus. Cancer 68:418–421, 1991.

361. Bolondi L, De Giorgio R, Santi V, et al: Primary non-Hodgkin's T-cell lymphoma of the esophagus. A case with peculiar endoscopic ultrasonographic pattern. Dig Dis Sci 35:1426–1430, 1990.

362. Mengoli M, Marchi M, Rota E, et al: Primary non-Hodgkin's lymphoma of the esophagus. Am J Gastroenterol 85:737–741, 1990.

363. Nagrani M, Lavigne BC, Siskind BN, et al: Primary non-Hodgkin's lymphoma of the esophagus. Arch Intern Med 149:193–195, 1989.

364. Williams MR, Chidambaram M, Salama FD, et al: Tracheo-oesophageal fistula due to primary lymphoma of the oesophagus. J R Coll Surg Edinb 29:60–61, 1984.

365. Doki T, Hamada S, Murayama H, et al: Primary malignant lymphoma of the esophagus. Endoscopy 16:189–192, 1984.

366. Weyand CM, Goronzy JJ, Huchzermeyer H: Presentation of an unrecognized lymphoma as esophageal tumor. Endoscopy 18:61–63, 1986.

367. Worgan P, Baldock CR: Lymphosarcoma of the oesophagus. J Laryngol Otol 90:207–210, 1976.

368. Okerbloom JA, Armitage JO, Zetterman R, et al: Esophageal involvement by non-Hodgkin's lymphoma. Am J Med 77:359–361, 1984.

369. Nissan S, Bar-Moar JA, Levy E: Lymphosarcoma of the esophagus: A case report. Cancer 34:1321–1323, 1974.

370. Sheahan DG, West AB: Focal lymphoid hyperplasia (pseudolymphoma) of the esophagus. Am J Surg Pathol 9:141–147, 1985.

371. Gervaz E, Potet F, Mahé R, et al: Focal lymphoid hyperplasia of the oesophagus: Report of a case. Histopathology 21:187–189, 1992.

372. Surks MI, Guttman AB: Esophageal involvement in Hodgkin's disease. Am J Dig Dis 11:814–818, 1966.

373. Chiolero J: Un cas d'un lymphogranulomatose primitive de l'oesophage. Ann Anat Pathol 12:305–310, 1935.

374. Stein HA, Murray D, Warner HA: Primary Hodgkin's disease of the esophagus. Dig Dis Sci 26:457–461, 1981.

375. Morris WT, Pead JL: Myeloma of the oesophagus. J Clin Path 25:537–538, 1972.

376. Ahmed N, Ramos S, Sika J, et al: Primary extramedullary esophageal plasmacytoma. First case report. Cancer 38:943–947, 1976.

377. Zarian LP, Berliner L, Redmond P: Metastatic endometrial carcinoma to the esophagus. Am J Gastroenteriol 78:9–11, 1983.

378. Boccardo F, Merlano M, Canobbio L, et al: Esophageal involvement in breast cancer. Report of 6 cases. Tumori 68:149–153, 1982.

379. Das Gupta T, Brasfield R: Metastatic melanoma: A clinicopathological study. Cancer 17:1323–1339, 1964.

380. Schneider A, Martini N, Burt ME: Malignant melanoma metastatic to the esophagus. Ann Thorac Surg 55:516–517, 1993.

381. Fisher MS: Metastasis to the esophagus. Gastrointest Radiol 1:249–251, 1976.

382. Gore RM, Sparberg M: Metastatic carcinoma of the prostate to the esophagus. Am J Gastroenterol 77:358–359, 1982.

383. Witzel L, Halter F, Gretillat PA, et al: Evaluation of specific value of endoscopic biopsies and brush cytology for malignancies of the oesophagus and stomach. Gut 17:375–377, 1976.

384. Prolla JC, Reilly RW, Kirsner JB, et al: Direct-vision endoscopic cytology and biopsy in the diagnosis of esophageal and gastric tumors: Current experience. Acta Cytol 21:399–402, 1977.

385. Kasugai T, Kobayashi S, Kuno N: Endoscopic cytology of the esophagus, stomach and pancreas. Acta Cytol 22:327–330, 1978.

386. Shu YJ: Cytopathology of the esophagus. An overview of esophageal cytopathology in China. Acta Cytol 27:7–16, 1983.

387. Young JA, Hughes HE, Lee F: Evaluation of endoscopic brush and biopsy touch smear cytology and biopsy histology in the diagnosis of carcinoma of the lower oesophagus and cardia. J Clin Pathol 33:811–814, 1980.

388. Shu Y-J: The Cytopathology of Esophageal Carcinoma. Precancerous Lesions and Early Cancer. New York, Masson Publishing USA, Inc., 1985.

389. Tim LO, Leiman G, Segal I, et al: A suction-abrasive cytology tube for the diagnosis of esophageal carcinoma. Cancer 50:782–784, 1982.

390. Lazarus C, Jaskiewicz K, Sumeruk RA, et al: Brush cytology technique in the detection of oesophageal carcinoma in the asymptomatic, high risk subject; a pilot survey. Cytopathology 3:291–296, 1992.

391. Jaskiewicz K, Venter FS, Marasas WF: Cytopathology of the esophagus in Transkei. J Natl Cancer Inst 79:961–967, 1987.

392. Robey SS, Hamilton SR, Gupta PK, et al: Diagnostic value of cytopathology in Barrett esophagus and associated carcinoma. Am J Clin Pathol 89:493–498, 1988.

393. Geisinger KR, Teot LA, Richter JE: A comparative cytopathologic and histologic study of atypia, dysplasia, and adenocarcinoma in Barrett's esophagus. Cancer 69:8–16, 1992.

394. Wang HH, Doria MI, Purohit-Buch S, et al: Barrett's esophagus. The cytology of dysplasia in comparison to benign and malignant lesions. Acta Cytol 36:60–64, 1992.

395. Selvaggi SM: Polypoid carcinoma of the esophagus on brush cytology. (Letter.) Acta Cytol 36:650–651, 1992.

20 PREMALIGNANT LESIONS OF THE ESOPHAGUS

Meade C. Edmunds and Richard W. McCallum

A premalignant lesion has a strong predisposition to undergo malignant degeneration. This does not guarantee neoplastic transformation; only the potential for such change is there. Until recently, little attention was paid to these premalignant conditions. In the past, emphasis was primarily placed on the treatment of esophageal cancer, with little attention given to etiology. Unfortunately, once esophageal cancer develops, the patient's overall prognosis is often very poor with few treatment options. The primary focus is comfort and not cure.

Those conditions associated with an increased risk of developing esophageal cancer have received some welcome investigation recently. Conditions such as Barrett's esophagus, achalasia, celiac disease, tylosis, and Plummer-Vinson syndrome (Paterson-Kelly syndrome) have acquired international recognition and respect as potential causes of esophageal cancer. Although much insight into the mechanism of disease and the malignant transformation has been gained, many questions remain unanswered. What activates these malignant capabilities? What factors are carcinogenic, and how do we identify them? Is the malignant transformation process reversible, and if so, at what stage do we need to intervene?

This chapter gives an in-depth view of those lesions within the esophagus that are believed to be premalignant conditions to both squamous and adenocarcinoma of the esophagus. Although the overall incidence of squamous cell cancer in the United States is approximately 3 per 100,000 population, its worldwide significance remains without question due to a much higher incidence in such areas as the Far East and Africa. Factors such as achalasia, celiac sprue, caustic ingestion, radiation and thermal injury, infection and chronic esophagitis have all been found to be associated with the development of squamous cell cancer and are discussed in detail in this chapter. Even more interesting is the dramatic rise in the incidence of esophageal adenocarcinoma over the past 10 years, which has resulted in an exponential rise in the investigation and understanding of Barrett's esophagus. Other, less common types of malignant conditions of the esophagus, namely adenoid cystic carcinoma, sar-comas, apudomas, and adenosquamous carcinomas, are not thought to be preceded by a premalignant lesion heralding the development of malignant degeneration and, therefore, are not considered any further.

BARRETT'S ESOPHAGUS

Barrett's esophagus, also called endo-brachy-esophagus, remains the prototype premalignant lesion resulting in esophageal cancer. Over the past couple of decades, its clinical significance has been increasingly recognized and has resulted in much research to clarify its role in chronic reflux esophagitis and, more important, the development of esophageal adenocarcinoma. Barrett's esophagus remains an enigma, and which patients will progress from metaplasia, to dysplasia, and to adenocarcinoma is poorly understood.

In the 1950s, Norman Barrett described a condition in which ulceration and columnar cell–lined epithelium were found distal to inflammatory strictures in patients who were thought to have congenital shortening of the esophagus.[1] Other clinicians also showed columnar cell–lined epithelium in the distal esophagus, and considered it to be due to gastroesophageal reflux disease.[2] Whether this condition represents an acquired or congenital abnormality, it is gaining worldwide importance owing to its association with the development of primary adenocarcinoma of the esophagus, one of the most rapidly growing cancers found today. In adults, this condition is thought to evolve through a direct effect from chronic gastrointestinal reflux, occurring in 10 to 15 per cent of patients with reflux esophagitis and resulting in metaplastic change in the esophageal epithelium.[3] Esophageal reflux in Barrett's esophagus is particularly severe; it affects more proximal parts of the esophagus than in reflux without esophagitis or esophagitis without Barrett's epithelium.

Definition

Much confusion and controversy has been associated with the actual definition of Barrett's esophagus because of the poor mucosal delineation between the stomach and the esophagus and the resulting difficulty in locating where normal gastric columnar mu-

---

cosa becomes pathologic in its location in the esophagus. In his initial report of this condition, Barrett described esophageal ulcers that were present in gastric epithelium and it was initially thought that these resulted from a mediastinal extension of the stomach in a congenitally short esophagus. In the 1960s, it was recognized that these ulcerations were actually in esophageal columnar epithelium, not gastric epithelium, and there was speculation that reflux may be partly responsible for this condition, resulting in the exchange of stratified columnar epithelium for stratified squamous epithelium in the esophagus. At present, it is believed that Barrett's esophagus results primarily from repeated chronic exposure of the esophageal mucosa to gastrointestinal refluxate, occurring in patients with gastroesophageal disease.

By definition, Barrett's esophagus is a condition in which normal esophageal columnar cell–lined stratified squamous mucosa is replaced by columnar mucosa that is normally fixed in the gastric or intestinal regions. Barrett's esophagus is considered to be present if at least 3 cm of the distal tubular esophagus is lined by columnar epithelium or if specialized epithelium can be found in the esophagus. Gastric mucosal epithelial remnants or proximal migration of normal gastric epithelium extending up to 2 cm from the gastroesophageal junction may represent aberrant fetal remnants of columnar epithelium; however, only in those in which specialized columnar epithelium is seen within the esophageal lumen is this thought to be clinically relevant and have a predisposition for malignant degeneration. Furthermore, the abnormal columnar epithelium seen in Barrett's esophagus consists of 1 of 3 cell types. (1) Gastric fundic epithelium resembles mucosa of the fundus of the stomach and contains chief and parietal cells. (2) Junctional-type epithelium resembles epithelium seen in the gastric cardia and contains mucous glands but no chief or parietal cells. (3) Specialized intestinal epithelium is found solely in Barrett's esophagus and is virtually pathognomonic for this condition. Intestinal epithelium has a villous structure that contains mucous glands and goblet cells, and represents the most common type of epithelium seen in Barrett's esophagus, as well as the type most likely to undergo malignant transformation. As previously mentioned, only the latter type of specialized intestinal epithelium is thought to be clinically relevant because of its potential ability to undergo malignant degeneration.

Endoscopically, it is more often difficult to delineate the actual border of the esophagus and the stomach. Common landmarks such as the Z-line, the diaphragmatic esophageal junction, or the lower esophageal sphincter are often poorly portrayed, making this identification even more difficult. Even when these landmarks are seen, marked variations in individual patients make identification of the gastroesophageal junction problematic. A hiatal hernia may further obscure this distinction.[4] Normal persons have been shown to have gastric columnar mucosa within the esophagus and this is considered to represent a condition resulting from embryologic development.[5] It is important to differentiate between the specialized epithelium of Barrett's esophagus and gastric mucosa seen in the hiatal hernia and aberrantly located gastric epithelium because the latter conditions are not thought to be premalignant in nature. Endoscopy shows that these gastric mucosal islands that remain from aberrant or embryologic progression are most commonly located in the proximal esophagus and are seen near the upper esophageal sphincter in 4% of patients.[6] Epithelium consistent with Barrett's epithelium has been found in very short tongues of atypical epithelium.[7]

Etiology

Barrett's esophagus is now considered to be an end result of chronic injury to the esophageal mucosa from gastroesophageal reflux. Norman Barrett, in his original description of Barrett's esophagus, thought that this condition most likely represented a congenital abnormality, whereas others such as Allison and Johnstone considered that Barrett's esophagitis represented the end result of gastroesophageal reflux disease, with subsequent replacement of normal stratified squamous mucosa with columnar epithelium. Although congenital causes cannot be totally excluded, the latter theory is currently most accepted.[3, 8–13]

Both congenital and genetic factors possibly play a role in the development of Barrett's esophagus. In prenatal development, the esophagus is initially lined by columnar epithelium that is subsequently replaced by squamous epithelium beginning in the midesophagus and extending both caudad and cephalad.[14] At birth, the entire esophageal mucosa is lined by stratified squamous epithelium. However, any disruption of this process may result in columnar epithelialization of the esophagus. Other factors, such as the presence of hiatal hernia and concomitant usage of toxic substances such as ethyl alcohol and tobacco, also have been found to be associated with Barrett's esophagus.[4, 9, 15, 16]

Gastroesophageal reflux disease (GERD) has been considered to be the premier etiology in the development of Barrett's esophagus: 10% to 15% of patients with reflux esophagitis develop the condition.[17] Supporting GERD's role in the development of Barrett's esophagus are a study of patients with GERD who have a much higher incidence of Barrett's esophagus compared with patients undergoing endoscopy for other reasons, and a study finding Barrett's esophagus in patients with achalasia who underwent a myotomy and were shown to have postsurgical chronic reflux.[3, 18] Experimentally, GERD's role in the etiology of Barrett's esophagus has been supported by the generation of columnar epithelium in the distal lower esophagus after surgically inducing reflux in dogs.[8] One hypothesis explaining the metaplastic changes occurring in Barrett's esophagus is that the repeated exposure of the esophageal squamous cells to an acidic environment from GERD leads to cellular destruction and replacement of these cells with multipotential, undifferentiated stem cells. As the exposure to acid and other constituents of reflux such as bile acids and pepsin occurs, these undifferentiated cells acquire the cellular characteristics of Barrett's esophagus.[19] Another theory is that the damaged esophagus is re-epithelialized by columnar cells that migrate cephalad from the gastric cardiac mucosa or the esophagogastric junction.

The role of bile salts in the possible development of Barrett's esophagus has been studied, and it has been shown that patients who have undergone gastrectomy with resultant esophagojejunostomy and free bile reflux have developed Barrett's.[20, 22] Bile as a possible etiologic factor has been supported by studies showing that dogs who had undergone cardioplasty with a cholecystogastrostomy to introduce bile reflux had columnar epithelium of the involved mucosa, and it also has been shown that bile and pancreatic enzymes can cause severe esophagitis in experimental animals.[21] In one retrospective analysis study, duodenal gastric reflux or alkaline reflux occurred frequently in patients with Barrett's esophagus, further supporting the possibility of alkaline-induced metaplastic change.[23] Some studies have found a concomitant infection of *Helicobacter pylori* in a significant number of patients with Barrett's esophagus.[24, 25] The presence of *H. pylori* within the columnar epithelium of Barrett's esophagus has resulted in a speculation that this organism may have a causative role in the development of Barrett's esophagus as well as its progression to adenocarcinoma; however, this relationship is not fully understood. Other studies have concluded that there was no association.[26, 27] Duodenal gastric reflux or alkaline reflux has been shown to occur frequently in patients with Barrett's esophagus, supporting the possibility that alkaline effects may also play some role in the metaplastic changes seen in this condition.[23]

Epidemiology

Symptomatic reflux disease is a common problem; on any day, an estimated 7% of the population suffer from it.[28] In symptomatic patients with reflux esophagitis undergoing endoscopy, the risk of developing Barrett's esophagus is between 2% and 15%.[29, 30] The actual prevalence of Barrett's esophagus is unknown because many patients are completely asymptomatic. In fact, there is estimated to be a 20-fold increase in the number of asymptomatic Barrett's esophagus patients in the general population for every case diagnosed by endoscopy.[31] In a study performed at the Mayo Clinic, the prevalence on autopsy was 376 cases per 100,000 population, compared with 22.6 cases per 100,000 population in the clinically diagnosed patients.[31] Men appear to be affected to a greater degree than women, in a ratio of 4:1.[32, 33] This disease occurs almost exclusively in the white population and is rarely seen in blacks.[15] A higher incidence of Barrett's esophagus is seen in elderly people with the average age at the time of diagnosis being 55 years. However, the peak occurrence of Barrett's esophagus occurs in a bimodal age distribution in patients from 0 to 15

years and 40 to 80 years old, with the greatest incidence seen during the latter time period.[9, 34] The increase in Barrett's esophagus during childhood and adolescence suggests a possible genetic predisposition to this condition, as does the finding of a high prevalence of the condition among certain families.[12, 13] However, factors such as tobacco and alcohol abuse in the setting of chronic reflux disease explain the development of Barrett's esophagus in older patients.[4, 9] The mechanisms by which these substances lead to the formation of Barrett's esophagus are unknown, but it may be by enhancing the gastroesophageal reflux or a direct toxic effect on the epithelial surface.[35] Their role in the subsequent development of adenocarcinoma is less clear. Other associations noted in patients with Barrett's esophagus include scleroderma (2%), colon cancer and polyps (4.5%) and previously diagnosed head and neck cancers. The association with colon cancer and polyps has been refuted by some.[36]

Adenocarcinoma of the esophagus resulting from Barrett's esophagus is a cancer that is rapidly increasing in incidence and occurs in an estimated 5% to 10% of patients with Barrett's esophagus.[3, 37, 39, 45] It accounts for 5% to 10% of all esophageal malignancies, and the rate of developing adenocarcinoma is approximately 30 to 40 times greater in patients who have Barrett's esophagus than in the general population.[16, 38] The overall prevalence and incidence data on the development of adenocarcinoma from Barrett's esophagus are difficult to fully quantify and may represent a marked overestimate because many patients with Barrett's esophagus are asymptomatic and do not seek medical attention. The development of adenocarcinoma from Barrett's esophagus most often occurs in the sixth to seventh decade, but a wide spectrum of ages has been reported.[9, 39, 40] Adenocarcinoma shows a male predominance, with a male-to-female ratio of 4:1 to 10:1.[39, 41, 42] Most commonly, adenocarcinoma associated with Barrett's esophagus is located in the distal esophagus but may occur anywhere in the esophagus.[43, 44] The presence of a hiatal hernia and reflux esophagitis strongly correlates with Barrett's metaplasia and subsequent carcinoma development.[9, 41]

Congenital Versus Acquired

To understand the possible role for congenital abnormalities leading to the development of Barrett's esophagus, one must first understand the embryologic development of the esophagus. The esophagus consists of a foregut derivative and in initial stages of development it is covered with stratified columnar epithelium. As development progresses, the columnar epithelium is replaced with stratified squamous epithelium by the 18th or 20th week of fetal development.[46] Even after this development, nearly 8% of cases have remaining gastric mucosa in the esophagus. The greatest amount is seen in the proximal esophagus, with less in the distal esophagus.[47] These remnants of gastric mucosa left in the esophagus are not thought to be associated with the development of Barrett's esophagus.[48]

Genetic factors are thought to play a possible role in the development of Barrett's esophagus. Numerous studies have emphasized a possible inheritable trait leading to its development.[49, 50] What is not clear at this point is whether this inherited trait is specific for Barrett's or whether it represents a propensity to have reflux disease that subsequently may lead to Barrett's formation. This inheritable nature of Barrett's esophagus is unclear, because there are few cases of Barrett's esophagus in neonates, and those that do have Barrett's at a young age have long-standing documented reflux.[51]

Current belief is that genetic predisposition to Barrett's esophagus plays less of a role in esophageal metaplastic change than does the effect of mucosal damage from chronic reflux disease. Most current opinion about Barrett's esophagus is that it is an acquired condition from long-standing GERD. This theory is supported by the fact that it usually occurs in people over 40 years old and in patients who have factors that enhance chronic reflux, such as decreased lower esophageal sphincter (LES) tone, hiatal hernia, and prior surgery, and by the fact that one may see regression of the condition after reflux is terminated either medically or surgically.[52] What predisposes one to the formation of Barrett's esophagus from reflux is not completely understood. Patients with Barrett's esophagus have lower LES pressures and more prolonged acid exposure.[53, 54] However, there is much overlap between the patients with reflux and those that develop Barrett's esophagus, so pH monitoring or manometry studies have found little usefulness in the diagnostic work-up. Gastric emptying rates are similar in patients with Barrett's esophagus and uncomplicated esophagitis patients. The esophageal segment involved in Barrett's esophagus has been found to have abnormal motility when compared with other noninvolved areas of the esophagus. Studies of the refluxate in Barrett's esophagus patients have shown no difference in acid or pepsin concentrations.[55] Often, patients show little regression of their Barrett's esophagus with marked acid suppression, suggesting that a nonacidic source is the possible cause. Studies looking at refluxate constituents in Barrett's esophagus patients have shown that higher postprandial gastric bile acid concentrations and increased esophageal alkaline exposures are present in patients with complications of Barrett's esophagus such as strictures and ulcerations compared with those Barrett's esophagus patients without complications.[56, 57] Trypsin, a pancreatic enzyme, has also been found to cause esophagitis, but its role in the formation of Barrett's esophagus is not well understood.[58] Case reports of esophageal trauma sustained from lye ingestion and chemotherapy associated with Barrett's esophagus have been published; however, the association between these problems and the development of Barrett's esophagus has not been substantiated in subsequent reports.[59, 60]

Clinical Presentation

As a rule, Barrett's esophagus alone does not cause symptoms. Most patients usually present with symptoms of reflux disease. These symptoms may be present for many years and may include heartburn (pyrosis), regurgitation, chest pain, dysphagia, respiratory complaints such as nighttime wheezing or hoarseness, or hematemesis. Heartburn is the most commonly seen symptom in Barrett's esophagus; however, its presentation is variable because Barrett's epithelium is thought to be less sensitive to acidic reflux. Therefore, patients with chronic reflux disease and long-standing pyrosis may develop a false sense of well-being after Barrett's esophagus develops in the setting of chronic reflux, even though esophageal disease continues to progress. Barrett's esophagus may also present in association with complications of reflux disease, including esophageal ulcers, stricture, bleeding, iron deficiency anemia, dysphagia, or adenocarcinoma.

Because of its often asymptomatic presentation, the diagnosis of Barrett's esophagus is usually made on endoscopic examination or at autopsy. Many patients with Barrett's esophagus remain completely asymptomatic because the columnar epithelium lining the metaplastic esophagus is thought to be less sensitive to acidic reflux. When the diagnosis of Barrett's esophagus is made, symptoms of reflux have usually been present for 6 to 8 years on average.[61] Weight loss and dysphagia are infrequent in uncomplicated Barrett's esophagus but may occur with stricture formation or the development of adenocarcinoma.

Once adenocarcinoma develops from Barrett's esophagus, the presenting symptoms depend on the size of the lesion. Dysphagia is the most common symptom and occurs later in the course, usually after at least 50% to 60% of the esophageal lumen is obliterated. Up to a third of patients with adenocarcinoma of the esophagus have no symptoms of GERD, although a long-standing history of heartburn is seen in two-thirds to three-quarters of patients with adenocarcinoma. Once adenocarcinoma develops, other symptoms, including malaise, fatigue, anemia, weight loss, or odynophagia occur. More than 50% of adenocarcinoma tumors are located in the distal one-third of the esophagus and the remainder in the middle third.[63] At the time of presentation and surgery, penetration of the tumor through the wall of the esophagus occurs in 70% of patients, and nodal involvement is present in approximately two-thirds. Previous studies have shown that tumor invasion and lymph node involvement are the most significant predictors of long-term survival in patients with Barrett's adenocarcinoma.[64]

Complications

There are five major complications in patients with Barrett's esophagus. Esophagitis, ulcerations, hemorrhages, and strictures are commonly benign complications associated with Barrett's esophagus. Adenocarcinoma, as previously mentioned, occurs in 5% to 10% of patients with Barrett's esophagus and in the majority of cases will be seen on the index endoscopy. At diagnosis, approximately 50% to 75% of patients present with one or more of these complications.[65, 66] Esophagitis may involve both columnar or squamous mucosa and may be superficial, deep, or erosive. Barrett's esophagus is frequently seen with ulcerated lesions in the esophagus. Clinically, Barrett's ulcers may be responsible for severe retrosternal pain with radiation to the back, odynophagia, or may represent a source of upper gastrointestinal bleeding. Dysphagia may occur from resultant scarring and contraction of the tissue surrounding the ulcer. Less commonly, one sees esophageal perforation or fistulization into adjacent structures. Esophageal ulcers occur less commonly than strictures, but they are serious conditions as a result of their associated complications such as bleeding and perforation.

There are two primary types of ulcer in Barrett's esophagus. Most common is a superficial linear ulcer on the squamous side of the squamous columnar junction, similar to ulcers in uncomplicated reflux disease. The second type is a deep, wide-mouthed circular ulcer lying on the columnar epithelium. It is similar in appearance to gastric ulcers; however, the mechanism by which these larger ulcers occur is unknown. One theory involves heterotopic epithelial secretion of acid and pepsin with subsequent formation of erosions of islands of squamous epithelium within the metaplastic columnar mucosa. The significance of H. pylori coinfection in patients with Barrett's esophagus is unknown. Its known stimulation of increased acid production of gastric mucosa may predispose the columnar epithelium or squamous epithelium within the columnar epithelium to ulcer formation. It has also been suggested that the metaplastic columnar epithelium in Barrett's esophagus is less resistant to acidic reflux.[67, 68]

Esophageal ulcers, especially with Barrett's esophagus, are unlike superficial ulcers seen in chronic reflux in that they appear to be more aggressive and have a higher propensity to bleed and perforate. They may penetrate the pericardium, pulmonary veins, pleural surfaces, and mediastinum.[69] The majority heal with medical management, which primarily consists of H_2-blockers, but in refractive cases, long-term and high dosages of omeprazole may be needed.[70] Healing rates of 85% have been reported with medical management.[71] Perforation, uncontrolled hemorrhage, and malignant degeneration of a Barrett's ulcer are indications for urgent surgical intervention. Surgical intervention should also be considered if the ulcer has not healed after 4 to 6 months of medical therapy. Patients should be considered for an antireflux operation to treat refractive cases of Barrett's ulceration. Resection of the involved mucosa should be considered when transmural penetration of the ulcer occurs. These ulcers are seen in both acid and alkaline reflux states. Studies of Barrett's ulcer formation have shown that in patients with complicated Barrett's esophagus including ulcers, strictures, and adenocarcinoma, there is a higher instance of alkaline reflux without an increase in acid exposure when compared with patients with Barrett's esophagus with no complications.[65]

Strictures have been found in approximately 25% to 84% of patients with Barrett's esophagus.[72–74] They are most commonly seen at the squamocolumnar junction rather than the esophageal gastric junction, as seen in reflux patients without Barrett's esophagus. A small percentage of Barrett's patients may develop a stricture in the middle of the columnar cell–lined esophagus or at its lower end due to the healing of ulcers with scar tissue. Once diagnosed, strictures should be routinely brushed for cytologic analysis to rule out concomitant adenocarcinoma. Rapid development of dysphagia and weight loss may mark the development of adenocarcinoma formation or strictures. If symptomatic relief is not obtained through dilation therapy, then surgical intervention will need to be considered.[75]

Hemorrhage is another complication seen in Barrett's esophagus and is often associated with the development of an esophageal ulcer.[61] Occult bleeding is frequent, and one-third of all patients with Barrett's esophagus have iron deficiency anemia. Gross bleeding may occur but is infrequent.

Dysplastic changes occur in 10% to 15% of patients with Barrett's esophagus and are thought to represent a premalignant condition, because numerous studies have outlined a metaplasia-dysplasia-carcinoma sequence, whereby Barrett's esophagus progresses to adenocarcinoma. Much less frequently, adenocarcinoma progresses from adenoma, which subsequently undergoes malignant transformation. Studies of the length of Barrett's esophagus in association with the formation of dysplasia and possible adenocarcinoma have suggested that dysplasia occurs only in longer segments of Barrett's esophagus; however, this idea has been highly debated.[76] Currently, dysplasia grading is borrowed from guidelines based on the outline by the inflammatory bowel disease study group.[77] Low-grade dysplasia is characterized by nuclei being located on the upper segments of the cell and is mostly associated with malignant degeneration. It is often difficult to differentiate low-grade dysplasia from inflammatory changes or high-grade dysplasia from carcinoma in situ. Many investigators believe that esophagectomy is warranted if high-grade dysplasia is found because of the frequency of high-grade dysplasia subsequently progressing to adenocarcinoma and the fact that many cases of resected high-grade dysplasia contain adenocarcinoma at the time of autopsy.[79, 80] The present goal in the management of dysplastic Barrett's esophagus is to resect all columnar esophageal tissue.

Adenocarcinoma remains the most clinically important complication of Barrett's esophagus. Barrett's esophagus may increase the patient's risk of adenocarcinoma 30 to 125 times that of the general population.[4, 16, 81] Factors leading to the progression of adenocarcinoma from dysplasia have not yet been identified. Tobacco and alcohol, which are thought to play a major role in the development of esophageal squamous cell cancer, are less conclusively shown to be a risk factor in the development of adenocarcinoma.[82] Once adenocarcinoma develops, surgical therapy is mandatory for acceptable surgical candidates.

The prognosis for patients with esophageal adenocarcinoma is very poor, with an overall 5-year survival rate of only 7%.[29, 38, 42]

Diagnosis

Radiologic evaluation of Barrett's esophagus is of limited usefulness. Its main utility is in detecting complications of Barrett's esophagus, such as strictures, ulcers, and adenocarcinoma; however, in uncomplicated cases Barrett's esophagus cannot be effectively assessed (Fig. 20–1). In one study, the sensitivity of contrast radiography in diagnosing Barrett's esophagus was only 24% with an overall specificity of 95%, suggesting that when radiographic features of Barrett's esophagus are found, the diagnosis is usually present.[17] Radiographically, the typical appearance of Barrett's esophagus is that of a hiatal hernia with the gastroesophageal junction lying above the hiatus. Hiatal hernia represents the most common radiographic abnormality associated with Barrett's esophagus, occurring in up to 90% of patients.[19] Radiographic evaluations of patients with Barrett's esophagus showed a somewhat characteristic entity of a high esophageal stricture with or without a solitary deep esophageal ulcer associated with a hiatal hernia and gastroesophageal reflux. Most lesions in Barrett's esophagus are located in the distal esophagus, with the mucosa ranging from normal to grossly abnormal. Radiographically, esophagitis in Barrett's esophagus presents as mucosal irregularity, nodularity, and thickening in 75% of patients. This process may be focal or diffuse. A reticular pattern in the columnar mucosa, occurring in up to 30% of patients with Barrett's esophagus, has not been found to be associated with any evidence of dysplasia nor has it been found to be specific for the diagnosis of Barrett's esophagus, because it is seen in other conditions such as glycogenic acanthosis and leukoplakia.[17] One may see discrete islands of squamous epithelium interspersed on the columnar epithelium, giving the radiographic appearance of pseudoulcerations. Radiographically, strictures most commonly occur at the squamocolumnar junction. The majority of strictures occur in the distal esophagus and are frequently associated with ulceration. At present, it is very difficult radiographically to distinguish benign from malignant strictures. The length of strictures is variable, ranging from a small ring to a long stricture, with progressive ascending strictures occurring with proximal migration of Barrett's esophagus.

Manometry and pH studies have shown some very interesting results in patients with Barrett's esophagus; however, their clinical usefulness in this condition is limited. All individuals have some element of reflux, but Patel and colleagues noted that in patients with Barrett's esophagus, the degree of reflux was higher when compared with controls having noncomplicated gastroesophageal reflux disease.[83] Esophageal motility studies have shown motor abnormalities in that portion of the esophagus affected by Barrett's esophagus. Failed peristalsis, tertiary contractions, and even aperistalsis have been seen, although normal peristaltic function is seen in segments of the esophagus not involved by Barrett's esophagus. Manometric studies have shown a decreased mean amplitude of contraction, particularly in the distal half of the esophagus and an increased frequency of nonpropulsive contractions of amplitudes less than 30 mm Hg. LES pressure is equally affected in patients with Barrett's esophagus. LES pressure in patients with Barrett's esophagus has been shown to be low, although some patients without associated peptic esophagitis may have normal LES pressures.[30] Stein and colleagues[84] have shown that the LES resting pressure, the overall length, and the abdominal length of the LES were markedly decreased in patients with Barrett's esophagus when compared with those of volunteers or patients with esophagitis. Gastric emptying is delayed in patients with esophagitis and Barrett's esophagus, but there is no difference between these two groups.[87] Together this increase in reflux and decrease in clearance of acid result in prolonged esophageal exposure time.

Esophageal pH monitoring has shown that in Barrett's esophagus patients, there is a change in the nature and amount of esophageal refluxate compared with patients with esophagitis. Twenty-four-hour pH monitoring of Barrett's patients reveals that exposure time of the esophageal mucosa to the acid constituents of the reflux is prolonged because the episodes occur frequently and last longer, and that clearance mechanisms are less effective.[85] Gastric hypersecretory states have also been associated in 40% of patients with Barrett's esophagus, and an increased acid response to gastrin stimulation has been shown.[65, 86]

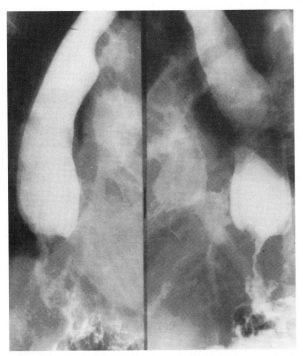

FIGURE 20–1. Barium swallow showing adenocarcinoma arising in Barrett's esophagus with extensive invasion of the mucosa with ulceration.

Also important is the fact that Barrett's esophagus has been shown to have prolonged exposure to alkaline reflux. In Barrett's esophagus, the amount of alkaline exposure is considered to be in the 95% percentile, particularly in those patients with complications like strictures, dysplasia, or ulcer formation.[65] Studies have shown that alkaline duodenal gastric reflux modifies the content and injurious effect of reflux gastric juice in the distal esophagus and may promote the development of adenocarcinoma.[57]

This increased frequency in both acidic and alkaline reflux episodes, the compromised esophageal appearance, gastric hypersecretion, and decreased LES tone all combine to give an increased esophageal exposure time to damaging and potentially carcinogenic substances. The resultant inflammation often leads to fibrosis, and once fibrosis is established, further decrease in motility is seen, allowing for the propagation of a vicious circle. Fibrosis may also lead to an insensitivity of the esophagus to further reflux, therefore making a false impression of clinical improvement. The fact that alkaline reflux can lead to complications in Barrett's esophagus indicates that the composition of the refluxate is also important in the pathogenesis of Barrett's esophagus.

Endoscopy remains the test of choice in diagnosing Barrett's esophagus. Histologic confirmation of the esophageal columnar mucosa is essential. Normally, the mucosa of Barrett's esophagus appears as a velvety salmon-pink color of columnar mucosa extending at least 3 cm up from the LES. The Z-line, or ora serrata, is placed proximally and elevates the junction between stratified squamous and metaplastic columnar epithelium. However, endoscopically perceived distinctions between Barrett's mucosa and normal gastric mucosa are often poorly delineated. Barrett's mucosa may present as detached islands, circumferential or finger-like projections protruding proximally. In cases of severe esophagitis and in children, it may be difficult to distinguish Barrett's epithelium from inflamed squamous epithelium.[88] It is thought that persons with the circumferential type of Barrett's esophagus may be more prone to stricture formation.[30] Barrett's mucosa is often congested, erythematous, and friable, with enlarged edematous folds, linear erosions, and necrotic pseudomembranes.[89] Twenty per cent of patients with Barrett's esophagus have endoscopic evidence of esophagitis, and 10% of columnar epithelium cases are missed by endoscopy.[90] Endoscopic visualization alone is not sufficient to make the diagnosis; only 34% of all histologically proved cases were discovered by endoscopy.[34]

To delineate Barrett's mucosa from normal esophageal squamous mucosa, certain methods can be implemented. Toluidine blue and Lugol's solution have been used to help differentiate Barrett's from normal squamous epithelium. These dyes are injected through the biopsy channel of the endoscope and stain columnar epithelium dark blue or black, leaving squamous mucosa unstained. Manometry and potential difference studies may be employed to localize the LES, but clinically these remain impractical.[91] Even with these techniques endoscopic differentiation between Barrett's and squamous epithelium is said to have a sensitivity of 89% and a specificity of 93%, with an overall accuracy of 91%; therefore, histologic diagnosis remains the gold standard.[92] One can see the extension of columnar gastric mucosa approximately 2 to 3 cm from the GE junction in normal patients, and when the GE junction is seen, it may be irregular, mimicking Barrett's esophagus.[93] The findings of gastric or fundic epithelium are not specific for the diagnosis of Barrett's esophagus. The presence of intestinal metaplasia or specialized metaplasia with accompanying goblet cells is absolutely necessary to make the diagnosis of Barrett's esophagus. Some authors believe that it remains noteworthy to make the diagnosis of both gastric and junctional-type epithelium because case reports have suggested a malignant potential in these tissue types. However, current belief is that adenocarcinoma developing from Barrett's esophagus occurs almost exclusively in the specialized intestinal epithelial type.

As mentioned, up to 90% of patients with Barrett's esophagus have a hiatal hernia.[90, 94] This often interferes with the delineation between the columnar and squamous epithelium. Hiatal hernias are lined by columnar epithelium, and it is very important not to obtain biopsies from the hiatal hernia sac for evaluation of Barrett's esophagus. The hiatal hernia is usually composed of fundic-type mucosa, whereas Barrett's mucosa usually consists of special metaplastic epithelium and is characterized by the presence of goblet cells. In equivocal cases, esophageal manometry often provides useful information by identifying the LES and correlating this with endoscopic findings. Manometry-guided suction biopsies are useful in the diagnosis of Barrett's esophagus because they ensure that tissue is being obtained above the LES through manometrically defined locations and not from the stomach. This method should be considered as a useful adjunctive method in diagnosing short tongues of Barrett's esophagus. These short tongues are also of great importance due to their possible malignant degeneration.[7] When junctional or gastric mucosa epithelium is found in these short tongues of aberrant mucosa, the diagnosis is not specific for Barrett's esophagus, but the finding of intestinal epithelium *is* considered to be diagnostic.[94]

If ulcers or strictures are encountered during endoscopy, then both biopsy and cytology should be performed because they are complementary diagnostic procedures and achieve almost a 100% sensitivity and specificity in the overall differentiation of benign and malignant cases.[88] The use of endoscopic brushings and biopsies increase the diagnostic yield for both dysplasia and adenocarcinoma; cytology has a sensitivity of 90% and a specificity of 80%.[95, 96] In studies reviewing the role of cytologic brushings in assessing Barrett's patients for adenocarcinoma and dysplasia, the overall diagnostic agreement between endoscopic biopsies and cytologic evaluation was 72%.[97] In a review of 65 specimens from 42 patients with known Barrett's esophagus, cytologic evaluation showed a higher grade lesion than that shown on histologic evaluation by biopsy, and in two cases, malignancy was seen only by cytology.[97] The rationale behind the increased diagnostic yield of cytologic evaluation is that a greater surface area of mucosa may be evaluated with less chance of missing small foci of dysplasia and adenocarcinoma. It should be emphasized that adenocarcinoma complicating Barrett's esophagus will most often be seen on the index endoscopy and it is believed that progression of low-grade dysplasia to high-grade dysplasia is not that common. Surveillance is still mandatory owing to the random sampling errors seen with esophageal biopsy and the difficulty in differentiating histologic grades.

Cancer and Surveillance

The incidence of cancer and the need for surveillance in patients with Barrett's esophagus has caused much debate.[15, 32, 98, 99] Many studies have shown a strong association between Barrett's esophagus and the development of adenocarcinoma. Adenocarcinoma in Barrett's esophagus accounts for 5% to 10% of all esophageal malignancies. The actual incidence and prevalence of adenocarcinoma in Barrett's esophagus is unknown due partly to the limited number of prospective studies, the limited number of patients studied, and the difficulty in delineating Barrett's adenocarcinoma from cancer arising in the gastric cardia as well as high-grade dysplasia. Spechler and colleagues were among the first to study the incidence and prevalence of adenocarcinoma and Barrett's esophagus.[16] Of 115 Barrett's patients, development of adenocarcinoma over an average of 3.3 years was one case per 175 person years.[81] Studies performed at the Mayo Clinic showed an incidence of one case per 441 years when 104 patients with Barrett's esophagus were followed for a period of up to 8.5 years. In a study performed by the American College of Gastroenterology, 220 patients were followed for a mean period of 4.1 years (902 person years) and were found to have an incidence of esophageal adenocarcinoma from Barrett's of one case per 150 person years.[78] In the 1970s and 1980s, adenocarcinoma arising from Barrett's esophagus had a more rapid rise in overall incidence compared with any other cancer in the United States. Larger prospective studies over many years are needed to find the incidence of adenocarcinoma transformation. It is also difficult to estimate the incidence in formation of adenocarcinoma due to the similarity of lower esophageal cancer to gastric cancer. Hamilton and Smith[101] showed Barrett's adenocarcinoma occurring near the GE junction beginning in short segments of Barrett's esophagus that were overgrown by tumor.[101] When compared with gastric cancer, Barrett's adenocarcinoma has been found to have many similarities, making the distinction even more difficult. Both tumor types occur predominantly in white men of the sixth and seventh decades with a long-standing history of smoking and reflux. Histologically they appear similar, although Barrett's adenocarcinoma patients do have a more frequent occurrence of dysplasia.[102, 103] The prevalence of Barrett's adenocarcinoma is said to vary between 7% and 46%[104, 105] although this is thought to be overestimated due to some patients being asymptomatic.[100] The risk of developing esophageal cancer is approximately 30 to 125 times above that of the general population.[81, 92, 106] Barrett's adenocarcinoma remains a disease of white men usually more than 50 years old, with half of patients having little symptomatic disease. The male-to-female ratio in adenocarcinoma is 6 to 10:1, which is higher than that seen in Barrett's esophagus.[32, 38, 62, 63, 81] The role of tobacco and alcohol usage in the formation of adenocarcinoma is thought to be less than in squamous cell esophageal cancer.[82] The extent of Barrett's esophagus does not seem to correlate with the development of malignancy, because malignant transformation occurs with equal frequency in limited and extensive Barrett's epithelium. Regression of Barrett's esophagus by either surgical or medical means is not thought to alter the subsequent risk of adenocarcinoma formation.

Surveillance is not thought to affect the overall mortality from cancer in Barrett's esophagus, but routine surveillance is thought to affect the overall survival. Streitz and colleagues[80] found that patients undergoing surveillance were able to be resected at an early stage of malignancy and also had an improved 5-year survival—62% for those undergoing surveillance and 20% for those with no surveillance. Studies of high-risk individuals in China have shown that through cytologic and endoscopic evaluation, patients with early stages of cancer and varying degrees of dysplasia may be detected. This allows identification of cancer at earlier stages prior to metastatic spread, as well as dysplastic changes that are thought by natural history to progress to malignant transformation. Reliable diagnostic markers of high-grade dysplasia and adenocarcinoma are not yet available, thus making endoscopic tissue sampling mandatory to detect early malignancy.

The World Congress of Gastroenterology suggested the following guidelines for surveillance in Barrett's esophagus: (1) Evaluation of newly diagnosed cases with close sampling on first diagnosis, with second opinion by an expert if high-grade dysplasia or adenocarcinoma is present. (2) If high-grade dysplasia or adenocarcinoma is seen, the patient should undergo resection as medically suitable. Six-month sampling is recommended for those not suitable for resection. (3) In patients with low-grade dysplasia, biopsies should be repeated after 12 weeks of aggressive medical therapy. (4) If no histologic evidence of dysplasia is present, repeat surveillance should be performed every 18 months to 2 years.[107] The rationale behind the increased diagnostic yield of cytologic evaluation is that a greater surface area of mucosa may be evaluated with less chance of missing small foci of dysplasia and adenocarcinoma.

Dysplasia, considered part of the natural progression of Barrett's epithelium, is thought to be a precancerous condition. The cellular dysplasia, which is characterized by changes in the cell's cytoplasmic and nuclear content as well as loss of autonomic regulatory function, occurs in all cellular types but is most commonly seen in specialized epithelium. It is thought to evolve through a sequence of metaplasia to low-grade dysplasia, then high-grade dysplasia, and finally to adenocarcinoma.[101, 108] Schmidt[108] and colleagues compared 23 patients with Barrett's esophagus and adenocarcinoma with 38 patients with benign Barrett's esophagus. They found dysplasia in 18 of the former, with dysplasia usually localized next to the invasive tumor, and in two of the benign cases.

Rabinovich and colleagues found multiple aneuploidal populations in these dysplastic areas, suggesting that malignancy in Barrett's esophagus is associated with genetic instability.[109] Cytometric flow studies used to assess neoplastic transformation detect aberrancies in DNA (aneuploidy). The prevalence of aneuploidy has been shown to correlate with increasing risk of malignancy.[110] Studies of cellular differentiation have shown that the risk of cancer is associated with increased S-phase functions as well as an increase in G_2 tetraploid fractions.[110]

Low-grade dysplasia is hard to differentiate from inflammation in regenerative epithelium and should be reconfirmed before aggressive therapy is undertaken. Numerous studies of subsequent progression show a high transformation rate from severe dysplasia to the development of adenocarcinoma. Unfortunately, there is no clear time period as to when this progression may occur. Nor are there any endoscopic criteria that suggest this ultimate transformation, because high-grade dysplasia has been reported to occur in endoscopically normal areas, with a high incidence of adenocarcinoma developing in these areas.[101] It may develop shortly after dysplastic changes, or it may remain without significant change for years. Hameeteman and colleagues prospectively studied 50 patients with known Barrett's esophagus without adenocarcinoma for a period of 1.5 to 14 years.[106] Over this time period, they found progression and dysplasia occurring primarily in the specialized columnar and intermediate types of epithelium, and the development of adenocarcinoma from these categories as well.[106]

In a series of patients who had esophagectomy because of high-grade dysplasia, most were found to have invasive carcinoma despite the absence of carcinoma on random biopsies.[104, 111]

Certain supplemental studies have arisen to help differentiate high-grade dysplasia from adenocarcinoma, such as mucin histochemistry. The presence of sulfomucins in the setting of specialized intestinal metaplasia marks a precancerous lesion in the stomach; however, when reviewed in Barrett's esophagus, sulfomucin specificity was a low 39% and was found to have little value in differentiating high-grade dysplasia from adenocarcinoma.[112] Flow cytometry examining the development of aneuploidy as a manifestation of genetic instability has also been used to detect early adenocarcinoma; however implementation of this into the clinical arena is still to be established.[113] O-Acetylated sulfomucins in the goblet cells of specialized intestinal metaplasia have been shown

to be markedly decreased or absent in dysplastic Barrett's tissue, suggesting that this may represent an early sign of malignancy.[114]

Rating the severity of dysplasia is often very difficult owing to interobserver variability.[115] Owing to its localized area, it may be entirely missed endoscopically. Once identified, dysplasia of varying degrees may progress at variable rates, with documented cases of Barrett's esophagus and high-grade dysplasia showing no progression over several years.[106, 111, 115] Increased ornithine decarboxylase has been shown to be a possible marker for dysplasia; however, due to its lack of specificity, its clinical usefulness is limited.[116]

Surveillance in patients with Barrett's esophagus is needed because of the significant risk of malignant transformation and the ability to detect and resect early carcinomas. Presently, no one knows how long it takes from progression to low-grade dysplastic changes to adenocarcinoma; therefore, the time course for surveillance is indeterminate. Patients with specialized epithelium or more extensive Barrett's esophagus seem to be at the greatest risk of the development of adenocarcinoma, so they should undergo more frequent screening.[117] However, adenocarcinoma may occur in all epithelial types, as well as in short segments of Barrett's esophagus. Both cytologic and endoscopic biopsying of patients with low-grade dysplasia every year is recommended, with surveillance performed every 3 to 4 months in those with high-grade dysplasia. Once adenocarcinoma has been documented, surgical intervention is mandatory for patients considered to be appropriate surgical candidates.

Factors such as expense and time need to be considered. Looking at the cost analysis for yearly endoscopic surveillance, the Cleveland Clinic estimated the cost at $62,000 with 78 lost work days per year to discover one cancer.[99] Some have questioned the role of periodic surveillance without evidence that overall morbidity and mortality for esophageal cancer are decreased with it.[118] Prior to committing someone to repeat endoscopies, brushings, and cytology, the overall clinical picture needs to be considered in reference to a patient's comorbid conditions and ability to tolerate surgery if adenocarcinoma is found.

In determining who should undergo surveillance endoscopy, we believe that certain patient profiles are at higher risk from adenocarcinoma and, therefore, strongly warrant routine surveillance. Factors such as male gender, white race, family history of either Barrett's esophagus or esophageal cancer, a history of tobacco abuse or history of head and neck cancer indicate the need for aggressive surveillance programs. Obviously, patients without these factors but who have Barrett's esophagus also require surveillance but may have an overall slightly decreased risk for the development of adenocarcinoma.

Treatment

The goal in the treatment of Barrett's esophagus is reducing associated symptoms of reflux disease such as pyrosis, odynophagia, and regurgitation; preventing complications; and promoting regression. No current therapy has proved to be effective in reducing the risk of malignant degeneration. Even complete suppression of reflux and acid production and surgical intervention have not been shown to prevent the development of cancer.

Until recently, the medical management of Barrett's esophagus has been somewhat limited, with the primary goal of prevention of further progression of Barrett's esophagus into adenocarcinoma. All patients with Barrett's esophagus should be treated for acid suppression, even though they may remain asymptomatic. Those patients with heartburn, regurgitation, pyrosis, or evidence of dysplasia should be educated in lifestyle modification and aggressively treated with H_2-blockers or H^+ pump inhibitors like omeprazole and lansoprazole. Simple measures thought to prevent reflux, such as elevating the head of the bed, weight loss, avoidance of foods late at night, small or more frequent meals, and avoidance of smoking, are often implemented.

Metoclopramide (Reglan) or other prokinetic agents have also been used periodically to help increase the pressure in the LES, as well as to improve gastric emptying. Cisapride, a newer prokinetic agent, has been used in the successful treatment of esophagitis, and studies have shown that it promotes healing and relieves symptoms of reflux esophagitis.[119–121] When H_2-blockers are used to treat Barrett's esophagus, they often need to be used in much higher dosages and for much longer periods of time than for peptic ulcer disease to achieve adequate results. Little evidence exists that H_2-blockers actually cause regression of Barrett's esophagus, although case reports do exist.[122] On the contrary, studies have shown progression of the disease even though symptomatic improvement occurs, thereby further supporting the need for close endoscopic follow-up.[123] Resistance to H_2 therapy may be secondary to the gastric hypersecretion or duodenal alkaline reflux seen in this condition.

Proton pump inhibitors like omeprazole and lansoprazole have revolutionized the treatment of esophagitis and Barrett's esophagus. Omeprazole has been the most extensively studied in Barrett's esophagus and has been found to be efficacious in healing patients refractory to standard H_2-blocker therapy.[124] Proton pump inhibitors have been associated with successful treatment of resistant Barrett's ulceration as well as actual regression of Barrett's epithelium.[125–129] Owing to the hypersecretion of gastric acid seen in Barrett's esophagus, 40 to 60 mg per day of omeprazole seem to be necessary to suppress acid production in nearly all patients, rather than the standard dosage of 20 mg per day.[130] Once regression of Barrett's epithelium occurs, often regeneration of squamous epithelium is seen in those areas that were previously Barrett's columnar epithelium. Even after regression of columnar epithelium and re-epithelialization of the esophageal lining with stratified squamous, epithelium, repeat endoscopy with histology and cytology

for surveillance for adenocarcinoma is thought necessary, because adenocarcinoma has been observed even in very short segments of glandular mucosa. The risk of malignant degeneration is unknown once columnar regression occurs.[7] Unfortunately, the use of high dosages as well as prolonged courses of proton pump inhibitors is limited by lack of knowledge regarding long-term side effects. This prevents using proton pump inhibitors in the prolonged treatment of Barrett's esophagus.

Newer developments in the treatment of Barrett's esophagus focus on intervening at levels of cellular differentiation. Compounds such as retinoic acid and inhibitors of decarboxylase such as difluoromethylornithine are currently being investigated.[131, 132]

Laser therapy also has been studied in the treatment of Barrett's esophagus. Barrett's patients undergoing laser therapy have been shown to have a temporary and transient regression when evaluated 6 weeks after laser therapy.[133] Before laser can be said conclusively to be beneficial in Barrett's esophagus, further prospective studies with a larger group of patients will need to be performed.

The presence of Barrett's metaplasia is not necessarily an indication for treatment unless the patient continues to have symptoms of reflux disease, at which time local antireflux measures, along with H_2-blockers or omeprazole, should be begun. Low-grade dysplasia should be aggressively treated with omeprazole, because evidence for regression is higher with this than with H_2-blockers. Even when patients are asymptomatic, low-grade dysplasia warrants aggressive medical therapy. The treatment of high-grade dysplasia remains controversial. When the patient is a poor surgical candidate, observation and aggressive medical management are preferred, but when the patient is thought to be able to tolerate surgical intervention, esophagectomy is recommended.

Surgical intervention is often necessary in the treatment of Barrett's esophagus, particularly when the complications of stricture, ulceration, dysplasia, and adenocarcinoma formation are present. Surgery has been deemed the treatment of choice in those patients with high-grade dysplasia and adenocarcinoma, deep-penetrating ulcers resistant to medical therapy, multiple previous operations, and inability to dilate a stricture.[69, 134] Less clear indications for surgery are nondysplastic Barrett's esophagus, inability to differentiate high-grade dysplasia from adenocarcinoma histologically, and young patients refusing long-term surveillance with poor medical compliance.[135, 136] Surgical intervention is often used in patients who have failed medical therapy, as defined by lack of response after 4 to 6 months of medical regimens.

In patients with metaplastic Barrett's epithelium who show no symptomatic improvement with aggressive medical management, antireflux surgery should be considered.[33] Indications for antireflux surgery include the persistence of erosive and ulcerative esophagitis that is refractory to medical therapy, reflux symptoms not responsive to medical therapy and local antireflux measures, and reflux complications including refractive Barrett's ulcers, strictures, and aspiration during medical therapy.[105, 134] Antireflux surgery has had variable effects on regression of Barrett's esophagus and progression to adenocarcinoma.[104, 105, 134, 137, 138] It does not cause a complete regression of Barrett's esophagus, nor does it prevent the development of adenocarcinoma. However, when compared with medical therapy aimed at acid suppression alone, surgery has been associated with better control of patients' symptoms as well as lower rates of development of complications.[105, 139] An effective antireflux procedure may also halt the progression of columnar epithelium and possibly prevent the development of strictures and ulcers; this may slow the progression of low-grade to high-grade dysplasia and the subsequent formation of adenocarcinoma.[65]

Once a patient undergoes a surgical antireflux procedure, the squamocolumnar junction may relocate several centimeters distally, and squamous epithelium may spread on top of and into areas of Barrett's epithelium, both incorrectly suggesting epithelial regression. Therefore, in benign Barrett's esophageal disease, the indications for surgery are similar to those of standard reflux disease. In symptomatic patients with Barrett's esophagus but no complications, intensive medical management is warranted, but in patients with recurrent symptoms or complications during medical management, an antireflux procedure needs to be considered.

Any reflux operation may be used, but in patients with poor peristalsis, a 360-degree fundoplication should not be used because of the increased likelihood of postoperative dysphagia. Patients with esophageal shortening or strictures may require a Collis gastroplasty. In patients with endoscopically documented Barrett's ulceration, antireflux surgery should be considered after healing of the ulceration with aggressive medical management. In patients with Barrett's stricture with esophageal stenosis, the strictured site should be dilated prior to any antireflux procedure. If peristalsis is intact, then a Nissen fundoplication should be considered, because this has been shown to provide relief of severe reflux symptoms in 90% of patients for over 10 years.[140, 141] Once an antireflux operation is performed, early endoscopy to reassess the location of the aberrant epithelium is needed, along with 24-hour pH studies and manometry to document adequate reflux prevention. Repeat endoscopy, manometry, and pH studies have been recommended 1.2 to 5 years after antireflux surgery, along with yearly cytologic brushings to assess for malignant degeneration.[142]

Even with previously documented minimal complications in Barrett's esophagus, antireflux procedures do not necessarily cure the patient or bring complete remission, nor do they prevent the development of adenocarcinoma.[143] In a study at the Leahy Clinic, only 4 of 37 (11%) Barrett's patients who underwent antireflux operations showed evidence of partial regression of the aberrant mucosa.[134] No patients exhibited complete regression, and surgery was found to have no benefit on patients with pre-existing dys-

plasia. In fact, there was progression of dysplasia in five patients, with three of five patients developing carcinoma despite anatomically documented successful surgery.[134] Adenocarcinoma is an indication for surgical intervention as long as the patient is able to tolerate the procedure. The proper management of patients with high-grade dysplasia but no evidence of carcinoma and Barrett's esophagus remains unsettled, although early surgical intervention with esophagectomy is emerging as the standard of care. Factors such as small foci of adenocarcinoma being missed with biopsy sampling, considerable intraobserver disagreement over severe dysplastic changes compared with early adenocarcinoma, and the rapidity with which dysplastic changes progress to invasive carcinoma set the stage for early surgical intervention in patients with high-grade dysplasia. In localized disease, esophagectomy is performed; however, nonsurgical palliative intervention such as chemotherapy or radiation is often given, with marginal success, for an unresectable lesion or metastatic disease. All columnar cell–lined esophageal areas should be resected with the goal of reanastomosing the stomach or isoperistaltic colonic segment to normal esophageal squamous mucosa. This reanastomosis helps reduce the incidence of complications as well as the recurrence of Barrett's esophagus, which is seen in up to a third of patients after esophageal gastrostomy. These complications are notably less when the cervical esophagus is used to perform a cervical esophageal gastric reanastomosis.[143]

Summary

Barrett's esophagus remains a fascinating and potentially lethal condition. Its marked variability in clinical presentation often allows malignant transformation to occur prior to medical or surgical intervention. Endoscopic surveillance, newer and more aggressive medical therapies, and earlier surgical intervention are some of the modalities currently being used to try to lower morbidity and mortality. An increase in patient awareness; persistent surveillance for the development of adenocarcinoma, particularly in those patients with high-risk profiles; and aggressive treatment of reflux disease are warranted.

SQUAMOUS CELL CANCER

No chapter regarding esophageal cancer is complete without discussing squamous cell cancer of the esophagus. Squamous cell cancer represents 90% of all cancers of the esophagus and remains a worldwide concern as high-endemic areas have been shown to exist in such places as Israel, China, and Iran.[212] It remains clinically significant because incidence and death rates have remained relatively unchanged in the past 30 years. Five-year survival data for white patients range from 8% to 10%, whereas those for black patients are even more dismal, at 4% to 6%.[213] Through studies investigating patients in high endemic areas, numerous etiologic factors have been found to lead to the development of squamous cell cancer. The development of squamous cell cancer is believed to be multifactorial in etiology because certain risk factors are found in high-endemic areas and not in others. In Western society, tobacco and alcohol are believed to be the major etiologic agents in esophageal squamous cell cancer; however, these agents are thought to play less of a role in less developed countries. Other factors, such as nutrition, certain carcinogens like nitrosamine, methods of food preparation, and regional differences in the environment, have been speculated to have an effect on the development of esophageal cancer.

Environmental factors are thought to play a role in the marked regional variability seen in esophageal cancer. In these areas, esophageal cancer is thought to possibly develop through chronic esophagitis, which occurs in up to 80% of the population. In Western countries, the incidence of esophagitis is only 10% based on historical studies,[217] and this type of esophagitis appears to be different from that seen leading to cancer formation in less developed countries. Through research investigation, it has been speculated that squamous cell cancer developing from chronic esophagitis in high endemic areas occurs through an atrophy-dysplasia-carcinoma sequence.

Nutritional factors also are thought to play a significant role in the development of squamous cell cancer. Patterns of micronutrient intake in endemic regions of esophageal cancer have demonstrated that nutritional deficiencies of riboflavin, vitamin C, vitamin E, nicotinic acid, magnesium, zinc and molybdenum are closely correlated with numerous occurrences of premalignant and malignant neoplasms of the esophagus.[219] Common dietary habits seen in high-endemic areas include low intake of fat and animal protein; high intake of carbohydrates from corn, wheats, rice, and sweet potatoes, and very low consumption of fresh fruits and vegetables.[219] Nitrosamine has generated interest as an etiologic possibility in the formation of esophageal cancer. Nitrosamine is a well-known carcinogen and is produced in the soil where there is molybdenum deficiency. Deficiency of vitamin A has been known to be associated with hyperkeratinization, metaplasia, dysplasia, and epithelial tissue tumors. Furthermore, there is an inverse relationship between vitamin A intake and carcinoma. However, not all studies have supported the role of vitamin A in the development of esophageal cancer. In a study conducted by Groenewald and associates, excessive vitamin A intake was found in high esophageal cancer endemic areas of South Africa and France.[218] In high-risk areas of China, high rates of *Candida* infection, which is known to have the ability to produce nitrosamine, may be one link in the high incidence of esophageal cancer.[158, 159, 160] Pickled vegetables in high-risk populations such as in Iran and China have been found to promote high concentrations of nitrosamine. These studies have shown a direct correlation between the absolute amounts of consumption of the pickled products and the mortality rates of esopha-

geal cancer.[161] Aflatoxin is yet another known powerful carcinogen produced from known fungal agents such as *Aspergillus*.

Genetic predisposition remains controversial as a factor in the development of esophageal cancer. Crespi and colleagues showed an increased familial incidence of 28% from studies examining high-endemic areas of Iran.[153] Tylosis, an autosomal recessive condition characterized by hyperkeratosis of the palms and soles, has been associated with esophageal cancer development. In spite of these findings, current belief is that genetic factors play little or no part in the etiology of this disease.

ACHALASIA

The term *achalasia* is from the Greek word that means "failure to relax." The term reflects only one small aspect of the disease: the lower esophageal sphincter (LES) dysfunction. Achalasia represents the prototype of esophageal motility disorders. It is characterized by the complete absence of esophageal peristalsis as well as the loss of lower esophageal sphincter relaxation. These factors result in esophageal obstruction and its associated complications, including mucosal erosions from stagnation, aspiration, and most important, the potential development of esophageal cancer. Generally the esophagus is entirely involved in achalasia, but in certain cases, only the distal two-thirds, the portion containing smooth muscle, is involved.

Achalasia is characterized by the loss of normal progressive peristalsis due to degeneration and subsequent loss of the ganglionic cells in Auerbach's plexus. Clinically, the course is often indolent but progressive and presents the patient with lifelong problems regarding nutrition, recurrent aspiration, and the risk of developing malignancy. The association of achalasia and malignancy has been debated for years.[144–148] Achalasia-associated malignancy occurs in the middle third of the esophagus and is most often of the squamous cell type, compared with adenocarcinoma in the distal or middle third of the esophagus seen in Barrett's esophagus. Malignancy from achalasia is rare, and thus, formal recommendations regarding endoscopic cancer surveillance have not been established. When malignancy does occur, it is often many years after the initial diagnosis and most often in patients who have received therapy late in the course of their disease or who have been treated ineffectively initially. The mechanism by which this malignant degeneration occurs is unknown; however, chronic irritation of esophageal mucosa from chronic stagnation and prolonged exposure to foodstuffs, and bacterial toxins may play a role.

CAUSTIC AND LYE-INDUCED INJURIES

Caustic substances are a prominent and common material in the household. Their wide use as cleaning agents and their easy availability propagate their role in esophageal injury. Legislation and reform have tried to address this problem, but still these substances are subject to accidental ingestion as well as deliberate ingestion and suicide attempts. The federal government has mandated the use of childproof containers and has restricted the sale of highly concentrated caustic materials. Even with these measures, more than 5000 cases of caustic ingestion occur each year in this country.

In cases of milder caustic injury to the esophagus, treatment consists of medical management, with no need for surgical intervention. However, when severe injury occurs or complication such as refractive strictures or perforation occurs, esophagectomy with possible colonic interposition is the treatment of choice. Replacement of the affected esophageal segment with a colonic interposition has been used effectively to treat patients with severe caustic esophageal burns. When colonic interposition is employed, concomitant esophagectomy is warranted because caustic esophageal injury produces a 1000-fold increase in the patient's risk of developing esophageal cancer, predominantly of the squamous cell type. There is also an increased risk of hiatal hernia, reflux esophagitis, and peptic strictures if the injured esophagus is left intact. Others believe that the postoperative mortality and morbidity from removal of the esophagus, which is 5% or more, outweigh the risk of subsequent esophageal cancer formation.[149]

CELIAC DISEASE

Celiac sprue is a disease involving the mucosa of the small intestines and is elicited by gluten and other cereal grain proteins that result in destruction of the small bowel mucosa and loss of normal villous structure. This condition, which was not well understood until the 1950s, has a marked variability in its clinical presentation. It is characterized by a malabsorptive state involving the small intestines that is activated by wheat gluten and associated products. Symptoms most often present early in life as failure to thrive or as complications resulting from chronic malabsorption and malnutrition. There is a bimodal age distribution, with the first incidence peak occurring when cereals are initially introduced into the diet and the second peak occurring in the third decade of life. Celiac disease has been said to occur in as many as 5% to 15% of first-degree relatives of celiac patients.[150]

Association with Malignancy

Celiac disease has long been known to be associated with malignancy.[151-152] The most common malignancy seen with celiac disease remains lymphoma, but esophageal malignancy has been shown to be associated with celiac disease in numerous studies. Neoplastic disease occurs in 10% to 15% of patients with celiac disease and usually involves older patients. It may present after a period of up to 30 years from the patient's first symptom. The increase in overall malignancy is two times normal in patients with celiac disease, with the increase in gastrointestinal malignancy much greater.

VIRAL INFECTIONS

Viral infections have long been associated with the development of malignancy. Human papilloma virus, herpes virus, Epstein-Barr virus, and cytomegalovirus have been associated with squamous cell carcinoma, cervical neoplasms, oral cancer, colon cancer, and Kaposi's sarcoma lesions.

Human Papilloma Virus

Human papilloma virus (HPV) probably has received the most extensive evaluation for the development of esophageal cancer. It is a double-stranded DNA virus with more than 60 subtypes. Clinically, HPV causes hyperplastic lesions, papillomas, or squamous cell lesions that involve the anal-genital area, urethra, esophagus, or skin. Most of these subtypes are tissue specific.[165] The association of HPV with the development of malignancy has been well established, as in anal-genital carcinomas, squamous cell carcinomas, and cervical neoplasms.[166-168] Recently, attention has focused on HPV as causing a premalignant state leading to esophageal cancer. Early studies in animal models showed an association between bovine papillomatous virus Type 4 (BPV 4) and squamous carcinoma of the esophagus.[169] This malignant transformation depends on concomitant environmental factors such as bracken fern exposure, and without these factors, the occurrence of malignancy is less likely. It is unknown whether the HPV causes the initial premalignant lesion or acts as a synergistic factor in the development of esophageal cancer. In human esophageal cancer, this association was initially speculated on when histologic changes seen in esophageal cancer were noted to be similar to those seen in genital condylomatous lesions.[170] HPV antigens and DNA have been found in esophageal squamous cell lesions by DNA hybridization and polymerase chain reaction methodology.[171-173] Using these methods, HPV DNA was isolated in 43.1% and 49% of precancerous and cancerous lesions, respectively, in patients from high-risk areas of Iran and China.[173, 174] In these studies, HPV DNA was increasingly detected as the level of dysplasia increased ranging from 22.2% of patients without cytologic atypia to 66.7% of patients with invasive carcinoma.[175] As a result of these studies, it is suggested that HPV is associated with precancerous lesions of the esophagus.

HPV is known to be linked to cancer of the larynx, cervix, lungs, and colon. Cells infected with HPV show cytologic abnormalities. Two recent reports have stressed the association between HPV and the development of squamous papilloma.[176-177] HPV has been shown to be present in squamous epithelium adjacent to and within esophageal cancer[177, 178] and is associated with the development of esophageal squamous papilloma, which is usually considered to be a benign condition. Squamous papillomas in general are asymptomatic, but they may spread rapidly. They occur two times as often in men as they do in women, with a peak incidence at 40 to 70 years of age.[179] Endoscopically, they have characteristically fleshy, pink color with a warty, lobulated texture and are either pedunculated or sessile. They usually are less than 5 mm in size and may be solitary or seen in clusters. They occur preferentially in the distal one-third of the esophagus. When squamous papillomas are present, they should be removed with as little manipulation as possible because of potential seeding. At endoscopy, a biopsy is mandatory as squamous papillomas have a similar appearance to acanthosis nigricans or verrucous squamous cell cancer. These three lesions are differentiated through histologic examination. The cause of squamous papillomas is currently unknown, but they are thought to develop through an association with gastroesophageal reflux disease, given their location in similar segments of the esophagus. They have been shown to be associated with tylosis.

Squamous papillomas have been shown to undergo malignant degeneration when associated with the human papilloma virus.[180] Initial studies performed in cattle show confirmed malignant degeneration of esophageal squamous papillomas.[169]

The association between esophageal papillomas and the development of esophageal malignancy is not yet firmly established in humans, but similar papillomas of the larynx and cervix have been shown to be precursors to malignancy in these organs.[181, 182] Chang, looking at the presence of HPV in patients with a previous diagnosis of squamous cell dysplasis, found that 58 of 80 patients (66.3%) demonstrated HPV DNA positivity.[173] Another study of patients with established invasive squamous cell carcinoma of the esophagus showed that 33% had epithelial changes consistent with HPV infection and approximately 30% of these patients had HPV antigens.[172] It is interesting that the detection rate of HPV in actual carcinomas is much lower (3.9%) than that seen in hyperplastic or dysplastic epithelium adjacent to the carcinoma (22.2%).[174] This suggests that HPV may be the initial factor in the development of malignancy, being dependent on synergistic actions from other factors before malignancy can occur. Other such factors seen in patients with a high rate of infectivity with HPV and in high endemic areas include physical trauma, chemical carcinogens, and associated nutritional deficiencies.[156]

Immunosuppressed States

Acquired Immunodeficiency Syndrome (AIDS)

Acquired immunodeficiency syndrome (AIDS) was first described in male homosexuals in the United States in 1981 and is characterized by immunosuppression with a predilection for opportunistic infections and malignant degeneration, particularly Kaposi's sarcoma, and lymphoma. The esophagus serves as a location of significant pathologic disease in those patients with AIDS. Opportunistic infection with such organisms as Candida, cytomegalovirus, herpesvirus, Epstein-Barr virus, and Mycobacterium have all been associated with esophageal infection in patients with AIDS. Cytomegalovirus has been found to be associated with disorders such as colon cancer, capacious lesions, and herpetic esophagitis.[186] The long-term sequelae from these often chronic infections remain unknown, and at present, it is not understood what significance these chronic, recurrent infections have, if any, on subsequent tumor development.

ESOPHAGOCUTANEOUS SYNDROMES

Epidermolysis Bullosa

Epidermolysis bullosa is a relatively rare hereditary skin disorder characterized by excessive cutaneous blistering at sites of local trauma. Blisters develop after local injury and subsequently rupture, leading to scar formation and the potential for infection. The esophagus is one of the most common gastrointestinal sites affected in epidermolysis bullosa. Esophageal involvement appears to be most common in the recessive type of dystrophic epidermolysis bullosa.[207] Esophageal strictures, webs, and ulcerations have all been observed in this condition. Esophageal disease may become symptomatic at any age, but most studies show symptomatic occurrences primarily between infancy and the third decade.[209] Most commonly the esophageal stricture is in the cervical region of the esophagus, where the intraluminal diameter is the narrowest, although more distal esophageal strictures have been reported.[208] Esophageal webs occur, particularly in dystrophic epidermolysis bullosa, and may be related to local trauma or chronic blood loss. The recessive form of dystrophic epidermolysis bullosa is frequently associated with extensive lesions of the esophagus; however, the autosomal dominant form of the disease is not associated with esophageal erosions or strictures. Disorganized and poor esophageal peristalsis has also been seen during radiographic examinations in these patients.[210] Although it is believed that there is an increased risk of esophageal cancer in patients with epidermolysis bullosa, the relationship between this condition and the development of esophageal cancer has yet to be fully defined, and to date, no formal recommendations have been made regarding cancer surveillance.

Tylosis

Tylosis palmaris et plantaris is a rare, autosomally dominant inherited disorder characterized by striking hyperkeratosis of the palms of the hand and the soles of the feet and by papillomatous lesions of the esophagus. Tylosis has been found to have a strong association with the subsequent development of squamous cell esophageal cancer. It is estimated that up to 95% of patients with this condition will develop squamous cell carcinoma of the esophagus by 65 years of age.[187]

Most esophageal tumors in patients with tylosis occur in the lower one-third of the esophagus, and nearly all are the squamous cell type. This is interesting because esophagitis of various degrees was shown to occur in nearly 50% of tylosis patients and involve all levels of the esophagus.[188] Chronic esophagitis associated with tylosis has been found to be a poor predictor of the development of esophageal cancer.[188] Hyperkeratosis also may serve as a mechanism by which tylosis leads to esophageal cancer. Hyperkeratosis has been seen in the webs of Plummer-Vinson syndrome and in esophageal strictures, both of which have been associated with esophageal malignant degeneration. Clinically, patients have varying degrees of keratinization; some have only mild involvement of the soles.

Hereditary tylosis occurs equally in men and women, and there is no ethnic predilection. There are two types of hereditary tylosis, which are differentiated by the age at onset, variation in the cutaneous keratinization, and the degree of fissuring. The most prominent clinical findings are marked thickening and fissure formation on the palms and soles. Esophageal cancer with tylosis develops through the occurrence of dysplastic cellular changes. Histologically, abnormalities in maturation with the presence of prominent basophilic inclusions and clear cell acanthosis with inflammation are seen in 50% of cases.[188]

Lichen Planus

Lichen planus is a skin disorder manifested by a tiny flat-topped skin lesion most commonly seen as a violaceous-colored papule with a network of delicate lines on its surface (Wickham's striae). Lesions are usually distributed symmetrically and bilaterally over flexor surfaces on the forearms, wrists, neck, legs, and lower back; however, esophageal disease is commonly seen. Esophageal lesions may present in the form of papular lesions, ulcerations, or benign strictures. In one recent study, it was shown that one quarter of patients with lichen planus had esophageal involvement in the form of papular lesions.[211] Although the overall risk for the development of esophageal cancer is ill-defined at present, it is known that oral lichen planus is associated with an increased risk of malignant degeneration. Therefore, aggressive treatment with steroids should be employed for chronic erosive changes of lichen planus in the esophagus in order to decrease potentially the risk of malignant transformation.

Plummer-Vinson Syndrome (Paterson-Kelly Syndrome)

Plummer-Vinson syndrome is characterized by the development of esophageal webs in association with koilonychia, angular stomatitis,[189] and glossitis, and is also considered to be a premalignant lesion of the esophagus. It was initially thought to be associated with cervical cancer.[190] It is most commonly seen in middle-aged women. The hypopharyngeal webs consist of normal esophageal tissue, with 50% having inflammatory changes and 10% having cytologic atypia.[191] Clinically, patients present with symptoms secondary to iron deficiency or symptoms of dysphagia or esophageal obstruction secondary to the esophageal webs (Fig. 20–2).

RADIATION

Esophageal cancer resulting from radiation damage to the esophageal mucosa usually occurs within a prolonged time period from the time of radiation. The majority of esophageal cancers following radiation develop within 8 to 12 years; the average age is during the sixth decade. This is essentially the same time period the general population is at highest risk for the development of esophageal cancer; however, those patients with radiation succumb at a slightly younger age.

The mechanism by which esophageal cancer develops after radiation is currently unknown; however, the radiation is thought to result in significant mucosal damage leading to malignant transformation.[192] Shimizu and colleagues[193] reviewed 24 patients with radiation-induced esophageal cancer. The study found that the mean latent period between the initial radiation and the diagnosis of esophageal cancer was 29 years. No clear association was found between the cumulative dose of radiation and the diagnosis of esophageal cancer. The most common site of radia-

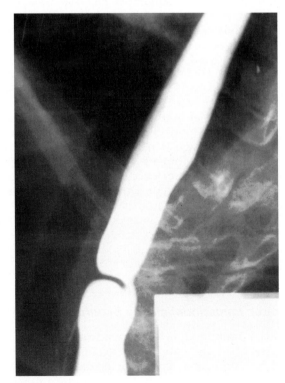

FIGURE 20–2. Hypopharyngeal web, a smooth linear intraluminal filling defect arising from the anterior wall of the hypopharynx just above the pharyngeo-esophageal junction characteristically seen in Plummer-Vinson syndrome.

tion-induced cancer is the cervical esophagus, followed by the middle intrathoracic esophagus.

The criteria suggesting the diagnosis of radiation-induced malignancy are (1) history of prior radiation, (2) appearance of the malignancy within the irradiated area, (3) observable chronic radiation damage, and (4) a long interval between the radiation exposure and the development of malignancy.[194] The latter two are not necessary for the diagnosis of radiation-induced malignancy. The overall survival with a radiation-induced esophageal cancer is expected to be better than that with esophageal cancer from other causes.

Mucosal damage from endoscopic injection of varices has been reported as a premalignant condition of the esophagus. Eight cases have been reported in the literature, with the majority of esophageal cancers being the squamous cell type.[195, 196] Whether the natural cause of the esophageal cancer was the sclerosant that was used or the ulcer that was induced from the injection of the varices with surrounding inflammation is not well established. Nearly all the patients had marked histories of both tobacco and alcohol use, making the cause of esophageal cancer less clear.

Historically, numerous other medical conditions have been associated with the development of esophageal cancer. Although these are not necessarily associated with premalignant lesions of the esophagus, in the past, it was believed that they potentially predisposed the patient to the development of esophageal cancer. Such conditions as esophageal diverticula, dyskeratosis congenita, ectodermal dysplasia, porokeratosis of Mibelli, Torre's syndrome, and Fanconi's anemia, as well as the effects of sclerosing therapy, have been reported to be associated with esophageal cancer; however, these associations are weak, and at present require further investigation.

Conclusion

Esophageal cancer remains a prominent and devastating medical condition. Although much work has been performed to find the underlying mechanism of disease and to prevent the high morbidity and mortality associated with esophageal cancer, the overall prognosis has been only slightly improved and remains dismal. Study of conditions associated with esophageal cancer, such as Barrett's esophagus, achalasia, caustic injury, and others, have resulted in programs that stress not only primary prevention but also surveillance strategies and modification of treatment regimens. Increased public awareness and education are needed to decrease the overall incidence of the disease and allow early intervention in both diagnosis and therapy.

SELECTED REFERENCES

Cooper BT, Holmes GKT, Ferguson R, et al: Celiac disease and malignancy. Medicine 59:249, 1980.
Informative review of the clinical manifestations of lymphoma and other malignant tumors seen in patients with celiac disease. Specific emphasis is on lymphoma associated with celiac disease, particularly in regard to time of onset, clinical presentation, and aids to diagnosis.

Eckardt VF, Aignherr C, Bernhard G: Predictors of outcome in patients with achalasia treated by pneumatic dilation. Gastroenterology 103:1732, 1992.
Prospective study investigating various patient characteristics predicting long-term clinical response in achalasia patients treated with pneumatic dilation. Postdilation LES pressure is highly predictive of long-term outcome, whereas young age, small-diameter dilating bag, and high postdilational LES pressures are unfavorable factors.

Reynolds JC, Parkman HP: Achalasia. Gastroenterol Clin North Am 18(2):233, 1989.
Extensive review regarding the clinical manifestations, pathophysiology, diagnosis, and different therapeutic options in patients with achalasia.

Spechler SJ, Goyal RK: Barrett's esophagus. N Engl J Med 315:362, 1986.
Thorough review investigating the effects of growth factors and genetic alterations in patients with Barrett's esophagus. Dysplasia and endoscopic surveillance are discussed in regard to the development of adenocarcinoma.

Wong RKH, Maydonowitch CL: Achalasia—new knowledge about an old disease. Semin Gastrointest Dis 3(3):156, 1992.
Concise summary of achalasia, with particular emphasis on diagnosis and therapeutic intervention. Contains an extensive table of secondary causes of achalasia.

REFERENCES

1. Barrett NR: Chronic peptic ulcer of the esophagus and esophagitis. Br J Surg 38:175, 1950.
2. Allison PR, Johnstone AS: The oesophagus lined with gastric mucous membrane. Thorax 8:87, 1953.
3. Naef AP, Ozzello L: Columnar lined lower esophagus: An acquired lesion with malignant predisposition. J Thorac Cardiovasc Surg 70:826, 1975.
4. Spechler SJ, Goyal RK: Barrett's esophagus. N Engl J Med 315:362, 1986.
5. Rector LE, Connerley ML: Aberrant mucosa in the esophagus in infants and in children. Arch Pathol 31:285, 1941.
6. Jabbari M, Goresky CA, Lough J, et al: The inlet patch: Heterotopic gastric mucosa in the upper esophagus. Gastroenterology 89:352, 1985.
7. Schnell TG, Sontag SJ, Chejfec G: Adenocarcinoma arising in tongues or short segments of Barrett's esophagus. Dig Dis Sci 37:137, 1991.
8. Bremner CG, Lynch VP, Ellis FH Jr: Barrett's esophagus: Congenital or acquired? An experimental study of esophageal mucosal regeneration in the dog. Surgery 68:209, 1970.
9. Borrie J, Goldwater L: Columnar cell-lined esophagus: Assessment of etiology and treatment. J Thorac Cardiovasc Surg 71:826, 1975.
10. Goldman MC, Beckman RC: Barrett's syndrome: Case report with discussion about concepts of pathogenesis. Gastroenterology 39:104, 1960.
11. Halvorsen JF, Semb BKH: The Barrett syndrome (the columnar-lined lower oesophagus): An acquired condition secondary to reflux esophagitis; a case report with discussion of pathogenesis. Acta Chir Scan 141:683, 1975.
12. Everhart CW Jr, Holtzapple PG, Humphries TJ: Barrett's esophagus: Inherited epithelium or inherited reflux? J Clin Gastroenterol 5:357, 1983.
13. Crabb DW, Berk MA, Hall TR, et al: Familial gastroesophageal reflux and the development of Barrett's esophagus. Ann Intern Med 103:52, 1985.
14. Johns BAE: Developmental changes in the oesophageal epithelium in man. J Anat 86:431, 1952.
15. Smith RRL, Hamilton SR, Boitnott JK, et al: The spectrum of carcinoma arising in Barrett's esophagus: Clinicopathologic study of 26 patients. Am J Surg Pathol 8:563, 1984.
16. Spechler SJ, Robbins AH, Rubins HB, et al: Adenocarcinoma and Barrett's esophagus: An overrated risk. Gastroenterology 87:927, 1984.

17. Winters C Jr, Spurling JJ, Chobonian SJ, et al: Barrett's esophagus: A prevalent, occult complication of gastroesophageal reflux disease. Gastroenterology 92:118, 1987.

18. Kortan P, Warren RE, Gardner J, et al: Barrett's esophagus in a patient with surgically treated achalasia. J Clin Gastroenterol 3:357, 1981.

19. Hamilton SR: Pathogenesis of columnar-cell lined (Barrett's) esophagus. *In* Spechler SJ, Goyal RK (eds): Barrett's Esophagus: Pathophysiology, Diagnosis, and Management. New York, Elsevier Science, 1985, pp 29–37.

20. Meyer W, Vollmar F, Bar W: Barrett esophagus following total gastrectomy: A contribution to its pathogenesis. Endoscopy 11:121, 1979.

21. Gillen P, Keeling P, Byrne PJ, et al: Experimental columnar metaplasia in the canine oesophagus. Br J Surg 75:113, 1988.

22. Lillimore KP, Johnson LF, Harmon JW: Alkaline esophagitis: A comparison of the ability of gastroduodenal components to injure the rabbit esophagus. Gastroenterology 85:621, 1983.

23. Waring JP, Legrand J, Chinichian A, et al: Duodenogastric reflux in patients with Barrett's esophagus. Dig Dis Sci 35:759, 1990.

24. Paull G, Yardley JH: Gastric and esophageal *Campylobacter pylori* in patients with Barrett's esophagus. Gastroenterology 95:216, 1988.

25. Tally NJ, Cameron AJ, Shorter RG, et al: *Campylobacter pylori* and Barrett's esophagus. Mayo Clin Proc 63:1176, 1988.

26. Houck J, Lucas J: Absence of *Campylobacter*-like organisms and Barrett's esophagus. Arch Pathol Lab Med 113:470, 1989.

27. Paull G, Yardley J: Gastric and esophageal *Campylobacter pylori* in patients with Barrett's esophagus. Gastroenterology 95:216, 1988.

28. Nebel OT, Fornes MF, Castell DO: Symptomatic gastroesophageal reflux: Incidence and precipitating factors. Dig Dis Sci 21:955, 1976.

29. Enterline H, Thompson J: Barrett's metaplasia and adenocarcinoma. *In* Enterline H, Thompson J (eds): Pathology of the Esophagus, New York, Springer-Verlag, 1990, pp 109–126.

30. Herliby KJ, Orlando RC, Bryson JC, et al: Barrett's esophagus: Clinical, endoscopic, histologic, manometric and electrical potential difference characteristics. Gastroenterology 86:436, 1984.

31. Cameron AJ, Zinsmeister AR, Ballard DJ, et al: Prevalence of columnar lined (Barrett's) esophagus: Comparison of population based on clinical and autopsy findings. Gastroenterology 99:918, 1990.

32. Van der Veen AH, et al: Adenocarcinoma in Barrett's esophagus: An overrated risk. Gut 30:14, 1989.

33. Polepalle SC, McCallum RW: Barrett's esophagus: Current assessment and future perspectives. Gastroenterol Clin North Am 19:733, 1990.

34. Sarr MG, Hamilton SR, Marrione GC, et al: Barrett's oesophagus: Its prevalence and its association with adenocarcinoma in patients with symptoms of gastroesophageal reflux. Am J Surg 149:187, 1985.

35. Kahrilas PJ, Gupta RR: Mechanism of acid reflux associated with cigarette smoking. Gut 31:4, 1990.

36. Post AB, Achkar E, Carey WD: Prevalence of colonic neoplasia in patients with Barrett's esophagus. Am J Gastroenterol 88:877, 1993.

37. Blot WJ, Devesa SS, Kneller RW, et al: Rising incidence of adenocarcinoma of the esophagus and gastric cardia. JAMA 265:1287, 1991.

38. Haggitt RC, Dean PJ: Adenocarcinoma in Barrett's epithelium. *In* Spechler SJ, Goyal RK (eds): Barrett's Esophagus: Pathophysiology, Diagnosis, and Management. New York, Elsevier Science, 1985, pp 153–166.

39. Poleynard GD, Marty AT, Birnbaum WB, et al: Adenocarcinoma in the columnar lined (Barrett) esophagus. Arch Surg 112:997, 1977.

40. Haggitt RC, Tryzelaur J, Ellis FH Jr, et al: Adenocarcinoma complicating columnar epithelium-lined (Barrett's) esophagus. Am J Clin Pathol 70:1, 1978.

41. Webb JN, Busuttil A: Adenocarcinoma of the oesophagus and the oesophageal junction. Br J Surg 65:475, 1978.

42. Bosh A, Friaz Z, Caldwell WL: Adenocarcinoma of the esophagus. Cancer 43:1557, 1979.

43. Messian RA, Hermos JA, Robbins AH, et al: Barrett's esophagus: Clinical review of 26 cases. Am J Gastroenterol 69:458, 1978.

44. Paull A, Trier JS, Dalton MD, et al: The histological spectrum of Barrett's esophagus. N Engl J Med 295:476, 1976.

45. Belladonna JA, Hajdu SI, Bains MS, et al: Adenocarcinoma in situ of Barrett's esophagus diagnosed by endoscopic cytology. N Engl J Med 291:895, 1974.

46. Johns BAE: Developmental changes in the oesophageal epithelium in man. J Anat 86:431, 1952.

47. Mangla JC: Barrett's esophagus: An old entity rediscovered. J Clin Gastroenterol 3:347, 1981.

48. Jabbari M, Goresky CA, Lough J, et al: The inlet patch: Heterotopic gastric mucosa in the upper esophagus. Gastroenterology 89:352, 1985.

49. Gelfand MD: Barrett's esophagus in sexagenarian identical twins. J Clin Gastroenterol 5:251, 1983.

50. Jochem VJ, Fuerst PA, Fromkes JJ: Familial Barrett's esophagus associated with adenocarcinoma. Gastroenterology 102:1400, 1992.

51. Hassall E, Weinstein WM, Ament ME: Barrett's esophagus in childhood. Gastroenterology 89:1331, 1985.

52. Hassel E, Weinstein WM: Partial regression of childhood Barrett's esophagus after fundoplication. Am J Gastroenterol 87:1506, 1992.

53. Iascone C, DeMeester TR, Little AG, et al: Barrett's esophagus: Functional assessment, proposed pathogenesis and surgical treatment. Arch Surg 118:543, 1983.

54. Gillen P, Keeling P, Byrne PJ, et al: Barrett's esophagus: pH profile. Br J Surg 74:774, 1987.

55. Richter JE: Barrett's esophagus: Too much acid, alkali or both? Gastroenterology 98:798, 1990.

56. Gillen P, Keeling P, Byrne PJ, et al: Implications of duodenogastric reflux in the pathogenesis of Barrett's esophagus. Br J Surg 75:540, 1988.

57. Attwood SEA, DeMeester TR, Bremner CG, et al: Alkaline gastroesophageal reflux: Implications in the development of complications in Barrett's columnar-lined lower esophagus. Surgery 106:764, 1989.

58. Johnson LF, Harmon JW: Experimental esophagitis in a rabbit model. J Clin Gastroenterol 8:26, 1986.

59. Spechler SJ, Schimmel EM, Dalton JW, et al: Barrett's epithelium complicating lye ingestion with sparing of the distal esophagus. Gastroenterology 81:580, 1981.

60. Sartori S, Neilsen I, Indelli M, et al: Barrett's esophagus after chemotherapy with cyclophosphamide, methotrexate and 5-fluorouracil (CMF): An iatrogenic injury. Ann Intern Med 114:210, 1991.

61. Burgess JN, Payne WS, Anderson HA, et al: Barrett's esophagus. Mayo Clin Proc 46:728, 1971.

62. Sanfey H, Hamilton SR, Smith RRL, et al: Carcinoma arising in Barrett's esophagus. Surg Gynecol Obstet 161:570, 1985.

63. Altorki NK, Skinner DB: Adenocarcinoma in Barrett's esophagus. Semin Surg Oncol 6:274, 1990.

64. Skinner DB, Dowaltshahi KD, DeMeester TR: Potentially curable cancer of the esophagus. Cancer 50:2571, 1985.

65. DeMeester TR, Attwood SE, Smyrck TC, et al: Surgical therapy in Barrett's esophagus. Ann Surg 212:528, 1990.

66. DeMeester TR, Stein HJ: Gastroesophageal reflux disease. *In* Moody FG, Jones RS, Kelly KA, et al (eds): Surgical Treatment of Digestive Diseases, 2nd ed. Chicago, Yearbook Medical Publishers, 1989, pp 65–108.

67. Ustach TJ, Tobon F, Schuster MM: Demonstration of acid secretion from esophageal mucosa in Barrett's ulcer. Gastrointest Endosc 16:98, 1969.

68. Fontolliet CH, Wellinger J, Monnier P, et al: Barrett's ulcer: A heterogeneous group of disorders. Presented at the 4th World Congress of the International Society for diseases of the Esophagus, Chicago, IL, September, 1989.

69. Altorki N, Skinner DB, Segalin A, et al: Indications for esophagectomy in nonmalignant Barrett's esophagus: A ten-year experience. Ann Thorac Surg 49:724, 1990.

70. Pearson FG, Cooper JD, Patterson GA, et al: Peptic ulcer in acquired columnar lined esophagus: Results of surgical treatment. Ann Thorac Surg 43:241, 1987.

71. Williamson WA, Ellis FH Jr, Gibb SP, et al: Barrett ulcer: A surgical disease? J Thorac Cardiovasc Surg 103:2, 1992.

72. Naef AP, Savary M: Conservative operations for peptic esophagitis with stenosis in columnar lined lower esophagus. Ann Thorac Surg 13:543, 1972.

73. Robbins AH, Vincent ME, Saini M, et al: Revised radiologic concepts of the Barrett esophagus. Gastrointest Radiol 3:337, 1978.

74. Savary M, Ollyo JB, Monnier P: Frequency and importance of endobrachyesophagus in reflux disease. *In* Siewart JR, Holscher AH (eds): Diseases of the Esophagus. Berlin, Springer-Verlag, 1988, pp 529–536.

75. Henderson RD: Management of the patient with benign oesophageal strictures. Surg Clin North Am 63:805, 1983.

76. Iftikhar SY, James PD, Steele RJC, et al: Length of Barrett's oesophagus: An important factor in the development of dysplasia and adenocarcinoma. Gut 33:1155, 1992.

77. Riddell RH, Goldman H, Ransohoff DF, et al: Dysplasia in inflammatory bowel disease: Standardized classification with provisional clinical applications. Hum Pathol 14:931, 1983.

78. Schnell T, Sontag S, Chejfec G: Adenocarcinoma arising in Barrett's esophagus. Dig Dis Sci 34:1336, 1989.

79. Pera M, Trastek VF, Carpenter HA, et al: Barrett's esophagus with high grade dysplasia: An indication for esophagectomy? Ann Thorac Surg 54:193, 1992.

80. Streitz JM, Andrews CW Jr, Ellis FH Jr: Surveillance endoscopy for Barrett's esophagus. Does it help? J Thorac Cardiovasc Surg 105:383, 1993.

81. Cameron AJ, Ott BJ, Payne WS: The incidence of adenocarcinoma in the columnar lined (Barrett's) esophagus. N Engl J Med 313:857, 1985.

82. Martini GA: Ethanol abuse and Barrett's esophagus. N Engl J Med 295:1322, 1976.

83. Patel GK, Clift SA, Read RC: Mechanism of gastroesophageal reflux (GER) in patients with Barrett's esophagus. Gastroenterology 82:1146, 1982.

84. Stein HJ, Hoeft S, DeMeester TR: Barrett's esophagus: A functional foregut disorder. Acta Endosc 23:83, 1993.

85. Gillen P, Byrne PJ, Heally M, et al: Implications of duodenogastric reflux in the pathogenesis of Barrett's esophagus. Br J Surg 75:540, 1988.

86. Collen MJ, Ciarleglio CA, Stanczak VJ, et al: Basal acid output in patients with gastroesophageal reflux disease. Gastroenterology 92:1350A, 1987.

87. Johnson DA, Winters C, Drane WE, et al: Solid phase gastric emptying in patient with Barrett's esophagus. Dig Dis Sci 11:1217, 1986.

88. Hassell E, Weinstein WM, Ament ME: Barrett's esophagus in childhood. Gastroenterology 89:1331, 1985.

89. Desbaillets L, Mangla J: Endoscopic diagnosis of Barrett's esophagus. Endoscopy 8:67, 1976.

90. Levine MS: Barrett's oesophagus: A radiologic diagnosis. Progress in radiology. Am J Radiol 151:433, 1988.

91. Vidius EI, Beck I: Transmural potential difference (PD) in the body of the esophagus in patients with esophagitis, Barrett's epithelium, and carcinoma of the esophagus. Am J Dig Dis 16:991, 1971.

92. Spechler SJ: Complications of GE reflux disease. *In* Castell DO: The Esophagus. Boston, Little, Brown, 1992, p 543.

93. Hayward J: The lower end of the esophagus. Thorax 16:36, 1961.

94. Agha FP: Radiologic diagnosis of Barrett's esophagus: Critical analysis of 65 cases. Gastrointest Radiol 11:123, 1986.

95. Dowaltshahi KD, Skinner DB, DeMeester TR, et al: Evaluation of brush cytology as an independent technique for detection of esophageal carcinoma. J Thorac Cardiovasc Surg 89:848, 1985.

96. Robey SS, Hamilton SR, Gupta PK, et al: Diagnostic value of cytopathology in Barrett's esophagus and associated adenocarcinoma. Am J Clin Pathol 89:493, 1988.

97. Geisinger KR, Teot LA, Richter JE: A comparative cytopathologic and histologic study of atypia, dysplasia, and adenocarcinoma in Barrett's esophagus. Cancer 69:8, 1992.

98. Thompson JJ, Zinsser KR, Enterline HT: Barrett's metaplasia and adenocarcinoma of the esophagus and gastroesophageal junction. Hum Pathol 14:42, 1983.

99. Achkar E, Carey W: The cost of surveillance for adenocarcinoma complicating Barrett's esophagus. Am J Gastroenterol 83:291, 1988.

100. Monnier PH, Frontoilliet C, Savary M, et al: Barrett's esophagus or columnar epithelium of the lower esophagus. Baillieres Clin Gastroenterol 1:769, 1987.

101. Hamilton SR, Smith RRL: The relationships between columnar epithelial dysplasia and invasive adenocarcinoma arising in Barrett's esophagus. Am J Clin Pathol 87:301, 1987.

102. Kalish RJ, Clancy PE, Orringer MB, et al: Clinical, epidemiologic and morphologic comparison between adenocarcinomas arising in Barrett's esophageal mucosa and in the gastric cardia. Gastroenterology 86:461, 1984.

103. Wang HH, Antonioli DA, Goldman H: Comparative features of esophageal and gastric adenocarcinoma: Recent changes in type and frequency. Hum Pathol 17:482, 1986.

104. Skinner DB, Walther BC, Riddell RH, et al: Barrett's esophagus: Comparison of benign and malignant cases. Am Surg 198:554, 1983.

105. Starnes VA, Adkins RB, Ballinger JF, et al: Barrett's esophagus: A surgical entity. Arch Surg 119:563, 1984.

106. Hameeteman W, Tygat GN, Houthoff HT, van den Tweel JG: Barrett's esophagus: Development of dysplasia and adenocarcinoma. Gastroenterology 96:1249, 1989.

107. Dent J, Bremner CG, Collen MJ, Haggitt RC, et al: Barrett's esophagus. *In* Working Party Reports, World Congress of Gastroenterology. Melbourne, Blackwell Scientific Publications, 1990, pp 17–26.

108. Schmidt HG, Riddell RH, Walter B, et al: Dysplasia in Barrett's esophagus. J Cancer Res Oncol 110:145, 1985.

109. Rabinovich PS, Reid BJ, Haggitt RC, et al: Progression to cancer in Barrett's esophagus in association with genomic instability. Lab Invest 60:65, 1988.

110. Reid BJ, Haggitt RC, Rubin CE, et al: Barrett's esophagus: Correlation between flow cytometry and histology in detection of patients at risk for adenocarcinoma. Gastroenterology 93:1, 1987.

111. Lee RG: Dysplasia in Barrett's esophagus. A clinicopathologic study of six patients. Am J Surg Pathol 9:845, 1985.

112. Haggitt RC, Reid BJ, Rabinovich PS, et al: Barrett's esophagus: Correlation between mucin histochemistry, flow cytometry, and histological diagnosis for predicting increased Cancer risk. Am J Pathol 131:53, 1988.

113. Rabinovich PS, et al: Progression to cancer in Barrett's esophagus is associated with genomic instability. Lab Invest 60:65, 1988.

114. Chejfec G, Schnell T, Sontag S: Barrett's esophagus: A preneoplastic disorder. Am J Clin Pathol 98:5, 1992.

115. Reid BJ, Haggitt RC, Rubin CE, et al: Observer variation in the diagnosis of dysplasia in Barrett's esophagus. Hum Pathol 19:166, 1988.

116. Garewell HS, Sampliner R, Gerner E, et al: Ornithine decarboxylase activity in Barrett's esophagus: A potential marker for dysplasia. Gastroenterology 94:819, 1988.

117. Reid BJ, Rubin GE: When is the columnar lined esophagus premalignant? Gastroenterology 88:1552, 1985.

118. Spechler JS: Endoscopic surveillance for patients with Barrett's esophagus: Does the cancer risk justify the practice? An Intern Med 106:902, 1987.

119. Robertson CS, Evans DF, Ledingham SJ, et al: Cisapride in the treatment of gastroesophageal reflux disease. Aliment Pharmacol Therap 7:181, 1993.

120. McCallum RW: Gastric emptying in gastroesophageal reflux and the therapeutic role of prokinetic agents. Gastroenterol Clin North Am 19:551, 1990.

121. Galmiche JP, Frailag B, Filoche B, et al: Double blind comparison of cisapride and cimetidine in treatment of reflux esophagitis. Dig Dis Sci 35:649, 1990.

122. Lee FI, Isaacs PE: Barrett's ulcer: Response to standard dose ranitidine, high dose ranitidine and omeprazole. Am J Gastroenterol 83:914, 1988.

123. Saltzman M, Barwick K, McCallum RW: Progression of cimetidine-treated reflux esophagitis to a Barrett's stricture. Dig Dis Sci 27:181, 1982.

124. Fiorucci S, Santucci L, Farroni F, et al: Effect of omeprazole on gastroesophageal reflux in Barrett's esophagus. Am J Gastroenterol 84:1263, 1989.

125. Hameeteman W, Tytgat GN: Healing of chronic Barrett's ulcer with omeprazole. Am J Gastroenterol 81:764, 1986.

126. Deviere J, Buset M, Dumonceau JM, et al: Regression of Barrett's epithelium with omeprazole. N Engl J Med 320:1497, 1989.

127. Gore S, Sutton R, Eyre Brook IA, et al: Regression of columnar epithelium in Barrett's oesophagus with omeprazole. Gut 31:A1191, 1990.

128. Deviere J, Buset M, Dumonceau JM, et al: Regression of Barrett's epithelium with omeprazole. N Engl J Med 320:1497, 1989.

129. Sampliner RE, Mackel C, Jennings D, et al: Effect of 12 months of a proton pump inhibitor (lansoprazole) on Barrett's esophagus. A randomized trial (abstract). Gastroenterology 102:A157, 1992.

130. Fiorucci S, Santucci L, Morelli A: Effect of omeprazole and high doses of ranitidine on gastric acidity and gastroesophageal reflux in patients with moderately severe esophagitis. Am J Gastroenterol 85:1458, 1990.

131. Sampliner RE, Garewal HS: Phase II trials of 13-*cis*-retinoic acid (isotretinoin) in Barrett's esophagus. Gastroenterology 94:A396, 1988.

132. Garewal HS, Sampliner RE, Fennerty MB, et al: Low dose difluoromethylornithine (DFMO) produces significant change in polyamine content of upper GI mucosa in patients with Barrett's esophagus. Gastroenterology 100:A364, 1991.

133. Brandt LJ, Kauvar DR: Laser-induced transient regression of Barrett's epithelium. Gastrointest Endosc 38:619, 1992.

134. Williamson WA, Ellis FH Jr, Gibb SP, et al: Effect of antireflux operations on Barrett's mucosa. Ann Thorac Surg 49:537, 1990.

135. Iascone C, DeMeester TR, Little AG, et al: Barrett's esophagus: Functional assessment, proposed pathogenesis and surgical therapy. Arch Surg 118:543, 1983.

136. Ellis FH Jr: Indications for surgery in Barrett's esophagus. Acta Endosc 23:101, 1993.

137. Harle IA, Finley RJ, Belsheim M, et al: Management of adenocarcinoma in columnar lined esophagus. Ann Thorac Surg 40:330, 1985.

138. Naef AP, Savary M, Ozzello L: Columnar lined esophagus—an acquired lesion with malignant predisposition: Report of 140 cases of Barrett's esophagus with 12 adenocarcinomas. J Thorac Cardiovasc Surg 70:826, 1975.

139. Attwood SEA, Barlow AP, Norris TL, el: Barrett's oesophagus: Effect of antireflux surgery on symptom control and development of complications. Br J Surg 79:1050, 1992.

140. Spechler SJ and the Department of Veterans Affairs Gastroesophageal Reflux Group: Comparison of medical and surgical therapy for complicated gastroesophageal reflux disease in veterans. N Engl J Med 326:786, 1992.

141. Siewert JR, Feussner H, Walker SJ: Fundoplication: How to do it? Periesophageal wrapping as a therapeutic principle in gastroesophageal reflux prevention. World J Surg 16:326, 1992.

142. Skinner DB: Controversies about Barrett's esophagus. Ann Thorac Surg 49:523, 1990.

143. Orringer MB, Stirling MC: Cervical esophagogastric anastomosis for benign disease. J Thorac Cardiovasc Surg 96:887, 1988.

144. Carter R, Brewer LA: Achalasia and esophageal carcinoma studies in early diagnosis for improved surgical management. Am J Surg 130:114, 1975.

145. Meijssen NAC, et al: Achalasia complicated by squamous cell carcinoma: A prospective study of 195 patients. Gut 33:155, 1992.

146. Rake G: Epithelioma of the esophagus in association with achalasia of the cardia. Lancet 2:682, 1931.

147. Carter R, Brewer LA: Achalasia and esophageal carcinoma. Am J Surg 130:114, 1975.

148. Proctor DO, Fraser JL, Mangona MM, et al: Small cell carcinoma of the esophagus in a patient with long-standing primary achalasia. Am J Gastroenterol 87:664, 1992.

149. Tucker JA, Yarrington CT: The treatment of caustic ingestion. Otolaryngol Clin North Am 12:343, 1979.

150. MacDonald WC, Dobbins WO, Rubin CE: Studies on the familial nature of celiac sprue using biopsy of the small intestines. N Engl J Med 272:448, 1968.

151. Cooper BT, Holmes GKT, Ferguson R, et al: Celiac disease and malignancy. Medicine 59:249, 1980.

152. Holmes GK, Stokes PL, McWalter R, et al: Celiac disease, malignancy and gluten-free diet. Gut 15:339A, 1974.

153. Crespi M, Munioz N, Grassi A: Precursor lesions of esophageal cancer in high-risk populations in Iran and China. *In* Pfeiffer CJ: Cancer of the Esophagus. Boca Raton, Florida, CRC Press, 1982, p 111.

154. Castelletto R, Munoz N, Landoni N, et al: Precancerous lesions of the oesophagus in Argentina: Prevalence and association with tobacco and alcohol. Int J Cancer 51:34, 1992.

155. Day N, Munoz N: Esophagus. *In* Schottenfeld D, Fraumeni JF (eds): Cancer; Epidemiology and Prevention. Philadelphia, WB Saunders, 1982, pp 596–623.

156. Chang-Claude J, Wahrendorf J, Liang QS, et al: An epidemiological study of precursor lesions of esophageal cancer among young persons in a high-risk population in Huixian, China. Can Res 50:2268, 1990.

157. Xia QJ: Carcinogens in the esophagus. *In* Huang GJ, Kai WY (eds): Carcinoma of the Esophagus and Gastric Cardia. New York, Springer-Verlag, 1984, pp 54–77.

158. Xia QJ, Zhan Y: Fungal invasion in esophageal tissue and its possible relation to esophageal carcinoma. Chin Med J 58:392, 1978.

159. Goff JS: Infectious causes of esophagitis. Annu Rev Med 39:163, 1988.

160. Li MX, Lu SX, Ji C, et al: Formation of carcinogenic N-nitroso compounds in cornbread inoculated with fungi. Sci China 22:471, 1979.

161. Li M, Li P, Li B: Recent progress in research on esophageal cancer in China. Adv Cancer Res 33:173, 1980.

162. Yang CS: Research on esophageal cancer in China: A review. Can Res 40:2633, 1980.

163. Xia QJ, Cao SK, Zing TS, et al: Studies on the relation of *Candida* infection and esophageal carcinoma. Chin J Oncol 6:168, 1984.

164. Xia QJ, Sun ZT, Wang YY, et al: Enhancement of formation of the esophageal carcinogen benzylmethylnitrosamine from its precursors by *Candida albicans.* Proc Natl Acad Sci USA 78:1878, 1981.

165. Zur Hausen H: Papillomaviruses as carcinoma virus. Adv Viral Oncol 8:1, 1989.

166. Kilander AF, Nilsson LA, Gillberg R: Serum antibodies to gliadin in coeliac disease after gluten withdrawal. Scand J Gastroenterol 22:29, 1987.

167. Gissmann L: Papillomaviruses and their association with cancer in animals and in man. Cancer Surv 3:161, 1984.

168. Chang F, Syrjanen S, Kellokoski J, et al: Human papillomavirus (HPV) infections and their association with oral disease. J Oral Pathol Med 20:305, 1991.

169. Campo MS: Papillomas and cancer in cattle. Cancer Surv 6:39, 1987.

170. Syrjanen KJ: Histological changes identical to those of condylomatous lesions found in esophageal squamous cell carcinoma. Arch Geschwulstforsch 52:283, 1982.

171. Chang F, Shen Q, Zhou J, et al: The etiology for esophageal cancer: Searching for clues. Scand J Gastroenterol 25:383, 1990.

172. Hille JJ, Margolius KA, Markowitz S, et al: Human papillomavirus infection related to oesophageal carcinoma in black South Africa. S Afr Med J 69:417, 1986.

173. Chang F, Shen Q, Zhou J, et al: Detection of human papillomavirus DNA in cytologic specimens derived from esophageal pre-cancer lesions and cancer. Scand J Gastroenterol 25:383, 1990.

174. Chang F, Syrjanen S, Shen Q, et al: Human papillomavirus (HPV) involvement in esophageal precancer lesions and squamous cell carcinomas as evidenced by microscopy and different DNA techniques. Scand J Gastroenterol 27:553, 1992.

175. Fong LYY, Sivak A, Newberne PM: Zinc deficiency and methylenzylnitrosamine-induced esophageal cancer in rats. J Natl Cancer Inst 61:145, 1978.

176. Politoske EJ: Squamous papilloma of the esophagus associated with the human papillomavirus. Gastroenterology 102:668, 1992.

177. Hordine M, Hording U, Daugaard S, et al: Human papillomavirus type 11 in a fatal case of esophageal and bronchial papillomatosis. Scand J Infect Dis 21:229, 1989.

178. Kuski J, Demeter T, Sterrett G, et al: Human papillomavirus DNA in esophageal cancer. Lancet 2:683, 1986.

179. Livestone EM, Skinner DB: Tumors of the esophagus. *In* Berk

JE, Hanbreich WS, Kaiser ME, et al (eds): Bockus Gastroenterology, Vol. 2. 4th Ed. Philadelphia, W.B. Saunders, 1985, p 818.

180. Van Cutsem E, Gebes K, Vantrappen G: Malignant degeneration of esophageal squamous papilloma associated with the human papillomavirus. Gastroenterology 103:1119, 1992.

181. Toso G: Epithelial papillomas: Benign or malignant? Interesting findings in laryngeal papillomas. Laryngoscope 81:1524, 1971.

182. Qizilbash AH: Papillary squamous tumors of cervix. Am J Clin Pathol 61:508, 1974.

183. Zur Hausen H: The role of viruses in human tumors. Adv Cancer Res 33:77, 1980.

184. McDougall JK, Nelson JA, Myerson D, et al: HSV, CMV and HPV in human neoplasia. J Invest Dermatol 83:72, 1984.

185. Spence IM: Electron microscopic evidence of herpes virus in association with oesophageal carcinoma. South Afr Med J 68:103, 1985.

186. Young LS, Sixby JW: Epstein-Barr virus and epithelial cells: A possible role for the virus in the development of cervical carcinoma. Cancer Surv 7:507, 1988.

187. Howel-Evans AW, McConnell RB, Clark CA, et al: Carcinoma of the oesophagus with keratosis palmaris et plantaris (tylosis): A study of two families. Q J Med 27:413, 1958.

188. Ashworth MT, Nash JRG, Ellis A, et al: Abnormalities of differentiation and maturation in the oesophageal squamous epithelium of patients with tylosis: Morphological features. Histopathology 19:303, 1991.

189. Goyal RK: Diseases of the esophagus. In Braunwald E, Isselbacher KJ, et al. (ed): Harrison's Principles of Internal Medicine. 12th Ed. New York, McGraw-Hill, 1991, pp 1231–1238.

190. Ahlbom HE: Simple achlorhydria anemia, Plummer-Vinson syndrome, and carcinoma of the mouth, pharynx, and oesophagus in women: Observations at Radiumhemmett, Stockholm. Br Med J 2:331, 1936.

191. Entwistle CC, Jacobs A: Histological findings in the Paterson-Kelly syndrome. J Clin Pathol 18:408, 1965.

192. Vanaguna A, Jacob P, Olinger E: Radiation-induced esophageal injury: A spectrum from esophagitis to cancer. Am J Gastroenterol 85:808, 1990.

193. Shimizu T, Matsui T, Kimura O, et al: Radiation-induced esophageal cancer: A case report and a review of the literature. Jpn Surg 20:97, 1990.

194. Goolden AWG: Radiation cancer: A review with special reference to radiation tumors in the pharynx, larynx, and thyroid. Br J Radiol 30:626, 1957.

195. Bochna GS, Harty RF, Harned RK, et al: Development of squamous cell carcinoma of the esophagus after endoscopic variceal sclerotherapy. Am J Gastroenterol 83:564, 1988.

196. Kokudo N, Sanjo K, Umekita N, et al: Squamous cell carcinoma after endoscopic injection sclerotherapy for esophageal varices. Am J Gastroenterol 85:861, 1990.

197. Clements JL, Abernathy J, Weens HS: Atypical esophageal diverticuli associated with progressive systemic sclerosis. Gastrointest Radiol 3:383, 1978.

198. Bowdler DA, Stell PM: Carcinoma arising in posterior pharyngeal pulsion diverticulum (Zenker's diverticulum). Br J Surg 74(7):561, 1987.

199. Huang BS, Unni KK, Payne WS: Long-term survival following diverticulectomy for cancer in pharyngoesophageal (Zenker's) diverticula. Ann Thorac Surg 38:207, 1984.

200. Hefu C, Hua R, Hongquan Y, et al: Esophageal diverticulum associated with carcinoma of the esophagus—a report of four cases. Chin Med Sci J 6:244, 1991.

201. Huang B, Payne WS, Cameron AJ: Surgical management for recurrent pharyngoesophageal (Zenker's) diverticulum. Ann Thorac Surg 37:189, 1984.

202. Schottenfeld D: Epidemiology of cancer of the esophagus. Semin Oncol 11:92, 1984.

203. Maeta M, Koga S, Shimizu M, et al: Possible association between gastrectomy and subsequent development of esophageal cancer. J Surg Oncol 44:20, 1990.

204. Shearman DJC, Finlayson NDC, Arnott SJ, et al: Carcinoma of the oesophagus after gastric surgery. Lancet 1:581, 1970.

205. Sherman DJC, Finlayson NDC, Arnott SJ, et al: Carcinoma of the esophagus after gastric surgery. Lancet 647:581, 1970.

206. MacDonald JB, Waissbluth JG, Langman MJS: Carcinoma of the esophagus and gastric surgery. Lancet 1:19, 1971.

DIAGNOSIS AND STAGING

21 CANCER OF THE ESOPHAGUS: CLINICAL PRESENTATION AND STRICTURE MANAGEMENT

Carolyn E. Reed

The clinical presentation of esophageal cancer is highly characteristic, but unfortunately the signs and symptoms leading to diagnosis occur late in the disease process. The biology of this disease leads to tumor manifestations that challenge surgical treatment.

At present the general inability to detect early disease results in 50% to 75% of patients needing palliation at presentation. For those with obstructing unresectable tumors, the form of palliation is of utmost importance since life span is measured in weeks to months. It is incumbent upon the thoracic oncologist to become familiar with the various methods of managing these advanced malignant strictures.

CLINICAL PRESENTATION

Symptoms

The most common symptoms of carcinoma of the esophagus are dysphagia, weight loss, pain, anorexia, and vomiting. Table 21–1 relates the symptoms to tumor location. The majority of patients seek medical attention within a few weeks of the onset of symptoms, although Ojala and colleagues reported an average duration of symptoms of 3.1 months before first presentation.[1]

Dysphagia occurs in greater than 80% to 90% of reported series. Dysphagia, from the Greek *phagein* (to eat) and *dys* (difficult or disordered), refers to the sensation of food being hindered in its normal passage from the mouth to the stomach. A patient may report that food "sticks," "hangs up," "gets caught," or "will not go down."[2] Because it is such a dominant characteristic of esophageal cancer, every patient complaining of true dysphagia deserves evaluation. Initial inquiry should include whether the dysphagia is to liquids or solids, whether it is intermittent or progressive, and whether there is associated heartburn. Because of the distensibility of the wall of the esophagus, up to two-thirds of the circumference must be involved with tumor to produce obstruction.[3, 4] Patients often intentionally or unconsciously change their eating habits by eliminating coarse foods, chewing more thoroughly, or drinking more with meals, and thereby delay seeking help.[3] Once dysphagia to solids occurs, symptoms quickly become progressive. If impaction occurs, the patient must regurgitate for relief. The site at which a patient localizes the obstruction is seldom of value, and frequently dysphagia localized to the neck is referred from below.[2]

Weight loss occurred in 42% of patients with esophageal cancer reported by Ojala and colleagues[1] and in 71% of patients in the Cleveland Clinic series.[5] The degree of weight loss may be of prognostic significance and certainly affects performance status and tolerance to therapeutic maneuvers. A significantly longer survival has been reported in patients who suffered a weight loss of less than 10% of their premorbid weight or who had improved their nutritional status on therapy.[6]

Pain may be related to swallowing (odynophagia); bony metastases; local tumor growth into the chest wall, vertebral bodies, or mediastinum; or periesophageal inflammation. Epigastric pain is reported in approximately half of patients with distal esophageal

TABLE 21–1. Symptoms of Esophageal Carcinoma

| SYMPTOMS | PATIENTS BY LOCATION OF TUMOR (%) | | | TOTAL NUMBER OF PATIENTS (%) |
	Upper Esophagus	Middle Esophagus	Lower Esophagus	
Dysphagia	90	98	94	96
Weight loss	45	30	55	42
Pain				
Retrosternal	18	16	24	20
Epigastric	0	11	34	20
Cachexia	9	8	4	6
Cough or hoarseness	18	4	1	4

Modified from Ojala K, Sorri M, Jokinen K, et al: Symptoms of carcinoma of the oesophagus. Med J Aust 1:384, 1982. © Copyright 1982. The Medical Journal of Australia. Reproduced with permission.

cancer. It may be the result of metastases to the celiac axis and lesser curvature lymph nodes. Pain may radiate to the neck, shoulders, jaw, or ears.[3]

Respiratory symptoms may be due to aspiration or local invasion of tumor. Hoarseness can result from recurrent laryngeal nerve involvement or chronic aspiration. Both cough and hoarseness occur most frequently in tumors of the upper esophagus (18%).[1] Cough after swallowing may herald the onset of a tracheoesophageal fistula (TEF). The incidence of TEF was reported to be 4.9 percent in a large series of patients with esophageal cancer.[7] The site of malignant communication is tracheoesophageal in 52 percent to 57% of patients and bronchoesophageal in 37% to 40%.[8] Disease may still be confined to the thorax in up to half of these patients. Once a TEF is established, death is hastened by repetitive bouts of aspiration pneumonitis.

Bleeding from an esophageal cancer is rare (4 to 7%). Although widespread dissemination is present in a large number of patients at the time of presentation, extraesophageal metastases are seldom the initial complaint or finding. Symptoms in patients with adenocarcinoma developing within Barrett's esophagus are discussed later.

Tumor Characteristics

Location

The frequency of location of the tumor is related to the histology (Table 21–2). Tumors of the upper third of the esophagus are almost always squamous cell, whereas 74% to 81% of lower third tumors are adenocarcinoma.[5, 9] With the rising increase in adenocarcinoma among white men,[9, 10] an increased frequency of gastroesophageal junction tumors is to be expected in this population. Adenocarcinoma remains rare in the African-American population.

Size

The length of a tumor has been shown to correlate with the extent of disease. For squamous cell carcino-

mas 5 cm or less in length, 40% are localized, 25% extend beyond the esophagus, and 35% are unresectable or have distant metastases. For tumors greater than 5 cm in length, 75% will be unresectable or have distant metastases, only 10% will be localized, and 15% extend beyond the esophageal wall.[11, 12] There is a progressive relationship between depth of invasion and the incidence of nodal metastases.[13]

Intraesophageal and Submucosal Spread

It is well recognized that both squamous cell carcinoma and adenocarcinoma can extend mucosally and submucosally for considerable distances from the apparent macroscopic tumor limits. Sixty-four per cent of specimens examined may be found to have tumor 3 cm beyond the visible lesion, and in 22% microscopic spread may be 6 cm from visible tumor.[14] Microscopic inferior extension is less than superior spread and rarely exceeds 5 cm.[3] Tumor emboli may result in satellite nodules 2 cm or more from the main tumor.

Local Invasion

Extraesophageal spread into neighboring structures is facilitated by lack of a serosa. For lesions of the upper and middle esophagus, either of the main bronchi or trachea may be invaded, mandating bronchoscopy in the staging evaluation. The left main bronchus is most frequently involved. The aorta may be abutted or invaded at any level, but vessel penetration is rare. One

TABLE 21–2. Location of Esophageal Tumors

SITE	SQUAMOUS CELL (%)	ADENOCARCINOMA (%)
Upper third	19	3
Middle third	50	18
Lower third	31	79

Data from Yang PC, Davis S: Incidence of cancer of the esophagus in the US by histologic type. Cancer 61:612–617, 1988.

in every five cancers of the distal esophagus had invasion of neighboring mediastinal structures, most frequently the pleura or lung (19%), trachea (10.7%), and bronchi (9%), followed by the aorta (6%) and pericardium (3%).[15]

Lymphatic Spread

Lymphatic drainage of the esophagus is longitudinal rather than segmental and results in the common presentation of nodal metastases distal to the location of the primary tumor. Upper esophageal lesions also drain to external and internal jugular nodes,[16] and cervical lymph node involvement may be more frequent than previously realized in patients with thoracic esophageal cancer (26% in one series).[17] In a careful analysis of lymph node involvement, Akiyama and colleagues demonstrated a wide distribution of positive lymph nodes regardless of tumor location.[18] There was essentially no difference in the rate of positivity for tumors in the upper, middle, or lower esophagus, but there was a relation between the frequency of positive nodes in each station or group and the anatomic location of the primary tumor (Table 21–3). It should be noted that upper esophageal cancers may have positive abdominal lymph nodes in 32% of cases, whereas tumors of the lower esophagus may have positive superior mediastinal lymph nodes in 10% of cases.

Organ Metastases

Hematogenous spread may be present in 25% to 30% of patients at the time of presentation. In an autopsy study, 50% of all patients with squamous cell carcinoma had visceral metastases, and the rate increased as the tumor became less differentiated (from 40 percent for well-differentiated tumors to 87% for poorly differentiated ones).[19] The most common organs involved, in order of decreasing frequency, were lung,

liver, pleura, bone, kidney, and adrenal gland. Metastases to the brain are rare. In an autopsy study of patients with cancer of the distal esophagus, hematogenous metastases were present in 35%, with lung (22%) and liver (23.5%) being most frequent, followed by peritoneum (12%), kidney (9%), bone (7.4%), and adrenal gland (6%).[15]

Adenocarcinoma in Barrett's Esophagus

Comment has already been made regarding the rising incidence of adenocarcinoma of the esophagus and the significant features of a high male-to-female ratio and higher incidence among whites.[9] Although dysphagia continues to be the dominant presenting complaint in patients with adenocarcinoma arising in Barrett's esophagus,[20–23] other symptoms may vary. Heartburn is reported in 38% to 89% of series.[21, 22, 24, 25] However, symptoms of gastroesophageal reflux do not have to be present and are often chronic and not the chief complaint. It has been suggested that the lack of the universal finding of reflux symptoms is due to the decreased acid sensitivity in Barrett's epithelium.[23] Approximately 11% to 12% of patients will present with bleeding.[20, 23] Unlike squamous cell carcinoma, a history of heavy smoking or alcohol consumption has not been a predominant clinical feature,[21, 23] although some have reported an association varying from 50% to 80%.[22, 25]

Diagnosis

Once suspicion has been aroused by clinical signs and symptoms, the diagnosis is easily achieved by esophagoscopy and biopsy or brush cytology. Accuracy should approach 100%. For dense fibrotic strictures or deep submucosal lesions without obvious mucosal neoplasm, a rigid esophagoscope can provide a more satisfactory specimen.

In the usual patient, no objective findings are present on physical examination to aid in the diagnosis. However, sites of metastatic spread should be examined (i.e., palpation of cervical and supraclavicular lymph nodes). Visceral metastases (e.g., liver) are seldom palpable. Occasionally clubbing of the fingers and toes may be seen. During an initial careful examination, the assessment of cardiac and pulmonary function, the presence of concomitant disease, and assessment of nutritional status are critically important. All too often cachexia, added to the ravages of heavy alcohol and cigarette consumption, dominates the clinical picture. Further staging maneuvers are discussed elsewhere.

The presence of synchronous carcinomas has been reported in 2.5% to 20% of patients with squamous carcinoma of the esophagus.[5, 26–28] Because of the known occurrence of simultaneous carcinomas of the head and neck and esophagus, a thorough head and neck examination is mandatory.[29, 30]

The laboratory examination is not specific. It may reveal anemia, hypoproteinemia, or abnormal liver

TABLE 21–3. Geographic Location of Malignant Lymph Nodes

	Upper (67%)*	Middle (51%)*	Lower (71%)*
Thoracic			
Superior mediastinal	29†	11†	10†
Middle mediastinal	27	21	14
Lower mediastinal	29	18	27
Abdominal			
Superior gastric	32	33	62
Celiac axis	0	4	21
Hepatic artery	0	2	10
Splenic artery	0	6	15

*Percentage of patients with positive lymph nodes for tumor in the upper, middle, or lower esophagus.
†Columns indicate percentage of patients with tumor at a given location having specific node groups positive.
Modified from Akiyama H, Tsurumaru M, Kawamura T, et al: Principles of surgical treatment for carcinoma of the esophagus. Analysis of lymph node involvement. Ann Surg 194:438–446, 1981.

function tests. Hypercalcemia may be present in up to 15% of patients.[31]

MANAGEMENT OF MALIGNANT ESOPHAGEAL OBSTRUCTION

Goals of Palliation

Although some of the techniques for managing malignant strictures discussed in the following section may be employed for temporary relief prior to definitive resection, the major use is the palliation of advanced, unresectable, obstructing cancers. The goal of such palliation is the relief of dysphagia and restoration of oral alimentation by the least invasive means possible. The procedure should be easy and reproducible, have low morbidity and mortality, and preferably be of low cost. Time in the hospital and in treatment (including retreatment) should be minimized, since life span is usually measured in weeks to months. Since radiotherapy of esophageal cancer is discussed elsewhere, the focus of this chapter will be on endoscopic methods of palliation.

Dilatation of Malignant Esophageal Strictures

Dilation of malignant strictures is both successful at relieving symptoms and safe in a high percentage of cases. In two large series,[32, 33] the success rate was 92% and 98%, respectively, and with a mortality of 0% and 1.5%.

Despite its effectiveness, dilation is seldom used alone because of its short duration of effect. However, it is often an important first step in the majority of alternative palliative techniques.

There are two basic types of dilators: (1) the push-type dilator, which can be divided into those that are passed over a guide wire and those used without a guide wire, and (2) the balloon-type dilator (Table 21–4). It is theorized that balloon dilators are safer than push-type bougies because the radial force delivered to the stricture waist by the balloon is more evenly distributed circumferentially than the shearing axial force by the bougie dilator.[34] This has not been proved clinically. One must be familiar with several methods.

Mercury-filled rubber bougies, either the blunt-tipped Hurst or tapered-tip Maloney, are most effective for short, relatively soft, larger diameter (>12 to 14 mm) symmetric strictures. Smaller sizes are usually too flexible to dilate a malignant stricture. The Malo-

ney dilator (available in size 12 to 60 Fr) is preferred because the flexible 14 Fr tip allows easy insinuation into the ostium of a stricture. Peroral dilation with a Maloney dilator is safe, easy, and inexpensive and does not require fluoroscopy. Morbidity is in the range of 0.4%, and perforation is rare (0.1%).[35]

For many years, the preferred method for dilating complicated malignant strictures was the passage of olive-tipped metallic Eder-Puestow dilators over a guide wire. Over the past decade, the Savary-Gilliard dilators have replaced the Eder-Puestow system. The Savary dilator is a semiflexible polyvinyl chloride bougie with a graduated tip, similar in shape to the Maloney dilator.[36] A standard set ranges from 15 to 54 French. A central core allows the dilator to be passed over a guide wire. Using endoscopic visualization from above and fluoroscopic guidance, the guide wire is passed well into the stomach (especially important for strictures near the gastroesophageal junction). Fluoroscopy reduces the risk of complication by assuring the position of the guide wire tip and assessing dislodgement during the exchange of dilators. Resistance at the stricture site is determined by tactile sensation as the dilator is passed through the obstruction, and it is advised to pass no more than three dilators of progressive size once resistance is felt.[37] A true French size is obtained with dilating.

Balloon dilators may be passed over a guide wire or under direct vision through the endoscope (through-the-scope [TTS]) and are useful for long, tight asymmetric strictures. Balloons are made from a polymer that will not stretch beyond a defined French size without rupturing, and they range from 18 to 60 Fr. The TTS balloon dilator can be passed through a 2.8-mm biopsy channel and passed across the stricture under direct endoscopic vision. A controlled pressure and volume syringe that delivers a fixed pressure is available, and balloons are distended for 1 minute and released several times. The over-the-wire balloon dilator is passed over a guide wire and placed in the stomach under fluoroscopic guidance; the deflated balloon is withdrawn and positioned within the stricture, using radiopaque markers. Controlled dilatation is provided by visualizing the disappearance of the balloon waist at fluoroscopy. Balloon dilators are more cumbersome than the Savary system and lack tactile sensation, and a true French size is not obtained in tight strictures.[37] Hydrostatic balloon dilation of malignant esophageal stenoses was reported in a national survey to be a technical success in 75% of cases, with immediate symptomatic relief in 68%.[38]

The ease of dilatation will depend upon the location, length, degree of elasticity, and angulation of the tumor. To relieve dysphagia, dilatation to at least 40 Fr is usually required.[39] For preparation of an endo-esophageal prosthesis, dilatation to 45 Fr to 50 Fr is required. Dilatation for subsequent endoscopic palliation (intubation or laser ablation) is frequently performed at the same session. However, gradual dilation (no more than three sizes at one sitting) may be associated with less risk of perforation.[40] Perforation of a very rigid tumor may result from fracturing or asymmetric splitting on initial passage of a dilator.

TABLE 21– 4. Esophageal Dilators

Push-type	Balloon-type
Without guide wire	Over-the-wire
Maloney	Through-the-scope
Hurst	
With guide wire	
Eder-Puestow	
Savary-Gilliard	

TABLE 21–5. Esophageal Endoprostheses

	PROCTER-LIVINGSTONE	ATKINSON (KEYMED)	CELESTIN (MEDOC)	WILSON-COOK
Material	Latex rubber, armored nylon	Silastic rubber nylon spiral	Latex rubber, nylon spiral	Silicone, stainless steel spiral
Internal diameter (mm)	12	11.6(M), 12.9(L)	11	9, 12
Outer diameter (mm)	18	—	15	13, 16
Length (cm)	10, 15, 19	M: 10.9, 14.1, 19 L: 13.9, 18.9	9.5, 12.5, 15, 21	4.4, 6.4, 8.4, 10.4, 12.4, 14.4, 16.4
Comments	Fishmouth proximal and distal ends	29-mm proximal funnel, distal shoulder	Proximal inkwell funnel, umbrella-shaped distal flange	Proximal 28-mm funnel, distal shoulder

M = medium, L = large.

Esophageal Intubation

Historical Perspective

The use of an endoesophageal prosthesis to stent an obstructing tumor dates back to 1845 (decalcified ivory tube). The history and characteristics of various tubes have been reviewed by Earlam and Cunha-Melo.[41] An ideal prosthesis was described by Sir Henry Souttar in 1924 as "a flexible, incompressible, non-traumatic and compact tube that had an adequate lumen and remained in place."[42] At first tubes were inserted blindly, and later under direct vision using a rigid esophagoscope. The Mousseau-Barbin tube, developed in 1956[43] and modified by Celestin,[44] was designed to be pulled down through a malignant stricture in the esophagus or cardia via a gastrotomy and fixed into position. However, the need for laparotomy in a severely compromised group of patients resulted in high mortality (up to 29 percent) and morbidity (25%)[40] when compared with the peroral push-through or pulsion technique. With the development of various introducing devices and pushers, the peroral pulsion technique became easier and is used almost exclusively today.

Indications

The indications for using an endoesophageal prosthesis instead of other techniques include a long, asymmetric or tortuous stricture, extrinsic compression of the esophagus by tumor, and a tracheoesophageal fistula (TEF). Placement of a prosthesis is often done as salvage therapy after other methods (i.e., radiotherapy, laser treatment) have failed. A relative contraindication to stenting is a tumor less than 3 cm from the cricopharyngeus muscle. However, the proximal funnel of a tube can be cut to a length less than 2 cm, and low-profile tubes are commercially available (Wilson-Cook) to accommodate a tumor and still be below the cricopharyngeus. The Celestin (Medoc) endoprosthesis has been modified for high cervical lesions by amputation of its funnel 3 mm proximal to the shaft and replacement with a distal flange from another tube. This floppy funnel has been placed in the hypopharynx above the cricopharyngeus, with 75% of patients reporting no foreign body sensation.[45] Intubation of bulky tumors in the cervical esophagus can lead to respiratory distress secondary to tracheal compression, and urgent removal may be necessary. Patients undergoing intubation should have an expected life span of at least 6 weeks, unless a TEF is present. A prerequisite for insertion of a prosthesis is the ability to pass a guide wire through the tumor and achievement of adequate dilatation.

The Prosthesis

The majority of frequently used tubes have internal diameters varying from 9 to 13 mm. The thickness of the tube wall is usually 1 to 2 mm. The shaft of the prosthesis ranges from approximately 40 Fr to 48 Fr, and several lengths are available (Table 21–5). The proximal end of the tubes is fashioned to be anchored on the shelf of tumor, to direct food into the tube, and to prevent downward migration. Proximal shapes have varied between collar, funnel, cup, and tulip.[41] Commonly used tubes have a distal flange or shoulder to prevent proximal migration (Fig. 21–1).

Technique of Insertion

Endoprosthesis insertion entails proper sedation and/or anesthesia, a suitable prosthesis, preliminary endoscopy with dilatation of the malignant stricture,

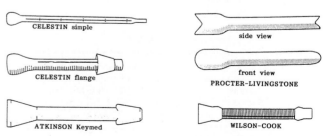

Figure 21–1. Commercially available endoesophageal prostheses.

positioning of the prosthesis with an introducing device, and confirmation of position with postinsertion endoscopy and fluoroscopy. Intravenous sedation techniques employed for routine dilatations can be used. Many surgeons prefer to perform the entire procedure under general anesthesia.

A key step is dilatation to appropriate size, usually 45 Fr to 50 Fr. A pediatric esophagoscope is then passed through the tumor to assess its position and length. A steel guide wire (which has probably been used for guided dilation) is left well into the stomach. A suitable prosthesis is mounted on an introducing device. One popular device is the Nottingham KeyMed introducer, which grips the internal end of the prosthesis by expansion of a distal metal olive. A pusher or positioning tube is passed over the introducer and engaged in the proximal funnel of the prosthesis (Fig. 21–2). The whole assembly is passed along the guide wire over the stricture under fluoroscopic control until the base of the funneled end touches the proximal part of the tumor. The tube is released and the introducer and guide wire removed while the tube is held in position by the pusher, which is itself finally removed. The positioning is checked with a final endoscopic examination.

Tube position should be confirmed by radiography (Fig. 21–3). Preferably, tube patency and function are confirmed with a Gastrografin or thin barium swallow, especially for a TEF. The patient is instructed to eat while upright, masticate thoroughly, and take plenty of fluids during and after eating.

Complications

The incidence of complications after esophageal intubation in major series is summarized in Table 21–6. The most dangerous complication is perforation. It may result from dilatation prior to tube insertion or occur during placement or later secondary to pressure necrosis. When recognized immediately, perforation is best handled by completing the insertion of the tube in an attempt to seal the perforation. Conservative management of small leaks is often successful. Recent

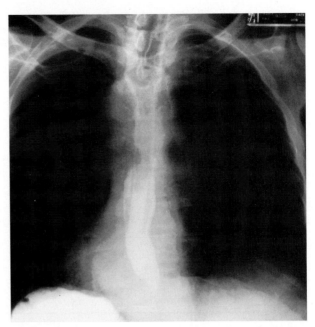

Figure 21–3. Endoprosthesis is confirmed by radiography and barium swallow.

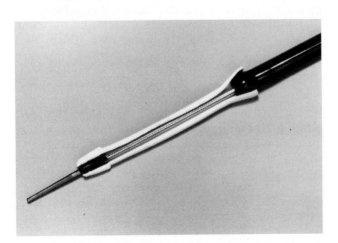

Figure 21–2. Atkinson tube and Nottingham introducer and pusher, which is passed over a guide wire.

mortality from perforation has ranged from 27% to 50%.[61, 62]

The most frequent late complications are tube migration and obstruction. Proximal displacement can occur when the tube is not well seated on the tumor. Distal migration can occur if additional therapy, i.e., radiation therapy, is added to the tumor.[63] Removal of the tube can be accomplished using an introducing device, biopsy forceps through a rigid esophagoscope, or various prosthesis extractors. Food impaction can occur easily if patients are not thoroughly instructed to chew their food carefully and "flush" the tube with excess intake of carbonated beverages. Items such as steak, leafy vegetables, and bread, which stick to the tube, may cause problems. Unrelieved blockage often can be corrected by ingesting meat tenderizer, by drinking a small quantity of hydrogen peroxide diluted in water, or by endoscopic removal. Overgrowth by tumor is best avoided by placing a tube that is 3 cm longer than the malignant stricture.

Whenever possible, the endoesophageal prosthesis should be placed above the gastroesophageal junction in order to avoid reflux and aspiration.[64] Successful use has been reported of an antireflux mechanism consisting of a 7-cm latex device attached to the distal end of the tube, which allows food to pass but bends in decubitus position.[56]

Results

The advantages of esophageal intubation include its simplicity, one-stage technique, and short hospitalization (average 3 to 5 days). Failure to intubate the patient ranges from 0 percent to 15 percent. Reasons include the inability to pass a guide wire through the malignant stricture, inadequate dilation of the steno-

TABLE 21–6. Complications of Esophageal Endoprostheses

SERIES	YEAR	TOTAL NO. OF PATIENTS	FAILURE RATE (%)	IMMEDIATE COMPLICATIONS (%)*			LATE COMPLICATIONS (%)*	
				Perforation	Hemorrhage	Death	Displacement	Obstruction
Palmer[46]	1973	93	0	0	0	0	0	1
Den Hartog[47]	1979	200	3.5	8.3	1.6	2.1	22.8	18.1
Balmes[48]	1980	72	2.7	0	1.4	—	—	6.9
Bergerault[49]	1980	35	0	0	8.5	5.7	14.3	8.6
Dunham[50]	1981	43	9	2.3	4.6	0	41.8	4.6
Jones[51]	1981	55	12.7	8.5	—	12.5	8.3	6.2
Ogilvie[52]	1982	121	2.5	12.7	3.4	11	13.5	28
Seifert[53]	1983	26	0	11.5	3.8	—	11.5	11.5
Lux[54]	1983	66	9	7.6	1.5	3	18.2	4.5
Rose[55]	1983	100	7	9.8	—	11.8	12.9	11.8
Valbuena[56]	1984	40	—	0	5	5	2.5	—
Chavy[57]	1986	91	15	14	5	4	15.5	15.5
Buset[58]	1987	116	5.2	8.2	3.6	4.3	19.1	6.4
Gasparri[59]	1987	248	0	2	—	7.6	3.2	14.5
Angorn[60]	1988	2446	1.5	—	—	15	3.8	0.4
Függer[61]	1990	105	10.5	6.3	5.3	16.8	11.6	9.5
Cusumano[62]	1992	445	8.1	6.4	2.0	3.4	12.7	4.4
AVERAGE			5.4	6.1	3.5	6.8	13.2	9.5

*Based on successful intubations.

sis, sharp angulation of the tumor, or an inadequate proximal "shelf" to hold the prosthesis. In one report, failure of push-through intubation was significantly greater for tumors at the gastroesophageal junction (18.2%) than in the thoracic esophagus (6.7%).[62]

If late complications are considered, the morbidity of esophageal intubation may range from 22% to 60%.[57, 58, 61, 64] Hospital mortality averages 10 percent. Length of survival is not really an end point in this group of patients, but the median is about 3 months. A statistical analysis of risk factors indicated that there was a significant rise in postoperative mortality with increasing age, poor general health, and the presence of distant metastases.[61] In approximately 80% to 90% of patients, successful esophageal intubation results in improved food intake, although many patients eat only a semisolid diet.[57, 59, 61] Overall, general status is not improved in the majority of patients because tumor growth has not been modified by esophageal tube placement.

Expandable Metallic Stents

The use of expandable metallic stents has been successfully applied to the biliary system, and both the Wallstent (Medinvent SA, Lausanne, Switzerland) and the Gianturco or Z stent (Wilson-Cook) have been used for malignant esophageal strictures in small series.[65–68] Problems with tumor ingrowth,[67, 69] dislodgement, and prosthesis extraction are being investigated. Advantages of the expandable stent are the potential for a larger lumen, need for more modest dilatation and therefore ease of insertion, the lack of need for general anesthesia, less shearing force at the time of placement, and ability to easily overlap stents.

Laser Ablation

The neodymium:yttrium-aluminum-garnet (Nd:YAG) laser was first employed for the endoscopic palliation

of obstructing esophageal cancer in the early 1980s. The Nd:YAG laser is a solid-state laser consisting of a crystalline rod grown by combining yttrium, aluminum, and garnet and doping it with neodymium ions, which form the active laser medium. The emitted wavelength of light is 1064 nanometers, which is in the infrared portion of the electromagnetic spectrum. A white or colored aiming beam is coupled into the system to visualize the target. The flexible quartz monofilament laser fiber can be introduced through the working channel of a flexible endoscope. The high thermal energy possible with this laser can produce gradual vaporization, coagulative necrosis, and coagulative hemostasis.

Indications

Tumors that are in the mid or distal esophagus, relatively short ($\leq$ 5 cm), exophytic, and nonangulated are most amenable to laser ablation.[70] A tracheoesophageal fistula is a contraindication to this technique, as is predominantly extrinsic compression of the lumen by tumor.

Technique

The procedure is commonly performed in an outpatient setting using topical anesthesia and intravenous sedation. There are two standard techniques of laser ablation: the prograde and retrograde approaches. As originally described by Fleischer and colleagues,[71, 72] the endoscope is passed to the proximal tumor margin, and ablation is started centrally and applied circumferentially using high (80 to 100 watts) power settings and short power durations (< 1 second) at a distance of 0.5 to 1 cm from the tumor. The initial effect is vaporization of the upper portion and coagulation of deeper portions of a 1- to 2-cm length of

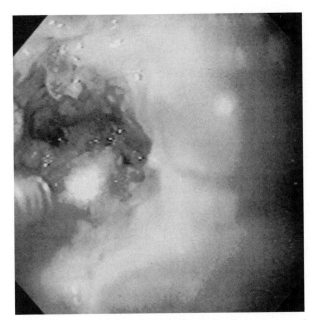

Figure 21–4. Laser ablation of exophytic, obstructing esophageal tumor.

laser fiber, a contact method of delivering laser energy has become available. The theoretic advantage of this method is the ability to ablate tumor at lower power settings with more precision. In a prospective comparison of contact and noncontact laser therapy for inoperable esophageal carcinoma, the contact method offered no advantage in respect to number of treatment sessions, relief of dysphagia, or occurrence of complications.[75] Lessening of mucosal edema or smoke production did not occur. The benefit of contact laser ablation might be in very short and tight strictures or tumor overgrowth of an endoprosthesis.[76]

Complications

In 14 reported series,[58, 70, 74, 77–87] the major complication rate per total number of patients was 13.2%, and the per treatment number was less than 10%. The patient mortality rate was 2.6%, with a treatment mortality about half this value. The major early complications of perforation—significant hemorrhage and tracheoesophageal fistula—have been low (≤ 3%).[88] It is sometimes difficult to attribute death or a complication to laser therapy versus progression of disease. In an international inquiry of 1359 patients treated with laser ablation, there was a complication rate of 4.1% and mortality of 1%.[89]

Results

The results of Nd:YAG laser therapy for obstructing esophageal carcinoma are summarized in Table 21–7. In the majority of series, successful palliation exceeds 80%. However, technical success does not assure functional success. Mellow and Pinkas reported a 97% success rate, but dysphagia was improved in only 87% of patients, and all necessary calories were ingested by only 73%.[77] The best prediction of functional outcome was the pretreatment performance status.

tumor (Fig. 21–4). Over the next 48 hours the coagulated tumor undergoes liquefaction, and necrotic debris can be removed at the subsequent treatment session. The number of laser sessions depends upon the length of the malignant stricture. Using the alternative retrograde approach, an attempt is made to treat the entire tumor in one treatment session.[73, 74] This technique requires preliminary dilatation. Tumor destruction is then begun at the distal margin, and vaporization is continued proximally in a circumferential fashion. When possible, the retrograde technique is favored secondary to reduced treatment time and better visualization of the lumen.

By adding a synthetic sapphire tip to the quartz

TABLE 21–7. Results of Nd:YAG Laser Therapy for Obstructing Esophageal Carcinoma

SERIES	NUMBER OF PATIENTS	PREDOMINANT TECHNIQUE	MEAN TUMOR LENGTH (CM)	MEAN DRUG SESSIONS	MEAN DURATION OF DRUGS (DAYS)	SUCCESSFUL PALLIATION (%)	MEAN TIME TO RETREATMENT (WEEKS)	MEAN SURVIVAL (WEEKS)
Mellow and Pinkas[77]	30	Retrograde	7.9	3.3	7	83	7	NS
Lightdale et al[78]	50	Both	8	2.5	NS	69	NS	NS
Fleischer and Sivak[70]	60	Prograde	7.0	3.4	7.1	92	NS	NS
Buset et al[58]	28	Retrograde	5.6	2.6	8.2	100	NS	27.2
Pietrafitta et al[74]	20	Retrograde-10	8.9	1.6	2.9	90	NS	NS
		Prograde-10	4.8	2.7	7.8	100	NS	NS
Murray et al[79]	26	Retrograde-17 Prograde-17 Both-2	7	3.4	NS	96	NS	16
Jensen et al[80]	14	Retrograde	6.6	NS	NS	86	6-10	16
Krasner et al[81]	76	Retrograde	8	4	NS	86	NS	19
Goldberg and King[82]	15	Prograde	5.6	3.5	9.2	93	NS	NS
Bown et al[83]	34	Retrograde	8	2.7	9	85	6	NS
Cello et al[84]	12	Prograde	5	3.3	18.5	100	NS	NS
Jung and Wieman[85]	16	Retrograde	7	2.5	NS	88	4	23.2
Wolf et al[86]	25	Prograde	8.2	3.6	NS	100	6.6	30.0
Ahlquist et al[87]	25	Retrograde	6*	2*	NS	80	12.8*	20.3*

NS = not stated; * = median
From Pass HI, Reed CE: Lasers in the management of upper aerodigestive malignancies. *In* DeVita VT, Hellman S, Rosenberg SA (eds): Important Advances in Oncology, 1990. Philadelphia, J.B. Lippincott, 1990, p 159, with permission.

Ahlquist and colleagues noted that patients with the best pretreatment appetite had the greatest amelioration of their dysphagia, and this variable was more closely associated with dysphagia response rather than any treatment or tumor variable.[87] Lightdale and colleagues reported that in 33 patients with improved swallowing after laser therapy, anorexia continued to be a problem in 90%.[78]

A carcinoma of the proximal cervical esophagus is particularly difficult to palliate.[78, 90] The tumor may invade the cricopharyngeus muscle and prevent normal opening of the upper esophageal sphincter secondary to disruption of neurogenic reflex activity or spastic closure by residual functioning musculature. Despite the lower success rate, laser therapy is often attempted since placement of a prosthesis is not generally advocated when tumor is within 3 cm of the cricopharyngeus.

The need for retreatment and time to retreatment has been variable. Some have reported that 30% to 45% of patients require repeat laser therapy within 3 to 4 months.[58, 87] However, others have reported a shorter time from initial session to repeat intervention (4 to 6 weeks).[77, 80, 85, 86] A policy of monthly endoscopic examinations to check tumor status has been advocated.[84] There is no maximum dose of laser therapy.

Laser ablation has been equivalent to prosthesis insertion in restoring esophageal patency.[58] In a prospective randomized trial, laser ablation followed by radiotherapy was equal to esophageal intubation in relieving dysphagia and had a lower complication rate and retreatment requirement.[63]

Although the advantages of laser therapy include its efficiency, option of avoiding general anesthesia, and low complication rate, equipment is costly. Patients with TEF or tumors with extrinsic obstruction are not suitable candidates.

Brachytherapy

Intracavitary irradiation is an attractive modality because it is directed only to the obstructing component. The technique is relatively simple and can be performed in the outpatient setting. The source most frequently used is iridium-192 with a high activity (high-dose-rate brachytherapy).

Technique

After appropriate dilatation, a pediatric endoscope is passed through the tumor to assess tumor position and length. A guide wire is passed into the stomach and a flexible plastic brachytherapy afterloading catheter is passed over the wire and fixed in place. The patient is transported to the radiotherapy suite, and the radioactive source is connected to the catheter (Fig. 21–5). Computer-generated isodose curves are optimized to the patient's tumor geometry. The source is programmed to the correct number of dwell positions and dwell time. Iridium-192 is automatically afterloaded by remote control while the patient is monitored. Treatment time depends on the activity of the

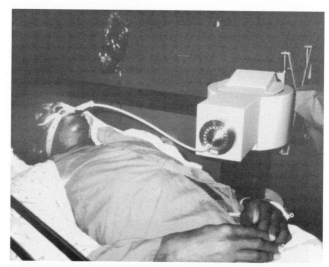

Figure 21–5. Brachytherapy catheter has been passed through the tumor, has been fixed to a mouth guard, and is afterloaded by remote control.

iridium-192 source and length of the tumor but is generally under 15 minutes. A dose of 7 to 7.5 Gy at one session and repeated two or three times is a common regimen, although a single dose of 15 Gy can be used.

Complications and Results

Reported complications of brachytherapy are low.[91, 92] Transient dysphagia may last from 3 to 7 days in up to one-third of patients.[92] The procedure is well tolerated and easy to perform by clinicians familiar with standard endoscopic techniques. The equipment costs represent a substantial financial investment for an institution.

The improvement in swallowing ability appears equivalent to laser ablation. In a randomized study, dysphagia relief and duration of success after laser ablation or brachytherapy were equivalent.[92] Hospital time was minimized.

Photodynamic Therapy

Photodynamic therapy (PDT) employs a photosensitizing chemical (porfimer sodium or dihematoporphyrin ethers) that is selectively retained by tumor and activated by light of a specific wavelength (630 nm) in the presence of molecular oxygen, resulting in tumor necrosis. The patient receives the photosensitizer intravenously and 2 to 3 days later undergoes laser light treatment. A cylindric diffusing fiber is placed through the biopsy channel of an endoscope, embedded in the tumor, and connected to an argon-pumped dye laser. The degree of PDT cytotoxicity depends on the rate at which the dose of energy is given. Patients are re-endoscoped 48 to 72 hours after treatment for debridement and evaluation.

Several researchers have reported successful palliation of advanced obstructing esophageal carcinoma using PDT.[93–96] Patients with total esophageal obstruction (guide wire cannot be passed)[95] and patients who have tumors just below the cricopharyngeus, angulated lesions, or largely infiltrating tumors can be candidates for this modality.

The major complication of PDT is skin photosensitivity, and strict compliance with precautions is required. Other complications include pleural effusion, tracheoesophageal fistula, late strictures, and full-thickness esophageal wall necrosis.[94, 96, 97]

The advantages of PDT include the ability to perform the procedure in an outpatient setting with minimal operative risks, the applicability to patients who have exhausted other forms of therapy or who are not candidates for them, and no limitation on retreatment. The method is potentially more controllable than laser ablation. The eventual role of PDT in palliation of esophageal cancer awaits further study.

Other Methods of Palliation

Bipolar electrocoagulation (BICAP) probes were developed to improve endoscopic thermal palliation of obstructing lesions by allowing treatment of long tumors with reduced cost and greater ease. Tumor probes are similar to metal olive dilators and available in several diameters. After dilatation and determination of the upper and lower distances of the stricture, the BICAP tumor probe is passed over a guide wire and stationed within the tumor. Coagulation of the stricture is carried out in overlapping fashion by both the prograde and retrograde techniques. Depth of tissue heating varies directly with energy density and appositional force. In a pilot study, BICAP treatment produced significant improvement in channel patency and relief of dysphagia.[98] The treatment was fast, efficient, and technically easy. However, there was a major complication rate of 20% (delayed hemorrhage and tracheoesophageal fistula). In a comparison study of laser ablation and electrocoagulation, endoscopic palliation efficacy and safety for circumferential lesions were similar.[80] BICAP tumor probes can be used for submucosal circumferential tumors, long lesions, and

cervical tumors. Asymmetric or noncircumferential strictures are better treated with the laser. It may be best to consider the BICAP tumor probe as a complementary technique to Nd:YAG laser therapy.

The use of endoscopic chemical necrolysis for palliation has been reported.[99] Local injection via a sclerotherapy needle of 3% pilodocanol into the neoplastic mass resulted in improvement of dysphagia in 13 of 16 cases (81%). Benefits of this method include its low cost and simplicity.

Selection of Method of Palliation

It is clear that no one method of managing malignant strictures is ideal for all cases. Thoracic oncologists must be familiar with several techniques of palliation and often individualize treatment. Equipment will vary from institution to institution. PDT is not readily available and still considered experimental. Although several studies have compared various methods of palliation,[58, 63, 92, 100] no consensus has been reached regarding the best first option. An algorithm of management based upon tumor characteristics is illustrated in Figure 21–6.

SELECTED REFERENCES

Boyce WH: Palliation of advanced esophageal cancer. Semin Oncol 11:186–195, 1984.
The experienced author reviews the nonsurgical alternatives for palliation of advanced esophageal carcinoma with special emphasis on dilatation.

Chavy AL, Rougier MD, Pieddeloup SA, et al: Esophageal prosthesis for neoplastic stenosis. Cancer 57:1426–1431, 1986.
A review of the French experience with endoprostheses insertion is presented and the literature summarized in tables.

Earlam R, Cunha-Melo JR: Malignant oesophageal strictures: A review of techniques for palliative intubation. Br J Surg 69:61–68, 1982.
This is a superb review of the history of esophageal intubation, tube designs, and possible complications.

Ojala K, Sorri M, Jokinen K, et al: Symptoms of carcinoma of the oesophagus. Med J Aust 1:384–385, 1982.
A succinct review of the most common symptoms in 162 patients with cancer of the esophagus.

Pass HI, Reed CE: Lasers in the management of upper aerodigestive malignancies. In DeVita VT, Hellman S, Rosenberg SA (eds): Important Advances in Oncology 1990. Philadelphia, JB Lippincott, 1990, pp 159–179.
The authors review the use of lasers in the treatment of advanced esophageal cancer. Results and complications of previous studies are summarized in tables.

Webb WA: Esophageal dilation: Personal experience with current instruments and techniques. Am J Gastroenterol 83:471–475, 1988.
Based on a personal experience with 2000 esophageal dilations, the author discusses current dilators, technique, and indications for their use.

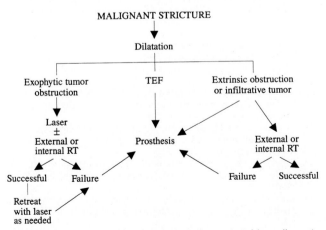

MALIGNANT STRICTURE

Figure 21–6. Algorithm of management of unresectable malignant strictures based on tumor characteristics.

REFERENCES

1. Ojala K, Sorri M, Jokinen K, et al: Symptoms of carcinoma of the oesophagus. Med J Aust 1:384, 1982.
2. Cattau EL, Castell DO: Symptoms of esophageal dysfunction. Adv Intern Med 27:151, 1982.
3. Postlethwait RW: Surgery of the Esophagus, 2nd ed. Norwalk, Connecticut, Appleton-Century-Crofts, 1986, pp 369–442.

4. Stair JM, Brian JE: The spectrum of esophageal carcinoma. J Arkansas Med Soc 82:107, 1985.

5. Galandiuk S, Hermann RE, Gassman JJ, et al: Cancer of the esophagus. The Cleveland Clinic experience. Ann Surg 203:101, 1986.

6. Pedersen H, Hansen HS, Cederqvist C, et al: The prognostic significance of weight loss and its integration in stage-grouping of oesophageal cancer. Acta Chir Scand 148:363, 1982.

7. Martini N, Goodner JT, D'Angio GJ, et al: Tracheoesophageal fistula due to cancer. J Thorac Cardiovasc Surg 59:319, 1970.

8. Duranceau A, Jamieson GG: Malignant tracheoesophageal fistula. Ann Thorac Surg 37:346, 1984.

9. Blot WJ, Devesa SS, Kneller RW, et al: Rising incidence of adenocarcinoma of the esophagus and gastric cardia. JAMA 265:1287, 1991.

10. Yang PC, Davis S: Incidence of cancer of the esophagus in the US by histologic type. Cancer 61:612, 1988.

11. Fleming JAC: Carcinoma of the thoracic oesophagus. Some notes on its pathology and spread in relation to treatment. Br J Radiol 16:212, 1943.

12. Rosenberg JC, Franklin R, Steiger Z: Squamous cell carcinoma of the thoracic esophagus: An interdisciplinary approach. Curr Probl Cancer 5:1, 1981.

13. Watson A: Pathologic changes affecting survival in esophageal cancer. In Delarue NC, Wilkins EW, Wong J (eds): Esophageal Cancer. International Trends in General Thoracic Surgery, Vol 4. St Louis, CV Mosby, 1988, pp 90–97.

14. Miller C: Carcinoma of thoracic oesophagus and cardia. A review of 405 cases. Br J Surg 49:507, 1962.

15. Sons HU, Borchard F: Cancer of the distal esophagus and cardia. Ann Surg 203:188, 1986.

16. Akiyama H: Surgery for Cancer of the Esophagus, 1st ed. Baltimore, Williams & Wilkins, 1990, pp 143–174.

17. Kato H, Watanabe H, Tachimori Y, et al: Evaluation of neck lymph node dissection for thoracic esophageal carcinoma. Ann Thorac Surg 51:931, 1991.

18. Akiyama H, Tsurumaru M, Kawamura T, et al: Principles of surgical treatment for carcinoma of the esophagus. Ann Surg 194:438, 1981.

19. Mandard AM, Chasle J, Marnay J, et al: Autopsy findings in 111 cases of esophageal cancer. Cancer 48:329, 1981.

20. Witt TR, Bains MS, Zaman MB, et al: Adenocarcinoma in Barrett's esophagus. J Thorac Cardiovasc Surg 85:337, 1983.

21. Kalish RJ, Clancy PE, Orringer MB, et al: Clinical, epidemiologic, and morphologic comparison between adenocarcinoma arising in Barrett's esophageal mucosa and in the gastric cardia. Gastroenterology 86:461, 1984.

22. Sanfey H, Hamilton SR, Smith RR, et al: Carcinoma arising in Barrett's esophagus. Surg Obstet Gynecol 161:570, 1985.

23. Streitz JM, Ellis FH, Gibb SP, et al: Adenocarcinoma in Barrett's esophagus. Ann Surg 213:122, 1991.

24. Achkar E, Carey W: The cost of surveillance for adenocarcinoma complicating Barrett's esophagus. Am J Gastroenterol 83:291, 1988.

25. Duhaylongsod FG, Wolfe WG: Barrett's esophagus and adenocarcinoma of the esophagus and gastroesophageal junction. J Thorac Cardiovasc Surg 102:36, 1991.

26. Adelstein DJ, Forman WB, Beavers B: Esophageal cancer. A six-year review of the Cleveland Veterans Administration Hospital experience. Cancer 54:918, 1984.

27. Shibuya H, Takagi M, Horiuchi J, et al: Carcinomas of the esophagus with synchronous or metachronous primary carcinoma in other organs. Acta Radiol Oncol 21:39, 1982.

28. Stone R, Rangel DM, Gordon HE, et al: Carcinoma of the gastroesophageal junction. A ten-year experience with esophagogastrectomy. Am J Surg 134:70, 1977.

29. Shapshay SM, Hong WK, Fried MP, et al: Simultaneous carcinomas of the esophagus and upper aerodigestive tract. Otolaryngol Head Neck Surg 88:373, 1980.

30. McGuirt WF, Matthews B, Koufman JA: Multiple simultaneous tumors in patients with head and neck cancer. Cancer 50:1195, 1982.

31. Shields TW: Squamous cell carcinoma of the esophagus. In Shields TW (ed): General Thoracic Surgery, 3rd ed. Philadelphia, Lea and Febiger, 1989, pp 1041–1059.

32. Heit HA, Johnson LF, Siegel SR, et al: Palliative dilation for dysphagia in esophageal carcinoma. Ann Intern Med 89:629, 1978.

33. Cassidy DE, Nord HJ, Boyce HW: Management of malignant esophageal strictures: Role of esophageal dilation and peroral prosthesis. Am J Gastroenterol 76:173, 1981.

34. Graham DY, Tabibian N, Schwartz JT, et al: Evaluation of the effectiveness of through-the-scope balloons as dilators of benign and malignant gastrointestinal strictures. Gastrointest Endosc 33:431, 1987.

35. Mandelstam P, Sugawa C, Silvis SE, et al: Complications associated with esophagogastroduodenoscopy and with esophageal dilation. Gastrointest Endosc 23:16, 1976.

36. Monnier PH, Hsiek V, Savary M: Endoscopic treatment of esophageal stenosis using Savary-Gilliard bougies: Technical innovations. Acta Endosc 15:119, 1985.

37. Webb WA: Esophageal dilatation: Personal experience with current instruments and techniques. Am J Gastroenterol 83:471, 1988.

38. Kozarek RA: Hydrostatic balloon dilation of gastrointestinal stenoses: A national survey. Gastrointest Endosc 32:15, 1986.

39. Boyce HW: Nonsurgical measures to relieve distresses of late esophageal carcinoma. Geriatrics 28:97, 1973.

40. Boyce HW: Palliation of advanced esophageal cancer. Semin Oncol 11:186, 1984.

41. Earlam R, Cunha-Melo JR: Malignant oesophageal strictures: A review of techniques for palliative intubation. Br J Surg 69:61, 1982.

42. Souttar HS: Method of intubating the oesophagus for malignant stricture. Br Med J 1:782, 1924.

43. Mousseau M, LeForestier J, Barbin J, et al: Place de l'intubation a demeure dans le traitement palliative du cancer de l'oesophage. Arch Mal Appar Digest 45:208, 1956.

44. Celestin LR: Permanent intubation in inoperable cancer of the oesophagus and cardia. A new tube. Ann R Coll Surg Engl 25:165, 1959.

45. Loizou LA, Rampton D, Bown SG: Treatment of malignant strictures of the cervical esophagus by endoscopic intubation using modified endoprosthesis. Gastrointest Endosc 38:158, 1992.

46. Palmer ED: Peroral prosthesis for management of incurable carcinoma. Am J Gastroenterol 59:487, 1973.

47. Den Hartog J, Bartelsman JFWM, Tytgat GNJ: Palliative treatment of obstructing esophagogastric malignancy by endoscopic positioning of a plastic prosthesis. Gastroenterology 77:1008, 1979.

48. Balmes JL, Adda M, Michel H: Traitement endoscopique des stenoses de l'oesophage par prosthese endoluminale. Rev Fr Gastroenterol 161:27, 1980.

49. Bergerault P, Denez B, Mahe J, et al: Prostheses endoesophagiennes de Celestin posees par voie endoscopique: Experience de 35 cas de cancers de l'oesophage. Ann Gastroenterol Hepatol 16:37, 1980.

50. Dunham F, Bourgeois N, Toussaint J, et al: Non-surgical plastic prosthesis as palliative treatment for inoperable gastro-esophageal malignant strictures. In Gerard A (ed): Progress and Perspectives in the Treatment of Gastrointestinal Tumors. New York, Pergamon Press, 1981, p 16.

51. Jones DB, Davies PS, Smith PM: Endoscopic insertion of palliative oesophagogastric neoplasm. Br J Surg 68:197, 1981.

52. Ogilvie AL, Dronfield MW, Ferguson R, et al: Palliative intubation of oesophagogastric neoplasms at fibreoptic endoscopy. Gut 23:1060, 1982.

53. Seifert E, Reinhard A, Luke A, et al: Palliative treatment of inoperable patients with carcinoma of the cardia region. Gastrointest Endosc 29:6, 1983.

54. Lux G, Groitl H, Riemann JR, et al: Tumor stenosis of the upper gastrointestinal tract; Nonsurgical therapy by bridging tubes. Endoscopy 15:207, 1983.

55. Rose JDR, Smith PM: Fibre endoscopic insertion of palliative oesophageal tubes with the Nottingham introducer. J R Soc Med 76:266, 1983.

56. Valbuena J: Endoscopic palliative treatment of esophageal and cardiac cancer: A new antireflux prosthesis. Cancer 53:993, 1984.

57. Chavy AL, Rougier MD, Pieddeloup SA, et al: Esophageal prosthesis for neoplastic stenosis. Cancer 57:1426, 1986.

58. Buset M, des Marez B, Baize M, et al: Palliative endoscopic management of obstructive esophagogastric cancer: Laser or prosthesis? Gastrointest Endosc 33:357, 1987.

59. Gasparri G, Casalegno PA, Camandona M, et al: Endoscopic insertion of 248 prostheses in inoperable carcinoma of the esophagus and cardia: Short-term and long-term results. Gastrointest Endosc 33:354, 1987.

60. Angorn IB, Haffejee AA: Endoesophageal intubation for palliation in obstructing esophageal carcinoma. *In* Delarue NC, Wilkins EW, Wong J (eds): Esophageal Cancer. International Trends in General Thoracic Surgery, Vol 4. St. Louis, CV Mosby, 1988, p 410.

61. Függer R, Niederle B, Jantsch H, et al: Endoscopic tube implantation for the palliation of malignant esophageal stenosis. Endoscopy 22:101, 1990.

62. Cusumano A, Ruol A, Segalin A: Push-through intubation: Effective palliation in 409 patients with cancer of the esophagus and cardia. Ann Thorac Surg 53:1010, 1992.

63. Reed CE, Marsh WH, Carlson LS, et al: Prospective, randomized trial of palliative treatment for unresectable cancer of the esophagus. Ann Thorac Surg 51:552, 1991.

64. Kratz JM, Reed CE, Crawford FA, et al: A comparison of endoesophageal tubes: Improved results with the Atkinson tube. J Thorac Cardiovasc Surg 97:19, 1989.

65. Kozarek RA, Ball TJ, Patterson DJ: Metallic self-expanding stent application in the upper gastrointestinal tract: Caveats and concerns. Gastrointest Endosc 38:1, 1992.

66. Neuhaus H: Metal esophageal stents. Semin Intervention Radiol 8:305, 1991.

67. Schaer J, Katon RM, Ivancev K, et al: Treatment of malignant esophageal obstruction with silicone-coated metallic self-expanding stents. Gastrointest Endosc 38:7, 1992.

68. Song H-Y, Choi K-C, Cho B-H, et al: Esophagogastric neoplasms: Palliation with a modified Gianturco stent. Endoscopy 180:349, 1991.

69. Knyrim K, Wagner HJ, Pausch J, et al: Expandable metal stents for the palliative treatment of esophageal obstruction. Gastrointest Endosc 36:236, 1990.

70. Fleischer D, Sivak MB: Endoscopic Nd:YAG laser therapy as palliation for esophagogastric cancer: Parameters affecting initial outcome. Gastroenterology 89:827, 1985.

71. Fleischer D, Kessler F, Haye O: Endoscopic Nd:YAG laser therapy for carcinoma of the esophagus: A new palliative approach. Am J Surg 143:280, 1982.

72. Harrell JH: Nd:YAG laser therapy in pulmonary medicine. West J Med 149:113, 1988.

73. Pietrafitta JJ, Dwyer RM: New laser technique for the treatment of malignant esophageal obstruction. J Surg Oncol 35:157, 1987.

74. Pietrafitta JJ, Bowers GJ, Dwyer RM: Prograde versus retrograde endoscopic laser therapy for treatment of malignant esophageal obstruction: A comparison of techniques. Lasers Surg Med 8:288, 1988.

75. Redford CM, Ahlquist DA, Gostout CG: Prospective comparison of contact with noncontact Nd:YAG laser therapy for palliation of esophageal carcinoma. Gastrointest Endosc 35:394, 1989.

76. Ell C, Hochberger J: Contact versus noncontact laser therapy. Gastrointest Endosc 33:125, 1987.

77. Mellow MH, Pinkas H: Endoscopic laser therapy for malignancies affecting the esophagus and gastroesophageal junction: Analysis of technical and functional efficacy. Arch Intern Med 145:1443, 1985.

78. Lightdale CJ, Zimbalist E, Winawer SJ: Outpatient management of esophageal cancer with endoscopic Nd:YAG laser. Am J Gastroenterol 82:46, 1987.

79. Murray FE, Bowers GJ, Birkett DH, et al: Palliative laser therapy of advanced esophageal carcinoma: An alternative approach. Am J Gastroenterol 83:816, 1988.

80. Jensen DM, Machicado G, Randall G, et al: Comparison of low-power YAG laser and BICAP probe for palliation of esophageal cancer strictures. Gastroenterology 94:1263, 1988.

81. Krasner N, Barr H, Skidmore C, et al: Palliative laser therapy for malignant dysphagia. Gut 28:792, 1987.

82. Goldberg SJ, King KH: Endoscopic Nd:YAG laser coagulation as palliative therapy for obstructing esophageal carcinoma. Am J Gastroenterol 81:629, 1986.

83. Bown SG, Hawes R, Matthewson K, et al: Endoscopic laser palliation for advanced malignant dysphagia. Gut 28:799, 1987.

84. Cello JP, Gerstenberger PD, Wright T, et al: Endoscopic Nd:YAG laser palliation of non-resectable esophageal malignancy. Ann Intern Med 102:610, 1985.

85. Jung SS, Wieman TJ: Endoscopic Nd:YAG laser therapy for advanced esophageal cancer. J Kent Med Assoc 86:405, 1988.

86. Wolf EL, Frager J, Brandt LJ, et al: Radiographic appearance of the esophagus and stomach after laser treatment of obstructing carcinoma. AJR 146:519, 1986.

87. Ahlquist DA, Gostout CJ, Viggiano TR, et al: Endoscopic laser palliation of malignant dysphagia: A prospective study. Mayo Clin Proc 62:867, 1987.

88. Pass HI, Reed CE: Lasers in the management of upper aerodigestive malignancies. *In* DeVita VT, Hellman S, Rosenberg SA (eds): Important Advances in Oncology 1990. Philadelphia, JB Lippincott, 1990, pp 159–179.

89. Ell CH, Deming L: Laser therapy of tumor stenoses in the upper gastrointestinal tract: An international enquiry. Lasers Surg Med 7:491, 1987.

90. Rontal E, Rontal M, Jacob HJ: Laser palliation for esophageal carcinoma. Laryngoscope 96:846, 1986.

91. Bader M, Dittler HJ, Ultsch B, et al: Palliative treatment of malignant stenoses of the upper gastrointestinal tract using a combination of laser and afterloading therapy. Endoscopy 18:27, 1986.

92. Low DE, Pagliero KM: Prospective randomized clinical trial comparing brachytherapy and laser photoablation for palliation of esophageal cancer. J Thorac Cardiovasc Surg 104:173, 1992.

93. McCaughan JS, Williams TE, Bethel BH: Palliation of esophageal malignancy with photodynamic therapy. Ann Thorac Surg 40:113, 1985.

94. McCaughan JS, Nims TA, Guy GT, et al: Photodynamic therapy for esophageal tumors. Arch Surg 124:74, 1989.

95. Likier HM, Levine JG, Lightdale CJ: Photodynamic therapy for completely obstructing esophageal carcinoma. Gastrointest Endosc 37:75, 1991.

96. Thomas RJ, Abbott M, Bhathal PS, et al: High-dose photoirradiation of esophageal cancer. Ann Surg 206:193, 1987.

97. Heier SK, Rothman K, Rosenthal WS, et al: Photodynamic therapy for obstructing esophageal malignancies: Efficacy and light dosimetry analysis. Gastrointest Endosc 36:225, 1990.

98. Johnston JH, Fleischer D, Petrini J: Palliative bipolar electrocoagulation therapy of obstructing esophageal cancer. Gastrointest Endosc 36:349, 1987.

99. Angelini G, Pasni AF, Ederle A, et al: Nd:YAG laser versus polidocanol injection for palliation of esophageal malignancy: A prospective, randomized study. Gastrointest Endosc 37:607, 1991.

100. Sander R, Hagenmuellar F, Sander C, et al: Laser versus laser plus afterloading with iridium-192 in the palliative treatment of malignant stenosis of the esophagus: A prospective, randomized, controlled study. Gastrointest Endosc 37:433, 1991.

22 DIAGNOSTIC IMAGING OF ESOPHAGEAL CANCER

Gerald D. Dodd and Marvin H. Chasen

RADIOLOGIC DIAGNOSIS

Conventional Radiography

Most esophageal cancers are moderately well advanced when first seen, and virtually all patients are symptomatic. Approximately 50% of symptomatic individuals have abnormal chest radiographs. The most frequent finding is an abnormal azygoesophageal recess followed by widening of the mediastinum or posterior tracheal indentation, or both (Fig. 22–1). Associated complications may include bronchoesophageal fistula, tracheoesophageal fistula, and aortic erosion.[1]

The azygoesophageal recess is readily demonstrable by computed tomography (CT). It is seen as an arc with the convexity directed to the left and extending in a caudal direction from the azygos arch. When the convexity is directed toward the right, one should suspect an abnormality in the mediastinum (Figs. 22–2A, B). Causes include esophageal cancer, enlarged subcarinal lymph nodes, bronchogenic cysts, massive left pleural effusion, and atrial enlargement.

The radiologic anatomy of the retrotracheal soft tissue stripe has been described by Bachman and Teixidor[2] and Putman and associates.[3] According to Bachman, the posterior tracheal stripe may be observed on the lateral chest radiograph in 91% of normal individuals, usually as a band not more than 3 mm in thickness. It is seen as the result of the interface between the right posterior tracheal wall and the pleura covering that portion of the upper lobe that lies in the retrotracheal recess (Fig. 22–3). Thickening may be due to infiltrating cancer (Fig. 22–4). According to Putman, this thickening may antedate symp-

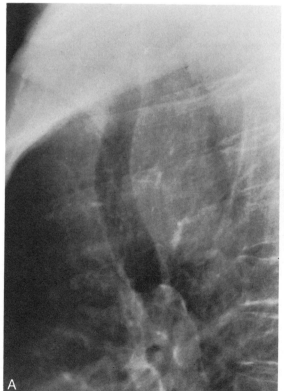

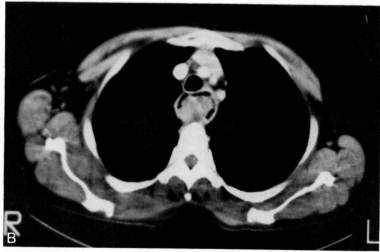

FIGURE 22–1. Leiomyosarcoma of the esophagus. *A,* Lateral chest film. The trachea is bowed anteriorly by mass in the esophagus. *B,* CT scan. The esophagus is dilated by a multilobular mass with anterior displacement of the trachea.

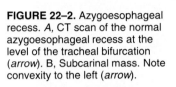

FIGURE 22–2. Azygoesophageal recess. *A*, CT scan of the normal azygoesophageal recess at the level of the tracheal bifurcation (*arrow*). B, Subcarinal mass. Note convexity to the left (*arrow*).

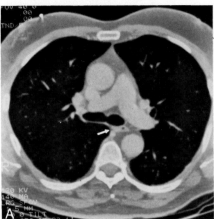
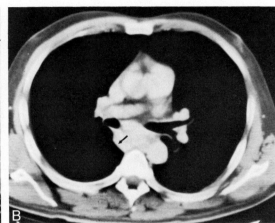

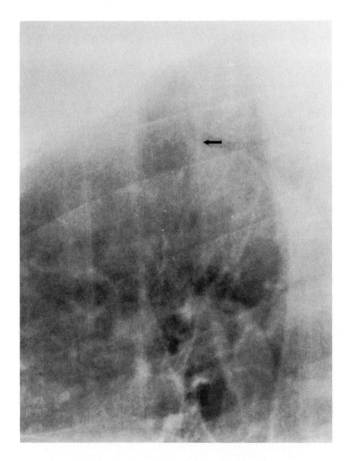

FIGURE 22–3. Retrotracheal stripe. Lateral chest film. The retrotracheal stripe is a thin structure immediately behind the tracheal air column (*arrow*).

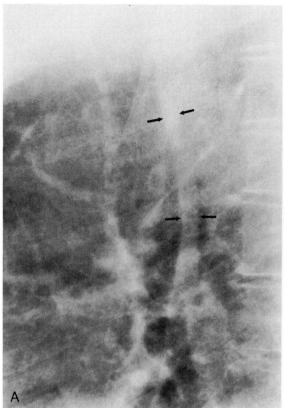

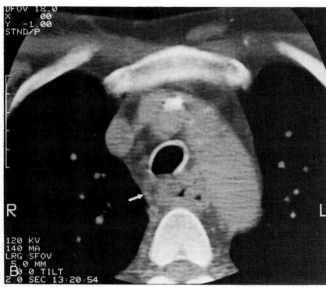

FIGURE 22–4. Carcinoma of the esophagus. *A,* Lateral chest film. The posterior tracheal stripe is thickened. Thickening of the tracheoesophageal stripe is also present (*arrows*). *B,* Computed tomography. There is irregular thickening of the esophageal wall with obliteration of the tracheoesophageal recess of the right upper lobe (*arrow*).

toms by as much as 6 months. In Lindell's series, absence of the above-mentioned signs did not indicate a better prognosis.

Patients with complications may have normal chest films or parenchymal infiltrates in various locations. Tracheoesophageal and bronchoesophageal fistulas are suggested by the clinical symptoms and are readily demonstrated by contrast studies of the esophagus (Fig. 22–5).

Contrast Esophagography

Contrast examination of the esophagus is a sensitive technique but requires careful attention to detail.[4] A routine must be devised and carefully followed if a reasonable proportion of lesions is to be detected. Once an abnormality is identified, an effort must be made to obtain the following:

1. Views of the lesion in different degrees of obliquity, taking care to include en face as well as profile projections.
2. A sufficient number of films to show the mucous membrane of the entire esophagus with emphasis on the mucosa surrounding the lesion. Early manifestations of neoplasia may be subtle and may require detailed inspection of the entire mucous membrane.
3. Films in all projections with complete distention of the esophagus.
4. If a malignant lesion is present, an attempt should be made to elicit criteria of resectability, such

as the presence of lymph node metastases, involvement of the major airways, paralysis of the recurrent laryngeal nerve, and diaphragmatic paralysis (Fig. 22–6).

Double-contrast esophagography has proved useful in securing maximum distention and in elucidating the morphologic characteristics of obvious lesions. It is particularly valuable in the diagnosis of small abnormalities and in differentiating mucosal masses from those arising in the extramucosal layers.

In general, double-contrast studies are best performed with the patient in the upright position, but a complete examination should include fluoroscopy and single-contrast radiographs in the prone position. This biphasic approach affords maximum information with regard to morphology and function.

It is usually possible to distinguish between nonadherent extrinsic masses and those that arise from the wall of the esophagus. The differentiation of true intramural tumors from adherent extraesophageal masses may be more difficult. The distinction between mucosal and extramucosal tumors is critical and is based primarily on mucosal integrity; with very small lesions, a differential diagnosis by radiologic means may not be possible. The differential diagnosis of mucosal and extramucosal lesions is based on the marginal appearance of a mass, including the angle formed with the wall of the esophagus. With benign intramural or adherent extraesophageal masses, the edges of the defect are usually smooth and semicir-

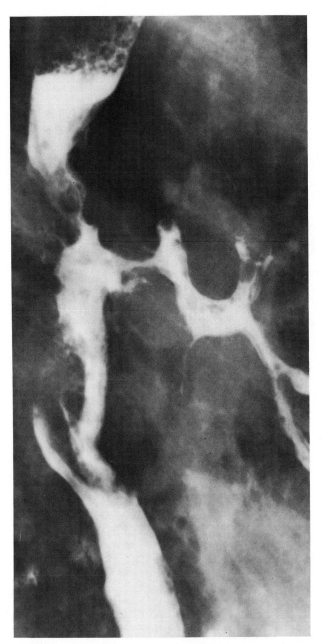

FIGURE 22–5. Carcinoma of the esophagus with bronchoesophageal fistula. A long, ulcerating cancer has eroded into the left main bronchus.

cular, forming a right or slightly obtuse angle with the esophageal wall (Fig. 22–7A).[5] Occasionally, an extra-esophageal soft tissue component can be visualized. This depends on the esophageal tissue layer from which the tumor arose or its origin external to the esophagus.

Ulceration is uncommon with benign extramucosal masses and the smooth integrity of the mucous membrane is best demonstrated by the double-contrast techniques. Conversely, irregularities or defects in the mucosa can be readily appreciated, a finding usually indicative of a proliferative process that has either arisen from the mucous membrane or invaded it (Fig. 22–7B).

Benign polypoid masses arising from the mucous membrane commonly occur in the upper third of the esophagus and may be multiple. Very large, pedunculated mucosal tumors have been reported that have caused obstruction (Fig. 22–8A), have been aspirated, or have been regurgitated through the mouth. The presence of a stalk is usually sufficient to identify the mucosal origin of the mass, but if it is sessile, differentiation from a carcinoma or leiomyosarcoma may be difficult (Fig. 22–8B).

The gross pathologic forms of epidermoid carcinoma of the esophagus vary considerably, but three major types have been described[6, 7]:

1. Polypoid: This form is most common, occurring in about 60% of patients.[7] Initially, a nodular or fungating lesion protrudes into the lumen, with interruption of the normal mucous membrane pattern at the point of origin. The outline of the mass is usually irregular owing to superficial erosion or frank ulceration, or both (Fig. 22–9). The tumor may eventually encircle the esophageal wall or obstruct the lumen by its sheer bulk (Fig. 22–10) So-called varicoid carcinoma may represent a form of polypoid disease (Fig. 22–11) or, alternatively, infiltrative disease.

2. Ulcerative: Approximately 25% of esophageal cancers present as a deeply excavating ulcer.[7] There is abrupt transition from normal to abnormal mucous membrane, usually with a steeply rolled margin of

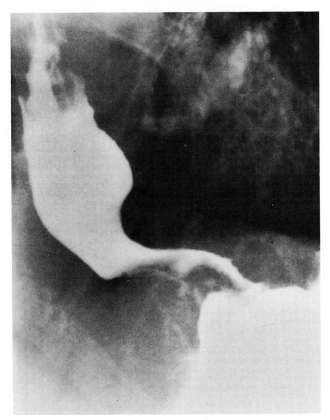

FIGURE 22–6. Carcinoma of the distal esophagus with subdiaphragmatic node involvement. The subdiaphragmatic portion of the esophagus is elevated and compressed by an enlarged node. There is also compression of the gastric fundus.

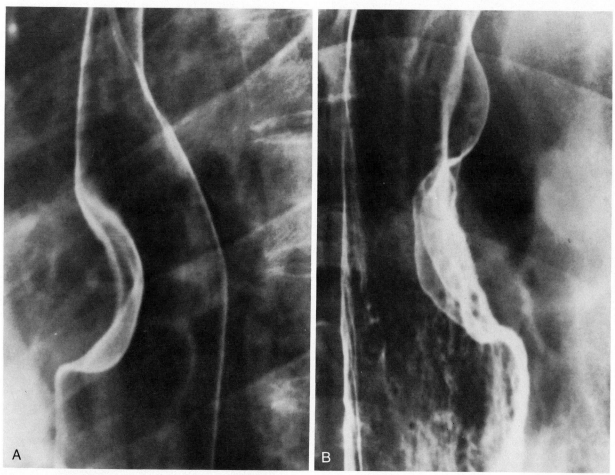

FIGURE 22–7. Differentiation of mucosal and extramucosal lesions. *A,* Leiomyoma of the esophagus. The mass is covered by smooth, intact mucosa with sharp delineation from the adjacent normal esophagus. *B,* Adenocarcinoma of the esophagus. The intraluminal margin appears smooth owing to submucosal extension, but there is central irregularity and ulceration.

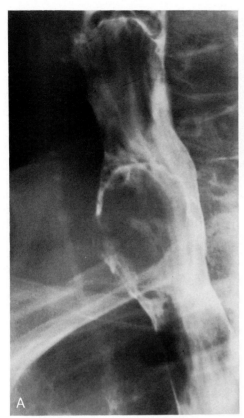

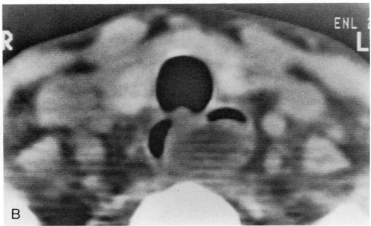

FIGURE 22–8. Epithelial polyps with early malignant degeneration. *A*, Esophagram. Dilatation and partial obstruction of the esophagus by a lobulated mass. *B*, CT scan. The esophagus is distended by a large soft tissue mass. A pedicle is clearly shown opposite the posterior tracheal wall.

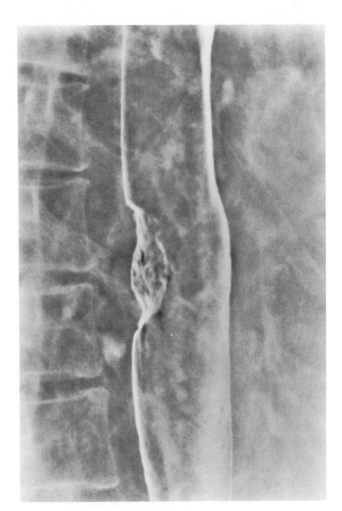

FIGURE 22–9. Polypoid epidermoid carcinoma of the esophagus.

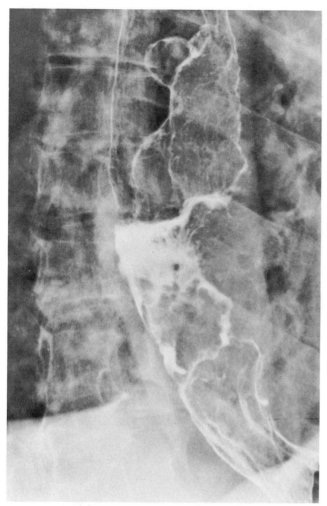

FIGURE 22–10. Adenocarcinoma of the esophagus. The lumen of the lower one-third is filled with tumor. A hiatal hernia is present with early retrograde invasion of the stomach.

tumor about the edge of the ulcer (Fig. 22–12) The margins may or may not be nodular depending on the propensity of the tumor to extend submucosally. Usually, there are mucosal abnormalities about the ulceration, and the overall appearance of the cancer may meet the criteria of the classic Carman-Kirklin complex (Fig. 22–13). The ulcerations may be extremely large and may erode into the respiratory tree or aorta (see Fig. 22–5).

3. Infiltrative or stenosing: The infiltrative forms produce a tapered narrowing not unlike that seen in benign inflammatory processes. The mucosa in the area of primary involvement may be relatively normal or show fine serrations or distortions that are useful for differential diagnostic purposes. These are best shown with double-contrast techniques (Fig. 22–14). Frank ulceration may occur.

Annular constrictions are common presenting forms of esophageal cancer. In general, they are late manifestations of one of the basic morphologic types and are similar in appearance to annular cancers elsewhere in the gastrointestinal tract. The mucosa of the

involved area is characteristically destroyed, producing an irregular nodular pattern. The area of involvement may be long, and the edges of the cancer are frequently characterized by shelving margins.

Although these are the classic morphologic presentations of carcinoma of the esophagus, they represent advanced disease, and one form often overlaps another. The patients are usually symptomatic, and the overall survival rate is less than 5%.

Double-contrast techniques permit the identification of much smaller cancers (Fig. 22–15) These diagnoses, in patients with no symptoms or minimal symptoms, do improve survival but not to the extent that might be hoped. It is important to recognize that the descriptive terms small or early as used radiologically do not necessarily correspond to early carcinoma in the histopathologic sense. Zornoza and Lindell[8] reported on a series of 11 patients with cancers ranging from 0.8 cm to 3.5 cm on representative films. One individual declined treatment, and a second died from a myocardial infarction. In the remaining nine,

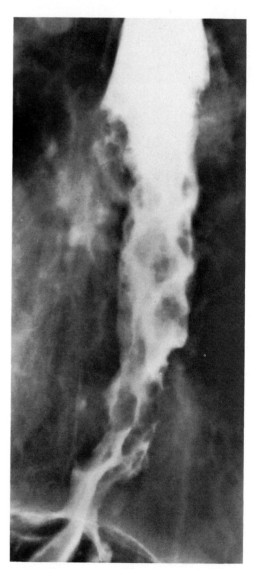

FIGURE 22–11. Varicoid epidermoid carcinoma.

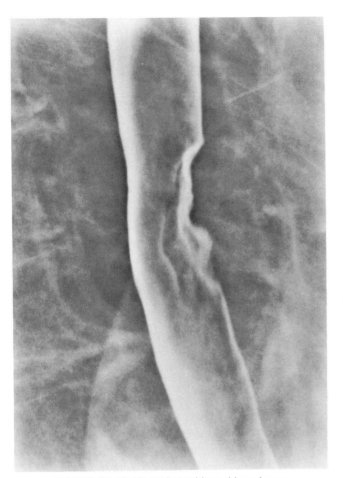

FIGURE 22–12. Ulcerating epidermoid carcinoma.

lated to the esophagus or as a survey in patients known to be at increased risk, usually because of a history of squamous cell carcinoma elsewhere in the head and neck area.[11] In Sugimachi's series of patients with early stage lesions, seven patients with cancer confined to the epithelium or muscularis mucosa were without symptoms. However, of the 35 patients with submucosal spread of the cancer, 26 or 74.3% had subjective symptoms such as slight dysphasia, chest discomfort or pyrosis.[9]

The incidence of adenocarcinoma of the esophagus has been estimated to be between 1% and 19%.[10, 12] According to Blot and colleagues,[13] there has been a steady rise in the rate of adenocarcinoma from 1966 to 1987. The increase among men ranges from 4% to 10% per year, exceeding any other type of cancer. By contrast, the incidence of squamous cell carcinoma of the esophagus has been relatively stable. The disease has been disproportionately observed in white men and rarely in women. Although up to 76% of these tumors are of gastric origin, the remainder arise predominantly from esophageal columnar (Barrett's esophagus) epithelium. As noted, primary adenocarcinomas rarely originate from esophageal mucus-secreting glands.[14, 15] Grossly, adenocarcinoma of the proximal esophagus is indistinguishable from the

the average survival time was 12.5 months. All deaths in the latter group were directly related to metastatic disease. By contrast, Sugimachi and colleagues[9] have reported a 56.7% 5-year survival rate in patients with early-stage esophageal carcinomas histologically confined to the intraepithelium, mucosa, or submucosa. In patients with invasion of the muscularis propria or deeper, the same author found a 15.6% 5-year survival rate. In general, the early-stage cancers described by Sugimachi and his coworkers were smaller than those reported by Zornoza and Lindell, but Levine and coworkers have reported instances of histologically early cancer in masses as large as 4.5 cm.[10]

It is interesting that the morphologic appearance of the smaller lesions tends to parallel that of the larger cancers, i.e., plaquelike or polypoid intraluminal defects, and depressed or infiltrating lesions with or without central ulceration and without a significant mass component (see Fig. 22–12). Superficial disease may not be apparent radiologically in the earlier stages but eventually exhibits a granular pattern without encroachment on the lumen. Such lesions are difficult, if not impossible, to detect consistently with conventional solid-column techniques and, in the absence of symptoms, would not normally be subject to endoscopic examination. In three of the four instances illustrated, the lesions were incidental to a gastrointestinal examination performed for symptoms unre-

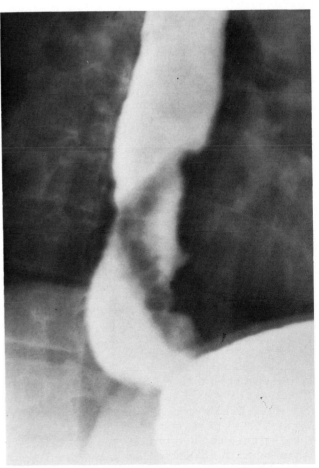

FIGURE 22–13. Ulcerating epidermoid carcinoma. The large, plaquelike ulcer is surrounded by a cuff of tumor, producing a typical Carman-Kirklin sign.

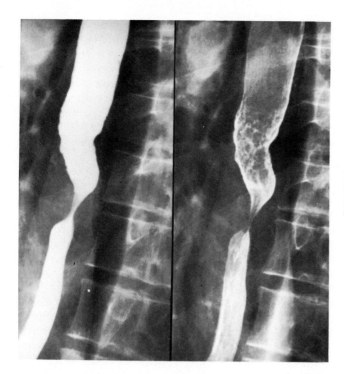

FIGURE 22–14. Infiltrating epidermoid carcinoma. There is no mass component, but slight marginal irregularities are seen in the single-contrast study. Marked mucosal distortion is apparent in the double-contrast image.

squamous cell variety, and when the esophagogastric junction is involved, there is no radiologic means of differentiating between gastric and esophageal tumors. However, in each instance, the prognosis is the same for tumors of a similar stage.

In a series of 17 cases of adenocarcinoma of the esophagus reported from the University of Texas M. D. Anderson Cancer Center,[16] hiatal hernia was the most frequently associated finding, followed by esophageal stricture, gastroesophageal reflux, and severe esophagitis with or without ulceration (Fig. 22–16). Ulceration was present in approximately one-third of patients. Despite the often repeated statement that Barrett's epithelium is prone to occur in the middle third of the esophagus, involvement of the esophagogastric junction is more common. In the M. D. Anderson Cancer Center series, nine of the adenocarcinomas arose from the region of the esophagogastric junction. Only one was seen in the proximal esophagus (immediately below the crycopharyngeus), four in the middle esophagus, and two at the junction of the middle and distal thirds of the esophagus. Mass or wall infiltration was demonstrable in all cases. The proximal tumors were grossly similar to epidermoid carcinomas, and the possibility of adenocarcinoma could only be suggested on the basis of secondary findings. Levine and his coworkers[17] have described a villous mucosal pattern that may be found in approximately one-third of cases of columnar dysplasia. This may have the same significance as villous tumors elsewhere in the gastrointestinal tract and is helpful in suggesting the histologic type of an associated tumor. It is also useful as an indicator of premalignant disease or early malignancy. (Fig. 22–17).

Carcinosarcoma of the esophagus is a reputedly un-

common tumor in which both epithelial and connective tissue components can be demonstrated.[18, 19] The lesion commonly presents in the lower third of the esophagus as a bulky, polypoid growth that can expand and obstruct the esophageal lumen. The surfaces are frequently irregular. The configuration and location of these tumors may suggest the histologic diagnosis, but in general, they resemble bulky carcinomas and a precise radiologic diagnosis is not possible (Fig. 22–18). Indeed, the histologic demonstration of transition from typical squamous carcinoma to a sarcomatous component in resected specimens, as well as related ultrastructure observations, has led to the suggestion that the sarcomatous component may represent mesenchymal metaplasia of the squamous epithelium.[20]

Primary small cell carcinomas comprise approximately 2.5% of all esophageal cancers. The tumors are often large and frequently occur in the middle or lower thirds of the esophagus. There are no radiologic features which clearly distinguish small cell carcinomas from the more common types of esophageal cancer (Fig. 22–19).[6]

Extrinsic lymphomatous masses may displace the esophagus but seldom cause significant dysphagia. The lymphoid tissue of the esophagus is sparse, and therefore primary or secondary involvement by lymphoma is rare. All histologic varieties may occur, and as with lymphomas elsewhere in the gastrointestinal tract, a wide morphologic spectrum occurs. Any segment of the esophagus may be involved, and appearances may include nodular forms, thickened folds, or bulky mass. Ulceration is relatively uncommon (Fig. 22–20).[21]

The esophagus can be involved by neoplasms that

FIGURE 22–15. Small epidermoid cancers. *A,* Small, elevated plaquelike defect *(arrow)* on the anterior esophageal wall. *B,* Multiple intraluminal defects with wall invasion. *C,* Superficial posterior wall cancer with a small area of ulceration. *D,* Multiple cancers (four) with central ulceration.

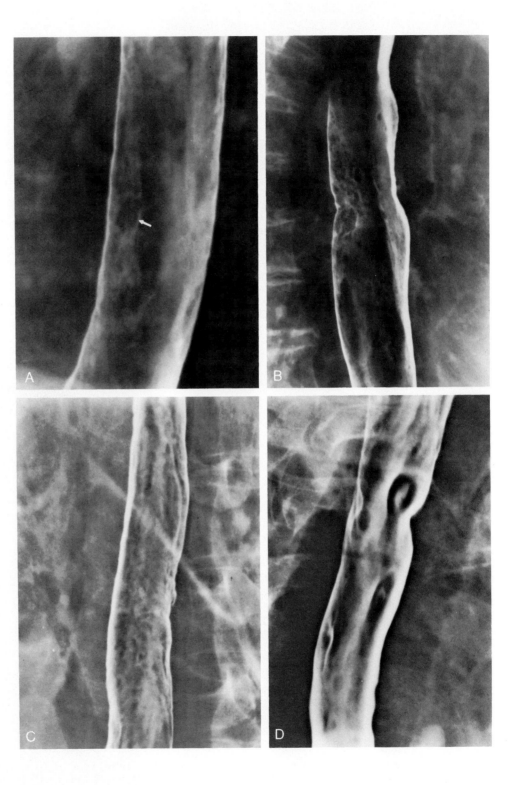

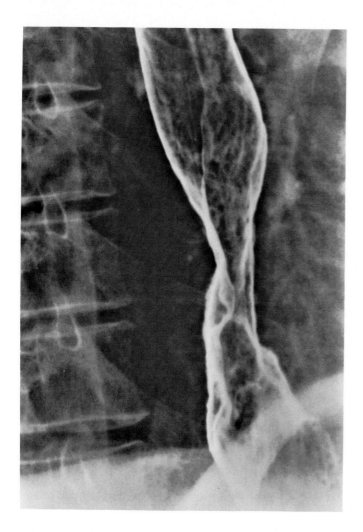

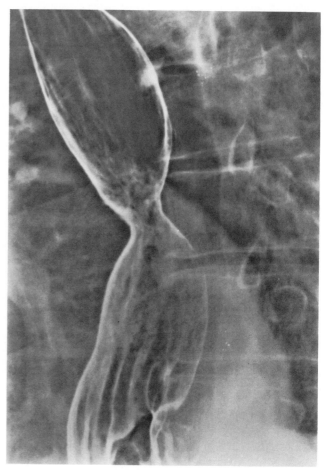

FIGURE 22–16. Extensive adenocarcinoma of the esophagogastric junction. Infiltrating tumor involves both the distal esophagus and herniated stomach.

FIGURE 22–17. Adenocarcinoma of the esophagogastric junction. Hiatal hernia with stricture and Barrett's epithelium at the esophagogastric junction. Histologically, early malignant degeneration was present in the metaplastic epithelium.

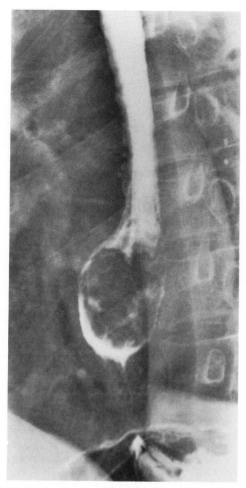

FIGURE 22–18. Carcinosarcoma of distal esophagus. The mass is irregular; it expands and partially obstructs the lumen.

plicable because lymph nodes cannot be adequately assessed prior to a surgical procedure. Moss et al.[22] have therefore introduced a modified staging classification based on CT capabilities, with Stage 1 represented by intraluminal mass; Stage 2, by mass with wall thickening; Stage 3, by direct local invasion; and Stage 4, by distant metastases. Stages 1 and 2 are considered potentially curable, whereas Stages 3 and 4 are candidates for palliation.

In 60% of scans, the esophagus is seen by virtue of intraluminal air.[23] The wall should be less than 3 mm in thickness.[24] If it is not distended, an estimate of the wall thickness is difficult, but the external margins of the esophagus are usually demarcated by fat from the surrounding mediastinal structures. Blurring of these margins coupled with thickening of the wall beyond 5 mm are reliable indicators of esophageal disease (Fig. 22–22).[25] Extension of tumor through the muscle coat is classified as a Stage 3 tumor. Other criteria of

originate in other organs. Involvement via the mediastinal nodes is relatively common in patients with carcinoma of the lung and carcinoma of the breast and may also occur with tumors of the ovary, testes, and cervix and with melanoma. The possibility of involvement by mediastinal nodes can be suggested by the large extramural component, coupled with localized breakdown of the mucous membrane (Fig. 22–21). If diffuse invasion of the mucous membrane has occurred, differentiation from primary carcinoma of the esophagus may not be possible by radiologic means and endoscopic biopsy is necessary for diagnostic purposes.

STAGING

Computed Tomography

CT is of limited value in the detection and diagnosis of carcinoma of the esophagus. The procedure is expensive and time consuming and is not useful in detecting or resolving the morphologic characteristics of smaller cancers. The examination is, however, of value for pretreatment staging. The TNM system is not ap-

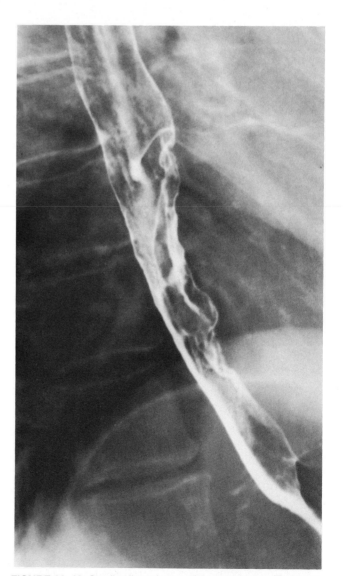

FIGURE 22–19. Small cell carcinoma of the esophagus. There are mixed mucosal and submucosal elements, but the radiologic findings are not specific.

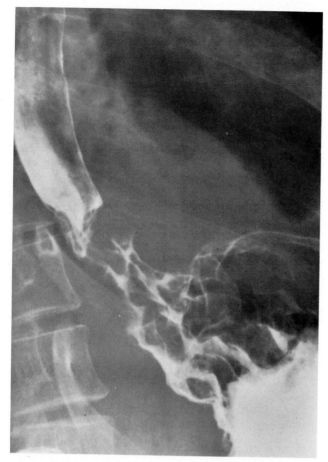

FIGURE 22–20. Lymphoma of the gastroesophageal junction. Thickened nodular folds are present in both the distal esophagus and the stomach, and the caliber of the esophagus is decreased. The findings are nonspecific.

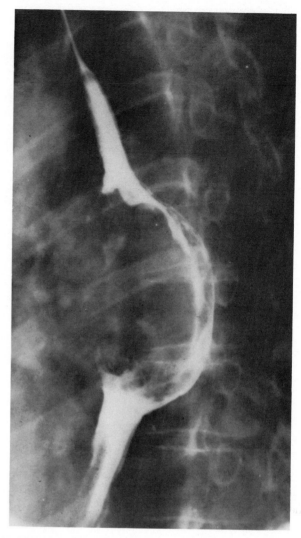

FIGURE 22–21. Carcinoma of the cervix metastatic to mediastinal nodes. The roentgen characteristics are similar to those of an intramural tumor indicating invasion of the esophageal wall.

Stage 3 disease include bowing of the posterior wall of the trachea or left main bronchus or disruption of the fat plane (Fig. 22–23).

Obliteration of the fat plane between the esophagus and aorta for a distance equal to 90 degrees of the circumference of the aorta is considered suggestive of invasion of the aortic wall. Below 45 degrees is normal, whereas 45 to 90 degrees is indeterminate. Aortic invasion is found in only 2% of patients at postmortem and hence is an uncommon radiologic observation.[26]

The assessment of lymph node metastases is of great importance, but CT has proved a disappointment in this respect. It cannot identify tumor in lymph nodes of normal size, nor can it differentiate between nodes enlarged by metastatic tumor and those that are hyperplastic. However, CT can demonstrate infiltration of soft tissues (Fig. 22–23), erosion of vertebral bodies, and the presence of liver metastases with reasonable specificity.

The reported accuracy of CT in the staging of carcinoma of the esophagus varies considerably and has been summarized by Rankin.[27] Early studies were encouraging with a sensitivity for tracheobronchial invasion ranging between 83% and 100%; specificity,

75% to 100%; and accuracy, 88% to 93%. The corresponding figures for aortic invasion were 92% to 100%, 83% to 89% and 90% to 94%.[26, 28–31]

Results were less satisfactory with mediastinal

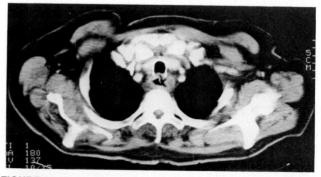

FIGURE 22–22. Wall thickening in esophageal carcinoma. CT scan of the thick, irregular esophageal wall with poor definition of some aspects of surrounding fat.

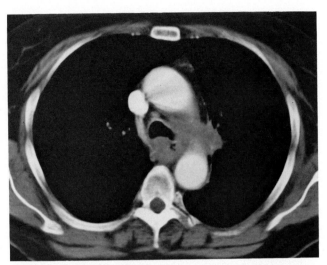

FIGURE 22–23. Stage 3 esophageal carcinoma. CT scan of esophageal carcinoma invading into surrounding structures. Note bowing of posterior tracheal wall and tumor infiltration into the aorticopulmonic window obliterating normal fat in the area.

nodes; sensitivity was 61%, specificity was 60%, and accuracy was 61%.[27] Results were somewhat better for abdominal lymphadenopathy, with reported accuracies between 78% and 85%.[30, 32, 33]

Other studies, including those conducted more recently, have been less encouraging, with 61% of tumors incorrectly staged according to the Moss classification and 44% incorrectly staged on the basis of the TNM classification. An accuracy of only 39% was obtained for the abdominal nodes.[31] Quint and associates[33] also found a low accuracy for lymph node status and aortic invasion with numerous indeterminate results. There was little difference between CT and magnetic resonance imaging (MRI).[34]

In general, CT is less accurate in assessing tumors of the gastroesophageal junction, with accuracy increasing with the more proximal position of a tumor. Rankin[27] has concluded that the examination is best employed to separate patients into three groups. The first consists of those without evidence of extraesophageal disease; the second, those with obvious mediastinal involvement or distant metastases; and third, those with indeterminate scans who require exploratory surgery. In summary, the use of CT has added an additional parameter to the preoperative assessment of patients with esophageal carcinoma. Despite its limitations, it has, for practical purposes, replaced older imaging procedures such as azygography, pneumomediastinum, and conventional tomography.

Magnetic Resonance Imaging

MRI suffers from the same limitations as CT in the detection and diagnosis of esophageal cancer. Reports dealing with MRI as a staging modality are few in number but do provide an indication of its usefulness. Initial reports were pessimistic, possibly because of the lack of cardiorespiratory gating and the inclusion of gastroesophageal cancers in the series.[34, 35]

Recent series have been more optimistic. Petrillo and coworkers[36] have applied interpretive criteria similar to those used with CT. Tracheobronchial infiltration is assumed when interruption of the fat plane can be demonstrated in conjunction with a concave profile of the posterior tracheal wall due to extrinsic compression. The presence of both criteria is considered more reliable than either criterion alone (Fig. 22–24).

The aortic wall is presumed to be infiltrated when the angle of contact between its circumference and the tumor is over 90 degrees. Invasion of the periesophageal adipose tissue is assumed in the presence of esophageal profile irregularities and the absence of regional fat.

Mediastinal lymph nodes with diameters exceeding 10 mm are considered metastatic. Esophageal diameters are considered normal up to 28 mm in the transverse plane and 20 mm in the anteroposterior aspect.

In the experience of Petrillo and his coworkers, all esophageal masses with a transverse diameter of more than 40 mm had extraluminal extension at surgery and they suggest that this dimension can be used as a predictor of extraluminal disease despite the lack of other criteria.

The authors found MRI to provide good results in the evaluation of resectability in 75% of cases. In four false-negative cases, which resulted from minimal adipose infiltration, the histologic result did not prevent radical surgery. The addition of these cases increased the accuracy of the prediction of resectability to 84%.

Overall accuracy was found to be 91% as compared with previously published results of 65% to 75%.[35] The worst results were obtained with lymph node metastases. Interpretation was based on size alone; the hoped for tissue-differentiating capability of MRI has not been found useful in the evaluation of lymph nodes.

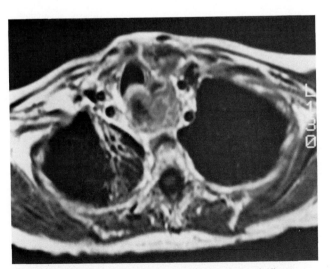

FIGURE 22–24. MRI of esophageal carcinoma. Large bulky esophageal mass bowing the posterior tracheal wall and obliterating aspects of surrounding fat. The trachea was found to be infiltrated by tumor at bronchoscopy.

Takashima and colleagues[37] have reported a prospective study of CT and MRI, comparing their ability to determine resectability in patients with carcinoma of the esophagus. The same criteria were used for both imaging modalities and were essentially the same as the criteria used by Petrillo and associates.[36] Sensitivity, specificity, and accuracy for resectability were 100%, 84%, and 87%, respectively, for MRI; for CT, the comparable figures were 100%, 80%, and 84%. It was concluded that MRI and CT have nearly the same accuracy.

Overall, it would appear that CT and MRI have essentially the same capabilities in staging carcinoma of the esophagus. Both have limitations in the staging of tumors involving the esophagogastric junction and, with the exception of one reported series,[29] neither modality is considered optimum for staging purposes in this area.

Although technical improvements continue in both CT and MRI systems, they have not significantly affected the staging capabilities of either modality.[38] Both are most effective when used in conjunction with barium contrast studies and endoscopic ultrasound.

Endoscopic Ultrasound

Using a specially adapted side-viewing endoscope, an ultrasound probe can now be applied directly to the esophageal wall. Alternatively, the probe can be wrapped in a balloon, which is inflated with water to provide uniform contact with the esophagus.[39]

Five sonic layers have been identified that correspond with the interface between the transducer balloon and mucosa; the mucosa, the submucosa, the muscularis propria, and the adventitia (Fig. 22–25).[39, 40] A tumor appears as a sonically homogeneous area with evidence of disruption of the normal esophageal layers (Fig. 22–26). The examination is not intended for diagnostic purposes but serves as a staging modality. Multiple series have now been reported,

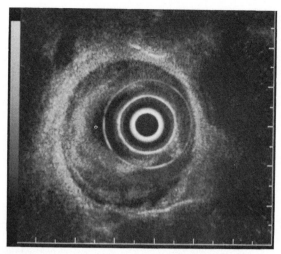

FIGURE 22–26. Endoscopic ultrasound showing infiltrating adenocarcinoma. The submucosa and muscularis propria are thickened with loss of distinct layering. (Compare with Figure 22–25.)

several of which compare endoscopic ultrasound and CT. Botet[41] staged 42 patients with both modalities. All results were compared with the surgical pathology examinations of resected specimens. In staging depth of tumor, endoscopic ultrasound was significantly more accurate (46 of 52 tumors, 88%) than CT (25 of 42 tumors, 60%). It was also more accurate in staging regional lymph nodes (44 of 50 patients, 88%) than CT (31 of 42 patients, 74%).

CT was found to be more accurate in staging for distant metastases, but the superior overall agreement with the pathologic specimens was obtained with the combined use of CT and ultrasound.

Tio and colleagues[40] accurately predicted resectability in 24 of 26 patients and correctly assessed local and distant lymph nodes in 17 of 19 patients with resectable tumors (Fig. 22–27).

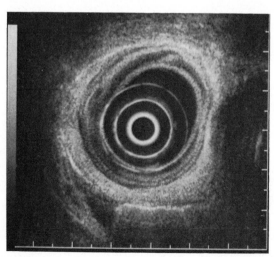

FIGURE 22–25. Endoscopic ultrasound of normal esophageal wall. The five-layered internal structure is depicted. The aorta lies at the 3 o'clock position.

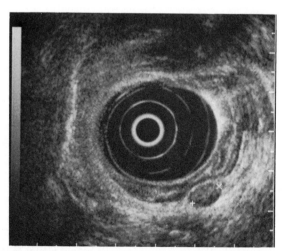

FIGURE 22–27. Endoscopic ultrasound showing infiltrating adenocarcinoma with node involvement. The node is bracketed by a cursor. Note granular quality with intermediate echogenicity. Vessels may appear similar but are distinguishable by being more hypoechoic and elongated.

Vilgrain and coworkers[42] compared the results of endoscopic sonography and CT in the preoperative staging of 46 patients. A total of 51 tumors were found in 46 patients. Sonographic estimation of tumor extension through the different layers of the esophagus was correct in 73% of all 51 tumors and in 22 of the 26 tumors in which the examination was complete. The endoscopic instrument could not pass through the tumor area in 23 cases (50%). Infiltration of adjacent organs was found in 15 patients at surgery; in four of which the extension was detected by CT as opposed to seven detected sonographically. False-negative findings occurred in those cases in which the probe could not be passed beyond the tumor, but there were no false-positive results with either CT or endoscopic sonography.

For detection of mediastinal lymph node involvement, the sensitivity of CT was 48%, as opposed to 50% for sonography. If those cases in which the endoscope could not be passed are excluded, the sensitivity rises to 84%. Statistically, sonography was superior to CT for the detection of lymph node metastases. It is evident, however, that both modalities are necessary owing to the inability of the endoscope to be maneuvered past the tumor in all cases.

Baker and Kopecky[43] have found endoscopic ultrasound to be superior to CT in its ability to define the extent of wall invasion. Because this is an important prognostic indicator, the increasing use of this modality is anticipated.

Image-Guided Fine-Needle Aspiration Biopsy

Early lymphatic spread through the nonsegmental drainage patterns of the esophagus is common, involving nodes from the neck to the abdomen. Frequently, there is a disparity between the location of the primary tumor and the group of nodes that are involved. Overhagen and associates[44] have noted a high percentage of supraclavicular metastases in patients with squamous cell carcinoma of the esophagus (22%), and others have reported an incidence as high as 31.8% when nodes were systematically dissected. Rankin[27] has noted that 32% of upper-third cancers metastasize to the abdominal lymph nodes. In the series reported by van Overhagen and colleagues,[44] supraclavicular metastases were not associated with mediastinal and abdominal adenopathies in 25% of patients. In their experience, the detection of supraclavicular metastases by palpation is unreliable, but they can readily be detected by either CT or ultrasound in the majority of patients. They found the predictive value of supraclavicular node metastases to be 0.74 by ultrasound and 0.85 by CT. Nodes with metastasis had a round configuration with a statistically significant greater short axis–to–long axis ratio than benign nodes. It is their conclusion that patients with carcinoma of the esophagus and gastroesophageal junction require examination of the supraclavicular area by imaging techniques as well as palpation. Cytologic

confirmation of metastasis can be safely obtained by means of ultrasonically guided fine-needle aspiration. This confirmation has a significant impact on the treatment regimen.

REFERENCES

1. Lindell MM, Jr. Hill, CA, and Libshitz, HI: Esophageal cancer: Radiographic chest findings and their prognostic significance. AJR Am J Roentgenol 133:461–465, 1979.
2. Bachman AL, Teixidor HS: The posterior trachael band: A reflector of local superior mediastinal abnormality. Br J Radiol 48:352–359, 1975.
3. Putman CE, Curtis AM, Westfried, M, McLoud T: Thickening of the posterior tracheal stripe: A sign of squamous cell carcinoma of the esophagus. Radiology 121:533–536, 1976.
4. Halpert RD, Feczko PJ, Spickler EM, et al: Radiological assessment of dysphagia with endoscopic correlation. Radiology 157:599–602, 1985.
5. Schatzki R, Hawes, LE: The roentgenological appearance of extramucosal tumors of the esophagus. Analysis of intramural extramucosal lesions of the gastrointestinal tract in general. AJR Am J Roentgenol 8:11–15, 1941.
6. Morsun BC, Dawson IMP, Day DW, et al: Gastrointestinal Pathology. 3rd Ed. London, England, Blackwell Scientific, 1990, pp 59–60.
7. Robbins SL, Cotran RS, Kumar V: Pathologic Basis of Disease. 3rd Ed. Philadelphia, W.B. Saunders Company, 1984, p 805.
8. Zornoza J, Lindell MM: Radiologic evaluation of small esophageal carcinoma. Gastrointest Radiol 5:107–111, 1980.
9. Sugimachi K, Ohno S, Matsuda H, et al: Clinicopathologic study of early stage esophageal carcinoma. Surgery 105:706–710, 1988.
10. Levine MS, Caroline D, Thompson JJ, et al: Adenocarcinoma of the esophagus: Relationship to Barrett mucosa. Radiology 150:305–309, 1984.
11. Goldstein H and Zornoza J: Association of squamous cell carcinoma of the head and neck with cancer of the esophagus. AJR Am J Roentgenol 131:791–794, 1978.
12. Ellis FH Jr: Carcinoma of the esophagus. Cancer J Clin 33:264–281, 1983.
13. Blot WJ, Devesa SS, Kneller RW, et al: Rising incidence of adenocarcinoma of the esophagus and gastric cardia. JAMA 265:1287–1289, 1991.
14. Raphael HA, Ellis FH Jr, Dockerty MB: Primary adenocarcinoma of the esophagus: 18-year review and review of the literature. Ann Surg 164:785, 1966.
15. Smith JL Jr: Pathology of adenocarcinoma of the esophagus and gastrointestinal region. *In* Strohlein JR, Romsdahl MM (eds): Gastrointestinal Cancer. New York, Raven Press, 1981, pp 125–135.
16. Keen SJ, Dodd GD, Smith JL: Adenocarcinoma arising in Barrett esophagus: Pathologic and Radiologic Features. Mt Sinai J Med, 51:442–450, 1984.
17. Levine MS, Kressel HY, Caroline DF, et al: Barrett esophagus: Reticular pattern of the mucosa. Radiology 146:663–667, 1983.
18. McCort JJ: Esophageal carcinosarcoma and pseudosarcoma. Radiology 102:519–524, 1972.
19. Moore TC, Batterby JS, Vellios F, et al: Carcinosarcoma of the esophagus. J Thorac Cardiovasc Surg 45:281–288, 1963.
20. Battifora H: Spindle cell carcinoma. Ultrastructural evidence of squamous origin and collagen production by tumor cells. Cancer 37:2275, 1976.
21. Carnovale RL, Goldstein HM, Zornoza J, et al: Radiologic manifestations of esophageal lymphoma. AJR Am J Roentgenol 128:751–754, 1977.
22. Moss AA, Schnyder PA, Thoeni RF, Margulis AR: Esophageal carcinoma: Pretherapy staging by computed tomography. AJR Am J Roentgenol 136:1051–1056, 1981.
23. Halber MD, Daffner RH, Thompson WM: CT of the esophagus. I. Normal appearance, AJR Am J Roentgenol 133:1047–1050, 1979.

24. Reining, JW, Stanley JH, Schabel SI: CT evaluation of thickened esophageal walls. AJR Am J Roentgenol 140:931–934, 1983.
25. Halvorson R, Thompson W: Computed tomographic evaluation of esophageal carcinoma. Semin Oncol 11:113–126, 1984.
26. Picus D, Balfe DM, Koehler RE, et al: Computed tomography in staging of esophageal carcinoma. Radiology 146:433–438, 1983.
27. Rankin S: The role of computed tomography in the staging of oesophageal cancer. (Editorial.) Clin Radiol 40:152–153, 1990.
28. Thompson WM, Halvorsen RA, Foster WL, et al: Computed tomography for staging esophageal and gastroesophageal cancer: Reevaluation. AJR Am J Roentgenol 141:951–958, 1983.
29. Freeny PC, Marks WM: Adenocarcinoma of the gastroesophageal junction: Barium and CT examination. AJR Am J Roentgenol 138:1077–1084, 1982.
30. Daffner RH, Haslber MD, Postlethwait RW, et al: CT of the esophagus II. Carcinoma. AJR Am J Roentgenol 133:1051–1055, 1979.
31. Lea JW, Prager RL, Bender HW: The questionable role of computed tomography in the preoperative staging of esophageal cancer. Ann Thoracic Surg 19:228–232, 1984.
32. Becker CD, Barbier P, Porcellini B: CT evaluation of patients undergoing transhiatal esophagectomy for cancer. J Comput Assist Tomogr 10:607–611, 1986.
33. Quint LE, Glazer GM, Orringer MB, Gross BH. Esophageal carcinoma: CT findings. Radiology 155:171–175, 1985.
34. Quint L, Glazer GM, Orringer MB: Esophageal imaging by MR and CT: Study of normal anatomy and neoplasms. Radiology 156:727–731, 1985.
35. Lehr L, Rupp N, Siewert JR: Assessment of resectability of esophageal cancer by computed tomography and magnetic resonance imaging. Surgery 103:344–350, 1987.
36. Petrillo R, Balzarini L, Bidoli P, et al: Esophageal squamous cell carcinoma: MRI evaluation of the mediastinum. Gastrointest Radiol 15:275–278, 1990.
37. Takashima S: Carcinoma of the esophagus: CT vs MR imaging in determining resectability. AJR Am J Roentgenol 156:297–302, 1991.
38. O'Donovan PB: The radiographic evaluation of the patient with esophageal carcinoma. Surg Clin N Am 4:241–256, 1994.
39. Bolondi CL, Zani L, Labo G: Technique of endoscopic ultrasonography investigation: Esophagus, stomach and duodenum. Scand J Gastroenterol 21(Suppl 123):1–5, 1986.
40. Tio TL, Tytgat GNJ: Endoscopic ultrasonography in the assessment of intra- and transmural infiltration of tumours in oesophagus, stomach and papilla of Vater and in the detection of extraoesophageal lesions. Endoscopy 16:203–210, 1984.
41. Botet JB, Lightdale CJ: Endoscopic sonography of the upper gastrointestinal tract. AJR Am J Roentgenol 156:63–68, 1991.
42. Vilgrain V, Mompoint D, Palazzo L, et al. Staging of esophageal carcinoma: Comparison of results with endoscopic sonography and CT. AJR Am J Roentgenol 155:277–281, 1990.
43. Baker MK, Kopecky KK: Endoscopic US in the staging of esophageal and gastric cancer. Radiology, 181:242–343, 1991.
44. van Overhagen H, Laméris JS, Berger MY, et al: Supraclavicular lymph node metastases in carcinoma of the esophagus and gastroesophageal junction: Assessment with CT, US and US-guided fine-needle aspiration biopsy. Radiology 179:155–158, 1991.

23 DIAGNOSIS AND STAGING OF ESOPHAGEAL CARCINOMA

Thomas W. Rice

The diagnosis and staging of esophageal carcinoma are slowly evolving from clinical art to precise science. This is the result of the ever-increasing understanding of the disease and the continued development of diagnostic modalities that provide assessment of the tumor, surrounding tissues, and distant sites. This evolution has not yet translated into improved survival because the majority of patients present with advanced disease and current therapy is inadequate for late-stage esophageal carcinoma.

If survival is to improve, identification and aggressive management of early-stage disease and potent therapy for late-stage carcinoma are needed. The identification of premalignant conditions and early-stage carcinomas allows treatment of these potentially curable conditions with increased survival expected with early surgical intervention. However, screening is in its infancy, and treatment of early-stage disease is not presently possible in the majority of patients. If successful treatment of advanced disease is to be realized, better staging before and after nonsurgical or induction therapy is essential. This will allow accurate evaluation of the treatment and will direct future modifications of therapy for advanced disease. In addition, the timely diagnosis and staging of recurrent disease are necessary for treatment evaluation. Continued improvements in diagnosis and staging are required if therapeutic advances in the treatment of esophageal carcinoma are to be achieved.

DIAGNOSIS

Flexible esophagoscopy is the procedure of choice for the diagnosis of esophageal carcinoma. The introduction of video technology has allowed simple and easy documentation of upper gastrointestinal (GI) malignancies (Fig. 23–1). Improvements in optics and instrument flexibility and the reduction of endoscope size have provided unexcelled visualization of the entire esophagus, particularly areas that have been previously difficult to examine: the cervical esophagus, the esophagogastric junction, and the gastric cardia. Also, flexible endoscopy permits assessment of the GI tract distal to obstructing esophageal carcinomas in approximately 80% of patients.[1] Inspection of the mucosa, distant from the primary tumor site, allows de-

tection of intramural metastases, which are associated with advanced tumor stage (increased incidence of regional lymph node and liver metastases) and decreased survival. Intramural metastases have been reported to occur in 11.9% of patients with squamous cell carcinoma of the esophagus.[2]

The clinical diagnosis of esophageal carcinoma requires tissue confirmation before treatment. The inadequacy of biopsies obtained with the original flexible endoscopy equipment had been a shortcoming. However, improved equipment and techniques have increased the diagnostic capabilities of fiberoptic endoscopic biopsy from a range of 70% to 80% to nearly 100%.[3–6] The number of biopsy specimens obtained increases the diagnostic yield from 93% for one specimen to 98% to 100% with six or seven specimens. Lusink and colleagues[7] reported flexible endoscopy to be unsatisfactory in the diagnosis of adenocarcinoma of the lower esophagus due to inflammation of the mucosa and tumor infiltration of the submucosa. Lal and colleagues[6] reported that neither site nor type of malignancy adversely affects diagnostic yield. The area biopsied within an esophageal lesion has not been reported to influence diagnostic accuracy. However, if an esophageal ulcer is encountered, experience with gastric ulcers shows the combination of biopsies from the rim of the ulcer and the ulcer crater provides a diagnostic accuracy of 95%.[8]

Endoscopic cytology brushings of esophageal lesions are easily obtained and should be considered for all lesions. In the diagnosis of gastroesophageal malignancy, brush cytology has a reported accuracy of 80% to 97% and a false-positive rate of 0.3% to 2.0%.[3, 4, 9–11] O'Donoghue and colleagues[11] analyzed both endoscopic brush cytology and biopsy and reported sensitivities of 81% and 87%, specificities of 98% and 99%, and positive predictive values of 92% and 96%, respectively, in the diagnosis of esophageal malignancies. Brush cytology is particularly helpful when adequate biopsies are difficult to obtain, such as with small, superficial cancers or strictures. It has been reported that when obstructing lesions preclude biopsy, cytology may provide a diagnosis in 75% of patients.[12] The diagnostic yield of endoscopic biopsy is increased with the addition of brush cytology by as much as 20.8%.[12] Cytology specimens should be obtained before biopsies. The accuracy of brush cytology

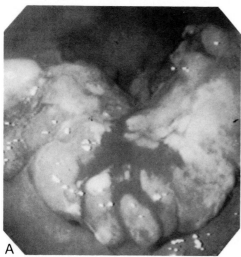
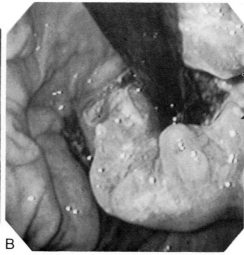

FIGURE 23–1. *A*, A polyploid adenocarcinoma involves one half of the luminal circumference of the esophagus, just proximal to the esophagogastric junction. *B*, Endoscopic documentation of invasion of the cardia by the same carcinoma. This view was obtained from the gastric body by retroflexing the endoscope.

is reduced from 93.5% to 82.6% if it is performed after biopsy.[13] The accuracy of endoscopic biopsy is not altered by preceding brush cytology. Brush cytology is complementary to biopsy and may be used to improve diagnostic yield.

Endoscopic fine-needle aspiration may be helpful in the diagnosis of mucosal and submucosal esophageal lesions. This procedure should be reserved for deeper lesions and those that remain undiagnosed by both biopsy and brush cytology.[14, 15]

Rigid esophagoscopy allows large biopsy specimens to be obtained and may permit assessment of fixation of an esophageal carcinoma. Without insufflation and magnification, the esophageal assessment may be difficult and incomplete. However, examination of the entire esophagus with rigid esophagoscopy has been reported in 79% of patients with esophageal carcinoma.[16] It has been reported that the passage of the rigid scope through a tumor increases the risk of perforation from negligible levels to 1.13%.[17] Although rigid esophagoscopy may be as likely as flexible esophagoscopy to allow passage of the instrument through the carcinoma, examination of the esophagogastric junction is inferior and examination of the stomach and duodenum is not possible with rigid esophagoscopy. Also, a general anesthetic is usually required for this examination. Because flexible endoscopy provides more information, is easier and safer to perform, and is better tolerated than rigid esophagoscopy, rigid esophagoscopy should be reserved for failures of flexible endoscopy.

Barium esophagram, once the premier test and the initial procedure performed for the diagnosis of esophageal carcinoma, has been relegated to a secondary role. The need for an esophagram to guide endoscopic examination has been eliminated by flexible endoscopes that allow visual passage and controlled advancement of the instrument. The determination of tumor length, radiologic tumor type, and esophageal axis in the radiographic assessment of esophageal carcinoma has been rendered obsolete by advanced diagnostic and staging techniques.[18, 19] Furthermore, barium esophagram does not have an adequate diag-

nostic accuracy in problem cases. Eastman and colleagues[20] reported an accuracy of 59% in the diagnosis of malignant esophageal strictures. In the diagnosis of early esophageal carcinoma, barium esophagram has been able to detect early lesions in approximately one-half of patients.[21] The barium esophagram and upper GI are an adjunct to upper GI endoscopy in the evaluation of esophageal carcinoma, most notably for the study of an obstructing tumor and the GI tract distal to it.

Early Diagnosis and Screening

The majority of the patients with esophageal carcinoma present late in the course of their disease with symptoms of dysphagia and weight loss. Because effective treatment of advanced disease does not exist, the diagnosis of early-stage disease in the asymptomatic patient is one treatment strategy that may improve survival. Occasionally, patients with early-stage cancers are serendipitously identified while being investigated for other medical conditions that require esophagoscopy or barium esophagram. Also, some patients present with atypical symptoms, such as chest or abdominal pain, odynophagia, anemia, or upper GI bleeding, which prompt investigations and lead to the diagnosis of early-stage esophageal carcinoma. However, these are uncommon events, and the diagnosis of early carcinoma in the asymptomatic patient is a chance occurrence.

The key to early diagnosis is the identification of precursors of malignancy in the patient at risk. Dysplasia is the best marker to date for the potential development of carcinoma of the esophagus. Dysplasia is intraepithelial neoplasia, and it is recognized histologically using well-defined cytologic criteria.[22] Dysplasia itself may be an early carcinomatous change that will progress to invasive cancer. Although most cancers arise in association with high-grade dysplasia (carcinoma-in-situ), all grades of dysplasia have been reported to give rise to invasive cancers. There need not be an orderly progression from low-grade dysplasia to invasive carcinoma. The evidence for the dysplasia-carcinoma sequence is compelling, but not all patients will progress to invasive carcinomas. The time course of these changes is variable. A confounding problem is that dysplasia may mimic inflammatory and reparative changes, and it is sometimes difficult to distinguish among these changes during screening.

Screening for esophageal carcinoma is the surveillance of a high-risk population for the development of dysplasia and early invasive carcinoma. For surveillance to be practical, a population at risk for the disease must submit to an accurate screening test. This test must be palatable with minimal morbidity, it must have a high sensitivity (ability to detect disease when present) and a high specificity (ability to determine absence of disease). The best screening tests provide esophageal mucosal specimens, which may be examined by cytology or histology for the presence of dysplasia or carcinoma.

In select groups, screening may improve survival by allowing earlier intervention and thus a greater probability of cure. The screening of high-risk groups for dysplasia or early esophageal carcinoma has proved difficult.

Screening for Squamous Cell Carcinoma

The incidence of squamous cell carcinoma is extremely variable, but a band of exceedingly high incidence exists. This belt starts in eastern Turkey; stretches through the Caspian littoral, Iraq, and Iran; and ends in northern China.[23] Mortality rates in excess of 100 deaths per 100,000 population, more than 10 times that of the United States, are seen in these areas. There also are isolated pockets of endemic disease in South Africa and France. This geographic distribution is attributed to environmental, dietary, and personal factors. No common agent or carcinogen has been identified, but the interplay of multiple factors in these areas allow for these peculiarly high incidences of squamous cell carcinoma of the esophagus. Surveillance programs for squamous dysplasia have used brush, balloon, and plastic loop cytology and endoscopy and biopsy with or without Lugol's staining for screening.[24–32] Preselection of patients for dysplasia screening has been suggested. The passage of a blood bead detector and the finding of occult upper GI bleeding have been used to determine which high-risk patients require further examination.[33] It has been difficult to interpret the results of these programs and to define their impact on survival. Presently, there are no recommendations for screening in areas of high incidence of squamous cell carcinoma of the esophagus.[34]

In addition to a geographic association, squamous cell carcinoma of the esophagus is related to certain medical conditions, in which screening should be considered. The theory of field cancerization states that a carcinogen applied to a large epithelial surface will initially cause neoplastic changes in the area of maximal stimuli, but eventually these changes will be manifested in neighboring areas.[35] Field cancerization may account for the increased incidence of aerodigestive malignancies in patients with head and neck cancers. The incidence of second primary cancers in this group of patients ranges from 5% to 21%.[36, 37] Synchronous lesions have a reported incidence of 1% to 11%.[38] Second primary malignancies are more likely in patients with glottic and floor of mouth tumors and in patients whose head and neck tumors were well- or moderately well-differentiated Stage I or Stage II cancers.[39] In this study, the 1- and 5-year survival rates were 75% and 25%, respectively, and the average time from diagnosis of the second primary cancer to death was 2.3 years. These multiple primary tumors are most often head and neck, lung, and esophageal carcinomas. From 1% to 8% of patients with head and neck primaries have a synchronous esophageal cancer.[40, 41] For synchronous primary tumors, the practice of screening by panendoscopy or triple endoscopy (laryngoscopy, bronchoscopy, and esophagoscopy) is considered by many to be the standard of care,[42–47] although some dispute its efficacy and cost effectiveness.[48–51] The incidence of metachronous tumors is equal to or greater than that of synchronous tumors and depends on the curative treatment of the head and neck primary and the duration of follow-up. The preferred method of surveillance of these patients has not been identified,[52] and there may be no survival advantage in the screening of these high-risk patients.[53]

Chronic inflammation may account for the reported increased incidence of squamous cell carcinoma in patients with achalasia and caustic strictures. Although not supported by all reports, there is a potential 5- to 33-fold increase in the incidence of cancer of the esophagus in patients with achalasia.[54, 55] Myotomy does not prevent the development of carcinoma. Therefore, screening of all patients, despite prior treatment, with long-standing achalasia should be considered. From 1% to 7% of patients with caustic strictures may develop squamous cell carcinomas of the esophagus.[56, 57] Although the interval between caustic injury and the development of carcinoma can average 40 years, some have suggested the early resection of these patients.[58] However, surveillance for cancer may be more effective in the long-term management of patients with caustic strictures.

The association of esophageal squamous cell cancer with tylosis and iron-deficiency anemia is frequently mentioned but is rarely seen. Tylosis is an autosomal dominant genetic defect that causes hyperkeratosis of the palms of the hands and the soles of the feet. There is a significant association with squamous cell carcinoma of the esophagus, with a 95% probability of developing carcinoma of the esophagus by age 65.[59, 60] The Plummer-Vinson (Paterson-Kelly) syndrome is the association of iron-deficiency anemia, esophageal webs, and atrophic changes of the nails and upper GI tract with esophageal carcinoma. If a patient with this rare syndrome is encountered, surveillance for squamous cell carcinoma of the esophagus is indicated.

Screening for Adenocarcinoma

The columnar cell–lined esophagus was first reported to be associated with carcinoma in 1953, 2 years after Barrett's first report.[61] Patients with Barrett's esophagus are at increased risk for esophageal adenocarcinoma; however, the exact magnitude of this risk is unknown. The incidence of adenocarcinoma in patients with Barrett's esophagus has been reported to vary from one carcinoma in 16 patient-years of surveillance to one carcinoma in 441 patient-years of follow-up.[62, 63] This is 30 to 180 times the incidence of esophageal carcinoma in the general population.

A recent report confirms the speculation that surveillance and surgery for early carcinoma in patients with Barrett's esophagus result in improved survival.[64] In this study, 58% of esophageal adenocarcinomas in surveillance patients were Stage 0 or I, whereas 17% of carcinomas were early-stage tumors in those patients with Barrett's esophagus who presented with cancer. The 5-year survival was 62% in the former patients versus 20% in latter patients.

Screening for dysplasia and early carcinoma must be considered the standard of care in patients with Barrett's esophagus (see Chapter 19). Endoscopic surveillance with directed biopsy is the presently accepted screening technique. Although brush cytology has been shown to be satisfactory in the screening for esophageal carcinoma and may be more cost effective, its role in the surveillance of Barrett's esophagus remains to be defined.[65–67] The surveillance interval must also be clarified. Routine endoscopic screening every 1 to 2 years, with reduction of the interval to 3 to 6 months when low-grade dysplasia, is detected is an accepted practice.

Scleroderma, another disease associated with reflux, has not been found to be a precursor of cancer.[68]

STAGING

The stage of an esophageal carcinoma, as defined by its anatomic extent, is the best prognosticator available for patients with esophageal carcinoma. Recent refinements in the staging of esophageal carcinoma has resulted in the present staging system, which is TNM based (Table 23–1). The primary tumor (T) is defined only by the depth of invasion. T1 tumors are confined to the submucosa or more superficial esophageal layers. T2 tumors invade into but do not breach the muscularis propria. T3 tumors invade beyond the esophageal wall and into the paraesophageal tissue but do not invade adjacent structures. T4 tumors directly invade structures in the vicinity of the esophagus.

Regional lymph nodes (N) are characterized only by the presence (N1) or absence (N0) of metastases. These regional lymph nodes must be in the area of the primary tumor. Although regional lymph nodes are easy to conceptualize, they are difficult to define. As with the esophagus, regional nodes can be divided into five regions: cervical, upper thoracic, middle tho-

TABLE 23–1. TNM Classification of Esophageal Carcinomas

T: PRIMARY TUMOR
- TX The primary tumor cannot be assessed
- T0 No evidence of a primary tumor
- Tis Carcinoma-in-situ (high-grade dysplasia)
- T1 The tumor invades the lamina propria, muscularis mucosae, or submucosa but does not breach the boundary between the submucosa and muscularis propria
- T2 The tumor invades the muscularis propria but does not breach the boundary between the muscularis propria and periesophageal tissue
- T3 The tumor invades the periesophageal tissue but does not invade adjacent structures
- T4 The tumor invades adjacent structures

N: REGIONAL LYMPH NODES
- NX Regional lymph nodes cannot be assessed
- N0 No regional lymph node metastasis
- N1 Regional lymph node metastasis

M: DISTANT METASTASIS
- MX Presence of distant metastasis cannot be assessed
- M0 No distant metastasis
- M1 Distant metastasis

racic, lower thoracic, and abdominal. However, no esophageal carcinoma is located exactly in the middle of any one region, and there is inevitable overlap of regions. There is no dispute that a lower thoracic lymph node metastasis from a cervical esophageal cancer is not a regional lymph node metastasis but is a distant metastasis. However, many dispute that a celiac axis lymph node metastasis from an abdominal or lower thoracic esophageal carcinoma is not a distant metastasis (as presently defined) but is a regional lymph node metastasis. The definition of a regional lymph node depends on the surgeon's appreciation of the lymphatic drainage of the esophagus. The determination of regional lymph node status (N) requires consistent and accurate nodal mapping during a careful lymph node dissection or lymphadenectomy.

Distant sites (M) are characterized by the presence (M1) or absence (M0) of metastases. These TNM descriptors can be grouped into stages with similar behavior and prognosis (Table 23–2).

The stage of an esophageal carcinoma may be determined at four periods during the course of the disease.[69] Before any treatment, the clinical stage (cTNM) is determined by a combination of physical examination, diagnostic imaging, endoscopy, and biopsy. Pathologic stage (pTNM) is determined at surgery

TABLE 23–2. Stage Groupings

Stage 0	Tis	N0	M0
Stage I	T1	N0	M0
Stage IIa	T2	N0	M0
	T3	N0	M0
Stage IIb	T1	N1	M0
	T2	N1	M0
Stage III	T3	N1	M0
	T4	Any N	M0
Stage IV	Any T	Any N	M1

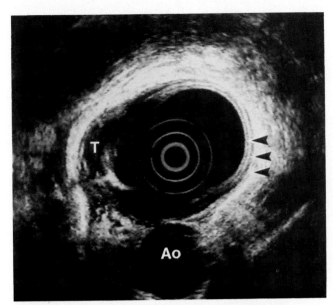

FIGURE 23-2. The esophageal wall as seen at endoscopic esophageal ultrasound (EUS). The esophagus is seen as five distinct layers. The first layer *(upper arrow)* is hyperechoic (white) and represents the interface between the EUS balloon and the superficial mucosa. The second layer is hypoechoic (black) and represents the deep mucosa. The third layer *(middle arrow)* is hyperechoic (white) and represents the submucosa. The fourth layer is hypoechoic (black) and represents the muscularis propria. The fifth layer *(lower arrow)* is hyperechoic (white) and represents the periesophageal tissue. Ao = aorta; T = hypoechoic tumor. (Reprinted with permission from Rice TW, Boyce GA, Sivak MV Jr: Esophageal ultrasound and the preoperative staging of carcinoma of the esophagus. J Thorac Cardiovasc Surg 101:536, 1991.)

and is based on the clinical stage modified by information obtained at surgery and pathology examination. Retreatment stage (rTNM) is the stage before additional treatment. The treatment may be the continuation of planned multimodality therapy or it may be further therapy for a documented recurrence. Postmortem stage (TNM) is determined at autopsy.

Clinical Stage

Endoscopic esophageal ultrasound (EUS) is the most accurate modality for the determination of depth of

tumor invasion (T) before treatment.[70-75] This is the result of the definition of the esophageal wall and the periesophageal tissue afforded by EUS (Fig. 23-2). Five ultrasound layers are seen in the examination of the esophagus and periesophageal tissues; however, it is the fourth ultrasound layer, which represents the muscularis propria, that must be carefully examined to differentiate T1, T2, and T3 tumors (Figs. 23-3 to 23-5). The same definition of the esophageal wall is not offered by computed tomography (CT). The thickened esophageal wall, the principal CT finding in esophageal carcinoma, is not specific for esophageal carcinoma and lacks the definition required to distinguish T1, T2, and T3 tumors.[76]

In the differentiation of T3 from T4 tumors, EUS is superior to CT (Figs. 23-6 and 23-7). The evaluation of fat planes is used to define local invasion at CT examination. The obliteration or lack of fat planes is not sensitive in the prediction of local invasion; however, the preservation of these planes is specific for the absence of T4 disease.[77-83] In the evaluation of aortic invasion, obliteration of the smooth contour of a fourth or more of the circumference of the aorta and an angle of contact between the tumor and the aorta of more than 45 degrees are the CT criteria for aortic invasion. Compared with CT, EUS provides a more sensitive and reliable determination of vascular involvement.[84]

Despite its superiority, there are shortcomings of EUS in the determination of depth of tumor invasion. There is a learning curve for EUS—with improved technical and interpretative skills, the accuracy of determination of depth of tumor invasion increased from 59% to 81% at our institution.[85, 86] The loss of definition of the first three ultrasound layers and their merging into one layer in the cervical esophagus or with overdistension of the EUS balloon make the identification of early-stage carcinoma difficult and may lead to the overstaging of these tumors.[85] The inability to pass the EUS probe through a malignant stricture occurs in 21% to 44% of patients.[85, 87] Attempts to stage the tumor in the region above the stenosis is inaccurate.[88, 89] Despite this incomplete examination, the inability to advance the EUS probe through the malignant stricture is a finding that is

FIGURE 23-3. *A,* A T1 tumor invades the submucosa but does not breach the boundary between the submucosa and muscularis propria. *B,* A T1 tumor as seen at EUS. The hypoechoic (black) tumor invades the hyperechoic (white) third ultrasound layer (submucosa) but does not breach the boundary between the third and fourth layers *(arrows).* (Reprinted with permission from Rice TW, Boyce GA, Sivak MV Jr: Esophageal ultrasound and the preoperative staging of carcinoma of the esophagus. J Thorac Cardiovasc Surg 101:536, 1991.)

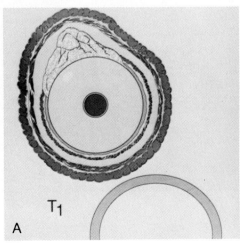

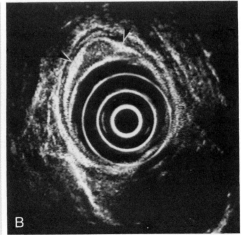

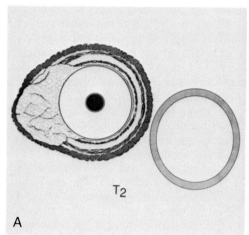

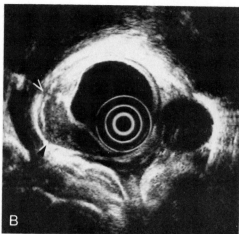

FIGURE 23–4. *A,* A T2 tumor invades the muscularis propria but does not breach the boundary between the muscularis propria and the periesophageal tissue. *B,* A T2 tumor as seen at EUS. The hypoechoic (black) tumor invades the hypoechoic (black) fourth ultrasound layer but does not breach the boundary between the fourth and fifth layers *(arrows).* (Reprinted with permission from Rice TW, Boyce GA, Sivak MV Jr: Esophageal ultrasound and the preoperative staging of carcinoma of the esophagus. J Thorac Cardiovasc Surg 101:536, 1991.)

FIGURE 23–5. *A,* A T3 tumor invades the periesophageal tissue but does not involve adjacent structures. *B,* A T3 tumor as seen at EUS. The hypoechoic (black) tumor breaches the boundary between the fourth and fifth ultrasound layers *(arrows)* and invades the hyperechoic (white) fifth ultrasound layer (periesophageal tissue). (Reprinted with permission from Rice TW, Boyce GA, Sivak MV Jr: Esophageal ultrasound and the preoperative staging of carcinoma of the esophagus. J Thorac Cardiovasc Surg 101:536, 1991.)

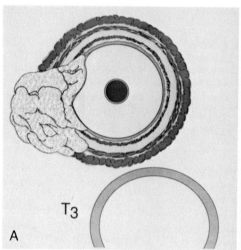

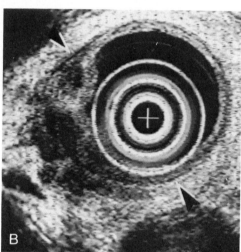

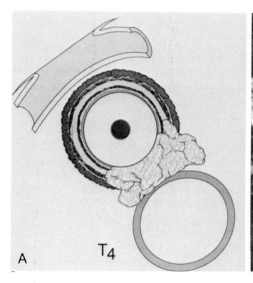

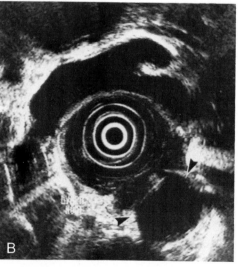

FIGURE 23–6. *A,* A T4 tumor invades the aorta. *B,* A T4 tumor as seen at EUS. The hypoechoic (black) tumor invades the aorta. The tumor breaches the boundary between the periesophageal tissue and the aorta *(arrows).* (Reprinted with permission from Rice TW, Boyce GA, Sivak MV Jr: Esophageal ultrasound and the preoperative staging of carcinoma of the esophagus. J Thorac Cardiovasc Surg 101:536, 1991.)

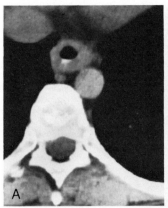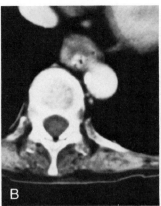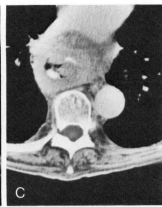

FIGURE 23–7. CT determination of T4 disease. *A,* The fat plane between an esophageal carcinoma (thickened esophageal wall) and the aorta is maintained. The angle of contact of the tumor and the aorta is less than 45 degrees. These are accurate predictors of absence of T4 disease. *B,* The fat plane between an esophageal carcinoma and the aorta is obliterated. The angle of contact between the tumor and the aorta is greater than 45 degrees. CT criteria predict aortic invasion (T4). The aorta was not invaded at resection. *C,* The fat planes between an esophageal carcinoma and the aorta, and the esophageal carcinoma and the pericardium are obliterated. The angle of contact between the tumor and the aorta is greater than 45 degrees. CT criteria predict aortic and pericardial invasion (T4). There was no invasion of local structures at resection.

highly predictive of advanced disease. Ninety-one per cent of patients in whom the malignant stricture was severe enough to prevent passage of the ultrasound probe had Stage III or IV tumors.[89]

In the assessment of T4 disease, other modalities are available. Compared with CT, magnetic resonance imaging (MRI) offers no advantages in the staging of esophageal carcinoma.[90–92] Most notably, detection of aortic invasion is no better with MRI than with CT. Bronchoscopic assessment of the airways is mandatory for tumors of the cervical and upper thoracic esophagus and should be considered with all esophageal tumors. Twelve and one-half per cent of lower thoracic esophageal tumors and 5% of abdominal esophageal tumors have abnormalities of the airway detected at bronchoscopy.[93] Airway invasion may be difficult to demonstrate by biopsy; in these situations, brush cytology is helpful in detecting airway invasion.[94] A more common finding is encroachment on the airway by the tumor. This may appear as a bulging of the posterior wall of the trachea or bronchus, widening of the carina, deviation of the trachea or bronchus, or narrowing of the airways. The majority of patients with airway encroachment are resectable.[1, 95]

Thoracoscopy allows visual inspection of the thoracic cavity, but the esophageal tumor may not always be seen.[96] The inability of thoracoscopy to routinely visualize the area of suspected involvement and to visually differentiate inflammatory from malignant fixation limits the usefulness of thoracoscopic inspection in distinguishing T3 from T4 disease. Thoracoscopic dissection to determine local invasion is similarly restricted. Limited exploration, the loss of bimanual palpation to assess fixation, and the danger of thoracoscopic biopsies of potentially invaded structures make thoracoscopic assessment of T4 disease undesirable.[97]

In the assessment of regional lymph nodes (N), CT relies solely on lymph node size to predict metastatic disease. Studies of mediastinal lymph nodes of normal patients show that N0 nodes are usually less than 1.0 cm and not larger than 1.6 cm in largest dimension.[98, 99] Regional lymph nodes of larger than 1.5 cm are considered suspicious for N1 disease. In addition to size, EUS evaluates nodal shape, border, and internal echo characteristics in regional lymph node assessment (Fig. 23–8). These additional factors account for the superiority of EUS in the determination of regional lymph node status.[70, 72–75] The major shortcomings of EUS in the determination of N are its inabilities to detect micrometastasis, which may not display detectable EUS changes, and to differentiate large inflammatory nodes from nodal metastases, which sometimes share the same EUS findings. These problems may be overcome by EUS-directed fine-needle aspiration of indeterminate nodes.[100] The prediction of regional lymph node metastases may be extrapolated from the EUS determination of depth of tumor invasion. The incidence of lymph node metastases increases with increasing depth of tumor invasion.[70, 101] This association of T with N may be one of the most sensitive indicators of regional lymph node metastases (Table 23–3).[102, 103]

Lymphoscintography has been used to examine the regional lymph nodes in patients with esophageal carcinoma. This examination requires the injection of a radioisotope into the esophageal submucosa in the area of the tumor.[104, 105] False-positive results are common and limit the usefulness of this experimental study. Gallium scanning has a low sensitivity, ranging from 25% to 61%, in the detection of regional lymph

TABLE 23–3. Association of T and N

STUDY	TUMORS WITH N1 DISEASE (%)				
	Tis	T1	T2	T3	T4
Catalano et al[102]	0	14.3	33.3	73.3	85.7
Dittler et al[103]	—	4	52	82	91

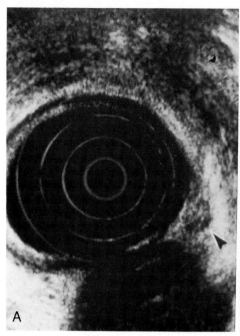

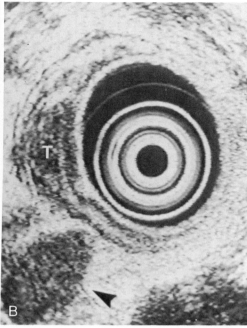

FIGURE 23–8. *A*, A N0 node *(arrow)* as seen at EUS. The node is 5 mm in diameter, has an ill-defined border, and a hyperechoic (white) internal structure. *B*, A N1 node *(arrow)* as seen at EUS. The large node, which is 12 mm in diameter, has a sharply demarcated border. The internal structure is hypoechoic (black) and is similar to that of the primary tumor (T). (Reprinted with permission from Rice TW, Boyce GA, Sivak MV Jr: Esophageal ultrasound and the preoperative staging of carcinoma of the esophagus. J Thorac Cardiovasc Surg 101:536, 1991.)

node metastases. However, the sensitivity may be increased to acceptable levels if lateral thoracic views are used.[106]

Depending on the clinical situation, regional lymph nodes may be sampled by percutaneous fine-needle aspiration or biopsy. In the cervical region, palpable nodes may be biopsied or aspirated. However, ultrasound assessment and ultrasound guided biopsy has proved to be superior in the assessment of cervical nodes and should be considered in the evaluation of patients with cervical esophageal cancer.[107–109] Mediastinoscopy may be used to biopsy nodes about the trachea and may be useful in the assessment of patients with upper and midthoracic esophageal tumors. Anterior mediastinotomy, thoracoscopy, and laparoscopy may also be used for regional lymph node sampling.

EUS is of limited value in the assessment of sites of distant metastases (M). Endoscopic ultrasound is use-

ful only if the distant organ is in direct contact with the upper GI tract (Fig. 23–9). The celiac axis and left lateral segment of the liver are two such sites. Intraabdominal assessment may be afforded by CT, ultrasound, or laparoscopy.[110] Laparoscopy is superior to either CT or surface ultrasound in the assessment of peritoneal and hepatic metastases. The accuracy of CT in the detection of liver metastases increases with the size of the nodules, and CT is very sensitive for metastases larger than 2 cm in diameter.[111] In the assessment of intra-abdominal lymph nodes, laparoscopy is no better than CT, and the shortcomings of surface ultrasound may be overcome by endoscopic ultrasound assessment of these nodes.

CT provides excellent evaluation of the lungs and pleura; however, CT is very sensitive but not specific in the assessment of pulmonary nodules. Percutaneous fine-needle aspiration or transbronchial biopsy is necessary to differentiate benign from malignant

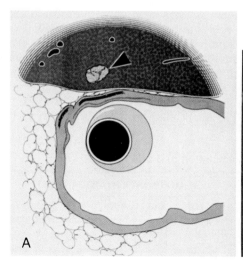

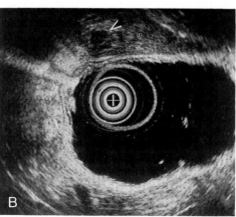

FIGURE 23–9. *A*, A hepatic metastasis *(arrow)* in the left lateral segment of the liver. The esophageal ultrasound probe is seen in the gastric cardia. *B*, A hepatic metastasis *(arrow)* as seen from the gastric cardia by esophageal ultrasound. The metastasis was imaged only by esophageal ultrasound. (Reprinted with permission from Rice TW, Boyce GA, Sivak MV, et al: Esophageal carcinoma: Esophageal ultrasound assessment of preoperative chemotherapy. Ann Thorac Surg 53:972, 1992.)

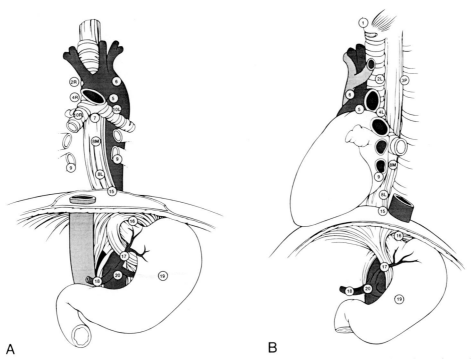

A   B

FIGURE 23–10. Lymph node map for esophageal carcinoma. *A,* Anterior view. *B,* Left lateral view. Lymph node stations: 1 = supraclavicular, 2 = paratracheal, 3P = posterior mediastinal, 4 = tracheo-bronchial angle, 5 = subaortic window, 6 = para-aortic, 7 = subcarinal, 8M = middle paraesophageal, 8L = lower paraesophageal, 9 = inferior pulmonary ligament, 10 = hilar, 15 = diaphragmatic, 16 = paracardial, 17 = left gastric, 18 = common hepatic, 19 = splenic, 20 = celiac axis.

nodules. Thoracoscopy provides superb visualization of the pleura and lung surface, but deeper pulmonary lesions are difficult to locate and assess. Thoracoscopy is an adjunct to CT in the evaluation of the pleural surfaces for distant metastatic disease.

Routine nuclear scanning has not proved useful in the search for distant metastases. Bone scanning may detect silent bone metastases,[112] but it lacks the sensitivity to be used routinely and should be reserved for the detection of bone involvement that is suspected clinically.

Pathologic Stage

The pathologic stage is the clinical stage modified by the findings at surgery and pathologic review of all excised tissue. The depth of tumor invasion can be assessed from the resection specimen if adequate soft tissue margins are included and marked. In suspected cases of T4 disease, care must be taken to ensure that adequate biopsies are taken from the invaded structures to confirm this status. However, pathologic proof of T4 disease cannot always be safely obtained. In these situations, intraoperative assessment, which is inferior to tissue confirmation, must be used. Regional lymph node excision with careful mapping should be performed in all resections and explorations (Fig. 23–10). All sites of potential distant metastases that are exposed at surgery should be assessed to confirm or modify the information obtained from clinical staging.

Retreatment Stage

Retreatment staging should be conducted with the same methods and tools used in clinical staging. EUS has been used to assess induction therapy and to restage patients before resection.[113] In patients receiving palliative therapy who will not have a pathologic stage, EUS has proven useful in retreatment staging.[114]

If therapy is successful it may be difficult to differentiate fibrosis and necrosis from viable tumor by EUS examination.[87] EUS has been useful in the diagnosis and restaging of patients with anastomotic recurrences that are not endoscopically visible.[115]

Postmortem Stage

Every effort should be made to obtain an autopsy and to determine the postmortem stage of patients with esophageal carcinoma. This approach will allow therapeutic assessment in treated patients and a record of the natural history in untreated patients.[116–119]

SELECTED REFERENCES

Beahrs OH, Henson DE, Hutter RVP, et al: Manual for Staging of Cancer. 4th Ed. Philadelphia, JB Lippincott, 1992, pp 57–59.
The guidelines for the staging of esophageal cancer are clearly outlined in this manual.
Chamberlain J, Day NE, Hakama M, et al: UICC Workshop of the Project on Evaluation of Screening Programs for Gastrointestinal Cancer. Int J Cancer 37:329, 1986.
Included in this workshop on screening programs are suggestions for screening esophageal squamous cell carcinoma.

Souquet JC, Napoleon B, Pujol P, et al: Endosonography-guided treatment of esophageal carcinoma. Endoscopy 24(suppl 1):324, 1992.
This article provides an overview of endoscopic esophageal ultrasound and its role in the management of esophageal carcinoma.

REFERENCES

1. Cheung HC, Siu KF, Wong J: A comparison of flexible and rigid endoscopy in evaluating esophageal cancer patients for surgery. World J Surg 12:117, 1988.
2. Takubo K, Sasajima K, Yamashita K, et al: Prognostic significance of intramural metastasis in patients with esophageal carcinoma. Cancer 65:1816, 1990.
3. Prolla JC, Reilly RW, Kirsner JB, et al: Direct-vision endoscopic cytology and biopsy in the diagnosis of esophageal and gastric tumors: Current experience. Acta Cytol 21:399, 1977.
4. Witzel L, Halter F, Grétillat PA, et al: Evaluation of specific value of endoscopic biopsies and brush cytology for malignancies of the esophagus and stomach. Gut 17:375, 1976.
5. Graham DY, Schwartz JT, Cain GD, et al: Prospective evaluation of biopsy number in the diagnosis of esophageal and gastric carcinoma. Gastroenterology 82:228, 1982.
6. Lal N, Bhasin DK, Malik AK, et al: Optimal number of biopsy specimens in the diagnosis of carcinoma of the esophagus. Gut 33:724, 1992.
7. Lusink C, Sali A, Chou ST: Diagnostic accuracy of flexible endoscopic biopsy in carcinoma of the oesophagus and cardia. Aust NZ J Surg 53:545, 1983.
8. Hatfield ARW, Slavin G, Segal AW, et al: Importance of the site of endoscopic gastric biopsy in ulcerating lesions of the stomach. Gut 16:884, 1975.
9. Kasugai T, Kobayashi S, Kuno N: Endoscopic cytology of the esophagus, stomach, and pancreas. Acta Cytol 22:327, 1978.
10. Chambers LA, Clark WE: The endoscopic diagnosis of gastroesophageal malignancy: A cytologic review. Acta Cytol 30:110, 1986.
11. O'Donoghue J, Waldon R, Gough D, et al: An analysis of the diagnostic accuracy of endoscopic biopsy and cytology in the detection of oesophageal malignancy. Eur J Surg Oncol 18:332, 1992.
12. Cussó X, Monés-Xiol J, Vilardell F: Endoscopic cytology of cancer of the esophagus and cardia: A long term evaluation. Gastrointest Endosc 35:321, 1989.
13. Zargar SA, Khuroo MS, Jan GM, et al: Prospective comparison of the value of brushings before and after biopsy in the endoscopic diagnosis of gastroesophageal malignancy. Acta Cytol 35:549, 1991.
14. Graham DY, Tabibian N, Michaletz PA, et al: Endoscopic needle biopsy: A comparative study of forceps biopsy, two different types of needles, and salvage cytology in gastrointestinal cancer. Gastrointest Endosc 35:207, 1989.
15. Layfield LJ, Reichman A, Weinstein WM: Endoscopically directed fine needle aspiration biopsy of gastric and esophageal lesions. Acta Cytol 36:69, 1992.
16. Bacon CK, Hendrix RA: Open tube versus flexible esophagoscopy in adult head and neck endoscopy. Ann Otol Rhinol Laryngol 101:147, 1992.
17. Ritchie AJ, McManus K, McGuigan J, et al: The role of rigid oesophagoscopy in oesophageal carcinoma. Postgrad Med J 68:892, 1992.
18. Akiyama H, Kogure T, Itai Y: The esophageal axis and its relationship to the resectability of carcinoma of the esophagus. Ann Surg 176:30, 1972.
19. Mori S, Kasai M, Watanabe T, et al: Preoperative assessment of resectability for carcinoma of the thoracic esophagus. Ann Surg 190:100, 1979.
20. Eastman MC, Gear MWL, Nicol A: An assessment of the accuracy of modern endoscopic diagnosis of oesophageal stricture. Br J Surg 65:182, 1978.
21. Moss AA, Koehler RE, Margulis AR: Initial accuracy of esophagograms in detection of small esophageal carcinoma. Am J Roentgenol 127:909, 1976.
22. Riddell RH, Goldman H, Ransohoff DF, et al: Dysplasia in inflammatory bowel disease: Standardized classification with provisional clinical information. Hum Pathol 14:931, 1983.
23. Muir CS, McKinney PA: Cancer of the esophagus: A global overview. Eur J Cancer Prevent 1:259, 1992.
24. Coordinating Group for Research on Esophageal Cancer: Early diagnosis and surgical treatment of esophageal cancer under rural conditions. Chin Med J 2:113, 1976.
25. Li FP, Shiang EL: Screening for oesophageal cancer in 62,000 Chinese. Lancet 2:804, 1979.
26. Dowlatshahi K, Daneshbod A, Mobarhan S: Early detection of cancer of oesophagus along Caspian littoral: Report of a pilot project. Lancet 1:125, 1978.
27. Guojun H, Lingfang S, Dawei Z, et al: Diagnosis and surgical treatment of early esophageal carcinoma. Chin Med J 94:229, 1981.
28. Shu Y-J: Cytopathology of the esophagus: An overview of esophageal cytopathology in China. Acta Cytol 27:7, 1983.
29. Crespi M, Grassi A, Amiri G, et al: Esophageal lesions in Northern Iran: A premalignant condition? Lancet 1:217, 1979.
30. Zaridze DG, Blettner M, Trapeznikov NN, et al: Survey of a population with a high incidence of oral and oesophageal cancer. Int J Cancer 36:153, 1985.
31. Lazarus C, Jaskiewicz K, Sumeruk RA, et al: Brush cytology technique in the detection of oesophageal carcinoma in the asymptomatic, high risk subject: A pilot survey. Cytopathology 3:291, 1992.
32. Qin D, Zhou B: Elastic plastic tube for detecting exfoliative cancer cells in the esophagus. Acta Cytol 36:82, 1992.
33. Qin D, Wang G, Zuo JH, et al: Screening of esophageal and gastric cancer by occult blood bead detector. Cancer 71:216, 1993.
34. Chamberlain J, Day NE, Hakama M, et al: UICC Workshop of the Project on Evaluation of Screening Programs for Gastrointestinal Cancer. Int J Cancer 37:329, 1986.
35. Slaughter DP, Southwick HW, Smejkal W: "Field cancerization" in oral stratified squamous epithelium: Clinical implications of multicentric origin. Cancer 6:963, 1953.
36. Odette J, Szymanowski RT, Nichols RD: Multiple head and neck malignancies. Trans Am Acad Ophthalmol Otolaryngol 84:805, 1977.
37. Gluckman JL, Crissman JD, Donegan JO: Multicentric squamous-cell carcinoma of the upper aerodigestive tract. Head Neck Surg 3:90, 1980.
38. Gluckman JL: Synchronous multiple primary lesions of the upper aerodigestive system. Arch Otolaryngol 105:597, 1979.
39. Larson JT, Adams GL, Fattah HA: Survival statistics for multiple primaries in head and neck cancer. Otolaryngol Head Neck Surg 103:14, 1990.
40. Thompson WM, Oddson TA, Kelvin F, et al: Synchronous and metachronous squamous cell carcinomas of the head, neck and esophagus. Gastrointest Radiol 3:123, 1978.
41. McGuirt WF: Panendoscopy as a screening examination for simultaneous primary tumors in head and neck cancer: A prospective sequential study and review of the literature. Laryngoscope 92:569, 1982.
42. Weaver A, Fleming SM, Knechtges TC, et al: Triple endoscopy: A neglected essential in head and neck cancer. Surgery 86:493, 1979.
43. Maisel RH, Vermeersch H: Panendoscopy for second primaries in head and neck cancer. Ann Otol Rhinol Laryngol 90:460, 1981.
44. McGuirt WF, Matthews B, Koufman JA: Multiple simultaneous tumors in patients with head and neck cancer. Cancer 50:1195, 1982.
45. Atkins JP, Keane WM, Young KA, et al: Value of panendoscopy in determination of second primary cancer. Arch Otolaryngol 110:533, 1984.
46. Leipzig B, Zellmer JE, Klug D, et al: The role of endoscopy in evaluating patients with head and neck cancer: A multi-institutional prospective study. Arch Otolaryngol 111:589, 1985.
47. Abemayor E, Moore DM, Hanson DG: Identification of synchronous esophageal tumors in patients with head and neck cancer. J Surg Oncol 38:94, 1988.
48. Atkinson D, Fleming S, Weaver A: Triple endoscopy: A valuable procedure in head and neck surgery. Am J Surg 144:416, 1982.

49. Schuller DE, Fritsch MH: An assessment of the value of triple endoscopy in the evaluation of head and neck cancer patients. J Surg Oncol 32:156, 1986.

50. Shaha A, Hoover E, Marti J, et al: Is routine triple endoscopy cost-effective in head and neck cancer? Am J Surg 155:750, 1988.

51. Hordijk GJ, Bruggink T, Ravasz LA: Panendoscopy: A valuable procedure? Otolaryngol Head Neck Surg 101:426, 1989.

52. Bundrick TJ, Cho SR: Evaluation of the esophagus in patients with head and neck cancer. Am J Roentgenol 142:1082, 1984.

53. Atabek U, Mohit-Tabatabai MA, Rush BF, et al: Impact of esophageal screening in patients with head and neck cancer. Am Surg 56:289, 1990.

54. Choung JJ, DuBovik S, McCallum RW: Achalasia as a risk factor for esophageal carcinoma: A reappraisal. Digest Dis Sci 29:1105, 1984.

55. Meijssen MAC, Tilanus HW, van Blankenstein M, et al: Achalasia complicated by oesophageal squamous cell carcinoma: A prospective study in 195 patients. Gut 33:155, 1992.

56. Appelqvist P, Salmo M: Lye corrosion carcinoma of the esophagus: A review of 63 cases. Cancer 45:2655, 1980.

57. Csikos M, Horvath O, Petri A, et al: Late malignant transformation of chronic corrosive esophageal strictures. Langenbecks Arch Chir 365:231, 1985.

58. Imre J, Kopp M: Argument against long-term conservative treatment of oesophageal strictures due to corrosive burns. Thorax 27:594, 1972.

59. Howel-Evans W, McConnell RB, Clarke CA, et al: Carcinoma of the oesophagus with keratosis palmaris et plantaris (tylosis): A study of two families. Q J Med 27:413, 1958.

60. Shine I, Allison PR: Carcinoma of the esophagus with tylosis (keratosis palmaris and plantaris). Lancet 1:951, 1966.

61. Morson BC, Belcher JR: Adenocarcinoma of the esophagus and ectopic gastric mucosa. Br J Cancer 6:127, 1953.

62. Iftikhar SY, James PD, Steele RJC, et al: Length of Barrett's oesophagus: An important factor in the development of dysplasia and adenocarcinoma. Gut 33:1155, 1991.

63. Cameron AJ, Ott BJ, Payne WS: The incidence of adenocarcinoma in columnar lined (Barrett's) esophagus. N Engl J Med 313:857, 1985.

64. Streitz JM Jr, Andrews CW, Ellis FH Jr: Endoscopic surveillance of Barrett's esophagus: Does it help? J Thorac Cardiovasc Surg 105:383, 1993.

65. Robey SS, Hamilton SR, Gupta PK, et al: Diagnostic value of cytopathology in Barrett's esophagus and associated carcinoma. Am J Clin Pathol 89:493, 1988.

66. Geisinger KR, Teot LA, Richter JE: A comparative cytopathologic and histologic study of atypia, dysplasia, and adenocarcinoma in Barrett's esophagus. Cancer 69:8, 1992.

67. Wang HH, Doria MI Jr, Purohit-Buch S, et al: Barrett's esophagus: The cytology of dysplasia in comparison to benign and malignant lesions. Acta Cytol 36:60, 1992.

68. Segel MC, Campbell WL, Medsger TA, et al: Systemic sclerosis (scleroderma) and esophageal adenocarcinoma: Is increased patient screening necessary? Gastroenterology 89:485, 1985.

69. Beahrs OH, Henson DE, Hutter RVP, et al: Manual for Staging of Cancer. 4th Ed. Philadelphia, JB Lippincott, 1992, pp 6–9.

70. Tio TL, Cohen P, Coene PP, et al: Endosonography and computed tomography of esophageal carcinoma: Preoperative classification compared to the new (1987) TNM system. Gastroenterology 96:1478, 1989.

71. Date H, Miyashita M, Sasajima K, et al: Assessment of adventitial involvement of esophageal carcinoma by endoscopic ultrasonography. Surg Endosc 4:195, 1990.

72. Vilgrain V, Mompoint D, Palazzo L, et al: Staging of esophageal carcinoma: Comparison of results with endoscopic sonography and CT. Am J Roentgenol 155:277, 1990.

73. Botet JF, Lightdale CJ, Zauber AG, et al: Preoperative staging of esophageal cancer: Comparison of endoscopic US and dynamic CT. Radiology 181:419, 1991.

74. Heintz A, Höhne U, Schweden F, et al: Preoperative detection of intrathoracic tumor spread of esophageal cancer: Endosonography versus computed tomography. Surg Endosc 5:75, 1991.

75. Ziegler K, Sanft C, Zeitz M, et al: Evaluation of endosonography in TN staging of oesophageal cancer. Gut 32:16, 1991.

76. Reinig JW, Stanley JH, Schabel SI: CT evaluation of thickened esophageal walls. Am J Roentgenol 140:931, 1983.

77. Duignan JP, McEntee GP, O'Connell DJ, et al: The role of CT in the management of carcinoma of the oesophagus and cardia. Ann R Coll Surg Engl 69:283, 1987.

78. Ruol A, Rossi M, Ruffatto A, et al: Reevaluation of computed tomography in preoperative staging of esophageal and cardial cancers: A prospective study. In Siewert JR, Hölscher AH (eds): Diseases of the Esophagus. 1st Ed. Berlin, Springer-Verlag, 1988, pp 194–197.

79. Kasbarian M, Fuentes P, Brichon PY, et al: Usefulness of computed tomography in assessing the extension of carcinoma of the esophagus and gastroesophageal junction. In Siewart JR, Hölscher AH (eds): Diseases of the Esophagus. 1st Ed. Berlin, Springer-Verlag, 1988, pp 185–188.

80. Markland CG, Manhire A, Davies P, et al: The role of computed tomography in assessing the operability of oesophageal carcinoma. Eur J Cardio-Thorac Surg 3:33, 1989.

81. Kirk SJ, Moorehead RJ, McIlrath E, et al: Does preoperative computed tomography scanning aid assessment of oesophageal carcinoma? Postgrad Med J 66:191, 1990.

82. Søndenaa K, Skaane P, Nygaard K, et al: Value of computed tomography in preoperative evaluation of resectability and staging of oesophageal carcinoma. Eur J Surg 158:537, 1992.

83. Consigliere D, Chua CL, Hui F, et al: Computed tomography for oesophageal carcinoma: Its value to the surgeon. J R Coll Surg Edinb. 37:113, 1992.

84. Ginsberg GG, Al-Kawas FH, Nguyen CC, et al: Endoscopic ultrasound evaluation of vascular involvement in esophageal cancer: A comparison with computed tomography. Gastrointest Endosc 39:276, 1993.

85. Rice TW, Boyce GA, Sivak MV Jr: Esophageal ultrasound and the preoperative staging of carcinoma of the esophagus. J Thorac Cardiovasc Surg 101:536, 1991.

86. Rice TW, Sivak MV Jr, Kirby TJ: Ultrasound staging of esophageal carcinoma. Can J Surg 34:399, 1991.

87. Souquet JC, Napoleon B, Pujol P, et al: Endosonography-guided treatment of esophageal carcinoma. Endoscopy 24:(suppl 1)324, 1992.

88. Hordijk ML, Zander H, van Blankenstein M, et al: Influence of tumor stenosis on the accuracy of endosonography in preoperative T staging of esophageal cancer. Endoscopy 25:171, 1993.

89. Van Dam J, Rice TW, Catalano MF, et al: High-grade malignant stricture is predictive of esophageal tumor stage: Risks of endosonographic evaluation. Cancer 71:2910, 1993.

90. Quint LE, Glazer GM, Orringer MB: Esophageal imaging by MR and CT: Study of normal anatomy and neoplasms. Radiology 156:727, 1985.

91. Lehr L, Rupp N, Siewert JR: Assessment of resectability of esophageal cancer by computed tomography and magnetic resonance imaging. Surgery 103:344, 1988.

92. Takashima S, Takeuchi N, Shiozaki H, et al: Carcinoma of the esophagus: CT vs MRI imaging in determining resectability. Am J Roentgenol 156:297, 1991.

93. Choi TK, Sui KF, Lam KH, et al: Bronchoscopy and carcinoma of the esophagus. I: Findings of bronchoscopy in carcinoma of the esophagus. Am J Surg 147:757, 1984.

94. Watanabe A, Saka H, Sakai S, et al: Bronchoscopic and cytopathological findings of tracheobronchial involvement in esophageal carcinoma. Endoscopy 22:273, 1990.

95. Choi TK, Siu KF, Lam KH, et al: Bronchoscopy and carcinoma of the esophagus. II: Carcinoma of the esophagus with tracheobronchial involvement. Am J Surg 147:760, 1984.

96. Fiocco M, Krasna MJ: Thoracoscopic lymph node dissection in the staging of esophageal carcinoma. J Laparoendo Surg 2:111, 1992.

97. Rice TW: Thoracoscopy and the staging of thoracic malignancies. In Daniel TM, Kaiser LR (eds): Thoracoscopic Surgery. 1st Ed. Boston, Little, Brown & Co, 1993, pp 153–162.

98. Genereux GP, Howie JL: Normal mediastinal lymph node size and number: CT and anatomic study. Am J Roentgenol 142:1095, 1984.

99. Glazer GM, Gross BH, Quint LE, et al: Normal mediastinal lymph nodes: Number and size according to American Thoracic Society mapping. Am J Roentgenol 144:261, 1985.

100. Wiersema MJ, Kochman ML, Chak A, et al: Real-time endoscopic ultrasound-guided fine-needle aspiration of a mediastinal node. Gastrointest Endosc 39:429, 1993.

101. Tio TL, Coene PPLO, Luiken GJHM, et al: Endosonography in the clinical staging of esophagogastric carcinoma. Gastrointest Endosc 36:S2, 1990.

102. Catalano MF, Sivak MV Jr, Rice TW, et al: Depth of tumor invasion of esophageal carcinoma (ECA) is predictive of lymph node metastasis: Role of endoscopic ultrasonography (EUS). Am J Gastroenterol 87:1245A, 1992.

103. Dittler HJ, Rösch T, Lorenz R, et al: Failure of endoscopic ultrasonography to differentiate malignant from benign nodes in esophageal cancer. Gastrointest Endosc 38:240A, 1992.

104. Terui S, Yamaguchi H, Kato H, et al: A new method of visualizing the lymph nodes of esophageal carcinoma using superimposed lymphoscintigraphy. *In* Siewert JR, Hölscher AH (eds): Diseases of the Esophagus. 1st Ed. Berlin, Springer-Verlag, 1988, pp 140–142.

105. Saito T, Kuwahara A, Kaketani K, et al: Preoperative assessment of cervical lymph node involvement in esophageal cancer. Jpn J Surg 21:145, 1991.

106. Sostre S, Romero I, Rivera JV, et al: Gallium imaging of esophageal carcinoma: Increased sensitivity with lateral views of the thorax. Clin Nucl Med 15:163, 1990.

107. Tohnosu N, Onoda S, Isono K: Ultrasonographic evaluation of cervical lymph node metastases in esophageal cancer with special reference to the relationship between the short to long axis ratio (S/L) and the cancer content. J Clin Ultrasound 17:101, 1989.

108. van Overhagen H, Laméris JS, Zonderland HM, et al: Ultrasound and ultrasound-guided fine needle aspiration biopsy of supraclavicular nodes in patients with esophageal carcinoma. Cancer 67:585, 1991.

109. Eftekhari F, Fornage BD, Mahon TG: Carcinoma of the cervicothoracic esophagus: Sonographic findings and guided percutaneous needle biopsy. J Clin Ultrasound 20:632, 1992.

110. Watt I, Stewart I, Anderson D, et al: Laparoscopy, ultrasound, and computed tomography in cancer of the oesophagus and gastric cardia: A prospective comparison for detecting intra-abdominal metastases. Br J Surg 76:1036, 1989.

111. Wernecke K, Rummeny E, Bongartz G: Detection of hepatic masses in patients with carcinoma: Comparative sensitivities of sonography, CT, and MR imaging. Am J Roentgenol 157:731, 1991.

112. Inculet RI, Keller SM, Dwyer A, et al: Evaluation of noninvasive tests for the preoperative staging of carcinoma of the esophagus: A prospective study. Ann Thorac Surg 40:561, 1985.

113. Rice TW, Boyce GA, Sivak MV, et al: Esophageal carcinoma: Esophageal ultrasound assessment of preoperative chemotherapy. Ann Thorac Surg 53:972, 1992.

114. Nousbaum JB, Robaszkiewicz M, Cauvin JM, et al: Endosonography can detect residual tumor infiltration of oesophageal cancer in the absence of endoscopic lesions. Gut 33:1459, 1992.

115. Lightdale CJ, Botet JF, Kelsen DP, et al: Diagnosis of recurrent upper gastrointestinal cancer at the surgical anastomosis by endoscopic ultrasound. Gastrointest Endosc 35:220, 1989.

116. Attah EB, Hajdu SI: Benign and malignant tumors of the esophagus at autopsy. J Thorac Cardiovasc Surg 55:396, 1968.

117. Anderson LL, Lad TE: Autopsy findings in squamous cell carcinoma of the esophagus. Cancer 50:1587, 1982.

118. Cilley RE, Strodel WE, Peterson RO: Cause of death in carcinoma of the esophagus. Am J Gastroenterol 84:147, 1989.

119. Soares FA, Magnani Landell GA, Mello de Olivera JA: Pulmonary tumor embolism from squamous cell carcinoma of the oesophagus. Eur J Cancer 27:495, 1991.

THERAPY

24 SURGERY FOR CARCINOMA OF THE ESOPHAGUS

Jack A. Roth and Joe B. Putnam, Jr.

Surgical resection of esophageal carcinomas has played a prominent role in attempts both to palliate dysphagia and to cure. The success of surgical resection of esophageal tumors has been closely linked with the development of perioperative and intraoperative improvements in the care of thoracic surgical patients.

The first successful resection of an esophageal carcinoma was performed by Czerny in 1877.[1] A cervical esophageal carcinoma was removed, and the patient was fed through a distal cervical esophagostomy. The patient lived for 15 months.[2] During the next 30 years, surgeons focused their efforts primarily on bypassing unresectable obstructions. Tubes were developed to carry food from an esophageal fistula to a gastrostomy opening, and skin tubes and jejunal loops were used as conduits.[3] The first intrathoracic esophagectomy was performed by Torek in New York;[4] the cervical esophagostomy was connected to the stomach by a rubber tube. In 1933, Turner reported the first extrathoracic esophagectomy.[5] Two months later a reconstruction was performed with a skin tube and jejunal loop. The patient, a 58-year-old miner, lived 19 months. The modern era of resection and immediate reconstruction was initiated by Adams and Phemister in 1938 with their report of the first transpleural esophagectomy followed by esophagogastrostomy performed through a left thoracoabdominal incision.[6]

Following World War II, the principles of transthoracic resection and immediate reconstruction had become accepted, and debate centered on the best operative approach. Sweet favored a left-sided thoracoabdominal incision and presented one of the first series of successful resections that used this technique.[7] Lewis described the combined laparotomy and right thoracotomy approach.[8] The merits of each have been hotly debated.[9] These operations, plus the Turner extrathoracic esophagectomy recently advocated by Orringer,[10] are the mainstays of thoracic surgery for cancer of the esophagus. The relative merits of each approach will be discussed in a subsequent section.

Although effective palliation of dysphagia and a low operative mortality rate have been achieved for esophagectomy, the rate of survival following resection alone remains poor. Recent clinical trials have focused on the addition of other therapeutic modalities, including radiation therapy and chemotherapy, to surgical resection. These adjuvant therapies are discussed in Chapter 26.

ANATOMIC AND TECHNICAL CONSIDERATIONS

The esophagus is a muscular tube that consists of an outer longitudinal muscle layer and an inner circular muscle layer lined with squamous epithelium. The outer layer is invested with a thin adventitia, but there is no true serosal layer. The esophagus extends from the cricopharyngeus to the histologic gastroesophageal (squamous-columnar) junction (Fig. 24–1A). The average length of the esophagus is 25 cm but may vary.[2] The distance from the incisors to the cricopharyngeus (the beginning of the cervical esophagus) is about 15 cm in men and 14 cm in women. The distance from the incisors to the carina averages 26 cm in men and 23.9 cm in women. Thus, the total length measured on endoscopy from incisors to cardioesophageal junction is approximately 40 cm. The diameter

A

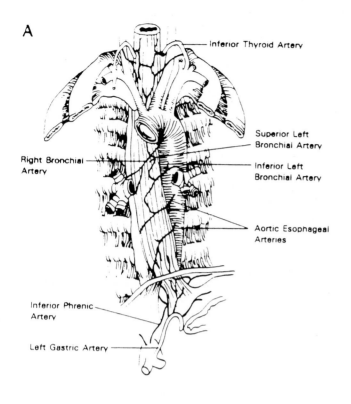

B

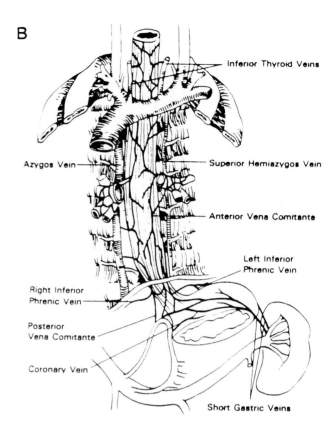

C

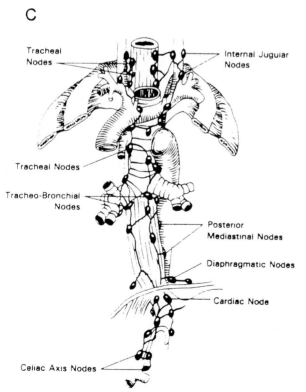

D

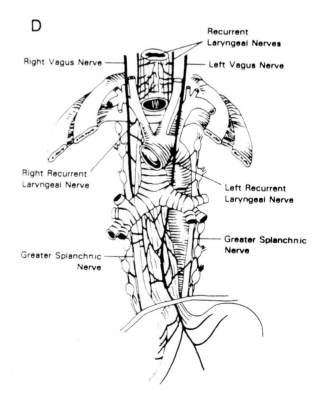

Figure 24–1. Anatomy of the esophagus illustrating arteries *(A)*, veins *(B)*, lymphatics *(C)*, and nerves *(D)*. (From Postlethwait RW: Surgery of the Esophagus. 2nd Ed. Norwalk, Connecticut, Appleton-Century-Crofts, 1986.)

of the esophagus varies from 2.3 to 2.5 cm in the sagittal plane and from 1.7 to 2.4 cm in the transverse plane.

The cervical esophagus begins at the sixth cervical vertebra and extends to the third thoracic vertebra, a length of approximately 5 cm. It is bordered ventrally by the membranous portion of the trachea, laterally by the recurrent laryngeal nerve, and dorsally by the deep cervical fascia. Tissue planes are easiest to develop around the more distal portion of the cervical esophagus.

After transversing the thoracic inlet, the supra-aortic esophagus lies behind and just to the left of the trachea and is bordered on the left by the vagus nerve, the left common carotid and subclavian arteries, and the left paratracheal lymph nodes. It is located between the aorta and the azygos vein. Division of the azygos vein will allow the entire esophagus to be dissected from its intrathoracic bed. At the tracheal bifurcation, the esophagus lies behind the junction of the subcarinal and left tracheobronchial lymph nodes as well as the left main-stem bronchus with the carina. A tumor arising in this location, within the midesophagus, may form a tracheoesophageal fistula with the left main-stem bronchus. Even small tumors arising in this area may invade the trachea, bronchus, or aorta, making complete resection impossible. The thoracic duct courses from right to left at the fifth thoracic vertebra and is at risk for injury during right-sided dissections below this level.

Distal to the carina, the esophagus lies behind the pericardium and the left atrium and ventricle of the heart. At the level of the ninth thoracic vertebra, the esophagus passes through the diaphragmatic foramen. The left vagus nerve becomes ventral and the right vagus nerve becomes dorsal at the cardioesophageal junction.

For the purpose of classification and description, the esophagus is arbitrarily divided into sections. This system is clinically useful because treatment options for tumors of the cervical and upper thoracic esophagus may be quite different from those for tumors of the intrathoracic or intra-abdominal esophagus. However, there are currently no standard divisions. The American Joint Committee for Cancer Staging and End Results Reporting divides the esophagus into three sections: the cervical esophagus extending from the pharyngoesophageal junction to the thoracic inlet 18 cm from the incisors; a second portion extending from the thoracic inlet to 10 cm above the esophagogastric junction; and a third region comprising the distal 10 cm of esophagus. It is probably most useful clinically to divide the esophagus into thirds: the upper, consisting of the cervical esophagus and upper thoracic esophagus; the middle, from the superior position of the aortic arch to the inferior pulmonary vein; and the lower, from the pulmonary vein to the gastroesophageal junction. Describing the positions of tumors relative to these locations informs the surgeon of the major anatomic structures that may be involved and suggests potential difficulties with resection.

Arterial Supply. The cervical and upper thoracic portion of the esophagus is supplied by the inferior thyroid artery as well as by branches of the subclavian, common carotid, superior thyroid, costocervical, superficial cervical, and vertebral arteries (Fig. 24–1B). The esophagus from the thoracic inlet to the carina is supplied by the bronchial arteries and other aortic branches. Below the carina, arteries to the esophagus arise directly from the aorta. Two or three unpaired branches are usually found. The abdominal portion is supplied by branches of the left gastric and inferior phrenic arteries. The arteries are segmentally arranged, although there are anastomoses between them.[11] Extensive trauma from dissection of the esophagus without intent to resect should be avoided because the blood supply to a surgical anastomosis may be interrupted.

Veins. The esophageal veins originate from the periesophageal plexus (Fig. 24–1C). In the cervical region, these empty into the inferior thyroid vein or vertebral vein. In the thorax, they drain into the bronchial veins, pericardial veins, superior diaphragmatic vein, or the azygos system.

Innervation. The cervical and upper thoracic portions are innervated by branches of the recurrent laryngeal nerve (Fig. 24–1D). The thoracic and abdominal esophagus is supplied by the vagus nerve with a contribution from the sympathetic trunk.

Lymphatics. The esophagus has a rich mucosal and submucosal lymphatic network that is independent of blood vessels.[2] Injection studies have demonstrated that spread is always greater in the longitudinal direction than in the transverse (6:1 ratio). The submucosal lymphatics may run particularly long courses. This plexus drains into the internal jugular, peritracheal, hilar subcarinal, paraesophageal, para-aortic, paracardial lesser curvature, left gastric, and celiac nodes (Fig. 24–1C). Thus, this extensive lymphatic network permits longitudinal spread of tumors to remote sites in unpredictable fashion. In one series, 12 of 27 patients with tumors at 25 to 34 cm from the incisors had metastases in the celiac lymph nodes.[12] Skip areas also may be present within the esophagus at a distance from the primary tumor (see Chapter 21). Thus, careful evaluation of the entire esophagus and lymphatic drainage is required during resection to avoid leaving residual gross tumor. Surgical resection of the total esophagus may be required for maximal mechanical extirpation of tumor.

PATIENT SELECTION AND PREOPERATIVE PREPARATION

The extremely poor long-term survival rates following surgical resection for carcinoma of the esophagus have fostered pessimism with respect to any attempts at curative treatment. Many clinicians have adopted the attitude that palliation is all that can be hoped for, but others have stated that since the percentage of

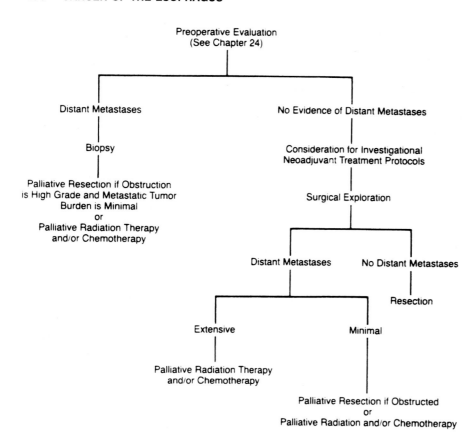

Figure 24–2. Preoperative evaluation and treatment options for patients with esophageal carcinoma.

patients alive 5 years after surgery exceeds the current operative mortality rate, curative surgery should be undertaken. Pessimism with respect to curative surgical procedures has stemmed from early reports of high mortality rates,[13, 14] but operative mortality rates of 5% are now being achieved. Thus, the goals of palliation and potential cure can frequently be achieved within the context of the surgical resection. A curative resection may not only eradicate the tumor but also relieve dysphagia, the primary goal of palliation. Thus, the division of surgical therapies into palliative and curative is to a large extent artificial.

Preoperative determination of the resectability of an esophageal carcinoma is difficult, and noninvasive studies are not completely reliable. Inculet and associates found that chest and abdominal computed tomographic scans were the most reliable noninvasive tests.[15] In their study, compression of the tracheobronchial tree was noted for all five patients with unresectable middle third tumors. However, only five of the ten patients with locally unresectable tumor in this area had this compression. Other degrees of abutment or separation of the tumor from the trachea or aorta were unreliable indicators of resectability. In our experience, computed tomography is more accurate than barium swallow in assessing the size and local extension of the primary tumor. Bronchoscopy is critical to assessing bronchial invasion. Preoperative determination of the presence of distant metastases is useful in that patients may be spared an attempt at extensive resection, although other surgical procedures to restore swallowing may be indicated. Syn-

chronous bone metastases are seen in fewer than 10% of cases, but a bone scan should be obtained in any patient with a history of bone pain. A flow diagram illustrating treatment options appears in Figure 24–2.

Patients with esophageal carcinoma frequently present with significant weight loss. Nutritional metabolic deficits have been documented.[16] Obvious dehydration and blood volume deficits should be corrected preoperatively. Patients who can still swallow liquids can be given one of the commercially available high-calorie and protein liquid supplements while they are undergoing preoperative evaluation. The value of long or short (5- to 10-day) preoperative courses of enteral or total parenteral nutrition has not been determined. Correction of nutritional deficits theoretically could reduce operative morbidity. In a retrospective analysis, patients who received at least 5 days of total parenteral nutrition had a lower rate of postoperative complications than patients who received none.[17] However, a number of complications have been associated with total parenteral nutrition, including fluid overload, catheter-related sepsis, and venous thrombosis.[18] Prospective randomized clinical trials are needed to determine the value of this approach.

Normal swallowing should be restored as soon as possible. Usually, the most debilitated patients are those with complete obstruction. While alimentation for several weeks may correct some of the nutritional deficit, the additional delay places these patients at increased risk for aspiration and sepsis. A gastrostomy should be avoided if possible, since the stomach is a useful conduit for reconstruction.

Preoperative assessment of pulmonary function is important. Patients with squamous cell carcinomas frequently have a long history of cigarette smoking, and cessation of smoking is critical. Smoking cessation for a minimum of 2 weeks is required. Instruction in the use of the incentive spirometer will assist in postoperative pulmonary hygiene. Poor pulmonary function per se should not be a contraindication for resection but may influence the decision to perform a thoracotomy. Preoperative placement of a nasogastric tube may help avoid aspiration. Cardiac and hepatic functions should be carefully assessed preoperatively. Good oral hygiene should be established or maintained, and dental extractions performed preoperatively if needed. Because the oral/esophageal bacterial flora in patients with esophageal carcinoma consists of both aerobic and anaerobic species,[19] third-generation cephalosporins are appropriate for use as preoperative prophylactic antibiotics. Aminoglycosides are to be avoided if the patient has impaired renal function or has received cisplatin chemotherapy preoperatively.

OPERATIVE CONSIDERATIONS

Surgical resection and reconstruction are reliable means of achieving normal swallowing and restoring gastrointestinal continuity in patients with esophageal cancer, which are the primary goals of palliation. As discussed previously, these goals can be achieved with an acceptable rate of operative mortality. A potential added benefit is that a small percentage of patients will survive long-term following surgical resection. Resection and reconstruction are accomplished in a single-stage procedure. Multiple-stage procedures with bypass during one operation and subsequent resection are to be avoided.

Laparotomy is a useful first step in all operative procedures. Noninvasive staging is not completely reliable in determining resectability or the presence of distant metastases. The finding of unresectable local celiac lymph node metastases or extensive hepatic metastases precludes attempts at an aggressive curative resection. If the tumor cannot be resected completely, it may still be beneficial to remove the bulk of the tumor and mark the residual tumor by metal clips to guide radiation therapy. Large bulky tumors often cause symptoms. Bypass procedures that leave the primary tumor and a "blind" esophageal pouch have high rates of operative mortality and complications.[20, 21] Extensive resection involving the lung, main-stem bronchi, or trachea should be avoided.

An additional rationale for aggressive resection is that occasional patients with positive regional lymph nodes or histologically positive margins may enjoy long-term survival following resection. In Postlethwait's series, 7% of patients (3 of 44) with positive regional lymph nodes were alive 5 or more years following resection.[2] Three of 12 patients with positive margins were also alive for 5 or more years. Because the rich submucosal lymphatic plexus favors longitu-dinal spread of tumors within the esophagus, total or subtotal esophagectomy is usually the preferred approach. Segmental resection frequently results in microscopic residual tumor at the surgical margin and a high incidence of local recurrence. This finding was emphasized by Scanlon and colleagues who found the incidence rate of positive margins or local recurrence to be 45.6% in 79 patients undergoing segmental resection.[22]

TECHNIQUES OF ESOPHAGECTOMY

A number of technical approaches have been described for resecting cancers of the esophagus. They vary in one or more of the following: type of incision, extent of resection, conduit for reconstruction, and type of anastomosis. Because few controlled clinical trials have been done to compare these technical differences, it is not possible to make definitive statements regarding the advantages of one technique over another. Comparison of different series is also difficult because results are not presented in a standardized format. Inclusion of varying proportions of different histologic types and stages can make comparisons among series misleading. Claims concerning resectability are also difficult to interpret: "resectable" may mean tumor-free margins in one series and removal of the bulk of the tumor with residual gross tumor in another. Similarly, survival rates can be altered depending on the denominator used. Survival can be expressed as a percentage of all patients with esophageal cancer seen at an institution, all patients who were operative candidates, or all patients actually undergoing surgery, or as actuarial survival. A difference of only 5% to 10% may result in a significant apparent improvement in overall survival. Clearly, then, treatment decisions must therefore be made on the basis of incomplete data. In this chapter, we will summarize the most comparable results from recent series.

APPROACHES TO ESOPHAGEAL RESECTION

Esophagectomy for carcinoma of the esophagus poses considerable physiologic and technical challenges to both the surgeon and the patient. Esophagectomy for carcinoma of the esophagus provides excellent palliation from dysphagia that is unsurpassed by any other modality, including chemotherapy and radiation therapy. Surgery remains the primary treatment of esophageal tumors that are confined to the esophagus and paraesophageal tissues and provides local control and survival rates superior to those afforded by any nonsurgical modality, either single or combined.

Various techniques are used to resect the esophagus. In all procedures a laparotomy is done first to mobilize the gastric conduit. In the Lewis procedure (Ivor Lewis esophagectomy), the esophagus is resected through a right thoracotomy incision and an intrathoracic esophagogastric anastomosis is performed, usually at the level of the azygos vein. In the total thoracic esophagectomy, the gastric conduit is brought either substernally or through the posterior mediastinum, and the esophagogastrostomy is completed in the left neck. The intrathoracic esophagus is resected through a right thoracotomy.

The transhiatal resection of the esophagus was first described by Turner and later reintroduced by Orringer,[23] Kirk,[24] and Akiyama and associates.[25] A transhiatal esophagectomy consists of resection of the intrathoracic esophagus performed through the esophageal hiatus and the thoracic inlet without an open thoracotomy. The esophagus is dissected bluntly from both cervical and abdominal incisions. Much of the operation can be done under direct vision by dividing the esophageal hiatus. Dissection of midesophageal tumors must be accomplished in part without direct vision.[10] The gastric conduit is placed into the posterior mediastinum and a cervical anastomosis is performed.

Indications for this procedure remain controversial. Disadvantages include the possibility that some patients will be denied cure because of inadequate resection. Because it is difficult to perform a complete lymph node dissection with this technique, patients may be understaged, denying them access to clinical trials for which they should be eligible. Finally, there is some increased risk of tracheobronchial or vascular tears when this approach is used for large tumors. This technique is probably most useful in patients with cervical tumors or distal third tumors for removal of residual normal esophagus. In our experience, it is also useful in patients with severe respiratory compromise in whom thoracotomy would be hazardous.

Few series have directly compared right and left thoracotomies for resecting the esophagus. In general, the left thoracoabdominal incision is used for tumors located between the aortic arch (inferior) and the cardia. In a series reported by Launois and associates, the operative mortality and survival rates did not differ significantly for the two approaches.[26] Table 24–1 summarizes the operative mortality and survival rates for several recent series employing one or more of the approaches just described.[23, 26–31]

The extensive and unpredictable longitudinal extension of esophageal carcinomas makes total intrathoracic esophagectomy prudent in many cases. For very distal lesions that involve only the stomach, it is possible to determine the proximal extent of the tumor by quadrant biopsies of the esophagus during endoscopy. If no tumor is present in the biopsies, anastomosis can be performed provided there is no extraesophageal spread at that level. However, reflux can be a severe problem with lower intrathoracic anastomoses. An anastomotic leak within the thorax is also much more difficult to treat than a leak from a cervical anastomosis following total esophagectomy. We reviewed a series of 248 patients who underwent one of the three types of esophagectomies and found that operative morbidity and mortality were similar for the three operations but that patients with a cervical anastomosis had a higher anastomotic leak rate (11%) than those with an intrathoracic anastomosis (6%).[32] The stage-specific survival was similar for the three operations. Survival from esophageal cancer is still dependent on resectability and the stage of disease and appears not to be altered by differences in any of the techniques currently used for resection.

Extensive and radical surgical procedures for resection of esophageal tumors have been advocated by some.[33, 34] Logan described removing the esophagus and tumor in a sheath of normal mediastinal tissue.[34] The surrounding pleura, azygos system, thoracic duct, lymphatics, and segments of the pericardium and diaphragm are taken with the tumor. Skinner reported on a series of 80 patients who underwent en bloc esophagectomy with an operative mortality rate of 11% and an actuarial survival rate of 18% at 5 years.[33] It seems unlikely that a relatively extensive local procedure would salvage patients with extensive local spread, nodal involvement, or both, since the majority of patients do have systemic metastases at the time of resection. Patients with early stage tumors probably would not benefit from en bloc esophagectomy as these tumors could be completely resected by a less radical operation. The high operative mortality rate associated with the more extensive procedures also would negate any small benefit from the salvage of late-stage patients. Survival following more extensive operations (also called en bloc esophagectomy)[35] is no greater than that for any other techniques of esophagectomy, and the operative mortality rate is higher.[23]

RECONSTRUCTION FOLLOWING RESECTION

The stomach, colon, and jejunum have all been successfully used as replacement conduits following esophagectomy. No controlled clinical trials have compared these techniques, and thus there has been no definitive demonstration of superiority of one technique over the others. However, there are practical considerations that favor the use of the stomach for

TABLE 24–1. Comparison of Operative Morbidity and Mortality and Survival for Different Techniques of Surgical Resection for Epidermoid Carcinoma of the Esophagus

SERIES	TECHNIQUE	OPERATIVE MORTALITY (%)	SURVIVAL*
Launois[26]	Left thoracoabdominal	26/147 (17.7)	6
Launois[26]	Right thoracotomy	10/58 (17.2)	14
Launois[26]	Akiyama	1/27 (3.2)	—
Hankins[27]	Right thoracotomy	0/11 (0)	—
Hankins[27]	Left thoracoabdominal	0/6 (0)	—
Carey[28]	Right thoracotomy	0/37 (0)	13 months mean
Roth[29]	Right thoracotomy	1/34 (2.9)	9 months median
Katlic[30]	Right thoracotomy	7/67 (10.4)	18
Putnam[32]	Right thoracotomy	10/134 (9.6)	24
Putnam[32]	Akiyama	2/45 (4.2)	16
Putnam[32]	Transhiatal	2/42 (4.8)	24
Orringer[23]	Transhiatal	6/100 (6)	17 (4 yr)
Yonezawa[31]	Transhiatal	0/31 (0)	NA

*Actuarial 5-year per cent survival unless otherwise stated.

TABLE 24–2. Comparison of Operative Morbidity and Mortality and Overall Survival for Different Conduits Used for Surgical Reconstruction for Epidermoid Carcinoma of the Esophagus

SERIES	CONDUIT	OPERATIVE MORBIDITY (%)	OPERATIVE MORTALITY (%)	SURVIVAL*
Hoffman[56]	Stomach	14/44 (32)	7/44 (16)	11.5 months mean
Wang[93]	Stomach	59/193 (26)	8/193 (4)	—
Wang[93]	Colon	41/114 (36)	8/114 (7)	—
Nishihira[43]	Stomach	—	23/181 (13)	28
Nishihira[43]	Jejunum	—	8/78 (11)	34
Bernstein[94]	Stomach	15/20 (75)	4/20 (20)	30 (2 yr)
Bernstein[94]	Colon	14/18 (78)	4/18 (22)	33 (2 yr)
Wilkins[95]	Colon	40/100 (40)	9/100 (9)	7
Postlethwait[96]	Colon	—	62/367 (17)	—
Akiyama[25]	Stomach	6/130 (5)	1/130 (0.8)	—
Launois[26]	Stomach	—	1/27 (3)	—

*Actuarial 5-year per cent survival unless otherwise stated.

reconstruction in patients with esophageal malignancies.

The stomach is easily mobilized and has an excellent vascular supply. An extensive network of intramural vessels supplies the fundus even when the left gastric and left gastroepiploic vessels are divided during mobilization. In our experience, the stomach is adequate in length to reach the neck and the base of the tongue in all individuals. For distal third tumors, a 5-cm margin can be excised radially from the distal end of the tumor, leaving the fundus, where the single cervical anastomosis is performed.[10] Use of the gastric conduit is generally accompanied by a pyloroplasty or pyloromyotomy to prevent gastric stasis induced by vagotomy. There is no universal agreement that this drainage procedure is necessary,[36] but evidence indicates that an inadequate pyloromyotomy or omission of the pyloroplasty can result in significant delay in gastric emptying.

In patients undergoing total esophagectomy, the stomach may be placed in one of three different locations: subcutaneous, retrosternal, or mediastinal. Posterior mediastinal placement is probably the most popular. This position gives the shortest distance to the neck,[37] but the retrosternal route is only 2 cm longer.[38] Nor does the posterior mediastinal position require widening of the thoracic inlet by resection of the medial clavicle, manubrium, and portion of first rib as does retrosternal placement. The stomach can be positioned either anteriorly or posteriorly to the hilum. A disadvantage of the anterior approach is compression of the lung from gastric distention, which increases the risk of pulmonary complications in the postoperative period. When a total intrathoracic esophagectomy is performed, and it is likely that postoperative radiation therapy is needed, our preference is for the substernal placement of the gastric conduit as described by Akiyama and associates.[25] The theoretic advantage of this conduit location is that it reduces the risk and degree of radiation injury if postoperative radiation therapy is required, because the conduit is not in the radiation field. This position interferes little with lung function, and the widened

thoracic inlet allows a tension-free anastomosis. Reflux through the gastric conduit may occur, since the drainage occurs by gravity only. Patients are instructed not to recline during or for one hour after eating and should sleep with the head of the bed elevated 30° to 45°. Ward and Collis interviewed 23 patients an average of 5 years following esophagogastrectomy and elicited no reports of clinical symptoms of reflux esophagitis, although reflux of barium could be demonstrated in all patients.[39]

If patients have had a previous partial or total gastrectomy or if the stomach is extensively involved with tumor, it may not be long enough to serve as a conduit replacement. The colon is the most commonly used alternative to the stomach. Either the right or left colon can be used, although the segment of the left and transverse colon supplied by the left colic artery is longer. In addition, an intact marginal artery is present more often for the left colon.[40] It is essential to obtain a preoperative arteriogram to delineate the arterial anatomy in the segment to be used for replacement. A barium enema should also be obtained to rule out a synchronous colon carcinoma or inflammatory changes in the colon. The operative mortality rate following colon interposition is generally higher than that for a gastric conduit (Table 24–2). The difference in mortality rates, the need for two additional anastomoses (colojejunostomy and colocolostomy) with colon interposition and the frequency of atherosclerosis noted in the intestinal arteries of the older patient population with cancer have persuaded us to use the stomach for replacement whenever possible. However, long-term function of colon conduits in patients with esophageal replacement for benign disease has been excellent.[41, 42]

Jejunal loops have also been used for conduit replacement. The restricted mobility of these loops and the unpredictability of their vascular supply have limited their popularity in patients with carcinoma, although successful series have been reported.[43]

Tubes formed from the greater curvature of the stomach have also been used as gastric conduits.[44] This procedure has been evaluated by only a small number of investigators. The additional complexity of the procedure is a significant disadvantage in debilitated patients.

More recently, free jejunal graft interposition has been used successfully for conduit replacement following resection for carcinoma of the upper cervical esophagus or hypopharynx that does not extend past the thoracic inlet. Once the esophagus is resected, the proximal and distal anastomoses are completed to stabilize the graft. Vascular access is usually obtained from the external carotid artery and the internal jugular vein. Up to 15 to 20 cm of jejunum may be used as a free graft.

ESOPHAGEAL ANASTOMOSIS

A variety of suture materials and techniques have been described for esophageal anastomosis. Technique rather than type of suture material is probably the most critical factor in achieving a successful anastomosis. Tension on the anastomosis must be avoided, and this can be done by securing the proximal stomach to mediastinal tissue or prevertebral fascia. Anastomotic narrowing will be minimized by using interrupted sutures. For intrathoracic anastomosis, a two-layer 3-0 silk anastomosis is used. The first row of the inner layer includes submucosal sutures anchoring the esophagus to the stomach. The stomach is then incised, and sutures encompassing the full thickness of the esophageal and gastric walls are placed as an inner layer with knots tied on the inside. The final outer row consists of horizontal mattress sutures that invaginate the anastomosis in a cuff of stomach.

Automatic stapling devices have been used for esophagogastric anastomoses,[45-48] but stapling and handsewn techniques have not been compared in appropriately controlled clinical trials. The need for gastrotomy and precise placement of pursestring sutures obviates any time advantage that use of the stapler might have in actual performance of anastomosis. Errors in staple placement are also difficult to correct. The late stricture incidence of 16 percent in one series of stapled anastomoses is higher than the 5 percent to 10 percent usually reported for handsewn anastomoses.[48] Cervical anastomoses also may be constructed with interrupted absorbable braided sutures. The risk of leak may be as low as 10 percent.[49]

DESCRIPTION OF SURGICAL TECHNIQUES

Abdominal Approach to Mobilize Conduit

If a total thoracic esophagectomy (TTE) or transhiatal esophagectomy (THE) is to be performed, the patient is positioned as follows. After appropriate lines are placed for intravenous fluids and for monitoring, a small roll is placed under the patient's shoulders, and the head is placed on a head rest and turned to the right so that the left neck is extended. The hands are

tucked at the patient's side. The patient is prepped from the angle of the jaw and chin to the pubis. An iodine-impregnated plastic drape is placed over the abdomen and lower third of the chest. Staples may be used to secure the drapes to the patient's chin and jaw.

The abdominal approach is common to all operations for carcinoma of the esophagus. An upper midline incision is used for the exploratory celiotomy. The abdomen is explored thoroughly, with particular attention to the liver and celiac axis, which are common sites of metastases and unresectable nodal disease. Celiac lymph nodes are considered to be in the regional lymph drainage for lower third lesions. Unresectability relative to celiac nodal disease is considered a contraindication for resection. If no metastases are identified, the stomach is mobilized by freeing the greater curvature. The right gastroepiploic artery is identified and preserved throughout its entire length. The viability of the stomach is based on the vascular supply from right gastric and right gastroepiploic arteries (Fig. 24–3). The greater omentum is separated from the greater curvature (preserving the gastroepiploic artery) to the level of the short gastrics. The short arteries are individually ligated and divided. Sponges may be packed behind the spleen to elevate it for better visualization of the short gastric vessels. This maneuver may be helpful in obese patients. The gastroesophageal junction may also be completely mobilized and encircled with a Penrose drain so that the short gastric vessels may be better visualized from the distal esophagus to the spleen. The paracardial lymph nodes are dissected with the specimen.

The left gastric artery and vein are identified by elevating the stomach toward the patient's right side to expose the posterior aspect of the vessels. Care is taken to determine whether an aberrant hepatic artery is arising from the left gastric artery. If the aberrant artery appears to represent a significant portion of hepatic blood flow, it should be preserved, but a small accessory aberrant hepatic artery can be safely ligated. The left gastric artery and vein are divided. The left gastric artery is divided close to its take-off from the celiac axis to preserve collateral circulation to the stomach. The celiac and left gastric lymph nodes are carefully dissected with the specimen. The lesser curve is then mobilized by dividing the lesser omentum close to the liver, and nodes within the gastrohepatic ligament are taken with the specimen. The gastroesophageal junction is then completely encircled and the paracardial lymph nodes are dissected with the specimen. The omentum is mobilized to a point 2 cm proximal to the pylorus so as not to injure the right gastroepiploic artery or the pylorus. This dissection is easily performed from an anterior approach. A Kocher maneuver is done to the level of the third portion of the duodenum, freeing the duodenum inferiorly and medially to the level of the inferior vena cava. The gallbladder is examined at this point. If cholelithiasis is noted, the gallbladder is removed.

With the stomach completely mobilized, a pyloromyotomy or pyloroplasty may be performed to de-

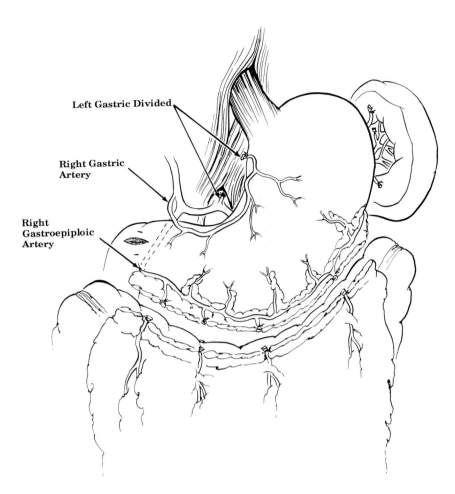

Left Gastric Divided

Right Gastric Artery

Right Gastroepiploic Artery

Figure 24–3. Mobilization of the stomach. The stomach is used primarily as a conduit for esophageal replacement. The blood supply is based on the right gastric artery and gastroepiploic artery. The left gastric and the short gastric arteries are divided. Notice the pyloromyotomy.

crease the likelihood of gastric outlet obstruction, which occurs in only about 20% of patients. Some surgeons use no drainage procedure, but we recommend it because postoperative problems requiring gastric drainage cannot be predicted, and complications are more frequent when a drainage procedure is not used.[50] Fine silk sutures on an atraumatic needle are used to mark the superior and inferior aspects of the pyloric ring to minimize venous bleeding. The pylorus is scored from the very proximal duodenum, through the pylorus, onto the stomach. The muscles are split using a microvascular mosquito clamp with a needle tip electrocautery on a low cut setting. With careful dissection and spreading of the cut edges of the serosa, the muscle fibers can be easily identified. The duodenal mucosa rises almost vertically from the distal portion of the pylorus; care must be taken not to injure it. If the duodenal mucosa is opened, it should be repaired with interrupted fine prolene sutures (5-0 or 6-0) and patched with paraduodenal or omental fat. Clips are used to mark either side of the pyloromyotomy or pyloroplasty and serve as landmarks for the postoperative barium swallow. Alternatively, a single-layer Heineke-Mikulicz pyloroplasty can be performed. A 16-Fr red rubber feeding tube is placed 20 cm distal to the ligament of Treitz for patients having a cervical anastomosis or those who may require longer-term nutritional supplementation.

At this point, the hiatus is briefly explored to determine the extent of tumor. If the tumor is in the distal third, its relationship to the spine, the aorta, and other adjacent structures should be determined. It is convenient at this point to complete the reconstruction for the TTE by placing the gastric conduit substernally. A cervical esophagogastrostomy is fashioned in the left neck following removal of the medial third of the clavicle, the manubrium, and a portion of the first rib to widen the thoracic inlet.

Intrathoracic Resection

The two most commonly used operative approaches to resection of esophageal tumors are a combined laparotomy and right thoracotomy or a left thoracoabdominal incision. The left thoracoabdominal incision begins as an upper midline abdominal incision and continues across the costal margin through the bed of the seventh or eighth rib. The diaphragm is divided. This incision gives excellent exposure for the lower portion of the esophagus. Problems arise when the tumor extends beyond or posterior to the aortic arch. Dissection of the tumor in this area becomes hazardous, particularly if the azygos vein is involved. High anastomoses are difficult with this approach, which may lead to inadequate resection of the esophagus and a greater chance of local recurrence.[51] Other disadvantages of the left thoracoabdominal incision include less than complete esophagectomy and the potential for infection in the costal cartilage and respiratory compromise following division of the diaphragm.

An approach incorporating a right thoracotomy eliminates these problems and exposes the upper intrathoracic esophagus. This exposure permits resection of the entire intrathoracic esophagus, extensive dissection of lymph nodes, and anastomoses at any level. Combining this thoracic incision with an initial exploratory laparotomy to assess intra-abdominal metastases and mobilization of the bypass conduit is expedient and avoids division of the diaphragm and costal cartilage.

Both the Lewis procedure and TTE require a right thoracotomy for esophageal resection. The patient is positioned in a left lateral decubitus position with the operating room table flexed to expand the curvature of the right chest and enhance exposure. A right posterolateral thoracotomy incision is used. A muscle-sparing incision (preserving the latissimus dorsi and serratus anterior muscles) or standard thoracotomy (dividing the latissimus dorsi and mobilizing the serratus anterior muscle anteriorly) provides access to the chest wall. The chest is entered through the fifth intercostal space. The mediastinal pleura overlying the esophagus is incised ventrally and dorsally. After the tumor is identified, the esophagus is encircled above and below the tumor with Penrose drains and completely mobilized.

Lewis Procedure

In the Lewis procedure, the esophageal hiatus is further mobilized to provide easy egress of the stomach into the chest. If not already done, the esophagus is resected with a 5-cm radial margin of the gastric lesser curvature with GIA staplers to elongate the gastric conduit if desired. The suture line is oversewn. The esophagus is then resected as far cephalad as is possible in the chest. The mediastinal lymph nodes are dissected. Usually the thoracic anastomosis is placed at or beyond the level of the azygos vein (Fig. 24–4). Higher intrathoracic anastomoses have been described, but if additional esophageal resection is required to achieve a 5-cm margin, we prefer a total intrathoracic esophagectomy with cervical anastomosis.

The stomach is sutured to the prevertebral fascia. We prefer a handsewn two-layer silk for an intrathoracic anastomosis. However, the EEA stapler may be used. A gastrotomy is made and an EEA stapler is inserted through the gastrotomy and out of the apical portion of the gastric conduit. The anvil is placed into the esophagus, the EEA is fired, and the anastomosis is completed. The gastrotomy is oversewn, and a nasogastric tube is then placed under the direct guidance of the surgeon.

The anastomosis should have no tension and should be at least 25 mm in diameter. The suture line is reinforced and the thoracic cavity irrigated. Two

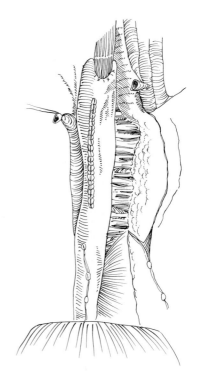

Figure 24–4. Intrathoracic anastomosis following the Lewis esophagectomy. The anastomosis pictured is performed with two layers of interrupted silk sutures placed at the level of the azygous vein.

chest tubes are placed for drainage and are not removed until the patient is eating.

Total Thoracic Esophagectomy

The abdominal exploration and gastric mobilization are done as previously described. The cervical dissection for mobilization of the esophagus in the neck (see Transhiatal Esophagectomy to follow) includes resection of the head of the left clavicle and a portion of the manubrium and first rib to enlarge the thoracic outlet (Fig. 24–5). The stomach, prepared as a tube, is placed retrosternally and brought out through the thoracic inlet. Next the cervical esophagus is mobilized. An L-shaped incision is made from just above the sternal notch (at the level of the left supraclavicular head) approximately four to five fingerbreadths obliquely along the anterior border of the sternocleidomastoid muscle. The platysma is divided, and the sternocleidomastoid muscle and the carotid sheath are retracted laterally. The assistant uses his or her finger to retract the trachea medially and gain exposure to the esophagus. No metal retractor is placed at the level of the tracheoesophageal groove, since this could injure the recurrent laryngeal nerve and cause transient vocal cord paresis or permanent damage. The omohyoid muscle is divided and the vertebral fascia identified; the esophagus is encircled gently with a finger at a site approximately 3 to 4 cm inferior to the cricoid. Care must be taken to stay lateral and posterior to the tracheoesophageal groove and the recurrent laryngeal nerve, which must not be incorporated

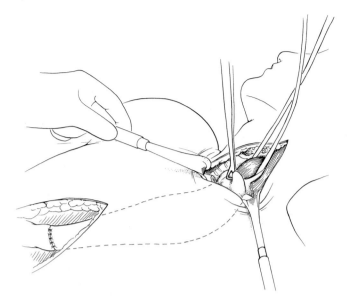

Figure 24–5. Re-establishment of alimentary continuity. The stomach is placed in a retrosternal position, and a cervical anastomosis is fashioned. The proximal third of the clavicle and lateral portion of the manubrium are resected. A pyloroplasty has been created.

into the surgical specimen. The inferior thyroid artery may be divided. A 3/4-inch Penrose drain is placed around the esophagus. The vagus nerve is visualized and protected. The stomach (prepared as a tube) is placed retrosternally and brought out through the thoracic inlet. An anastomosis is handsewn between the end esophagus and the "side" stomach, and a nasogastric tube is placed by direct visual guidance before completing the anastomosis (Fig. 24–6). When the anastomosis is completed, the neck wound is irrigated and a closed-system drain is placed.

The patient is then positioned for a right thoracotomy to resect the esophagus. The chest is entered as described earlier. Because gastrointestinal continuity has already been established, only the esophagus needs to be resected. The esophagus has been stapled closed at its proximal and distal ends. The pleura is incised at a 2-cm distance from the anterior and posterior aspects of the esophagus so that the esophagus is resected with a strip of pleura. It is mobilized from both ends along with the tumor. The arteries supplying the esophagus arise from the aorta and are ligated with clips. The adventitia of the aorta is removed en bloc with the resected esophagus. The thoracic duct is identified, and if it is incised or transected during the procedure, it must be ligated. The esophagus is resected, and the mediastinal lymph nodes, including the paraesophageal, subcarinal, and paratracheal nodes, are dissected. Two chest tubes are placed for drainage.

Transhiatal Esophagectomy

The abdominal and cervical dissections are performed as described earlier. The bony thoracic inlet is not enlarged or resected. A nasogastric tube or an esoph-

ageal stethoscope may then be placed to aid in encircling the esophagus. When the esophagus has been encircled with the Penrose drain in the neck, the loose tissues surrounding the esophagus in the upper thorax are freed circumferentially. This maneuver is accomplished by gently placing the finger on the esophagus and pushing downward while exerting mild tension on the esophagus with the Penrose drain. The nasogastric tube should be removed before freeing the esophagus in the chest. When all circumferential tissue has been gently dissected away from the esophagus, attention is turned back to the abdomen.

The hiatus is exposed and elevated with two small retractors. With the hiatus opened, the esophagus is mobilized posteriorly from the prevertebral fascia and aorta (Fig. 24–7). From the surgeon's side, with the left hand holding the stomach, the right hand is placed posterior to the esophagus and in the midline. Posterior to the hand lie the vertebral column and the aorta. The hand is inserted to the level of the carina. If the hand deviates from the midline and the esophagus, it is quite easy to tear the aorta, the bronchial branches off the aorta, the membranous trachea, or the azygos vein. The esophagus is then dissected from the prevertebral fascia in the neck.

During the abdominal exploration, the tumor may be found to be attached to the prevertebral fascia or to the aorta so that it is unresectable (gross tumor would remain). If a question exists as to the tumor's resectability, then a right thoracotomy will allow further assessment. If resectable, the esophagus may be completely freed from all attachments in the chest. The stomach is mobilized, and a cervical or thoracic anastomosis is performed. Should the tumor be unresectable, the extent of tumor could be marked with metal clips for subsequent radiation therapy.

The anterior portion of the esophagus is mobilized next. The hand is placed flat along the ventral surface of the esophagus. The index and middle fingers are pulled gently alongside the esophagus to mobilize the lateral attachments. Distally, the right and left vagus

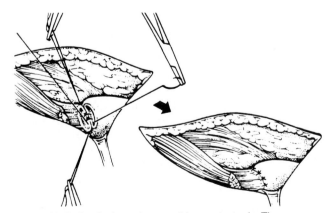

Figure 24–6. Cervical esophagogastric anastomosis. The sternocleidomastoid and omohyoid muscles have been divided. The fundus of the substernal stomach is shown. A two-layer silk anastomosis is performed.

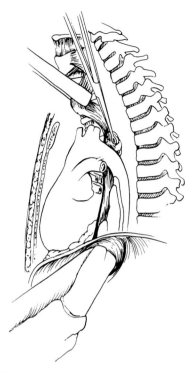

Figure 24–7. Transhiatal esophagectomy. The surgeon's hand may be used to dissect the esophagus off the prevertebral fascia posteriorly in the midline. When the esophagus is completely mobilized, it is divided in the neck with a surgical stapling device and is removed. A single-layer cervical anastomosis is created.

nerves are ligated and divided. Lateral attachments are freed bluntly or encircled with clamps, divided, and tied to minimize mediastinal blood loss, which often is less than 600 to 800 ml for the surgery. Using retractors, it is usually possible to visualize up to the subcarinal area, but if visualization is not possible, the diaphragm may be divided in the midline, ventrally, to provide for additional exposure and mobilization. Mobilization of the esophagus alternates between the abdomen and the neck. After complete mobilization, the esophagus is divided using a GIA stapling device in the neck above the tumor but with as much normal esophagus as possible remaining proximally. The esophagus is then pulled through the posterior mediastinum, with a Penrose drain remaining in the newly created posterior mediastinal tunnel.

The mediastinum is inspected for bleeding. The cervical dissection is also examined. The only area that cannot be well visualized is the area behind the left main-stem bronchus. Mediastinal lymph nodes are resected when encountered. Paraesophageal and subcarinal lymph nodes are readily identified from the abdominal hiatus. Paratracheal lymph nodes are not accessible from the esophageal hiatus but may be identified by palpation from the cervical dissection.

Pleural entry occurs in over 50% of patients, and chest tubes are placed when the pleural tear is discovered. A chest radiograph is obtained in the operating room at the conclusion of the procedure to assess placement of the chest tubes and the nasogastric tube.

The stomach is routinely lengthened. The distal aspect of the right gastric artery along the lesser curvature is identified at least 5 cm from the gastroesophageal junction. Five to six applications of the GIA stapler are usually needed to unfold the gastric fundus and create a long gastric tube. The suture line is oversewn. The gastric conduit can reach to the base of the tongue if a cervical exenteration or laryngectomy is required. The gastric conduit is placed into the posterior mediastinum, advanced to the neck, and secured to the prevertebral fascia. The esophageal anastomosis is constructed after the abdomen is closed.

The distal stomach is secured to the hiatus with silk sutures to avoid herniation of abdominal contents. The jejunostomy tube is secured. The abdomen is closed and the incision draped before beginning the neck anastomosis. The neck, having been covered previously with a moistened saline sponge, is examined and the viability of the stomach is inspected. The cervical anastomosis is then performed to connect the end of the esophagus to the "side" of the stomach (greater curvature).

Laryngoesophagectomy with Anterior Mediastinal Tracheostomy

Patients with carcinoma of the esophagus involving the larynx or upper trachea will require laryngectomy and esophagectomy for local control of their disease. The extent of the tumor will determine the extent of the resection and the reconstruction required. These patients will require either (1) laryngectomy with an anterior cervical tracheostomy, esophagectomy, and gastric conduit interposition ("gastric pull-up")[52, 53] or jejunal interposition, or (2) laryngectomy with upper tracheal resection and anterior mediastinal tracheostomy, esophagectomy, and gastric interposition.[54, 55] Patients with esophageal tumors that do not extend past the thoracic inlet may be ideal candidates for jejunal interposition following laryngectomy and upper (cervical) esophagectomy. The patients' physical response to jejunal interposition is minimized with the extensive mediastinal and intra-abdominal dissection for total esophagectomy and gastric interposition. A prerequisite for superior results with this procedure is the availability of a microvascular surgical team with expertise in this technique.

Patients with prior head and neck neoplasms requiring laryngectomy may develop recurrent cancer at their tracheal stoma site. The tracheal stoma may be resected and an anterior mediastinal tracheostomy created (without esophagectomy) provided that at least 5 cm of normal trachea are present above the carina. This length is the minimum amount of trachea necessary for creation of a viable anterior mediastinal tracheostomy.

The cervical dissection is performed first to identify the extent of the tumor and the degree of involvement of carotid arteries. A curvilinear cervical incision is made, and a superior flap is created to expose the tumor. If the tumor can be resected safely in the neck, an inferior flap is created and attention is then turned to resecting the breastplate.

The breastplate is composed of the proximal two-thirds of the clavicles and clavicular heads, the manubrium, and the medial first and second ribs. The clavicles are divided to expose the first and then the second ribs. Care is taken not to injure the underlying vascular structures. The internal mammary artery may be divided. The clavicles, ribs, and sternum are divided with a Gigli saw or with an oscillating saw. The sternum is divided just superior to the costosternal junction of the third rib. The carina is located at this level. The trachea is rotated anteriorly (vertically) to create the tracheostoma. A 45° oblique cut to the trachea, leaving the posterior aspect longer, allows the stoma to be flush with the anterior chest. Chest tubes should be inserted if the pleura is entered. With the breastplate removed, the tumor is resected and a site for the stoma is identified and created. The tracheal remnant should be positioned above the innominate artery but may be positioned below this artery if necessary.

In patients with a recurrent tumor at an anterior cervical tracheostomy site, 5 cm of skin in all directions must be removed. A pectoralis myocutaneous flap may be fashioned and advanced to cover the defect.

Of all complications resulting from this procedure, hypoparathyroidism is the most severe. At least one parathyroid gland should be preserved, if possible. If all the glands must be removed, then a diligent effort must be made to find one or two glands in the specimen and reimplant them into a forearm muscle.

OPERATIVE PROCEDURES FOR PALLIATION

In some cases, it is clear before exploration that an esophageal carcinoma is unresectable. Most of these patients, however, have high-grade partial or complete esophageal obstruction, and some palliative therapy is necessary to restore swallowing. Only patients who cannot tolerate an extensive surgical procedure or who have metastases and therefore a short life expectancy are excluded from operation. Bypass of the obstructing tumor has been advocated as a relatively nonextensive procedure that affords effective palliation. Bypass is usually accomplished with the stomach placed substernally. The esophagus and tumor are excluded by suturing or stapling both ends, but dysphagia can be relieved in more than 90% of patients with this procedure.[21, 56] The operative mortality rate for this procedure is greater than 20%,[21, 57] and long-term survival is often measured in months.

The complications of this procedure are generally either pulmonary or related to sepsis from the residual tumor and esophageal pouch. We have experienced a high complication rate from this procedure and believe that if the tumor cannot be partially or completely resected, palliation should be nonoperative.

For patients with malignant tracheoesophageal fistula, the least invasive means of palliation should be considered. Various tubes may minimize soilage of the tracheobronchial tree. Bypass may be the only therapeutic alternative; however, rarely patients who undergo bypass for tracheoesophageal fistula survive for long periods.[58] Cervical esophagostomy and gastrostomy offer poor palliation, since swallowing is not restored and these patients generally require extensive nursing care.

Jejunostomy is favored for palliative care if nutritional support is needed during therapy; patients with jejunostomy require less care than those receiving total parenteral nutrition, and the procedure permits the stomach to be used for bypass if necessary.

In general, surgical removal of the tumor and restoration of alimentary tract continuity provide rapid and effective relief of dysphagia, optimal local control of the tumor, and potential for cure. In patients with unresectable tumors or a short life expectancy because of extensive metastases or compromised cardiopulmonary function, means of palliation other than surgical bypass should be tried. These other palliative modalities are discussed in Chapter 20 and in the chapters on radiation therapy (Chapter 25) and chemotherapy for advanced disease (Chapter 26).

POSTOPERATIVE CARE AND COMPLICATIONS

It is important to anticipate the complications that may result from esophagogastrectomy. Prevention of these complications is considerably easier than treatment of the complications once they are established. The major causes of morbidity are pulmonary or related to an anastomotic leak.[59, 60]

Meticulous preoperative pulmonary preparation and postoperative pulmonary care will prevent many complications. Patients have difficulty clearing their secretions and maintaining airway patency. Suctioning through the flexible bronchoscope is useful for removing secretions and probably safer than blind suctioning with a nasotracheal catheter, which could disrupt the anastomosis if inadvertently passed into the esophagus. Patients may require overnight assisted ventilation to optimize pulmonary hygiene. The inspired oxygen concentration is kept at the minimum necessary to maintain oxygen saturation at 95%.

Intra-operative monitoring of fluid and electrolytes is critical. Appropriate intravascular volumes are maintained with a combination of crystalloid or colloid solutions or blood when needed. A Swan-Ganz catheter or continuous mixed venous oxygen saturation (SvO_2) may be helpful in monitoring cardiac function and filling pressures in patients with compromised cardiac function. Daily chest roentgenograms are necessary to assess lung expansion, pulmonary hygiene, and the presence of pleural effusions.

Cardiac complications related to myocardial infarction or arrhythmias may occur, but maintenance of electrolyte balance and adequate oxygenation will help prevent them. Arrhythmias are treated with the appropriate agents when they occur. Prophylactic treatment with digitalis is not used.

A nasogastric tube should be inserted at the time of the operation and kept on suction until the tube ceases to function or until bowel function returns. It is critical to avoid gastric distention, which can disrupt the esophagogastric anastomosis. Feeding via the jejunostomy may be started as early as 2 days following surgery. Between 7 and 10 days following surgery, a contrast study is performed to assess integrity of the anastomosis. Oral feeding begins immediately if the anastomosis is intact. Feedings should begin with liquids and be advanced slowly; the diet adjusted, if necessary; and frequent small meals given if the patient experiences early satiety. No dietary restrictions are placed on the patient. Patients should be instructed to eat in the upright position and sleep with the head of the bed elevated.

Septic complications other than those related to anastomotic leaks can occur, including empyema and mediastinitis. Most small intrathoracic leaks will heal with appropriate drainage, antibiotics, and alimentation. Larger leaks can cause life-threatening mediastinitis, and if identified early in the postoperative course, should be closed operatively.[61] Cervical anastomotic leaks will heal readily with simple drainage and rarely cause major septic complications.

Other frequently encountered complications include thrombophlebitis and pulmonary emboli, chylothorax,[62] and injury to the recurrent nerve. Simple chest tube drainage or pleuroperitoneal shunting is a useful technique for treatment of chylothorax refractory to thoracentesis. Injury to the recurrent nerve can occur during the cervical anastomosis and can be prevented by careful intraoperative identification of the nerve so that direct traction or inadvertent division can be avoided.[60]

Anastomotic strictures are a common late complication of gastroesophageal surgery. Most are not severe and can be managed with passage of graded dilators. Diarrhea and dumping may follow division of the vagus nerves and pyloroplasty. Symptomatic reflux esophagitis is rare in our experience.

RESULTS OF SURGICAL RESECTION

Comparison of the end results of surgical treatment of patients with carcinoma of the esophagus is extremely difficult. In addition to the variety of operative techniques, most series include a mixture of histologies and do not provide adequate staging information. Overall survival for some selected recent series is shown in Tables 24–1 and 24–2.

Contemporary series of patients undergoing a Lewis esophagectomy have an operative mortality rate of less than 5% and postoperative complication rates ranging from 10% to 27%.[63–68] Survival is stage-dependent and ranges from 68% to 85% for Stage I

and Stage II patients to 15% to 28% for Stage III patients.

In one study, 21 patients who underwent TTE were compared with 25 patients who underwent the Lewis procedure. The overall mortality rate was 22%. The 5-year survival rate was 20%. No differences in long-term survival between the two groups were noted, but there was better reflux control in patients undergoing TTE.[69]

Orringer and associates reported the results of THE in 583 patients, including 417 patients with carcinoma.[23, 70] Operative mortality for patients with carcinoma was 5%. The anastomotic leak rate was 9%. For all patients, complications included pleural entry (74%), left recurrent laryngeal nerve injury (59 patients, 9%; 40 resolved, 19 permanent paralysis), chylothorax (2%), tracheal laceration (4 patients), splenectomy (4%), and bleeding (4 patients who required intraoperative thoracotomy for control; three other patients explored following surgery). Another series described 40 patients with a 30-day mortality rate of 12%.[71] Complications included intraoperative pneumothorax in 71% (treated by tube thoracostomy), transient hoarseness in 19%, leak in 17%, and pulmonary complications in 7%.[71] In another report of 54 patients who underwent THE, respiratory complications were common (41%) and caused all six postoperative deaths (11%).[72] Atrial fibrillation occurred in 26% and transient palsy of the recurrent laryngeal nerve in 11%. The overall 3-year survival was 10%. All patients had normal swallowing, but 11 (20%) had strictures requiring dilation at some point following surgery.[72]

A possible disadvantage of THE is that patients who undergo this procedure may have a higher probability of local recurrence because a complete lymph node dissection and open resection are not done. When the patterns of recurrence after THE were examined in 35 patients, 13 patients (37%) had no evidence of disease after 18 months, and the other 22 (63%) developed recurrent esophageal cancer within 14 months. Thirteen of the 22 patients were asymptomatic. The recurrence comprised local and distant metastases in half the patients and local recurrence only in the other half. Computed tomography was better than barium studies in detecting early recurrence.[73] The local recurrence rate following THE is higher than those reported for the Lewis procedure or TTE. Longer follow-up and prospective randomized trials are required to determine whether these represent real differences in the operation's effectiveness in controlling the local tumor.

TTE and transthoracic esophagectomy (Lewis procedure or TThE) have also been compared in several studies. In one study, 52 patients underwent TThE, and 26 patients underwent THE. Five anastomotic leaks occurred in the THE group (only one required hospitalization longer than 14 days). Three leaks occurred in the TThE group, but each of these patients was hospitalized for an extended stay of several weeks. The overall morbidity was high: 75% for TThE and 85% for THE (p = ns). Overall mortality rates were similar: 6% (3 of 52) for TThE, 8% (2 of 26) for THE. This study concluded that the results of the procedures with respect to operative mortality and morbidity are equivalent.[72]

Another study compared THE and thoracoabdominal esophagectomy in 72 patients.[74] Thoracoabdominal esophagectomy was performed in 43 patients and THE in 29. The demographic characteristics of the two groups were similar. Complications occurred in 48% of the THE patients and in 86% of the other patients (P < 0.05). Transhiatal esophagectomy had significantly better mortality rates (7% versus 14%, P < 0.05), intra-operative blood loss (1187 ml versus 2150 ml, P < 0.05), and postoperative hospitalization duration (12.3 days versus 22.2 days, P < 0.05). There was no difference in length of survival.[74]

In one series, 210 patients with middle or distal esophageal carcinoma underwent resection with THE (n = 38) or TTE (n = 172).[75] More complications occurred in the THE group: seven patients (18%) had excessive bleeding and perforation of the esophagus at the tumor, and five had injury of the recurrent laryngeal nerve. The TTE group of patients survived longer. The less frequent use of THE may be the reason for the higher number of complications.[75]

Because none of the studies presented here used a random allocation study design, definitive conclusions regarding a comparison of the two procedures cannot be made. The available data do not appear to indicate significant differences in the operative mortality, morbidity, or survival rates of THE, TThE, and TTE.

Radical resection for esophageal cancer can be compared with radical resection for breast cancer. The value of surgical resection is local control of the neoplasm. Although surgery may be considered curative for early-stage disease in either instance, surgery cannot control the systemic spread or wide local extent of lymphatic spread in either disease.

DeMeester and associates proposed an extended en bloc resection of carcinoma of the esophagus.[76] A curative resection consisted of en bloc thoracic esophagectomy, mediastinal lymph node dissection, and gastrectomy with abdominal (celiac) lymph node dissection. Gastrointestinal continuity was re-established using the left colon. The operative mortality rate was 7% and the actuarial survival rate was 53% at 5 years (Stage I and Stage II).[76]

In 111 patients treated with en bloc esophagectomy, the operative mortality rate was 11%, and complications occurred in 49 patients (44%). No recurrences were noted after 3 years. The duration of survival was dependent on stage.[77] The survival rate for comparable stage patients undergoing radical en bloc esophagectomy[33] is no better than for other types of resections.[70]

BARRETT'S ESOPHAGUS AND ADENOCARCINOMA

Adenocarcinomas generally arise in the lower third of the esophagus and are frequently difficult to distinguish from esophageal extensions of gastric cancers. Many of these tumors arise in columnar cell–lined lower esophagus, a premalignant lesion usually called Barrett's esophagus.[78] If reflux is present, an antireflux procedure may minimize the changes.[79] Careful follow-up with periodic endoscopy is mandatory (see Chapter 20). The surgical treatment of invasive adenocarcinoma is no different from that for epidermoid carcinoma. Longitudinal spread is frequently encountered, and esophagectomy is necessary to remove all tumor.[51]

CONCLUSION

Surgical resection continues to provide good palliation with acceptable morbidity and mortality rates. Surgical resection alone infrequently results in long-term survival and has stimulated the search for a combined modality therapy to control micrometastatic disease present at the time of primary treatment. In the following chapter, we will discuss attempts to combine surgery and adjuvant chemotherapy to improve long-term survival.

SELECTED REFERENCES

Akiyama H, Hiyama M, Hashimoto C: Resection and reconstruction for carcinoma of the thoracic oesophagus. Br J Surg 63:206–209, 1976.
This paper describes a useful technique for reconstruction following total esophagectomy, using cervical esophagogastromy with retrosternal placement of the stomach.

Orringer MB: Transhiatal blunt esophagectomy without thoracotomy. In Modern Technics in Surgery: Cardiac Thoracic Surgery. Mt. Kisco, New York, Futura Publishers, 1983, pp 62-0–62-21.
The technique of transhiatal blunt esophagectomy is described and illustrated in this chapter.

Postlethwait RW: Surgery of the Esophagus, 2nd ed. Norwalk, Connecticut, Appleton-Century-Crofts, 1986.
This comprehensive and well-illustrated book summarizes the natural history and operative approaches to carcinoma of the esophagus. A large single institutional experience is also described.

Putnam JB, Suell DM, Natarajan G, Roth JA: Three techniques of esophagectomy. Ann Thorac Surg 57:319–325, 1994.
This paper describes the results from a single institution where the Lewis procedure, total thoracic esophagectomy, and transhiatal esophagectomy were performed concurrently for resection of esophageal cancer.

REFERENCES

1. Czerny J: Neue Operationen. Zentralbl Chir 4:433, 1877.
2. Postlethwait RW: Surgery of the Esophagus. New York, Appleton-Century-Crofts, 1979.
3. Roux C: Esophagojejunogastrostomy, a new operation for intractable obstruction of the esophagus. Semin Med 27:37, 1907.
4. Torek AF: The first successful case of resection of the thoracic portion of the oesophagus for carcinoma. Surg Gynecol Obstet 16:614, 1913.
5. Turner G: Excision of thoracic esophagus for carcinoma with construction of extrathoracic gullet. Lancet 2:1315–1316, 1933.
6. Adams WE, Phemister DB: Carcinoma of the lower thoracic esophagus. Report of successful resection and esophagogastrostomy. J Thorac Surg 7:621–632, 1938.
7. Sweet RH: Surgical management of carcinoma of the mid thoracic esophagus. N Engl J Med 233:1–7, 1945.

8. Lewis I: The surgical treatment of carcinoma of the esophagus: Special reference to a new operation for growths of the middle third. Br J Surg 33:19–31, 1946.

9. Kent EM, Harbison SP: The combined abdominal and right thoracic approach to lesions of the middle and upper thirds of the esophagus. J Thorac Surg 19:559–571, 1950.

10. Orringer MB: Transhiatal blunt esophagectomy without thoracotomy. In Modern Technics in Surgery. Mt. Kisco, New York, Futura Publishers, 1983. pp 62-0–62-21.

11. Kubik S: Surgical Anatomy of the Thorax. Philadelphia, WB Saunders, 1970, p 187.

12. Guernsey JM, Knudsen DF: Abdominal exploration in the evaluation of patients with carcinoma of the thoracic esophagus. J Thorac Cardiovasc Surg 59:62–66, 1970.

13. Berman EF: Carcinoma of the esophagus: A new concept in therapy: 60 collected cases using the polyethylene tube; Report of 10. Surgery 35:822, 1954.

14. Ravitch MN, Bahnson HT, Johns TMP: Carcinoma of the esophagus: Consideration of curative and palliative procedures. J Thorac Surg 24:256, 1952.

15. Inculet RI, Keller SM, Dwyer A, et al: Evaluation of noninvasive tests for the preoperative staging of carcinoma of the esophagus: A prospective study. Ann Surg 40:561–565, 1985.

16. Burt ME, Gorschboth CM, Brennan MF: A controlled prospective randomized trial evaluation of the metabolic effects of enteral and parenteral nutrition in the cancer patient. Cancer 49:1092–1105, 1982.

17. Daly JM, Massar E, Giacco G, et al: Parenteral nutrition in esophageal cancer patients. Ann Surg 196:203–208, 1982.

18. Weiner RS, Kramer BS, Klamon GH: Effects of intravenous hyperalimentation during treatment in patients with small-cell lung cancer. J Clin Oncol 3:949–957, 1985.

19. Finlay IG, Wright PA, Menzies T: Microbial flora in carcinoma of the oesophagus. Thorax 37:181–184, 1982.

20. Orringer MB: Esophageal carcinoma: What price palliation? Ann Thorac Surg 36:377–379, 1983.

21. Conlan AA, Nicolaou N, Hammond CA, et al: Retrosternal gastric bypass for inoperable esophageal cancer: A report of 71 patients. Ann Thorac Surg 36:396–401, 1983.

22. Scanlon EF, Morton DR, Walker JM: The case against segmental resection for esophageal carcinoma. Surg Gynecol Obstet 101:290–296, 1955.

23. Orringer MB: Transhiatal esophagectomy without thoracotomy for carcinoma of the thoracic esophagus. Ann Surg 200:282–288, 1984.

24. Kirk RM: Palliative resection of esophageal carcinoma without formal thoracotomy. Br J Surg 61:689–690, 1974.

25. Akiyama H, Hiyama M, Hashimoto C: Resection and reconstruction for carcinoma of the thoracic oesophagus. Br J Surg 63:206–209, 1976.

26. Launois P, Lygidakis C, Malledant G, et al: Results of the surgical treatment of carcinoma of the esophagus. Surg Gynecol Obstet 156:753–760, 1983.

27. Hankins JR, Colen EN, Ward A, et al: Carcinoma of the esophagus: The philosophy for palliation. Ann Thorac Surg 14:189–197, 1972.

28. Carey JS, Plested WG, Hughes RK: Esophagogastrectomy. Ann Thorac Surg 14:59–68, 1972.

29. Roth JA, Pass HI, Flanagan MM, et al: Randomized trial of pre- and post-operative cisplatin, vindesine and bleomycin (DVB) chemotherapy in epidermoid carcinoma of the esophagus. In Ishigami J (ed): Proceedings of the 14th International Congress of Chemotherapy. Tokyo, University of Tokyo, 1985, pp 1158–1159.

30. Katlic MR, Wilkins EW, Grillo HC: Three decades of treatment of esophageal squamous carcinoma at the Massachusetts General Hospital. J Thorac Cardiovasc Surg 99:929–938, 1990.

31. Yonezawa T, Tsuchiya S, Ogoshi S, et al: Resection of cancer of the thoracic esophagus without thoracotomy. J Thorac Cardiovasc Surg 88:146–149, 1984.

32. Putnam JB Jr, Suell DA, Natarajan G, et al: A comparison of three techniques of esophagectomy for carcinoma of the esophagus from one institution with a residency training program. Ann Thorac Surg 57:319–325, 1994.

33. Skinner DB: En bloc resection for neoplasms of the esophagus and cardia. J Cardiovasc Thor Surg 85:59–71, 1983.

34. Logan A: The surgical treatment of carcinoma of the esophagus and cardia. J Thorac Cardiovasc Surg 46:150–161, 1963.

35. Pearson JG: Carcinoma of the esophagus—operation or radiation. Arch Chir 337:739–743, 1974.

36. Angorn IB: Oesophagogastrostomy without a drainage procedure in oesophageal carcinoma. Br J Surg 62:601–604, 1975.

37. McKeown KC: Trends in oesophageal resection for carcinoma. J R Coll Surg 51:213–239, 1972.

38. Ngan SYK, Wong J: Lengths of different routes for esophageal replacement. J Thorac Cardiovasc Surg 91:791–792, 1986.

39. Ward AS, Collis JL: Late results of oesophageal and oesophagogastric resection in the treatment of oesophageal cancer. Thorax 26:1–5, 1971.

40. Ventemiglia R, Khalil KG, Frazier OH, et al: The role of preoperative mesenteric arteriography in colon interposition. J Thorac Cardiovasc Surg 74:98–104, 1977.

41. Kelly JP, Shackelford GD, Roper CL: Esophageal replacement with colon in children: Functional results and long-term growth. Ann Thorac Surg 36:634–643, 1983.

42. Neville WE, Najem A: Colon replacement of the esophagus for congenital and benign disease. Ann Thorac Surg 36:626–633, 1983.

43. Nishihira T, Watanabe T, Ohmori N, et al: Long-term evaluation of patients treated by radical operation for carcinoma of the thoracic esophagus. World J Surg 8:775–785, 1984.

44. Gavriliu D: Aspects of esophageal surgery. Curr Probl Surg 12:1, 1975.

45. Chassin JL: Stapling technique for esophagogastrostomy after esophagogastric resection. Am J Surg 136:399–403, 1978.

46. Dorsey JS, Esses S, Goldberg M, et al: Esophagogastrectomy using the autosuture EEA surgical stapling instrument. Ann Thorac Surg 30:308–312, 1980.

47. Steichen FM, Ravitch MM: Mechanical sutures in esophageal surgery. Ann Surg 191:373–381, 1980.

48. West PN, Marbarger JP, Martz MN, et al: Esophagogastrostomy with EEA stapler. Ann Surg 193:76–81, 1981.

49. Orringer MB, Marshall B, Stirling MC: Transhiatal esophagectomy for benign and malignant disease. Cardiovasc Surg 105:265–277, 1993.

50. Cheung HC, Siu KF, Wong J: Is pyloroplasty necessary in esophageal replacement by stomach? A prospective, randomized controlled trial. Surgery July:19–24, 1987.

51. Molina JE, Lawton BR, Myers WO, et al: Esophagogastrectomy for adenocarcinoma of the cardia. Ann Surg 195:146–151, 1982.

52. Mansour KA, Picone AL, Coleman JD: Surgery for high cervical esophageal carcinoma: Experience with 11 patients. Ann Thorac Surg 49:597–601, 1990.

53. Goldberg M, Freeman J, Gullance PJ, et al: Transhiatal esophagectomy with gastric transposition for pharyngolaryngeal malignant disease. J Thorac Cardiovasc Surg 97:327–333, 1989.

54. Grillo HC, Mathisen DJ: Cervical exenteration. Ann Thorac Surg 49:401–409, 1990.

55. Orringer MB, Sloan H: Anterior mediastinal tracheostomy: Indications, techniques, and clinical experience. J Thorac Cardiovasc Surg 78:850–859, 1979.

56. Hoffman TH, Kelly JR, Grover FL, et al: Carcinoma of the esophagus. J Thorac Cardiovasc Surg 81:44–49, 1981.

57. Robinson JC, Isa SS, Spees EK, et al: Substernal gastric bypass for palliation of esophageal carcinoma: Rationale and technique. Surgery 91:305–311, 1982.

58. Ong GB, Lam KH, Wong J: Factors influencing morbidity and mortality in esophageal carcinoma. J Thorac Cardiovasc Surg 76:745–754, 1978.

59. Postlethwait RW: Complications and deaths after operations for esophageal carcinoma. J Thorac Cardiovasc Surg 85:827–831, 1983.

60. Ellis FH, Gibb SP, Watkins E: Esophagogastrectomy. A safe, widely applicable and expeditious form of palliation for patients with carcinoma of the esophagus and cardia. Ann Surg 198:531–540, 1983.

61. Hermreck AS, Crawford DG: The esophageal anastomotic leak. Am J Surg 132:794–798, 1976.

62. Milsom JW, Kron IL, Rheuban KS: Chylothorax: An assessment of current surgical management. J Thorac Cardiovasc Surg 89:221–227, 1985.

63. Shahian DM, Neptune WB, Ellis FH, et al: Transthoracic versus

extrathoracic esophagectomy: Mortality, morbidity and long-term survival. Ann Thorac Surg 41:237–246, 1986.

64. Mathisen DJ, Grillo HC, Wilkins EWJ, et al: Transthoracic esophagectomy: A safe approach to carcinoma of the esophagus. Ann Thorac Surg 45:137–143, 1988.

65. Shao L, Gao Z, Yang N, et al: Results of surgical treatment in 6123 cases of carcinoma of the esophagus and gastric cardia. J Surg Oncol 42:170–174, 1989.

66. King RM, Pairolero PC, Trastek VF, et al: Ivor Lewis esophagogastrectomy for carcinoma of the esophagus: Early and late functional results. Ann Thorac Surg 44:119–122, 1987.

67. Lozac'h P, Topart P, Etienne J, et al: Ivor Lewis operation for epidermoid carcinoma of the esophagus. Ann Thorac Surg 52:1154–1157, 1991.

68. Mitchell RL: Abdominal and right thoracotomy approach as standard procedure for esophagogastrectomy with low morbidity. J Thorac Cardiovasc Surg 93:205–211, 1987.

69. Plukker JT, Van Slooten EA, Joosten HJ: The Akiyama procedure in the surgical management of oesophageal cardiacarcinoma. Eur J Surg Oncol 14:33–40, 1988.

70. Orringer MB: Transhiatal esophagectomy without thoracotomy for carcinoma of the esophagus. Adv Surg 19:1–49, 1986.

71. Gupta NM: Transhiatal esophagectomy. Acta Chem Scand 156:149–152, 1990.

72. Gotley DC, Beard J, Cooper MK, et al: Abdominocervical (transhiatal) oesophagectomy in the management of oesophageal carcinoma. Br J Surg 77:815–819, 1990.

73. Richmond J, Seydel HG, Bae Y, et al: Comparison of three treatment strategies for esophageal cancer within a single institution. Int J Radiat Oncol Biol Phys 13:1617–1620, 1987.

74. Goldfaden D, Orringer MB, Appelman HD, et al: Adenocarcinoma of the distal esophagus and gastric cardia: comparison of results of transhiatal esophagectomy and thoracoabdominal esophagogastrectomy. J Thorac Cardiovasc Surg 91:242–247, 1986.

75. Fok M, Siu KF, Wong J: A comparison of transhiatal and transthoracic resection for carcinoma of the thoracic esophagus. Am J Surg 158:414–419, 1989.

76. DeMeester TR, Zaninotto GJ, Johansson KE: Selective therapeutic approach to cancer of the lower esophagus and cardia. J Thorac Cardiovasc Surg 95:42–54, 1988.

77. Altorki NK, Skinner DB: En bloc esophagectomy: The first 100 patients. Hepatogastroenterology 37:360–363, 1990.

78. Kalish RJ, Clancy PE, Orringer MB, et al: Clinical, epidemiologic and morphologic comparison between adenocarcinomas arising in Barrett's esophageal mucosa and the gastric cardia. Gastroenterol 86:461–467, 1984.

79. Starnes VA, Adkins RB, Ballinger JF, et al: Barrett's esophagus: A surgical entity. Arch Surg 119:563–567, 1984.

80. Sampliner RE, Garewal HS, Fennerty MB, et al: Lack of impact of therapy on extent of Barrett's esophagus in 67 patients. Dig Dis Sci 35:93–96, 1990.

25 DEFINITIVE RADIATION THERAPY AND COMBINED MODALITY THERAPY FOR CANCER OF THE ESOPHAGUS

Theodore L. Phillips and Bruce Minsky

The prognosis for patients with carcinoma of the esophagus remains discouraging despite advances in surgical and radiotherapeutic techniques and the advent of chemotherapeutic agents. Soon after the discovery of radium, in 1909 Jean Giusez used radium bougienage in the treatment of esophageal carcinoma.[1] There was little evidence that this changed the natural history of the disease, although it provided palliation in some cases. In the 1920s, radiation therapy was introduced for this malignancy using radium bougies and external irradiation, often with disappointing results. Equipment in the range of 250 KeV was used. Orthovoltage machines were poorly suited for such deep-seated lesions, and skin reactions and damage to the lungs and other structures close to the esophagus were frequent. In the 1930s and 1940s, radiation therapy was often chosen as a means of controlling the growth and spread of esophageal malignancy.

In the 1960s, the advent of megavoltage machines raised hopes for improved treatment of esophageal cancer. The poor results obtained with surgical procedures persuaded many clinicians to resort to radiation therapy, especially in view of its lower morbidity and mortality. At that time, neither of these two forms of therapy demonstrated superiority.

There are a number of approaches to the use of radiation therapy in the treatment of esophageal cancer, including radiation therapy in the adjuvant setting (before or after surgery, or both) or as a primary treatment modality (alone or in conjunction with chemotherapy). Intraluminal brachytherapy may be combined with external beam irradiation. In general, the results of external beam radiation therapy alone in the treatment of esophageal cancer have been as discouraging as those with surgery alone. Depending on the series, the median survival is generally less than 1 year, and 5-year survival rates range from 2% to 20%.

Although the overall results of surgery and radiation therapy are similar, the patient population selected for treatment with each modality is different. First, poor prognostic patients are commonly selected for treatment with radiation therapy; these patients include those who are not surgical candidates due to medical contraindications and/or locally advanced or metastatic disease. Second, nonsurgical series report results based on clinically staged patients, whereas surgical series report results based on pathologically staged patients. Pathologic staging has the advantage of excluding some patients with metastatic disease. Third, because many patients treated with radiation therapy alone are approached in a palliative rather than a potentially curative fashion, the doses and techniques of radiation therapy often are suboptimal. Despite these adverse selection factors, the use of radiation therapy offers a defined cure rate and has a significant impact on the palliation of dysphagia.

This chapter focuses on the role and techniques of external beam radiation therapy, in both the primary and adjuvant setting. Much of the discussion focuses on the results of randomized trials. Where randomized trials are not available, selected nonrandomized trials are discussed. Radiation therapy can also be delivered by brachytherapy, and the techniques and results of brachytherapy alone for palliation or combined with external beam irradiation for definitive treatment are presented. Although the use of chemotherapy with radiation therapy is discussed in Chapter 26, aspects also are presented here because chemotherapy is an effective enhancer of radiation response.

ANATOMIC CONSIDERATIONS

Lesions of the cervical esophagus may extend to the carotid arteries, pleura, recurrent laryngeal nerves, and trachea. Lesions of the middle third may invade the mainstem bronchi, thoracic duct, aortic arch, subclavian artery, intercostal vessels, azygos vein, and right pleura. Tracheoesophageal or bronchoesophageal fistulae are most common in lesions of the middle third and develop in 15% of patients with esophageal cancer. With rare exceptions, a pre-existing fistula is a contraindication for radiation therapy. Tumors of the lower third may extend into the pericardium, left pleura, and descending aorta. These tumors can spread and perforate the mediastinum, causing mediastinitis or massive hemorrhage if there is extension to mediastinal vessels.

Tumors in the upper third will metastasize to abdominal nodes in approximately 10% of patients—25% in the middle third and 45% in the lower third.[2] Supraclavicular and infraclavicular nodes will be positive 10% of the time with upper third lesions (classified as metastatic disease). Mediastinal nodes are positive in about 50% to 60% of all patients, and 30% to 40% of patients have liver involvement. The esophagus is not covered by a serosal lining except for the most distal portion, an anatomic feature that reduces curability of the tumor by surgery and increases the importance of radiation therapy. All of these anatomic factors influence the choice of radiation therapy portals and treatment volumes.

EXTERNAL BEAM RADIATION THERAPY ALONE

Squamous cell carcinoma of the esophagus tends to spread early to adjacent mediastinal nodes and structures. Extension along lymphatics is common. Squamous cell carcinoma of the esophagus is, on the average, moderately radioresponsive[3] (Fig. 25–1). The use of radiation therapy in the potentially curative setting requires doses of at least 50 Gy at 1.8 to 2 Gy per fraction. Given the large size of many unresectable esophageal cancers, doses of more than 60 Gy are probably required.

There are no randomized studies to compare the use of radiation therapy alone with the use of surgery alone for resectable disease. Advocates of radiation therapy point out the substantial surgical morbidity and mortality that occur in these often debilitated patients. Radiation therapy is frequently recommended for cervical esophageal lesions because of the functional and cosmetic impairment that accompanies laryngopharyngoesophagectomy. In theory, the ability of radiation therapy to treat tumor invasion beyond the esophageal wall with preservation of structural integrity of adjacent vital structures is a clear benefit.

For *cervical esophageal* lesions, cure rates with surgery range from 10% to 20%; survival rates for radiation therapy alone are comparable. The University of Florida[4] reported 2-year disease-free survival for 25% of 16 patients, with two additional patients dying of intercurrent illness without tumor less than 2 years after treatment. Between 1933 and 1963, a Royal Marsden study[5] reported 3-year and 5-year survival rates of 11% and 7%, respectively, for 263 patients with cervical esophageal carcinoma.

The prognosis for carcinoma of the *thoracic esophagus* treated with radiation alone is poor (Table 25–1). Earlam and Cunha-Melo[6] reported that 8489 patients treated between 1954 and 1979 had 2-year and 5-year survival rates of 9% and 6%, respectively, although they concluded that these results were not different from published results for surgery and that neither surgery nor irradiation appears to significantly alter the natural history of the disease, except in a small number of patients. In a similar review of the litera-

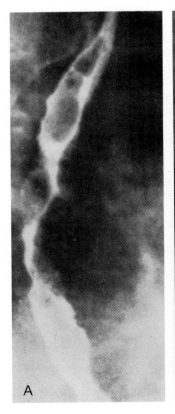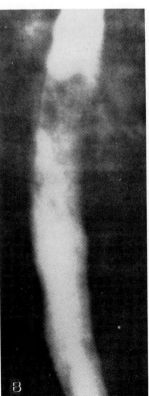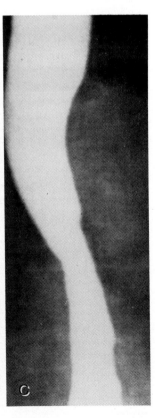

FIGURE 25–1. *A*, Barium esophagram showing a constricting carcinoma before treatment. *B*, Esophagram after 5040 cGy. *C*, Esophagram after 6500 cGy.

TABLE 25–1. Results of Radiation Therapy Alone for Esophageal Cancer

STUDY	DATE	NO. OF PATIENTS	DOSE (Gy)	SURVIVAL (%) 2-yr	SURVIVAL (%) 5-yr
Leborgne et al[10]	1963	294	50/5 wk to 60/6 wk	3.5	3
Pearson[8]	1969	208	50/4 wk	27	20
Beatty et al[11]	1979	146	40 to 50/4 wk	21	0
Earlham and Cunha-Melo[6]	1980	8489	Various	8	6
Newaishy et al[9]	1982	444	50 to 55/4 wk	19	9
Okawa et al[12]	1989	288			9
De-Ren[14]	1989	678			8

ture of patients treated with irradiation alone, Hancock and Glatstein[7] reported that of 9511 patients, 550 were alive at 5 years, for a survival rate of 5.8%. No one has been able to duplicate the 20% 5-year survival rate reported by Pearson[8] in 1969. Newaishy and associates[9] updated this experience in Edinburgh and reported 2-year and 5-year survival rates of 19% and 9%, respectively. The differences between the earlier and later series are not explained by the authors.

At University of California, San Francisco (UCSF) (Table 25–2), Wara and associates[13] reported only one 5-year survivor of 129 patients who completed definitive treatment with radiation only between 1950 and 1971. Recently, we have updated (unpublished observations) the UCSF experience with radiation therapy alone for esophageal carcinoma. Between 1971 and 1985, we treated 76 patients with curative intent. No patient had evidence of metastatic spread or mediastinal invasion at the initiation of treatment. Eight patients did not complete therapy owing to poor preexisting condition or noncompliance. Sixty-eight patients received doses between 50 and 70 Gy at 1.8-Gy fractions. Of these 68 patients, four (6%) survived with no evidence of disease for 5 years, and two are alive without disease at 8 and 9 years. We attributed the slight improvement in survival to improvements in radiotherapeutic techniques.

Additional recent series have reported the results of external beam radiation therapy alone for esophageal carcinoma. The majority of these series include patients with unfavorable features such as clinical T4 lesions, positive lymph nodes, and unresectable dis-

ease. For example, in the series by De-Ren,[14] 184 of 678 patients had Stage IV disease. The results of selected recent series of patients treated by radiation therapy alone are given in Table 25–3 as a function of stage. Overall, the 5-year survival rate for patients with carcinoma of the esophagus treated with radiation therapy alone is approximately 10%.

These results have led many to explore combinations of radiation therapy and surgery. Certainly, with the possible exception of cervical lesions, radiation therapy alone should be reserved for palliation or unresectable disease.

PREOPERATIVE RADIATION THERAPY

The rationale for using preoperative radiation therapy is to reduce marginal tumors to resectable size, reduce the risk of spread of viable tumor by surgical manipulation, and treat extension of the tumor beyond the surgical specimen. On the other hand, surgery can remove the central, more radioresistant primary tumor mass.

This combined approach seemed promising in light of the study by Akakura and associates.[15] Two hundred twenty-nine patients underwent surgery alone between 1956 and 1968, and 117 received preoperative radiation between 1963 and 1968 in this nonrandomized study. The radiation dose was 50 to 60 Gy at 1.5- to 2.0-Gy fractions followed by surgery after a 2- to 4-week break. Of the 229 patients receiving surgery only, 91 (39.7%) had resectable disease.

TABLE 25–2. The UCSF Experience: Carcinoma of the Esophagus

GROUP AND TYPE OF THERAPY	NO. OF PATIENTS	DOSE (Gy)	RESECTED (%)	SURVIVAL Median (mo)	SURVIVAL 2-yr (%)	SURVIVAL 5-yr (%)
Definitive						
1950–1971	103	50–60		7	8	1
1971–1985	68	50–70		9	15	6
Preoperative						
1950–1971	17	50–60	67	11	24	24
1971–1985	10	44–55	70	20	10	10
Postoperative						
1950–1971	8	30–60		6	25	25
1971–1985	17	22–65		9	18	18
Palliative						
1971–1985	55	9–52		4	0	0

TABLE 25–3. Radiation Therapy Alone for Esophageal Cancer

STUDY	HISTOLOGY	STAGE	NO. OF CASES	5-YR SURVIVAL (%)
Okawa et al[12]	Squamous	I	43	20
		II	130	10
		III	92	3
		IV	23	0
		T1	47	18
		T2	147	10
		T3	94	3
		Total	288	9
De-Ren[14]	Various	II	177	22
		III	501	28
		<5 cm	59	25
		5 cm	115	25
		>5 cm	504	6
		Total*	678	8
Newaishy et al[9]	Squamous	Inoperable	444	9

*Includes 184 patients with Stage IV disease.

Among those receiving combined treatment, 96 of 117 (82.1%) underwent resection. Pathologic review of the resected specimen indicated very effective cell kill in 51% of the irradiated group. Five-year survival for the surgery-only group was 13.6% versus 25% for the combined modality treatment, although it is not clear if these survival rates included all patients entered in the study.

Equally encouraging but somewhat biased was the 1966 report by Nakayama and Kinoshita[16] of a lengthy three-stage surgical procedure after presurgical irradiation. They used a rapid fractionation radiation course of 20 to 25 Gy over 3 to 4 days. Surgery involved a laparotomy and then esophagectomy, followed at a later time by reconstruction. They reported the best survival rates in the literature—38% at 2 years and 37.5% at 5 years—although they had only eight patients at risk for 5 years. They have been criticized for excluding patients who died or developed distant disease before completion of the 6- to 12-month three-stage surgical procedure.

Perhaps the most aggressive presurgical attempt was reported by Doggett and associates[17] at Stanford in 1962. After an extensive work-up including laparotomy, 42 patients were found to have disease limited to the local-regional area. The radiation dosage was 50 to 66 Gy over 7 weeks. Of these 42 patients, 29 completed radiation therapy and esophagectomy was attempted. Only 22 patients completed radiation therapy, esophagectomy, and interposition. In four patients (18%) no tumor was found in the resected esophagus. The surgical mortality rate was 28% (8 patients). Of the 21 patients who survived surgery, four died from radiation pericarditis and myocarditis 7 to 69 months after the initiation of therapy and one died from radiation pneumonitis, for a radiation complication rate of 12.5%. At autopsy, 11 of 22 resected patients (50%) were free of disease. The overall treatment-related mortality was 31% (12 of 42 patients). At their final report, only two of 42 patients (5%) were still alive.

The Rotterdam experience reported by Van Andel and associates[18] has shown that of patients judged to be clinically operable and resectable on the basis of physical examination, chest radiography, upper and lower gastrointestinal radiography, liver scan, endoscopy, and bronchoscopy, 42% had unresectable disease at surgery after receiving 40 Gy, and none of these patients survived 5 years despite additional postsurgical irradiation to total doses of 60 to 66 Gy. Among the 81 clinically operable, curable patients who completed radiation therapy and had resectable disease, the 5-year actuarial survival rate was 21%.

Hancock and Glatstein[7] reviewed a group of preoperative studies with a total of 1181 patients, of whom 85 survived 5 years, for a survival rate of 6%. For the highly select group of 616 patients who completed preoperative irradiation and esophageal resection, the 5-year survival rate was 14%. In what is one of the largest preoperative studies in the United States (332 patients), Marks and associates[19] reported 2-year and 5-year survival rates of 23% and 14%, respectively, using 45 Gy in 18 fractions. However, only 101 of 332 patients (30%) were resectable.

In the patients treated (see Table 25–2) at the UCSF, there were four long-term (5-year) survivors among 18 patients who completed irradiation and surgery. All four were in a subgroup of patients who received planned combined treatment rather than radiation alone followed by surgical salvage at the time of recurrence. In the latter group, there were no long-term survivors. In our review (unpublished) of 10 preoperative patients treated between 1971 and 1985, two patients are still alive without evidence of malignancy. However, only one patient (10%) has survived longer than 5 years without disease. The median survival was 20 months. In the preoperative group, one of the 10 had no viable tumor found in the resected specimen (10% sterilization), and one had only microscopic disease. Seventy per cent were resectable at surgery, and only one perioperative death occurred.

There are six randomized trials of preoperative radiation therapy for esophageal cancer (Table 25–4). The series from Launois and associates,[20] Gignoux and associates,[21] and Nygaard and associates[22] are limited to patients with squamous cell carcinoma. Patients with both squamous cell carcinoma and adenocarcinoma are included in the series by Arnott and associates.[23] The series reported by Huang and associates[24] and Mei and associates[25] do not mention the histologies.

Overall, there were no differences in the resectability rates between patients who underwent presurgical radiation therapy compared with those who underwent surgery alone. Only two of the six series reported local failure rates. Mei and associates[25] reported no difference in local failure; however, Gignoux and associates[21] reported a significant decrease in local failure (46% versus 67%) in patients who received presurgical radiation therapy compared with those who received surgery alone.

Two series have reported an improvement in survival with presurgical radiation therapy. In the series from Nygaard and associates,[22] patients who received

TABLE 25–4. Randomized Trials of Preoperative Radiation Therapy for Esophageal Cancer

STUDY	HISTOLOGY	NO. OF PATIENTS	DOSE (Gy)	FRACTION (cGy)	RESECTED (%)		LOCAL FAILURE		5-YR SURVIVAL	
					Surgery	RT	Surgery	RT	Surgery	RT
Launois et al[20]	Squamous cell	109	40	NA	70	76	NA	NA	10	10
Arnott et al[23]	Squamous cell and adenocarcinoma	176	20	2	NA	NA	NA	NA	17	9
Huang et al[24]	NA	160	40	2	90	92	NA	NA	25	46†
Mei et al[25]	NA	206	40	NA	85	93	12	13	30	35
Gignoux et al[21]	Squamous cell	229	33	3.3	58	47	67	46*	8	10
Nygaard et al[22]	Squamous cell	186	35‡	1.75	NA	NA	NA	NA	5	18*

RT = radiation therapy; NA = information not available in article; * = statistically significant; † = statistical analysis not performed; ‡ = with or without chemotherapy.

presurgical radiation therapy had a significant improvement in overall 5-year survival (18% versus 5%). However, all patients received chemotherapy, which may have had an impact on these results. A similar improvement in survival was reported by Huang and associates[24] (46% versus 25%). Unfortunately, a statistical analysis was not performed.

In summary, it is difficult to reach firm conclusions regarding the impact of presurgical radiation therapy on the incidence of local failure since only two of the six series report local failure rates. Regarding the impact on survival, four of the six series report no advantage in overall 5-year survival.

There have been substantial local tumor responses to presurgical irradiation. Tumor response, and in some cases sterilization of the tumor, has been shown in combined modality series. As mentioned, the presurgical regimen used at Stanford[17] resulted in no tumor in seven of 29 resected specimens, and at autopsy, no tumor was found in 11 of 23 patients. In a small series at the National Cancer Institute, there was no tumor in two of seven patients receiving 40 Gy before surgery.[26] Goodner[27] found no evidence of tumor in seven of 85 resected specimens (8%) from patients treated at Memorial Sloan Kettering in New York with 45 Gy over 4 to 6 weeks. Parker and Gregorie[28] found no residual cancer in six of 61 patients treated with a 45-Gy presurgical dose. In the UCSF series, no disease was present in one of 10 patients and only microscopic disease was present in another patient after a presurgical dose of 44.2 to 55.2 Gy, using 1.8-Gy fractions.

The variation in results of preoperative irradiation is in large part due to the techniques used in many series, which resulted in high doses to the lung and caused high perioperative mortality. In other series, the preoperative dose was too low or the volume was too small. Although only two randomized studies show a benefit of preoperative radiation, we do not believe that optimal preoperative treatment was delivered in most studies. In view of the improved resectability and survival obtained in preoperative nonrandomized studies and the 8% to 25% sterilization rate of resected specimens, we remain convinced that careful preoperative irradiation to 50 Gy, which avoids lung irradiation and covers the esophagus beyond the surgical margins, may improve local control.

POSTOPERATIVE RADIATION THERAPY

Radiation is commonly used after surgery to sterilize residual, microscopic disease and to control bulky local-regional tumor. In other malignancies, postoperative rather than preoperative irradiation is used to avoid subjecting all patients with surgically resectable disease to irradiation.

Goodner[27] reported on 260 patients treated surgically between 1940 and 1966 at Memorial Sloan-Kettering. Of these, 30 received postoperative radiation after esophagectomy followed by esophagogastrostomy. The average survival for these patients was 9.9 months. No mention was made of the locoregional control. At the Mayo Clinic, Gunnlaugsson and associates[29] noted that of 17 patients with esophageal cancer who received postoperative therapy, six survived for more than 3 years.

Among the eight patients treated after surgery in the early series at UCSF (see Table 25–2), two (20%) were 10-year survivors, both of whom received postoperative treatment when the tumor was found at the resection margin. There were no long-term survivors among patients irradiated after recurrence was documented. In our review (Table 25–2) of cases between 1971 and 1985 at UCSF, 17 patients were irradiated after surgery, and four patients are still alive without disease. Three patients (18%) were disease free at 5 years. The median survival for our group was 9 months.

An interesting retrospective review was reported by Kasai and associates[30] in Japan. A dose of 60 Gy over 6 weeks improved 5-year survival to 35% in 20 patients who had evidence of tumor in resected mediastinal nodes. (The fact that nearly two-thirds developed disseminated disease despite resection of the primary, negative nodes, and wide-field irradiation to 60 Gy is proof of the aggressive nature of this disease.) Five-year survival in 19 node-negative patients treated with surgery only was 16%. It was demonstrated that the use of postoperative irradiation did not improve survival for patients with lymph node involvement but did improve local control. In only two of 14 patients with recurrence after combined therapy did the tumor recur in the mediastinum. In a group of 18 patients who did not receive postopera-

TABLE 25–5. Randomized Trials of Postoperative Radiation Therapy for Esophageal Carcinoma

STUDY	NO. OF PATIENTS	SURVIVAL			LOCAL FAILURE (%)		LOCAL FAILURE OVERALL	DISTANT FAILURE (%)
		Median (mo)	(%) DFS	Total	LN+	LN−		
Teniere et al[31]								
Radiation	119		85	19	30	10		
Surgery	102		70	19	38	35		
Fok et al[32]								
Radiation	30	15					10	40
Surgery	30	21					13	30

DFS = disease-free survival; LN+ = lymph node positive; LN− = lymph node negative.

tive irradiation, 14 had recurrence in the locoregional area.

Despite many trials of postoperative radiation therapy, there are only two randomized trials (Table 25–5). Teniere and associates[31] reported results of 221 patients with squamous cell carcinoma randomized to surgery alone versus postsurgical radiation therapy (45 to 55 Gy at 1.8 Gy per fraction). The minimum follow-up period was 3 years. For the total patient group, the addition of postsurgical radiation therapy had no significant impact on survival. However, patients with negative lymph nodes had a significant decrease in local failure (35% for surgery alone versus 10% for postsurgical radiation therapy).

The series by Fok and associates[32] included patients with both squamous cell carcinoma and adenocarcinoma. It should be emphasized that patients with both curative and palliative resections were included in this series. Although the total dose of radiation therapy was conventional, the dose per fraction (3.5 Gy per fraction) was unconventional. There was no significant improvement in median survival, local failure, or distant failure with the addition of postoperative radiation therapy. Therefore, based on the limited randomized trials, although postoperative radiation therapy may improve local control, there is no impact on survival.

PREOPERATIVE PLUS POSTOPERATIVE VERSUS POSTOPERATIVE RADIATION THERAPY

Iizuka and associates[33] randomized 364 patients with a variety of histologies to receive preoperative plus postoperative radiation therapy (30 Gy followed by surgery followed by postoperative radiation therapy

up to 54 Gy) or postoperative radiation therapy alone (50 Gy). Based on analysis limited to the 207 eligible patients, there was a significant improvement in 4-year survival (33% versus 20%) as well as median survival (22 versus 13 months) in patients who received postoperative radiation therapy compared with preoperative plus postoperative radiation therapy. The major criticisms of this trial are that only 207 of 364 randomized patients were eligible for analysis and a higher percentage of patients who received preoperative plus postoperative radiation therapy had tumors of more than 7 cm (56% versus 39%).

COMBINED MODALITY THERAPY FOR ESOPHAGUS CANCER

Given the limited success of radiation therapy when used as either a single modality or in the adjuvant setting (preoperative or postoperative), a number of investigators have explored the use of systemic chemotherapy in conjunction with radiation therapy. There is good rationale for combining systemic chemotherapy with radiation therapy for the treatment of esophageal cancer, including an objective response rate of 40% to 60% in patients with metastatic disease, the observation that most patients with esophageal cancer die of distant metastasis, and that some of the active agents in esophageal cancer (i.e., 5-fluorouracil [5-FU], cisplatin, mitomycin C) are radiation enhancers (see Chapter 26).

In a randomized trial from Memorial Sloan-Kettering Cancer Center (Table 25–6), 96 patients with potentially resectable squamous cell carcinoma of the esophagus were randomized to either preoperative radiation therapy (5500 cGy) or preoperative chemotherapy (5-FU and cisplatin).[34] There were no signifi-

TABLE 25–6. Randomized Trial of Preoperative Radiation Therapy Versus Chemotherapy for Esophageal Cancer

TREATMENT	NO. OF PATIENTS	RESECTED (%)	OBJECTIVE RESPONSE (%)	LOCAL FAILURE (%)	MEDIAN SURVIVAL (MO)
Radiation	48	65	64	15	12
Chemotherapy	48	58	55	6	10

Data from Araujo CMM, et al: A randomized trial comparing radiation therapy versus concomitant radiation therapy and chemotherapy in carcinoma of the thoracic esophagus. Cancer 67:2258–2261, 1991.

cant differences in the resectability rates, overall objective response rates, and the local failure rates between the two preoperative therapies. Since there was a cross-over postoperatively, it was not possible to compare the survival rates. The overall survival rate for both arms was 20% at 5 years and the median survival was 10 to 12 months. Based on this trial, the Intergroup trial #0112 (ECOG PE-289, RTOG 91-12) of neoadjuvant chemotherapy followed by concurrent chemotherapy and radiation therapy was designed.

A comprehensive review of the results of systemic chemotherapy in esophageal cancer is beyond the scope of this chapter (see Chapter 26). The following discussion focuses on those trials that have integrated chemotherapy with radiation therapy.

PREOPERATIVE COMBINED MODALITY THERAPY

In general, there are two approaches to preoperative combined modality therapy. Patients either have a planned operation (Table 25-7) or, for a variety of reasons, are selected to undergo an operation (Table 25-8). It is important to analyze the data from these two approaches separately because the selection factors for surgery may have an impact on the results.

The results of selected series in which patients undergo planned preoperative combined modality therapy followed by a planned operation are seen in Table 25-7. Initial studies from Leichman and colleagues from Wayne State University reported the results of 21 patients with squamous cell carcinoma.[35] Patients received 3000 cGy at 200 cGy/fraction with two cycles of concurrent 5-FU and cisplatin. If there was residual tumor in the specimen, patients received an additional 2000 cGy postoperatively. Of the 21 patients, 19 underwent an operation. The pathologic complete response rate was 37% and the median survival was 18 months. The operative mortality was 27%. In addition to the substantial mortality, 48% of patients required hyperalimentation during the preoperative therapy.

Although the morbidity and mortality rates were high, because complete response rates were encouraging, this pilot trial was expanded to a Southwest Oncology Group trial (SWOG 8037). The results were reported by Poplin and colleagues in 1987.[36] A total of 113 patients with squamous cell carcinoma underwent the preoperative therapy designed by Leichman. Of the 113 patients, only 71 underwent operation. The pathologic complete response rate was 16%, and the operative mortality was 11%. Despite a 3-year actuarial survival rate of 16%, all patients were dead of disease by 4 years.

Naunheim and associates reported the results of 47 patients who received preoperative radiation therapy (3000 to 3600 cGy) and concurrent 5-FU/cisplatin followed by esophagectomy.[37] Of the 47 patients, 39 underwent surgery and the pathologic complete response rate was 21%. The overall mortality rate was 5%. The median survival was 23 months, and the 3-year actuarial survival was 40%.

At the University of Michigan, two separate series have been reported. Forastiere and colleagues reported on a group of 39 patients with both squamous cell cancer and adenocarcinoma who received preoperative 5-FU, vinblastine, cisplatin, and concurrent radiation therapy.[38, 39] Radiation therapy was delivered with either large fractions (250 cGy) or with hyperfractionation (150 cGy bid). Patients received the therapy on an inpatient basis for 21 days. Following the preoperative therapy, a transhiatal esophagectomy was performed. The pathologic complete response rate was 27%, the 3-year actuarial survival rate was 46%, and the operative mortality rate was only 2%. A randomized trial of this approach is being performed at the University of Michigan. Urba and associates reported the results of 24 patients with adenocarcinoma of the esophagus who underwent preoperative continuous infusion 5-FU and concurrent radiation therapy followed by a transhiatal esophagectomy.[40] Although patients received 4900 cGy, it was delivered at 350 cGy/fraction. The pathologic complete response rate was 11%, and the median survival was only 11 months. The operative mortality rate was 16%. The large radiation fraction sizes may have contributed to the morbidity and mortality rates reported in this series.

It is unclear whether the addition of surgery following combined modality therapy is of benefit (Table 25-8). In a nonrandomized trial by Gill and coworkers, patients received two cycles of 5-FU, cisplatin, and radiation therapy.[41] Patients who were treated either palliatively or were medically inoperable were excluded from surgery. Therefore, the better prognostic

TABLE 25-7. Planned Preoperative Combined Modality Therapy for Esophageal Cancer

STUDY	NO. OF PATIENTS	HISTOLOGY	NO. OF PATIENTS WHO UNDERWENT SURGERY	COMPLETE RESPONSE (%)	SURVIVAL MEDIAN/ 3 YEAR % 18 MONTHS	MORTALITY (%)
Leichman et al[35]	21	Squamous	19	37	18 mo	27
Poplin et al[36]	113	Squamous	71	16	12 mo 16%	11
Naunheim et al[37]	47	Squamous and adenocarcinoma	39	21	23 mo 40%	5
Forastiere et al[38, 39]	43	Squamous and adenocarcinoma	39	27	29 mo 46%	2
Urba et al[40]	24	Adenocarcinoma	19	10	11 mo	16

TABLE 25–8. Preoperative Combined Modality Therapy With or Without Surgery for Esophageal Cancer

| STUDY | NO. OF PATIENTS | LOCAL FAILURE (%) | DISTANT FAILURE (%) | MEDIAN SURVIVAL (MO) | | |
				All Histology	Squamous Cell Carcinoma	Adenocarcinoma
Gill et al[41]						
Surgery	46	25	36		36	14
No surgery	36	17	12		26	15
Kavanagh et al[*42]						
Surgery	72	24	39	9†		
No surgery	71	44	38	15‡		

* = Results limited to the 103 of 143 patients who had no clinical evidence of metastatic disease at the time of preoperative assessment; † = all dead of disease by 5 yrs; ‡ = all dead of disease by 3.5 years.

patients were selected for surgery. Although the differences were not statistically significant, the local failure and distant failure rates were higher in the patients who underwent surgery compared with those who did not undergo surgery.

A similar trial was reported by Kavanagh and associates.[42] Patients received 4400 to 4600 cGy plus chemotherapy with either VP-16, 5-FU, cisplatin, or carboplatin. Following re-evaluation, those who were potentially operable underwent surgery and if they had positive margins, received postoperative radiation therapy. Patients who were either medically or technically inoperable also received additional radiation therapy to a total dose of 6000 to 6400 cGy. The patients who underwent surgery had a lower local failure rate (44% versus 24%), but there was no difference in distant failure or median survival. However, regardless of the type of treatment, all patients were dead of disease within 3½ to 5 years.

As with preoperative irradiation, it has not been proved that preoperative chemoradiation is superior to surgery alone.

RADIATION THERAPY ALONE VERSUS COMBINED MODALITY THERAPY

There are four randomized trials comparing radiation therapy alone with combined modality therapy (Table 25–9). Unfortunately, in three of the four trials, inadequate doses of systemic chemotherapy were delivered. For example, in the small trial reported by Araujo and associates,[43] patients received only one cycle of 5-FU, mitomycin C, and bleomycin. In the EORTC trial reported by Roussel and associates,[44] subcutaneous methotrexate was used. In the Scandinavian trial reported by Hatlevoll and associates,[45] patients received inadequate doses of chemotherapy (20 mg/m² cisplatin and 10 mg/m² bleomycin for a maximum of two cycles).

The only trial that was designed to deliver adequate doses of systemic chemotherapy with concurrent radiation therapy was reported by Herskovic and associates[46] from the Radiation Therapy Oncology Group (RTOG 8501). In this trial, patients received four cycles of 5-FU (1000 mg/m² for 4 days) and cisplatin (75 mg/m² on day 1). Radiation therapy (50 Gy) was given concurrently with chemotherapy beginning on day 1. A higher dose of radiation (64 Gy) was used in the radiation therapy control arm. At 2 years, patients who received combined modality therapy had a significant improvement in survival (38% versus 10%) as well as a significant decrease in local failure (44% versus 65%) and distant failure (12% versus 26%). With longer follow-up, the 3-year actuarial survival rate of patients who received combined modality therapy was 31%. There were no 3-year survivors in the radiation therapy control arm.[47]

TABLE 25–9. Randomized Trials of Radiation Therapy Versus Combined Modality Therapy for Esophageal Cancer

STUDY	NO. OF PATIENTS	COMPLETE RESPONSE (%)	SURVIVAL (%)	LOCAL FAILURE (%)	DISTANT FAILURE (%)
Herskovic et al[46]					
Radiation	60	NA	10 (2 yr)	65	26
Chemoradiation	61	NA	38 (2 yr)*	44*	12*
Araujo et al[43]					
Radiation	31	58	6 (5 yr)	84	23
Chemoradiation	28	75	16 (5 yr)	61	32
Roussel et al[44]					
Radiation	69	NA	6 (3 yr)	NA	NA
Chemoradiation	75	NA	12 (3yr)	NA	NA
Hatlevoll et al[45]					
Radiation	51	NA	6 (3 yr)	NA	NA
Chemoradiation	46	NA	0	NA	NA

* = Statistically significant; NA = information not available in article.

A similar randomized trial of radiation therapy alone versus combined modality therapy was performed by the Eastern Cooperative Oncology Group (ECOG EST-1282).[48] However, because patients had the option of surgery after receiving 40 Gy, the results are more difficult to interpret. An interim analysis revealed a significant improvement in median survival (14.9 versus 9 months) in patients who received combined modality therapy. Final results of this trial have not been published.

Based on the positive results from the RTOG 8501 trial, the conventional nonsurgical treatment for esophageal carcinoma in the United States is combined modality therapy rather than radiation therapy alone. A replacement intergroup trial (ECOG PE-289, RTOG 91-12) has been activated to determine if there is an advantage of neoadjuvant chemotherapy as well as higher doses of radiation therapy. In this Phase II trial, patients with squamous cell carcinoma receive three cycles of neoadjuvant 5-FU and cisplatin followed by two additional cycles of 5-FU and cisplatin and concurrent radiation therapy (64.8 Gy). Results are pending.

There are a number of single-arm trials of combined modality therapy alone for esophageal cancer. The trial reported by Coia and associates is the only combined modality therapy trial in which patients with clinically early stage esophageal cancer (Stages I and II) were treated and analyzed separately.[49] Patients received 5-FU, mitomycin C, and 6000 cGy of radiation therapy. Combining clinical Stages I and II, the local failure rate was 25%, the 5-year actuarial survival rate was 30%, and the 5-year actuarial local relapse-free survival rate was 70%. The series reported by John and associates included 30 patients with clinical Stages I to III disease and reported a similar local failure rate of 27%.[50] In this trial, the radiation dose was limited to 4000 to 5000 cGy. The 2-year actuarial survival rate was 29%.

It should be emphasized that combined modality therapy is associated with acute toxicity. In a separate toxicity analysis from Coia and associates,[49] an additional 33 patients with Stage III or IV disease were included. For the total group of 90 patients, the incidence of Grade III toxicity was 22% and of Grade IV toxicity was 6%. There was no treatment-related mortality. A similar increase in toxicity was noted in the RTOG 8501 trial. Compared with radiation therapy alone, the use of combined modality therapy was associated with a higher incidence of Grade III toxicity (44% versus 25%) and Grade IV toxicity (20% versus 3%). There was one treatment-related death in the combined modality arm.

ADENOCARCINOMA VERSUS SQUAMOUS CELL CARCINOMA

Given the increasing incidence of adenocarcinoma of the esophagus compared with squamous cell carcinoma, treatment results need to be examined by histology. In the series by Coia and associates,[49] patients with adenocarcinoma had improved survival compared with patients with squamous cell carcinoma. In contrast, Gill and associates[41] and Forastiere and associates[38, 39] reported that patients with squamous cell carcinoma had improved survival compared with those with adenocarcinoma. Naunheim and associates[37] reported no survival difference with histology. Until randomized trials are performed with adequate numbers of patients with each histology and in which patients are stratified, the impact of histology cannot be adequately assessed.

PALLIATION

The majority of patients with esophageal cancer present with unresectable disease or are poor surgical candidates owing to their underlying medical problems. In addition, as Hancock and Glatstein[7] point out, relapse occurs in at least 80% of patients who receive aggressive combined therapy, making palliation an important consideration in management of this malignancy. Those patients whose disease recurs after surgery and irradiation are more likely to have better and longer palliation before recurrence than are patients treated with other approaches.

Among the 103 patients completing irradiation at UCSF,[13] 11% achieved no palliation and 60% had an improvement in symptoms that lasted longer than 2 months. The average duration of palliation was 6 months, and the median duration was 3 months. El-Domeiri and associates[51] studied 74 patients who underwent a colon bypass procedure for palliation. Of those who survived surgery, 51% had a good palliative response and were able to eat regular food with minimal discomfort for the remainder of their lives. Transient results were obtained in 17% of the patients; the remaining 32% did not benefit from the bypass procedure. At the Princess Margaret Hospital,[11] gastrostomy tubes provided poor palliation. However, a physiologic retrosternal bypass with interposed colon or gastric tube resulted in average survival in six of eight patients (who survived the procedure) of 266 days with excellent palliation. Dysphagia recurred in 27% of patients who underwent esophageal resection and physiologic bypass with either esophagogastrostomy or colonic interposition. Only 20% of patients treated with approximately 50 Gy in 4 weeks remained locally free of tumor or had only benign stricture of the esophagus after eradication of their primary tumor. One-third of the patients had sustained palliation during the remainder of their lives.

Either palliative physiologic bypass surgery or radiation therapy to near-radical doses may constitute equally reasonable therapy for the patient with unresectable disease without distant metastatic disease and without tracheoesophageal fistulae. Radiation therapy can provide substantial local responses, good local palliation, and a small but finite possibility of cure. As many as one-third of patients may have effective palliation of their dysphagia for life.

Laser resection with or without intraluminal brachytherapy can also provide palliation. Sander and associates[52] compared laser resection alone in 20 patients with laser plus intraluminal brachytherapy at high dose rate (HDR) in 19 patients. The brachytherapy consisted of three intraluminal treatments of 7 Gy each. Patients with squamous cell carcinoma had a significant prolongation of their obstruction-free interval from 30 to 65 days (p ≤ .03). Holting and associates[53] also found that the addition of endoluminal brachytherapy improved the stenosis-free interval from 20 to 36 weeks after laser resection.

RADIATION THERAPY TECHNIQUE

It is important for the radiation oncologist first to evaluate the patient's medical condition and then decide whether the patient will be able to tolerate radiation and, if so, whether it will be for cure or palliation. Careful computer-assisted treatment planning and treatment delivery are imperative when treating the esophagus with high doses in view of the deep-seated location of the esophagus and the adjacent normal vital structures. Of special concern to the radiation oncologist are the normal structures that lie in proximity to the esophagus, i.e., the spinal cord, heart, and lungs. The dose received by the spinal cord should not exceed 45 Gy in 1.8- to 2-Gy fractions. Doses to the heart and lung depend to a large extent on the volume of these organs in the treatment field. Whole-heart irradiation should be limited to 25 to 30 Gy at standard fractionation. In the thorax, radiation fields frequently traverse substantial volumes of lung, especially with oblique or lateral fields. Decreased pulmonary function frequently occurs after irradiation, particularly if large volumes of lung are treated to doses of more than 20 Gy. There is progressive, decreased ventilatory and diffusing capacity as a result of endothelial degeneration and interstitial fibrosis. Fields that include such substantial volumes of lung should be limited to 20 Gy at standard fractionation. This dose must be reduced to 13 Gy when combined with chemotherapy. However, it is acceptable for small volumes of lung tissue in immediate proximity to the esophagus to receive the minimum tumor dose of 60 to 65 Gy.

If the patient is to receive presurgical irradiation, the radiographic extent of the primary tumor should be treated with large margins in the cephalocaudal direction (i.e., almost the entire esophagus) and 1.5 to 2 cm of margin lateral to the tumor extent with anteroposterior fields each day at a 1.8-Gy midplane dose to 45 to 50 Gy (Fig. 25–2A). Generally, port dimensions are from 15 to 25 cm long × 7 to 8 cm wide. The cumulative dose to the spinal cord is recorded, and compensating filters are used. Coverage of the celiac nodes is used for T3 and T4 lesions of the middle and lower third. For lesions of the cervical esophagus and upper thoracic esophagus, the supraclavicular nodes should be included (Fig. 25–3). The spinal cord is shielded at 45 Gy, and the final 5 Gy is given

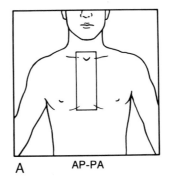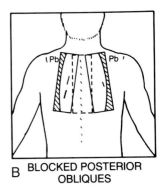

A AP-PA	B BLOCKED POSTERIOR OBLIQUES

FIGURE 25–2. Portals used for *A*, the preoperative and initial AP–PA portal for definitive radiation therapy and *B*, oblique boost sparing the spinal cord.

with oblique or lateral ports (see Fig. 25–2B). The planned surgical margins should be irradiated to sterilize microscopic tumors. Limited boost fields that elevate the total dose to 65 Gy are used after delivery of 45 Gy to the large volume when radiation alone is used. Esophageal cancer has spread more than 6 cm from the primary site in approximately 15% of cases.[2]

If doses of more than 45 Gy (spinal cord tolerance) are desired for curative intent using radiation therapy alone, for postoperative positive margins and/or nodes, or for palliation, a computer-assisted treatment plan is used. During conventional simulation, barium is given to the patient to outline the esophagus. Three contours (upper, midplane, and lower) are taken. The tumor volume is reproduced from a computed to-

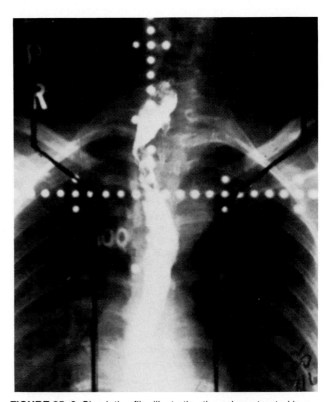

FIGURE 25–3. Simulation film illustrating the volume treated in a patient with carcinoma of the upper thoracic esophagus.

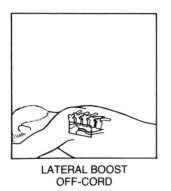
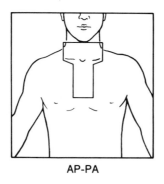

LATERAL BOOST
OFF-CORD

AP-PA

FIGURE 25–4. Ports used for the treatment of lesions of the upper third of the esophagus, including the lateral off cord boost and the anterior field.

mography (CT) scan on each contour. Other vital structures, such as the spinal cord and lungs, are also shown on the contours. This is typical two-dimensional planning. Recently, three-dimensional conformal therapy using CT scans of the entire volume have become available. Dose-volume histograms for each organ and the tumor are calculated, and the number of beams and the shape of each port are optimized to increase tumor dose and reduce normal tissue dose.

Approaches to treating lesions in the upper third of the esophagus depend on the contour of the patient and the location of the tumor and vital structures. A significant problem encountered in treatment planning is the sloping surface of the chest with decreased separation in the upper thoracic and cervical esophagus as well as the changing thickness at the junction of the neck and shoulders. To correct for the slope of the chest, tissue compensators are used when the maximum dose exceeds the tumor dose by 10%. Usually with the upper third lesions, the patient is treated to 45 Gy in an anteroposterior fashion (margins similar to those used in the preoperative approach mentioned previously) to include the supraclavicular and lower cervical nodes (see Figs. 25–3 and 25–4). Lateral fields, usually smaller and off the spinal cord to cover the primary with limited margins, are then used to boost the tumor to the desired dose (see Fig. 25–4). Bolus, or a compensator to accomplish the same effect

as bolus, is used above the shoulders to in effect increase the thickness of the neck. Sometimes, anterior obliques are used with wedges (Fig. 25–5), using compensators above the shoulders.

For the tumors in the middle third of the esophagus, posterior oblique fields (see Figs. 25–2 and 25–6 to 25–8) are generally used in addition to anteroposterior fields in a four-field plan (Fig. 25–9). A four-field box with anteroposterior and lateral fields can also be used. Radiation energies of 6 MeV and higher and source-to-axis distance of 100 cm are desirable. The entire length of the esophagus is included in the irradiated volume. The decreased attenuation of the radiation beam through the lung can lead to increased dose delivery to more deeply seated structures. Lung corrections are used for any four-field plan to take into account the tissue inhomogeneities.

These plans use CT information in a two-dimensional planning system. When three-dimensional planning and CT scans of the entire volume are available, a conformal plan can be generated and optimized. The target volume is outlined, and multiple shaped portals are designed. Figure 25–10 demonstrates sagittal, coronal, and axial views as well as the shape of one of the ports. Although a simple pair of portals using 18-MeV x-rays was optimal, these portals must be conformed to the target at each slice level. The dose volume histogram (Fig. 25–11) indicates that

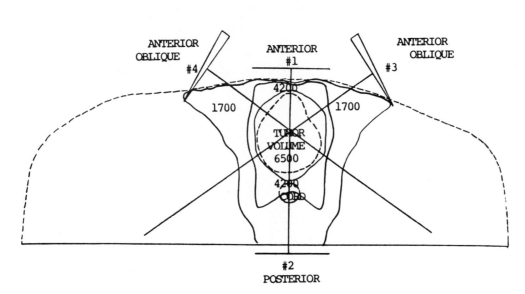

FIGURE 25–5. Three-field treatment plan using anterior oblique ports with wedge filters and a posterior field for carcinoma of the upper third of the esophagus. (Total doses in cGy.)

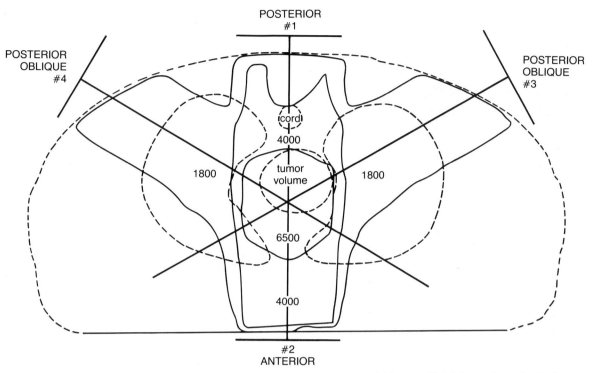

FIGURE 25–6. Four-port treatment plan using posterior oblique ports and AP ports. (Total doses shown in cGy.)

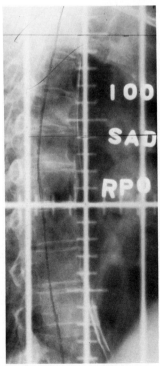

FIGURE 25–7. Simulation film of port for posterior oblique treatment used in three- and four-port plans.

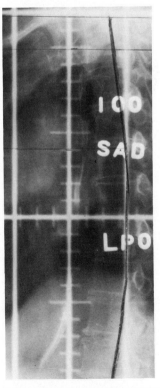

FIGURE 25–8. Simulation film of right posterior oblique port.

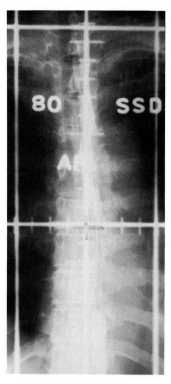

FIGURE 25–9. Simulation film of anterior port used for the treatment of tumors of the middle third of the esophagus.

the tumor is completely enclosed in the 95% isodose line, whereas 90% of the cord receives less than 30% of the dose and 60% of the lung receives less than 40% of the dose. This type of three-dimensional plan gives excellent tumor coverage and prevents cord and lung injury.

With tumors located in the distal third of the thoracic esophagus, we routinely irradiate the gastroesophageal junction and celiac-axis nodes. Usually, the entire field is treated to 45 Gy in an AP-PA fashion (Figs. 25–12 and 25–13). If the celiac nodes are negative, the primary tumor is boosted with laterals (Figs. 25–14 and 25–15). If the celiac nodes are positive, they are sometimes taken to higher doses.

The dose of radiation varies from institution to institution and ranges from 50 Gy in 20 treatments over 4 weeks to 66 Gy in 33 treatments over 7 weeks. Although no dose regimen has proved to be superior, available data suggest that tumor response does increase with increasing dose.

BRACHYTHERAPY FOR ESOPHAGEAL CANCER

Intraluminal therapy with radioactive sources has long been available as a boost or as palliative treatment. The limited penetration of radiation because of

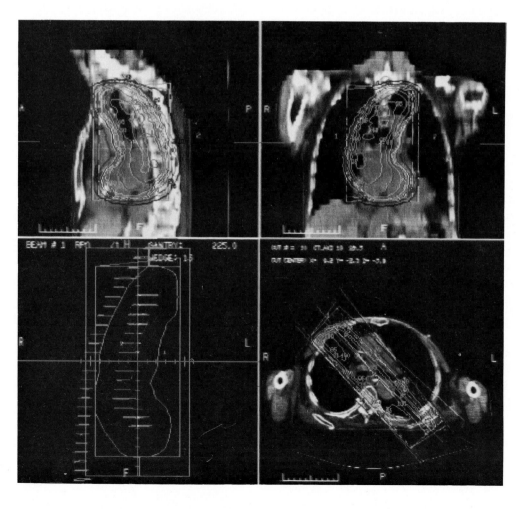

FIGURE 25–10. Computer screen output of a three-dimensional treatment plan for middle-third tumors. Sagittal, coronal, and axial views are shown, as well as the block outline for one of the two shapes of ports used. Isodose curves and clinical target volumes are shown.

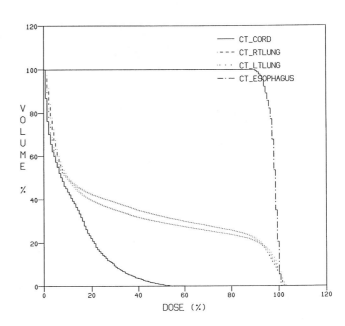

FIGURE 25–11. Dose volume histogram showing per cent of the total volume treated on the vertical axis and per cent of the maximum dose on the horizontal axis. Plots for spinal cord (lower line), lungs (middle lines), and tumor (upper line) are shown.

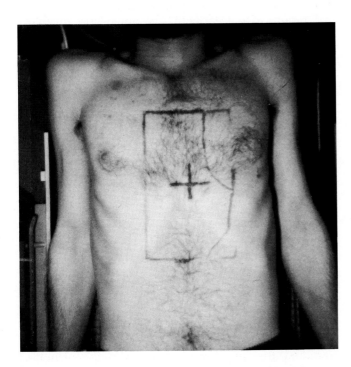

FIGURE 25–12. Anterior field for treatment of a tumor of the lower third of the esophagus including the GE junction and the celiac nodes.

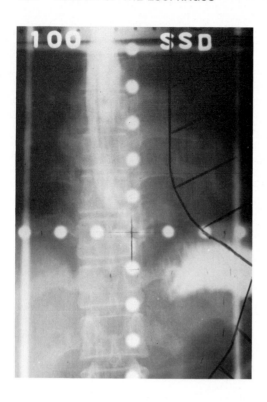

FIGURE 25–13. Simulation film of the anterior port shown on the patient in Figure 25–12.

inverse-square law falloff in dose, difficulty in placing tubes of sufficient diameter, and prolonged placement limited the application. The advent of laser endoscopic resection, new tube designs, guide wire techniques, and HDR remote afterloading led to a new evaluation of this technique. Remote afterloading can be a low dose rate (LDR) that delivers 0.3 to 1.0 Gy per hour, intermediate dose rate (IDR) that delivers 2 to 6 Gy per hour, or HDR that delivers 10 to 40 Gy per hour. The radioactive source is multiple cesium or iridium pellets for LDR and a single intense iridium source for HDR. The catheter is placed in the esophagus under fluoroscopic guidance, and contrast is used to determine the portion of the esophagus to be irradiated. The patient is then attached to a guide cable from the remote safe and the source inserted and removed automatically from a remote control. Doses of 5 to 20 Gy are given 1 cm from the center of the catheter.

Palliative treatment for patients with metastatic disease or for whom external beam radiation therapy was a failure is of definite but limited value. An adequate lumen must be provided by either dilatation or laser resection. The tube containing the sources must be at least 5 mm in diameter and is preferably 1 cm in diameter. The dose is usually prescribed to be 1 cm from the center of the catheter. Using a single HDR treatment of 15 Gy, Jager[54] found that 22 of 32 patients surviving 6 weeks experienced improvement in dysphagia. As discussed earlier, under palliation intraluminal treatment also prolongs the relief of obstruction achieved with laser resection.

The use of HDR or LDR intraluminal treatment as a boost after external beam treatment has been widely

explored (Table 25–10). In Stage I disease, survival rates as high as 43% at 5 years were reported by Hareyama and associates[55] from Japan. Treatment consisted of 60-Gy external beam plus 15 to 20 Gy in two or three HDR intraluminal treatments. In 161 patients of all stages, 53% achieved a complete response at 1 month after treatment. Five long-term survivors had strictures. There are no randomized trials comparing the results of brachytherapy boost to external alone, but in a comparison study Sur and associates[56] treated 50 patients with 35 Gy in 3 weeks and then gave 25 patients a boost of 20-Gy external beam irradiation in 10 fractions and an additional 25 patients an intraluminal boost of 12 Gy in two HDR fractions. Both local control and actuarial survival rates were better in the brachytherapy group.[50] In the future, intraluminal boost should be considered for patients with Stage I or II cancer. A randomized trial is indicated.

FUTURE CONSIDERATIONS

It was hoped that hypoxic-cell radiation sensitizers would improve tumor response and survival, but they did not. One obstacle in these studies has been peripheral neuropathy, which limits the dose of the nitroimadazole that can be given.

Another area of investigation has been hyperfractionation, the use of more than one daily fraction of less-than-conventional size. Cell survival theory based on the alpha/beta model suggests that hyperfractionation should spare late-reacting healthy tissues while allowing higher cell kill in the tumor. Several large

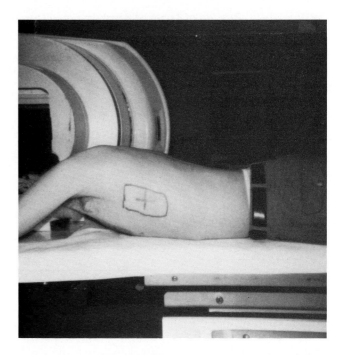

FIGURE 25–14. Lateral boost field off cord for a patient with a lower-third esophageal tumor.

studies are under evaluation for squamous cancers of the head and neck. If they show a benefit for altered fractionation, it should be explored in the treatment of esophageal cancer.

As discussed earlier, intraluminal boost may offer added local control for superficial lesions. This approach should be tested in a randomized trial. Particle beam radiation therapy is radiobiologically attractive because it could overcome the radioresistance of hy-

poxic cells. At the Bevalac facility at Berkeley, Castro and associates[61] reported no advantage to helium ion irradiation in a small series of patients. There was substantial healthy tissue injury with particle irradiation. Studies by the RTOG[62] with neutrons or combinations of neutrons and external beam irradiation have shown no survival advantage or improvement in local control.

Other investigational approaches involve intraoper-

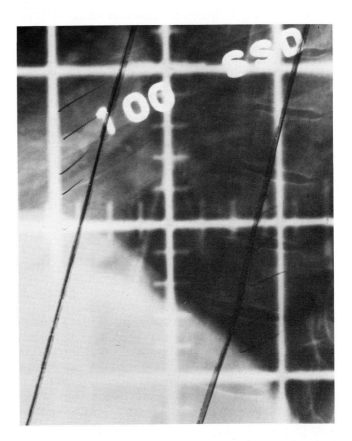

FIGURE 25–15. Simulation film of the lateral boost field shown in Figure 25–14.

TABLE 25–10. Results of Trials of Brachytherapy Combined with External Beam Irradiation in Esophageal Carcinoma

STUDY	NO. OF PATIENTS	EXTERNAL DOSE (Gy)	BRACHY DOSE (Gy/Dose Rate)	PALLIATION (%)	SURVIVAL Median (mo)	SURVIVAL 1 yr (%)	SURVIVAL Multiple Years
Pakisch et al[57]							
Stage I/II	32	50–60	12.4/HDR	96	19	66	
Stage III/IV	16	50–60	12.4/HDR	96	7	0	
Caspers et al[58]	35	50–60	15–20/LDR	91	11	42	10% (2 yr)
Hareyama et al[55]	161						
Stage I	30	48–70	4–20/LDR			80	43% (5 yr)
Stage II	71	48–70	4–20/LDR			70	21% (5 yr)
Stage III/IV	60	48–70	4–20/LDR			28	0% (5 yr)
Agrawal et al[59]	67	20–50	10/IDR	92		42	
Sur et al[56]							
External RT	25	55	None	60		44	
External and Brachy	25	35	20/HDR	91		78	
Hishikawa et al[60]							
Limited	66	60	12/HDR			37 (2 yr)	18% (5 yr)
Extensive	82	60	12/HDR			7 (2 yr)	None

LDR = low dose rate; IDR = intermediate dose rate; HDR = high dose rate.

ative radiation therapy and the use of hyperthermia with radiation and/or chemotherapy. Both hyperthermia and intraoperative radiation appear to be promising for local control. New intraluminal ultrasound irradiators in combination with intraluminal diagnostic ultrasound should be tested.

SUMMARY

The prognosis for patients with carcinoma of the esophagus treated with surgery and/or radiation therapy remains discouraging despite advances in techniques and technology. Radiation alone or combined with surgery has the ability to cure a small minority of patients. There is a significant cure rate when tumors do not penetrate the esophageal wall and when lymph nodes are negative and lesions are smaller than 5 cm. However, in most centers, the 5-year survival rate is less than 5% when palliative cases are included. A careful screening before aggressive intervention is warranted. Intraluminal ultrasound is helpful.

Our current recommendations for the treatment of patients with locoregional disease are to follow the regimen of the chemoradiation arm of the successful RTOG study.[46] The patients start chemotherapy and irradiation on day 1. The chemotherapy consists of 5-FU (4-day infusion of 1000 mg/m^2 on weeks 1, 5, 8, and 11) and cisplatin (75 mg/m^2 on the first day of weeks 1, 5, 8, and 11). Radiation consists of 2-Gy fractions to 30 Gy followed by a 20-Gy boost. The radiation-alone arm consists of 50 Gy (2-Gy fractions) followed by a 14-Gy boost. The preferred alternative is to enter patients into a national protocol if available.

Owing to selection bias, it is difficult to determine the best treatment for esophageal cancer. From the available data, there is no clear survival advantage when radiation therapy is delivered in the adjuvant setting (preoperative or postoperative) versus when radiation therapy is used as a primary modality, com-

bined with adequate doses of systemic chemotherapy. Trials are in progress that are examining the effectiveness of neoadjuvant chemotherapy and higher doses of radiation therapy as well as the role of surgery after combined modality therapy.

SELECTED REFERENCES

Coia LR, et al: Long-term results of infusional 5-FU, mitomycin C, and radiation: A primary management of esophageal cancer. Int J Radiat Oncol Biol Phys 20:29–36, 1991.
  A very well-conducted and adequately followed trial of chemoradiation in a single institution.
De-Ren S: Ten year follow-up of esophageal cancer treated by radical radiation therapy: Analysis of 869 patients. Int J Radiat Oncol Biol Phys 16:329–334, 1989.
  A well-documented large single series of patients treated with definitive radiation therapy.
Hancock SL, Glatstein E: Radiation therapy of esophageal cancer. Semin Oncol 11:144–158, 1984.
  An excellent review of multiple large series of patients treated with radiation therapy alone in the era before combined modality therapy.
Herskovic A, et al: Combined chemotherapy and radiotherapy compared with radiotherapy alone in patients with cancer of the esophagus. N Engl J Med 326:1593–1598, 1992.
  The first report of the RTOG randomized trial, which demonstrated a large and statistically significant benefit for radiation therapy combined with cisplatin and 5-FU chemotherapy compared with radiation therapy alone.
Hishikawa Y, et al: High-dose-rate intraluminal brachytherapy for esophageal cancer: 10 years experience in Hyogo College of Medicine. Radiother Oncol 21:107–114, 1991.
  A large trial of combined external beam irradiation and intraluminal brachytherapy boost for the definitive treatment of esophageal cancer.

REFERENCES

1. Guisez J: Essais de traitement de quelques cas d'epithelioma de l'oesophage par les applications locales directes de radiu. Bull Soc Med Hop Paris 27:717–722, 1909.
2. Fletcher GH: Textbook of Radiotherapy. 3rd Ed. Philadelphia, Lea & Febiger, 1980, pp 688–703.
3. Fajardo LF: Pathology of Radiation Injury. New York, Masson, 1982, pp 50–53.
4. Mendenhall WM, et al: Carcinoma of the cervical esophagus

treated with radiation therapy using a four-field box technique. Int J Radiat Oncol Biol Phys 8:1435–1439, 1982.

5. Lederman M: Carcinoma of the oesphagus, with special reference to the upper third: Part I. Clinical considerations. Br J Radiol 39:193–294, 1982.

6. Earlam R, Cunha-Melo JR: Oesophageal squamous cell carcinoma: II. A critical review of radiotherapy. Br J Surg 67:457–461, 1980.

7. Hancock SL, Glatstein E: Radiation therapy of esophageal cancer. Semin Oncol 11:144–158, 1984.

8. Pearson JG: The value of radiotherapy in the management of esophageal cancer. Am J Roentgenol 105:500–513, 1969.

9. Newaishy GA, Rad GA, Duncan W: Results of radical radiotherapy of squamous cell carcinoma of the oesophagus. Clin Radiol 33:347–352, 1982.

10. Leborgne R, Leborgne JF, Barlocci L: Cancer of the esophagus: Results of radiotherapy. Br J Radiol 36:806–811, 1963.

11. Beatty JD, et al: Carcinoma of the esophagus: Pretreatment assessment, correlation of radiation treatment parameters with survival, and identification and management of radiation treatment failure. Cancer 43:2254–2267, 1979.

12. Okawa T, et al: Results of radiotherapy for inoperable locally advanced esophageal cancer. Int J Radiat Oncol Biol Phys 17:49–54, 1989.

13. Wara WM, et al: Palliation for carcinoma of the esophagus. Radiology 121:717–720, 1976.

14. De-Ren S: Ten year follow-up of esophageal cancer treated by radical radiation therapy: Analysis of 869 patients. Int J Radiat Oncol Biol Phys 16:329–334, 1989.

15. Akakura I, et al: Surgery of carcinoma of the esophagus with pre-operative radiation. Chest 57:47–57, 1970.

16. Nakayama K, Kinoshita Y: Cancer of the gastrointestinal tract. II. Esophagus: Treatment—localized and advanced. Surgical treatment combined with pre-operative concentrated irradiation. JAMA 227:178–181, 1974.

17. Doggett RLS, Guernsey JM, Bagshaw MA: Combined radiation and surgical treatment of carcinoma of the thoracic esophagus. Front Radiat Ther Oncol 5:147–154, 1970.

18. Van Andel JG, et al: Carcinoma of the esophagus: Results of treatment. Ann Surg 190:684–689, 1979.

19. Marks R, Scrugs H, Wallace K: Pre-operative radiotherapy for carcinoma of the esophagus. Cancer 38:84–89, 1976.

20. Launois B, et al: Pre-operative radiotherapy for carcinoma of the esophagus. Surg Gynecol Obstet 153:690–692, 1981.

21. Gignoux M, et al: The value of pre-operative radiotherapy in esophageal cancer: Results of a study of the EORTC. World J Surg 11:426–432, 1987.

22. Nygaard K, et al: Pre-operative radiotherapy prolongs survival in operable esophageal carcinoma: A randomized, multicenter study of pre-operative radiotherapy and chemotherapy. The Second Scandinavian Trial in Esophageal Cancer. World J Surg 16:1104–1109, 1992.

23. Arnott SJ, et al: Low dose pre-operative radiotherapy for carcinoma of the oesophagus: Results of a randomized clinical trial. Radiother Oncol 24:108–113, 1992.

24. Huang GJ, et al: Combined pre-operative irradiation and surgery for esophageal carcinoma. In International Trends in General Thoracic Surgery. St Louis, CV Mosby, 1988, pp 315–318.

25. Mei W, et al: Randomized clinical trial on the combination of pre-operative irradiation and surgery in the treatment of esophageal carcinoma: Report on 206 patients. Int J Radiat Oncol Biol Phys 16:325–327, 1989.

26. Schwade JG, et al: Clinical experience with intravenous misonidazole for carcinoma of the esophagus: Results in attempting radiosensitization of each fraction of exposure. Cancer Invest 2:91–95, 1984.

27. Goodner JT: Surgical and radiation treatment of cancer of the thoracic esophagus. Am J Roentgenol 105:523–528, 1969.

28. Parker EF, Gregorie HB: Carcinoma of the esophagus: Long-term results. JAMA 235:1018–1020, 1976.

29. Gunnlaugsson GH, et al: Analysis of the records of 1657 patients with carcinoma of the esophagus and cardia of the stomach. Surg Gynecol Obstet 130:997, 1970.

30. Kasai M, Mori S, Watanabe T: Follow-up results after resection of thoracic esophageal cancer. World J Surg 2:543–551, 1978.

31. Teniere P, et al: Postoperative radiation therapy does not increase survival after curative resection for squamous cell carcinoma of the middle and lower esophagus as shown by a multicenter controlled trial. French University Association for Surgical Research. Surg Gynecol Obstet 173:123–130, 1991.

32. Fok M, et al: Postoperative radiotherapy for carcinoma of the esophagus: A prospective, randomized controlled study. Surgery 113:138–147, 1993.

33. Iizuka T, et al: Preoperative radioactive therapy for esophageal carcinoma: Randomized evaluation trial in eight institutions. Chest 93:1054–1058, 1988.

34. Kelsen DP, et al: Pre-operative therapy for esophageal cancer: A randomized comparison of chemotherapy vs. radiation therapy. J Clin Oncol 8:1352–1361, 1990.

35. Leichman L, et al: Pre-operative chemotherapy and radiation therapy for patients with cancer of the esophagus: A potentially curative approach. J Clin Oncol 2:75–79, 1984.

36. Poplin E, et al: Combined therapies for squamous-cell carcinoma of the esophagus, a Southwest Oncology Group Study (SWOG 8037). J Clin Oncol 5:622–628, 1987.

37. Naunheim KS, et al: Preoperative chemotherapy and radiotherapy for esophageal carcinoma. J Thorac Cardiovasc Surg 5:887–895, 1992.

38. Forastiere A, et al: Concurrent chemotherapy and radiation therapy followed by trans-hiatal esophagectomy for local-regional cancer of the esophagus. J Clin Oncol 8:119–127, 1990.

39. Forastiere A: Treatment of local-regional esophageal cancer. Sem Oncol 19:57–63, 1992.

40. Urba SG, et al: Concurrent pre-operative chemotherapy and radiation therapy in localized esophageal adenocarcinoma. Cancer 69:285–291, 1992.

41. Gill PG, et al: Patterns of treatment failure and prognostic factors associated with the treatment of esophageal carcinoma with chemotherapy and radiotherapy either as sole treatment or followed by surgery. J Clin Oncol 10:1037–1043, 1992.

42. Kavanagh B, et al: Patterns of failure following combined modality therapy for esophageal cancer, 1984–1990. Int J Radiat Oncol Biol Phys 24(4):633–642, 1992.

43. Araujo CMM, et al: A randomized trial comparing radiation therapy versus concomitant radiation therapy and chemotherapy in carcinoma of the thoracic esophagus. Cancer 67:2258–2261, 1991.

44. Roussel A, et al: Controlled clinical trial for the treatment of patients with inoperable esophageal carcinoma: A study of the EORTC Gastrointestinal Tract Cancer Cooperative Group. In Recent Results in Cancer Research. Berlin, Springer-Verlag, 1988, pp 21–30.

45. Hatlevoll R, et al: Bleomycin/cis-platin as neoadjuvant chemotherapy before radical radiotherapy in localized, inoperable carcinoma of the esophagus: A prospective randomized multicentre study: The second Scandinavian trial in esophageal cancer. Radiother Oncol 24:114–116, 1992.

46. Herskovic A, et al: Combined chemotherapy and radiotherapy compared with radiation therapy alone in patients with cancer of the esophagus. N Engl J Med 326:1593–1598, 1992.

47. Al-Sarraf M, et al: Progress report of combined chemo-radiotherapy (CT-RT) vs radiotherapy (RT) alone in patients with esophageal cancer: An intergroup study. Proc ASCO 12:197, 1993.

48. Sischy B, et al: Interim report of EST 1282 phase III protocol for the evaluation of combined modalities in the treatment of patients with carcinoma of the esophagus. Proc ASCO 9:105, 1990.

49. Coia LR, et al: Long-term results of infusional 5-FU, mitomycin C, and radiation: A primary management of esophageal cancer. Int J Radiat Oncol Biol Phys 20:29–36, 1991.

50. John MJ, et al: Radiotherapy alone and chemoradiation for non-metastatic esophageal carcinoma: A critical review of chemoradiation. Cancer 63(12):2397–2403, 1989.

51. El-Domeiri O, Matini N, Beattie EJ: Esophageal reconstruction by colon interposition. Arch Surg 100:358–362, 1970.

52. Sander R, et al: Laser versus laser plus afterloading with iridium-192 in the palliative treatment of malignant stenosis of the esophagus: A prospective, randomized, and controlled study. Gastrointest Endosc 37:433–440, 1991.

53. Holting T, et al: Palliation of esophageal cancer—Operative resection versus laser and afterloading therapy. Surg Endosc 5:4–8, 1991.

54. Jager JJ, et al: Palliation in esophageal cancer with a single session of intraluminal irradiation. Radiother Oncol 25:134–136, 1992.
55. Hareyama M, et al: Intracavitary brachytherapy combined with external-beam irradiation for squamous cell carcinoma of the thoracic esophagus. Int J Radiat Oncol Biol Phys 24:235–240, 1992.
56. Sur RK, et al: Radiation therapy of esophageal cancer: Role of high dose rate brachytherapy. Int J Radiat Oncol Biol Phys 22:1043–1046, 1992.
57. Pakisch B, et al: Iridium-192 high dose rate brachytherapy combined with external beam irradiation in non-resectable oesophageal cancer. Clin Oncol 5:154–158, 1993.
58. Caspers RJ, et al: Combined external beam and low dose rate intraluminal radiotherapy in oesophageal cancer. Radiother Oncol 27:7–12, 1993.
59. Agrawal RK, Dawes PJ, Clague MB: Combined external beam and intracavitary radiotherapy in oesophageal carcinoma. Clin Oncol 4:222–227, 1992.
60. Hishikawa Y, et al: High-dose-rate intraluminal brachytherapy for esophageal cancer: 10 years experience in Hyogo College of Medicine. Radiother Oncol 21:107–114, 1991.
61. Castro JR, et al: Treatment of cancer with heavy charged particles. Int J Radiat Oncol Biol Phys 8:2191–2198, 1982.
62. Laramore GE, et al: RTOG phase I study on fast neutron teletherapy for squamous cell carcinoma of the esophagus. Int J Radiat Oncol Biol Phys 9:465–473, 1983.

26 CHEMOTHERAPY AND COMBINED MODALITY THERAPY FOR SQUAMOUS CELL CARCINOMA AND ADENOCARCINOMA OF THE ESOPHAGUS AND GASTROESOPHAGEAL JUNCTION

Jaffer A. Ajani, David P. Kelsen, Tyvin A. Rich, and Jack A. Roth

Carcinoma of the esophagus and gastroesophageal junction is relatively uncommon, accounting for approximately 1% of all malignancies in the United States.[1] Approximately 11,300 new cases and 10,200 deaths are estimated in 1993 due to carcinoma of the esophagus and gastroesophageal junction.[1] Nearly half of the patients present with locoregional disease and thus can be treated with combined modality therapy. Prognosis of these patients remains poor, and the 5-year survival rates for the past 4 decades for patients with even locoregional disease have remained under 10%.

The incidence of adenocarcinoma of the esophagus and proximal stomach has increased dramatically in the past 15 years,[2] whereas that of squamous carcinoma of the esophagus has proportionately declined. This alarming rate of increase in adenocarcinoma of the esophagus has afflicted predominantly males of Caucasian descent and those who do not necessarily abuse alcohol and tobacco. The reasons for this rapid rise in the incidence of adenocarcinoma at these two sites remains elusive and is a subject of intense evaluation. An increase in adenocarcinoma of the upper gastrointestinal tract has also been reported in Europe.[3–5]

Autopsy series suggest that carcinoma of the esophagus is a systemic carcinoma.[6,7] This would imply that therapeutic strategies emphasizing predominantly locoregional therapy or suboptimal systemic therapies are less likely to improve patient survival time or cure rate than more optimal strategies that address locoregional and systemic carcinoma. Because of the systemic nature of this illness from the outset, chemotherapy has deservedly occupied an important place in the evolving research strategies for carcinoma of the esophagus and gastroesophageal junction. Chemotherapy has been combined with surgery, radiotherapy, or both. We will review a variety of therapeutic options, including chemotherapy, radiotherapy, and both together or also in combination with surgical treatment.

ROLE OF CHEMOTHERAPY

Before 1976, there was little information regarding chemotherapy because few studies had been performed in patients with esophageal cancer. By 1993, many single-agent studies have been completed and at least five agents with modest activity have been identified. A large number of multidrug combinations have had at least preliminary evaluation. In addition to its use as palliative therapy for patients with advanced incurable cancer, chemotherapy is becoming an established part of the nonoperative treatment of local regional epidermoid cancers.

Assessment of Response to Chemotherapy

Evaluating the response to chemotherapy in patients with advanced metastatic disease is usually not difficult. These patients have measurable tumor masses on physical or radiographic examination. Standard criteria of response, as outlined by Miller and associates,[8] are usually employed. However, if the patients have locoregional disease only, evaluating the patient's response after chemotherapy can be difficult. Improvement in swallowing function is not a reliable indicator. This parameter can be misleading because minor tumor shrinkage can lead to a marked improvement in dysphagia. This may be a result of a decrease in resistance to flow as predicted in Laplace's law: Small changes in radius cause a major increase or decrease in resistance. On the other hand, several studies have demonstrated that by using serial barium contrast esophagograms, objective assessment of response can

433

be performed in patients with locoregional disease.[9–11] Additional assessment of the effectiveness of chemotherapy involves endoscopic or surgical confirmation, with complete pathologic remission requiring histologic confirmation, in addition to a normal esophagogram. In some cases with measurable tumor mass, computed tomography proves useful in quantifying changes in tumor volume. The use of endoscopic ultrasonography to measure response to chemotherapy is under study. Preliminary data in gastric cancer suggests that endoscopic ultrasonography cannot yet be considered a reliable tool for this parameter.

Single-Agent Chemotherapy of Esophageal Cancer

Although a major drawback of many of the earlier studies conducted during the 1970s is the absence of strict response criteria, as well as small numbers of patients entered on these trials requiring pooling of data from several studies, more recent studies have used stricter response criteria and more adequate patient numbers. Table 26–1 summarizes the single-agent chemotherapy data in esophageal cancer.

Bleomycin was one of the first drugs to be studied in esophageal cancer. The initial studies were performed in the late 1960s and early 1970s.[11–17] Overall, it has a response rate of 15% in 80 evaluable patients. Bleomycin has been given both intramuscularly and intravenously, and different schedules have been employed. There are no data to suggest that one dose or schedule is superior to another. The median duration of response is brief, being 2 to 3 months. There are no studies evaluating continuous infusion bleomycin being given without other drugs in esophageal cancer.

Mitomycin C has been tested as a single agent in three Phase II trials.[18–20] In all, 15 of 58 evaluable patients (26%) had major tumor regression with mitomycin C. However, most of these remissions were included in one trial using a dose schedule of mitomycin that is very toxic. Furthermore, response durations were brief.

Cisplatin is among the most active single agents based on the results of nonrandomized, Phase II studies. Fifty-three of 167 (32.4%) patients treated with cisplatin as a single agent had a major response.[18, 21] However, in a random assignment trial in patients with advanced disease comparing cisplatin alone to cisplatin plus 5-fluorouracil (5-FU), the response rate to cisplatin alone was much lower (11%).[22] Toxicity has generally been tolerable and, as anticipated, includes nausea, emesis, nephrotoxicity, and ototoxicity.

Because cisplatin alone is modestly effective, and cisplatin-based combination chemotherapy has activity but also modest toxicity, there has been intense interest in newer, less toxic platinum analogues. In a series of trials performed at Memorial Sloan-Kettering Cancer Center, New York, NY, carboplatin was used in the treatment of both epidermoid and adenocarcinomas of the esophagus and stomach. Carboplatin was given alone and in combination with vinblastine.[23, 24] Although it was less toxic, carboplatin also appears to be less effective than cisplatin-based therapy. Carboplatin is not a substitute for cisplatin in this disease.

TABLE 26–1. Esophageal Cancer Single-Agent Chemotherapy

DRUG	EVALUABLE PATIENTS	CELL TYPE	RESPONSE RATE (%)	95% CONFIDENCE LIMITS (%)
Antibiotics				
Bleomycin	80	E	15	7–23
Mitomycin C	58	E	26	15–37
Doxorubicin	38	E	18	6–31
4DMDR	16	A	6	0–18
Heavy Metals				
Cisplatin	167	E	32	25–39
Carboplatin	30	E	7	0–16
Cisplatin	12	A	8	0–24
Carboplatin	11	A	9	0–26
Plant Alkaloids				
Vindesine	86	E	22	13–31
Etoposide	20	A + E	0	<14
Antimetabolites				
Methotrexate	67	E	34	23–46
5-Fluorouracil	36	A + E	42	26–58
Dichloromethotrexate	22	E	0	<14
Trimetrexate	24	E	13	0–26
Alkylating Agents				
Lomustine	19	E	16	0–32
Ifosfamide	28	E	7	0–17
Miscellaneous				
Mitoguazone	45	E	20	8–32

4DMDR = 4 demethoxydaunorubriacin; E = epidermoid; A = adenocarcinoma.
From Kelsen D, Atiq OT: Therapy of upper gastrointestinal tract cancers. Curr Probl Cancer 5:239–294, 1991.

Vindesine, an investigational vinca alkaloid, has undergone four trials in patients with esophageal cancer.[25–28] Overall, the response rate in 86 evaluable patients is 22%. In each trial, the major side effects of vindesine were peripheral neuropathy and myelosuppression. In general, the drug was well tolerated. Although two other vinca alkaloids, vinblastine and vincristine, have been used in combination regimens, neither have been studied in phase II trials as single agents in the treatment of epidermoid carcinoma of the esophagus.

Methotrexate, an antimetabolite, induced responses in 34% of 67 evaluable patients. In an ECOG trial, methotrexate, given at a dose of 50 mg/m² every week, had a response rate of 12%.[29] In contrast, when given at a dose of 200 mg/m² as an intravenous infusion on Days 1 and 10 by Advani and associates, a response rate of 48% was seen.[30] The marked difference in the response rate noted in these two studies at different dosage schedules remains unexplained. It may have been related to the extent of disease among the patients studied (locoregional versus metastatic) and differences in performance status.

Two trials of 5-FU as a single agent in esophageal cancer have been reported with a cumulative response rate of 42% in 36 evaluable patients. In one trial, 5-FU was given as a bolus injection at a dose of 500 mg/m² daily for 5 days at 5-week intervals.[29] Only four of 23 previously untreated patients responded (17%). In the second study, 13 patients were given 5-FU at a dose of 300 mg/m²/day as a continuous 24-hour intravenous infusion for 6 weeks, followed by radiation therapy. The reported response rate was 85%.[31] The marked difference using the same agent given on different schedules remains unexplained but again may, in part, reflect the extent of disease and performance status.

Other chemotherapeutic agents have been studied, with lower reported response rates. They are summarized also in Table 26–1.

Combination Chemotherapy

With the identification of at least modest antitumor activity for five single agents, and based on data showing that combination chemotherapy is more effective than single-agent therapy in some tumors (such as the leukemias, lymphomas, and breast and testicular cancers), combination chemotherapy has been used in esophageal cancer. Phase II single-arm trials involving combination chemotherapy that have been conducted in the last few years are outlined in Table 26–2.[32–40] Almost all combination regimens include cisplatin.

Although commonly used in combination chemotherapy, it has not been determined that cisplatin is an essential element in the treatment of esophageal cancer. Although toxicities of most cisplatin-containing regimens are tolerable, they should not be underestimated. Because no random assignment comparisons have been performed, it is not known whether one regimen is superior to another. Commonly used

TABLE 26–2. Esophageal Cancer Combination Chemotherapy

DRUGS	EVALUABLE PATIENTS	RESPONSE RATE (%)	95% CONFIDENCE LIMITS (%)
CDDP-Bleo	115	26	18–34
CDDP-Bleo-VDS	192	48	41–55
CDDP-FU	134	49	41–58
CDDP-MTX	42	76	63–89
CDDP-VDS-MGBG	39	41	26–56
CDDP-MTX-Bleo	41	32	17–46
CDDP-FU-Bleo	38	61	45–76
CDDP-FU-VDS	32	53	36–70
CDDP-FU-MTX	34	71	55–86
CDDP-FU-VP-16	35	49	32–65
CDDp-FU-Adria	21	33	13–53
Carbo-VLB	19	0	<15

CDDP = Cisplatin; Bleo = bleomycin; VDS = vindesine; FU = fluorouracil; MTX = methotrexate; MGBG = mitoguazone; VP-16 = etoposide; VLB = vinblastine; Adria = adriamycin; Carbo = carboplatin.
From Kelsen D, Atiq OT: Therapy of upper gastrointestinal tract cancers. Curr Probl Cancer 5:239–294, 1991.

regimens include cisplatin plus 5-FU or cisplatin and vinblastine, with or without 5-FU. The dose of cisplatin is usually 100 mg/m², most often given as a rapid infusion on Day 1. 5-FU is delivered at 1000 mg/m² by continuous 24-hour intravenous infusion on Days 1 to 4 or 1 to 5. Each cycle is repeated every 29 days. Careful attention to dose attenuation for renal, auditory, gastrointestinal, and myelotoxicity is mandatory. Responses, when seen, usually occur within 6–8 weeks.

There has been substantial interest in the combination of interferon plus 5-FU in a number of gastrointestinal malignancies. Two Phase II trials in the treatment of esophageal cancer have been reported. In the first, Kelsen and colleagues[41] reported an overall response rate of 27% in a group of 37 evaluable patients with advanced unresectable esophageal cancer. The median duration of response was 6 months. Toxicity was tolerable and primarily manifested as fatigue. A second trial performed by Wadler and associates yielded a similar result (25% response rate).[42] Although these response rates are comparable to those seen with cisplatin-containing combinations, the use of interferon and 5-FU in the treatment of this disease should still be considered investigational.

Response Rates For Adenocarcinoma Or Epidermoid Cancer

As noted earlier, the marked increase in adenocarcinomas of the esophagus and gastroesophageal junction has raised the question as to whether adenocarcinomas have the same response rate to chemotherapy as epidermoid cancers do. Shown in Table 26–3 are data from three separate studies in which the same group of investigators, using the same response criteria, prospectively evaluated patients with both adenocarcinoma and epidermoid cancer who were receiving the same chemotherapy regimen. Dose atten-

TABLE 26–3. Response to the Same Chemotherapy Regimen: Epidermoid Versus Adenocarcinoma

AUTHOR	REGIMEN	ADENOCARCINOMA	EPIDERMOID
Forastiere et al[49, 69]	C-V-MGBG	7/19 (37%)	11/18 (61%)
Kelsen et al[41]	INF-FU	6/16 (38%)	4/21 (21%)
Wadler et al[42]	INF-FU	1/8 (12%)	4/13 (31%)

C = Cisplatin; V = vinblastine; FU = fluorouracil; INF = interferon-alpha.

uation schedules and toxicity assessment were identical. In two of these studies, involving a cisplatin-containing combination, patients with epidermoid carcinoma were more likely to have major objective responses than were those with adenocarcinomas. These differences, however, are not statistically significant at this point. In the study by Kelsen and associates (using interferon and 5-FU without cisplatin), patients with adenocarcinoma had a slightly higher response rate than did with those with epidermoid tumors, but the study conducted by Wadler and co-workers had the opposite result. Thus, to date, the data available do not indicate a statistically significant difference in outcome for chemotherapy on the basis of histologic cell type. In the Intergroup neoadjuvant chemotherapy trial (see below), patients are stratified on the basis of histology. This trial should allow a better assessment of a difference in outcome of adenocarcinoma versus epidermoid carcinoma.

It is now clear that chemotherapy can result in palliation of symptoms in a modest but reproducible number of patients with advanced disease. However, the duration of response is brief and the impact on survival uncertain. These findings may arise because none of the chemotherapy regimens developed so far result in complete remissions in more than 2% to 5% of patients. Early data suggest that adenocarcinomas of the esophagus and the gastroesophageal junction respond to regimens similar to those employed for epidermoid carcinoma.

PREOPERATIVE CHEMOTHERAPY

The use of preoperative chemotherapy is based on the premise that most patients even with localized carcinoma have occult widespread metastases. In addition, the curative resection rate (defined as negative proximal, distal, and radial margins by histopathology) in patients with potentially resectable carcinoma is less than 60%. Thus, the use of preoperative chemotherapy can favorably influence these factors. However, there are two major considerations worth emphasizing: (1) effective chemotherapeutic regimens would be necessary to eliminate or delay the appearance of occult metastatic disease, and (2) to have an impact on survival, one must consider delivering more than two courses of chemotherapy (preferably five or six courses) without inflicting significant toxic effects on patients undergoing surgery.

The initial studies involved patients predominantly or exclusively with squamous cell carcinoma histology because of the relative rarity of adenocarcinoma histology in the 1960s and 1970s. Investigators at the Memorial Sloan-Kettering Cancer Center initiated preoperative chemotherapy trials in patients with squamous cell carcinoma of the esophagus.

One of the earlier studies was reported by Coonley and colleagues[38] in which 43 patients with locoregional squamous cell carcinoma were treated with one or two courses of combination chemotherapy consisting of cisplatin and bleomycin either prior to surgery or radiotherapy. The response rate to this regimen was rather low (17%), the median survival time was 10 months, and the 5-year survival rate was 10%. Bleomycin was considered the culprit drug for increasing postoperative morbidity and mortality.

Kelsen and associates[37] subsequently reported their results with one or two courses of a preoperative three-drug chemotherapy regimen consisting of cisplatin, vindesine, and bleomycin administered to 34 patients with locoregional squamous cell carcinoma. The major response rate secondary to preoperative chemotherapy was 63%, and the curative resection rate was 47%. There was no complete pathologic response. The median survival time for this group of patients was 16.2 months. There was no increase in the rates of operative morbidity or mortality observed. In addition to leukopenia as the dose-limiting toxicity, bleomycin was also considered to have caused lethal pulmonary toxicity.

Kelsen and colleagues,[43] in a subsequent study, substituted bleomycin for mitoguazone, thus combining mitoguazone, vindesine, and cisplatin. Among a total of 44 patients, 22 had a locally advanced squamous cell carcinoma of the esophagus. The overall response rate was 42% (similar for patients with localized disease and metastatic disease), the duration of response for patients with metastatic disease was brief (approximately 3 months). Among the 19 evaluable patients with localized disease, there was one complete pathologic response. The median survival time for all patients was 4.8 months and that for patients with localized disease was 8.5 months. The authors concluded that, although there were no pulmonary toxic effects and leukopenia remained as the dose-limiting toxicity, they did not observe an increase in therapeutic activity by substituting bleomycin with mitoguazone.

Forastiere and associates[44] reported their results with a similar combination consisting of vinblastine (in place of vindesine), cisplatin, and mitoguazone in 36 patients with carcinoma of the esophagus. Among the 29 patients with locoregional disease, 18 had adenocarcinoma and 11 had squamous cell carcinoma. Patients received two preoperative chemotherapy courses, and the overall response was 44%. Response rate in patients with adenocarcinoma was less than that in patients with squamous cell carcinoma histology. The curative resection rate was not stated. The median survival time for patients with localized disease was 14 months. There were four treatment-related deaths, and patients did not tolerate planned postoperative therapy.

Hilgenberg and colleagues[45] treated 35 patients with squamous cell carcinoma of the esophagus using a combination of 5-FU and cisplatin. Patients received two courses of preoperative chemotherapy, and some patients were offered postoperative chemotherapy. The majority of patients (57%) responded to preoperative chemotherapy. The curative resection rate is not clearly stated, and there was one complete pathologic resection. Postoperative chemotherapy could not be administered in the majority of the patients who were eligible because of poor nutritional condition or patient refusal. Although the median survival time is not stated, 56% of patients were alive at 1 year.

Although, there appears to be a good theoretical rationale for preoperative chemotherapy, however, the validity of the concept in theory could only be proved by controlled clinical trials in which patients with potentially resectable carcinoma of the esophagus would be randomized to surgery alone versus chemotherapy and surgery. Roth and associates[46] attempted to resolve this issue in patients with squamous cell carcinoma. A total of 39 patients were randomized to either surgery alone (n = 20) or preoperative chemotherapy with vindesine, cisplatin, and bleomycin (n = 19). The response to preoperative chemotherapy was 47%. The overall resection rate was similar in both groups. There was no difference in overall survival time among the two group of patients. However, patients responding to chemotherapy had a significantly longer survival compared with those who did not respond. In addition, loss of more than 10% of total body weight was determined as a poor prognostic factor irrespective of the therapy rendered. Because of a low denominator used in this study, it does not conclusively reject a potential value of chemotherapy for patients with carcinoma of the esophagus.

Studies in a substantial number of patients with adenocarcinoma using preoperative chemotherapy started to appear in late 1980s and early 1990s, and this increase in studies paralleled the increasing number of cases with this histology. Ajani and coworkers[47] studied 35 patients with adenocarcinoma of the esophagus or gastroesophageal junction. All patients received two courses of preoperative chemotherapy with a combination of 5-FU, etoposide, and cisplatin, and patients who demonstrated any evidence of objective response to preoperative chemotherapy received an additional three or four courses of the same type of chemotherapy postoperatively. Seventeen (49%) of patients responded to preoperative chemotherapy. The median number of courses was five (range, 1 to 6). Among 32 patients who underwent surgery, the curative resection rate was 78%; one patient had a pathologic complete response. The median survival time for all patients was 23 months (range 6 months to 33 months). This regimen was well tolerated, and there were no deaths related to chemotherapy, surgery, or radiotherapy. The role of more than two courses of chemotherapy was emphasized. The authors also concluded that chemotherapy regimens that resulted in 5% to 10% complete pathologic response should be developed.

Carey and colleagues[48] treated 15 patients with potentially resectable adenocarcinoma of the esophagus with two courses of preoperative chemotherapy consisting of 5-FU and cisplatin. Eleven of 15 patients had a curative resection, but none had a complete pathologic response. The median survival time for the entire group was 18.5 months.

Based on a report of a 15% pathologic complete response rate due to a combination of etoposide, cisplatin, and doxorubicin (EAP) in patients with unresectable gastric carcinoma,[49] Ajani and colleagues[50] used two courses of high-dose EAP followed by colony-stimulating factor in 26 patients with resectable adenocarcinoma of the esophagus or with gastroesophageal junction. Patients who responded to preoperative chemotherapy were to receive three courses of reduced-dose EAP. The response rate to preoperative high-dose EAP was observed in 50% of patients. The curative resection rate was, however, rather low (56%), and there were no complete pathologic responses. This regimen incorporating high doses of chemotherapy with colony-stimulating factor proved particularly toxic. The median number of courses was only three (range 1 to 5), and the median survival time was 12.5 months for the entire group, again suggesting that more effective and less toxic regimens need to be defined if one wishes to eliminate or delay the appearance of micrometastases.

Various investigators have experienced difficulty in administering postoperative chemotherapy in patients with potentially resectable upper gastrointestinal carcinoma, suggesting that postoperative chemotherapy is more toxic.[44, 47, 48, 50, 51] The reason for poor tolerance is unclear, but it might be related to patients' poor nutritional status, weight loss, impact of a major surgical procedure, associated complications, and emotional difficulties. Ajani and colleagues[52] studied the feasibility of administering all chemotherapy preoperatively and omitting postoperative chemotherapy. Thirty-two patients with potentially resectable adenocarcinoma of the esophagus or gastroesophageal junction were studied in a stepwise fashion in which combination chemotherapy with cisplatin, high-dose arabinoside, and 5-FU was administered. In the first part, 15 patients were to receive three chemotherapy courses preoperatively and two chemotherapy courses postoperatively. In the second part, the next 15 patients were to receive all five chemotherapy courses preoperatively, provided there was an objective response after three courses. All of the 14 assessable patients in the first group tolerated all three courses of preoperative chemotherapy, and 86% of patients in this group completed all protocol chemotherapy. In the second group, 9 of 18 (50%) assessable patients tolerated all five courses of preoperative chemotherapy and 100% of patients in this group received all protocol chemotherapy. The median number of chemotherapy courses for the entire group (32 patients) was five (range, 1 to 5). Forty-one per cent had a major response to chemotherapy. Sixty-nine per cent (or 76% of 29 patients taken to surgery) had a curative resection. One patient had a pathologic complete response. The median survival time of 32 patients was 17 months (range, 2 months to 36+ months). Fourteen patients (37%) remain alive at a median follow-up time of 26+ months. Thus it has been possible to administer five courses of cisplatin-based chemotherapy to patients with potentially resectable adenocarcinoma of the esophagus or gastroesophageal junction.

CONCURRENT CHEMOTHERAPY AND RADIATION THERAPY

Several early studies began by using chemoradiation for nonresected patients in whom chemoradiation produced excellent palliation.[38, 53, 54] Steiger and coworkers reported on palliative chemoradiation administered to 25 patients; 11 (44%) achieved local tumor control and were able to swallow until their death.[55] The chemotherapeutic regimens used have varied (Table 26–4), but the mainstay of drug therapy has been 5-FU administered by short (5-day) or protracted (30- to 40-day) infusion. The series by Coia and associates,[56, 57] Keane and colleagues,[58] and Leichman and coworkers[59] substantiate an optimistic outlook for radical chemoradiation for patients with carcinoma of the esophagus. These authors administered 5-FU by infusion, 1000 mg/m² over 24 hours for 4 to 5 days, plus mitomycin C (typically 10 mg/m²) with high-dose external beam radiotherapy (ExBRT). The

trial from the Princess Margaret Hospital, Toronto, which used a similar program, reported an actuarial 73% local control rate at 2 years.[58] This local control rate was significantly better than that for age- and stage-matched historic controls. These investigators also demonstrated the superiority of continuous irradiation (45 to 50 Gy, total dose) over split course irradiation (22.5 to 25 Gy/10 fractions in 2 weeks × 2). This observation fits with the possibility of a detrimental effect by protracting the overall ExBRT treatment time caused by tumor repopulation during the treatment break.

An interesting report on adenocarcinoma of the esophagus and gastroesophageal junction using radical chemoradiation (60 Gy plus 5-FU, 1000 mg/m²/24 hrs and mitomycin C, 10 mg/m²) indicates the potential utility of this combined-modality approach for this histologic type.[60] Eleven of 20 patients had advanced disease, and nine were Stage I or II. In eight evaluable patients, seven achieved a complete response, yielding an overall median relapse-free survival of 10 months and a median survival time of 15 months.

The survival data for groups treated with 5-FU alone or in combination with cisplatin are interesting.[61, 62] In one of the first reports of cisplatin and 5-FU chemoradiation, Richmond and associates reported on a superior median survival duration of 12 versus 5 months for chemoradiation compared with the use of radiation alone in patients treated with 40 to 60 Gy.[62] Survival differences, however, were not

TABLE 26–4. Esophageal Cancer Chemoradiation

STUDY	CHEMOTHERAPY			RADIATION DOSE (GY/FRACTIONS/ DAYS)	NO. OF PTS	LOCAL CONTROL (%)	SURVIVAL
	5-FU	Mitomycin C	Cisplatin				
Byfield et al[65]	20–30 mg/kg × 5 days (5–6 cycles)	—	—	50–60/20–24/ 70–80	6	83	66%
Steiger et al[55]	1 g/m² × 4 days (2 cycles)	10 mg/m² × 1	—	50–60/ 30/42	25	44†	2 pts at 9 and 12.5 mos
Coia et al[57]	1 g/m² × 4 days (2 cycles)	10 mg/m² × 1	—	60/30 48–49	50	75 (Stages I and II)	68% 1 yr, 47% 2 yrs, 32% 5 yrs (Stages I & II)
Coia et al[56]	—	—	—	—	30	—	18 mos (median) 29% (3 yrs), 18% (5 yrs)
Keane et al[58]	1 g/m² × 4 days (1–2 cycles)	10 mg/m² × 1 or 2	—	35–50/† 14–20/28	15	73	48% 2 yrs§
				22.5–50‡ 9–20/56	20	29	13% 2 yrs§
Richmond et al[62]	1 g/m² × 4 days (3 cycles)	—	100 mg/m²	40–65/33 49	17	—	38% 2 yrs
Leichman et al[59]	1 g/m² × 4 days (2 cycles)	10 mg/m² + Bleomycin "sandwiched"	100 mg/m²	60/30/110	21	60	22 mos (median)
Lokich et al[67]	300 mg/m²‖	—	—	44–60	13	—	16 mos (median) 22% (3 yrs)
Ajani et al[66]	300 mg/m² × 30–40 days (protracted infusion with XRT only)		¶	30–60/30	8	66	23 mos (median)
Seitz et al[70]	1 gm/m²	—	70 mg/m²	20/5/5 × 2	35	—	17 mos (median) 41% (2 yrs)
Gill et al[68]	1 gm/m²	—	80/mg/m²	36–54**	117	—	12 mos (median)
Herskovic et al[61]	1 gm/m²	—	75 mg/m²	50††	121	—	12.5 mos (median) 33% (2 yrs)

5-FU = 5-Fluorouracil; NED = no evidence of disease; XRT = radiotherapy.
*Per cent esophageal cancer palliated.
†Single course.
‡Split course.
§Actuarial survival.
‖Protracted infusion prior to and following XRT.
¶All patients treated with 2 to 67 cycles systemic 5-FU (1 g/m²/day × 5 days) and cisplatin (20 mg/m²/day × 5 days) prior to radiation.
**Survival better in patients receiving high XRT doses; clinical complete responders had a median survival of 27 months.
††Randomized study-control group received 64 Gy with chemotherapy.

seen between the groups receiving preoperative chemoradiation (30 Gy) and high-dose radiotherapy (40 to 60 Gy). Two-year survival rates are as high as 45% to 50%. Others have used a slightly different treatment philosophy regarding the so-called radiosensitization by chemotherapeutic agents. Because experimental data suggest an increased radioenhancement when 5-FU is administered by continuous intravenous infusion when the duration of drug exposure exceeds the cell cycle time, 5-FU alone may be sufficient.[63, 64] Results of a pilot study using 5-FU infusion alone in doses of 1000 mg/m^2/24 hrs $\times$ 4 days and concomitant cyclic ExBRT indicated a striking improvement in survival for six patients with squamous cell carcinoma of the esophagus compared with the historical control group treated at the University of California, San Diego.[65] An alternative treatment schedule to cyclic irradiation and 5-FU infusion is that reported by Ajani and associates[66] using protracted intravenous 5-FU infusion (300 mg/m^2/24 hrs) combined with a 1.8 to 2.0 Gy/day for 5 to 7 weeks. Complete tumor responses seen on barium swallow in 11 of 14 patients. The local control rate was 50%, with a median survival duration of 23 months; 14% were alive without disease 3 years after treatment. All patients also received between 3 to 5 cycles of systemic 5-FU and cisplatin in addition to chemoradiation. Similar results were reported by Lokich and colleagues using protracted intravenous infusion before and after 5-FU chemoradiation.[67]

Recent studies using chemoradiation have demonstrated that survival of patients with either squamous cell carcinoma or adenocarcinoma of the esophagus treated with 5-FU and cisplatin can be improved remarkably. In the study by Gill and associates, a significant improvement in survival time was found for those patients who completed a full course of chemoradiation compared with preoperative chemoradiation (54 to 50 Gy compared to 36 Gy).[68] These data indicate the importance of using doses of ExBRT over 50 Gy. They also found a highly significant improved median survival time for those patients with a clinical complete response compared with those with less response, so that the benefit of chemoradiation may be only a selection phenomena. In another study using 5-FU, cisplatin, and vinblastine, a resectability rate of 84% was found, resulting in a median survival time of 29 months and a 5-year survival of 34%.[69] These exciting results appear to be better than surgery alone and are being confirmed by a randomized trial.

In another study by Herskovic and colleagues, the use of chemoradiation in a prospective randomized trial was evaluated for patients with unresectable disease. 50 Gy plus 5-FU and cisplatin was compared with 64 Gy alone.[61] These data show a significant improvement in local control, disease-free survival, and overall survival time for those treated with chemoradiation. The use of chemoradiation as the new standard of practice for locally advanced, unresectable esophageal cancer is indicated by these data. These results, however, cannot be generalized for patients with adenocarcinoma, because this trial predominantly was composed of patients with squamous cell carcinoma.

New studies will be needed to assess this drug combination with ExBRT, to evaluate alternate methods of drug administration (short versus protracted continuous infusion), and to determine optimal ExBRT fractionation schedules in conjunction with chemotherapy in order to improve local control survival further.

CONCLUSIONS

There is increasing interest in the treatment of localized carcinoma of the esophagus. Two major approaches involving local therapies, for example, surgery and radiotherapy, are evolving simultaneously. Chemotherapy, however, has occupied an ever-increasing role in the newer strategies. It is also clear that in most strategies, more than two courses of chemotherapy are being used for these systemic diseases. Better chemotherapeutic agents and better radioenhancers are necessary in the future to improve on the modest current efforts. The future is exciting, in that the intergroup mechanism is in full momentum and we can now embark on perhaps two multi-institutional trials simultaneously in the United States. Surgery remains the best local therapy for patients with potentially resectable carcinoma of the esophagus and gastroesophageal junction, whereas chemoradiotherapy has demonstrated definite benefit for a fraction of these patients. Whether chemoradiotherapy can predictably replace surgery in some cases is an unanswered question and will require significant refinement and advances in therapy to make it more effective and less toxic. Development of effective new drugs is crucial for future advances.

The future challenges lie in developing cost-effective, less high-technologic methods of therapies that will provide effective palliation or improve cure rates for patients with carcinoma of the esophagus.

REFERENCES

1. Boring CC, Squires TS, Tong T: Cancer statistics, 1993. CA Cancer J Clin 43:7–26, 1993.
2. Blot WJ, Devesa SS, Kneller RW, Fraumeni JF: Rising incidence of adenocarcinoma of the esophagus and gastric cardia. JAMA 265:1287–1289, 1991.
3. Levi F, La Vecchia C: Adenocarcinoma of the esophagus in Switzerland (letter). JAMA 265:2960, 1991.
4. Powell J, McConkey CC: Increasing incidence of adenocarcinoma of the gastric cardia and adjacent sites. Br J Cancer 62:440–443, 1991.
5. Reed PI: Changing pattern of esophageal cancer. Lancet 338:178, 1991.
6. Anderson LL, Lad TE: Autopsy findings in squamous-cell carcinoma of the esophagus. Cancer 50:1587–1590, 1982.
7. Bosch A, Frias Z, Caldwell WL, Jaeschke WH: Autopsy findings in carcinoma of the esophagus. Acta Radiologica Oncology 18:103–112, 1979.
8. Miller AB, Hoogstraten B, Staquet M, et al: Reporting of cancer treatment toxicity. Cancer 47:207–214, 1981.
9. Agha FP, Gennis MA, Orringer MB, Forastiere AA: Evaluation of response to preoperative chemotherapy in esophageal and gastric cardia cancer using biphasic esophagrams and surgical-pathologic correlation. Am J Clin Oncol 9:227–232, 1986.
10. Kelsen DP, Heelan R, Coonley C, et al: Clinical and pathological

evaluation of response to chemotherapy in patients with esophageal carcinoma. Am J Clin Oncol 6:539–546, 1983.

11. Kolaric K, Maricic Z, Dujmovic I, et al: Therapy of advanced esophageal cancer with bleomycin, irradiation and combination bleomycin and irradiation. Tumori 62:255–262, 1976.

12. Tancini G, Bajetta E, Bonadonna G: Terapia con bleomycin da sola o in associazione con methotrexate nel carcinoma epidermoids dell'esofago. Tumori 60:65–71, 1974.

13. Ravry M, Moertel CG, Schutt AJ, et al: Treatment of advanced squamous cell carcinoma of the gastrointestinal tract with bleomycin (NSC 125066). Cancer Chemother Rep 57:493–495, 1973.

14. Stephens F: Bleomycin—a new approach in cancer chemotherapy. Med J Aust 1:1277–1283, 1973.

15. Bonadonna G, de Lena M, Monfardini S, et al: Clinical trial with bleomycin in lymphomas and in solid tumors. Eur J Cancer 8:205–215, 1972.

16. Yagoda A, Mukherji B, Young C, et al: Bleomycin, an antitumor antibiotic: Clinical experience in 274 patients. Ann Intern Med 77:861–870, 1972.

17. Clinical Screening Group. Study of the clinical efficiency of bleomycin in human cancer. BMJ 2:643–645, 1970.

18. Engstrom PF, Lavin PT, Klaassen DJ: Phase II evaluation of mitomycin and cisplatin in advanced esophageal carcinoma. Cancer Treat Rep 67:713–715, 1983.

19. Whittington R, Close H: Clinical experience with Mitomycin-C. Cancer Chemother Rep 54:195–198, 1970.

20. Desai P, Borges E, Vohrs V, et al: Carcinoma of the esophagus in India. Cancer 23:979–989, 1969.

21. Panettiere FJ, Leichman LP, Tilchen EJ, Chen TT: Chemotherapy for advanced epidermoid carcinoma of the esophagus with single-agent cisplatin: Final report on a Southwest Oncology Group study. Cancer Treat Rep 68:1023–1024, 1984.

22. Bleiberg H, Jacob J, Bedenne L, et al: Randomized phase II trial of 5-fluorouracil and cisplatin versus cisplatin alone in advanced esophageal cancer (abstract). Proc Am Soc Clin Oncol 10:145, 1991.

23. Bajorin D, Kelsen D, Heelan R: Phase II trial of dichloromethotrexate in epidermoid carcinoma of the esophagus. Cancer Treat Rep 70:1245–1246, 1986.

24. Sternberg C, Kelsen D, Dukeman M, et al: Carboplatin: A new platinum analog in the treatment of epidermoid carcinoma of the esophagus. Cancer Treat Rep 69:1305–1307, 1985.

25. Bezwoda WR, Derman DP, Weaving A, Nissenbaum M: Treatment of esophageal cancer with vindesine: An open trial. Cancer Treat Rep 68:783–785, 1984.

26. Bedikian A, Valdivieso M, Bodey G, et al: Phase II evaluation of vindesine in the treatment of colorectal and esophageal tumors. Cancer Chemother Pharmacol 2:263, 1979.

27. Kelsen DP, Bains MS, Cvitkovic E, Golbey R: Vindesine in the treatment of esophageal carcinoma: a phase II study. Cancer Treat Rep 63:2019–2021, 1979.

28. Popkin J, Bromer R, Byrne R, et al: Continuous 48-hour infusion of vindesine in squamous cell carcinoma of the upper aerodigestive tract (abstract). Proceedings of the 13th International Cancer Congress 40, 1983.

29. Ezdinli EZ, Gelber R, Desai DV, et al: Chemotherapy of advanced esophageal carcinoma: Eastern Cooperative Oncology Group experience. Cancer 46:2149–2153, 1980.

30. Advani SH, Saikia TK, Swaroop S, et al: Anterior chemotherapy in esophageal cancer. Cancer 56:1502–1506, 1985.

31. Lokich JJ, Shea M, Chaffey J: Sequential infusional 5-fluorouracil followed by concomitant radiation for tumors of the esophagus and gastroesophageal junction. Cancer 60:275–279, 1987.

32. Kelsen DP, Minsky B, Smith M, et al: Preoperative therapy for esophageal cancer: A randomized comparison of chemotherapy versus radiation therapy. J Clin Oncol 8:1352–1361, 1990.

33. Schlag P, Herrmann R, Raeth V, et al: Preoperative chemotherapy in esophageal cancer. A phase II study. Acta Oncol 27:811–814, 1988.

34. Kies MS, Rosen ST, Tsang TK, et al: Cisplatin and 5-fluorouracil in the primary management of squamous esophageal cancer. Cancer 60:2156–2160, 1987.

35. De Besi P, Sileni VC, Salvagno L, et al: Phase II study of cisplatin, 5-FU, and allopurinol in advanced esophageal cancer. Cancer Treat Rep 70:909–910, 1986.

36. Dinwoodie WR, Bartolucci AA, Lyman GH, et al: Phase II evaluation of cisplatin, bleomycin, and vindesine in advanced squamous cell carcinoma of the esophagus: A Southeastern Cancer Study Group Trial. Cancer Treat Rep 70:267–270, 1986.

37. Kelsen D, Hilaris B, Coonley C, et al: Cisplatin, vindesine, and bleomycin chemotherapy of local-regional and advanced esophageal carcinoma. Am J Med 75:645–652, 1983.

38. Coonley CJ, Bains M, Hilaris B, et al: Cisplatin and bleomycin in the treatment of esophageal carcinoma. A final report. Cancer 54:2351–2355, 1984.

39. Elster K, Carson W, Eidt H, Thomasko A: Significance of gastric polypectomy (histological aspect). Endoscopy 15(Suppl 1):148–149, 1983.

40. Bosset J, Hurteloup P, Bontemas P, et al: A phase II trial of bleomycin and cisplatin in advanced oesophagus carcinoma (abstract). Proceedings of the 13th International Cancer Congress 41, 1983.

41. Kelsen D, Lovett D, Wong J, et al: Interferon alfa-2a and fluorouracil in the treatment of patients with advanced esophageal cancer. J Clin Oncol 10:269–274, 1992.

42. Wadler S, Fell S, Haynes H, et al: Treatment of carcinoma of the esophagus with 5-fluorouracil and recombinant alfa-2a-interferon. Cancer 71:1726–1730, 1993.

43. Kelsen DP, Fein R, Coonley C, et al: Cisplatin, vindesine, and mitoguazone in the treatment of esophageal cancer. Cancer Treat Rep 70:255–259, 1993.

44. Forastiere AA, Gennis M, Orringer MB, Agha FP: Cisplatin, vinblastine, and mitoguazone chemotherapy for epidermoid and adenocarcinoma of the esophagus. J Clin Oncol 5:1143–1149, 1987.

45. Hilgenberg AD, Carey RW, Wilkins EW, et al: Preoperative chemotherapy, surgical resection, and selective postoperative therapy for squamous cell carcinoma of the esophagus. Ann Thor Surg 45:357–363, 1988.

46. Roth JA, Pass HI, Flanagan MM, et al: Randomized clinical trial of preoperative and postoperative adjuvant chemotherapy with cisplatin, vindesine, and bleomycin for carcinoma of the esophagus. J Thorac Cardiovasc Surg 96:242–248, 1988.

47. Ajani JA, Roth JA, Ryan B, et al: Evaluation of pre- and postoperative chemotherapy for resectable adenocarcinoma of the esophagus or gastroesophageal junction. J Clin Oncol 8:1231–1238, 1990.

48. Carey RW, Hilgenberg AD, Choi NC, et al: A pilot study of neoadjuvant chemotherapy with 5-fluorouracil and cisplatin with surgical resection ad postoperative radiation therapy and/or chemotherapy in adenocarcinoma of the esophagus. Cancer 68:489–492, 1991.

49. Wilke H, Preusser P, Fink U, et al: Preoperative chemotherapy of locally advanced and non-resectable gastric carcinoma. J Clin Oncol 7:1318–1326, 1989.

50. Ajani JA, Roth JA, Ryan MB, et al: Intensive preoperative chemotherapy with colony-stimulating factor for resectable adenocarcinoma of the esophagus or gastroesophageal junction. J Clin Oncol 11:22–28, 1993.

51. Ajani JA, Mayer RJ, Ota DM, et al: Preoperative and postoperative combination chemotherapy for potentially resectable gastric carcinoma. J Natl Cancer Inst, 1993, in press.

52. Ajani JA, Roth JA, Putnam JB, et al: Feasibility of five courses of preoperative chemotherapy in patients with resectable adenocarcinoma of the esophagus or gastroesophageal junction. Eur J Cancer, in press.

53. Earle JR, Gelber RD, Moertel CG, Hahn RG: A controlled evaluation of combined radiation and bleomycin therapy for squamous cell carcinoma of the esophagus. Int J Radiat Oncol Biol Phys 6:821–826, 1980.

54. Fujimaki M: Role of preoperative administration of bleomycin and radiation in the treatment of esophageal cancer. Jpn J Surg 5:48–50, 1975.

55. Steiger Z, Franklin R, Wilson RF, et al: Eradication and palliation of squamous cell carcinoma of the esophagus with chemotherapy radiotherapy and surgical therapy. J Thoracic Cardiovascular Surg 5:713–719, 1981.

56. Coia LR, Engstrom PF, Paul A: Nonsurgical management of esophageal cancer: Report of a study of combined radiotherapy and chemotherapy. J Clin Oncol 5:1783–1790, 1987.

57. Coia LR, Engstrom PF, Paul AR, et al: Long-term results of infusional 5-FU, Mitomycin-C, and radiation as primary man-

agement of esophageal carcinoma. Int J Radiat Oncol Biol Phys 20:29–36, 1991.

58. Keane TJ, Harwood AR, Elhakin T, et al: Radical radiation therapy with 5-Fluorouracil infusion and Mitomycin-C for esophageal carcinoma. Radiother Oncol 4:205–210, 1985.

59. Leichman L, Herskovic A, Leichman CG, et al: Nonoperative therapy for squamous-cell cancer of the esophagus. J Clin Oncol 5:365–370, 1987.

60. Coia LR, Paul AR, Engstrom PF: Combined radiation and chemotherapy as primary management of adenocarcinoma of the esophagus and gastroesophageal junction. Cancer 61:643–649, 1988.

61. Herskovic A, Martz K, Al-Sarraf M, et al: Combined chemotherapy and radiotherapy compared with radiotherapy alone in patients with cancer of the esophagus. N Engl J Med 326:1593–1598, 1992.

62. Richmond J, Seydel HG, Bae Y, et al: Comparison of three treatment strategies for esophageal cancer within a single institution (abstract). Int J Radiat Oncol Biol Phys 12:119, 1986.

63. Rich TA, Lokich JJ, Chaffey JT: A pilot study of protracted venous infusion of 5-Fluorouracil and concomitant radiation therapy. J Clin Oncol 3:402–406, 1985.

64. Byfield JE: Useful interactions between 5-fluorouracil and radiation in man: 5-fluorouracil as a radiosensitizer. *In* Hill BT, Bellamy AS (eds): Antitumor Drug-Radiation Interactions. Boca Raton, Florida, CRC Press, 1990, p 87.

65. Byfield JR, Barone R, Mendelsohn J: Infusional 5-fluorouracil and x-ray therapy for non-resectable esophageal cancer. Cancer 45:703–708, 1980.

66. Ajani JA, Ryan B, Rich TA, et al: Prolonged chemotherapy for localized squamous carcinoma of the esophagus. Eur J Cancer 28A:880–884, 1992.

67. Lokich JJ, Shea M, Chaffey J: Sequential infusion of 5-Fluorouracil followed by concomitant radiation for tumors of the esophagus and gastroesophageal junction. Cancer 60:275–279, 1987.

68. Gill PG, Denham JW, Jamieson GG, et al: Patterns of treatment failure and prognostic factors associated with the treatment of esophageal carcinoma with chemotherapy and radiotherapy either as sole treatment or followed by surgery. J Clin Oncol 10:1037–1043, 1992.

69. Forastiere AA, Orringer MB, Perez-Tamayo C, et al: Preoperative chemoradiation followed by transhiatal esophagectomy for carcinoma of the esophagus: Final report. J Clin Oncol 11:1118–1123, 1993.

70. Seitz JF, Giovannini M, Padaut-Cesana J, et al: Inoperable nonmetastatic squamous cell carcinoma of the esophagus managed by concomitant chemotherapy (5-fluorouracil and cisplatin) and radiation therapy. Cancer 66:214–219, 1990.

Part III

MALIGNANCIES OF THE MEDIASTINUM

27 GENERAL PRINCIPLES AND SURGICAL CONSIDERATIONS IN THE MANAGEMENT OF MEDIASTINAL MASSES

Garrett L. Walsh

The mediastinum provides a diagnostic and surgical challenge as the site of a myriad of tumors both benign and malignant with a wide range of clinical and radiologic presentations. The thoracic surgeon must be well versed in the embryology, anatomy, physiology, and pathology of all structures within the mediastinum. A consistent and organized approach is required to avoid poorly timed or inappropriate and potentially dangerous surgical procedures. When evaluating a mediastinal mass, the surgeon must first review possible congenital, infectious, developmental, and traumatic etiologies before considering the differential diagnostic subgroup of neoplastic lesions.

Neoplasms must be evaluated as primary or secondary mediastinal tumors. An appropriate laboratory and radiologic work-up must precede biopsy or excision if surgical disasters are to be avoided (e.g., biopsy of a saccular aneurysm of the aorta believed to be a neoplasm).[1] Close cooperation and deliberation among the thoracic surgeon, radiologist, pathologist, cytologist, hematologist, oncologist, and anesthesiologist are required in managing patients with mediastinal masses.

Previous textbooks and articles have recommended a direct surgical approach to all lesions in the mediastinum. If a lesion was found during surgery to be unresectable, then a biopsy or debulking and simple closure was recommended. This philosophy subjected many patients to unnecessary thoracotomies or sternotomies. Today, although surgery is not recommended for all masses, because of a high incidence of malignancy in mediastinal tumors and local problems even from benign neoplasms, lesions should not be passively observed. The surgeon must recognize when an aggressive surgical approach, which may even entail cardiopulmonary bypass and reconstruction of great vessels, is warranted and when it is absolutely contraindicated.[2, 3]

With advances in neoadjuvant chemotherapy, some tumors previously considered unresectable with poor prognosis can be cured through appropriately timed chemotherapy followed by surgery. The use of fine-needle aspiration (FNA) and cytopathologic analysis can minimize unnecessary open biopsies.[4] At present, minimally invasive thoracoscopic techniques have expanded our surgical armamentarium for directed biopsies and resection of some tumors. This chapter provides a brief outline of and diagnostic approach to the lesions of the mediastinum, both benign and malignant. It emphasizes the similarities of clinical presentations, which may lead to diagnostic pitfalls. The various imaging modalities for the presurgical radiologic assessment of these masses and the appropriate surgical techniques to gain access to the mediastinum for tumor biopsy or resection are discussed.

ANATOMY OF THE MEDIASTINUM

Boundaries

The mediastinum is the space in the median portion of the chest between the two pleura. It extends from the thoracic inlet superiorly to the cephalad portion of the diaphragm inferiorly and from the inner aspect of the sternum anteriorly to the vertebral bodies (anterior longitudinal spinal ligament) posteriorly. The bilateral paravertebral sulci (the costovertebral regions) are not truly within the mediastinum, but lesions arising in these posterior regions classically have been grouped with tumors of the mediastinum and are discussed as such in this chapter and textbook. The mediastinum contains all of the thoracic viscera except the lungs (Fig. 27–1).

Compartments

The arbitrary divisions of the mediastinum seen in various anatomy, surgery, and radiology textbooks and journals have been somewhat confusing. As rightly pointed out by Shields,[5] this has led to an illogical scheme in which one organ may be in two or more regions of the mediastinum. Attempts to subdivide the mediastinum by radiologic classification of lesions may not be clinically useful to the surgeon. Because many masses can extend into two compart-

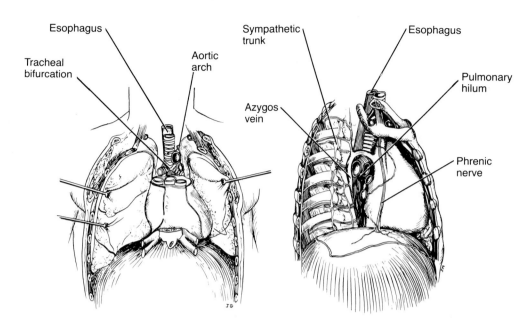

Esophagus

Tracheal
bifurcation

Aortic
arch

Sympathetic
trunk

Esophagus

Pulmonary
hilum

Azygos
vein

Phrenic
nerve

FIGURE 27–1. Frontal and right lateral view of the mediastinum illustrating the major normal structures. (Modified from Hardy JD, Ewing HP: *In* Glenn WWL, Baue AE, Geha AS, et al [eds]: Thoracic and Cardiovascular Surgery. 5th Ed. East Norwalk, Connecticut, Appleton-Century-Crofts, 1982, p 182.)

ments, the epicenter of the tumor or the bulk of the lesion is used to judge the compartment of origin. A few methods of mediastinal compartmentalization are reviewed.

Anatomic purists[6] have divided the mediastinum into the superior and inferior compartments (Fig. 27–2*A*). The superior mediastinum includes the area above the upper level of the pericardium, bounded by the plane from the angle of Louis to the fourth thoracic vertebrae (T4) posteriorly. It contains the origins of the strap muscles (sternohyoid, sternothyroid), arch of the aorta, innominate artery and thoracic portion of the left carotid and subclavian arteries, upper half of the superior vena cava, innominate veins, trachea, upper esophagus, upper portion of the thoracic duct, thymus, paratracheal and pretracheal lymph nodes and lymphatics, and upper portions of the phrenic nerves and the left recurrent laryngeal nerve.

The inferior mediastinum includes the area below the upper level of the pericardium and the imaginary dividing line from the angle of Louis to T4 posteriorly. The inferior mediastinum is further divided into three subcompartments: (1) an anterior mediastinum, bounded in front by the sternum, laterally by the pleura, and behind by the pericardium; (2) the middle mediastinum, containing the heart enclosed in the

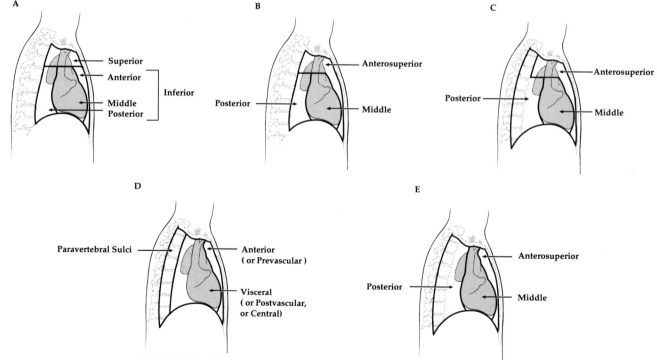

FIGURE 27–2. Various methods for dividing the mediastinum into compartments.

pericardium, the ascending aorta, the lower half of the superior vena cava with the azygos vein, the bifurcation of the trachea and the two bronchi, main pulmonary artery dividing into its two branches, the phrenic nerves, and some bronchial lymphatic vessels; and (3) the posterior mediastinum, bounded in front by the pericardium and the roots of the lungs and behind by the vertebral column from the lower border of the fourth thoracic vertebrae and containing the descending aorta, the azygos and hemiazygos veins, the splanchnic nerves, and the lower portion of the thoracic duct and esophagus.

Many surgery texts, in an effort to improve the clinicoanatomic correlation of tumors with surgical approaches, have grouped the superior mediastinum with the anterior portion of the inferior mediastinum (sometimes called the anterosuperior compartment) (Fig. 27–2B, C). This has worked well for the discussion of tumors of the anterosuperior mediastinum such as thymomas, substernal thyroids, and teratomas but inappropriately divides organs such as the esophagus and trachea (both of foregut embryologic origin) into two compartments. A simpler scheme with better clinical applications[5] divides the mediastinum into three compartments oriented vertically: (1) the anterior (prevascular) compartment, (2) the visceral (middle, postvascular, or central) compartment, and (3) the paravertebral sulci (costovertebral or posterior compartment). Each compartment extends the full length of the mediastinum from the inlet to the diaphragm and, again, is bounded laterally by the respective mediastinal pleura (Fig. 27–2D).[5]

The anterior or prevascular compartment is bounded by an imaginary line formed by the anterior surfaces of the great vessels and the pericardium and the undersurface of the sternum. The innominate vessels limit the space superiorly so that this anterior compartment does not communicate with the thoracic inlet directly; it can, however, be reached surgically by a suprasternal incision with dissection immediately behind the sternum. The visceral compartment extends from this imaginary line in front of the great vessels and pericardium to the ventral surface of the vertebral column. This compartment has the highest concentration of lymphatic vessels and lymph nodes and therefore the highest concentration of lymphomas. The incidence of mediastinal cysts is highest in this compartment as well. The paravertebral sulci or costovertebral regions, again, are not truly mediastinal but rather are potential spaces that lie along each side of the vertebral column and adjacent portions of the proximal ribs. Because this area contains the highest concentration of nerves (intercostal and sympathetic), it has the greatest number of neurogenic tumors in the mediastinum.

Some other classifications use these three vertical compartments but move the junction between the middle and the posterior compartments more anteriorly to the back of the pericardium such that the esophagus, descending aorta, and thoracic duct are included in the posterior compartment (Fig. 27–2E).[7] The compartmentalization of the mediastinum, al-

though arbitrary, allows an organized approach to the classification of mediastinal tumors. A surgeon must, however, develop a three-dimensional perspective of the anatomy of the chest and mediastinum, which is important for the diagnostic evaluation of these masses and crucial for the ultimate surgical resection.

TUMORS OF THE MEDIASTINUM

Incidence

What is the most common mediastinal tumor? The true incidence of mediastinal tumors is unclear. In a review of the literature, reports claiming thymomas, neurogenic tumors, or foregut cysts[8] as the most common mass can all be found. There has been an increase in the incidence of both lymphoproliferative disorders over the past 20 years[9] and asymptomatic thymic lesions discovered on routine chest radiographs and computed tomography (CT) or as part of the evaluation of a patient with newly diagnosed myasthenia gravis. Some tertiary referral centers with a special interest in neuromotor disorders therefore will report an even higher incidence of thymomas in their reviews.

Thymic lesions are extremely rare in patients less than 20 years of age, whereas neurogenic tumors are the most common posterior mediastinal tumor in both children and adults. Combined series that include a higher proportion of children will have a higher overall incidence of neurogenic tumors. Many lymphomas, which may involve the chest as part of a systemic disorder (43% for non-Hodgkin's to 67% for Hodgkin's),[10] have been included in some reviews and skew the statistics to a higher incidence of lymphomas. In fact, primary mediastinal lymphomas affect only a small group (5% to 10%) of patients with lymphomas. Nine series from the past four decades (comprising approximately 600 children and 2200 adults) have been combined in an effort to gain an overall perspective on the true incidence of mediastinal tumors (Fig. 27–3).[11] Neurogenic tumors appear to be the most common mediastinal tumor in both children and adults. In future reviews, the incidence of thymic lesions in adults may surpass that of neurogenic tumors. Surprisingly, the overall incidence of lymphomas, germ cell tumors, and cysts are about equal in the two groups. The differences in tumor incidence in the anterior mediastinum are shown by age (Fig. 27–4).[12] Examples of the wide variety of tumors and lesions that can occur in mediastinal structures in each of the three mediastinal compartments are listed (Tables 27–1 to 27–3) as well as lesions that originate from a nonmediastinal site, which can mimic a primary mediastinal neoplasm (Table 27–4).[13]

Symptoms and Signs

Lesions within the mediastinum are often detected on routine chest radiography.[14] Symptomatic lesions are more likely to have a malignant etiology, but with the

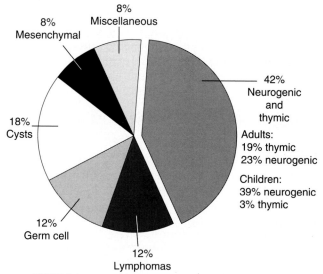

FIGURE 27–3. Overall incidence of mediastinal tumors.

8% Miscellaneous

8% Mesenchymal

18% Cysts

12% Germ cell

12% Lymphomas

42% Neurogenic and thymic

Adults:
19% thymic
23% neurogenic

Children:
39% neurogenic
3% thymic

increasing use of screening chest radiography there is a higher detection rate of asymptomatic malignant lesions.[8] The lack of symptoms, therefore, does not guarantee benignity. Because of the smaller size of their chest cavities, lesions in children tend to be

TABLE 27–1. Lesions Arising in Mediastinal Structures—Anterior Compartment

STRUCTURE	TUMOR
Thymus	Thymoma
	Thymolipoma
	Thymic carcinoid
	Thymic cyst
	Thymic hyperplasia
	Thymic carcinoma
Thyroid	Substernal goiter
	Ectopic thyroid without connection to neck
Parathyroid	Ectopic parathyroid adenoma
	Parathyroid carcinoma
Fat	Lipoma
	Liposarcoma
Lymph nodes	Malignant diseases
	Hodgkin's lymphoma
	Non-Hodgkin's lymphoma
	Metastatic carcinoma
	Benign processes
	Castleman's disease (nodal hyperplasia)
	Infectious mononucleosis
	Granulomas
	Fungal
	Histoplasmosis
	Coccidioidomycosis
	Tuberculosis
	Sarcoidosis
	Wegener's granulomatosis
Germ cell rests	Benign
	Teratomas (dermoids)
	Malignant
	Seminomas
	Nonseminomatous germ cell tumors
	Embryonal carcinoma
	Choriocarcinoma
	Endodermal sinus tumor (yolk sac)
	Teratocarcinoma

TABLE 27–2. Lesions Arising in Mediastinal Structures—Visceral Compartment

STRUCTURE	TUMOR
Trachea	Bronchogenic cyst
	Bronchial adenoma
	Adenocystic carcinoma
	Carcinoid tumor
	Mucoepidermoid
	Bronchial mucous gland adenoma
	Mixed salivary gland tumor
	Squamous cell carcinoma of trachea
Esophagus	Primary malignancies of esophagus
	Adeno or squamous cell carcinoma
	Small cell carcinoma
	Mesenchymal tumors
	Leiomyosarcoma
	Rhadomyosarcoma
	Lymphoma
	Benign lesions
	Duplication cyst
	Leiomyoma
	Esophageal diverticulum (pulsion or traction)
Pericardium	Pericardial cyst
	Pericardial diverticulum
	Hemangiopericytoma
Heart	Fibroma
	Rhabdomyosarcoma
Aorta and arch vessels	Aneurysms (saccular and diffuse)
	Coarctation
	Arch anomalies
	Double aortic arch
	Right arch with left ligamentum
	Left arch with aberrant right subclavian
	Leiomyosarcomas, leiomyomas
Veins	Ectasia and aneurysm formation
	Venous anomalies
	Persistent left superior vena cava
	Anomalous pulmonary venous drainage
	Azygos continuation of the inferior vena cava
	Leiomyomas, leiomyosarcomas
Lymph nodes	Sarcoidosis
	Lymphomas
	Metastatic carcinoma
Phrenic and vagus nerves	Nerve sheath tumors
Sympathetic nerves	Paraganglionomas (chemodectomas)
Thoracic duct	Cysts
Lymphatic vessels	Lymphangiomas (cystic hygromas)
	Lymphangiopericytomas

symptomatic when first detected (i.e., in 50% to 85%).[15, 16] Mediastinal tumors are also more likely to be malignant in children (more than 50%). Remarkably, however, some slow-growing benign or malignant lesions can reach an enormous size, with gradual compensation by the individual, relatively little awareness, and few symptoms. When they arise, symptoms occur locally (by distortion, compression, superinfection, or invasion of thoracic organs) or systemically. Systemic manifestations can be related to the constitutional, endocrinologic, or autoimmune effects or associations of these tumors. Physical examination cannot be limited solely to the cardiopulmonary system; a detailed history and physical examination are essential. Examples of symptoms and

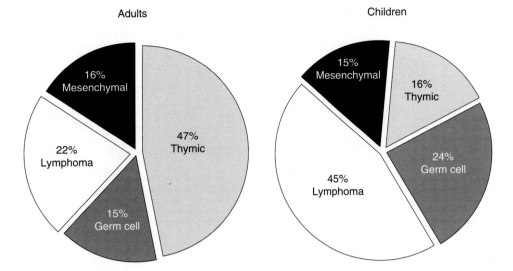

FIGURE 27–4. Anterior mediastinal tumors in adults and children.

signs caused by different etiologies are given to highlight the scope of these clinical presentations (Tables 27–5 and 27–6). Laboratory investigations that may be useful in the evaluation of these patients are listed (Table 27–7).

RADIOLOGIC EVALUATION OF MEDIASTINAL MASSES

Over the past decade, there have been many significant advances in radiology, including the development of high-resolution CT scanners, magnetic resonance imaging (MRI) scanners, nuclear radioisotope scans, transesophageal ultrasonography, and color flow Doppler techniques. These techniques have supplanted many tests previously used in the work-up of patients with mediastinal pathology, including conventional tomography, oblique chest radiography, the creation of pneumomediastinum, bronchography, and myelography. Some of these tests may still be of value where the more advanced technologies are not available.

Chest Radiography

The routine chest radiograph remains one of the most important tests in the evaluation of patients with mediastinal masses. In more than 50% of adults with mediastinal lesions, a chest radiograph is the mode by which an asymptomatic abnormality is discovered. The overlying radiopacity of the sternum in the frontal view can obscure the mass. A lateral radiograph is often important to both visualize a lesion and accurately localize the abnormality to a mediastinal compartment. The surgeon must become familiar with five areas on the plain radiograph that represent boundaries between lung and normal mediastinal structures. Distortion or loss of these lines implies anatomic abnormalities or pathology (Fig. 27–5, on p

TABLE 27–3. Lesions Arising in Mediastinal Structures—Posterior Compartment

STRUCTURE	TUMOR

Peripheral intercostal nerve	Benign
	   Neurofibroma
	   Neurilemmoma (Schwannoma)
	Malignant
	   Neurosarcoma

Sympathetic ganglia	Benign
	   Ganglioneuroma
	Malignant
	   Ganglioneuroblastoma
	   Neuroblastoma

Paraganglia	Pheochromocytoma Chemodectoma (paraganglioma)

TABLE 27–4. Radiographic Pseudotumors of the Mediastinum Presenting as a "Mediastinal Mass"

NONMEDIASTINAL SITE OF ORIGIN	EXAMPLES

Abdomen	Hernias
	   Morgagni (anterior)
	   Bochdalek (posterior)
	   Hiatus hernia
	   Paraesophageal
	Pseudocyst of the pancreas

Neck	Thyroid goiter (with downward migration into anterior or visceral compartments) Cervicomediastinal cystic hygroma
Thoracic cage and vertebrae	Sternal sarcomas Chondroma or chondrosarcoma of a rib Vertebral body chordoma Paravertebral abscess (tuberculosis)
Lung	Primary bronchogenic carcinoma (medial location with mediastinal invasion) Extralobar sequestration
Meninges	Meningocele
Ectopic hematopoietic tissue	Intrathoracic extramedullary hematopoiesis (usually a paraspinal mass)

TABLE 27–5. Local Symptoms (Compression or Invasion)

STRUCTURE	SYMPTOMS/SIGNS	EXAMPLE
Airway	Cough, wheeze, stridor (may be positional) Obstructive pneumonia Expectorating hair or subaceous material	Large thymic tumor or substernal thyroid Bronchogenic cyst with or without airway communication Teratoma with airway invasion
Blood vessels		
Superior vena cava	Distended veins of neck, arms and anterior chest wall, breast enlargement, facial flushing, headaches	Lymphomas, histoplasmosis with fibrosing mediastinitis, small cell carcinoma of lung with extensive mediastinal lymphadenopathy
Aorta and branches	Anterior chest/neck pain (ascending aorta and arch branches) Back and interscapular pain (descending aorta) Hemoptysis or hematemesis (herald bleed or major exsanguinating hemorrhage)	Saccular aneurysm of arch or Type A dissection Type B aortic dissection Invasive carcinoma of the esophagus
Pulmonary artery	Dyspnea, right ventricular failure	Invasive thymic malignancy
Heart and pericardium	Acute tamponade, arrythmias, chronic congestive heart failure (right side more than left side)	Primary cardiac tumor or any mediastinal tumor with pericardial or cardiac invasion
Esophagus	Dysphagia, odynophagia, hematemesis, weight loss	Carcinoma of the esophagus, duplication cysts
Thoracic duct	Chylous pleural effusion	Lymphomas, tuberculosis
Nerves		
Recurrent	Voice hoarseness, aspiration with or without pneumonia Mild dysphonia	Lymphomas, any vascular lesion in region of ligamentum arteriosus (aneurysms, coarctation), metastatic carcinoma to left aortopulmonary window nodes (5)
Phrenic	Dyspnea, hiccups, elevation hemidiaphragm	Involvement of left prevascular nodes (6)
Sympathetic chain or stellate ganglion	Horner's syndrome (enophthalmus, meiosis, anhidrosis)	Neurogenic tumors Superior sulcus tumors
Spinal cord	Leg weakness, hyperreflexia, paraplegia	Neurogenic tumors (especially pediatric patients), dumbbell tumors
Bones		
Vertebrae	Back pain and scoliosis	Neurogenic tumors (benign and malignant)
Chest wall and sternum	Pain, mass	Lymphomas (involving internal mammary lymph nodes with chest wall invasion) Germ cell tumors Mediastinal infections that can invade the chest wall (actinomycetes, blastomycetes, Cryptococcus)

452), including the paratracheal stripe, the aortopulmonary window, the azygoesophageal recess, the paraspinal line, and the retrosternal airspace.[17] A conventional chest radiograph, when properly processed and interpreted by an experienced radiologist, is 97% accurate in detecting mediastinal masses.[18] Previous chest radiographs must always be reviewed, if possible, because these may supply valuable information on tumor growth and organ of origin. A subtle mass may be evident only after close comparison to old films. Calcification of tumors can often be appreciated on plain films. Vertebral body abnormalities and scoliosis, which can be associated with duplication cysts and posterior mediastinal masses in children, can be recognized on plain radiographs.

Computed Tomography

Besides the routine chest radiograph, CT represents the gold standard for the assessment of the mediastinum and should be performed on virtually every patient who presents with a mediastinal abnormality.[19–22] CT scanning allows precise anatomic localization of lesions and rapid determination of the primary nature of a mass as either vascular, fat, cystic, or soft tissue.[23] The degree and pattern of tumor calcification, enhancement characteristics, homogeneity, and continuity with other intrathoracic structures can also be assessed. In any patient with a mass that is associated with the aorta or its branches, a CT scan should be done before any biopsies.[24] Congenital vascular anomalies such as a right-sided aortic arch or an aberrant right subclavian artery can mimic a right paratracheal soft tissue mass on plain radiographs that could easily be misinterpreted as a neoplasm without appropriate cross-sectional imaging and vascular assessment.[1]

With CT, a good differential diagnosis can be formulated before any surgical intervention or biopsy. Hounsfield units (HU) constitute a scale from -1000 HU (air) to $+1000$ HU (cortical bone), with pure water (as seen in a pericardial cyst) equal to 0 HU, fat equal to -70 HU, soft tissue equal to $+30$ HU, and calcified tissue equal to more than 165 HU. Use of this scale allows for detailed analysis of the lesion and its contents.[23] Contrast medium (100 ml) should be injected at a rate of approximately 2 ml/sec for adequate comparison and delineation of the vascular structures. Contrast enhancement will aid in differentiating vascular compression, encasement, and venous obstruction (with collateral development) and may

TABLE 27–6. Systemic Symptoms

SYMPTOMS/SIGNS	EXAMPLE
Constitutional	
Fever and night sweats	B symptoms of lymphomas
	Infectious etiology of mediastinal mass (fungal, bacterial, tuberculosis)
	Obstructive pneumonia from mechanical effects of mediastinal tumor
	Superinfection of mediastinal tumor (i.e., bronchogenic cyst)
Weight loss and anorexia	Advanced mediastinal malignancy with systemic metastases
	Hyperthyroidism
	Chronic infection
	Mechanical difficulty with swallowing
Endocrine	
Hypercalcemia	Ectopic mediastinal parathyroid adenoma, bone metastases
Hypertension	Mediastinal pheochromocytoma
Watery diarrhea	Neuroblastomas with VIP secretion
Gynecomastia	Germ cell tumors with β-hCG production
Cushing's syndrome	Thymomas, bronchial carcinoids
Autoimmune disorders	
Myasthenia gravis	Thymomas
Red cell hypoplasia	
Hypogammaglobulinemia	

clearly show vascular invasion. Obliteration of fat planes around major vascular structures implies invasion by the tumor. Two sites that are difficult to assess by plain chest radiography—the pretracheal and left paratracheal regions—are clearly seen with CT. The longitudinal orientation of many of the structures passing through the mediastinum en route to the abdomen and neck allows good perpendicular imaging for most lesions. Mural calcifications are best identified by CT scans. Some lesions that are known to contain calcium include goiters, thymomas, treated lymphomas, carcinoid tumors, inflammatory masses (tuberculosis and histoplasmosis), aneurysms, some neurogenic tumors, and esophageal leiomyomas.[17] Modern helical CT scanners are capable of imaging the entire thorax in minutes and therefore are excellent for use with patients who are very ill or who are restless or uncomfortable in the supine position. CT scanning can simultaneously detect small pulmonary metastases (which may not be visible on the chest

TABLE 27–7. Diagnostic Laboratory Tests Useful in the Evaluation of Patients with Mediastinal Masses

TEST	EXAMPLE
Blood	
Complete blood cell count	Assessing chronic or acute blood loss (esophageal malignancy)
	Anemia of chronic disease related to malignancy or infectious etiology (tuberculosis)
	Red blood cell hypoplasia associated with thymomas
	Thrombocytopenia associated with some germ cell tumors
	Nonlymphocytic leukemia associated with some nonseminomatous germ cell tumors
Lactate dehydrogenase	Elevated in lymphomas, seminomas, yolk sac tumors
Alkaline phosphatase	May indicate metastatic disease to liver or bones; may be elevated with parathyroid tumors
Glucose	Some teratomas can produce insulin with secondary hypoglycemia
Calcium	May be increased in hyperparathyroidism or metastatic disease to bone
β-human chorionic gonadotropin, α-fetoprotein	Should be done in any young male with an anterior mediastinal mass
	Benign teratomas are marker negative; negative markers do not guarantee benignity, however α-fetoprotein is normal in pure seminomas; β-human chorionic gonadotropin may be increased
	Elevation in α-fetoprotein indicates a nonseminomatous component to germ cell tumor
	Important markers to follow for treatment effects
Thyroid function tests	Usually normal with substernal and ectopic thyroids although 10% hyperfunctioning
Urine	
Vanillylmandelic acid	Urinary screening of catecholamines for the evaluation of pheochromocytomas
Normetanephrine	
Metanephrine	
Bone marrow	
Aspirates and biopsies	Assessment of marrow involvement in patients with lymphomas, neuroblastomas, and carcinomas

radiograph) and pericardial or pleural effusions and can assess the upper abdomen for liver and abdominal metastases.

Magnetic Resonance Imaging

MRI technology has the advantage of requiring no ionizing radiation and no iodinated contrast agents and therefore is ideal for patients with known allergies to these agents. MRI is particularly valuable for the assessment of vascular structures and anomalies and is better for demonstrating vascular invasion by tumors than is CT.[25] Soft tissues can be easily distinguished from blood vessels on MRI. The ability of MRI to image coronally and sagittally and to gate the scan to cardiac motion allows excellent discrimination in the areas of the aortic root, the subcarina, the aortopulmonary window, the brachial plexus, and the spinal cord. MRI is the procedure of choice when there is a concern that the tumor extends posteriorly through the intervertebral canal to the epidural space and spinal cord (Fig. 27–6). These scans have a distinct disadvantage compared with CT scan in that they do not show calcification of lesions. However, MRI is excellent in assessing the characteristics of fluid collections. Lesions such as radiation fibrosis (which contains little water and therefore will be dark on T2 imaging) can be distinguished from tumor by MRI but probably not by CT scan.[26, 27]

Because the cost of this technology is high, scanning times are long, and the process is labor intensive, MRI is not suitable for the routine evaluation of mediastinal masses or for the patient who is claustrophobic or too ill to lie flat for an extended period of time. Most mediastinal masses do not require MRI for evaluation. Patients with metallic intracranial clips or pacemakers cannot be placed in the strong magnetic field of these scanners.

Fluoroscopy

Fluoroscopy is used primarily to guide the FNA of larger neoplasms, which can be visualized on the routine chest radiograph. It may also be helpful in observing movement of a mediastinal mass in relation to other dynamic structures within the mediastinum and chest, which may indicate the origin of the tumor or invasion of these structures by the tumor. The following are examples of these relative movements: (1) The upward movement of a substernal mass with deglutition implies thyroid, laryngeal, or tracheal association. (2) Diminished diaphragmatic excursion with inspiration may imply phrenic nerve paresis or paralysis from an invasive tumor or process. (3) Medial movement during inspiration suggests a lung primary with secondary invasion or abutment of the mediastinum. A mediastinal primary tumor that invades the lung would tether the lung at that point and inhibit movement. (4) Pulsations can occasionally be appreciated if the mass represents a true or false aneurysm of the aorta or left ventricle. (5) Some venous struc-

tures change in size with position; the lesion will increase in size when the patient is supine.[28]

Barium Studies

The esophagogram is an important road map for the surgeon to have before endoscopic evaluation of the esophagus and therefore is needed before esophagoscopy. The incidental finding of a Zenker's diverticulum may prevent an iatrogenic perforation on introduction of the esophagoscope. The mucosal pattern is important in distinguishing mucosal, intramural, and extrinsic lesions. Some duplication cysts in the mediastinum have connections with the upper intestinal tract and demonstrate delayed opacification on follow-up films.[29]

A barium swallow can also be very useful in the evaluation of congenital vascular rings in pediatric patients. Anomalies such as double aortic arches, right aortic arches with retroesophageal left subclavian ar-

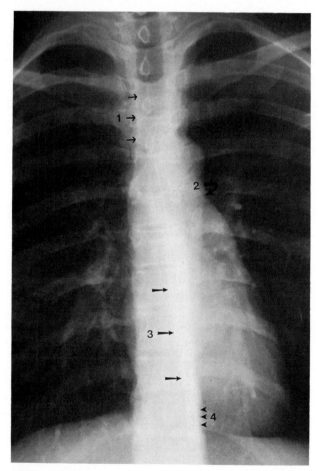

FIGURE 27–5. Important radiographic junction lines between mediastinal structures and lung. Widening, distortion, or deviation of any of these boundary lines indicates a mediastinal process: (1) Right paratracheal stripe (right upper lobe against the right wall of the trachea). (2) Aortopulmonic window (left upper lobe against the superior aspect of the left pulmonary artery and the inferior aspect of the transverse arch of the aorta). (3) Azygoesophageal recess (right lung against the azygos venous arch and descending along groove between azygos and esophagus). (4) Paraspinal line (above the diaphragm, the right lower lobe adjacent to the spine).

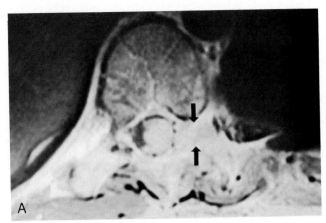 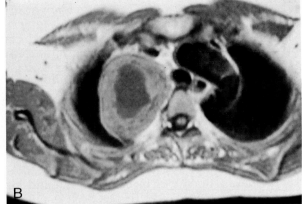

FIGURE 27–6. Magnetic resonance imaging of neurogenic tumors. *A,* MRI demonstrating intervertebral extension (arrows) of a neurofibrosarcoma, which required a combined thoracotomy and posterior neurosurgical approach for resection. *B,* A large encapsulated neurilemmoma of the T1 nerve root resected by right posterolateral thoracotomy.

teries, and pulmonary arterial slings (anomalous origin of left pulmonary artery from right pulmonary artery with a retrotracheal course) each have a characteristic esophageal wall indentation.[30] MRIs have replaced this study in many centers. A barium swallow, however, is a relatively inexpensive test and can be extremely valuable when properly interpreted. Barium enemas may be helpful if a suspected mass is from a morgagnian hernia; this may demonstrate colon within the chest. Administration of barium during routine CT scanning may make further barium studies unnecessary.

NUCLEAR RADIOLOGY

Nuclear medicine is rarely required in the evaluation of mediastinal masses, but for certain tumors it may prove to be helpful in diagnosis and for follow-up.

Thyroid and Parathyroid Scanning

Thyroid scanning (technetium-99m pertechnetate, iodine-123, and, less frequently, iodine-131) is a sensitive method of detecting functioning thyroid tissue within the mediastinum. The uptake by a substernal thyroid, however, is variable and can be altered by the prior administration of intravenous contrast.[31] Therefore, if thyroid scanning is to be performed, it should be done before the CT scan. Because substernal thyroids are often nonfunctional, a negative scan does not rule out a thyroid origin to a retrosternal or mediastinal mass. In a case of a suspected true ectopic thyroid, scanning should be performed to confirm that this is not the patient's only functioning thyroid tissue. This so-called abnormal mediastinal mass may represent the patient's only normal thyroid tissue that is simply malpositioned.

The technetium (technetium-99m) and thallium (thallium-201) digital subtraction technique (technetium-99m is taken up by thyroid tissue only, whereas thallium-201 is taken up by both thyroid and para-

thyroid tissue) is useful for the localization of ectopic parathyroids in the evaluation of primary hyperparathyroidism.[32, 33] The technetium-99m pertechnetate test can also be used to identify the 50% of esophageal cysts that contain gastric mucosa.[34]

Gallium Scanning

Gallium-67 can be useful in distinguishing gallium-avid tumors, such as active lymphomas, from an area of fibrosis that may persist after treatment of a mediastinal lymphoma. Gallium will also localize to inflammatory processes in the lungs and mediastinum. Lung cancer, mesotheliomas, and germ cell tumors have been shown to take up gallium.[35]

Metaiodobenzylguanidine Scanning

Iodine-131 metaiodobenzylguanidine is an analogue of norepinephrine and has a special affinity for adrenal medullary tumors. It is used to identify mediastinal pheochromocytomas (paragangliomas) and neuroblastomas.[36, 37]

Bone Scans

Bone scans are sensitive for cortical bone destruction by tumor and therefore are useful for the evaluation of any tumor located near bone (sternum, ribs, or vertebrae) in a patient with localized pain. The finding of diffuse bony metastases suggests that the mediastinal tumor under evaluation may be a secondary mediastinal growth or a primary tumor that is advanced and should be managed nonsurgically.

Nuclear Venography

Nuclear venography is occasionally used to document a site of venous obstruction by a mediastinal mass.

Ventilation Perfusion Scan

Xenon-133 and technetium-99m have been used to demonstrate ventilation and perfusion mismatches as seen in pulmonary emboli.[38] They can also demonstrate hypoperfusion secondary to compression or invasion of the pulmonary arterial or venous system by primary mediastinal tumors. Selective ventilation and perfusion scanning coupled with pulmonary function testing are valuable in the preoperative assessment and postoperative prediction of remaining pulmonary function if a pulmonary resection is anticipated.[39]

ULTRASOUND

Ultrasound technology is very helpful in differentiating solid from cystic lesions in many organs and locations throughout the body.[40] It has been useful in assessing the substernal extent of thyroid goiters in adults, and prenatal ultrasonography has even been used to identify a bronchogenic cyst and teratoma in utero.[41] The noninvasive echocardiographic examination of a child may reveal a mediastinal mass to be a vascular anomaly. Transesophageal echocardiography in adults may be helpful in assessing pericardial effusions, pericardial cysts, and extension of tumors into cardiac chambers. The central mediastinal location of the esophagus avoids the problem of acoustic shadowing by the lungs, which in adults can interfere with the anterior ultrasonographic examination.[42] Flexible esophagoscopes, in conjunction with intraluminal ultrasound probes, can be used to examine a submucosal or intramural esophageal mass and help in the differential diagnosis of an enteric cyst or leiomyoma. It is also helpful for assessing transmural extension of esophageal carcinomas and possible paraesophageal nodal extension or aortic wall abutment or invasion.

ANGIOGRAPHY

The use of angiography can often be avoided now with the use of dynamic CT scanning and MRI, although many thoracic surgeons still prefer or require angiography for preoperative planning. Angiographic embolization has been used in managing some tumors as part of a diagnostic and therapeutic intervention, and angiography is still important in the assessment of a suspected pulmonary sequestration, which may mimic a mediastinal mass.[17] Digital subtraction techniques can minimize the contrast load, particularly in patients with a degree of renal insufficiency. Angiography of the chest can be associated with transient ischemic attacks induced by particle embolization as a result of catheter manipulation in the great vessels. Transverse myelitis and paraplegia have resulted from injection into bronchial arteries, as these vessels have branches that also supply the spinal cord.[43]

Angiograms may give a false sense of security that a mass is not vascular, as an aneurysm may contain extensive thrombus with a relatively normal appearing lumen, resulting in a relatively normal angiogram. CT scanning with contrast infusion or MRI would help in distinguishing this. Angiography has been used in the evaluation of angiomatous tumors in the pediatric population. Left-sided and right-sided cardiac catheterizations are required for the evaluation of many congenital heart lesions, which may be vital in the work-up of a mediastinal lesion that is suspected of having a vascular origin.[44]

Venography

Venography can be used to document precise sites of venous obstruction (intrinsic or extrinsic) and map collateral pathways. This can be useful in planning major thoracic resections that may entail the sacrifice of a major venous structure such as the superior vena cava or innominate vein. The preoperative finding of complete obstruction with collateralization through the azygos or hemiazygos system means that reconstruction after resection may not be required, because the patient has already developed anatomic and physiologic venous bypasses.

PREOPERATIVE PULMONARY FUNCTION TESTING IN PATIENTS WITH MEDIASTINAL MASSES

Patients with large anterior and middle mediastinal masses should undergo preoperative pulmonary function testing to assess lung function and reserve. Surgery may entail en bloc resections of pulmonary segments, lobes, or even an entire lung and occasionally sacrifice of a phrenic nerve. Flow volume loops in the supine and upright positions may show a degree of airway obstruction that cannot be appreciated on symptom review or clinical examination.[45] Baseline lung diffusion capacity for carbon monoxide should be tested before the initiation of chemotherapy with bleomycin and prior to surgery as this drug is recognized to cause pulmonary fibrosis and secondary oxygen-sensitive lungs.[46] Xenon scans and arterial blood gases in conjunction with these basic pulmonary function tests may be invaluable in predicting surgical limitations, postoperative weaning, and future cardiopulmonary restrictions in these patients.

SURGICAL APPROACHES TO THE MEDIASTINUM

Before proceeding to any interventional study, the surgeon must review the clinical presentation and radiologic evaluation and formulate a differential diagnosis. Once vascular, congenital, and infectious etiologies have been ruled out, the surgeon should ask the following questions in determining the course of treatment.

1. Is my role in treating this patient to obtain tissue for diagnosis or to resect for cure?
2. Is this a primary or secondary mediastinal neoplasm? Should a further search be made for a primary tumor at another site (e.g., use of testicular ultrasound)? Do CT scans of the chest and upper abdomen

show pulmonary parenchymal metastases, liver or retroperitoneal metastases (germ cell tumors), or adrenal metastases (in the case of an occult primary bronchogenic tumor)? Are serum markers negative?

3. According to radiologic criteria, is this lesion resectable? Is the tumor well encapsulated, and are fat planes preserved? If so, does the patient have any medical contraindications to a direct surgical approach?

4. Does the tumor appear to be locally advanced? Does it appear to abut or invade vascular structures? Are fat planes obliterated? Is there clinical or radiologic evidence of other intrathoracic organ invasion? Are there pleural or pericardial effusions that may be amenable to aspiration and cytologic analysis for diagnosis?

5. If the lesion is locally advanced, how can a diagnosis be made in the safest, most cost-effective, and most expeditious manner? Should FNA be performed before an open surgical biopsy?

6. If the initial attempt at obtaining a diagnosis is unsuccessful, is there a second minimally invasive procedure that might be effective?

7. If a surgical biopsy is to be undertaken, has the case been discussed with the pathologist before the operation so that appropriate preparations can be made for frozen section analysis, sterile collection, and proper tissue handling? Is the pathologist satisfied with the amount of tissue supplied for all immunohistochemical tests, electron microscopy, and cultures?[47]

The final histologic assessment should be awaited before proceeding to an aggressive resection. Frozen sections are helpful in supplying a preliminary diagnosis and in judging whether the tissue sampled is sufficient for a detailed histologic analysis, but basing a major resection on a frozen section report is dangerous.[48] An initial interpretation of a "thymoma" on frozen section may turn out to be a lymphoma once permanent stains are available. When possible, the surgeon should incise the tumor to remove a specimen rather than use biopsy forceps, which can cause crush artifacts and make it difficult for the pathologist to tell the architecture of the specimen. A surgeon should also avoid using electrocautery on the base of the biopsy site until the pathologist is satisfied with the tissue provided should additional, deeper biopsies be required. Cautery artifacts can also make histologic interpretation difficult.

Fine-Needle Aspiration

As the practitioners of FNA, the interventional radiologist and cytopathologist can play a very important role in the work-up of patients with mediastinal lesions.[49, 50] Their skills can avoid the use of many unnecessary general anesthetics and open surgical procedures. In fact, the skills of the radiologist and cytopathologist in an institution are often inversely related to the number of open procedures required for diagnosis. Most FNAs can be performed on an out-patient basis. Critically ill patients, who may be a prohibitive anesthetic risk for an open diagnostic procedure, can usually undergo FNA. Patients with extremely limited pulmonary function may require the prophylactic insertion of a Heimlich valve before the biopsy. Pneumothorax (in 15% to 20% of patients) and bleeding (self-limited hemoptysis) are the main complications. Serious hemorrhagic complications and tamponade are extremely rare. Follow-up chest films are done 4 hours after the procedure, or sooner if symptoms develop. Because small-caliber needles (nos. 20, 22, and 25) are used, most lesions can be biopsied even if a major vessel must be punctured to access the lesion. Most radiologists require coagulation parameters before performing a biopsy near major hilar structures. The shortest route from the skin to the lesion is usually chosen.[51, 52]

The shortcomings of FNA for the diagnosis of lymphoma are related to the limited number of cells, the requirement for architectural analysis, and the necessity for special staining. Some tumors are surrounded by an intense inflammatory process, making it difficult to interpret. Similar difficulties in obtaining a histologic diagnosis can be encountered during surgery. Desmoplastic tumors that overlie major vascular structures, creating a solid pulsatile wall of tumor without clear anatomic landmarks, can be technically dangerous to biopsy.

FNA is most helpful for the diagnosis of metastatic carcinomas to the mediastinum (90% sensitive). Larger lesions are aspirated under fluoroscopic guidance, whereas smaller lesions require CT guidance of the needle. Needle-tip localization is better with CT and may improve sampling by avoiding the center of a necrotic tumor and selecting the rim of more active growth. Under CT guidance, FNA is a slower process, often requiring movement of the patient in and out of the scanner for needle repositioning.

In the management of a suspected pericardial cyst, FNA can be both diagnostic and therapeutic. Fluid aspirated from cysts can be analyzed for mesothelium (as in pericardial cysts) or bronchial epithelium (as in bronchogenic cysts). Aspirated fluid should always be sent for cytologic analysis. With advances in immunohistochemistry, in the future even problematic diagnoses such as subtyping of lymphomas will be improved. Contamination, or seeding, of the needle track with tumor is exceedingly rare and therefore should not be used as a reason not to aspirate a lesion.

Bronchoscopy

Flexible and rigid bronchoscopic techniques can be used for the diagnosis and palliative management of airways that are compressed or invaded by mediastinal tumors. Any patient with a history of a suspicious cough, wheeze, or stridor without a clear radiologic abnormality must undergo bronchoscopy to rule out an endobronchial tumor. An erroneous diagnosis of adult-onset asthma can be made if a bronchoscopy is not performed. Bronchoalveolar lavage (BAL) and bronchial brushings may be helpful in obtaining a

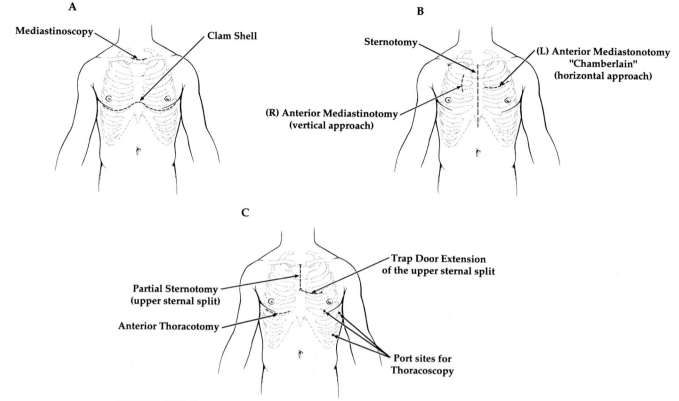

FIGURE 27–7. Surgical approaches to the mediastinum with the patient in the supine position.

cytologic diagnosis. Fluorescent endoscopy (now in early clinical trials) uses diagnostic lasers and spectroscopic analysis of mucosal autofluorescent and exogenously administered dye-enhanced fluorescence and may soon be helpful in localizing occult lung primaries in cases in which the BAL shows metastatic carcinoma with no radiologically apparent primary.[53] The palliative placement of Gianturco or Dumont stents may significantly relieve airway obstruction in patients with unresectable extrinsic tumors that compress or invade the airway.[54–57] Resection and cauterization with carbon dioxide and yttrium-aluminum-garnet (YAG) lasers or coring with the rigid bronchoscope can re-establish an airway if there is an endobronchial primary tumor or metastases.[58–60] Paratracheal and subcarinal masses can be biopsied through the airway with Wang needles.[61, 62]

Esophagoscopy

A barium swallow should precede the endoscopic evaluation of the esophagus. Esophageal ultrasound may be performed during the endoscopy. The surgeon can perform a biopsy of obvious mucosal lesions but must avoid lesions that are submucosal in origin (e.g., suspected duplication cyst or leiomyoma), because this breaching of the mucosa may greatly complicate an otherwise straightforward surgical enucleation. Bronchoscopy and esophagoscopy can be easily performed with the patient under one topical pharyngeal and tracheal anesthetic by repositioning the patient in a lateral position after the bronchoscopic evaluation.

The diagnosis of a tracheoesophageal fistula can be made quickly.

Mediastinoscopy

Mediastinoscopy was first described by Carlens in 1959.[63] An incision is made in the base of the neck, and the dissection is carried in between the strap muscles down to the trachea (Fig. 27–7A). The pretracheal fascia is incised, and blunt digital dissection and palpation are performed as distally as possible before the introduction of the mediastinoscope. Unlike performing a tracheostomy, this maneuver does not require division of the isthmus of the thyroid; a more posterior angulation of the trachea behind the innominate artery allows dissection into the visceral compartment.[64] This allows easy access to paratracheal (American Thoracic Society nodal stations 2R and 2L, 4R and 4L[65]), anterior subcarinal (7), and tracheobronchial angle nodes (10R and 10L).

Some mediastinal cysts have been removed or aspirated through this approach. Mediastinoscopy into the visceral compartment often is not performed in children. Videoassisted mediastinoscopy has recently been described by attaching a fiberoptic system to the standard mediastinoscope to magnify and improve the visualization of this area. In experienced hands, mediastinoscopy is a safe procedure, but an in-depth knowledge of the three-dimensional anatomy of the visceral compartment is mandatory before this approach is used to perform a biopsy of suspected nodes or tumors. Each biopsy should be preceded by needle aspiration, and lymph nodes should be bluntly dissected until practically free before a biopsy is taken. Nodes may be densely adherent to a vascular structure and tear the vessel when removed. All major vascular structures, including the aorta, the innominate artery, the superior vena cava, the azygos vein, and the right pulmonary artery, are at risk. Structures such as the esophagus, the main trachea, the right upper lobe bronchus, and the lung have been accidentally biopsied. The patient should be widely prepped whenever a mediastinoscopy is performed in case an emergency sternotomy or thoracotomy is required because of severe bleeding.

Extended or Substernal Mediastinoscopy

As described by Ginsberg and colleagues,[66] a modification of the standard mediastinoscopy called extended or substernal mediastinoscopy has been used to access the anterior compartment. The usual neck incision for mediastinoscopy is performed with lateral retraction of the strap muscles. The cervical extension of the thymus can be identified and the scope advanced anterior to the thymus, thus entering the prevascular or anterior mediastinal compartment. The mediastinoscope can be advanced anterior to the great vessels, which allows biopsy of aortopulmonary window (5) and prevascular (6) nodal station without using the standard anterior mediastinotomy approach. With this substernal approach, the angle of the mediastinoscope is more horizontal and the tissue planes are often less amenable to digital dissection, as seen in the visceral compartment with standard mediastinoscopy.[67] Care must be taken not to injure the innominate vein. With proper preoperative radiologic assessment, large masses clearly in the anterior compartment can be approached for biopsy in this manner. This cervical approach to the anterior or prevascular compartment of the mediastinum is the approach preferred by some surgeons for thymectomies in children and adults who have myasthenia gravis.[68] A cervical thymectomy is not indicated if a thymoma is known to be present.

Anterior or Parasternal Mediastinotomy

Anterior or parasternal mediastinotomy was described and used by Chamberlain in 1965 and has been used most frequently for staging of the left-sided (aortopulmonary [5] and prevascular [6]) mediastinal nodes in patients with lung cancer (see Figure 27–7B). It is also a safe approach for anterior mediastinal or retrosternal masses in which a histologic diagnosis is required and FNA has been unsuccessful.[69, 70] A transverse incision is made in the skin and underlying pectoralis major fascia. The muscle fibers are retracted, and dissection in an interspace or removal of a portion of the second or third rib with disarticulation of the cartilage from the sternum allows access to the anterior compartment and nodes in the visceral compartment.[69] Because of its proximity to the subclavian vessels, the first interspace is not used. The inter-

nal mammary artery and vein can be individually ligated if further medial exposure is required. A blunt extrapleural dissection against the sternum can be performed to access the mediastinum. A transpleural approach and reincision of the mediastinal pleura to return to the mediastinum proper are sometimes safer in visualizing the phrenic nerve. By removing a portion of the second or third rib, the surgeon can easily palpate the mediastinal structures and directly aspirate the lesion before biopsy. The procedure can be extended into a limited anterior thoracotomy should greater exposure be required or difficulties encountered.

A right-sided Chamberlain procedure allows access for biopsy of right-sided anterior mediastinal tumors that are retrosternal or extend toward the right hemithorax. Biopsies of lymph nodes in the tracheobronchial angle (10R) and paratracheal (4R) positions can also be made. These nodes require some mobilization of the superior vena cava, which can be performed from this approach.

Vertical incisions with removal of two costocartilages have been used, although the cosmetic outcome of this approach is less desirable than those of other approaches (Fig. 27–7B). The patient can often be discharged the same day if an extrapleural dissection is performed or if the transpleural route is chosen and the air is evacuated with a catheter during closure. If cartilage is removed, there will be minor, local paradoxical movement of the skin and muscle with respiration, but this improves within a few weeks or may not be discernible if the patient has bulky pectoralis musculature.

Simultaneous mediastinoscopy and mediastinotomy incisions with palpation through both incisions can allow some tactile assessment of tumor fixation to mediastinal structures when large anterior lesions extend into the visceral compartment. An emergency Chamberlain procedure can be performed with the patient under local anesthesia in a critically ill patient who has a large mass that abuts or invades the chest wall or compresses the trachea. Performing the procedure with the patient breathing spontaneously and in an upright position minimizes the risk of loss of airway patency, which can occur with muscle paralysis, supine positioning, and general anesthesia.

Posterior Mediastinotomy

Posterior mediastinotomy is rarely used. It was used for the biopsy of posterior tumors but now is primarily reserved for the drainage of posterior mediastinal abscesses or empyemas. A vertical paraspinal incision approximately 4 cm from the midline vertebral spinous processes is made with the patient in the lateral or sitting position (Fig. 27–8). Two or three ribs are resected subperiosteally, and the intercostal vessels are ligated. An extrapleural dissection can be performed.[71] A large tube may be left in place to facilitate drainage. The ribs selected for resection should be the ones in the most dependent position of the abscess

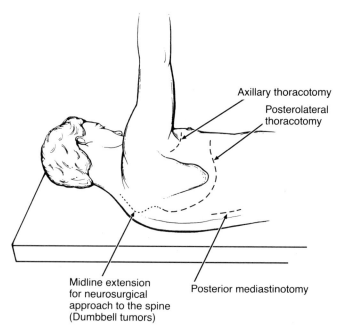

Axillary thoracotomy

Posterolateral thoracotomy

Midline extension for neurosurgical approach to the spine (Dumbbell tumors)

Posterior mediastinotomy

FIGURE 27–8. Surgical approaches to the mediastinum with the patient in the lateral position.

cavity; this can be outlined by a preoperative injection of the empyema or abscess cavity with contrast.

Video-Assisted Thoracic Surgery

Although thoracoscopic and pleuroscopic procedures have been performed for more than 70 years, recent advances in fiberoptics and endoscopic instruments, including expandable lung retractors, coagulation devices, scissors, graspers, and endoscopic stapling devices, allow excellent visualization of the thoracic cavity and mediastinum from a lateral approach. A visually guided aspiration or biopsy of lesions in any mediastinal compartment can be easily performed.[72–76] Simultaneously, the entire thoracic cavity can be assessed for visceral, pleural, or diaphragmatic tumor implants; pleural effusions; and associated surface pulmonary parenchymal lesions. Limited palpation of the pulmonary surface and chest wall is possible through the thoracoport sites (see Fig. 7C). Selective one-lung anesthesia is required for optimal visualization and mobility while performing video-assisted thoracoscopic techniques. Some critically ill patients with limited cardiorespiratory function may be unable to tolerate even short periods of one-lung ventilation and may require limited anterior or posterolateral thoracotomies for tissue procurement or resection with a single-lumen endotracheal tube.

The thoracoscopic evaluation of aortopulmonary window nodes as part of the staging of pulmonary malignancies is preferred by some surgeons to mediastinotomy, but mediastinoscopy remains the gold standard for paratracheal nodal staging.[77] Samples from these sites can also be taken for biopsy as part of the evaluation of mediastinal lymphadenopathy in the work-up of a primary mediastinal tumor and sus-

pected lymphomas. This requires a precise preoperative radiologic evaluation because the current technology does not allow adequate tactile assessment of the fixation of the tumor to the mediastinal structures. The development of virtual reality techniques may minimize this limitation.

Video-assisted thoracic surgical techniques have also been used recently to resect predominantly benign mediastinal tumors, including Stage I thymomas, esophageal leiomyomas, and bronchogenic cysts.[78–81] Larger tumors require a counterincision for removal from the chest cavity. Any tumor removed by these techniques must be placed in a protective endobag or glove before removal to avoid tumor spillage and contamination of the port sites and chest cavity.

Thoracotomy

Standard lateral and posterolateral thoracotomy allows excellent access to the posterior mediastinum and lesions behind the pulmonary hila. It is the optimal approach to posterior mediastinal tumors (see Fig. 27–8).

Thoracotomies can be performed by either dividing or sparing the latissimus dorsi musculature and similarly reflecting the serratus anterior.[82] Axillary or vertical thoracotomies can also give excellent exposure to the mediastinum.[83] If skin flaps are developed for muscle-sparing approaches, then subcutaneous closed drainage systems may be required to minimize postoperative seromas. Double-lumen endotracheal tubes are helpful in patients who undergo thoracotomies or sternotomies, as this allows selective collapse of the ipsilateral lung and improved visualization of the mediastinum. If the tumor should invade the lung and require a nonanatomic partial wedge resection, it is easier to apply staplers with the lung atelectatic. Care must be taken, however, not to resect an excessive amount of lung; the amount can be grossly underestimated when the lung is in the collapsed position. Full-lung atelectasis facilitates bimanual palpation of the pulmonary parenchyma for metastatic lesions.

A right thoracotomy is preferred for access in the regions of the carina and the right and proximal left mainstem bronchi and for masses that extend into the right hemithorax. The fourth or fifth interspace is preferred when dissecting around the carina. Lower interspaces can be used, depending on the location of the tumor. Two thoracotomies through two separate interspaces and the same skin incision can be easily performed with elevation of the latissimus dorsi muscle. Benign tumors involving the middle and upper esophagus are best approached from the right, whereas those in the distal esophagus may be better approached through the left chest. Malignant esophageal tumors, if resected through the chest, should be approached through a right thoracotomy. Thymomas, if they extend into one or the other hemithorax, may be better approached via thoracotomy than sternotomy.

Cardiopulmonary bypass through the right chest is possible by bicaval cannulation and aortic or femoral artery cannulation. Full cardiopulmonary bypass is more difficult from the left chest, although it is possible to cannulate the main pulmonary artery or the right ventricle for venous return if the need should arise. A bypass from the left atrium to the distal aorta or femoral artery with a centrifugal pump or aortic arch to distal aorta bypass with a heparin-bonded Gott shunt can be used if aortic reconstruction is required as part of a tumor resection (e.g., resection of a paraganglioma of the aorta or a sarcoma that invades a great vessel).[84, 85]

Partial Sternotomy

A partial sternotomy may be required should difficulty arise during the resection of substernal goiter. Most goiters that extend into the anterior compartment, however, can be removed through a cervical approach. A trap-door extension into the third or fourth interspace has also been described for resection of tracheal tumors (see Fig. 27–7C).[86, 87] If further exposure of the anterior mediastinum is required, a complete sternotomy improves exposure.

Sternotomy

Complete sternotomy allows excellent exposure to the entire anterior compartment and more anteriorly situated tumors arising in the visceral compartment (see Fig. 27–7B). This is an excellent approach for all lesions anterior to the pulmonary hila and is the preferred approach if resection of the tumor requires the use of cardiopulmonary bypass techniques. With mobilization of the ascending aorta and lateral dissection and retraction of the superior vena cava, access to the trachea and the subcarinal region can be obtained. If mediastinal tumors invade the pulmonary parenchyma, segmental resections or lobectomies (with the exception of the left lower lobe) are possible from this midline approach. The use of a mammary retractor can improve the exposure in both hemithoraces. The sternotomy incision can also be extended laterally into either hemithorax if required (e.g., invasive thymomas that extend laterally). Closure of the sternotomy and repositioning of the patient for a posterolateral thoracotomy with the patient under the same anesthetic may occasionally be required for very extensive tumors.

The standard sternotomy incision heals well and is well tolerated by the patients. It is more comfortable than a thoracotomy, which entails rib and ligament stretching. For cosmesis, the vertical skin incision can be short, starting well below the angle of Louis with undermining of the skin up to the sternal notch to perform the sternotomy. The skin incision can also be placed transversely in the submammary creases in female infants, girls, and women with relatively short sternums. This requires more extensive elevation of skin flaps with the increased incidence of postoperative seromas.

Bilateral Anterior Thoracotomy: The Clam Shell Incision

The combination of a bilateral anterior thoracotomy and a transverse sternotomy gives superb exposure to the anterior compartment and both pulmonary hila, the phrenic nerves, both lung apices, and regions of the posterior mediastinum (see Fig. 27–7A). Cardiopulmonary bypass can be easily implemented. The submammary placement of the skin incision makes this a cosmetic approach without compromising chest or mediastinal exposure.

Combined Thoracotomy and Neurosurgical Approach to the Spine

Should a clinical assessment or radiologic evaluation suggest or indicate that a posterior mediastinal tumor invades the intervertebral foramina and extends into the epidural space, then a combined thoracic and neurosurgical resection may be required with access to the spinal cord from the back and the front. Patients are positioned laterally, held in place by a bean bag, and taped. Patients with tumors high in the mediastinum, which may require lower cervical or upper thoracic vertebrae resection, may require additional immobilization of the cervical spine with skull tongs during the procedure. A posterior midline vertical incision can be combined with a separate thoracotomy, or a single midline incision curving into a thoracotomy is possible (see Fig. 27–8). Usually, the area of tumor is marked, and a skin incision is made extending 5 cm above and below the lesion. The thoracotomy should be planned to enter an interspace above or below the tumor should rib resections be required. After laminectomies, ultrasound guidance during resection of the tumor from the thecal sac and spinal cord is possible. Extensive resections and reconstruction of several vertebral bodies are possible because immediate anterior and posterior stabilization can be performed through the same incision.

SURGICAL INDICATIONS: WHEN TO AND WHEN NOT TO OPERATE

Thymomas

Well-encapsulated anterior mediastinal tumors (determined by CT scan) suspected of being thymomas can be removed without FNA confirmation or biopsy. Pathologists have difficulty distinguishing benign and malignant thymomas on the basis of microscopy; it is believed that the two can be distinguished only by the lesion's invasiveness, which can be judged only by the surgeon. Adherence observed at surgery, however, does not necessarily mean invasiveness. It is easier to view all thymomas as having malignant potential for both local recurrence and distant spread. A direct surgical approach rather than needle aspiration or open biopsy is preferred to avoid the potential problem of mediastinal and pleural seeding, which appears to be more frequently associated with thymomas than other malignancies. (Pleural seeding may be related to the biology of thymomas rather than fine needle aspiration.) Thymic tumors that appear to be very advanced or invasive by initial CT scan assessment should be treated with preoperative chemotherapy.[88, 89]

Localized invasion of nonvital structures should entail resection of that structure (e.g., pericardium, wedge resection of lung). There have been long-term survivors with resection and reconstruction of the superior vena cava.[90] Resection of one phrenic nerve is permissible provided the patient's pulmonary function is adequate and there is no evidence of contralateral phrenic nerve paresis.[91] A surgeon should not be hesitant to open the pericardium, as this can simplify dissection from the great vessels and quickly determine transpericardial invasion of the tumor by direct palpation and inspection of the parietal pericardium. Routine opening of the pleural space improves intraoperative exposure of the phrenic nerves and allows for the simultaneous examination of the pulmonary parenchyma and diaphragm for tumor implants. Caution should be exercised in the dissection of the left phrenic nerve, which courses medially as the dissection continues more cephalad.

In the dissection of extensive tumors, the surgeon should gain as much tumor mobility as possible before the dissection at the site of maximum adherence should vascular control be required. If the tumor invades the pulmonary parenchyma, the final resection may involve simply placing a stapler at an appropriate margin on the lung and transecting the lung and removing the specimen with the lung en bloc. If it is impossible to remove all of the tumor, marking the periphery of the remaining tumor with clips may be very helpful for the radiotherapist in planning postoperative radiation therapy; these tumors can be relatively radiosensitive.[92] Some groups have advocated postoperative radiotherapy (35 to 45 Gy) for all thymomas to minimize postoperative local recurrences, although the risk of this is less than 2% for a completely resected, encapsulated tumor.[93, 94] It is believed that wide resection is adequate for thymomas, but some advocate radical thymectomy with combined sternotomy and neck incision with dissection of both pleura and extension of the thymic tails into the neck similar to the "maximal" thymectomy that they perform for myasthenia gravis.[95] Resection of the thymus by a cervical approach is possible but should be reserved for patients with thymic hyperplasia or myasthenia gravis and not thymomas. Thymomas have also been removed thoracoscopically, although future outcome analysis of tumor recurrence and patient survival will be required before this method can be recommended. In summary, because surgery is the treatment for malignant and symptomatic thymomas and because the benignity of tumors of the thymus cannot be ensured solely on radiologic grounds, then all thymomas should be removed.[96]

Germ Cell Tumors

All marker-negative and encapsulated tumors believed to be benign teratomas should be removed. The diagnosis of benignity can only be determined by complete removal of the tumor and a thorough histologic assessment of the specimen. Resection of these benign lesions can be difficult, however, because of the associated local adhesions and the neovascularity that develops in these tumors. However, even an incomplete resection of a benign teratoma is associated with excellent survival rates.[97]

Malignant germ cell tumors with elevated markers must be treated before surgery with cisplatin-based chemotherapy protocols.[98, 99] Before 1978, only 3% of patients survived longer than 16 months after surgery. Today, with very aggressive chemotherapy followed by surgery, as many as 58% of patients can expect 5 years of disease-free survival; complete responses are seen now in 50% to 70% of patients. Patients who are too ill to undergo any diagnostic procedure, including FNA, can begin aggressive chemotherapy based solely on positive markers. There are rare cases of marker-positive non–small cell lung cancer, however, that can resemble these tumors. Heroic attempts at an initial aggressive resection or "debulking" is contraindicated. Surgery is indicated for the resection of a residual mass after several cycles of chemotherapy and marker normalization (Fig. 27–9).[100–103] Four to 6 weeks is required after completion of chemotherapy to recover from the blood count nadir. Remaining benign teratomas, non–germ cell elements, or areas of fibrosis are usually found in the resected specimen. If the resected specimen is found on histologic evaluation to be an active tumor, further postoperative chemotherapy is mandated. However, these patients with chemoresistant tumors generally do poorly despite aggressive salvage chemotherapy. Residual teratoma or necrosis usually does not require further chemotherapy. If the patient had mediastinal nodal disease or supraclavicular nodes before chemotherapy, then these areas must also be resected at the time of surgery. Attempts should be made to preserve vital structures. Often, a dense fibrotic capsule adheres to the major vascular structures, which can be removed by dissection in the periadventitial plane of the vessels. Simultaneous resection of the pericardium may be required and can facilitate the dissection by establishing a vascular plane over the superior vena cava, aorta, and pulmonary artery. During surgery, a surgeon cannot assume that if one area of tumor shows only fibrosis on frozen section, then the remainder of the mass will be free of active tumor. All known sites of disease therefore must be resected.[104]

A combined sternotomy-laparotomy or thoracoabdominal procedure may be required in cases of secondary mediastinal germ cell lesions with evidence of retroperitoneal nodal involvement. Patients who have received bleomycin as part of their chemotherapeutic regimen must be monitored closely since they have oxygen-sensitive, fibrotic lungs that do not handle well high oxygen concentrations or fluid volumes. Serious postoperative pulmonary insufficiency may result if these patients are overtransfused or overloaded with fluids. Early extubation should be undertaken with caution. Recurrent masses that develop in pa-

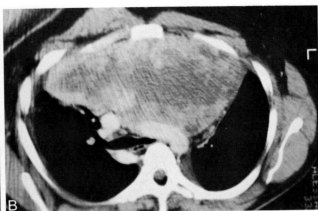

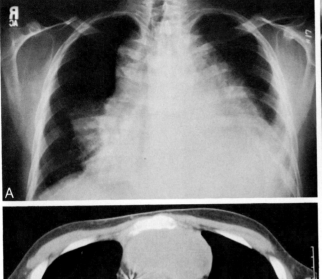

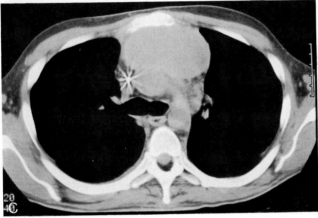

FIGURE 27–9. Patient with an advanced non-seminomatous (endodermal sinus) germ cell tumor. *A,* Chest radiograph (PA). *B,* CT scan at time of this presentation showing a large mediastinal mass with airway compression. The patient could not lie supine for this examination. *C,* Residual mass following adriamycin-based chemotherapy that was subsequently completely resected by sternotomy. Final histologic examination showed no viable tumor, with 100% necrosis.

tients who remain marker negative require re-exploration and re-excision. When tumor markers have not normalized and masses are present despite aggressive chemotherapy, caution should be used in approaching these patients surgically. Although potentially resectable lesions can be removed, these patients do not do well.[105]

Seminomas

Seminomas, which are sensitive to radiotherapy and chemotherapy, should be treated by these methods.[104] Like gonadal seminomas, their exquisite radiosensitivity allows a long-term survival rate of 60% to 80% in patients treated with radiotherapy alone. Chemotherapy now plays a more important role in the management of patients with large primary mediastinal seminomas that invade intrathoracic structures and expand over broad areas of the lung and hilum. They require large-volume radiotherapy fields that could lead to significant pulmonary damage.[106] The drugs used (cisplatin, bleomycin, and etoposide or vinblastine) are similar to those used in the treatment of nonseminomatous germ cell tumors. Residual tumor after chemotherapy is now usually treated with radiotherapy. Surgery has little role in the management of these patients.[107] Very rarely, a patient may undergo surgery if he or she presents with a localized mediastinal lesion that is small and resectable and proves to be a seminoma on final pathologic analysis.

Lymphomas

The role of surgery in lymphomas is primarily initial biopsy and work-up (Fig. 27–10). The very rare presentation of an isolated anterior mediastinal mass may justify a complete surgical resection as part of an intended diagnostic and therapeutic approach.[9] The usual presentation, however, is an advanced lesion that may simulate an invasive Stage II or III thymoma, germ cell tumor, or small cell lung carcinoma with extensive mediastinal lymphadenopathy. The pathologist usually requires more tissue (at least 1 cm³) than can be obtained by FNA or core biopsy to distinguish lymphomas from thymomas. Because these tumors often have a dense sclerotic capsule that is not helpful for diagnosis, deeper incisional biopsies may be required. Open biopsies allow for the proper architectural assessment and subtyping of the lymphomas, flow cytometry, electromicroscopy, and chromosomal analysis.[47]

Occasionally, a thoracic surgeon may be requested to obtain a sample for biopsy of a persistent or recurrent mass after treatment or may be involved in managing the complications of the medical therapy of patients with lymphomas, such as constrictive pericarditis or associated premature coronary artery disease, which may be related to mantle irradiation. This requires a cautious approach, as the tissue planes may be obliterated and the vasculature more fragile secondary to chemotherapy and radiotherapy effects.[108, 109]

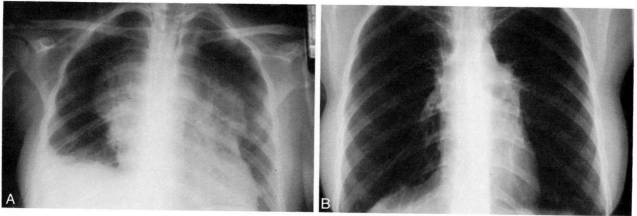

FIGURE 27–10. *A,* Twenty-two-year-old woman who presented with extensive mediastinal lymphadenopathy and pleural and pericardial effusions, who required a Chamberlain procedure for a diagnosis of non-Hodgkin's lymphoma. *B,* Chest radiograph following chemotherapy and radiation therapy showing a normal mediastinal width following a complete response.

Bronchogenic Cysts

In children, all bronchogenic cysts should be removed because they have a tendency to enlarge and may eventually become symptomatic.[110] Some have advocated a conservative approach to cysts in adults who are asymptomatic and who agree to be followed regularly. These cysts should be in the middle or posterior mediastinal compartment; showing a cyst only by CT imaging, with no solid or soft tissue components; and have a negative cytologic assessment. Other surgeons, however, have recommended removal of all cysts to avoid future complications that would make subsequent resection more difficult, and they point out that the aspiration of a cyst determined by cytologic analysis to be benign does not guarantee that the lining of the cyst contains only benign epithelium. Eighty-five per cent of asymptomatic cysts become symptomatic with long-term follow-up.[111]

Interventional radiologists have occasionally managed bronchogenic cysts by instilling sclerosing agents to destroy the secretory cyst lining.[112] Acutely symptomatic cysts can also be initially decompressed before surgery to optimize the patient's pulmonary function.[113] Transbronchial aspiration during bronchoscopy has been used[114] but may lead to superinfection of these lesions. Cysts can be removed using video-assisted thoracic surgical techniques.[78]

Most bronchogenic cysts involve the subcarinal region and therefore are most easily approached through a right thoracotomy (Fig. 27–11).[115] A complicated cyst that has become infected may be impossible to dissect from vital structures. In these situations, the cyst should be opened and stripped of the mucosa to avoid a recurrence. A chronically infected cyst usually has nonfunctional epithelium.

Enteric Cysts

Similar direct surgical management and universal excision are recommended for enteric cysts. A surgeon or endoscopist must resist the temptation to perform a biopsy or aspirate a submucosal soft mass appreci-

ated on esophagoscopy; this will avoid infection or a mucosal breach, which would make subsequent resection much more difficult.[116]

Pericardial Cysts

Pericardial cysts can be accurately diagnosed by CT scan and echocardiography. The finding of fluid resembling spring water on needle aspiration correlates with the water density on CT scan. These cysts do not require surgery unless they become symptomatic.

Substernal or Intrathoracic Thyroid

A thyroid goiter is considered by definition to be substernal if more than 50% of the lesion is below the thoracic inlet.[117, 118] They constitute less than 1% of all goiters but 5.3% of mediastinal tumors.[14] They should be resected to avoid future problems with tracheal malacia, hyperfunction, and sudden increase in size, which may be accompanied by acute respiratory compromise.[119] Most often, they can be removed from the neck through a collar incision.[120] Indications for an extension to partial or full sternotomy include the inability to identify or excessive traction on the recurrent nerves during the resection, previous intrathoracic goiter, suspicion of thyroid carcinoma or uncertain diagnosis, identification of a carcinoma during the neck dissection, suspicion of invasion of local structures or the superior vena cava, or emergency surgery for acute obstruction of the airway from extrinsic compression or incarceration in the inlet.[121]

A true ectopic thyroid has a vascular supply from the chest and therefore must be approached via a thoracotomy or sternotomy for control of the vascular pedicles.[122] Performance of a thyroid scan is of importance before removal of the thyroid to ensure that this is not the patient's only functioning thyroid tissue. A small percentage of ectopic thyroids harbor malignancy, further justifying resection in all medically fit individuals. Retrotracheal extension of some goiters may require a thoracotomy or trap-door incision

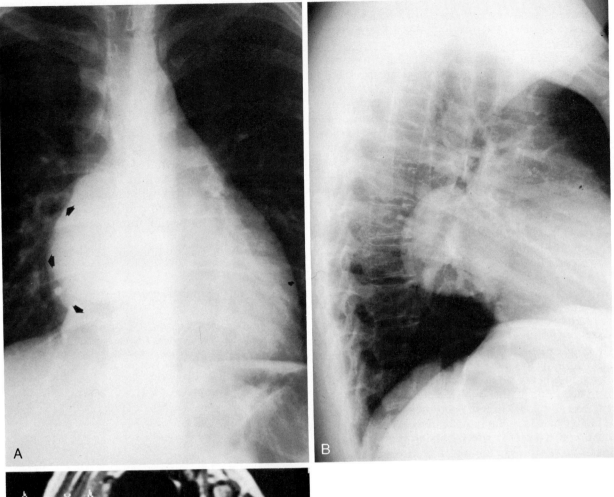

FIGURE 27–11. Mediastinal mass in visceral compartment that was identified as a bronchogenic cyst, which was subsequently resected through a right posterolateral thoracotomy. *A,* Chest radiograph (PA) showing subcarinal mass. *B,* Chest radiograph (lateral). *C,* Magnetic resonance imaging of bronchogenic cyst.

through partial sternotomy with extension into the second or third interspace. The anesthesiologist must be vigilant during induction in these patients, as the weight of the goiter may cause sudden airway collapse with the administration of paralytic agents.

Neurogenic Tumors

Some surgeons believe that close observation is the appropriate approach to asymptomatic neurogenic tumors in adults with no intraspinal extension or recent growth and no secondary hypertension. Although the incidence of malignancy is low (2% to 3%), in adults in whom a nonsurgical approach is chosen an FNA

should be performed. Other authors note the tendency of these tumors to increase in size with time, and even benign tumors can grow to compromise the spinal cord.[123] A surgical approach is justified unless the patient is elderly or in poor medical condition or it can be demonstrated through the review of old chest films that a prolonged period of dormancy exists in the lesion.[124] With video-assisted thoracic surgical techniques, many of these benign tumors can be resected without a thoracotomy.[74, 125] A direct surgical approach does not require a presurgical tissue diagnosis by FNA. The presurgical suspicion of intervertebral foramina extension must be high in any case of widening of the foramina on plain films or vertebral body erosion.[126] An MRI and preoperative neurosurgical consultation may be required. In children, these tumors have a higher incidence of malignancy, and all should be removed.[127]

Resection of some dumbbell tumors has been reported through a posterior neurosurgical approach without thoracotomy.[128] When a traditional thoracotomy is used, however, the surgeon should enter one or two interspaces above or below the lesion in case there is a need to resect ribs or lung. This will avoid broaching the tumor capsule at the time of thoracotomy.

Paragangliomas are highly vascular tumors that have a propensity to invade the aortic arch and heart and may require cardiopulmonary bypass for complete resection. This aggressive approach is justified, because complete resection is associated with cure, whereas chemotherapy and radiotherapy have little effect on incompletely resected tumors.[129]

Poorly Differentiated Carcinoma

Approximately 5% of patients evaluated for a mediastinal mass or lymphadenopathy will have the pathologic diagnosis of a "poorly differentiated carcinoma." Patients who are smokers or who have a past history of heavy smoking are often assumed to have an occult lung primary with mediastinal N2 or N3 nodal presentation. Curative resection of such tumors is not possible. The thoracic surgeon may be involved in obtaining additional tissue for special stains that can rule out a germ cell tumor, lymphoma, sarcoma, melanoma, or a poorly differentiated neuroendocrine tumor. Electron microscopy can be of importance in demonstrating neurosecretory granules. Serum markers for α-fetoprotein and β-human chorionic gonadotropin are required. Although these patients are not surgical candidates, a trial of cisplatin-based chemotherapy has resulted in a few cures in this subgroup of patients believed to be incurable.[130, 131]

SUMMARY

The wide variety of congenital and vascular anomalies and of benign and malignant neoplasms that present as symptomatic or asymptomatic mediastinal radiographic abnormalities requires a close and detailed review of the history, physical examination, and radiologic interpretation and ancillary tests before proceeding with any surgical intervention. The surgeon must take into account the age and sex of the patient and the anatomic location of the lesion and then make a decision to proceed with tissue procurement or directly to resection via sternotomy, thoracotomy, or a combination. Tissue for further analysis may be obtained by fine-needle or core-needle biopsy or by localized biopsy through limited approaches (e.g., mediastinoscopy, Chamberlain procedure, or thoracoscopy). In the future, better immunohistochemical analyses and improved determination of intracellular and intranuclear components by FNA will reduce the

role of surgery in diagnosis, but surgery will remain important for therapeutic interventions. Today, if a presurgical diagnosis cannot be made and the lesion appears resectable by radiologic criteria, then a direct surgical approach and resection are indicated. A direct surgical approach is also indicated for any cystic lesion of the mediastinum, except for an obvious pericardial cyst. For extensive tumors, a biopsy should be performed only so appropriate neoadjuvant chemotherapy or radiotherapy can begin. An aggressive surgical resection may subsequently be indicated after chemotherapy in advanced thymomas and nonseminomatous germ cell tumors but has little role at any time in patients with lymphomas and seminomas. Cooperation among health care providers is vital in the preoperative assessment, intraoperative management, postoperative care, and long-term follow-up of patients with mediastinal masses.

SELECTED REFERENCES

Faber LP, Benfield JR (eds): Chest Surgery Clinics of North America. Philadelphia, WB Saunders, February 1992.
Loop FD, Pearson FG (eds): Seminars in Thoracic and Cardiovascular Surgery, Vol 4, No 1, January 1992.
Shields TW (ed): Mediastinal Surgery. Philadelphia, Lea & Febiger, 1991.

REFERENCES

1. Bousamra M II, Wechsler AS, Henry DA, Olak J: Vascular lesions of the mediastinum. *In* Faber LP, Benfield JR (eds): Chest Surgery Clinics of North America. Philadelphia, WB Saunders, 1992, pp 57–87.
2. Darby C, Sinclair M, Westaby S: Treatment of a malignant bronchial carcinoid affecting the mediastinum and left atrium by radical two stage resection with cardiopulmonary bypass and somatostatin infusion. Br Heart J 63:55–57, 1990.
3. Shimizu N, Date H, Moriyama S, et al: Reconstruction of the superior vena cava in patients with mediastinal malignancies. Eur J Cardiothorac Surg 5:575–578, 1992.
4. Kohman LJ: Approach to the diagnosis and staging of mediastinal masses. Chest 103:328S–330S, 1993.
5. Shields TW: The mediastinum and its compartments. *In* Shields TW (ed): Mediastinal Surgery. Philadelphia, Lea & Febiger, 1991, pp 3–5.
6. Davies DV, Coupland RE (eds): The respiratory system. *In* Gray's Anatomy: Descriptive and Applied. London, Longmans, Green, and Co, 1958.
7. Fraser RG, Pare JAP, Pare PD, et al: The normal chest (the mediastinum). *In* Fraser RG, Pare JAP, Pare PD, Fraser RS, Genereux GP (eds): Diagnosis of Diseases of the Chest. Philadelphia, WB Saunders, 1988, pp 203–214.
8. Davis RD, Oldham HN, Sabiston DC: Primary cysts and neoplasms of the mediastinum: Recent changes in clinical presentation, methods of diagnosis, management, and results. Ann Thorac Surg 44:229–237, 1987.
9. Yellin A: Lymphoproliferative diseases. *In* Faber LP, Benfield JR (eds): Chest Surgery Clinics of North America. Philadelphia, WB Saunders, 1992, pp 107–120.
10. Filly R, Blank N, Castellino RA: Radiographic distribution of intrathoracic disease in previously untreated patients with Hodgkin's and non-Hodgkin's lymphoma. Radiology 120:277–281, 1976.
11. Shields TW: Primary mediastinal tumors and cysts and their diagnostic investigation. *In* Shields TW (ed): Mediastinal Surgery. Philadelphia, Lea & Febiger, 1991, pp 111–117.

12. Mullen B, Richardson JD: Primary anterior mediastinal tumors in children and adults. Ann Thorac Surg 42:338–345, 1986.
13. Shields TW: Lesions masquerading as primary mediastinal tumors or cysts. In Shields TW (ed): Mediastinal Surgery. Philadelphia, Lea & Febiger, 1991, pp 118–137.
14. Wychulis AR, Payne WS, Clagett OT, et al: Surgical treatment of mediastinal tumors: A 40-year experience. J Thorac Cardiovasc Surg 62:379–385, 1971.
15. Mogilner JG, Fonseca J, Davies MR: Life-threatening respiratory distress caused by a mediastinal teratoma in a newborn. J Pediatr Surg 27:1519–1520, 1992.
16. Azizkhan RG, Dudgeon DL, Buck JR, et al: Life-threatening airway obstruction as a complication to the management of mediastinal masses in children. J Pediatr Surg 20:816–822, 1985.
17. Moore EH: Radiologic evaluation of mediastinal masses. In Faber LP, Benfield JR (eds): Chest Surgery Clinics of North America. Philadelphia, WB Saunders, 1992, pp 1–22.
18. Harris GJ, Harman PK, Trinkle JK, et al: Standard biplane roentgenography is highly selective in documenting mediastinal masses. Ann Thorac Surg 44:238–241, 1987.
19. Brown K, Aberle DR, Batra P, Steckel RJ: Current use of imaging in the evaluation of primary mediastinal masses. Chest 98:466–473, 1990.
20. Heitzman ER: Computer tomography of the thorax: Current perspectives. Am J Roentgenol 136:2–12, 1981.
21. Kirks DR, Korobkin M: Computed tomography of the chest in infants and children: Techniques and mediastinal evaluation. Radiol Clin North Am 19:409–419, 1981.
22. Waller DA, Rees MR: Computed tomography in the pre-operative assessment of mediastinal tumours—Does it improve surgical management?. Thorac Cardiovasc Surg 39:158–161, 1991.
23. Hounsfield GN: Computed transverse axial scanning (tomography): Part 1. Description of system. Br J Radiol 46:1016, 1973.
24. Miller GA, Heaston DK, Moore AV, et al: CT differentiation of thoracic aneurysms from pulmonary masses adjacent to the mediastinum. J Comput Assist Tomogr 8:437–442, 1984.
25. Dooms GC, Higgins CB: The potential of magnetic resonance imaging for the evaluation of thoracic arterial disease. J Thorac Cardiovasc Surg 92:1088–1095, 1986.
26. Rholl KS, Levitt RG, Glazer HS: Magnetic resonance imaging of fibrosing mediastinitis. Am J Roentgenol 145:255–259, 1985.
27. Levitt RG, Glazer HS, Roper CL, et al: Magnetic resonance imaging of mediastinal and hilar masses: A comparison with CT. Am J Roentgenol 145:9–14, 1985.
28. Miller WT: Roentgenographic evaluation of the chest. In Shields TW (ed): General Thoracic Surgery. Philadelphia, Lea & Febiger, 1989, pp 127–130.
29. Dresler CM, Patterson GA, Taylor BR, et al: Complete foregut duplication. Ann Thorac Surg 50:306–308, 1990.
30. Arciniegas E: Vascular rings. In Arciniegas E (ed): Pediatric Cardiac Surgery. Chicago, Year Book Medical Publishers, Inc, 1985, pp 119–127.
31. Katlic MR, Wang C, Grillo HC: Substernal goiter. Ann Thorac Surg 39:391–399, 1985.
32. Stark DD, Gooding GA, Clark OH: Noninvasive parathyroid imaging. Semin Ultrasound Comput Tomogr Magn Reson 6:310–320, 1985.
33. Basarab RM, Manni A, Harrison TS: Dual isotope subtraction parathyroid scintigraphy in the preoperative evaluation of suspected hyperparathyroidism. Clin Nucl Med 10:302, 1985.
34. Kropp J, Emons D, Winkler C: Neurenteric cyst diagnosed by technetium-99m pertechnetate sequential scintigraphy. J Nucl Med 28:1218–1220, 1987.
35. Hoffer P: Gallium: Mechanisms. J Nucl Med 21:282, 1980.
36. Francis IR, Glazer GM, Shapiro B, et al: Complementary roles of CT and ^{131}I-MIBG scintigraphy in diagnosing pheochromocytoma. Am J Radiol 141:719, 1983.
37. Shapiro B, Sisson J, Kalff V, et al: The location of middle mediastinal pheochromocytomas. J Thorac Cardiovasc Surg 87:814, 1984.
38. Alderson PO, Rujanavech N, Sicker-Walker RH, et al: The role of ^{133}Xe ventilation studies in the scintigraphic detection of pulmonary embolism. Radiology 120:633, 1976.
39. Ali MK, Mountain CF, Ewer MS, Johnston D, Haynie TP: Predicting loss of pulmonary function after pulmonary resection for bronchogenic carcinoma. Chest 77:337–342, 1980.
40. Schiavone WA, Rice TW: Pericardial disease: Current diagnosis and management methods. Cleve Clin J Med 56:639–645, 1989.
41. Dumbell HR, Coleman AC, Pudifin JM, Winship WS: Prenatal ultrasonographic diagnosis and successful management of mediastinal teratoma: A case report. S Afr Med J 78:481–483, 1990.
42. Dawkins PR, Stoddard MF, Lindell NE, et al: Utility of transesophageal echocardiography in the assessment of mediastinal masses and superior vena cava obstruction. Am Heart J 122:1469–1472, 1991.
43. Hessel S, Adams D, Abrams H: Complications of angiography. Radiology 138:273, 1981.
44. Farooki ZQ, Green EW: Diagnostic procedures. In Arciniegas E (ed): Pediatric Cardiac Surgery. Chicago, Year Book Medical Publishers, Inc, 1985, pp 19–32.
45. Shaha AR, Burnett C, Alfonso A, et al: Goiters and airways problems. Am J Surg 158:378–381, 1989.
46. Waid-Jones MI, Coursin DB: Perioperative considerations for patients treated with bleomycin. Chest 99:993–999, 1991.
47. Sutcliffe SB: Primary mediastinal malignant lymphoma. In Loop FD, Pearson FG (eds): Seminars in Thoracic and Cardiovascular Surgery. Philadelphia, WB Saunders, 1992, pp 55–67.
48. Juttner FM, Fellbaum C, Popper H, et al: Pitfalls in intraoperative frozen section histology of mediastinal neoplasms. Eur J Cardiothorac Surg 4:584–586, 1990.
49. Herman SJ, Holub RV, Weisbrod GL, et al: Anterior mediastinal masses: Utility of transthoracic needle biopsy. Radiology 180:167–170, 1991.
50. Weisbrod GL, Lyons DJ, Tao LC, Chamberlain DW: Percutaneous fine-needle aspiration biopsy of mediastinal lesions. Am J Roentgenol 143:525–529, 1984.
51. Weisbrod GL: Percutaneous fine needle biopsy of the mediastinum. Clin Chest Med 8:27–41, 1987.
52. Weisbrod GL: Transthoracic percutaneous lung biopsy. Radiol Clin North Am 28:647–655, 1990.
53. Walsh GL: Lasers for the early detection of lung cancer. Semin Thorac Cardiovasc Surg 5:194–200, 1993.
54. Bolliger CT, Tschopp K, Perruchoud A: Silicone stents in the management of inoperable tracheobronchial stenoses. Chest 104:1653, 1993.
55. Dumon JF: A dedicated tracheobronchial stent. Chest 97:328–332, 1990.
56. Wallace MJ, Charnsangavej C, Ogawa K, et al: Tracheobronchial tree: Expandable metallic stents used in experimental and clinical applications. Radiology 158:309–312, 1986.
57. Varela A, Maynar M, Irving D, et al: Use of Gianturco self-expandable stents in the tracheobronchial tree. Ann Thorac Surg 49:806–809, 1990.
58. Toty L, Personne C, Colchen A, et al: Bronchoscopic management of tracheal lesions using neodymium YAG laser. Thorax 36:175, 1981.
59. Wolfe WG, Sabiston DC: Management of benign and malignant lesions of the trachea and bronchi with the neodymium-yttrium-aluminum-garnet laser. J Thorac Cardiovasc Surg 91:40, 1986.
60. Cavaliere S, Foccoli P, Farina PL: Nd:YAG laser bronchoscopy: A five-year experience with 1396 applications in 1000 patients. Chest 94:15–21, 1988.
61. Wang KP: Flexible transbronchial needle aspiration biopsy for histologic specimens. Chest 88:860, 1985.
62. Wang KP: Needle biopsy for the diagnosis of intrathoracic lesions: Transbronchial needle biopsy. In Kittle CF (ed): Current Controversies in Thoracic Surgery. Philadelphia, WB Saunders, 1986.
63. Carlens E: Mediastinoscopy: A method of inspection and tissue biopsy in the superior mediastinum. Chest 36:343, 1959.
64. Pearson FG: Mediastinoscopy: A method of biopsy of the superior mediastinum. J Thorac Cardiovasc Surg 49:11, 1965.
65. American Thoracic Society: Clinical staging of primary lung cancer. Am Rev Respir Dis 127:659, 1983.
66. Ginsberg RJ, Rice TW, Goldberg M, et al: Extended cervical mediastinoscopy—the best procedure for staging left upper lobe tumours. J Thorac Cardiovasc Surg 94:673, 1987.

67. Kirschner PA: Cervical substernal "extended" mediastinoscopy. *In* Shields TW (ed): Mediastinal Surgery. Philadelphia, Lea & Febiger, 1991, pp 81–83.
68. Cooper JD, Al-Jilaihawa AN, Pearson FG, et al: An improved technique to facilitate transcervical thymectomy for myasthenia gravis. Ann Thorac Surg 45:242, 1988.
69. McNeill TM, Chamberlain JM: Diagnostic anterior mediastinotomy. Ann Thorac Surg 2:532, 1966.
70. Elia S, Cecere C, Giampaglia F, Ferrante G: Mediastinoscopy vs anterior mediastinotomy in the diagnosis of mediastinal lymphoma: A randomized trial. Eur J Cardiothorac Surg 6:361–365, 1992.
71. Shields TW: Posterior mediastinotomy. *In* Shields TW (ed): Mediastinal Surgery. Philadelphia, Lea & Febiger, 1991, pp 92–94.
72. Kern JA, Daniel TM, Tribble CG, et al: Thoracoscopic diagnosis and treatment of mediastinal masses. Ann Thorac Surg 56:92–96, 1993.
73. Sugarbaker DJ: Thoracoscopy in the management of anterior mediastinal masses. Ann Thorac Surg 56:653–656, 1993.
74. Naunheim KS: Video thoracoscopy for masses of the posterior mediastinum. Ann Thorac Surg 56:657–658, 1993.
75. Ryckman FC, Rodgers BM: Thoracoscopy for intrathoracic neoplasia in children. J Pediatr Surg 17:521–524, 1982.
76. Landreneau RJ, Mack MJ, Hazelrigg SR, et al: The role of thoracoscopy in the management of intrathoracic neoplastic processes. Semin Thorac Surg 5:219–228, 1993.
77. Rendina EA, Venuta F, Giacomo TD, et al: Comparative merits of thoracoscopy, mediastinoscopy, and mediastinotomy for mediastinal biopsy. Ann Thorac Surg 57:992–995, 1994.
78. Naunheim KS, Andrus CH: Thoracoscopic drainage and resection of giant mediastinal cyst. Ann Thorac Surg 55:156–158, 1993.
79. Hazelrigg SR, Landreneau RD, Mack MJ, Acuff TE: Thoracoscopic resection of mediastinal cysts. Ann Thorac Surg 56:659–660, 1993.
80. Lewis RJ, Caccavale RJ, Sisler GE: Imaged thoracoscopic surgery: A new thoracic technique for resection of mediastinal cysts. Ann Thorac Surg 53:318–320, 1992.
81. Landreneau RJ, Dowling RD, Castillo WM, Ferson PF: Thoracoscopic resection of an anterior mediastinal tumor. Ann Thorac Surg 54:142–144, 1992.
82. Bethencourt DM, Holmes EC: Muscle-sparing posterolateral thoracotomy. Ann Thorac Surg 45:337, 1988.
83. Massimiano P, Ponn RB, Toole AL: Transaxillary thoracotomy revisited. Ann Thorac Surg 45:559–560, 1988.
84. Wolfe WG, Kleimman LH, Weschler AS, Sabiston DC: Heparin coated shunts for lesions of the descending thoracic aorta. Arch Surg 112:148, 1977.
85. Donahoo JS, Brawley RK, Gott VL: The heparin coated vascular shunt for thoracic aortic and great vessel procedures: A ten year experience. Ann Thorac Surg 23:507, 1977.
86. Grillo HC: Surgical approaches to the trachea. Surg Gynecol Obstet 129:374, 1969.
87. Grillo HC: Surgery of the trachea. Curr Probl Surg July:1, 1970.
88. Rea F, Sartori F, Loy M, et al: Chemotherapy and operation for invasive thymoma. J Thorac Cardiovasc Surg 106:543–549, 1993.
89. Cooper JD: Current therapy for thymoma. Chest 103:334S–336S, 1993.
90. Masuda H, Ogata T, Kikuchi K, et al: Total replacement of superior vena cava because of invasive thymoma: Seven years' survival. J Thorac Cardiovasc Surg 95:1083–1085, 1988.
91. Warren WH, Gould VE: Epithelial neoplasms of the thymus. *In* Faber LP, Benfield JR (eds): Chest Surgery Clinics of North America. Philadelphia, WB Saunders, 1992, pp 137–163.
92. Urgeis A, Monetti U, Rossi G, et al: Role of radiation therapy in locally advanced thymoma. Radiother Oncol 19:273–280, 1990.
93. Monden Y, Nakahara K, Iioka S, et al: Recurrence of thymoma: Clinical pathological features, therapy, and prognosis. Ann Thorac Surg 39:165–169, 1985.
94. Urgesi A, Monetti U, Rossi G, et al: Aggressive treatment of intrathoracic recurrences of thymoma. Radiother Oncol 24:221–225, 1992.
95. Jaretzki A III, Penn AS, Younger DS, et al: "Maximal" thymectomy for myasthenia gravis. J Thorac Cardiovasc Surg 95:747, 1988.
96. Rice TW: Benign neoplasms and cysts of the mediastinum. *In* Loop FD, Pearson FG (eds): Seminars in Thoracic and Cardiovascular Surgery. Philadelphia, WB Saunders, 1992, pp 25–33.
97. Lewis BD, Hurt RD, Payne WS, et al: Benign teratomas of the mediastinum. J Thorac Cardiovasc Surg 86:727–731, 1983.
98. Childs WJ, Goldstraw P, Nicholls JE, Dearnaley DP, Horwich A: Primary malignant mediastinal germ cell tumours: Improved prognosis with platinum-based chemotherapy and surgery. Br J Cancer 67:1098–1101, 1993.
99. Kantoff P: Surgical and medical management of germ cell tumors of the chest. Chest 103:331S–333S, 1993.
100. Toner GC, Panicek DM, Heelan RT, et al: Adjunctive surgery after chemotherapy for nonseminomatous germ cell tumors: Recommendations for patient selection. J Clin Oncol 8:1683–1694, 1990.
101. Knapp RH, Hurt RD, Payne WS, et al: Malignant germ cell tumors of the mediastinum. J Thorac Cardiovasc Surg 89:82–89, 1985.
102. Bajorin DF, Herr H, Motzer RJ, Bosl GJ: Current perspectives on the role of adjunctive surgery in combined modality treatment for patients with germ cell tumors. Semin Oncol 19:148–158, 1992.
103. Fujisawa T, Yamaguchi Y, Iwai N, et al: A case of mediastinal germ cell tumor radically operated on after neoadjuvant chemotherapy-combined resection of the superior vena cava and reconstruction with expanded-PTFE graft. Jpn J Surg 18:336–340, 1988.
104. Ginsberg RJ: Mediastinal germ cell tumors: The role of surgery. Semin Thorac Cardiovasc Surg 4:51–54, 1992.
105. Munshi N, Loehrer P, Williams S, et al: Ifosamide combination salvage chemotherapy in extragonadal germ cell tumors (EGGCT). Proc Am Soc Clin Oncol 10:182, 1991.
106. Nichols CR: Mediastinal germ cell tumors. *In* Loop FD, Pearson FG (eds): Seminars in Thoracic and Cardiovascular Surgery. Philadelphia, WB Saunders, 1992, pp 45–50.
107. Mencel PJ, Motzer RJ, Mazumdar M, et al: Advanced seminoma: Treatment results, survival, and prognostic factors in 142 patients. J Clin Oncol 12:120–126, 1994.
108. Ricci C, Rendina EA, Venuta F, et al: Surgical approach to isolated mediastinal lymphoma. J Thorac Cardiovasc 99:691–695, 1990.
109. Yellin A, Pak HY, Burke JS, Benfield JR: Surgical management of lymphomas involving the chest. Ann Thorac Surg 44:363–369, 1987.
110. DiLorenzo M, Collin PP, Vaillancourt R, et al: Bronchogenic cysts. J Pediatr Surg 24:988–991, 1989.
111. Allen MS, Payne WS: Cystic foregut malformations in the mediastinum. *In* Faber LP, Benfield JR (eds): Chest Surgery Clinics of North America. Philadelphia, WB Saunders, 1992, pp 89–106.
112. Whyte MKB: Central bronchogenic cyst: Treatment by extrapleural percutaneous aspiration. Br Med J 299:1457–1458, 1989.
113. McDougall JC, Fromme GA: Transcarinal aspiration of a mediastinal cyst to facilitate anesthetic management. Chest 97:1490–1492, 1990.
114. Schwartz AR, Fishman EK, Wang KP: Diagnosis and treatment of a bronchogenic cyst using transbronchial needle aspiration. Thorax 41:326–327, 1986.
115. Suen H, Mathisen DJ, Grillo HC, et al: Surgical management and radiological characteristics of bronchogenic cysts. Ann Thorac Surg 55:476–481, 1993.
116. Salo JA, Ala-Kulju KV: Congenital esophageal cysts in adults. Ann Thorac Surg 44:135–138, 1987.
117. Katlic MR, Grillo HC, Wang CA: Substernal goiter: Analysis of eighty Massachusetts General Hospital cases. Am J Surg 149:283–287, 1985.
118. Michel LA, Bradpiece HA: Surgical management of substernal goitre. Br J Surg 75:565–569, 1988.
119. Creswell LL, Wells SA Jr: Mediastinal masses originating in the neck. *In* Faber LP, Benfield JR (eds): Chest Surgery Clinic of North America. Philadelphia, WB Saunders, 1992, pp 23–55.
120. Allo MD, Thompson NW: Rationale for the operative management of substernal goiters. Surgery 94:969–977, 1983.
121. Sand ME, Laws HL, McElvein RB: Substernal and intrathoracic

goiter: Reconsideration of surgical approach. Am Surg 49:196–202, 1983.
122. Mitchell JD, Donnelly RJ: Retrosternal thyroid. *In* Loop FD, Pearson FG (eds): Seminars in Thoracic and Cardiovascular Surgery. Philadelphia, WB Saunders, 1992, pp 34–38.
123. Wain JC: Neurogenic tumors of the mediastinum. *In* Faber LP, Benfield JR (eds): Chest Surgery Clinics of North America. Philadelphia, WB Saunders, 1992, pp 121–136.
124. Ricci C, Rendina EA, Venuta F, et al: Diagnostic imaging and surgical treatment of dumbbell tumors of the mediastinum. Ann Thorac Surg 50:586–589, 1990.
125. Landreneau RJ, Dowling RD, Ferson PF: Thoracoscopic resection of a posterior mediastinal neurogenic tumor. Chest 102:1288–1290, 1992.
126. Akwari OE, Payne WS, Onofrio BM, et al: Dumbbell neurogenic tumors of the mediastinum. Mayo Clin Proc 53:353–358, 1978.
127. Adams GA, Shochat SJ, Smith EI, et al: Thoracic neuroblastoma: A Pediatric Oncology Group study. J Pediatr Surg 28:372–377, 1993.
128. Osada H, Aoki H, Yokote K, et al: Dumbbell neurogenic tumor of the mediastinum: A report of three cases undergoing single-staged complete removal without thoracotomy. Jpn J Surg 21:224–228, 1991.
129. Castanon J, Gil-Aguado M, de la Llana R, et al: Aortopulmonary paraganglioma, a rare aortic tumor: A case report. J Thorac Cardiovasc Surg 106:1232–1234, 1993.
130. Goldberg M: Metastatic tumors. Semin Thorac Cardiovasc Surg 4:68–70, 1992.
131. Greco FA, Vaughn WK, Hainsworth JD: Advanced poorly differentiated carcinoma of unknown primary site: Recognition of a treatable syndrome. Ann Intern Med 104:547–553, 1986.

MALIGNANCIES OF THE THYMUS

Eli Glatstein and Barry S. Levinson

The normal thymus gland is a primary site of immunologic development, where T-cell maturation and differentiation occur. The thymus functions early in life and normally involutes with age. The thymus also may serve as the site of origin of a vast array of tumors. Thymic epithelial cells may give rise to thymomas, the most common tumor of thymic origin. Other tumors such as lymphoblastic lymphomas or large cell lymphoma may arise from the lymphocyte population within the thymus. Neuroendocrine tumors such as carcinoid and small cell carcinoma may also originate within the thymus. Hodgkin's disease and germ cell tumors are also found as primary thymic malignancies. Because many of these tumors are amenable to a variety of therapies, it is imperative that accurate diagnoses are made when evaluating and treating malignancies of the thymus.

EMBRYOLOGY OF THE THYMUS

The mature functioning thymus contains two major cell populations, epithelial cells and lymphocytes. These two populations have their origin in separate embryologic compartments and come together to form the functioning organ.[1] In the third week of embryologic development, the primitive foregut develops into a series of pharyngeal arches separated by pharyngeal pouches. Proliferation of the endodermal cells that make up these pouches give rise to many of the structures of the head and neck in the adult. The third pharyngeal pouches migrate downward into the anterior mediastinum as they proliferate. There they give rise to two structures: the inferior parathyroid glands and the thymus. In forming the thymus, the lower portions of both pouches fuse, forming a single bilobed organ, which then severs its connection with the pharyngeal pouches and comes to lie on the anterior surface of the aorta. The endodermal cells, which had originally arisen as a hollow diverticulum, proliferate, forming a solid organ. Some of these cells will keratinize and undergo terminal differentiation to form aggregates called Hassall's corpuscles. These corpuscles are a characteristic histologic feature of the thymus.[2, 3] However, the endodermal cells also invade the surrounding mesenchyme, which differentiates, forming a capsule and trabeculae that divide the organ into lobules. The epithelial cells arising from the primitive foregut form a reticular framework within the organ; this framework becomes the medulla of the mature organ. During the third month of embryologic development, small lymphocytes begin to appear in the thymus. These are thought to arise from stem cells in the bone marrow and then migrate to the thymus,[4] where they undergo differentiation to form T cells. This process of differentiation occurs in the cortex of the mature gland.

The process of differentiation is partly under the control of thymic hormones produced by the epithelial cells of the thymus. These hormones include thymulin, alpha and beta thymosin, thymopoietin, and thymic humoral factors.[5, 6] Thymus-derived lymphocytes, or T cells, are responsible for a variety of humoral and and predominantly cellular immune functions of great importance throughout life; however, much of the process of differentiation of T cells occurs in late fetal and early postnatal life.[7]

At birth, the thymus is a large organ extending from the thyroid cartilage in the neck down to the surface of the pericardium. It continues to grow in postnatal life, reaching its maximum size of about 40 gm in adolescence, but it grows more slowly relative to the rest of the body. After adolescence, the thymus spontaneously involutes, becoming replaced largely by fatty tissue.

Congenital absence of the thymus (Di George's syndrome) or its removal early in life can result in severe, often fatal, immunologic abnormalities.[4] Removal of the thymus in the adult may lead to experimentally detectable abnormalities,[8] but they are rarely of major clinical consequence, probably because of the extremely long life of thymus-derived lymphocytes that have migrated to peripheral organs but have presumably retained their thymus-derived properties.

ANATOMY OF THE THYMUS

The thymus is a midline, pyramidal organ formed by two lobes. In most adults, it lies in the anterior mediastinum beneath the sternum at about the level of the third and fourth ribs. The level varies with some frequency because of migration to this site during embryologic development. In up to 30% of autopsy series, it may have a higher or lower location.[2] Rarely, however, is the main organ located above the manubrium or below the xyphoid process. In up to 20% of human beings, ectopic nodules of the thymic tissue are found, which may be important in the management of diseases such as myasthenia gravis. When present, these nodules are most frequently in the neck,[9] often close to or fused to the thyroid or parathyroid glands; however, they have been described at other sites, such as the base of the skull, root of a bronchus, and elsewhere in the mediastinum.[10] The blood supply of the thymus is derived from branches of the inferior thyroid arteries, the internal mammary arteries, and the pericardiophrenic arteries.

The size of the thymus relative to other structures of the body is greatest in the newborn. The normal thymus may appear as a significant mediastinal mass in the chest radiograph of a newborn or infant. This radiographic appearance gave rise to the theory that thymic enlargement is a possible cause of sudden infant death syndrome (SIDS). The appearance of an enlarged thymus on chest radiograph led to administration of mediastinal radiation to many infants, which effectively caused involution of the thymus. Because thymic enlargement is no longer thought to be the cause of SIDS, such therapy is no longer prescribed. Also, the treatment is now known to be associated with an increased risk of malignancy, particularly of the thyroid[11] and rarely of the thymus, later in life.[12]

THYMOMA

The term thymoma is now used to describe only those tumors derived from the epithelial component of the thymus, even though the thymus contains several types of cells.[2] There is little need for confusion in this regard except in the review of older literature, in which the term was used more freely in describing a number of other lesions, for example, granulomatous thymoma.[13, 14] These other neoplasms are now named to reflect their histogenesis; granulomatous thymoma is now recognized as thymic Hodgkin's disease. Thus, the identification of an epithelial component is necessary to correctly identify a tumor arising in the thymus as a thymoma. Germ cell tumors and lymphomas may also arise within the thymus but are not derived from thymic epithelium.

Strict criteria are important because of the possibility of misdiagnosis of thymic malignancies. For example, the nodular sclerosing subtype of Hodgkin's disease may have an obvious epithelial component and scant numbers of Reed-Sternberg cells, leading to the mistaken conclusion that it represents thymoma when it is seen arising in the thymus. Conversely, a true thymoma may have a large lymphoid component and only a few epithelial cells. Because many of the malignancies arising in the thymus are curable but require very different treatment strategies, depending on their histology, strict and reliable criteria for their identification are extremely important.

The distinction between benign and malignant thymomas cannot be made on histologic criteria because the vast majority of locally invasive or widely metastatic thymomas appear to be cytologically benign.

The distinction is usually determined by the surgeon at the time of operation, when careful examination of the thymic capsule may lead to a diagnosis of malignant or invasive thymomas.

Levine and Rosai[15] classified malignant thymomas on the basis of invasion, metastases, and cytologic atypia (Table 28–1).

Occurrence

About 20% of all mediastinal masses in the adult are thymomas.[2] They are the most common malignancy arising in the anterosuperior mediastinum. There is no evidence of any predilection for race, sex, or geographic distribution. Incidences in blacks and whites in the United States reflect the relative proportions of the two groups in the population. In many series, men slightly outnumber women but not to statistical significance.[2, 16–22] Over 70% of thymomas are seen in patients older than the age of 40, with most occurring in the fifth and sixth decades.[2, 16–22] Thymoma is less common in young adults and exceedingly rare in children.[23–25]

Gross Pathology

Ninety per cent of thymomas are surrounded by a fibrous capsule, which may be calcified.[2] The tumor surface may be smooth but more commonly is coarsely lobulated. The average size of the tumor is 150 gm, and it measures 5 to 10 cm; however, tumors as small as 1 mm have been found as incidental findings at autopsy, and the largest tumor described was close to 6 kg and measured 18 by 16 × 34 cm.[2] At surgery, 90% of the tumors are found arising in the anterior mediastinum, immediately above the pericardial sac, although they may extend up into the superior mediastinum. Fewer than 5% have been described as arising in the neck, and thymomas are virtually never found in the posterior mediastinum. At the time of surgery, a diligent search should be made for breaks in the capsule, a ragged outer surface, or invasion into adjacent tissues. These are all features that may indicate an invasive or malignant thymoma. Thymomas are one of the few tumors in which these features are more accurately determined operatively by the surgeon than histologically by the pathologist. Decisions regarding postoperative management of the

TABLE 28–1. Classification of Malignant Thymomas

I. With no or minimal cytologic atypia
   a. Locally invasive (usual form)
   b. With true lymphatic or hematogenous spread (rare)

II. Cytologically malignant (= thymic carcinoma)
   a. Squamous cell carcinoma
   b. Lymphoepithelioma like
   c. Clear cell carcinoma
   d. Sarcomatoid
   e. Undifferentiated

From Levine GD, Rosai J: Thymic hyperplasia and neoplasia: A review of current concepts. Hum Pathol 9:495–515, 1978.

patient may be based entirely on the surgeon's judgment.

Cysts may be found in up to 40% of tumors and are more common in larger masses. Foci of necrosis may also be seen in up to 25% of tumors. Neither cysts nor necrosis has been shown to correlate with the clinical behavior of the tumor.

Histopathology of Thymomas

Although thymoma is now strictly defined as a tumor arising from thymic epithelial cells, only 4% of thymomas consist of a pure population of epithelial cells. The rest contain varying mixtures of epithelial cells and lymphocytes. Indeed, the lymphocytes may appear to be the predominant cell type in the tumor. Nevertheless, to make the diagnosis, the pathologist should be convinced that the epithelial cells are the malignant cells in the population and that the remaining lymphocytes are normal or reactive.

The traditional subclassification of thymic epithelial tumors is based on the proportion of epithelial cells and lymphocytes present in the specimen. The subtypes are as follows: (1) lymphocytic—two-thirds of the cells are lymphoid, (2) mixed lymphocytic and epithelial—one-third to two-thirds of the cells are lymphoid, (3) epithelial—two-thirds of the cells are epithelial, and (4) spindled—two-thirds of the cells are epithelial and elongated or spindled.[26]

The clinicopathologic correlation with prognosis based on histopathologic subclassification has remained unclear. However, there are differences in the likelihood of association between histologic subclassification and the various autoimmune phenomena that accompany thymomas.

Myasthenia gravis is much more frequently seen with the lymphocytic or epithelial subtype of thymoma.[27–30] Conversely, red cell aplasia is seen more frequently with the spindle cell variant of thymoma.[31, 32]

A new histogenetic classification, originally described by Marino and Muller-Hermelink and co-workers, attempts to separate tumors into those derived from cortical epithelial cells from those which are derived from medullary epithelial cells.[33, 34] These investigators have noted that the spindled thymoma resembles the medullary epithelial cells of the normal thymus and believe that the cortical derived thymoma is associated with a worse prognosis than the medullary thymoma. The mixed cortical and medullary thymoma has an intermediate prognosis. This clinical pathologic correlation has been supported by Pescarmona and associates[35] and Nomori and colleagues.[36]

The use of flow cytometry has also introduced the DNA index in which aneuploid tumors (DI>1) appear to be correlated with a less favorable prognosis,[37, 38] although this has not been a consistent finding.[39]

Overall, the single most important independent variable in predicting prognosis remains the degree of tumor invasion described by the surgeon.

Presentation

Between one-third and one-half of all patients with thymoma present with an asymptomatic mass noted on a chest radiograph taken for some other reason. On a plain chest film, the mass is usually seen extending from the main mediastinal shadow into one of the lung fields. The outline of the mass is usually rounded and well demarcated but may be coarsely lobulated. Calcification is seen in up to 20% of cases; it is usually linear and peripheral, corresponding to the tumor capsule, although it may be scattered throughout the tumor mass. Calcification is more easily seen on CT scanning.

On computed tomography (CT), thymomas are usually seen as homogeneous soft tissue masses. Areas of decreased attentuation may correspond to foci of hemorrhage and necrosis within the mass. This is especially enhanced with intravenous contrast. As in radiography, the borders of the mass are usually smooth but may be lobulated. The mass may be completely or partially outlined by fat or may replace the anterior mediastinal fat. CT scanning is more sensitive than chest radiography in determining invasion into adjacent structures, such as the lung and pleura, or the extent of extrapleural seeding. Direct tumor invasion into mediastinal fat or vascular structures may be seen; however, absence of fat planes does not always indicate tumor invasion.[40, 41]

MRI may show involvement of surrounding structures in cases in which CT findings are equivocal. MRI may also show vascular involvement without the use of intravenous contrast.[42]

In the 50% to 70% of thymomas that are symptomatic, the symptoms may be vague, related only to the presence of a mass in the chest. Symptoms include cough, dyspnea, dysphagia, and chest pain. Patients may also have systemic symptoms of fever, weight loss, and anorexia. The large majority of patients, however, present with one or more of the variety of autoimmune or endocrine disorders known to be associated with thymomas (Table 28–2).

The presentation of a mediastinal mass associated with myasthenia gravis, hypogammaglobulinemia, or pure red cell aplasia is virtually diagnostic of thymoma.

In a group of 598 patients with thymoma reviewed by Souadjian and colleagues,[27] 71% had associated diseases. This figure is much higher than the incidence of only 12% in a group of 177 patients with parathyroid adenomas, which were chosen for comparison because these structures are also derived from the third pharyngeal pouch. Most of the associated diseases were autoimmune. Myasthenia gravis and pure red cell aplasia are classically associated with thymoma but Souadjian and colleagues[27] also found a variety of other abnormalities, especially leukopenia and thrombocytopenia, leading them to conclude that cytopenias in general were more common than the classically associated, but relatively rare, pure red cell aplasia.

TABLE 28–2. Incidences of Conditions Associated with Thymoma

	NUMBER	PERCENTAGE
All patients with thymoma	598	100
Patients with autoimmune diseases		
Myasthenia gravis	186	31
Cytopenias	89	15
Nonthymic cancer	70	12
Hypogammaglobulinemia	27	5
Polymyositis	20	3
Systemic lupus erythematosus	7	
Rheumatoid arthritis	5	
Thyroiditis	5	5
Sjögren's syndrome	4	
Ulcerative colitis	2	
Others	8	5
TOTAL	423	71
Patients with endocrine disorders		
Cushing's syndrome*	12	2
Hyperthyroidism	5	1
Others	3	1
TOTAL	20	3

*More commonly associated with thymic carcinoid than with thymoma.
Modified from Souadjian JV, Enriques P, Silverstein MN, et al: The spectrum of disease with thymoma. Arch Intern Med 134:374–379, 1974. Copyright 1974, American Medical Association.

Associated Disorders

Myasthenia Gravis

This is a disease of voluntary muscle weakness caused by circulating antibodies to the acetylcholine receptor, which is present on voluntary muscle at the neuromuscular end-plate.[28] Pathologic abnormalities in the thymus can be found in 75% to 85% of patients with myasthenia gravis. The most common abnormality is thymic lymphoid hyperplasia, referring to the appearance of germinal centers, which is not normally found in the thymus. The frequency of thymoma in patients with myasthenia gravis ranges from 8.5% to 15%. Conversely, the frequency of myasthenia gravis in thymoma patients range from 15% to 59% in published series.[18–22, 27] The wide range of frequency presumably reflects patterns of referral in the reporting institution.

The role of the thymus in the etiology of myasthenia gravis is not entirely understood. Several mechanisms have been proposed.[43] Thymic myoid cells, which resemble embryonic muscle cells, have acetylcholine receptors on their surface, and these cells may cause lymphocyte activation and the production of antibodies to acetylcholine receptors. Alternatively, the thymus may produce these antibodies. There may be a production of an abnormal proportion of T-cell subsets, or thymic hormones may be involved in the production of acetylcholine receptor antibodies.

The disease typically presents as weakness of the ocular muscles, with the patient complaining of diplopia. Difficulty with deglutition is also common. In more advanced cases, weakness of the larger extremity muscle groups may also be present, with proximal muscles being more commonly affected than distal ones.

A Tensilon test, in which administration of the drug provides rapid, although temporary clinical improvement, may confirm the diagnosis. In the case of nondiagnostic test results, more accurate neuromuscular testing with repetitive muscle stimulation may be necessary.

The initial management of the syndrome is frequently medical, with administration of acetylcholine esterase inhibitors, such as pyridostigmine or corticosteroids. As first noted by Blalock and associates[44] in a patient with a thymoma, myasthenia gravis may also respond to thymectomy. Overall, about 75% of patients with myasthenia gravis show some improvement after thymectomy, and about 30% achieve complete relief of symptoms. Patients with myasthenia gravis and thymoma do less well, showing only a 25% improvement in muscle weakness after thymectomy.

The age incidence of patients in the thymoma and the nonthymoma groups is different. The peak age of patients with nonthymoma myasthenia gravis is 30 years, whereas the peak age for the myasthenia gravis patients with thymomas is 40 to 50 years, the same age as that of all patients with thymomas.[2]

If surgery is to be attempted in a patient with myasthenia gravis and thymoma, it is important that all thymic tissue, not only the thymoma, be removed. Persistence of symptoms after surgery has been shown to be associated with residual normal thymus, as well as incomplete resection or regrowth of the tumor.[45]

Red Cell Aplasia

In red cell aplasia, there is an almost total absence of bone marrow erythroblasts and blood reticulocytes. Thirty per cent of the patients may also have depression of the leukocyte and platelet counts. This syndrome is seen in only 5% of thymoma patients, but 50% of the patients with red cell aplasia will have a thymoma. The cause of the syndrome is unknown. Two possible explanations are that thymoma may be a tissue that involves an antigen in common with erythroblastic cells or that thymomas may produce suppressor T cells, which inhibit erythroid differentiation. Approximately 20% to 40% of patients may show improvement after thymectomy.[32, 46]

Hypogammaglobulinemia

The association of acquired hypogammaglobulinemia with thymoma was first reported by Good and Gabrielson.[4] Only 5% of thymoma patients have the full syndrome, which may be associated with decreased cellular and humoral immunity. The most common clinical presentation is with bronchopulmonary disease[47]; however, diarrhea is also a common manifestation. Hypogammaglobulinemia rarely responds to thymectomy.[48, 32]

Staging Systems for Thymoma

The first commonly used staging system was proposed by Bergh and colleagues (Table 28–3).[49] This

TABLE 28–3. Bergh Staging System for Thymoma

STAGE	DEFINITION	PROPORTION OF CASES (%)
I	Intact capsule or growth within the capsule	40
II	Pericapsular growth into the mediastinal fat tissue	19
III	Invasive growth into the surrounding organs and/or intrathoracic metastases	41

Modified from Bergh NP, Gatzinsky P, Larsson S, et al: Tumors of the thymus and thymic region; I. Clinicopathologic studies on thymomas. Ann Thorac Surg 25:91–98, 1978. Reprinted with permission from the Society of Thoracic Surgeons (The Annals of Thoracic Surgery, 1978, 25, 91–98).

system distinguished between tumors with intact capsules and those with invasion into pericapsular fat or adjacent organs and distant metastases.

Masaoka and coworkers[50] in Japan proposed an alternative staging system that appears to predict outcome more accurately and has gained widespread acceptance (Table 28–4). This system separates those tumors that have spread into adjacent structures from the thymomas with noncontiguous spread, which may be intrapleural or via lymphatics or blood vessels.

The most important criterion in all the staging systems is to distinguish between invasive and noninvasive thymomas. No reliable histologic features distinguish malignant from benign or noninvasive thymoma. This distinction is made most reliably by the surgeon based on operative observations.

The Stage IIB tumors in the Masaoka staging system refer to microscopic invasion of the capsule, which cannot necessarily be determined at surgical examination and may require pathologic evaluation. The prognostic value of microscopic invasion into the capsule alone remains unresolved.[51]

Treatment

Surgery

Surgery is the principal initial therapy for thymoma. The removal of a well-encapsulated, noninvasive thymoma results in a recurrence rate of less than 2%.[52] Most surgeons also recommend that complete removal of the mediastinal mass be attempted, even in the face of invasion into neighboring structures. Some investigators have emphasized the prognostic significance of total resection. In a review of 36 patients, Pollack and colleagues[53] showed that when patients whose tumors were totally resected were subdivided into those with noninvasive and those with invasive disease, there was no difference in 5-year disease-free survival (75% and 74%, respectively). Nakahara and associates[54] reported a 5-year actuarial survival rate of approximately 95% for patients treated by total resection, even with Stage III disease.

Maggi and colleagues[55] reviewed 241 thymoma cases who underwent surgery. Fifty-five per cent had Stage I disease (by Masaoka classification). Overall,

TABLE 28–4. Masaoka Staging System for Thymoma

STAGE	DEFINITION	PROPORTION OF CASES (%)
I	Macroscopically, completely encapsulated; microscopically, no capsular invasion	40
IIA	Macroscopic invasion into surrounding fatty tissues or mediastinal pleura	14
IIB	Microscopic invasion into the capsule	
III	Macroscopic invasion into a neighboring organ, i.e., pericardium, great vessels, or lung	34
IVA	Pleural or pericardial dissemination	9
IVB	Lymphogenous or hematogenous metastases	3

Modified from Masaoka A, Monden Y, Nakahara K, et al: Follow-up study of thymomas with special reference to their clinical stages. Cancer 48:2485–2492, 1981.

87.5% underwent radical resection. The recurrence rates and actuarial survival by stage are shown in Table 28–5.

They found no significant difference in survival following total resection in patients with either invasive or noninvasive thymoma. In a review of 85 patients, Wilkins and associates[56] reported 20-year actuarial survival as follows: Stage I: 78.3%; Stage II: 74.7%; Stage III: 20.8%.

Every attempt should be made to remove all normal thymic tissue, especially when the patient has an associated autoimmune disease. Persistence of residual thymic tissue may be associated with continued symptoms of autoimmune diseases even if the thymoma is completely resected. The most common approach to resection of thymoma is via median sternotomy with complete resection of thymus and perithymic fat from sternum to pericardium. Lateral extension is handled by incision into the appropriate intercostal space. Other approaches may be necessary, as dictated by the extent of local disease.

Bergh and colleagues[49] reviewed the approach to the disease and the extent of resection in a series of 43 patients treated at the University of Goteberg, Sweden. They found that more advanced disease required extensive resection, including pericardiectomy, removal of the left innominate vein, partial or complete

TABLE 28–5. Data from Review by Maggi

STAGE	NO.	RECURRENCE (%)	ACTUARIAL SURVIVAL 5 year (%)	ACTUARIAL SURVIVAL 10 year (%)
I	133	1.5	89.2	86.9
II	34	12.5	71.9	59.9
III	53	29.7	71.3	64.3
IVa	21	25.0	59.4	39.6

Modified from Maggi G, Casadio C, Cavallo A, et al: Thymoma: Results of 241 operated cases. Ann Thorac Surg 51:152–156, 1991. Reprinted with permission from the Society of Thoracic Surgeons (The Annals of Thoracic Surgery, 1991, 51, 152–156).

pneumonectomy, and occasionally, sacrifice of the phrenic nerve or superior vena cava.

Most surgeons agree that resection of all gross disease is necessary even if the sacrifice of other organs is required. However, more extensive resections are associated with greater morbidity and mortality. Incomplete resection is associated with a poor prognosis, although some patients may still be salvaged by radiation therapy.[18, 57] Nevertheless, the death rate after surgery for thymoma has shown a progressive decline over the last 3 decades. One of the reasons for this decline clearly is the result of improvement in the perioperative management of patients with myasthenia gravis.

Earlier studies indicated that the presence of myasthenia gravis was a poor prognostic indicator in the treatment of thymoma. More recent investigators have not found this to be true uniformly.[56]

In a review of 103 patients with thymoma and myasthenia gravis, Crucitti and colleagues[58] reported a 4.85% mortality rate, with a 10-year survival of 78% and a recurrence rate of 3.06%. In part, this may be due to improvement in the pharmacologic therapy for myasthenia gravis that brings the patients to surgery in better clinical condition and reduces the postoperative ventilatory assistance period. Furthermore, the presence of myesthenia gravis is associated with earlier diagnosis and therapy of thymoma.

Radiation Therapy

Total surgical resection of completely encapsulated, or Stage I, thymoma is usually curative. Postoperative irradiation is not routinely advocated in such patients, with the possible exception of those who have persistent symptoms of myasthenia gravis that fail to respond to medical management.

Nakahara and associates[54] described four thymoma patients with Stage I to II disease who relapsed after complete resection. They suggest that even for early stage, totally resected patients, radiotherapy may be indicated in some circumstances, for example, for extensive pericardial or pleural adhesions.

The addition of postoperative radiation is recommended for all patients with evidence of invasive thymoma regardless of whether the tumor resection is judged to be complete. In several series the local failure rate for patients with Stage II or III disease who have undergone complete resection alone compares unfavorably to the intrathoracic tumor relapse in those patients who had complete resection plus postoperative radiation therapy or, in some cases, even those patients with incomplete resections and postoperative radiation therapy.[59–61]

In a review of 117 patients, Curran and coworkers[59] found a 53% mediastinal relapse rate in Stage II and III patients who had complete resection without follow-up radiotherapy. This compared unfavorably with the mediastinal relapse rate in same-stage patients who had complete resection and postoperative radiotherapy (0%), and subtotal resection with postoperative radiotherapy (21%).

There are few good dose-response or local recurrence data to guide radiation therapists in the selection of fields and doses. Penn and Hope-Stone[62] showed that doses of 40 Gy were inadequate for local control; however, given that much of the information in this paper is over 30 years old and antedates the modern era of radiotherapy, it is difficult to accept their further conclusions regarding doses and field sizes. In the absence of reliable dose-response data, it would seem reasonable to approach thymoma as one would epithelial malignancies. We would therefore recommend doses of 45 to 50 Gy for suspected areas of microscopic residual disease and dose of 60 Gy or more, where appropriate and possible, for regions of gross residual disease. This approach requires the closest possible cooperation between the surgeon and the radiotherapist. At a minimum, the surgeon should clearly mark all areas of original and especially residual disease with small radiopaque clips at the time of surgery to serve as a guide to radiation treatment planning. In difficult cases, the radiotherapist should consider being present in the operating room to give consideration to implanting areas of unresected disease with I^{125} seeds.

When the postoperative fields are planned, the original volume should cover the entire mediastinum, including the low mediastinum, because local drop metastases have been noted in this area. A shrinking field technique with CT directed treatment planning should be used to keep the radiation dose to the lungs and spinal cord within accepted tolerance limits. When possible, the hila may be included in the treatment fields, but it should also be recognized that nodal recurrence is not especially common in thymoma, which tends to spread by contiguous invasion. Care should be taken to minimize the dose to the lungs because radiation pneumonitis has been a cause of significant morbidity in several reported cases.[62–64] Pericarditis has also been reported as a less common complication of radiation therapy.

The use of preoperative radiation therapy is more controversial. It was at one time widely used in the treatment of patients with myasthenia gravis; however, improvements in medical management have now rendered this application unnecessary in most cases. Preoperative radiation therapy may still be considered in the patient whose disease is intractable to medical management and whose condition is too poor for immediate operation.

There is some literature on the use of radiation therapy in the patient with myasthenia gravis who has undergone surgery and who demonstrates none of the accepted indications for postoperation radiotherapy but whose disease remains refractory to conventional medical management. Phillips and Bushke[65] reported on their experience with radiating the thymic bed, and Engel and associates[66] reported on a small series of patients treated with either splenic irradiation or whole body irradiation. Yamanaka[67] also reported satisfactory control of three cases with unstable thymectomized myasthenia gravis by total body irradiation. Such an approach is not considered standard but may be useful for the rare patient in whom other modes of therapy have failed.

Chemotherapy

The low prevalence of thymoma and its comparatively infrequent tendency to metastasize contribute to a relative paucity of data regarding the role of chemotherapy in this disease. This tumor has been reported to respond to single agent and multiagent chemotherapy. However, the exact role of this treatment approach remains unclear.

The first attempt to collect and organize results from trials of chemotherapy in patients with invasive thymoma was reported by Boston in 1976.[68] More recently, Hu and Levine in their review of the chemotherapy of malignant thymomas concluded that as single agents, cisplatin and glucocorticoids have the highest response rates.[69]

In 1973, Talley and coworkers[70] described a single partial response to low-dose cisplatin. Since then, there were additional reports describing one[71] complete and two partial remissions[72, 73] in response to cisplatin treatment for thymoma. On the basis of anecdotal reports of cisplatin activity in this malignant neoplasm, the Eastern Cooperative Oncology Group initiated a Phase II trial of cisplatin given at a dosage of 50 mg/m^2 every 3 weeks. In the first 15 patients, two partial remissions were observed. Doxorubicin[68] and maytansine[74] have each produced short-term partial remissions as single agents.

In 1952, Sofer and associates[75] described regression of a thymoma following administration of adrenocorticotropic hormone. Subsequently, there have been at least 12 reported trials of corticosteroids, resulting in three complete remissions and seven partial remissions.[69] Because invasive thymomas consist of malignant epithelial cells and benign lymphocytes, it is uncertain whether the so-called tumor regressions are simply manifestations of a lympholytic rather than oncolytic effects. Reports have described the regression of thymomas and their metastases that have failed combination chemotherapy after surgery and radiation therapy and that have responded to glucocorticoid therapy in instances when myasthenia gravis is present or absent. This may lend credence to the theory that glucocorticoids indeed cause regression of the malignant element.[69] Anecdotal observations suggest that continuous glucocorticoid therapy may be necessary to achieve and maintain remission of thymic tumors.

The earliest experience with combination chemotherapy was reported by Boston,[68] who used two different four-drug regimens that included agents effective in treating lymphomas.

Subsequently, Evans and colleagues,[76] in a systematic effort to evaluate combination chemotherapy in invasive thymoma, used cyclophosphamide, vincristine, procarbazine, and prednisone. They observed four partial remissions in five patients, but the duration of response could not be determined because

each of the responding patients received radiation following one to three cycles of chemotherapy.

In 1980, Chahinian and associates observed two partial remissions in five patients treated with cisplatin, bleomycin, doxorubicin, and prednisone (BAPP).[77] Subsequently, they described one complete and five partial remissions in nine patients treated with BAPP. Their results represented the first experience with a cisplatin combination regimen in treating patients with invasive thymic tumors.

Goldel and colleagues[78] reviewed 22 patients with incompletely resected thymomas who received a variety of chemotherapeutic regiments, 12 of whom had received prior radiation therapy. Five of these 12 patients obtained a complete remission with a 5-year survival rate of 33%. There were 10 patients who received chemotherapy as initial therapy, and four of them obtained a complete remission with a 3-year survival rate of 34%. The regimens that yielded complete remissions included 5 of 13 who received cyclophosphamide, doxorubicin, vincristine and prednisone (CHOP) or CHOP/bleomycin; 3 of 6 receiving cyclophosphamide, vincristine and prednisone (COP) or COP plus procarbazine (COPP). One of two patients given COPP alternating with cisplatin/vinblastine/bleomycin (PVB) achieved complete remission. This group then began to use chemotherapy as their primary postoperative therapy. It was also found to be useful in the treatment of local or metastatic relapse after radiotherapy. The chemotherapy responders who remained free of relapse had subsequently received involved field radiation.

In an intergroup trial, Loehrer and associates[79] reported on 20 patients treated with cisplatin 50 mg/m^2, doxorubicin 50 mg/m^2 and cyclophosphamide 500 mg/m^2 on Day 1 every 21 days. There were three complete remissions and 11 partial remissions for an overall response rate of 70% with a median duration of remission of 13 months. The median survival time of all eligible patients was 59 months. Primary tumor regressions allowed the use of smaller radiotherapy ports for those with limited disease, using combined-modality therapy. The disparity between the relapse-free survival time and overall survival time raised some questions as to the curative potential of the regimen.

Fornasiero and coworkers[80] described the largest group of uniformly treated patients with Stage III or IV invasive thymomas. These 37 patients were given cisplatin, 50 mg/m^2, and doxorubicin, 40 mg/m^2, on Day 1; and vincristine, 0.6 mg/m^2, on Day 3 and cyclophosphamide, 700 mg/m^2, on Day 4 (ADOC). The overall response rate was 91.8% with a 43% complete remission rate. The median duration of response was 12 months and the median duration of survival was 15 months. Patients relapsing after ADOC received other chemotherapy regimens. Only those receiving cisplatin, etoposide, and ifosphamide (VIP) showed a response. This group has begun a neoadjuvant study, in which patients undergo surgery after four cycles of ADOC and have reported a pathologic remission in seven of 10 patients so treated. Nonetheless, despite a high remission rate, the long-term survival rate remains poor.

Another neoadjuvant protocol for seven Stage IIIA patients was reported by Macchiarini and associates.[81] The chemotherapy regimen consisted of cisplatin, 75 mg/m[2]; epirubicin, 100 mg/m[2], Day 1; etoposide, 120 mg/m[2], Days 1, 3, and 5 every 3 weeks. All patients had a partial remission. Complete resection was undertaken in four patients, of whom two had a negative histologic examination. These patients also received postoperative radiation therapy.

Interleukin-2 has been reported to generate a response in a patient who failed multiagent chemotherapy including prednisone as a therapy for a lymphoepithelial thymoma.[82]

Recurrence

Urgesi and associates[83] reviewed 21 patients with an intrathoracic recurrence of thymoma, of whom six patients were partially resected and five patients were totally resected prior to irradiation. In comparing radiation therapy alone with resection and radiotherapy, in relapsed patients, the 7-year survival was not markedly different (74% 7-year survival for surgery plus x-ray therapy; 65% for x-ray therapy alone). The conclusion was that for patients with good performance status, an aggressive approach to either surgery or radiation therapy or both is warranted if the disease is confined to the mediastinum or one hemithorax.

The largest report of reoperation for recurrent disease was conducted by Kirschner[84] and included 23 patients. There were four groups of patients, including (1) those who underwent complete thymectomy after initial thymomectomy alone or incomplete thymectomy, (2) those who underwent reoperation for recurrent thymoma after standard (complete) resection, (3) patients who underwent reoperation for initially unresectable thymoma after adjuvant therapy with chemotherapy, radiation therapy or both, and (4) miscellaneous. The conclusion of this group was that reoperation may be followed by tumor-free survival. Also, it was concluded that thymectomy should be abandoned in favor of complete thymectomy with wide operative exposure.

THYMIC CARCINOMA

Thymic carcinomas are histologically malignant neoplasms arising from thymic epithelial cells. They were originally described by Levine and Rosai[15] as Type II malignant thymomas. Compared with Type I malignant thymomas, these tumors have a malignant cytologic appearance with increased mitotic activity. The thymic carcinomas also have a high degree of central tumor necrosis that is generally lacking in malignant thymomas, as well as an absence of perivascular spaces commonly seen in thymomas.[85]

In one review,[86] thymic carcinomas appear to have more aggressive biologic behavior. Sixty-five per cent of these tumors were associated with widespread metastases and were not usually associated with autoimmune or endocrinologic paraneoplastic syndromes. These tumors may commonly be associated with symptoms attributable to an anterior mediastinal mass, such as chest pain, cough, or dyspnea.

Many histologic subtypes have been described and, as in thymomas, a varying degree of lymphoid population may occur in thymic carcinoma. In a review of 60 cases, Suster and Rosai divided these subtypes into low-grade and high-grade histology.[87] The low-grade category included well-differentiated squamous cell carcinoma, well-differentiated mucoepidermoid carcinoma, and basaloid carcinoma. The high-grade category included lymphoepithelioma-like carcinoma, small cell and neuroendocrine carcinoma, sarcomatoid carcinoma, clear cell carcinoma, and undifferentiated anaplastic carcinoma. They found that 85% of patients with a high-grade histology died of tumor, as compared with 0% with low-grade histology. This relatively good prognosis of squamous epidermoid carcinoma and poor prognosis of the lymphoepithelioma type carcinoma has also been reported by other observers.[88] Other favorable prognostic features included gross circumscription of the tumor, presence of a lobular growth pattern, and low mitotic activity.

Epstein-Barr viral genome has been identified in cells of several thymic lymphoepithelioma-like carcinomas[89]; this has not been a consistent finding,[88] and it is unclear whether or not this factor plays a role in the etiology of the disease.

As in thymomas, surgery is the main mode of therapy, as in thymomas. Radiotherapy may have potential benefit. The role of chemotherapy is unclear, although several patients have apparently achieved complete remissions with cisplatin-based combination chemotherapy.[90, 91]

Kirchner and associates[92] have described a well-differentiated thymic carcinoma. Such tumors have a degree of cytologic atypia that is intermediate between conventional thymoma and thymic carcinoma. They have histologic features suggestive of partial cortical differentiation with signs of organotypical differentiation. These tumors are often found in association with myasthenia gravis and are associated with low-grade malignant behavior. The authors suggest that some of the thymic carcinomas of the squamous type that have a good prognosis may fall into this subset.

THYMIC CARCINOID

Carcinoid tumors of the thymus were first described and differentiated from thymomas by Rosai and Higa in 1992.[93] They are rare tumors, and 90% of cases occur in men. The tumors are of neuroectodermal origin, derived from the primitive foregut, and are not associated with the carcinoid syndrome, which is common to carcinoid tumors derived from the midgut.

In distinguishing thymic carcinoid tumors from thymomas, staining for neuron-specific enolase may be helpful. Also, electron microscopy may reveal electron-dense neurosecretory granules.

These tumors are often discovered incidentally on chest radiograph. Symptoms may include, chest pain, dyspnea, shoulder pain or systemic symptoms, such as fatigue, fever, and night sweats. Thymic carcinoid is also associated with specific endocrinologic disorders.

In a review of 74 cases, Wick and associates[94] divided patients into three categories: (1) those with tumors associated with Cushing's syndrome with elevated production of adrenal corticotropic hormone, (2) those with tumors associated with multiple endocrine neoplasia Type I (MEN I), which is also associated with hyperparathyroidisim, and (3) those who are asymptomatic. The first group appears to have the worst prognosis. These tumors can also be seen as part of MEN II or in association with syndrome of inappropriate antidiuretic hormone (SIADH).

Surgery offers the best opportunity for cure. Radiotherapy has been used as adjuvant therapy and to control persistent and recurrent tumors. Chemotherapy agents, singularly or in a variety of combinations, may offer some palliation, although these therapies have not been shown to provide an overall advantage in survival.[96]

SMALL CELL CARCINOMA OF THE THYMUS

The thymus has been reported to be a primary site of extrapulmonary oat cell or small cell carcinoma.[97] These tumors reveal neuroendocrine differentiation and are included within the amine precursor uptake and decarboxylation (APUD) system (Please refer to Chapter 4 for an extensive discussion of these tumors.)

THYMOLIPOMA

Thymolipoma usually occurs as an asymptomatic mass and appears as a mixture of fat and a true hyperplasia of the thymus. These tumors may become very large (25% weigh over 2 kg).[2] They do not appear to metastasize, invade, or recur after resection. Case reports have associated thymolipomas with hypoplastic anemia and with myasthenia gravis.[98]

THYMIC HODGKIN'S DISEASE

The entity previously referred to as granulomatous thymoma is now recognized as Hodgkin's disease involving the thymus gland. When an anterior mediastinal mass is present in Hodgkin's disease, CT can help distinguish between a thymic mass and mediastinal lymph node involvement, or the two may appear simultaneously.[99] Keller and Castleman[100] found that half of the patients with mediastinal Hodgkin's disease had thymic involvement, and of those, half arose within the thymus gland. Mediastinal involvement is common in nodular sclerosing and mixed cellularity histologic subtypes and is unusual in lymphocyte predominant subtypes.

Mediastinal presentation of Hodgkin's disease was originally thought to be associated with a favorable prognosis. More recently, the presence of a large mediastinal mass (LMM) (maximum mediastinal width divided by the maximum intrathoracic diameter > 0.33) has demonstrated to be a risk factor for relapse. For this reason, combined-modality therapy with multiagent chemotherapy and radiotherapy has been used and reportedly has improved survival compared with the use of conventional radiation therapy alone.[101–104] Levitt and colleagues[105] advocate the use of radical radiotherapy and lung radiation without chemotherapy. Other researchers have found this approach to be complicated by frequent episodes of radiation pneumonitis.[102, 106]

Mediastinal involvement often is associated with a negative staging laparotomy. In some select cases of thymic Hodgkin's disease, therefore, such a staging operation may be obviated with a negative blind left scalene fat bed biopsy. This follows from Kaplan's theory of contiguous spread.[107] The communication between a mediastinal tumor and subdiaphragmatic sites would be via retrograde flow through the thoracic duct: If no positive nodes are found in the supraclavicular fossa, contiguous spread almost certainly has not occurred.[108]

Rebound thymic hyperplasia is a benign and transient condition that may occur as a consequence of chemotherapy for Hodgkin's disease and other tumors. Thymic hyperplasia should be considered in the differential diagnosis of an expanding anterior mediastinal mass in the postchemotherapy period. CT or gallium-67 scanning may help identify this process[109, 110] and distinguish it from active tumor. Serial follow-up scans help confirm this diagnosis.

THYMIC NON-HODGKIN'S LYMPHOMA

Most subtypes of non-Hodgkin's lymphomas, including Burkitt's lymphoma, mycosis fungoides, and small cleaved lymphoma, have been described as arising from the thymus.[2] The most common lymphomas to be derived from thymic lymphocytes are lymphoblastic lymphoma and large cell lymphoma of the thymus.

Lymphoblastic lymphoma (LBL) is postulated to be derived from thymic lymphocytes. The enzyme terminal deoxynucleotide transferase is found in virtually all LBL specimens.[111] It is commonly a disease of children and young adults. It has a bimodal peak of age distribution, the second peak occurring in adulthood.[112] There is a male predominance, and 45% to 75% of patients[112, 114] have a mediastinal mass at presentation. Bone marrow involvement occurs early in the disease and is associated with a leukemic blood picture. This clinical presentation, and the fact that the immature lymphocyte in lymphoblastic lymphoma may be indistinguishable from the lymphoblasts and prolymphocytes of acute lymphoblastic leukemia (ALL), make it difficult to distinguish de novo ALL from the leukemic conversion of lymphoblastic lymphoma.[113]

The disease is very aggressive and is associated with a high frequency of central nervous system and gonadal involvement during the course of the disease.

Progress has been made in the treatment of LBL with the advent of aggressive, prolonged multiagent chemotherapeutic regimens and central nervous system prophylaxis similiar to protocols for ALL.[114, 115] One successful regimen devised by Coleman and colleagues includes induction with cyclophosphamide, doxorubicin, vincristine, and methotrexate; central nervous system prophylaxis; four consolidation cycles with the drugs used in induction; and maintenance therapy with oral methotrexate and 6-mercaptopurine for 12 months.[114] The overall response rate was 100% (95% complete) with an actuarial 3-year freedom from relapse of 58% of the composite patient group.

Patients with Ann Arbor Stage IV disease with bone marrow or central nervous system involvement or an initial serum lactate dehydrogenase (LDH) concentration of greater than 300 IU/L have a very poor outcome.[114] Bone marrow transplantation is being evaluated in the treatment of these poor risk patients.[116]

Primary mediastinal lymphoma of B-cell lineage has been postulated to arise from the B-cell population within the thymus.[117] These cells are found within the medulla and the extraparenchymal septa. Clinically, these lymphomas present with symptoms of an anterior mediastinal mass or systemic symptoms of fatigue, fever, and weight loss. Superior venal caval syndrome has also been reported. They occur predominantly in young women who are 35 years of age or younger. The architecture is diffuse, and the cell type is predominately immunoblastic or large cell. Sclerosis is present in the majority of these cases. Immunohistochemical studies are helpful in differentiating these tumors from thymomas, thymic carcinomas, lymphoblastic lymphomas, Hodgkin's disease, and germ cell tumors.

These tumors have a more aggressive behavior and have reportedly involved the viscera such as the kidneys.[118, 119] The response to CHOP chemotherapy has been reported to be less favorable than the response to more aggressive chemotherapeutic combinations such as MACOP-B.[119] Radiation therapy may be a useful adjunct in the case of bulky medistinal adenopathy. The role of bone marrow transplantation in this disease is undergoing evaluation.[120]

There has been a report of a low-grade B-cell lymphoma of mucosa-associated lymphoid tissue (MALT) arising in the thymus. This appears to be an indolent tumor that responds well to surgery.[121]

GERM CELL TUMORS

Primary germ cell tumors of the anterior mediastinum usually develop in the thymus, and thymic remnants can be found in the vicinity of these tumors.[122] The etiology of these tumors in this site may be related to abnormal migration of germ cells during embryogenesis. These represent 5% to 10% of anterior mediastinal tumors. They occur predominantly in men in the second or third decade of life. All histologic subtypes

of gonadal germ cell tumors are found in the mediastinum: seminoma, embryonal carcinoma, teratoma, teratocarcinoma, choriocarcinoma and yolk sac tumors.[2] (Please refer to Chapter 29 for an extensive discussion of these tumors.)

SUMMARY

Understanding the embryology of the thymus has provided insight into the varied tumor types that originate in that organ. The natural history of these tumors differs, and therefore, different therapeutic approaches are necessary.

The most common of these tumors are thymomas. The quest for an optimal treatment is an evolving process because the roles for surgery, radiotherapy, and chemotherapy are constantly being re-evaluated.

SELECTED REFERENCES

Masaoka A, Monden Y, Nakahara K, et al: Follow-up of thymomas with special reference to their clinical stages. Cancer 48:2485–2492, 1981.
Outlines the clinical staging system for thymoma, which has gained widespread acceptance.

Rosai J, Levine GD: Tumors of the thymus. *In* Atlas of Tumor Pathology, Second Series, Fascicle 13. Washington, D.C., Armed Forces Institute of Pathology, 1976.
This authoritative work provides excellent detailed descriptions of pathology and clinical findings for the wide spectrum of thymic tumors.

Souadjian JV, Enriques P, Silverstein MN, et al: The spectrum of disease associated with thymoma. Arch Intern Med 134:374–379, 1974.
An extensive review of the many autoimmune and parathymic disorders associated with thymoma.

REFERENCES

1. Oppenheimer SB, Lefevre G Jr: Introduction to Embryonic Development. 2nd Ed. Boston, Allyn Bacon Inc., 1984.
2. Rosai J, Levine GD: Tumors of the thymus. *In* Atlas of Tumor Pathology, Second Series, Fascicle 13. Washington, D.C., Armed Forces Institute of Pathology, 1976.
3. Shier KJ: The thymus according to Schambacher. Cancer 48:1183–1199, 1981.
4. Good RA, Gabrielson AE: The Thymus in Immunobiology. New York, Hoeber, 1964.
5. Shulof RS, Goldstein AL: Thymosin and the endocrine thymus. Adv Intern Med 22:121–129, 1977.
6. Adkins B, Muller C, Okada C, et al: Early events in T cell maturation. Ann Rev Immunol 5:325–365, 1987.
7. MacFarlane-Burnet F: Role of the thymus and related organs in immunity. Br J Med 2:807–819, l963.
8. Claman HN, Talmage DW: Thymectomy, prolongation of tolerance in the adult mouse. Science 141:1193–1198, 1963.
9. Arnheim EE, Gemson BL: Persistent cervical thymus gland. Surgery 27:603–608, 1950.
10. Castleman B: Tumors of the thymus gland. *In* Atlas of Tumor Pathology, First Series, Fascicle 19. Washington, D.C., Armed Forces Institute of Pathology, 1955.
11. Shore RE, Woodard E, Hildreth N, et al: Thyroid tumors following thymus irradiation. J Natl Cancer Inst 74:1177–1184, 1985.
12. Jensen MO, Antonenko D: Thyroid and thymic malignancy following childhood irradiation. J Surg Oncol 50:206–208, 1992.

13. Katz A, Lattes R: Granulomatous thymoma or Hodgkin's disease of the thymus. Cancer 23:1–15, 1969.
14. Keller AR, Castleman B: Hodgkin's disease of the thymus gland. Cancer 33:1615–1623, 1974.
15. Levine GD, Rosai J: Thymic hyperplasia and neoplasia: A review of current concepts. Hum Pathol 9:495–515, 1978.
16. Wilkins EW, Castleman B: Thymoma: A continuing survey at the Massachusetts General Hospital. Ann Thorac Surgery 28:252–256, 1979.
17. Weissberg S, Goldberg M, Pearson FG: Thymoma. Ann Thorac Surgery 16:141–147, 1973.
18. Batata MA, Martini N, Huvos AG, et al: Thymomas: Clinicopathologic features, therapy and prognosis. Cancer 34:389–396, 1974.
19. Salyer WR, Eggleston JC: Thymoma, a clinical and pathological study of 65 cases. Cancer 37:229–249, 1976.
20. Sellors TH, Thackray AC, Thomson AD: Tumors of the thymus. Thorax 22:193–220, 1967.
21. LeGolvan DP, Abell MR: Thymomas. Cancer 39:2142–2157, 1977.
22. Gerein AN, Srivastava SP, Burgess J: Thymoma: A ten-year review. Am J Surgery 136:49–53, 1978.
23. Furman WL, Buckley PJ, Green AA, et al: Thymoma and myasthenia gravis in a 4-year-old child. Cancer 56:2703–2706, 1985.
24. Chatten J, Katz SM: Thymoma in a 12-year-old boy. Cancer 37:953–957, 1976.
25. Whittaker LD, Lynn HB: Mediastinal tumors and cysts in the pediatric patient. Surg Clin North Am 53:893–904, 1973.
26. Lewis JE, Wick MR, Scheithauer BW, et al: Thymoma: A clinicopathologic review. Cancer 60:2727–2743, 1987.
27. Souadjian JV, Enriques P, Silverstein MN, et al: The spectrum of disease associated with thymoma. Arch Intern Med 134:374–379, 1974.
28. Drachman DB: Myasthenia gravis. N Engl J Med 298:136–142, 186–193, 1978.
29. Alpert LI, Papatestas A, Kark A, et al: A histological reappraisal of the thymus gland in myasthenia gravis. Arch Pathol 91:55–61, 1971.
30. Verley JM, Hollmann KH: Thymoma—a comparative study of clinical stages, histologic features and survival in 200 cases. Cancer 55:1074–1086, 1985.
31. Zeok JV, Todd EP, Dillon M, et al: The role of thymectomy in red cell aplasia. Am Thorac Surg 28:257–260, 1979.
32. Masaoka A, Hashimoto T, Shibata K, et al: Thymomas associated with pure red cell aplasia. Cancer 64:1872–1878, 1989.
33. Marino M, Muller-Hermelink HK: Thymoma and thymic carcinoma: Relation of thymoma epithelial cells to the cortical and medullary differentiation of thymus. Virchows Arch (A) 407:119–149, 1985.
34. Muller-Hermelink HK, Marino M, Palestro G, et al: Immunohistological evidences of cortical and medullary differentiation in thymoma. Virchows Arch (A) 408:143–161, 1985.
35. Pescarmona E, Rendina EA, Venuta F, et al: The prognostic implication of thymoma histologic subtyping. A study of 80 consecutive cases. Am J Clin Pathol 93:190–195, 1990.
36. Nomori H, Ishihara T, Torikata C: Malignant grading of cortical and medullary differentiated thymoma by morphometric analysis. Cancer 64:1694–1699, 1989.
37. Davies SE, Macartney JC, Camplejohn RS, et al: DNA flow cytometry of thymomas. Histopathology 15:77–83, 1989.
38. Pollack A, El-Naggar AK, Cox JD, et al: Thymoma: The prognostic significance of flow cytometric DNA analysis. Cancer 69:1702–1709, 1992.
39. Sauter ER, Sardi A, Hollier LH, et al: Prognostic value of DNA flow cytometry in thymomas and thymic carcinomas. South Med J 83:656–658, 1990.
40. Fon GT, Bein ME, Mancuso AA, et al: Computed tomography of the anterior mediastinum in myasthenia gravis: A radiologic-pathologic correlative study. Radiology 142:135–141, 1982.
41. Hale DA, Cohen AJ, Schaefer P, et al: Computerized tomography in the evaluation of myasthenia gravis. South Med J 83:414–416, 1990.
42. Rosado-de-Christenson ML, Galobardes J, Moran CA: Thymoma: Radiologic-pathologic correlation. Radiographics 12:151–168, 1992.
43. Berrih-Akin S, Morel E, Raimoud F, et al: The role of the thymus in myasthenia gravis: Immunohistological and immunological studies in 115 cases. Ann NY Acad Sci 505:51–70, 1987.
44. Blalock A, Mason MF, Morgan HJ, et al: Myasthenia gravis and tumors of the thymic region. Ann Surg 110:544–561, 1939.
45. Rosenberg M, Jauregui WO, DeVega ME, et al: Recurrence of thymic hyperplasia after thymectomy in myasthenia gravis. Its importance as a cause of failure of surgical treatment. Am J Med 74:78–82, 1983.
46. Hirst E, Robertson TI: The syndrome of thymoma and erythroblastopenic anemia. Medicine 46:225–264, 1967.
47. Fox MA, Lynch DA, Make BJ: Thymoma with hypogammaglobulinemia (Good's syndrome): An unusual case of bronchiectasis. AJR Am J Roentgenol 158:1229–1230, 1992.
48. Rogers BHG, Manaligod JR, Blazek WV: Thymoma associated with pancytopenia and hypogammaglobulinemia. Am J Med 44:154–164, 1968.
49. Bergh NP, Gatzinsky P, Larsson S, et al: Tumors of the thymus and thymic region; I. Clinicopathological studies on thymomas. Ann Thorac Surg 25:91–98, 1978.
50. Masaoka A, Monden Y, Nakahara K, et al: Follow-up study of thymomas with special reference to their clinical stages. Cancer 48:2485–2492, 1981.
51. Kornstein MJ: Controversies regarding the pathology of thymomas. Pathol Annu 27:1–15, 1992.
52. Fechner RE: Recurrence of noninvasive thymomas. Cancer 23:1423–1427, 1969.
53. Pollack A, Komaki R, Cox JD, et al: Thymoma: Treatment and progress. Int J Radiat Oncol Biol Phys 23:1037–1043, 1992.
54. Nakahara K, Ohno K, Hashimoto J, et al: Thymoma: Results with complete resection and adjuvant post-operative irradiation in 141 consecutive patients. J Thorac Cardiovasc Surg 95:1041–1047, 1988.
55. Maggi G, Casadio C, Cavallo A, et al: Thymoma: Results of 241 operated cases. Ann Thorac Surgery 51:152–156, 1991.
56. Wilkins EW, Grillo HL, Scannell JG, et al: Role of staging in prognosis and management of thymoma. Ann Thorac Surg 51:888–892, 1991.
57. Couture MM, Mountain CF: Thymoma. Semin Surg Oncol 6:110–114, 1990.
58. Crucitti F, Doglietto GB, Bellantone R, et al: Effects of surgical treatment in thymoma with myasthenia gravis: Our experience in 103 patients. J Surg Oncol 50:43–46, 1992.
59. Curran WJ, Kornstein MJ, Brooks JJ, et al: Invasive thymoma: The role of mediastinal irradiation following complete or incomplete surgical resection. J Clin Oncol 6:1722–1727, 1988.
60. Arakawa A, Yasunaga T, Saitoh Y, et al: Radiation therapy of invasive thymoma. Int J Radiat Oncol Biol Phys 18:529–534, 1990.
61. Urgesi A, Monetti U, Rossi G, et al: Role of radiation therapy in locally advanced thymoma. Radiother Oncol 19:273–280, 1990.
62. Penn CR, Hope-Stone HF: The role of radiotherapy in the management of malignant thymoma. Br J Surg 59:553–539, 1972.
63. Ariaratnam LS, Kalnicki S, Mincer F, et al: The management of malignant thymoma with radiation therapy. Int J Radiat Oncol Biol Phys 5:77–80, 1979.
64. Jackson MA, Ball DL: Post-operative radiotherapy in invasive thymoma. Radiother Oncol 21:77–82, 1991.
65. Phillips TL, Bushke F: The role of radiation therapy in myasthenia gravis. Calif Med 106:282–289, 1967.
66. Engel WK, Lichter AS, Dalakas MC: Splenic and total-body irradiation treatment of myasthenia gravis. Ann NY Acad Sci 377:744–754, 1981.
67. Yamanaka N, Tanaka M, Kurihara T: Total body irradiation therapy for thymectomized myasthenia patients and immunological evaluations. Clin Neurol 23:467–472, 1983.
68. Boston B: Chemotherapy of invasive thymoma. Cancer 38:49–59, 1976.
69. Hu E, Levine J: Chemotherapy of malignant thymoma. Cancer 57:1101–1104, 1986.
70. Talley RW, O'Bryan RM, Gutterman JU, et al: Clinical evaluation of toxic effects of cis-diammine-dichloroplatinum—Phase I clinical study. Cancer Chemother 57:465–471, 1973.

71. Needles BM, Kemeny N, Urmacher C: Malignant thymoma: Renal metastases responding to cisplatinum. Cancer 48:223–226, 1981.

72. Shetty MR, Arora RK: Invasive thymoma treated with cisplatinum. Cancer Treatment Rep 65:531, 1981.

73. Cocconi G, Boni C, Cuomo A: Long-lasting response to cisplatinum in recurrent malignant thymoma. Cancer 49:1983–1987, 1982.

74. Jaffrey ZS, Denefrio JM, Chahinian P: Response to maytansine in a patient with malignant thymoma. Cancer Treat Rep 64:193–194, 1980.

75. Sofer LF, Gabrilove J, Wolff BS: Effect of ACTH on thymic masses. J Clin Endocrinol Metab 12:690–696, 1952.

76. Evans WK, Thompson DM, Simpson WJ, et al: Combination chemotherapy in invasive thymoma: Role of COPP. Cancer 46:1523–1527, 1980.

77. Chahinian AP, Holland JF, Bhardwaj S: Chemotherapy for malignant thymoma. Ann Intern Med 99:736, 1983.

78. Goldel N, Boning L, Fredrik A, et al: Chemotherapy of invasive thymoma—a retrospective study of 22 cases. Cancer 63:1493–1500, 1989.

79. Loehrer PJ, Perez CA, Roth LA, et al: Chemotherapy for advanced thymoma: Preliminary results of an intergroup study. Ann Intern Med 113:520–524, 1990.

80. Fornasiero A, Daniele O, Ghiotto C, et al: Chemotherapy for invasive thymoma: A 13-year experience. Cancer 68:30–33, 1991.

81. Macchiarini P, Chella A, Ducci F, et al: Neoadjuvant chemotherapy, surgery, and postoperative radiation therapy for invasive carcinoma. Cancer 68:706–713, 1991.

82. Berthaud P, LeChevalier T, Tursz T: Effectiveness of interleukin-2 in invasive lymphoepithelial thymoma. Lancet 335:1590, 1990.

83. Urgesi A, Monetti U, Rossi G, et al: Aggressive treatment of intrathoracic recurrences of thymoma. Radiother Oncol 24:221–225, 1992.

84. Kirschner PA: Reoperation for thymoma: Report of 23 cases. Ann Thorac Surg 49:550–555, 1990.

85. Walker AN, Mills SE, Fechner RE: Thomomas and thymic carcinomas. Sem Diag Pathol 7:250–265, 1990.

86. Wick M, Bernatz P, Carney J, et al: Primary thymic carcinomas. Am J Surg Pathol 6:613–630, 1982.

87. Suster S, Rosai J: Thymic carcinoma. Cancer 67:1025–1032, 1991.

88. Hartman CA, Roth C, Minck C: Thymic carcinoma—report of five cases and review of the literature. Cancer Res Clin Oncol 116:69–82, 1990.

89. Dimery IW, Lee JS, Blick M, et al: Association of Epstein-Barr virus with lymphoepithelioma of the thymus. Cancer 61:2475–2480, 1988.

90. Weide LG, Ulbright TM, Loehrer PJ, et al: Thymic carcinoma: A distinct clinical entity responsive to chemotherapy. Cancer 71:1219–1223, 1993.

91. Carlson RW, Dorfman RF, Sikic BI: Successful treatment of metastatic thymic carcinoma with cisplatin, vinblastine, bleomycin and etoposide chemotherapy. Cancer 66:2092–2094, 1990.

92. Kirchner T, Schalke B, Buchwald J, et al: Well-differentiated thymic carcinoma. Am J Surg Pathol 16:1153–1169, 1992.

93. Rosai T, Higa E: Mediastinal endocrine neoplasm of probably thymic origin, related to carcinoid tumor: Clinicopathologic study of 8 cases. Cancer 29:1061–1074, 1992.

94. Wick MR, Scott RE, et al: Carcinoid tumor of the thymus: A clinicopathologic report of seven cases with a review of the literature. Mayo Clin Proc 55:246–254, 1980.

95. Economopoulos GC, Lewis JW, Lee NW, et al: Carcinoid tumors of the thymus. Ann Thorac Surgery 50:58–61, 1990.

96. Zeiger MA, Swartz SE, Macgillivray DC, et al: Thymic carcinoid in association with MEN syndromes. Am Surgeon 58:430–434, 1992.

97. Remick SC, Hafez R, Carbone PP: Extrapulmonary small-cell carcinoma. Medicine 66:457–471, 1987.

98. Otto HF, Loning T, Lachenmayer L, et al: Thymolipoma in association with myasthenia gravis. Cancer 50:1623–1628, 1982.

99. Heron CW, Husband JE, Williams MP: Hodgkin disease: CT of the thymus. Radiology 167:647–651, 1988.

100. Keller AR, Castleman B: Hodgkin's disease of the thymus gland. Cancer 33:1615–1623, 1974.

101. Hoppe RT, Coleman CN, Cox RS, et al: The management of Stage I-II Hodgkin's disease with irradiation alone or combined modality therapy: The Stanford experience. Blood 59:455–465, 1982.

102. Hoppe RT: The management of bulky mediastinal Hodgkin's disease. Hematol Oncol Clin North Am 63:265–276, 1989.

103. Leopold KA, Canellos GP, Rosenthal D: Hodgkin's disease: Staging and treatment of patients with large mediastinal adenopathy. J Clin Oncol 7:1059–1065, 1989.

104. Dowling SW, Peschel RE, Portlock CS, et al: Mediastinal irradiation in combined modality therapy for Hodgkin's disease. Int J Radiat Oncol Biol Phys 19:543–546, 1990.

105. Levitt SH, Lee CK, Aeppli D, et al: The role of radiation therapy in Hodgkin disease: Experience and controversy. Cancer 70:693–703, 1992.

106. Tarbell NJ, Thompson L, Mauch P: Thoracic irradiation in Hodgkin's disease: Disease control and long-term complications. Int J Radiat Oncol Biol Phys 18:275–281, 1990.

107. Kaplan HS: Hodgkin's Disease. 2nd Ed. Cambridge, Massachusetts, Harvard University Press, l980.

108. Kinsella TJ, Glatstein E: Staging laparotomy and splenectomy for Hodgkin's disease: Current status. Cancer Invest 1:89–91, l983.

109. Kissin CM, Husband JE, Nicholas D, et al: Benign thymic enlargement in adults after chemotherapy: CT demonstration. Radiology 163:67–70, 1987.

110. Peylan-Ramu N, Haddy TB, Jones E, et al: High frequency of benign mediastinal uptake of gallium-67 after completion of chemotherapy in children with high-grade non-Hodgkin's lymphoma. J Clin Oncol 7:1800–1806, 1989.

111. Braziel RM, Kenklis T, Doulon JA, et al: Terminal deoxynucleotide transferase in non-Hodgkin's lymphomas. Am J Clin Pathol 80:655–659, 1983.

112. Nathwani BN, Diamond LW, Winberg CD, et al: Lymphoblastic lymphoma: A clinicopathologic study of 95 patients. Cancer 48:2347–2357, 1981.

113. Slater DE, Mertelsmann R, Koziner B, et al: Lymphoblastic lymphoma in adults. J Clin Oncol 4:57–67, 1986.

114. Picozzi VJ, Coleman CN: Lymphoblastic lymphoma. Semin Oncol 17:96–103, 1990.

115. Morel P, Lepage E, Brice P, et al: Prognosis and treatment of lymphoblastic lymphoma in adults: A report on 80 patients. J Clin Oncol 10:1078–1085, 1992.

116. Verdonck LF, Dekker AW, deGast GC, et al: Autologous bone marrow transplantation for adult poor-risk lymphoblastic lymphoma in first remission. J Clin Oncol 10:644–646, 1992.

117. Davis RE, Dorfman RF, Warnke RA: Primary large-cell lymphoma of the thymus: A diffuse B-cell neoplasm presenting as primary mediastinal lymphoma. Hum Pathol 21:1262–1268, 1990.

118. Haioun C, Gaulard P, Roudot-Thoraval F, et al: Mediastinal diffuse large-cell lymphoma with sclerosis: a condition with a poor prognosis. Am J Clin Oncol 12:425–429, 1989.

119. Todeschini G, Ambrosetti A, Meneghin V, et al: Mediastinal large-B-cell lymphoma with sclerosis: A clinical study of 21 patients. J Clin Oncol 8:804–808, 1990.

120. Kirn D, Mauch P, Shaffer K, et al: Large-cell and immunoblastic lymphoma of the mediastinum: Prognostic features and treatment outcome in 57 patients. J Clin Oncol 11:1336–1343, 1993.

121. Isaacson PG, Chan JK, Tung C, et al: Low-grade B-cell lymphoma of mucosa-associated lymphoid tissue arising in the thymus. Am J Surg Pathol 14:342–351, 1990.

122. Patcher MR, Lattes R: Germinal tumors of the mediastinum: A clinico-pathological study of adult teratomas, teratocarcinomas, choriocarcinomas and seminomas. Dis Chest 45:301–310, 1964.

29 MEDIASTINAL GERM CELL NEOPLASMS

John D. Hainsworth and F. Anthony Greco

Mediastinal germ cell tumors have been recognized as a distinct group of neoplasms, and elucidation of their biologic and clinical characteristics has occurred during the past two decades. Although uncommon, this group of neoplasms is of particular interest because young men are most often affected. In addition, mediastinal germ cell neoplasms have been added to the growing list of cancers that are potentially curable with systemic chemotherapy. This chapter is a review of the clinical and pathologic characteristics of benign and malignant germ cell tumors of the mediastinum and focuses on treatment of these neoplasms. An additional section addresses the evaluation and treatment of the patient with poorly differentiated carcinoma arising in the mediastinum. The origin of these poorly understood tumors and their possible relation to mediastinal germ cell tumors are also discussed.

BENIGN TERATOMAS OF THE MEDIASTINUM

Benign teratomas of the mediastinum (dermoid tumors) are rare neoplasms and account for 3% to 12% of all mediastinal tumors.[1-5] Most benign teratomas occur in young adults; however, these tumors have been described in patients ranging in age from 7 months to 65 years. The incidence rate in males and females is approximately equal.[5-7] Unlike malignant germ cell tumors of the mediastinum, no predisposing conditions or associated abnormalities have been described.

The pathologic appearance of benign mediastinal teratoma is identical to that of benign teratoma arising in the more common location, the ovaries. On gross examination, these tumors are usually well encapsulated and are composed of either a single large cystic cavity or several smaller intercommunicating cystic spaces. Mature tissue from ectodermal, mesodermal, and endodermal germ cell layers typically is present. The ectodermal component (i.e., skin, pilosebaceous tissue, neural tissue) is usually predominant; therefore, the term dermoid is used to describe these tumors.[7, 8] However, mature tissue that recapitulates the histology of any human organ can be found in these tumors.

Benign teratomas of the mediastinum grow slowly. Approximately 95% arise in the anterior mediastinum; the remainder arise in the posterior mediastinum.[5, 7, 9, 10] In recent years, 50% to 60% of patients have been asymptomatic at the time of diagnosis by routine chest roentgenography.[6, 7] When symptoms are present, substernal chest pain and dyspnea are most common. Cough productive of hair or sebum is pathognomonic of a benign mediastinal teratoma and occurs when the tumor ruptures into the tracheobronchial tree. However, except at late stages this distinctive symptom rarely occurs in the natural history of this condition. Superior vena cava syndrome is another late manifestation of these benign tumors. Physical examination usually contributes little to the diagnosis; most patients appear healthy. Similarly, laboratory evaluation is usually unremarkable. In particular, serum levels of human chorionic gonadotropin (hCG) and alpha-fetoprotein (AFP) are normal in patients with benign teratoma.

The chest radiograph typically reveals a well-encapsulated anterior mediastinal mass that often protrudes into one of the lung fields. These tumors are usually large at the time of diagnosis; in a recent series, the median size was $10 \times 8.5 \times 5.4$ cm.[7] Calcification is a distinctive radiographic feature of these tumors and occurs in approximately 25%. In addition to the pathognomonic radiographic finding of teeth within the tumor, calcification can occur in fragments of bone, within the tumor wall, or in nonspecific areas throughout the tumor. Computed tomography usually demonstrates cystic areas within the tumor but rarely provides additional diagnostic information.

Surgical excision is the treatment of choice for benign teratoma of the mediastinum. Median sternotomy is the preferred approach, although successful resection has also been achieved by thoractomy. Although these tumors are benign histologically, surgical removal is often difficult owing to their large size and frequent involvement of vital mediastinal structures. In decreasing order of frequency, mediastinal structures involved by these tumors include pericardium, lung, great vessels, thymus, chest wall, hilar structures, and diaphragm.[7] In 10% to 15% of patients, additional procedures (e.g., lobectomy, pericardiectomy) are necessary for successful complete tumor resection. Results with radiotherapy have been poor due to the radioresistance of these tumors, and this treatment should rarely, if ever, be used.

After complete surgical resection, tumor recurrence is rare.[5, 7, 11] Prolonged survival has also been reported in patients who receive only a subtotal resection due to involvement of vital mediastinal structures. In recent years, improved surgical technique and earlier diagnosis of these tumors have resulted in negligible surgical mortality.

MALIGNANT GERM CELL TUMORS

Etiology and Pathogenesis

The occurrence of choriocarcinoma and teratocarcinoma in the mediastinum was first reported more than 40 years ago.[12–14] Pure seminoma occurring in the mediastinum was first recognized by Friedman in 1951.[15] In 1946, Schlumberger[16] first speculated on the oncogenesis of extragonadal germ cell tumors. He postulated that these neoplasms arose from primitive rests of totipotential cells that had become detached from the blastula or morula during embryogenesis. Others subsequently hypothesized that extragonadal germ cell tumors arose from primitive germ cells from the endoderm of the yolk sac or from the urogenital ridge that had failed to completely migrate into the scrotum during development.[16, 17] Questions remain regarding the oncogenesis of extragonadal germ cell tumors, and both of these hypotheses remain unproved. Although either hypothesis can explain the occurrence of extragonadal neoplasms in the retroperitoneum or mediastinum, the occasional occurrence of these tumors in other locations (e.g., pineal, sacrococcygeal area) is best explained by Schlumberger's hypothesis.

A third hypothesis that was previously widely accepted proposes that extragonadal germ cell tumors are metastatic lesions from a gonadal primary that either remained small or spontaneously regressed. The occasional autopsy finding of small, unrecognized testicular primaries or fibrous scars (believed to represent sites of regressed primary tumors) supported this hypothesis.[18–20] However, much current evidence substantiates the extragonadal origin of these neoplasms. Several investigators have reported autopsy series in which the testes of patients with presumed extragonadal germ cell neoplasms were serially sectioned and carefully examined for microscopic neoplasms or fibrous scars; the great majority of patients had neither of these findings.[21–24] In addition, patients with primary testicular germ cell neoplasms rarely have isolated metastases to the anterior mediastinum.[25–28] In two large autopsy series, metastases to the anterior mediastinum were not found in 300 patients with testicular germ cell neoplasms.[25, 26] Finally, large numbers of patients with mediastinal germ cell tumors are long-term survivors after either mediastinal irradiation for pure seminoma or combination chemotherapy for nonseminomatous neoplasms. Testicular recurrences have not been observed in these patients. Because of this evidence, primary mediastinal germ cell neoplasms are now accepted as a distinct clinical entity. The coexistence of an occult testicular primary neoplasm is believed to be a very rare occurrence.

Incidence

Malignant germ cell tumors of the mediastinum are uncommon neoplasms. In most series, these tumors represent 3% to 10% of tumors originating in the mediastinum.[1–4, 29, 30] They are much less common than germ cell tumors arising in the testes and account for 1% to 5% of all germ cell neoplasms.[31–33] There is some indication that these incidence rates, which are derived from retrospective series reported between 1950 and 1975, underestimate the true incidence of mediastinal germ cell tumors. Difficulty in distinguishing these tumors from malignant thymomas was recognized by Lattes in 1961.[34] Several investigators have reported patients with clinical characteristics of extragonadal germ cell tumors in whom the initial pathologic diagnosis was either poorly differentiated carcinoma or another diagnosis.[35–37] A recent review of mediastinal malignancies in patients seen between 1970 and 1982 included 11 patients (28%) with germ cell tumors.[38] Although there is no doubt that these neoplasms are uncommon, increasing familiarity by both clinicians and pathologists should result in increased recognition.

Mediastinal germ cell tumors have been recognized in patients ranging in age from 2 to 70 years, but the great majority occur in patients between 20 and 35 years old. For unknown reasons, the great majority of these tumors occur in men. The very rare tumors that do occur in women (approximately 25 cases have been reported) appear to be histologically and biologically identical to those in their male counterparts.[11, 17, 23, 39–47] The relative rarity of extragonadal germ cell tumors in women parallels the rarity of gonadal germ cell tumors in women.

Pathology

Details of the histopathologic characteristics of mediastinal germ cell tumors are beyond the scope of this chapter. These tumors appear to be identical histologically to germ cell tumors that arise in the testis, and all histologic subtypes of testicular germ cell neoplasms have also been recognized in the mediastinum. The relative incidence of the various histologic subtypes also appears to be similar in mediastinal and testicular germ cell neoplasms. Table 29–1 is a summary of the incidence of the various histologic subtypes in published retrospective reviews involving more than 20 patients. Pure seminoma is the most common histology; although the relative incidence varies among reported series, seminomas account for 34% of all patients in these series. The remaining 66% of patients have neoplasms that contain nonseminomatous elements.

TABLE 29–1. Histology of Mediastinal Germinal Neoplasms

HISTOLOGY	NO. OF PATIENTS (%)				
	Martini et al[39]	Cox[23]	Luna and Valenzuela-Tamanz[24]	Economou et al[48]	Knapp et al[40]
Seminoma	10 (33)	6 (25)	3 (15)	11 (39)	24 (43)
Nonseminoma	18 (60)	14 (58)	14 (70)	13 (46)	29 (52)
Embryonal	4	5	3	2	9
Teratocarcinoma	10	7	3	4	5
Choriocarcinoma		2	2	2	3
Endodermal sinus				2	3
Mixed nonseminomatous histologies	4		6	3	9
Mixed seminoma/nonseminoma	2 (7)	4 (17)	3 (15)	4 (15)	3 (5)
Total	30	24	20	28	56

Pure endodermal sinus (yolk sac) tumor may be a histology that in men is found only in extragonadal tumors. These tumors are rare even among extragonadal germ cell tumors and have been reported to arise in either the mediastinum or the retroperitoneum. Although pure endodermal sinus tumor is a well-recognized entity arising in the ovary, similar tumors arising in the testis have not been reported, and it has been asserted that they do not exist.[49] The occurrence of testicular or extragonadal neoplasms containing endodermal sinus histology intermixed with other elements is well recognized.

Clinical Characteristics

Malignant mediastinal germ cell tumors are usually very large at the time of diagnosis and cause symptoms by compressing or invading local mediastinal structures, lungs, pleura, pericardium, or chest wall. Because pure seminomas are slower growing neoplasms with less potential for early metastasis than neoplasms with nonseminomatous elements, the initial presentation and subsequent course vary. Although these two subgroups are discussed separately, there is a great deal of overlap in their clinical characteristics.

Seminoma

Seminomas are usually slow growing and can become very large before causing symptoms; tumors 20 to 30 cm in diameter can exist with minimal symptomatology. From 20% to 30% of seminomas are detected by routine chest radiography while still asymptomatic.[42] Signs and symptoms are nonspecific and are identical to those seen with any slowly expanding mediastinal tumor. The initial symptom is usually a sensation of pressure or dull retrosternal chest pain. Other symptoms include exertional dyspnea, cough, hoarseness, and dysphagia.[41, 42, 50, 51] Approximately 10% of patients develop superior vena cava syndrome.[42] Systemic symptoms are not common, but some patients exhibit weight loss or easy fatiguability. Symptoms related to metastatic lesions are uncommon at diagnosis.

Some patients with mediastinal seminoma have tumor localized to the anterior mediastinum at the time of diagnosis. Most series reported before 1975 indicated that the majority of patients had localized disease[41, 48, 52, 53]; however, in recent series with larger numbers of patients, only 30% to 40% of patients have had localized disease.[40, 54] The lungs and other intrathoracic structures are the most common metastatic sites; early detection of metastases in these areas with the use of computed tomography may explain the recent apparent increase in patients with metastases. The skeletal system is the most frequently recognized extrathoracic metastatic site; the propensity of advanced testicular seminoma to metastasize to bone has also been recognized. The retroperitoneum is an uncommon site of metastases in patients with mediastinal seminoma, which is in contrast to the very common involvement of this area in patients with testicular primaries.[24, 51, 54]

The radiographic findings of primary mediastinal seminoma do not allow its distinction from other mediastinal masses, which can compress or deviate the trachea or bronchi if they are of sufficient size. Computed tomography of the chest typically shows a large, homogeneous anterior mediastinal mass, which obliterates fat planes surrounding the mediastinal vascular structures.[55]

Approximately 10% of mediastinal seminomas have elevated levels of hCG.[54] This incidence is similar to that reported in advanced testicular seminoma. The serum AFP level is always normal in patients with pure mediastinal seminoma; AFP elevation indicates the presence of nonseminomatous elements. Serum lactate dehydrogenase (LDH) is elevated in the majority of patients with mediastinal seminoma; in one series, LDH levels ranged from 176 to 5140 u/L (median, 365 u/L) and were elevated in 17 of 20 patients.[54]

Nonseminomatous Neoplasms

Mediastinal germ cell tumors with nonseminomatous elements are generally more rapidly growing than pure seminomas. Very few of these patients are asymptomatic at diagnosis. Symptoms caused by compression or invasion of local mediastinal structures are identical to those seen in patients with mediastinal seminomas. However, nonseminomatous neoplasms differ from pure seminomas in that 85% to

95% of patients have at least one site of metastatic disease at diagnosis, and presenting symptoms are frequently the result of metastases.[47, 49, 56] Common sites of metastases include lung, pleura, lymph nodes (supraclavicular, retroperitoneal), and liver. Bone, brain, and kidneys are less frequently involved. Gynecomastia is sometimes present in patients with high serum levels of hCG. Neoplasms with elements of choriocarcinoma have a marked hemorrhagic tendency; these patients may present with catastrophic events related to uncontrolled hemorrhage at a metastatic site (e.g., intracranial hemorrhage, massive hemoptysis).[57] Constitutional symptoms, including weight loss, fever, and generalized weakness, are more common in these patients than in those with pure seminoma.

Chest radiographic features of nonseminomatous germ cell tumors do not differ significantly from those of mediastinal seminomas. Computed tomography frequently shows an inhomogeneous mass with multiple areas of decreased attenuation representing necrosis and hemorrhage, which differs from the usually homogeneous appearance of mediastinal seminoma.[55] Approximately 90% of patients have elevated levels of hCG, AFP, or both.[47, 56] Serum LDH is elevated in 80% to 90% of patients.[56]

Syndromes Associated with Mediastinal Nonseminomatous Germ Cell Tumors

Klinefelter's Syndrome

Klinefelter's syndrome is a relatively common chromosomal abnormality characterized by hypogonadism, azoospermia, and elevated gonadotropin levels in association with an extra X chromosome. An increased incidence of breast cancer in males with this syndrome has been recognized,[58] but a general predisposition to other malignancies has not been observed. Multiple patients with Klinefelter's syndrome and mediastinal nonseminomatous germ cell tumors have been reported.[59–70] Four of 22 consecutive patients (18%) with mediastinal germ cell tumors seen at Indiana University had karyotypic confirmation of Klinefelter's syndrome, and a fifth patient had clinical features.[71] The average age of patients with Klinefelter's syndrome who develop extragonadal germ cell tumors is 18 years, 10 years younger than the median age of those developing these tumors in the absence of Klinefelter's syndrome. Most patients have mediastinal nonseminomatous germ cell tumors, particularly choriocarcinoma; testicular or retroperitoneal primary sites have rarely been associated with Klinefelter's syndrome.[72, 73]

The explanation for this peculiar association is unknown, but it is reasonable to assume that the chromosomal abnormality plays some role. Previous studies of both testicular and extragonadal germ cell tumors in healthy men have revealed the presence of nuclear chromatin and double Y bodies in a substantial proportion.[74] In addition, testicular tumor karyotypes are often hyperdiploid even when peripheral blood karyotypes are normal.[75] The presence of the extra X chromosome in individuals with Klinefelter's syndrome may confer on their germ cells an increased propensity to undergo aberrant chromosome dysjunction and therefore predispose these cells to malignant degeneration analogous to the germ cells in the dysgenetic undescended testicle.

One case of mediastinal choriocarcinoma has been described in a man with infertility, complete arrest of spermatogenesis with Leydig's cell hyperplasia, and an abnormal translocation of a segment of the short arm of chromosome 2 onto the short arm of chromosome 3.[76] Although this patient did not have Klinefelter's syndrome, the authors speculated that a similar genetic aberration predisposed to the development of neoplasia.

Hematologic Neoplasia

An association between hematologic malignancies and mediastinal nonseminomatous germ cell tumors has recently been recognized. A review of all patients with germ cell tumors seen between 1974 and 1983 at Indiana University and the Dana Farber Cancer Institute showed that three of 34 patients with primary mediastinal tumors developed hematologic malignancies (two patients with acute megakaryocytic leukemia and one patient with myelodysplastic syndrome), whereas none of the 654 patients with testicular primaries developed secondary hematologic malignancies.[77] Multiple patients with mediastinal nonseminomatous germ cell tumors and hematologic neoplasia have been reported.[77–84] The hematologic syndromes varied; diagnoses included acute nonlymphocytic leukemia, acute lymphocytic leukemia, erythroleukemia, myelodysplastic syndrome, and malignant histiocytosis. Most patients developed hematologic neoplasia after the diagnosis of mediastinal germ cell tumor, usually within 24 months. In several patients, the two diagnoses were simultaneous.

The cause of this association, which appears to be specific for mediastinal germinal malignancy, is unknown. The clinical features of these hematologic malignancies were not typical of chemotherapy-induced malignancies, since these patients did not exhibit the usual prodrome of refractory cytopenia. Two patients had acute lymphocytic leukemia, which is very unusual as a therapy-related disorder. In addition, the short time span between the two diagnoses is atypical of therapy-induced leukemia.

Most evidence points to a common origin of the malignant cells that produce the mediastinal germ cell tumor and the associated hematologic neoplasm. Through molecular chromosomal analysis, several patients with identical karyotypic abnormalities in malignant germ cells and leukemic cells have been identified.[85, 86] In most of these patients, the shared karyotypic abnormality was an isochromosome of the short arm of chromosome 12 (i[12p]), a cytogenetic marker found in extragonadal and testicular germ cell tumors.[87] The ability of germ cell tumors to produce a variety of histologic phenotypes is well recognized clinically; areas resembling sarcoma, adenocarcinoma, and neuroendocrine carcinoma have been well described.[88] Hematopoietic cells have rarely been described; however, a focus of lymphoblasts was recognized in the mediastinal germ cell tumor of one patient who subsequently developed acute lymphoblastic leukemia.[80] Although a common origin of these associated neoplasms seems likely, the specific association of hematopoietic malignancies and *mediastinal* germ cell tumors is unexplained.

In addition to hematologic malignancies, four cases of idiopathic thrombocytopenia have been reported in association with mediastinal germ cell tumors.[89, 90] In these patients, normal numbers of megakaryocytes were present in the bone marrow, but no immune destruction of platelets could be demonstrated. Prednisone and splenectomy were unsuccessful in increasing the platelet count; persistent thrombocytopenia caused significant morbidity in all patients and made treatment extremely difficult. The cause of this syndrome is unknown, but the authors postulated that a substance toxic to platelets was produced by the mediastinal germinal tumor.[89]

One patient with a mediastinal endodermal sinus tumor associated with the hemophagocytic syndrome has been reported.[91] In this patient, a proliferation of benign, mature-appearing macrophages with prominent hemophagocytosis was seen in the bone marrow. Treatment with chemotherapy produced a partial tumor response; however, the hemophagocytic syndrome persisted, and the patient subsequently died of progressive tumor.

Treatment

Pretreatment Evaluation

The diagnosis of mediastinal germ cell tumor should be considered in all young men who have a mediastinal mass. In addition to physical examination and routine laboratory studies, initial evaluation should include computed tomography of the chest and abdomen and determination of serum levels of hCG and AFP. Any symptoms suggestive of distant metastases should be evaluated with appropriate radiologic studies. If obvious metastases are present, histologic diagnosis should be made using the least invasive approach because surgical therapy does not play a role in the initial treatment of these patients and rapid institution of definitive systemic therapy is essential. In patients with tumors that appear to be localized to the mediastinum, exploration via thoracotomy with an attempt at tumor resection or debulking is sometimes appropriate. Exceptions to this approach include tumors that are obviously unresectable due to involvement of vital mediastinal structures or intrathoracic spread outside the anterior mediastinum (i.e., patients with superior vena cava syndrome, pericardial or pleural involvement) and patients with very high serum levels of hCG or AFP. In this second group of patients, the clinical presentation coupled with the elevated marker levels is diagnostic of a non-

seminomatous extragonadal germ cell tumor, and definitive systemic therapy should begin immediately.

The treatment and prognosis of mediastinal seminoma and nonseminoma differ; therefore, these tumors are discussed separately.

Seminoma

Because of the rarity of seminomas, most reports of therapy have been case reports or small patient series. It is therefore sometimes difficult to make definitive conclusions on the relative efficacy of therapies when more than one method exists. This section provides a review of existing data regarding the various treatment methods (surgical resection, radiotherapy, and chemotherapy) and concludes with our recommendations for optimal management of these neoplasms.

It has been recognized since the early 1950s that some patients with mediastinal seminoma are curable with surgical resection, radiotherapy, or both. Multiple case reports have described long-term survivors after complete surgical resection of mediastinal seminoma.[39, 41, 50, 52, 92–94] However, even in earlier series in which most patients had tumor localized to the anterior mediastinum, complete surgical resection was possible in fewer than 50% of patients owing to extensive local tumor involvement. More recently, improved staging methods have resulted in the recognition of metastases in more than 50% of patients with mediastinal seminoma; therefore, the opportunity for complete surgical resection exists in fewer than 25% of patients and is probably limited to patients who have had an asymptomatic mediastinal mass found on routine chest radiography. In addition, several reports have documented local recurrence after complete resection of mediastinal seminoma[95, 96]; for this reason, resection should never be used as the only therapeutic method in these patients.

Case reports of long-term survivors with mediastinal seminoma treated with radiotherapy as a single method have also appeared since the early 1950s.[18, 42, 97–101] Occasional long-term survivors have been described after radiotherapy of multiple metastatic lesions in addition to the primary lesion.[42, 52, 98, 102–104] Table 29–2 is a summary of the results of radiotherapy in reported series containing five or more patients. Radiotherapeutic techniques and dosages varied widely, with reported curative doses ranging from 2000 to 7000 cGy. In addition, some patients received radiotherapy after complete or partial surgical resection; these patients are indicated in Table 29–2, and results of treatment for this subset are indicated separately. As is evident from Table 29–2, treatment results using local therapeutic modalities are reasonably good; overall, 49 of 82 patients (60%) reported in these nine series achieved long-term disease-free survival. The majority of treatment failures were due to the appearance of distant metastases rather than failure to achieve local tumor control.

Specific recommendations for administering radiotherapy have varied and have been drawn more from experience in irradiation of metastatic testicular

TABLE 29–2. Mediastinal Seminoma: Results of Treatment with Radiotherapy

STUDY	YEAR	NO. OF PATIENTS	RADIOTHERAPY DOSE (Gy)	NO. OF PATIENTS WITH PRERADIOTHERAPY RESECTION (COMPLETE/PARTIAL)	NO. OF DISEASE-FREE SURVIVORS >24 MO IN TOTAL GROUP (%)	NO. OF DISEASE-FREE SURVIVORS >24 MO IN SUBGROUP WITH SURGICAL RESECTIONS (COMPLETE/PARTIAL)
El-Domeiri et al[41]	1968	8	30–50	2 (1/1)	3 (38)	1 (1/0)
Schantz et al[52]	1972	12	24–60	7 (2/5)	12 (100)	7 (2/5)
Martini et al[39]	1974	8	NA	1 (0/1)	2 (29)	0
Cox[23]	1975	6	20–40	0	6 (100)	—
Medini et al[102]	1979	5	35–45	3 (2/1)	3* (60)	3 (2/1)
Raghavan and Barrett[103]	1980	6	35–45	1 (1/0)	3 (67)	1 (1/0)
Bush et al[104]	1981	13	25–60	1 (0/1)	7† (54)	NA
Hurt et al[53]	1982	16	30–40	6 (4/2)	9 (56)	4 (3/1)
Jain et al[54]	1984	8	18.5–46	2 (2/0)	4 (50)	2 (2/0)

*One patient died of intercurrent illness; one patient had treatment delayed for 4 yr and subsequently died of distant metastases.
†Two patients with recurring illness are long-term survivors after salvage treatment with further radiotherapy plus chemotherapy.

seminomas than from experience with mediastinal seminomas. Mediastinal seminomas appear to be as exquisitely radiosensitive as testicular seminomas. Although doses as low as 2000 cGy have been curative in some patients, Bush and associates[104] observed local relapses when low doses were used but not when doses of at least 4700 cGY were administered. They therefore recommended the use of 4500 to 5000 cGy over 6 weeks delivered by external beam megavoltage irradiation to a shaped mediastinal field including both supraclavicular areas. Others have made similar recommendations, although some believe that a lower dose of radiotherapy (3500 to 4000 cGy) is sufficient.[53, 103] Owing to the low incidence of retroperitoneal involvement at diagnosis and the rare recurrence in this area after radiotherapy, routine irradiation of the retroperitoneum as part of primary therapy is not recommended.

Surgical debulking before definitive radiotherapy has also been recommended.[41, 105, 106] However, a review of the major reported series (see Table 29–2) indicates that there is benefit from a surgical procedure only when complete excision is performed. Only one treatment failure has been documented after complete excision and mediastinal irradiation; this patient developed distant metastases at multiple sites and subsequently died.[53] In contrast, when the size or location of tumor precludes complete excision, attempts at debulking can be detrimental because delay in the use of more effective treatment methods can result.

In recent years, systemic combination chemotherapy has become available as another treatment for mediastinal seminomas with the potential for cure. Intensive cisplatin-based combination regimens originally proved to be effective in metastatic nonseminomatous testicular neoplasms have subsequently proved to be effective in the treatment of advanced seminoma.[107, 108] The limited experience using optimal cisplatin-based combination regimens in mediastinal seminoma is summarized in Table 29–3. It is evident that a high percentage of reported cases have attained complete responses and long-term survival, even after radiotherapy failure. However, because most reports include very small numbers of patients, possible bias due to the selective reporting of favorable results must be considered.

Only one nonrandomized study compares results in patients treated initially with radiotherapy with those of patients treated initially with combination chemotherapy.[54] Five of nine patients treated initially with radiotherapy remain disease free (one received radiotherapy to metastatic bone lesions). In contrast, 10 of 11 patients treated initially with combination chemotherapy have remained continuously disease free since the completion of therapy. Because the results with radiotherapy are consistent with those achieved in other reported series, the conclusion is made that initial chemotherapy is the treatment of choice for patients with mediastinal seminoma. These excellent results with chemotherapy have been duplicated by the Southeastern Cancer Study Group.[112] Seven of nine patients achieved complete response with chemotherapy, seven of whom had relapsed after radiation therapy. Therefore, both studies suggest that chemotherapy is the superior treatment method. However, the lesser toxicity of radiotherapy coupled with the high chemotherapy salvage rate after radiotherapy failure makes the choice of initial therapy difficult in patients with locally advanced mediastinal seminoma.

Patients with bulky mediastinal seminoma frequently have residual radiographic abnormalities after chemotherapy. The management of such patients after completion of chemotherapy remains controversial; again, most experience has been with advanced testicular seminomas. Most evidence indicates that residual radiographic masses represent dense scirrhous reaction in 85% to 90% of cases, and viable seminoma or unexpected teratoma is uncommon.[112, 114–116] Because of the dense fibrosis, surgical resection in such patients is difficult and frequently incomplete and can be associated with a high mortality rate. Conflicting data have been reported from Memorial Sloan-Kettering Cancer Center; five of 20 patients undergoing postchemotherapy resection had residual seminoma.[117] All five patients had radiographic masses >3 cm in diameter. Therefore, patients with small residual masses (<3 cm) should be followed without biopsy; patients with masses >3 cm should be biopsied or followed very closely, with early biopsy of any enlarging tumor mass.

In summary, the majority of patients with medias-

TABLE 29–3. Mediastinal Seminoma: Results of Treatment With Cisplatin-Based Combination Chemotherapy

STUDY	YEAR	NO. OF PATIENTS	PREVIOUS TREATMENT	TREATMENT REGIMEN	NO. OF COMPLETE RESPONSES (%)	NO. OF LONG-TERM DISEASE-FREE SURVIVORS (MO)
Feun et al[83]	1980	2	2 RT	DDP/VLB/bleo*	0	0
van Hoesel and Piredo[109]	1980	1	RT, alkylating agents	DDP/VLB	1 (100)	1 (20+)
Einhorn and Williams[107]	1980	3	2 RT, 1 no therapy	PVB + A	2 (66)	2 (>24)
Hainsworth et al[47]	1982	4	3 RT, 1 no therapy	PVB	3 (75)	3 (>24)
Daugaard et al[110]	1983	1	1 RT	PVB	1 (100)	1 (>24)
Clamon[111]	1983	2	2 no therapy	PVB	2 (100)	2 (>24)
Jain et al[54]	1984	11	11 no therapy	VAB-6 8, PVB 1, DDP/CTX 2	10 (91)	10 (19+ to 46+)
Logothetis et al[49]	1985	4	NA	DDP/CTX 3, CISCA$_{II}$ 1	4 (100)	4 (follow-up not specified)
Loehrer et al[112]	1987	9	7 RT, 2 no therapy	PVB±A or BEP	8 (89)	7 (follow-up not specified)
Bukowski et al[113]	1993	8	None	PVB/EBAP	5 (63)	4 (>24)

*Used lower doses and longer intervals between doses than are currently considered optimal.

RT = radiotherapy, DDP = cisplatin, VLB = vinblastine, bleo = bleomycin, A = adriamycin, CTX = cyclophosphamide, PBV (Einhorn regimen) = cisplatin, vinblastine, and bleomycin, VAB-6 = multidrug regimen developed at Sloan-Kettering (Reference 108); CISCA$_{II}$ = multidrug regimen developed at M.D. Anderson (Reference 49), BEP = bleomycin 30 units weekly, etoposide 100 mg/m^2 IV × 5 days, cisplatin 20 mg/m^2 IV × 5 days; cycle repeated every 3 weeks × 4.

tinal seminoma can be cured with therapy, and all patients should be approached with this intent. All patients should have a careful pretreatment evaluation to look for evidence of distant metastases and to carefully determine the extent of involvement of mediastinal structures. Patients with small tumors (usually asymptomatic patients) that appear to be resectable should undergo thoracotomy and attempted complete resection. Radical debulking procedures for patients with extensive mediastinal involvement are not indicated. In the subset of patients who undergo complete excision, postoperative radiotherapy (3500 to 4500 cGy) is curative in almost all patients and clearly is the treatment of choice. The optimal treatment method for patients with distant metastases at the time of diagnosis is also clear; these patients should undergo combination chemotherapy with an intensive combination regimen containing cisplatin and etoposide. Although the optimal chemotherapy regimen for mediastinal seminoma is not defined, the combination of bleomycin, etoposide, and cisplatin (four courses) is considered standard therapy for testicular germ cell tumors with poor prognosis[118] and appears to be a good choice.

The optimal treatment for patients with locally advanced mediastinal seminoma who have no evidence of distant metastases is not clear. Approximately 60% of these patients can be cured with radiotherapy, and many of the patients who experience relapse can be successfully salvaged with combination chemotherapy.[47, 107, 109, 110, 112] Alternatively, first-line chemotherapy using cisplatin, etoposide, and bleomycin chemotherapy is curative in most patients. Whichever treatment option is selected, optimal therapy yields cures in the large majority of these patients.

Nonseminomatous Germ Cell Tumors

The futility of local treatment methods in the therapy of nonseminomatous mediastinal germ cell neoplasms has been recognized for more than 20 years. Not only are these tumors almost always metastatic at the time of diagnosis, but they are also relatively resistant to radiotherapy.[21, 23, 39, 48] In a review of the literature in 1975, Cox[23] found no reported survivors among 85 patients with mediastinal teratocarcinoma. Early attempts to treat these neoplasms with chemotherapy using single agents or combinations without cisplatin produced transient responses but had no meaningful impact on survival.

The application of intensive cisplatin-based chemotherapy regimens developed for the treatment of metastatic nonseminomatous testicular neoplasms to the treatment of their mediastinal counterparts has improved the formerly dismal outlook of these patients. Table 29–4 is a summary of the results of treatment with cisplatin-based combination chemotherapy regimens that are considered optimal. The overall long-term survival rate in these patients is 40% (50 of 125 patients). These results represent a marked improvement, but long-term survival rates of these patients are still lower than those in patients with metastatic testicular germ cell tumors. The large size of most mediastinal germ cell tumors at the time of diagnosis is the most likely explanation for these results; testicular germ cell tumors with far-advanced, bulky metastases have comparable long-term survival rates (approximately 40% to 50%) when treated with cisplatin-based regimens.[127]

Surgical therapy plays a significant role in the optimal treatment of nonseminomatous mediastinal germ

TABLE 29–4. Nonseminomatous Mediastinal Germ Cell Tumors: Results of Treatment With Cisplatin-Based Combination Chemotherapy

STUDY	YEAR	NO. OF EVALUABLE PATIENTS	PREVIOUS TREATMENT	CHEMOTHERAPY TREATMENT REGIMEN	NO. OF COMPLETE RESPONSES (%)	NO. OF LONG-TERM DISEASE-FREE SURVIVORS (%)
Funes et al[119]	1981	13	None	PVB	6 (46)	5 (38)
Vogelzang et al[120]	1981	7	2 RT	PVB (6)† VAB-6 (1)	3 (43)	3 (43)
Hainsworth et al[47]	1982	12	None	PVB ± A	7 (58)	7 (58)
Daugaard et al[110]	1983	5	None	PVB	1 (20)	1 (20)
Newlands et al[121]	1983	2	None	POMB/ACE	2 (100)	2 (100)
Garnick et al[122]	1983	8	None	PVB	3 (38)	1 (13)
Logothetis et al[49]	1985	11	None	CISCA$_{II}$ (6), CISCA/VB$_{IV}$ (5)	NA	4 (36)
Israel et al[56]	1985	11*	None	VAB-6	NA	4 (36)
Kay et al[123]	1987	11	None	PVB (5), BEP (6)	7 (64)	5 (45)
McLeod et al[124]	1988	7	None	VAB-6	2 (29)	2 (29)
Sham et al[125]	1989	7‡	None	PVB (2), BEP (1), BEVIP (3), EP (1)	3 (43)	3 (43)
Nichols et al[126]	1990	31	None	PVB ± A, BEP	18 (58)	13 (42)
Bukowski et al[113]	1993	16	None	PVB/EBAP	13 (81)	9 (56)
Total		141				59 (42)

*Includes patients with retroperitoneal tumors.
†Two patients received local radiotherapy after chemotherapy.
‡All seven patients had pure endodermal sinus tumors.
PVB (Einhorn regimen) = cisplatin, vinblastine, and bleomycin; A = adriamycin; POMB/ACE = cisplatin, vincristine, methotrexate, bleomycin, etoposide, actinomycin D, and cyclophosphamide; CISCA regimens = multidrug regimens developed at M.D. Anderson; VAB-6 = multidrug regimen developed at Memorial Sloan-Kettering; BEP = bleomycin 30 units weekly, etoposide 100 mg/m² IV × 5 days, cisplatin 20 mg/m² IV × 5 days; BEVIP = bleomycin, etoposide, vinblastine, and cisplatin.

cell tumors, as it does in the treatment of metastatic testicular neoplasms. Because of the high frequency of distant metastases or extensive mediastinal disease, initial surgical resection is seldom feasible, and no evidence exists that partial resection (debulking) is useful. However, surgical intervention is often necessary after the completion of initial chemotherapy. Surgical resection should be undertaken if combination chemotherapy produces normalization of serum tumor markers but only partial resolution of the mediastinal tumor. In this setting, 60% to 70% of patients have either necrotic tumor or benign teratoma and no evidence of active malignancy. The importance of completely resecting residual benign (mature or immature) teratoma in these patients has been recognized; unresected teratoma can cause further problems either by slow growth locally or by subsequent malignant degeneration. If viable carcinoma is resected after initial chemotherapy, patients should receive further chemotherapy with a salvage regimen[128–130] because long-term survival is unusual after resection alone,[120] even if complete tumor resection is performed. Patients with persistently elevated tumor markers after initial chemotherapy always have persistent carcinoma; attempts at surgical resection are almost never beneficial in this situation, and these patients should proceed directly to salvage chemotherapy. The management of patients with residual radiographic or tumor marker abnormalities after initial chemotherapy is presented as a diagram in Figure 29–1.

It has been suggested that certain histologic subtypes of nonseminomatous mediastinal germ cell neo-plasms are associated with a very poor therapeutic outcome. Kuzur and associates[131] reported on 10 patients with pure endodermal sinus tumor of the mediastinum, with only one long-term disease-free survivor. Six of these patients received initial cisplatin-containing combination chemotherapy, whereas three other patients received radiotherapy before chemotherapy. Other investigators have had better treatment results with patients with pure endodermal sinus tumor and do not believe this diagnosis implies a poor prognosis.[49, 125] Because these patients are rare, this controversy cannot be resolved. Clearly, patients with mixed tumors that include endodermal sinus elements have a prognosis similar to that of the group as a whole. Pure choriocarcinoma of the mediastinum has also been considered by some to have a poor prognosis.[47] Again, the small number of patients makes definitive statements very difficult to make.

Although the development of cisplatin-containing chemotherapy regimens has improved the prognosis of patients with nonseminomatous mediastinal germ cell tumors, these tumors continue to be fatal in the majority of patients. Further improvements in therapy are necessary; these improvements will probably parallel the development of increasingly effective treatment for patients with far advanced, testicular germ cell tumors with poor prognosis.

Poorly Differentiated Carcinoma of the Mediastinum

The patient with poorly differentiated (or anaplastic) carcinoma poses difficult problems for both clinician

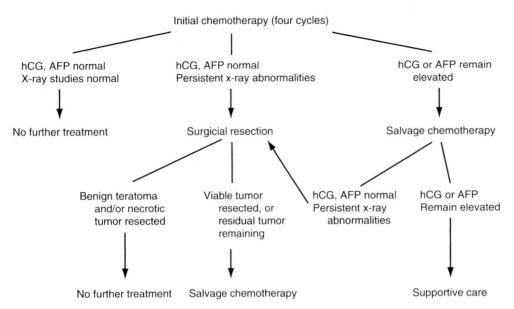

FIGURE 29–1. Management of nonseminomatous mediastinal germinal tumors after completion of initial chemotherapy.

and pathologist. Owing to the lack of definitive histopathologic features, the true nature of these neoplasms is usually not clear. The patient who develops a mediastinal mass and is found to have poorly differentiated carcinoma is often suspected of having metastatic lung cancer with an undetected primary lesion, and palliative radiotherapy is considered. Although an extensive discussion of poorly differentiated carcinomas is beyond the scope of this chapter, this brief section is included because some patients presenting in this manner have highly responsive, potentially curable neoplasms and should receive careful attention.

In 1979, a few patients with poorly differentiated carcinoma who had complete responses to cisplatin-based combination chemotherapy were reported by two groups of researchers.[36, 132] Four of five patients reported by Fox and associates[36] and eight of 12 patients reported by Richardson and associates[132] had tumor located primarily in the mediastinum. Four patients were later rediagnosed as having extragonadal germ cell tumors; all 12 patients responded to combination chemotherapy, and four of 12 are long-term disease-free survivors. Because most of these patients were young men with rapidly growing neoplasms and elevated serum levels of hCG and/or AFP, it was postulated by both groups that these patients had extragonadal germ cell neoplasms that were unrecognized histologically. They recommended that serum tumor markers be measured on all young patients with poorly differentiated carcinoma, particularly if the tumor is located in the mediastinum or retroperitoneum, and that these patients be treated with the same intensive cisplatin-containing combination chemotherapy regimens that are effective in the treatment of germ cell neoplasms.

Since that time, we have prospectively evaluated and treated patients with poorly differentiated carcinoma or poorly differentiated adenocarcinoma of unknown primary site. In a recent report, 220 such patients were treated with intensive cisplatin-based regimens effective in the treatment of germ cell tumors; 58 patients (26%) had a complete response, and 36 (16%) are long-term disease-free survivors.[133] Forty-three of these patients had predominant tumor location in the mediastinum; most of these patients were young (median age, 38 years), but only a few had elevated serum levels of hCG or AFP. Thirteen patients (30%) had a complete response, and seven (16%) had long-term disease-free survival.

The suspicion that some of the responsive tumors in this patient group may be histologically unrecognizable extragonadal germ cell tumors has been substantiated. With molecular genetic analysis, Motzer and associates[134] identified the i(12p) chromosomal abnormality specific for germ cell tumor in four of nine young men with midline poorly differentiated tumors. Three of these four patients had chemotherapy-sensitive tumors.

It is therefore firmly established that some patients have mediastinal germ cell tumors that cannot be diagnosed using standard pathologic techniques. The frequency of these tumors is unknown. This diagnosis should be considered in all young men with poorly differentiated mediastinal tumors of unknown origin. Chromosomal analysis, if available, should be considered to better define these tumors. All such patients should receive a trial of therapy with a cisplatin-based regimen, using the same guidelines outlined for the treatment of nonseminomatous mediastinal germ cell tumors.

SELECTED REFERENCES

Bush SE, Martinez A, Bagshaw MA: Primary mediastinal seminoma. Cancer 48:1877–1882, 1981.
This large retrospective series details radiotherapy techniques.
Hainsworth JD, Einhorn LH, Williams SD, et al: Advanced extragonadal germ cell tumors: Successful treatment with combination chemotherapy. Ann Intern Med 97:7–11, 1982.

A large series of extragonadal germinal tumors documents efficacy of cisplatin-based therapy.

Hainsworth JD, Johnson DH, Greco FA: Cisplatin-based combination chemotherapy in the treatment of poorly differentiated carcinoma and poorly differentiated adenocarcinoma of unknown primary site: Results of a 12-year experience. J Clin Oncol 10:912–922, 1992.

Large series documenting the efficacy of cisplatin-based regimens in patients with poorly differentiated carcinoma involving the mediastinum and other sites.

Jain KK, Bosl GJ, Bains MS, et al: The treatment of extragonadal seminoma. J Clin Oncol 2:820–827, 1984.

Retrospective comparison is of radiotherapy versus chemotherapy in mediastinal seminoma.

Lewis BD, Hurt RD, Payne WS, et al: Benign teratomas of the mediastinum. J Thorac Cardiovasc Surg 86:727–731, 1983.

This large review is of clinical, pathologic, and therapeutic aspects of benign teratoma of the mediastinum.

Nichols CR, Saxman S, Williams SD, et al: Primary mediastinal nonseminomatous germ cell tumors: A modern single institution experience. Cancer 65:1641–1646, 1990.

Largest series of mediastinal nonseminomatous germ cell tumors treated with modern chemotherapy regimens.

REFERENCES

1. Sabiston DC Jr, Scott HW Jr: Primary neoplasms and cysts of the mediastinum. Ann Surg 136:777–797, 1952.
2. Heimburger I, Battersby JS, Vellios F: Primary neoplasms of the mediastinum: A 15 year follow-up. Arch Surg 86:978–984, 1963.
3. Ringertz N, Lidholm SO: Mediastinal tumors and cysts. J Thorac Surg 31:458–487, 1956.
4. Rubush JL, Gardner IR, Boyd WC, et al: Mediastinal tumors: Review of 186 cases. J Thorac Cardiovasc Surg 65:216–222, 1973.
5. Wychulis AR, Payne WS, Clagett OT, et al: Surgical treatment of mediastinal tumors. J Thorac Cardiovasc Surg 62:379–391, 1971.
6. LeRoux BT: Mediastinal teratomata. Thorax 15:333–338, 1960.
7. Lewis BD, Hurt RD, Payne WS, et al: Benign teratomas of the mediastinum. J Thorac Cardiovasc Surg 86:727–731, 1983.
8. Adebonojo SA, Nicola ML: Teratoid tumors of the mediastinum. Am Surg 42:361–365, 1976.
9. Weinberg B, Rose JS, Efremidis SC, et al: Posterior mediastinal teratoma (cystic dermoid): Diagnosis by computerized tomography. Chest 77:694–695, 1980.
10. Philip WP, Harrison K, Cruickshank DB: A posterior mediastinal dermoid tumor with marked anatomical differentiation. Thorax 9:245–247, 1954.
11. Pachter MR, Lattes R: "Germinal" tumors of the mediastinum: A clinicopathologic study of adult teratomas, teratocarcinomas, choriocarcinomas and seminomas. Chest 45:301–310, 1964.
12. Kantrowitz AR: Extragenital chorionepithelioma in a male. Am J Pathol 10:531–543, 1934.
13. Laipply TC, Shipley RA: Extragenital choriocarcinoma in the male. Am J Pathol 21:921–933, 1945.
14. Caes HJ, Cragg RW: Extragenital choriocarcinoma of the male with bilateral gynecomastia: Report of a case. US Navy Med Bull 47:1072–1077, 1947.
15. Friedman NB: The comparative morphogenesis of extragenital and gonadal teratoid tumors. Cancer 4:265–276, 1951.
16. Schlumberger HG: Teratoma of anterior mediastinum in a group of military age: Study of 16 cases and review of theories of genesis. Arch Pathol 41:398–444, 1946.
17. Fine F, Smith RW Jr, Pachter MR: Primary extragenital choriocarcinoma in the male subject: Case report and review of the literature. Am J Med 32:776–794, 1962.
18. Meares EM, Briggs EM: Occult seminoma of the testis masquerading as primary extragonadal germinal neoplasm. Cancer 30:300–306, 1972.
19. Azzopardi JG, Mostofi FK, Theiss EA: Lesions of testes ob-

20. served in certain patients with widespread choriocarcinoma and related tumors. Am J Pathol 38:207–225, 1961.
20. Rather LJ, Gardiner WR, Frericks JB: Regression and maturation of primary testicular tumors with progressive growth of metastases: Report of six new cases and review of literature. Stanford Med Bull 12:12–25, 1954.
21. Oberman HA, Libcke JH: Malignant germinal neoplasms of the mediastinum. Cancer 17:498–507, 1964.
22. Johnson DE, Laneri JP, Mountain CF, Luna M: Extragonadal germ cell tumors. Surgery 73:85–90, 1973.
23. Cox JD: Primary malignant germinal tumors of the mediastinum. Cancer 36:1162–1168, 1975.
24. Luna MA, Valenzuela-Tamariz J: Germ-cell tumors of the mediastinum: Postmortem findings. Am J Clin Pathol 65:450–454, 1976.
25. Luna MA, Johnson DE: Postmortem findings in testicular tumors. In Johnson DE (ed): Testicular Tumors. New York, Medical Examination Publishing Co, 1975.
26. Lynch MJG, Blewitt GL: Choriocarcinoma arising in the male mediastinum. Thorax 8:157–161, 1953.
27. Nefzger MD, Mostofi FK: Survival after surgery for germinal malignancies of the testis: I. Rates of survival in tumor groups. Cancer 30:1225–1232, 1972.
28. Willis GW, Hajdu SI: Histologically benign teratoid metastasis of testicular embryonal carcinoma: Report of five cases. Am J Clin Pathol 59:338–343, 1973.
29. Hodge J, Aponte G, McLaughlin E: Primary mediastinal tumors. J Thorax Surg 37:730–744, 1959.
30. Boyd DP, Midell AI: Mediastinal cysts and tumors: An analysis of 96 cases. Surg Clin North Am 48:493–505, 1968.
31. Collins DH, Pugh RCB: Classification and frequency of testicular tumors. Br J Urol 36(suppl):1–11, 1964.
32. Surveillance, epidemiology and end results: Incidence and mortality data, 1973–77. Natl Cancer Inst Monograph 57:178–179, 1981.
33. Einhorn LH, Williams SD: Management of disseminated testicular cancer. In Einhorn LH (ed): Testicular Tumors: Management and Treatment. New York, Masson Publishing, 1980, pp 117–151.
34. Lattes R: Seminoma (dysgerminoma) of the thymus. Cancer Semin 2:221–224, 1961.
35. Richardson RL, Schoumacher RA, Fer MF, et al: The unrecognized extragonadal germ cell cancer syndrome. Ann Intern Med 94:181–186, 1981.
36. Fox RM, Woods RL, Tattersall MHN: Undifferentiated carcinoma in young men: The atypical teratoma syndrome. Lancet 1:1316–1318, 1979.
37. Greco FA, Vaughn WK, Hainsworth JD: Advanced poorly differentiated carcinoma of unknown primary site: Recognition of a treatable syndrome. Ann Intern Med 104:547–556, 1986.
38. Adkins RB Jr, Maples MD, Hainsworth JD: Primary malignant mediastinal tumors. Ann Thorac Surg 38:648–659, 1984.
39. Martini N, Golbey RB, Hajdu SI, et al: Primary mediastinal germ cell tumors. Cancer 33:763–769, 1974.
40. Knapp RH, Hurt RD, Payne WS, et al: Malignant germ cell tumors of the mediastinum. J Thorac Cardiovasc Surg 89:82–89, 1985.
41. El-Domeiri AA, Hutter RVP, Pool JL, et al: Primary seminoma of the anterior mediastinum. Ann Thorac Surg 6:513–521, 1968.
42. Polansky SM, Barwick KW, Ravin CE: Primary mediastinal seminoma. Am J Radiol 132:17–21, 1979.
43. Kersh CR, Hazru TA: Mediastinal germinoma: Two cases. Virginia Med 112:42–44, 1985.
44. Sandhaus L, Strom RL, Mukai K: Primary embryonal-choriocarcinoma of the mediastinum in a woman: A case report with immunohistochemical study. Am J Clin Pathol 75:573–578, 1981.
45. Poison B: Embryonal teratocarcinoma of the mediastinum in a woman with foci of anaplastic cells simulating choriocarcinoma. Chest 58:169–172, 1970.
46. Fanger H, MacAndrew R: Extragenital chorionepithelioma in a female arising from a mediastinal teratoma. Rhode Island Med J 35:259–260, 1952.
47. Hainsworth JD, Einhorn LH, Williams SD, et al: Advanced extragonadal germ cell tumors: Successful treatment with combination chemotherapy. Ann Intern Med 97:7–11, 1982.

48. Economou JS, Trump DL, Holmes EC, et al: Management of primary germ cell tumors of the mediastinum. J Thorac Cardiovasc Surg 83:643–648, 1982.

49. Logothetis CJ, Samuels ML, Selig DE, et al: Chemotherapy of extragonadal germ cell tumors. J Clin Oncol 3:316–325, 1985.

50. Kountz SL, Connolly JE, Cohn R: Seminoma-like (or seminomatous) tumors of the anterior mediastinum. J Thorac Cardiovasc Surg 45:289–301, 1963.

51. Bagshaw MA, McLaughlin WT, Earle JD: Definitive radiotherapy of primary mediastinal seminoma. Am J Radiol Radiother Biophys 105:86–94, 1969.

52. Schantz A, Sewall W, Castleman B: Mediastinal germinoma: A study of 21 cases with an excellent prognosis. Cancer 30:1189–1194, 1972.

53. Hurt RD, Bruckman JE, Farrow GM, et al: Primary anterior mediastinal seminoma. Cancer 49:1658–1663, 1982.

54. Jain KK, Bosl GJ, Bains MS, et al: The treatment of extragonadal seminoma. J Clin Oncol 2:820–827, 1984.

55. Levitt RG, Husband JE, Glazer HS: CT of primary germ cell tumors of the mediastinum. Am J Roentgenol 142:73–78, 1984.

56. Israel A, Bosl GJ, Golbey RB, et al: The results of chemotherapy for extragonadal germ cell tumors in the cisplatin era: The Memorial Sloan-Kettering Cancer Center experience (1975 to 1982). J Clin Oncol 3:1073–1078, 1985.

57. Sickles EA, Belliveau RF, Wiernik PH: Primary mediastinal choriocarcinoma in the male. Cancer 33:1196–1203, 1974.

58. Scheike D, Visfeldt J, Petersen B: Male breast cancer: 3. Breast carcinoma in association with the Klinefelter syndrome. Acta Pathol Microbiol Scand 81:352–358, 1973.

59. Richenstein LJ: Tumors of the Central Nervous System. Washington, DC: Armed Forces Institute of Pathology, 2nd series, fasc. 6, 1972, p 270.

60. Doll DC, Weiss RB, Evans H: Klinefelter's syndrome and extragenital seminoma. J Urol 116:675–676, 1976.

61. Sogge MR, McDonald SD, Cofold PB: The malignant potential of the dysgenetic germ cell in Klinefelter's syndrome. Am J Med 66:515–518, 1979.

62. Storm PB, Fallon B, Burge RG: Mediastinal choriocarcinoma in a chromatin-positive boy. J Urol 116:838–840, 1976.

63. Floret D, Renaud H, Monnet P: Sexual precocity and thoracic polyembryoma: Klinefelter syndrome? J Pediatr 94:163, 1979.

64. Curry WA, McKay CE, Richardson RL, et al: Klinefelter's syndrome and mediastinal germ cell neoplasms. J Urol 125:127–129, 1981.

65. McNeil MM, Leong AS, Sage RE: Primary mediastinal embryonal carcinoma in association with Klinefelter's syndrome. Cancer 47:343–345, 1981.

66. Turner AR, MacDonald RN: Mediastinal germ cell cancers in Klinefelter's syndrome. Ann Intern Med 94:279, 1981.

67. Chaussain JL, Lemerle J, Roger M, et al: Klinefelter syndrome, tumor and sexual precocity. J Pediatr 97:607–609, 1980.

68. Danon M, Weintraub BD, Kim SH, et al: Sexual precocity in a male due to thoracic polyembryoma. J Pediatr 92:51–53, 1978.

69. Weetman AP, Borysiewicz LK: Androgen production in a patient with Klinefelter's syndrome and choriocarcinoma. Br Med J 2:585–586, 1980.

70. Schimke RN, Madigan CM, Silver BJ, et al: Choriocarcinoma, thyrotoxicosis and the Klinefelter syndrome. Cancer Genet Cytogenet 9:1–8, 1983.

71. Nichols CR, Heerema NA, Palmer C, et al: Klinefelter's syndrome associated with mediastinal germ cell neoplasms. J Clin Oncol 5:1290–1294, 1987.

72. Isurugi K, Imao S, Hirose K, et al: Seminoma in Klinefelter's syndrome with 42, XXY, 15s+/karyotype. Cancer 39:2041–2047, 1977.

73. Gustavson KH, Gamstorp I, Meurling S: Bilateral teratoma of testis in two brothers with 47, XXY Klinefelter's syndrome. Clin Genet 8:5–10, 1975.

74. Kock F: The occurrence of sex chromatin in testicular tumors. Acta Pathol Microbiol Scand 70:45–49, 1970.

75. Martineau M: Chromosomes in human testicular tumours. J Pathol 99:271–282, 1969.

76. Hsueh Y, Tsung SH, Shamsai R, et al: Primary mediastinal choriocarcinoma in a man with an abnormal chromosome. South Med J 77:1466–1469, 1984.

77. Nichols CR, Roth B, Heerema N, et al: Hematologic neoplasia associated with primary mediastinal germ cell tumors: An update. N Engl J Med 322:1425–1429, 1990.

78. Sandberg AA, Abe S, Kowalczyk JR, et al: Chromosomes and causation of human cancer and leukemia: I. Cytogenetics of leukemias complicating other diseases. Cancer Genet Cytogenet 7:95–136, 1982.

79. Sales LM, Vontz FK: Teratoma and diGuglielmo syndrome. South Med J 63:448–450, 1970.

80. Larsen M, Evans WK, Shepherd FA, et al: Acute lymphoblastic leukemia: Possible origin from a mediastinal germ cell tumor. Cancer 53:441–444, 1984.

81. Johnson DC, Luedke DW, Sapiente RA, et al: Acute lymphocystic leukemia developing in a male with germ cell carcinoma: A case report. Med Pediatr Oncol 8:361–365, 1980.

82. Hoekman K, TenBokkelHuinink WW, Egers-Bogaards MA, et al: Acute leukemia following therapy for teratoma. Eur J Cancer Clin Oncol 20:501–502, 1984.

83. Feun LG, Samson MK, Stephens RL: Vinblastine (VLB), bleomycin (BLEO), cisdiamminedichloroplatinum (DDP) in disseminated extragonadal germ cell tumors: A Southwest Oncology Group study. Cancer 45:2543–2549, 1980.

84. Redman JR, Vugrin D, Arlin AZ, et al: Leukemia following treatment of germ cell tumors in men. J Clin Oncol 2:1080–1087, 1984.

85. Chaganti RSK, Landanyi M, Samaniego F: Leukemic differentiation of a mediastinal germ cell tumor. Genes Chromosomes Cancer 1:63–67, 1969.

86. Landanyi M, Samaniego F, Reuter VE, et al: Cytogenetic and immunohistochemical evidence for the germ cell origin of a subset of acute leukemias associated with mediastinal germ cell tumors. J Natl Cancer Inst 82:221–227, 1990.

87. Bosl GJ, Dmitrovsky E, Reuter V, et al: i(12p): A specific karyotypic abnormality in germ cell tumors. (Abstract.) Proc Am Soc Clin Oncol 8:131, 1989.

88. Ulbright TM, Loehrer PJ, Roth LM, et al: The development of non-germ cell malignancies within germ cell tumors: A clinicopathologic study of 11 cases. Cancer 54:1824–1833, 1984.

89. Garnick MB, Griffin JD: Idiopathic thrombocytopenia in association with extragonadal germ cell cancer. Ann Intern Med 98:926–927, 1983.

90. Helman LJ, Ozols RF, Longo DL: Thrombocytopenia and extragonadal germ cell neoplasm. Ann Intern Med 101:280, 1984.

91. Myers TJ, Kessimian N, Schwartz S: Mediastinal germ cell tumor associated with the hemophagocytic syndrome. Ann Intern Med 109:504–505, 1988.

92. Lattes R: Thymoma and other tumors of thymus: Analysis of 107 cases. Cancer 15:1224–1260, 1962.

93. Inada K, Kawasaki A, Hamazaki M: Germinoma of mediastinum: A critical review of classification of thymic neoplasms. Am Rev Resp Dis 87:560–567, 1963.

94. Besznyak I, Sebesteny M, Kuchar F: Primary mediastinal seminoma: A case report and review of the literature. J Thorac Cardiovasc Surg 65:930–934, 1973.

95. Pugsley WS, Carleton RL: Germinal nature of teratoid tumors of thymus. AMA Arch Pathol 56:341–347, 1953.

96. Woolner LB, Jamplis RW, Kirklin JW: Seminoma (germinoma) apparently primary in anterior mediastinum. N Engl J Med 252:653–657, 1955.

97. Iverson L: Thymoma: A review and classification. Am J Pathol 32:695–720, 1956.

98. Effler DB, McCormack LJ: Thymic neoplasms. J Thorac Surg 31:60–82, 1956.

99. Robinson BW: Germinal neoplasia of extragenital origin. J Natl Med Assoc 52:162–165, 1960.

100. Nazari A, Gagnon ED: Seminoma-like tumor of mediastinum: Case report. J Thorac Cardiovasc Surg 51:751–754, 1966.

101. Nickels J, Franssila K: Primary seminoma of the anterior mediastinum. Acta Pathol Microbiol Scand 80A:260–262, 1972.

102. Medini E, Levitt SH, Jones TK, et al: The management of extratesticular seminoma without gonadal involvement. Cancer 44:2032–2038, 1979.

103. Raghavan D, Barrett A: Mediastinal seminomas. Cancer 46:1187–1191, 1980.

104. Bush SE, Martinez A, Bagshaw MA: Primary mediastinal seminoma. Cancer 48:1877–1882, 1981.

105. Sterchi M, Cordell AR: Seminoma of the anterior mediastinum. Ann Thorac Surg 19:371–377, 1975.

106. Aygun C, Slawson RG, Bajaj K, et al: Primary mediastinal seminoma. Urology 23:109–117, 1984.

107. Einhorn LH, Williams SD: Chemotherapy of disseminated seminoma. Cancer Clin Trials 3:307–313, 1980.

108. Stanton GF, Bosl GJ, Whitmore WF Jr: VAB-6 as initial treatment of patients with advanced seminoma. J Clin Oncol 3:336–339, 1985.

109. van Hoesel QGCM, Piredo HM: Complete remission of mediastinal germ cell tumors with cis-dichlorodiammineplatinum (II) combination chemotherapy. Cancer Treat Rep 64:319–321, 1980.

110. Daugaard G, Rorth M, Hansen HH: Therapy of extragonadal germ cell tumors. Eur J Clin Oncol 19:895–899, 1983.

111. Clamon GH, River G, Loening S, et al: Successful treatment of mediastinal seminoma with vinblastine, bleomycin, and cisplatinum. Urology 22:640–642, 1983.

112. Loehrer PJ, Birch R, Williams SD, et al: Chemotherapy of metastatic seminoma: The Southeastern Cancer Study Group experience. J Clin Oncol 5:1212–1220, 1987.

113. Bukowski RM, Wolf M, Kulander BG, et al: Alternating combination chemotherapy in patients with extragonadal germ cell tumors. Cancer 71:2631–2638, 1993.

114. Schultz SM, Einhorn LH, Conces DJ, et al: Management of post-chemotherapy residual mass in patients with advanced seminoma: Indiana University experience. J Clin Oncol 7:1497–1503, 1989.

115. Peckham MJ, Horwich A, Hendry WF: Advanced seminoma: Treatment with cisplatinum-based combination chemotherapy or carboplatin. Br J Cancer 52:7–13, 1985.

116. Srougi M, Simon SD, Menezes de Goes G: Vinblastine, actinomycin-D, bleomycin, cyclophosphamide, and cisplatin for advanced germ cell testis tumors: Brazilian experience. J Urol 134:65–69, 1985.

117. Motzer R, Bosl G, Heclan R, et al: Residual mass: An indication for further therapy in patients with advanced seminoma following systemic chemotherapy. J Clin Oncol 5:1064–1070, 1987.

118. Williams SD, Birch R, Einhorn LH, et al: Treatment of disseminated germ cell tumors with cisplatin, bleomycin, and either vinblastine or etoposide. N Engl J Med 316:1435–1440, 1987.

119. Funes HC, Mendez M, Alonso E, et al: Mediastinal germ cell tumors treated with cisplatin, bleomycin and vinblastine (PVB). (Abstract.) Proc Am Assoc Cancer Res 22:474, 1981.

120. Vogelzang NJ, Raghavan D, Anderson RW, et al: Mediastinal nonseminomatous germ cell tumors: The role of combined modality therapy. Ann Thorac Surg 33:333–339, 1982.

121. Newlands ES, Begent RHJ, Rustin GJS, et al: Further advances in the management of malignant teratomas of the testis and other sites. Lancet 1:948–951, 1983.

122. Garnick MB, Canellos GP, Richie JP: Treatment and surgical staging of testicular and primary extragonadal germ cell cancer. JAMA 250:1733–1741, 1983.

123. Kay PH, Wells FC, Goldstraw P: A multi-disciplinary approach to primary nonseminomatous germ cell tumors of the mediastinum. Ann Thorac Surg 44:578–582, 1987.

124. McLeod DG, Taylor HG, Skoog SJ, et al: Extragonadal germ cell tumors: Clinicopathologic findings and treatment experience in 12 patients. Cancer 61:1187–1191, 1988.

125. Sham JST, Fu KH, Chiu CSW, et al: Experience with the management of primary endodermal sinus tumor of the mediastinum. Cancer 64:756–761, 1989.

126. Nichols CR, Saxman S, Williams SD, et al: Primary mediastinal nonseminomatous germ cell tumors: A modern single institution experience. Cancer 65:1641–1646, 1990.

127. Einhorn LH: Testicular cancer as a model for a curable neoplasm: The Richard and Hilda Rosenthal Foundation Award Lecture. Cancer Res 41:3275–3280, 1981.

128. Hainsworth JD, Williams SD, Einhorn LH, et al: Successful treatment of resistant germinal neoplasms with VP16 and cisplatin: Results of a Southeastern Cancer Study Group Trial. J Clin Oncol 3:666–671, 1985.

129. Loehrer PJ, Laver R, Roth BJ, et al: Salvage therapy in recurrent germ cell cancer: Ifosfamide and cisplatin plus either vinblastine or etoposide. Ann Intern Med 109:540–546, 1988.

130. Broun ER, Nichols CR, Kneebone P, et al: Long-term outcome of patients with relapsed and refractory germ cell tumors treated with high-dose chemotherapy and autologous bone marrow rescue. Ann Intern Med 117:124–128, 1992.

131. Kuzur ME, Cobleigh MA, Greco FA, et al: Endodermal sinus tumor of the mediastinum. Cancer 50:766–774, 1982.

132. Richardson RL, Greco FA, Wolff S, et al: Extra-gonadal germ cell malignancy: Value of tumor markers in metastatic carcinoma in young males. (Abstract.) Proc Am Assoc Cancer Res 20:204, 1979.

133. Hainsworth JD, Johnson DH, Greco FA: Cisplatin-based combination chemotherapy in the treatment of poorly differentiated carcinoma and poorly differentiated adenocarcinoma of unknown primary site: Results of a 12-year experience. J Clin Oncol 10:912–922, 1992.

134. Motzer RJ, Rodriguez E, Reuter VE, et al: Genetic analysis as an aid in diagnosis for patients with midline carcinoma of uncertain histologies. J Natl Cancer Inst 83:341–346, 1991.

30 MALIGNANT TUMORS INVOLVING THE HEART AND PERICARDIUM

Stephen A. Mills, Geoffrey M. Graeber, and Mark G. Nelson

CARDIAC AND PERICARDIAL TUMORS

Cardiac and pericardial malignant tumors are rare forms of heart disease. Despite this fact, many cardiologists and cardiothoracic surgeons will at some time encounter a patient with one of these two conditions. A high index of clinical suspicion is necessary for diagnosis. It is hoped that this review will be helpful to the clinician encountering either of these unusual tumors.

HISTORICAL ASPECTS

Cardiac tumors have been recognized since the report by Colombus in 1562.[1] In 1934, Barnes and associates[2] made the clinical diagnosis of a primary sarcoma of the heart. In 1942, Beck[3] removed an intrapericardial teratoma. Maurer[4] performed the first successful resection of a cardiac tumor. Angiocardiography was first used clinically in the demonstration of an intracardiac myxoma in 1951,[5] and in 1952, Crawford and associates[6] first used extracorporeal circulation for removal of a left atrial myxoma.

INCIDENCE

In two large postmortem series,[7, 8] primary tumors of the heart occurred in only 0.0017% to 0.03% of patients. Approximately 75% of all cardiac tumors are benign, and two-thirds of these benign tumors are myxomas.[9] Although modern techniques of diagnosis and surgical treatment have changed the benign cardiac tumor from a curiosity found at postmortem examination to an almost uniformly curable form of heart disease, unfortunately the same cannot be said for malignant cardiac tumors, which are more rare and almost always fatal.

In a 1979 Armed Forces Institute of Pathology (AFIP) review of 533 primary tumors and cysts of the heart and pericardium, approximately one-fourth of all tumors and cysts were malignant.[10] The type and occurrence rate of the 125 tumors that were malignant are shown in Table 30–1. Malignant tumors are rare in the pediatric age group, accounting for fewer than 10% of all tumors and cysts of the heart and pericardium in the AFIP series.[10]

CLINICAL SIGNS AND SYMPTOMS

Selzer and associates[11] noted that the clinical manifestations of cardiac tumors are protean. Cardiac tumors produce symptoms as a result of their mass effect, local invasion, embolization, and systemic constitutional manifestations. In a 1968 review of the clinical aspects of cardiac tumors, Harvey[12] suggested that the diagnosis be considered in any patient with one or a combination of the following symptom complexes.

Pericardial Involvement. Malignant infiltration of the pericardium can produce pericarditis with accompanying effusion and tamponade. The pericardium may become noncompliant, and the clinical picture may be indistinguishable from that of constrictive pericarditis from some other cause.

Congestive Heart Failure. The mass effect of an intracavitary tumor can obstruct blood flow to cardiac chambers or interfere with cardiac valvular function. Depending on the chamber and valve involved, the patient may develop syncope, angina, dyspnea,

TABLE 30–1. Malignant Tumors of the Heart and Pericardium

TYPE	NO.	%
Angiosarcoma	39	31.2
Rhabdomyosarcoma	26	20.8
Mesothelioma	19	15.2
Fibrosarcoma	14	11.2
Malignant lymphoma	7	5.6
Extraskeletal osteosarcoma	5	
Neurogenic sarcoma	4	
Malignant teratoma	4	
Thymoma	4	16.0
Leiomyosarcoma	1	
Liposarcoma	1	
Synovial sarcoma	1	
TOTAL	125	

From McAllister HA, Fenoglio JJ: Tumors of the cardiovascular system. *In* Atlas of Tumor Pathology, 2nd Series, Fascicle 15. Washington, DC, Armed Forces Institute of Pathology, 1978.

edema, ascites, and murmurs suggestive of valvular stenosis or incompetence. Myocardial infiltration by tumor may result in congestive heart failure similar to that of a cardiomyopathy.

Pulmonary Hypertension. Pulmonary hypertension often occurs as the result of pulmonary venous hypertension due to left heart obstruction by the tumor mass; rarely, elevated pulmonary artery pressures may be caused by tumor, emboli, or obstruction of the pulmonary artery. Embolization is commonly associated with left atrial myxoma but may occur with malignant cardiac tumors.

Dysrhythmias. Recurrent supraventricular or ventricular tachycardia, most likely due to irritation by an infiltrative tumor, may be the first sign of a malignant cardiac tumor or metastatic cardiac disease. Uncommonly, heart block and Stokes-Adams attacks may result.

Chest Pain. Chest pain is a common manifestation of malignant tumor. In rare instances, the pain may be the result of myocardial ischemia due to tumor embolization of the coronary arteries[13] or to extrinsic compression of the myocardial vessels, as was noted by Isner and associates[14] in a patient in whom a cardiac sarcoma simulated coronary artery disease.

Constitutional Symptoms. A variety of constitutional symptoms, including fever, malaise, weight loss, polymyositis, hepatic dysfunction, Raynaud's phenomenon, hyperglobulinemia, and an elevated erythrocyte sedimentation rate, have been described with both benign and malignant tumors but are more commonly associated with left atrial myxoma. Their cause is not known. Berkelbach van der Sprenkel and associates[15] reported the case of a 27-year-old woman whose polyarthritis was the presenting symptom and for 5 months the sole manifestation of a malignant fibrous histiocytoma of the heart. Signs of congestive heart failure then developed, leading to the diagnosis. Partial resection led to complete disappearance of joint symptoms. Further growth of the tumor was preceded by polyarthritis, and the patient died 6 months after surgery.

Hematologic Abnormalities. Polycythemia may be seen with right atrial tumors and is probably a response to tricuspid valve obstruction, elevation of right atrial pressure, and right-to-left shunting through a foramen ovale. Anemia and thrombocytosis were commonly seen in the Cleveland Clinic experience.[16]

DIAGNOSIS

Radiography. When the tumor contains calcium, the chest roentgenogram shows direct evidence of a cardiac tumor. Otherwise, the chest roentgenogram may be useful in reflecting the hemodynamic consequence of the tumor, such as pulmonary venous blood flow obstruction or obstruction of a valvular orifice.

Electrocardiography. The electrocardiogram, of course, provides only indirect evidence of a cardiac tumor. It may reveal enlargement of a cardiac chamber, or, more often, disturbances in rhythm such as atrial fibrillation.

Pohost and associates[17] have used gated radionuclide cardiac imaging to detect left atrial myxomas.

Cardiac Catheterization. Cardiac catheterization may result in tumor embolization. Although no reports of embolization of a malignant tumor following cardiac catheterization have been recorded, Pindyck and associates[18] reported embolization of a left atrial myxoma occurring after transseptal cardiac catheterization. In addition, intracavitary filling defects shown by angiography may represent thrombus, hematoma, or abscess or may be otherwise falsely positive. Pressure measurements are of great diagnostic help in assessing the functional status of the cardiac valves and heart. A mobile tumor may cause spontaneous variations in the end-diastolic gradient across a cardiac valve, probably due to movement of the tumor, which may result in varying degrees of valvular obstruction. An example of angiographic demonstration of a malignant tumor is given in Figure 30–1.

Major angiographic criteria for cardiac tumors are compression or displacement of cardiac chambers and great vessels, deformity of cardiac chambers, intracavitary filling defects, marked variation in myocardial thickness, pericardial effusion, and local alteration in myocardial wall motion.[19]

Echocardiography. The most valuable diagnostic tool in the imaging of a cardiac tumor, whether primary or metastatic, is echocardiography. Kutalek and associates[20] and Bulkley and Hutchins[21] have shown that it is the major contributing factor in the increasing accuracy of preoperative diagnosis of these tumors. The use of two-dimensional echocardiography for visualization of cardiac tumors has largely supplanted standard M-mode echocardiography because with two-dimensional echocardiography, the tumor size, shape, and motion as well as the cardiac function, both muscular and valvular, can usually be well documented. The two-dimensional echocardiogram will, in the vast majority of cases, provide information sufficient to avoid cardiac catheterization before any invasive diagnostic or therapeutic procedure (Fig. 30–2). The two-dimensional echocardiogram may also be valuable in assessing the response of a cardiac tumor to irradiation or chemotherapy. In patients with proven noninfective cardiac masses, precordial echocardiography was equally effective as transesophageal echocardiography (TEE) in the detection of left and right atrial myxomas. TEE was superior in identifying the tumor attachment point and additional morphological details such as cysts,[22] and in identifying masses located anterior to the heart or that had invaded the superior vena cava, pulmonary artery, or

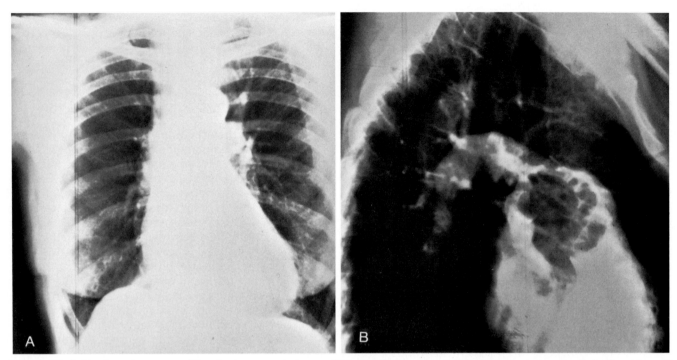

FIGURE 30–1. Chest roentgenogram *(A)* and pulmonary arteriogram *(B)* from following case. A 65-year-old woman presented with a 10-month history of dizziness and shortness of breath accompanied by intermittent episodes of cyanosis. On admission, a harsh pansystolic murmur was heard over the pericardium. The arterial blood gas value demonstrated on room air was 30 mm Hg. Chest roentgenogram showed the left pulmonary artery hilus to be displaced superiorly. A pulmonary arteriogram showed a large lobulated mass lesion in the outflow tract of the right ventricle and extending into the main and right pulmonary arteries. At surgery, the mass could be seen to involve the ventricular wall and to extend to the bifurcation of the main pulmonary artery; it was anchored to the pulmonary valve annulus and had destroyed the posterior valve leaflet. Histologic examination of the tumor showed it to be an undifferentiated sarcoma. (Courtesy of P.R.S. Kishore, M.D., Medical College of Virginia, Virginia Commonwealth University, Richmond.)

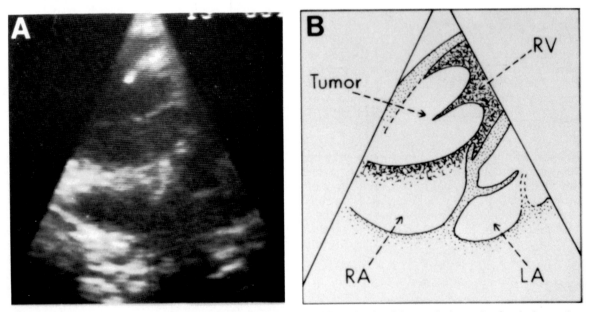

FIGURE 30–2. *A,* Two-dimensional echocardiogram of a primary lymphoma obliterating the right ventricular cavity. Surgical resection and adjuvant chemotherapy produced complete remission. *B,* Diagrammatic illustration of *A.* (RV = right ventricle; RA = right atrium; LA = left atrium.) (Courtesy of Joseph A. Kisslo, M.D., Duke University Medical Center, Durham.)

descending thoracic aorta.[22] TEE used in the follow-up of patients who have undergone excision of atrial myxoma demonstrated recurrent tumor in two of 14 patients that had been undetected in one patient by the precordial approach.[23] Despite the excellent sensitivity of TEE, it cannot displace computed tomography (CT) or magnetic resonance imaging (MRI) in planning the surgical approach because information concerning tumor extent and tissue characterization is often limited. In the operating room, TEE allows continuous monitoring of valve function and can aid in deciding between valve repair and replacement. In addition, the removal of renal cell tumor from the atrium and inferior vena cava can be monitored.

Computed Tomography. A CT scan of the chest can be of great value in documenting a primary cardiac tumor and can provide important information regarding regional invasiveness or lymph node metastases (Fig. 30–3). The cardiac chambers and interventricular septum are routinely demonstrated after injection of a bolus of contrast medium. In five patients with intracardiac tumors, each tumor and its relationship to the cardiac chambers, myocardial invasion, pericardial effusions, and lymphadenopathy were demonstrated with CT.[24] Reports of CT imaging of tumors that metastasized to the heart are isolated.[25]

Magnetic Resonance Imaging. MRI can define anatomic relationships and tissue characteristics and is a powerful noninvasive tool for evaluating suspected cardiac mass lesions.[26] Pizzarello and associates[27] used MRI to successfully visualize cardiac metastases from a liposarcoma. The images obtained compared favorably with a two-dimensional echocardiographic study and a postmortem examination. Fatty tissue is differ-

ent than other soft tissues in its relaxation time and spin density. Fatty cardiac tumors (lipomas and liposarcomas) can be identified with MRI. Becker and associates[28] used MRI to accurately localize an intracardiac rhabdomyosarcoma. Cine MRI can differentiate between stagnant blood and thrombus. In two patients with tuberous sclerosis, MRI was used to demonstrate three additional masses that had not been detected with two-dimensional echocardiography (one lipoma and two rhabdomyomas).[29] Examples of cardiac tumors demonstrated with MRI are given in Figures 30–4 and 30–5.

PRIMARY MALIGNANT TUMORS

Angiosarcoma

Angiosarcoma is the most frequently occurring primary malignant cardiac tumor, and it occurs two to three times more often in men than in women. All 39 patients with angiosarcoma in the AFIP series reported by McAllister[10] were young adults, ranging in age from 15 to 26 years.

Thirty of the 39 patients (77%) had clinical findings of right-sided heart failure or pericardial disease, including congestive heart failure, pericardial effusion, dyspnea, and pleuritic chest pain. Four, however, had had symptoms suggestive of malignancy (fever, weight loss, and malaise) before the onset of their cardiac symptoms. In six patients with evidence of right-sided heart failure, both systolic murmurs and atrial dysrhythmias were present. Eleven of the patients had distant metastases: in three, the metastases were confined to the central nervous system; in all others, there was local spread of the tumor to the adjacent pleura, the mediastinum, or both. Thirty-one

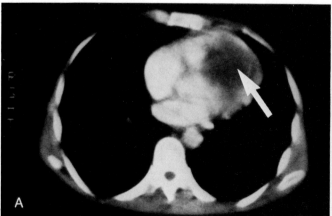
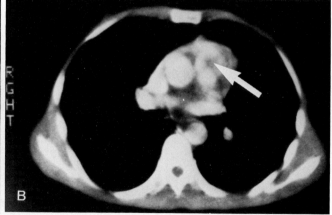

FIGURE 30–3. Cardiac computed tomographic scans from a 51-year-old man who 18 months earlier had been treated with a right radical neck dissection and radiation therapy for a squamous cell carcinoma of the right pharyngeal wall. Admission reports consisted of persistent chest pain, weakness, and anorexia. An electrocardiogram demonstrated markedly elevated ST segments in the anterior leads. Auscultation demonstrated a Grade III/VI systolic murmur along the left sternal border radiating into the pulmonic area. Chest roentgenogram showed a questionable calcium deposit in the pericardium of right ventricle. The tomograms demonstrate A, a large irregularly shaped filling defect involving the anterior part of the interventricular septum at the apex of the right ventricle (arrow), and B, extension of the filling defect into the right ventricle outflow tract and proximal portion of the main pulmonary artery (arrow). The filling defect was believed most likely to represent metastatic tumor. Cardiac catheterization confirmed the presence of a multilobulated filling defect occupying the entire right ventricular outflow tract with protrusion of this mass toward the pulmonary artery during systole. Autopsy confirmed the presence of squamous cell carcinoma in the right ventricle.

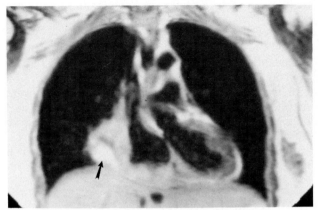

FIGURE 30–4. ECG-gated spin echo coronal MRI scan through the mid right atrium. There is an ill-defined mass along the right lateral and diaphragmatic aspects of the right atrium, which extends into the right lung. The irregular border and the obliteration of the pericardium are in keeping with a malignant tumor. The bright signal *(arrow)* within the right inferior aspect of the mass is due to subacute blood from a previous needle biopsy. The tumor was an angiosarcoma. (Courtesy of K. Link, M.D.)

of the 39 patients (79%) had tumors in the right atrium or pericardium. In the other eight patients, the angiosarcoma was intracavitary and obstructed the orifice of a valve—most often, the tricuspid valve, and less often, the pulmonary valve or mitral valve. An example is given in Figure 30–6.

Microscopically, cardiac angiosarcomas are composed of malignant cells forming vascular channels. There is considerable histologic variation within the same tumor. The vascular channels can vary markedly in size and configuration; pleomorphism and anaplasia can be marked, and mitoses are usual. Most angiosarcomas will contain foci of solid areas and spindle cells, but occasionally they are composed entirely of sheets of anaplastic or spindle cells. The most reliable indicators of angiosarcoma are anastomosing vascular channels, foci of endothelial tufting, and spindle cell areas.

Although cardiac angiosarcomas are commonly subclassified on the basis of microscopic appearance, their clinical courses and prognoses appear to be identical, irrespective of subclassification. The pericardial effusion associated with angiosarcoma involving the pericardium may wax and wane spontaneously, as it may with other malignant tumors of the pericardium, whether primary or secondary. Thus, spontaneous resorption of pericardial effusion does not exclude the possibility of malignant tumor.[30] A bone marrow may establish the diagnosis.

The prognosis for patients with cardiac angiosarcoma is grave; most patients die within 1 year of onset of symptoms. Radiation and chemotherapy are of only limited value.[31–33]

Rhabdomyosarcoma

Rhabdomyosarcoma is a tumor composed of malignant cells with features of striated muscle, and it is the second most common primary sarcoma of the heart. Although rare in the pediatric age group, it has been reported in patients ranging from 3 months to 80 years old. The 26 patients with rhabdomyosarcoma in the AFIP report ranged in age from 1 to 66 years, but only two were children.[10] The incidence of this tumor is slightly higher in men than in women.

In the AFIP series, the majority of patients with rhabdomyosarcoma had nonspecific symptoms of fever, anorexia, malaise, and weight loss. Findings of pericardial disease, including pleuritic chest pain, pleural effusion, dyspnea, and both pulmonary and cerebral embolic phenomena, were common. All patients demonstrated cardiomegaly on chest roentgenography and nonspecific electrocardiographic changes, including ST-segment and T-wave changes, low voltage, and varying degrees of bundle-branch block. One-half of the patients had unexplained systolic murmurs and/or intractable atrial or ventricular dysrhythmias. In the patients with cardiac murmurs, a large portion of the rhabdomyosarcomas were intra-

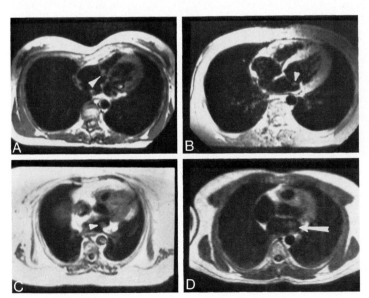

FIGURE 30–5. *A,* ECG-gated spin echo transaxial MRI through the tricuspid valve demonstrates a 1-cm oval mass on the septal leaflet *(arrowhead)* of the tricuspid valve. The tumor was a fibroelastoma. *B,* ECG-gated spin echo transaxial MRI through the mitral valve demonstrating mitral valve vegetation *(arrowhead). C,* ECG-gated spin echo transaxial MRI through the left atrium demonstrates a pedunculated mass arising from the posterior atrial wall *(arrowhead).* This is a surgically proved myxoma. *D,* ECG-gated spin echo transaxial MRI through the left atrium demonstrates an ill-defined mass arising from the posterior atrial wall *(arrow).* This was surgically proved to be a myxoma. (Courtesy of K. Link, M.D.)

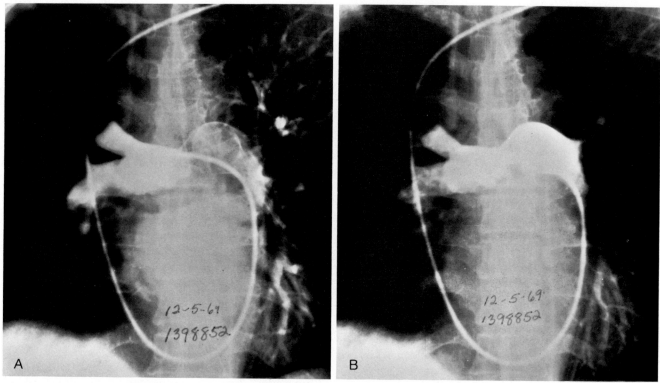

FIGURE 30–6. Pulmonary arteriograms *(A and B)* from following case. One month before admission to the hospital, this 57-year-old woman began experiencing pleuritic right chest pain and dyspnea. This pain did not resolve. On auscultation, a right pleural rub was noted. A lung scan showed no perfusion to the right lung. Pulmonary arteriograms showed complete occlusion of all branches of the right pulmonary artery. Heparin was administered, but a repeat arteriogram was unchanged. At surgery, a mass was seen involving the posterior wall of the pulmonary trunk, originating at the pulmonary valve and extending to the right pulmonary artery and its branches. The patient died in the early postoperative period. Autopsy demonstrated an angiosarcoma of the main pulmonary artery and valve with metastatic tumor emboli to the right pulmonary artery branches. (Courtesy of Jack Edeiken, M.D., Thomas Jefferson University Hospital, Philadelphia.)

cavitary and obstructed at least one valve orifice. The orifices of the mitral and pulmonary valves were most often obstructed; occasionally, the cardiac valves were invaded by tumor cells.

Rhabdomyosarcomas in the AFIP series occurred with equal frequencies on the left and right sides of the heart. In 60% of the patients, autopsy revealed tumor in multiple sites, with the pericardium being involved by direct extension in one-half of patients. The diffuse pericardial involvement characteristic of the cardiac mesotheliomas and angiosarcomas was not a feature of the cardiac rhabdomyosarcomas.

Microscopically, both juvenile and adult forms of cardiac rhabdomyosarcoma occur, with the latter being much more common. Diagnosis is made through identification of rhabdomyoblasts but can be difficult owing to the marked pleomorphism and anaplasia demonstrated by these tumors. Foci of necrosis and hemorrhage are common. A marked variation in the microscopic appearance of the tumor should precipitate a search for rhabdomyoblasts. Light microscopy can expose crossed striations in as many as one-third of these tumors.

Most patients with cardiac rhabdomyosarcoma die within 1 year of diagnosis. Various combinations of local excision, radiation, and chemotherapy have been tried but generally have not improved longevity in these patients.

Mesothelioma

Mesotheliomas are the most common malignant tumors of the pericardium and are derived from the mesothelial cells of either the visceral or the parietal pericardium. Approximately 120 cases of primary pericardial mesothelioma have been reported.[34] In a series of 84 pericardial tumors reported by Mahaim,[35] more than half of the 45 that were malignant were mesotheliomas. In the AFIP series, there were 19 cases of mesothelioma in patients ranging in age from 17 to 83 years. Patients in the pediatric age group have been reported. The male-to-female incidence ratio is 2:1. There is no evidence linking pericardial mesothelioma to asbestosis.[36]

Most pericardial mesotheliomas diffusely cover the pericardium and encase the heart; only rarely are they solitary or localized. Mesothelioma usually invades the heart only superficially; this is an important point in the differentiation of these tumors from other primary sarcomas, in which the intracavitary component may be common and functionally significant. Mesotheliomas frequently spread to adjacent pleura and mediastinum and involve the mediastinal lymph nodes; they may also spread through the diaphragm to involve the peritoneum, but distant metastases are unusual.

The most common clinical finding is dyspnea with

cough and other signs of pericardial effusion. The effusion may be recurrent, and cytologic examination of pericardial fluid may be of diagnostic value. Symptoms of pericarditis accompanied by nonspecific electrocardiographic changes have been noted; some patients have symptoms and signs of constrictive pericarditis with severe right-sided heart failure. Occasionally, the only clinical findings are nonspecific, consisting of fever, malaise, and weight loss. Chest roentgenography often shows cardiomegaly.

Diagnosis of the malignancy or its source is often difficult with echocardiography or cardiac CT.[37] Identification of the tumor cells in pericardial fluid may lead to the diagnosis, but differentiation between normal and malignant cells may be difficult. Mesothelial hyperplasia may be caused by radiotherapy or may be secondary to pericarditis after spread of carcinoma to the pericardium. Thus, the finding of mesothelial hyperplasia in a patient suspected of having metastatic pericardial carcinoma must not be used to exclude that diagnosis. Harrington and associates[38] reported that an elevated level of hyaluronic acid in the pleural fluid can aid in the diagnosis of pleural mesothelioma, and Takeda and associates[39] reported a case of pericardial mesothelioma in which elevated concentrations of hyaluronic acid were present in the pericardial effusion; they suggested that this finding may be of diagnostic value in future cases.

Fibrosarcoma and Malignant Fibrous Histiocytoma

These are malignant mesenchymal tumors that are primarily fibroblastic in differentiation. In the AFIP series, 14 such tumors were identified in patients ranging in age from younger than 1 year to 87 years.[10] Clinical findings were multiple and included systolic murmurs of variable intensity and recent onset, nonspecific electrocardiographic changes, atrial dysrhythmias, and symptoms of pericardial disease. Two patients had nonspecific symptoms suggestive of malignancy. Five of the 14 patients had distant metastases involving other viscera, and in two other patients, the tumor had spread directly to adjacent structures.

The tumors arose with equal frequencies on the left and right sides of the heart. They were nodular or infiltrated, gray-white, and firm. At autopsy, more than one-half of the cases showed multiple sites of involvement within the heart. The pericardium was involved in one-third of the patients, and intracavitary protrusion and valvular obstruction occurred in one-half.

In the AFIP series, surgery was attempted in three patients; however, excision was not feasible, and all three patients died after surgery. Others have noted that complete surgical excision usually is not possible, and radiation and chemotherapy have been tried with minimal success.[40–42] However, Eckstein and associates[43] reported the case of a 27-year-old woman who underwent surgical excision of a left atrial malignant fibrous histiocytoma, which recurred with enlargement of the right hilar lymph nodes. She was treated with chemotherapy, achieving a partial response, and resection of the residual tumor. The patient was reported alive and well without evidence of recurrent tumor 2 years after diagnosis. Stevens and associates[44] reported a similar patient who was treated with surgery and radiotherapy and followed with TEE. In general, however, the prognosis is poor, and in the AFIP series all patients with this type of tumor died within 2 years of the onset of symptoms.

Herhusky and associates[45] described two patients with primary cardiac fibrosarcoma and pleomorphic sarcoma in whom metastatic lesions were the first evidence of disease. One patient had fibrosarcoma of the tricuspid valve with pulmonary metastases. The second had a pleomorphic sarcoma of the mitral valve with renal and bony metastases. Thus, the possibility of a primary cardiac tumor should be considered in patients with occult metastatic carcinoma.

Malignant Lymphoma

Primary lymphoma of the heart is rare; only seven cases occurred in the AFIP series. The broad category of malignant lymphoma includes Hodgkin's disease, lymphosarcoma, reticulum cell sarcoma, and mycosis fungoides. Primary malignant lymphomas of the heart have been identified in patients ranging in age from 14 months to 77 years.[10] The incidences in men and women appear to be equal.

In patients with primary malignant lymphoma of the heart, radiotherapy associated with symptomatic remission has been reported. In the AFIP series, however, no cases were diagnosed antemortem, and all patients with symptoms died within 1 year of the onset of those symptoms.

Malignant lymphoma confined to the heart after renal transplantation has been reported.[46] Thus, this diagnosis should be considered in a renal transplant recipient with unexplained cardiomegaly.

Extraskeletal Osteosarcoma

Extraskeletal osteosarcoma was identified in five patients in the AFIP series.[10] Four of these patients were men, ranging in age from 16 to 58 years. Cardiac osteosarcoma most often arises from the posterior wall of the left atrium, close to the entrance of the pulmonary veins.

One patient in the AFIP series was treated with radiation and chemotherapy and survived 4 years after the onset of symptoms. The remaining four patients died within 2 years of diagnosis, despite various combinations of surgery, radiotherapy, and chemotherapy.

Malignant Nerve Sheath Tumor

The four patients in the AFIP series with malignant nerve sheath tumors were male and ranged in age from 9 to 52 years.[10] These tumors probably originate in the cardiac plexus or vagal innervation of the heart.

Two of the three patients with antemortem diagnoses died within 1 year of diagnosis despite surgical excision, radiotherapy, and chemotherapy. The third patient had evidence of recurrent disease at 1 year after surgery.

Malignant Teratoma

A malignant teratoma is a teratoma in which one of the elements has undergone malignant change, either metastasizing to or invading adjacent structures. This malignant portion may be a carcinoma or sarcoma. The most common malignant portion is embryonal carcinoma, but examples of choriocarcinoma and squamous cell carcinoma have been recognized.[47] When the malignant portion is embryonal carcinoma, the tumor is termed a teratocarcinoma. Most primary cardiac sarcomas occur in adults, but malignant cardiac teratomas occur most often in children. Like their benign counterparts, malignant teratomas of the heart are frequently primarily intrapericardial, attached to the base of the heart, and occur more often in females.

In the AFIP series, four malignant teratomas were found. The patients, three girls and a boy, ranged in age from 1 to 4 years. Symptoms of congestive heart failure were present in all four; all had cardiomegaly on chest roentgenography, two had dysrhythmias and nonspecific electrocardiographic findings, and one had a systolic murmur. Three of the tumors were primarily intrapericardial, being attached to the root of the aorta or pulmonary artery. In each, tumor elements derived from all three germ layers were identified. Two patients had metastases to the lungs and mediastinum, and one had extensive invasion of the left and right ventricular myocardia; the tumor in the fourth patient was situated over the anterior surface of the heart and had invaded the ventricular septum and right ventricle.

Surgical excision of the pericardial mass was attempted in one patient, but actual cardiac invasion made the procedure impossible. All four children died within 3 months of the onset of symptoms.

Thymoma

Although a thymoma in the pericardium is usually an anterior mediastinal tumor, it can be accepted as a primary tumor if there is no evidence of anterior mediastinal involvement. Presumably, in these cases the tumor is derived from thymic rests, which may be incidentally located in the parietal pericardium. In the AFIP series, four thymomas originating in the parietal pericardium were found. Iliceto and associates[48] reported the case of a 27-year-old woman with pericardial thymoma in whom two-dimensional echocardiography was used to demonstrate the tumor before biopsy and to follow the tumor response to chemotherapy.

Leiomyosarcoma

Only 25 cases of primary cardiac leiomyosarcoma have been reported in the literature. In only 11 of 25

was the diagnosis established premortem.[49] Only one leiomyosarcoma of the heart was reported in the AFIP series.[1] The patient, a 27-year-old man, developed atrial fibrillation, chest pain, and syncope. Angiography demonstrated a left atrial mass, and surgical excision was attempted but was not successful. No metastases were noted at autopsy.

A leiomyosarcoma is signified microscopically by the presence of elongated cells with blunt-ended nuclei growing interlacing cords. There may be a suggestion of nuclear palisading. Ultrastructurally, these cells contain haphazardly oriented bundles of myofibrils.

Fine and Raju[50] reported a 20-year cure in a 14-year-old boy who underwent excision of a pedunculated right atrial leiomyosarcoma. However, overall the prognosis is poor, with most cases not being operable, and death occurring soon after surgery.

Liposarcoma

Liposarcomas of the heart and pericardium are rare, with only one such tumor being noted in the AFIP collection. The patient was a 30-year-old woman with severe congestive heart failure who was diagnosed during life as having rheumatic heart disease. Autopsy showed a large tumor replacing the right atrium and extending to the pericardium, constricting the superior and inferior venae cavae. The tumor resembled embryonal adipose tissue, with signet-ring cells and stellate cells containing numerous tiny vacuoles.

The malignancy of liposarcomas is mainly local, with multiple recurrences being seen before blood and lymphatic metastases occur.[51] Mavroudis and associates[52] reported the successful surgical treatment of an intracavitary liposarcoma of the right ventricle. This patient had previously undergone three noncardiac procedures for removal of isolated foci of liposarcoma, each accompanied by extended tumor-free intervals.

Synovial Sarcoma

The AFIP series reported by McAllister[10] contains the only reported case of synovial sarcoma primary to the heart. The patient was a 30-year-old man who had progressive dyspnea and syncope with a systolic ejection murmur. At autopsy, a 10- by 15-cm tumor was found at the base of the heart, involving the pericardium and invading the outflow tract of the right ventricle and pulmonary artery. No metastases were found. Microscopically, the tumor had the classic properties of synovial sarcoma.

TREATMENT

Poole and associates[53] reviewed more than 60 reports of patients operated on for primary cardiac cancer, but only 28 of the cases had sufficient preoperative and postoperative data to be included in their review.

The most common histologic types to be treated surgically were rhabdomyosarcoma, fibrosarcoma, and angiosarcoma. The left atrium was the most commonly involved cardiac chamber (11 patients), followed in frequency by the right atrium (seven patients), right ventricle (six patients), pulmonary valve (two patients), root of the pulmonary artery at the pulmonary valve (one patient), and interatrial septum (one patient). This last tumor involved both atria in a dumbbell configuration.

The ages of the 14 male and 14 female patients ranged from 3 weeks to 70 years (mean, 31.4 years). Twenty-one of the patients (75%) were younger than 46 years.

Twenty-six patients were operated on with the use of cardiopulmonary bypass. One patient with an epicardial tumor arising on a pedicle from the right atrioventricular groove[54] and another with a tumor originating from the right atrial appendage[55] were not operated on. Rather, in each the tumor was resected by excluding the tumor from the remainder of the heart by vascular clamps. The only surgical death was that of a 3-week-old infant with a rhabdomyosarcoma of the interventricular septum, which had caused right ventricular outflow obstruction.[56]

Follow-up information was provided for 25 of the 27 survivors. Survival ranged from 2 to 55 months (mean, 14 months); 16 patients survived for 6 months or longer. Three of the seven patients still alive at the latest follow-up had known metastases, and a fourth had probable residual mediastinal disease. Death was caused by peripheral metastases in 11 patients and by local recurrence with blood flow obstruction in six patients. Two patients died of other causes, but both had persistent malignant cardiac disease.

The duration of symptoms before diagnosis was not related to the length of postoperative survival. Patients whose symptoms had been present for less than 3 months lived an average of 12.1 months after surgery, whereas patients whose symptoms had been present for 3 months or longer survived an average of 13.7 months after surgery. Female patients survived longer than male patients. Postoperative irradiation to the mediastinum might have helped prolong survival; even when patients who are alive but have a follow-up of less than 1 year are excluded from assessment, irradiated patients had more than twice (22.7 months) the duration of survival of nonirradiated patients (9.6 months). The average radiation dose administered was 52.2 Gy over approximately 30 days. No specific criteria for selection of these patients could be identified in a review of the charts.

Eight patients received postoperative chemotherapy, usually consisting of a combination of cyclophosphamide or methotrexate, dactinomycin or doxorubicin, and vincristine. However, adjunctive chemotherapy not only failed to improve the survival of patients receiving it but also correlated with shorter survival times than those of patients not receiving chemotherapy. This finding must be interpreted with caution, however, because the patients who received adjunctive chemotherapy may have had more advanced disease, although that possibility was not evident from available clinical data.

Because one-third of the deaths were due to local recurrence, it is conceivable that repeated operations or cardiac transplantations could have prolonged survival in selected patients. In fact, the four patients who underwent repeated operations for recurrent tumor had a mean survival of 36 months, although none lived longer than 55 months. One patient underwent five open-heart operations during a 31-month interval and survived 34 months after the onset of symptoms.[57] Although reoperation is not always feasible or appropriate, those findings demonstrate that an aggressive surgical approach can help prolong survival.

Cooley and associates[58] used autotransplantation of the heart to remove a paraganglioma of the left atrium. Removal of the heart allowed easy access to the tumor, and the excised atrial wall was repaired with an autologous pericardial patch.

Jamieson and associates[59] used cardiac transplantation to treat an unresectable left ventricular fibroma in a 17-year-old girl, who was alive and well 18 months after transplantation. Armitage and associates[60] reported the use of cardiac transplantation in 11 patients with malignant disease; in one patient with a primary cardiac angiosarcoma, there was no evidence of recurrence at 8 months. Aravot and associates[61] reported a patient with cardiac neurofibrosarcoma treated with cardiac transplantation who was well at 5.5 years after surgery with no evidence of recurrent disease. With the resurgence of cardiac transplantation and the improved survival of recipients, this therapy will be used more often in patients who have inoperable localized cardiac tumors.

SECONDARY METASTATIC AND NONINVASIVE CARDIAC AND PERICARDIAL TUMORS

In 1951, Prichard[9] reported that tumors that metastasized to the heart were 20 to 40 times more common than primary cardiac tumors. Primary sites, cell types, and the prevalence of cardiac metastases have changed over time as a result of chemotherapy,[62] increased survival of patients with cancer, increased incidence of lung carcinoma, and the rapid spread of acquired immunodeficiency syndrome (AIDS). In a recent series by Klatt and Heitz,[63] metastases to the heart were found in 10.7% of 1029 autopsy cases in which a malignant neoplasm was diagnosed. The lung was the most common primary site (36.4%) and adenocarcinoma was the most frequent cell type (36.4%) of neoplasms that metastasized to the heart. Nonepithelial tumors accounted for 22.7% of cardiac metastases. Epicardium was involved in 75.5% of metastatic lesions, and in this group, a pericardial effusion was present in 33.7%. Lymphomas associated with AIDS show extensive cardiac involvement. Melanoma appears to be the neoplasm with the greatest propensity for cardiac involvement, with more than 50% involving the heart. Although 10% to 20% of patients who die as a result of cancer have cardiac metastases, the incidence of clinical evidence of cardiac involvement before death ranges from 0% to 50%. Roberts and associates[64] reported secondary cardiac lymphoma in 24% of 196 autopsy cases. McDonnell and associates[65] proposed three mechanisms for cardiac involvement by a lymphoma that has arisen in another site, as follows. First, patients with lymphomatous involvement of mediastinal lymph nodes may have invasion of the pericardium by direct extension. Second, retrograde lymphatic spread from noncontiguous mediastinal lymph nodes may result in epicardial involvement, which then spreads into the adjacent myocardium. Third, hematogenous dissemination of tumor, as in cases of acute leukemia or lymphoma with a leukemic phase, may result in multifocal, predominantly perivascular involvement of the entire myocardium. In their series, Klatt and Heitz[63] found that the high-grade malignant lymphomas associated with AIDS represented 32% of all the noted lymphomas and nine of the 16 cardiac metastases with lymphoma. These lymphomas involve the heart (endocardium and myocardium) more extensively than other tumors, tend to be widespread, and respond poorly to therapy. Kaposi's sarcoma, which is vascular in origin and often widespread in patients with AIDS, had only a 4% incidence of cardiac involvement. In other series,[66] the incidence has ranged from 20% to 28%.

Metastatic cardiac tumors are more likely to cause symptoms when they involve the pericardium. However, symptoms may include dysrhythmias (including heart block), congestive heart failure due to myocardial replacement of intracavitary and valvular obstruction, myocardial infarction, peripheral embolism, and constitutional manifestations. Congestive heart failure and dysrhythmias in a patient with a known primary malignant tumor should raise the suspicion of cardiac metastasis.

Dysrhythmias associated with cardiac metastasis are often unresponsive to conventional medical therapy,[67] another sign that should raise the suspicion of a cardiac metastasis. When heart block is noted, permanent pacemakers may be required.[68] Survival of symptomatic patients with metastases may be prolonged with radiation therapy, chemotherapy, or both.

Although some patients with symptomatic myocardial infiltration by malignancy respond to irradiation,[69] in most cases, the treatment results in relentless congestive heart failure because of myocardial replacement by tumor. In contradistinction, chamber or valve obstruction by a tumor mass may be an indication for surgical intervention. The tumor may have invaded the myocardium, or it may exist as a purely intracavitary extension from the vena cava or a pulmonary vein.

Caution should be used, however, in undertaking surgical intervention in patients whose primary tumors are not adequately controlled or in whom insufficient time has elapsed after control of the primary cancer, because cryptic metastases may be present at other sites, thus nullifying the benefit of resecting the cardiac metastases.

Table 30–2 summarizes 11 reported cases of surgically resected secondary malignant cardiac tumors. Five of the 11 patients died in the perioperative period (45%). In two of the patients who died, the primary cancer had not been diagnosed or treated; a third patient died of widely disseminated disease; one patient died of a postoperative coagulopathy following cardiopulmonary bypass; and the fifth patient died of refractory low cardiac output. Three other patients died later. One death (at 5 months) was due to doxorubicin toxicity; that patient, who had had resection of a metastatic osteosarcoma, had no evidence of persistent cardiac tumor or other metastases at autopsy. The other two deaths (one at 14 months and one at 26 months) were due to extensive metastases. The remaining three patients, who had had surgical treatment of primary sarcomas 6, 11, and 25 years before the latest follow-up, were alive without evidence of other metastatic disease 9, 15, and 7 months, respectively, after their cardiac surgery.

Of tumors that grow into the right atrium from the vena cava without infiltrating the myocardium, the most common is renal cell carcinoma. Renal cell carcinoma extends into the inferior vena cava in 5% of cases and the right atrium in 1% of cases. Techniques described to excise these tumors include those with and without cardiopulmonary bypass as well as hypothermic circulatory arrest.[90-92] Intravascular ultrasound has been used in the preoperative evaluation of tumor extent and vessel wall adherence in the inferior vena cava.[93]

Choh and associates[94] reviewed six reports of patients with intracavitary renal cell carcinoma who had been operated on with cardiopulmonary bypass and added a case of their own. They concluded that extension of hypernephroma into the heart was not a hopeless situation, because surgery had effectively relieved symptoms in all seven patients and had resulted in the apparent cure of two patients. Thompson and associates[95] reported six patients with cavoatrial extension of Wilms' tumor that was successfully resected with cardiopulmonary bypass.

Other tumors that may extend into the heart from a major vein are listed in Table 30–3, which summarizes 11 cases that were treated surgically. There was no follow-up for one of the 11 patients. One patient (9%) died in the perioperative period; five died from 3 to 5 months after surgery (one of local recurrence). The remaining four patients were alive at 13 months to 6.5 years after surgery.

MALIGNANT PERICARDIAL EFFUSIONS

Patients with malignant pericardial disease may be asymptomatic or may have a number of clinical manifestations. The most common of these is pericardial effusion. Whether the pericardial effusion becomes hemodynamically significant and requires specific therapy depends on a number of factors. The presence of malignancy within the pericardium does not necessarily mean that a pericardial effusion will ensue.

TABLE 30–2. Clinical Data on 10 Patients with Surgically Resected Secondary Malignant Cardiac Tumors

CASE	AGE (yr)	SEX	SYMPTOMS	SITE	SOURCE	INTERVAL SINCE TREATMENT OF PRIMARY LESION	INTERVAL BETWEEN SYMPTOMS AND SURGERY	POSTOPERATIVE SURVIVAL	OUTCOME†
1	59	M	Chronic cough, dyspnea	RV	Liposarcoma, thigh	25 yr	2 mo	7 mo	Alive[52]
2	44	M	Chest pain	LA	Lung (direct extension)	NA	?	14 mo	Died of metastases[70]
3	45	F	Fever, cough	LA	Lung (direct extension)	NA	?	8 hr	Died in postoperative period[70]
4	46	F	Dyspnea, cough, SVC syndrome	RA	Leiomyosarcoma, uterus	NA	5 mo	hours	Died in postoperative period of pulmonary embolus; diagnosis made at autopsy[71]
5	58	M	Chest pain, dyspnea	RV	Renal cell carcinoma	NA	7 mo	2 wk	Died; diagnosis made postoperatively[72]
6	69	F	Dyspnea, palpitations	LA	Chondrosarcoma, pelvis	NA	2 mo	26 mo	Died of metastases[73]
7	12	F	Chest pain, syncope	LV	Rhabdomyosarcoma of leg	6 yr	2 mo	9 mo	Alive[74]
8	48	F	Dyspnea, fatigue, shoulder pain	RV	Leiomyosarcoma, uterus	11 yr	?	15 mo	Alive[75]
9	33	F	SOB, cough, hemoptysis, fever	RV	Squamous cell carcinoma, cervix	11 mo	3 mo	3 wk	Died of widespread metastases[76]
10	23	F	Dizziness, headache, palpitations, syncope	RV	Osteosarcoma, shoulder	4 yr	6 mo	5 mo	Died of doxorubicin toxicity[77]
11	30	F	Dyspnea, orthopnea, fatigue	LV	Leiomyosarcoma, uterus	1 yr	7 mo	48 hr	Died of refractory low cardiac output[78]

LA = left atrium; LV = left ventricle; NA = not applicable; RA = right atrium; RV = right ventricle; SOB = shortness of breath; SVC = superior vena cava syndrome.
†Superscript numbers refer to chapter references.
Modified from Poole GV Jr, Meredith JW, Breyer RH, et al: Surgical implications in malignant cardiac disease. Ann Thorac Surg 36:484–491, 1983.

The clinical picture associated with a pericardial effusion that progresses to tamponade depends on a number of factors, but the most important are the rate at which fluid accumulates in the pericardium and the propensity of the malignancy to involve the lymphatic drainage of the pericardium and heart.

Presentation in malignant pericardial effusions consists of a spectrum of symptomatologies, ranging from totally asymptomatic to relatively acute, florid cardiac tamponade with all its attendant manifestations. A number of malignancies are recognized as capable of causing malignant pericardial effusions, but those that have a predilection for the mediastinal lymphatics draining the heart and pericardium are the most likely offenders. Invasion of these lymphatics with retrograde progression of the malignancy toward the heart and pericardium is the most common cause of such effusions. Many different treatment methods have been tried, but the most successful regimens have been those that not only address the resolution of the effusion but also involve direct efforts to control the disseminated malignancy that is usually present. Obviously, the success of such therapy depends on the extent of the malignancy, its susceptibility to treatment regimens, and the general condition of the patient when therapy is undertaken.

ETIOLOGY AND PATHOGENESIS

Malignancy can be spread to the pericardium via direct growth from a nearby tumor, through the blood-stream, or by lymphatic channels.[96, 97] The predominant mode is via lymphatics.[96] Knowledge of the lymphatic drainage of the heart and pericardium is essential to understanding malignant pericardial effusions. Fraser and associates[98] summarized this information recently in their review of cardiac tamponade as the presenting symptom of extracardiac malignancy. The pericardium has relatively few lymphatics; most of its drainage occurs through the rich lymphatics in the heart. The precise location and distribution of the lymphatics in the pericardium remain somewhat controversial topics,[96] but most evidence suggests that the parietal pericardium contains a relatively unimportant lymphatic system.[96, 99]

Lymphatic drainage of the heart arises in the subendocardial plexus, which communicates with the more extensive subepicardial plexus.[98] The latter gives rise to the cardiac lymphatic trunks, which run with the coronary arteries to the base of the aorta (Fig. 30–7). Near the base of the aorta, the cardiac lymphatic trunks diverge by one of two routes from the coronary arteries and course to the cardiac node, which is located between the innominate artery and the superior vena cava. The primary route is directly to the cardiac node; the secondary route carries the lymph first to a pretracheal node and then to the cardiac node. The cardiac node drains into the mediastinal system.

An alternative and less important route of pericardial lymphatic drainage is the lymphatic plexus located in the pericardium, which communicates with

TABLE 30–3. Clinical Data on 11 Patients with Secondary Intracavitary (Noninvasive) Tumors of the Heart Removed During Cardiopulmonary Bypass

CASE	AGE (yr)	SEX	MAIN SYMPTOM	TUMOR	POSTOPERATIVE SURVIVAL	COMMENTS*
1	2	M	Abdominal distention	Wilms' tumor, right kidney	3 mo	Died of pulmonary insufficiency and sepsis secondary to radiation therapy and chemotherapy[79]
2	2	F	Fatigue, diarrhea, abdominal pain	Wilms' tumor, right kidney	3½ yr	Alive at follow-up[80]
3	9	M	Easy fatigue, dyspnea, cyanosis of lips and fingers	Wilms' tumor, right kidney	5 days	Died in immediate postoperative period[81]
4	14	M	Abdominal pain	Wilms' tumor, right kidney	6 mo	Died of lung and brain metastases[82]
5	7	M	Headache, fever, shortness of breath	Embryonal rhabdomyosarcoma of liver	5 mo	Died after attempted resection of primary liver tumor[83]
6	62	M	Back pain, weight loss	Liver cell carcinoma	1 yr	Alive with spinal metastases[84]
7	37	M	Dyspnea, chest pain, cough, hemoptysis; emboli to iliac artery	Chondrosarcoma of lung	4 mo	Died of widespread metastases; tumor entered left atrium via pulmonary vein[85]
8	28	M	Chest pain	Chondrosarcoma of lung	10 mo	Died of local recurrence; tumor entered left atrium via pulmonary vein[86]
9	52	M	Headache, hypertension, diabetes, episodic sweating	Pheochromocytoma	13 mo	Alive at follow-up; status 11 mo after resection of left adrenal for pheochromocytoma at time of cardiac operation[87]
10	47	M	Dyspnea, fever, cough, sudden hemiparesis and aphasia	Bronchogenic carcinoma, undifferentiated	?	No follow-up; primary tumor arose from right lower lobe and was unresectable[88]
11	31	F	Pedal edema, palpitations	Leiomyosarcoma	6½ yr	Alive at follow-up; hysterectomy performed 4 yr before diagnosis of cardiac involvement[89]

*Superscript numbers refer to chapter references.
Modified from Poole GV Jr, Meredith JW, Breyer RH, et al: Surgical implications in malignant cardiac disease. Ann Thorac Surg 36:484–491, 1983.

the plexus in the aortic adventitia. This superficial aortic plexus drains to the para-aortic nodes, which then drain to the thoracic duct or the paratracheal system.[98] Studies conducted on exposed human and canine hearts and radiologic studies of lymph flow in dogs have suggested that the more important of the two systems is the cardiac system.[100, 101] Therefore, lymphatic drainage of the heart and pericardium has a rather narrow zone (or "isthmus," as Fraser and associates[98] describe it), where metastases may block lymphatic drainage with little possibility for collateral flow.

Strong evidence suggests that many cardiac and pericardial metastases and pericardial effusions are a result of invasion of these lymphatics with retrograde progression of the disease to the heart and pericardium.[96, 98] Cardiac metastases are not uncommon, having a recognized incidence of from 5% to 15% in patients dying of cancer.[64, 102, 103] A recent large autopsy study revealed that 11.8% of patients with malignant disease had cardiac involvement by tumor.[104] Furthermore, the incidence of pericardial involvement by tumor in patients with cancer has been reported to be as high as 21%.[104, 105] Clinically apparent impairment of cardiac function, however, is not common.[106] In one study of 716 patients with malignancies, all 61 patients with cardiac metastases had mediastinal lymph node involvement, and tumor was often seen within the lymphatics of the pericardium as well as the lymphatics of the epicardium and the myocardium.[107] In an examination of 100 patients with pulmonary carcinomas, Onuigbo[108] found a similar mediastinal involvement associated with cardiac metastases and noted that epicardial lymphatic involvement was always associated with myocardial disease.

Malignant neoplasms that are commonly associated with pericardial effusions are those that invade the mediastinal lymphatics and obstruct lymphatic flow

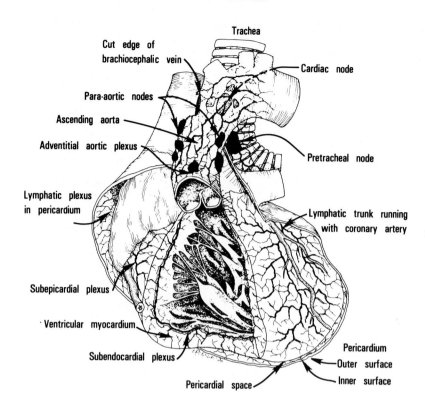

FIGURE 30–7. The lymphatic drainage of the heart and pericardium. The lymphatic channels are exaggerated in size to highlight their relations to the surrounding structures.

from the pericardium (Table 30–4). Metastatic carcinoma from the lung, breast, and hematologic malignancies account for three-fourths of all cases of neoplastic pericardial disease.[96, 109] Lung cancer (all histologic types) constitutes approximately one-third of cases of pericardial disease at autopsy.[96, 109] The next most common primary source is breast cancer (25%), followed by hematologic malignancies (15%).[96, 110, 111] Virtually all other types of cancer form the remainder of cases (except primary brain tumors), but special mention of metastatic malignant melanoma is relevant because the pericardium is involved in 50% of cases.[96]

CLINICAL PRESENTATION

As mentioned, in malignant pericardial effusion, presentation consists of a spectrum ranging from completely asymptomatic to florid cardiac tamponade.[98, 112–115] The development of symptoms depends on the rate of accumulation of pericardial fluid, volume of the fluid, and function of the underlying heart.[109] The severity of symptoms can vary so greatly because the pericardium distends over a period of time with the accumulation of fluid. When the fluid increases resistance to ventricular filling during diastole, symptoms begin to appear. With decreasing cardiac output, dyspnea appears, at first only with exertion and eventually even at rest. Numerous series report increasing dyspnea as the most common presenting symptom.[96, 107, 112] Finally, cardiac output can be reduced to such an extent that the patient has dyspnea and cyanosis at rest and becomes agitated and orthopneic.

DIAGNOSIS

Immediate evaluation of the patient with malignant pericardial effusion is directed not only at establishing the diagnosis but also at determining whether cardiac tamponade is present. Relatively simple measures allow the diagnosis of tamponade to be made in virtually any clinical setting. Examination of the patient reveals distended neck veins, evidence of hypoperfusion (including peripheral vasoconstriction, cool digits, diaphoresis, and poor capillary filling), dyspnea, and cyanosis in extreme cases. A blood pressure cuff enables determination of systolic and diastolic pres-

TABLE 30–4. Types of Tumors Reported to Cause Pericardial Effusion

PRIMARY SITE	RELATIVE FREQUENCY
Lung (three adenocarcinomas for every squamous cell carcinoma)	1
Breast	2
Lymphomas and leukemias (including Hodgkin's disease)	3
Other carcinomas and malignancies of unknown origin	4
Sarcomas	5

Assigning precise percentages is difficult because reported series are small and results vary depending on the extent of disease when diagnosed. In a number of cases the exact primary could not be determined. Several facts are clear: (1) adenocarcinomas are the most likely histologic type to cause malignant pericardial effusion; (2) sarcomas, because they spread more frequently by hematogenous than lymphatic routes, are less likely to cause malignant pericardial effusions; and (3) malignancies arising in tissues that have lymphatic drainage into the mediastinum are most likely to invade these lymphatics and to cause a malignant pericardial effusion.

sures, width of pulse pressure, and amount of pulsus paradoxus present. With tamponade, pulse pressure is narrowed, pulsus paradoxus is more than 10 mm Hg, diastolic pressure is elevated, and systolic pressure is depressed. There are marked variations in the quality of the sounds heard while taking the blood pressure. Auscultation of the heart occasionally reveals distant heart sounds and, rarely, a pericardial splash. The electrocardiogram reveals electrical alternans in many cases.[96] Atrial fibrillation may also be the presenting entity in malignant pericardial effusions.[116] With such findings, provisions should be made for immediate decompression of the pericardium. If an operating room is available, the patient should be prepared immediately and undergo surgery for decompression. If any significant delay (longer than 30 minutes) is anticipated, emergency pericardiocentesis should be contemplated.

Establishing the exact cause of a pericardial effusion in a patient who has malignant disease can be difficult because the patient may have received radiation therapy to the thorax and may now have pericarditis associated with that therapy. In essence, three diagnostic methods have been most helpful in evaluating malignant pericardial effusions and monitoring their progress (Fig. 30–8). Confirmation of malignant origin rests on identification of malignant cells in aspirated pericardial fluid, in direct biopsy specimens taken from the pericardium, or in masses found on exploration. An important feature of malignant pericardial disease is that metastatic deposits in the pericardium sometimes are not accompanied by cancer cells in the fluid.[11] Furthermore, sometimes malignant pericardial fluid cells do not invade pericardial tissue because of the lack of pericardial lymphatic pathways.[98]

In asymptomatic individuals, the diagnostic method that most frequently detects a pericardial effusion is the standard chest radiograph. The patient will pre-

sent with the classic water-bottle cardiac silhouette on the standard posteroanterior chest film that strongly suggests a pericardial effusion. Echocardiography may then be used to determine the presence and distribution of fluid within the pericardium.[115, 117] CT can be helpful, particularly in evaluating intrapericardial masses and their relation to pericardial effusions.[117] Glazer and associates[117] compared the efficacy of echocardiography with that of CT in evaluating intrapericardial masses in eight patients seen over 3 years and found that echocardiography was the method of choice in evaluating potential pericardial effusions. CT scan, however, was the preferred diagnostic test for evaluating suspected intrapericardial mass lesions. Other authors[118] have found that CT scan can be used to rapidly diagnose malignant pericardial effusions. Coplan and associates[119] noted that M-mode echocardiography has limitations in that it can misdiagnose a solid tumor as a pericardial effusion. Two-dimensional echocardiography and CT scanning accurately defined such a mass as an intrapericardial mesothelioma rather than an effusion. One can conclude, then, that serial chest roentgenograms may be useful in detecting changes in the cardiac silhouette that suggest a pericardial effusion, but echocardiography is required to confirm its presence.

The recent emergence of MRI offers a new diagnostic method of evaluating malignant pericardial disease and effusion. Experience with this method is limited in most institutions. The results are superior to CT in evaluating the myocardium but similar to CT in evaluating the pericardium. Radionuclide scans also can be helpful by showing accentuated uptake of isotope in metastatic disease to the pericardium, but the anatomic detail is much less than that rendered by CT or MRI.[96]

Pericardiocentesis has been advocated by some as a satisfactory method for obtaining the diagnosis of malignant pericardial effusion. Some have advocated the placement of a polytetrafluoroethylene cannula in the pericardium by first introducing a guide wire[120] or placing an 18-gauge catheter directly in the pericardium.[121, 122] Complications that have been reported with pericardiocentesis for diagnosis and treatment include puncture of the right ventricle, laceration of coronary vessels, arrhythmias, pneumothorax, and death.[113, 123] Therefore, many recommend ultrasound guidance for all patients with pericardial effusions to reduce the incidence of complications.[109, 123]

Other groups have found subxyphoid pericardiotomy to be more efficacious in establishing the diagnosis.[113, 124, 125] A subxyphoid window is definitive for both diagnosis and treatment of effusions of all causes.[113] Another useful diagnostic adjunct to open pericardial procedures is pericardioscopy.[96, 126] Millaire and associates[126] report a diagnostic sensitivity for surgical drainage that is 20% lower than that for drainage associated with pericardioscopy. This finding was believed to be related to the direct visualization of the pericardium and to the ability to perform guided biopsies.[126]

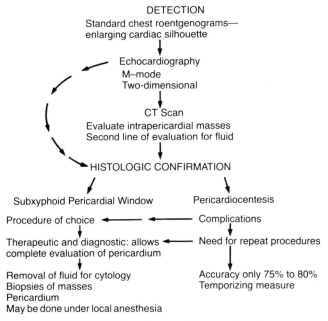

FIGURE 30–8. Flow diagram of diagnostic work-up.

TREATMENT

Therapy for malignant pericardial effusion has several goals: elimination of the pericardial fluid, prevention of reaccumulation and cardiac tamponade, and control of the malignancy. Historically, the most commonly used method of therapy is external radiation of the pericardium.[127, 128] Radiation therapy was useful only in patients who had not had prior radiotherapy. Results depended on the radiosensitivity of the tumor. Different methods are applied today, the results and liabilities of which are varied. Radiotherapy, however, has a role in cases of refractory malignant pericardial effusions and in patients with radiosensitive lymphomas.[98, 109, 125]

Pericardiocentesis is attractive in that it allows diagnosis and therapy to be conducted in the same procedure. The diagnostic yield of approximately 78% has been noted.[121, 122] Because many believe that open surgical procedures are not indicated in patients with end-stage disease, pericardiocentesis with drainage alone or in combination with a sclerosing agent has been advocated.[129, 130] Many patients will respond successfully with pericardiocentesis and drainage alone and will not reaccumulate fluid.[96] Many substances have been instilled into the pericardial space to promote pericardiodesis. Of these agents, the most commonly used substance has been tetracycline and is believed by some to be the treatment of choice for malignant pericardial effusions.[131] Instillation of tetracycline into the pericardium has been reported to be successful in 75% to 90% of cases.[96, 109] Attendant complications associated with its use include pain, arrhythmias, fever, and constrictive pericarditis.[96, 131, 132] The mechanism of action of tetracycline is most likely related to inherent acidity and direct cytotoxic action.[131] Perhaps somewhat less toxic but similarly efficacious is oxytetracycline.[131] There has been recent enthusiasm for the use of OK-432 in treating malignant pericardial effusions,[129] with no serious side effects reported. Other groups have instilled various agents into the pericardial sac with a range of results; these agents include bleomycin,[133] radioactive chromic phosphate,[134] antimetabolites,[135] and alkylating agents.[136]

Other groups have had problems with pericardiocentesis. Many report a high rate of recurrence of effusions.[137] Posner and associates[138] studied 31 patients with pericardial disease associated with various malignancies. Fifty-eight per cent of the patients had malignant pericardial involvement, 32% had idiopathic pericarditis, and 10% had pericarditis related to radiotherapy. Pericardiocentesis documented malignant disease in 85% of patients; in the remaining 15%, open biopsy was required for diagnosis. Wong and associates[122] reviewed 52 pericardiocenteses performed over a 3-year period in a cardiac catheterization laboratory. Thirty-five were successful and uncomplicated; 16 were nonproductive, one was nontherapeutic, and eight were complicated. The complications consisted of one death (a cardiac arrest), one aspiration of a subdiaphragmatic abscess,

and five ventricular punctures without clinically adverse sequelae. Laceration of coronary arteries, laceration of the internal mammary vessels, and puncture of the lung and resultant pneumothorax have also been reported as complications of pericardiocentesis.[139]

Because of the problems attending pericardiocentesis and the number of procedures that fail to give a definitive diagnosis or therapy, more groups are moving toward the use of subxyphoid pericardiotomy for definitive diagnosis and therapy of pericardial effusions. Some believe it is the procedure of choice for all malignant pericardial effusions.[113, 125] Little and associates[113] have had high diagnostic accuracy (100%) while encountering no significant complications; in the patients followed long term, the pericardial effusion did not recur. Alcan and associates[124] were able to relieve the tamponade in their 18 cases (both malignant and otherwise) without deaths and without reaccumulation of the fluid. In reviewing their experience with 17 patients with malignant pericardial effusions, Hankins and associates[125] found that a pericardial window relieved the effusion without deaths or significant complications. Thirteen had windows through the subxyphoid route, and four had either limited sternotomy or anterior thoracotomy. The subxyphoid pericardiotomy is advantageous in that it can be performed with the patient under local anesthesia.[124, 125] Exactly how creation of a pericardial window prevents subsequent effusions is unknown, but it probably occurs through fusion of the epicardium and pericardium.[113] As mentioned previously, use of pericardioscopy together with open surgical drainage can be beneficial, especially in cases where results of conventional drainage have been inconclusive.[126]

An alternative to the surgical pericardial window is the recently described percutaneous balloon pericardiotomy.[140, 141] Although the precise mechanism of action is unclear and further investigation is needed, this alternative may prove useful for recurrent pericardial effusions and may be used in conjunction with pericardioscopy.[140] Another alternative that has recently evolved is video-assisted thoracic surgery. This technique has been used successfully for diagnosis and treatment of malignant pericardial effusions.[142]

The ultimate survival of any patient with a malignant pericardial effusion depends on control of the systemic disease once evaluation of the effusion has been completed. Survival also depends on the histology since survival in patients with breast cancer is generally longer than for patients with other primaries.[138] Hankins and associates[125] noted that six of their patients died within 30 days of successful pericardiotomy because of extensive primary disease. Six of their patients successfully treated for pericardial effusions survived from 3 to 12 months, and two were alive at 8 and 21 months after surgery. Little and associates[113] reported that only two of six patients with malignant effusions had significant long-term survival. In the series reported by Davis and associates[121] in which the effusions were treated with intrapericardial tetracycline, survival ranged from 28 to 704 days and was directly related to the performance status and/or chemoradiosensitivity of the primary cancer. In a review by Fraser and associates,[98] survival ranged from days to 4 years and was related to the susceptibility of the primary tumors to therapeutic regimens.

Formal pericardiectomy has little place in the treatment of malignant pericardial disease or effusions; it is reserved for constrictive syndromes or failure of other measures.[138] In many cases, survival may be limited.[113] Pericardial window relieves symptoms, is easily performed, and yields a definitive diagnosis.[113, 124, 125] Reaccumulation of pericardial fluid and recurrence of symptoms are infrequent.[113, 124] In our experience, subxyphoid pericardiotomy has achieved all of the desired diagnostic and therapeutic goals without major complications or recurrence of symptoms.

For clinicians developing a treatment regimen for patients with malignant pericardial effusions, the accumulated data suggest that pericardiocentesis should be reserved for very specific needs in an acutely ill patient. Subxyphoid pericardiotomy offers the highest diagnostic and therapeutic yield with the least potential for complications and mortality because it can be conducted with the patient under local anesthesia. Pericardioscopy and percutaneous balloon pericardiotomy may play adjuvant therapeutic roles. The following treatment regimen recognizes these facts while presenting an approach that should yield the diagnosis, provide definitive therapy, and yet subject the patient to a low rate of morbidity and mortality (Fig. 30–9).

Therapeutic Approach

Before embarking on a diagnostic and therapeutic regimen for malignant pericardial disease and effusion, one must conduct a careful evaluation of the effects of previous diagnostic and therapeutic modalities on the heart and pericardium. This is particularly important in the patient who has had prior thoracic surgery or radiotherapy. Any surgical entrance into the pericardium will cause adhesions. Radiotherapy may cause pericarditis or pericardial effusions, or both, as a direct result of therapeutic radiation delivered to known intrathoracic malignancies.[143–145] Therefore, if a pericardial effusion occurs in a patient who has had radiation to an intrathoracic malignancy, further radiotherapy should be withheld until the exact etiology of the effusion can be demonstrated through analysis of the pericardium and any fluid it contains.

Pericardiocentesis

Although some groups have had success treating malignant pericardial effusions with pericardiocentesis,[120, 121] others have found the procedure inadequate because of its attendant complications, its relatively low yield in diagnosing the underlying cause of the pericardial effusion, and a frequent need for repeat pericardiocentesis to remove accumulations of fluid.[113] In the emergent situation with the patient in florid circulatory depression secondary to tamponade, pericardiocentesis should be considered as an emergency temporizing procedure performed to allow successful transport of the patient to the operating room. Conduct of pericardiocentesis is less likely to be attended by complications such as perforation of the right ventricle, laceration of a coronary artery, and injury to the right atrium if electrical alternans is present. Proper conduct of the procedure requires relatively few materials, most of which are available in hospital emergency departments and on many wards.

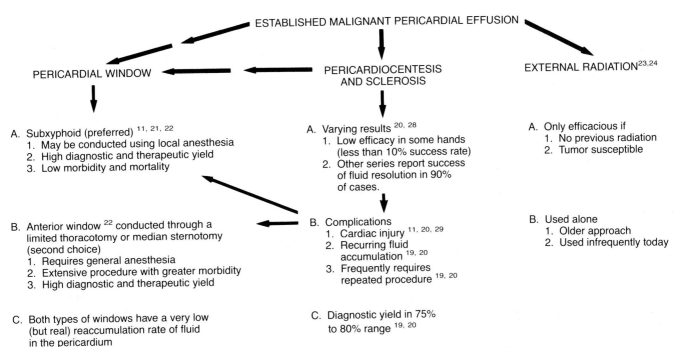

FIGURE 30–9. Flow diagram of therapy for established malignant pericardial effusion.

Preparation. The patient is placed on a stretcher, and the anterior abdominal wall and lower chest are prepared for surgery with sterile solutions and draped on all four sides to create a sterile field. An electrocardiograph is connected to the patient and set to record from the V lead. The V lead is attached to a sterile alligator clip that connects with a wire to a second clip, which, in turn, should be placed on the 22-gauge spinal needle that will be used to perform the pericardiocentesis.

Technique. A small wheal is created at the point of entry of the needle with 1% lidocaine (Xylocaine) local anesthesia. The point of entrance of the needle is at the right lateral margin of the xyphoid process near its tip. Once under the skin and underneath the xyphoid process, the needle should be directed toward the apex of the left shoulder.

Constant monitoring of the electrocardiogram is mandatory. The axis of the QRS complex often changes, and premature ventricular complexes are evoked when the needle touches the ventricle. The needle should be directed and advanced along a line established at the time of entrance. There should be no rotation or lateral motion of the needle once the tip is under the xyphoid, to avoid fracture and injury to the myocardium. Once fluid is aspirated, the needle should be fixed to the skin by the physician's hands, and 30 to 50 ml of the fluid is withdrawn through the needle.

The needle used should be the longest spinal needle available, so it can reach the pericardial sac in some robust and/or obese individuals. It may also be apparent that a 22-gauge needle is not strong enough to penetrate the tissues effectively. In these instances, a 20-gauge spinal needle may be used instead.

Failure to withdraw pericardial fluid should not prompt multiple attempts at pericardiocentesis. If nothing is obtained with three well-directed placements of the needle, the procedure should be abandoned, and an open pericardiotomy conducted.

Pericardiotomy

Some relief of the tamponade is mandatory before institution of general anesthesia. Attempts to place the patient under general anesthesia before the improvement in cardiac performance can cause severe arrhythmias and cardiac arrest. Therefore, the following approach using a subxyphoid pericardiotomy under local anesthesia should be conducted and the patient's hemodynamic status should be improved before venturing further.[124] Ideally, an anesthesiologist should be present to monitor the patient while the procedure is being performed.

Preparation. Intravenous access through two large-bore cannulas should be established before commencement of the procedure. If possible, an arterial line and a central line should be placed. Electrocardiographic monitoring is mandatory. The patient is usually maintained in a 45-degree upright position to facilitate oxygenation and ventilation, which are promoted by supplemental oxygen administered by face mask or nasal cannula. The entire anterior abdominal and chest wall is surgically prepared and draped for a median sternotomy in the relatively unlikely case that such a procedure might be required.

Technique. The midline is injected with 1% Xylocaine anesthesia, and an incision is made from 1 cm above the xyphoid process to a point 5 cm below its tip. The subcutaneous tissues and linea alba are opened using the electrocautery. At this time, the area around the xyphoid is heavily infiltrated with 1% lidocaine anesthesia, and the xyphoid process is excised using the electrocautery and heavy scissors. Occasionally, the base of the xyphoid will have to be cut with bone cutters. Once the xyphoid is excised, more local anesthesia is infiltrated into the inferior margin of the diaphragm, which should now be exposed in the incision. A small Richardson retractor is placed underneath the body of the sternum, and the sternum is elevated to expose the pericardium. Occasionally, a Kocher clamp will have to be placed on the diaphragm to provide caudad traction. The pericardium is then directly visible at the base of the wound (Fig. 30–10).

If there is any question as to whether the structure that has been visualized is the pericardium and whether it is free from the right ventricular wall, a needle should be introduced into the pericardium while the electrocardiogram is monitored. The needle is connected to a 50-ml syringe, and the pericardial space is aspirated. An improvement in hemodynamic performance should be reflected by a widening of the pulse pressure, an increase in systolic pressure, a decrease in diastolic pressure, and a concomitant fall in the central venous and pulmonary capillary wedge pressures. Once the patient's cardiac performance has improved, the anesthesiologist may institute general endotracheal anesthesia.

If the patient's condition remains poor and the level of cardiodynamic improvement does not allow institution of general anesthesia, a portion of the pericardium visible in the wound may be excised after it has been infiltrated with local anesthetic. The fluid that is present in the pericardium should be removed, and a portion of it should be sent for cytologic examination. A portion of the fluid should also be sent for standard bacteriologic cultures. The surgeon's fingers should be gently introduced into the pericardial space at this point to determine that all loculations present have been broken down and that no significant posterior effusion remains. Also, the surgeon should explore the pericardium to determine whether masses are present; if they are, they should be biopsied.

In some instances, when the patient cannot tolerate a general anesthetic, no further exploration of the pericardium is indicated or recommended. If further exploration of the pericardium is possible, it can be conducted not only by palpation but also by the placement of either a fiberoptic or rigid scope into the pericardium.[113] Both instruments have been used suc-

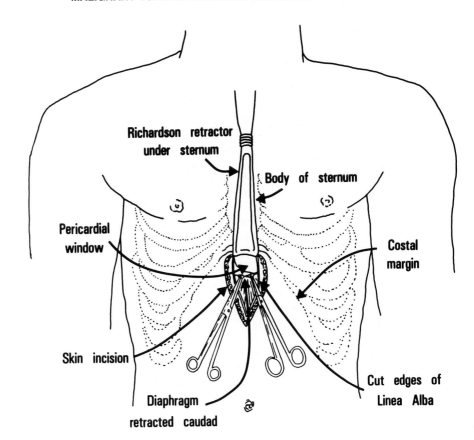

FIGURE 30–10. A completed subxyphoid pericardial window. The procedure may be conducted under local anesthesia until cardiac performance improves enough to allow initiation of general endotracheal anesthesia. A rigid mediastinoscope may also be introduced into the pericardium to evaluate any masses that may be present.

Labels in figure:
Richardson retractor under sternum
Body of sternum
Pericardial window
Costal margin
Skin incision
Cut edges of Linea Alba
Diaphragm retracted caudad

cessfully and have allowed drainage of posterior effusions as well as biopsy of pericardial nodules that may be present in the posterior recesses of the pericardium. The rigid mediastinoscope has been particularly useful.

After fluid has been evacuated, the biopsy specimens have been taken, and the extent of the disease has been determined, a single right-angle chest tube should be placed through a separate stab incision lateral to the primary incision and directed between the diaphragm and the heart. This tube should be secured to the skin by a heavy ligature and connected to suction drainage. A chest bottle or similar closed drainage system has proved very beneficial in maintaining drainage. Obviously, if either pleural space has been entered or explored, a chest drainage system with water seal will be mandatory. Closure is started by reconstructing the linea alba anterior to the pericardial tube with a heavy (such as a 0 polypropylene) running suture. The subcutaneous tissue and skin are reapproximated with running sutures. A sterile dressing is applied to the primary incision and to the chest tube site.

Postoperative Care. Pericardial drainage is maintained until the fluid removed is less than 100 ml in a 24-hour period. The pericardial drainage may be required anywhere from 2 to more than 8 days. Removal of the tube is based entirely on the judgment of the surgeon. If any questions arise as to whether the pericardium has been drained adequately, then a repeat echocardiogram should be obtained. Daily chest radiographs may be indicated to assess the res-

olution of the effusion and the proper position of the tube. The cardiac silhouette on chest radiography usually does not show much immediate improvement in size. Radiographic resolution may take several weeks even though the fluid has been properly drained. If there is any question of a remaining effusion, a repeat echocardiogram is indicated.

Results of Therapy

A summary of the results of the different modalities of therapy is presented in Figure 30–9. The foregoing discussion and the figure reflect our convictions that pericardiocentesis should be used early as a temporizing measure in the very acutely ill patient suffering from florid tamponade. Subxyphoid pericardiotomy is excellent in that it provides for high diagnostic accuracy, allows thorough assessment of pericardial disease, may be conducted with the patient under local anesthesia, and has a very high rate of therapeutic success (see Fig. 30–10). For these reasons, this procedure has become the technique of choice in our institution. Appropriate systemic treatment is organized and administered after control of the effusion has been achieved. The systemic therapeutic modalities are selected and administered on the basis of the histologic character of the primary tumor, extent of disease, and susceptibility of the neoplasm to the various regimens. Improvement and survival of the patient are directly related to the patient's general condition, the degree of neoplastic dissemination, and the response of the tumor to the therapeutic regimen chosen.

NEW DIRECTIONS

Because the majority of malignancies involving the heart are metastatic from other primary sites, any success in treating or preventing metastatic disease would translate into decreased mortality and morbidity from cardiac involvement. Treatment of primary tumors of the heart will benefit from advancing techniques in cardiac surgery, including transplantation. With respect to pericardial effusions, expanding roles for two-dimensional echocardiography and CT scanning can be anticipated. Two-dimensional echocardiography will be used to evaluate more accurately any loculations of fluid within the pericardium; CT will be used to evaluate neoplastic masses in the pericardium. The role of MRI in evaluating pericardial malignancies and effusions will be better defined as more data become available. Further use of endoscopy will undoubtedly enhance diagnostic and therapeutic capabilities. The expanding field of thoracoscopy also may contribute significantly to these capabilities. Advances in the therapy of neoplasms of the lung and breast, lymphomas, and leukemia will increase survival and improve the lifestyle of patients who have malignant pericardial involvement and effusions as a result of these diseases.

SELECTED REFERENCES

Bloor CM: Tumors of the endocardium and myocardium. *In* Bloor CM: Cardiac Pathology. Philadelphia, JB Lippincott, 1978.
This comprehensive review of the gross and histologic morphology of the most frequently encountered benign and malignant tumors is well illustrated and gives appropriate clinical correlations.

Davis S, Rambotti P, Grignani F: Intrapericardial tetracycline sclerosis in the treatment of malignant pericardial effusion: An analysis of thirty-three cases. J Clin Oncol 2:631–636, 1984.
An excellent account is given of the diagnosis and management of malignant pericardial effusions in 30 of 33 patients using an indwelling pericardial catheter. The results were good in the 30 successfully treated patients in that reaccumulation of the fluid was prevented. None of the patients had clinically significant complications associated with pericardiocentesis. Tetracycline infusion in the pericardium prevents reaccumulation of the effusion, but other therapy has to be used to control the systemic malignancy.

DePace NL, Soulen RL, Kotler MN, et al: Two dimensional echocardiographic detection of intra-atrial masses. Am J Cardiol 48:954, 1981.
The authors review the role of two-dimensional echocardiographic detection of masses in the atrium.

Fraser RS, Viloria JB, Wang N-S: Cardiac tamponade as a presentation of extracardiac malignancy. Cancer 45:1697, 1980.
The authors report on three cases of extracardiac malignancy that manifested initially as cardiac tamponade, review the literature for all cases of patients whose initial presentation included cardiac tamponade, and present an excellent discussion of the pathogenesis of malignant pericardial effusions, including a literature review.

Hancock EW: Neoplastic pericardial disease. Cardiol Clin 8:673, 1990.
This is an excellent overview of the signs and symptoms of malignant pericardial effusion as well as available diagnostic and therapeutic options. Surgical and nonsurgical methods are discussed.

Hankins JR, Satterfield JR, Aisner J, et al: Pericardial window for malignant pericardial effusion. Ann Thorac Surg 30:465, 1980.
Of 17 patients who had pericardial windows, in four, the windows were created by a limited median sternotomy or an anterior thoracotomy; in the remaining 13 patients, the windows were created via the subxyphoid route. Line drawings depict the subxyphoid approach.

Harvey WP: Clinical aspects of cardiac tumors. Am J Cardiol 21:328, 1968.
Signs and symptoms are emphasized that should alert the clinician to the presence of a cardiac neoplasm.

Little AG, Kremser PC, Wade JL, et al: Operation for diagnosis and treatment of pericardial effusions. Surgery 96:738, 1984.
In their experience with 32 consecutive patients with pericardial effusions, the authors emphasize the necessity for evaluating the etiology and the extent of pericardial effusions and stress the diagnostic and therapeutic efficacy of subxyphoid pericardiotomy. Photographs of the procedure are included.

McAllister HA Jr: Primary tumors and cysts of the heart and pericardium. Curr Probl Cardiol 4:1, 1979.
This is a comprehensive review of the vast experience of the Armed Forces Institute of Pathology with 533 primary cardiac tumors.

Poole GV Jr, Meredith JW, Breyer RH, et al: Surgical implications in malignant cardiac disease. Ann Thorac Surg 36:484, 1983.
This literature review presents 23 cases of primary cardiac tumors and of secondary tumors treated surgically; in selected patients, surgical treatment may be feasible.

REFERENCES

1. Colombus MR: De Re Anatomica. Paris, 1562, Libri XV, p 482.
2. Barnes AR, Beaver DC, Snell AM: Primary sarcoma of the heart: Report of a case with electrocardiographic and pathological studies. Am Heart J 9:480, 1934.
3. Beck CS: An intrapericardial teratoma and a tumor of the heart: Both removed operatively. Ann Surg 116:161, 1942.
4. Maurer ER: Successful removal of tumor of the heart. J Thorac Surg 23:479, 1952.
5. Goldberg HP, Glenn F, Dotter CT, et al: Myxoma of the left atrium: Diagnosis made during life with operative and postmortem findings. Circulation 6:762, 1952.
6. Crawford FA Jr, Selby JH Jr, Watson D, et al: Unusual aspects of atrial myxoma. Ann Surg 188:240, 1978.
7. Straus R, Merliss R: Primary tumor of the heart. Arch Pathol 39:74, 1945.
8. Benjamin HG: Primary fibromyxoma of the heart. Arch Pathol 27:950, 1939.
9. Prichard RW: Tumors of the heart: Review of the subject and report of one hundred and fifty cases. Arch Pathol 51:98, 1951.
10. McAllister HA Jr: Primary tumors and cysts of the heart and pericardium. Curr Probl Cardiol 4:1, 1979.
11. Selzer A, Sakai FJ, Popper RW: Protean clinical manifestations of primary tumors of the heart. Am J Med 52:9, 1972.
12. Harvey WP: Clinical aspects of cardiac tumors. Am J Cardiol 21:328, 1968.
13. Franciosa JA, Lawrinson W: Coronary artery occlusion due to neoplasm: Rare cause of acute myocardial infarction. Arch Intern Med 128:797, 1971.
14. Isner JM, Falcone MW, Virmani R, et al: Cardiac sarcoma causing "ASH" and simulating coronary heart disease. Am J Med 66:1025, 1979.
15. Berkelbach van der Sprenkel JW, Timmermans AJM, Elbers HRJ, et al: Polyarthritis as the presenting symptom of a malignant fibrous histiocytoma of the heart. Arthritis Rheum 28:944, 1985.
16. Bear PA, Moodie DS: Malignant primary cardiac tumors: The Cleveland Clinic experience, 1956–1986. Chest 92:860, 1987.
17. Pohost GM, Pastore JO, McKusick KA, et al: Detection of left atrial myxoma by gated radionuclide cardiac imaging. Circulation 55:88, 1977.
18. Pindyck F, Peirce EC II, Baron MG, et al: Embolization of left atrial myxoma after transseptal cardiac catheterization. Am J Cardiol 30:569, 1972.
19. Colucci WS, Braunwald E: Primary tumors of the heart. *In* Braunwald E (ed): Heart Disease: A Textbook of Cardiovascular Medicine, Vol 2. Philadelphia, WB Saunders, 1980.
20. Kutalek SP, Panidis IP, Kotler MN, et al: Metastatic tumors of the heart detected by two-dimensional echocardiography. Am Heart J 109:343, 1985.

21. Bulkley BH, Hutchins GM: Atrial myxomas: A fifty year review. Am Heart J 97:639, 1979.
22. Mugge A, Daniel WG, Haverich A, et al: Diagnosis of noninfective cardiac mass lesions by two-dimensional echocardiography. Circulation 83:70, 1991.
23. Waller DA, Scott PJ, Essop R, et al: The use of transesophageal echocardiography for detecting early recurrence of atrial myxoma. Int J Cardiol 35:235, 1992.
24. Gross BH, Glazer GM, Francis IR: CT of intracardiac and intrapericardial masses. Am J Roentgenol 140:903, 1983.
25. Hidalgo H, Korobkin M, Breiman RS, et al: CT of intracardiac tumor. Am J Roentgenol 137:608, 1981.
26. Menegus MA, Greenberg MA, Spindola-Franco H, et al: Magnetic resonance imaging of suspected atrial tumors. Am Heart J 123:1260, 1992.
27. Pizzarello RA, Goldberg SM, Goldman MA, et al: Tumor of the heart diagnosed by magnetic resonance imaging. J Am Coll Cardiol 5:989, 1985.
28. Becker RC, Hobbs RE, Ratliff NB: Cardiac rhabdomyosarcoma: Case report with review of clinical and pathologic features. Cleve Clin Q 51:83, 1984.
29. Yamashita K, Togashi K, Minami S, et al: Primary intracardiac tumors in magnetic resonance imaging. Radiol Med 9:127, 1991.
30. Brandenburg RO, Edwards JE: Cardiac Clinics CXLIII: Cardiac sarcoma: Report of case and comparison with a case of metastatic carcinoma of the pericardium. Mayo Clin Proc 29:437, 1954.
31. Poole-Wilson PA, Farnsworth A, Braimbridge MV, et al: Angiosarcoma of pericardium: Problems in diagnosis and management. Br Heart J 38:240, 1976.
32. Clancy DL, Morales JB Jr, Roberts WC: Angiosarcoma of the heart. Am J Cardiol 21:413, 1968.
33. Shackell M, Mitko A, Williams PL, et al: Angiosarcoma of the heart. Br Heart J 41:498, 1979.
34. Chun PKC, Leeburg WT, Coggin JT, et al: Primary pericardial malignant epithelioid mesothelioma causing acute myocardial infarction. Chest 77:559, 1980.
35. Mahaim I: Les Tumeurs et les Polypes du Coeur: Etude Anatomoclinique. Paris, Masson, 1945.
36. Sytman AL, MacAlpin RN: Primary pericardial mesothelioma: Report of two cases and review of the literature. Am Heart J 81:760, 1971.
37. Moncada R, Baker M, Salinas M, et al: Diagnostic role of computed tomography in pericardial heart disease: Congenital defects, thickening, neoplasms, and effusions. Am Heart J 103:263, 1982.
38. Harrington JS, Wagner JC, Smith M: The detection of hyaluronic acid in pleural fluids of cases with diffuse pleural mesotheliomas. Br J Exp Pathol 44:81, 1963.
39. Takeda K, Ohba H, Hyodo H, et al: Pericardial mesothelioma: Hyaluronic acid in pericardial fluid. Am Heart J 110:486, 1985.
40. Cayley FE, Bijapur HI: Fibrosarcoma of left atrium. Br Med J 1:1134, 1963.
41. Baldelli P, De Angeli D, Dolara A, et al: Primary fibrosarcoma of the heart. Chest 62:234, 1972.
42. Shah AA, Churg A, Sbarbaro JA, et al: Malignant fibrous histiocytoma of the heart presenting as an atrial myxoma. Cancer 42:2466, 1978.
43. Eckstein R, Gossner W, Rienmuller R: Primary malignant fibrous histiocytoma of the left atrium: Surgical and chemotherapeutic management. Br Heart J 52:354, 1984.
44. Stevens CW, Sears-Rogan P, Bitterman P, et al: Treatment of malignant fibrous histiocytoma of the heart. Cancer 69:956, 1992.
45. Herhusky MJ, Gregg SB, Virmani R, et al: Cardiac sarcomas presenting as metastatic disease. Arch Pathol Lab Med 109:943, 1985.
46. Rodenburg CJ, Kluin P, Maes A, et al: Malignant lymphoma confined to the heart, 13 years after a cadaver kidney transplant (letter to the editor). N Engl J Med 313:122, 1985.
47. Berry CL, Keeling J, Hilton C: Teratomata in infancy and childhood: A review of 91 cases. J Pathol 98:241, 1969.
48. Iliceto S, Quagliara D, Calabrese P, et al: Visualization of pericardial thymoma and evaluation of chemotherapy by two-dimensional echocardiography. Am Heart J 107:605, 1984.
49. Takamizawa S, Sugimoto K, Tanaka H, et al: A case of primary leiomyosarcoma of the heart. Intern Med 31:265, 1992.
50. Fine G, Raju BU: Leiomyosarcoma of the heart: A twenty-year cure. Henry Ford Hosp Med J 33:41, 1985.
51. Nzayinambaho K, Noel H, Brohet C, et al: Primary cardiac liposarcoma simulating a left atrial myxoma. Thorac Cardiovasc Surg 33:193, 1985.
52. Mavroudis C, Way LW, Lipton M, et al: Diagnosis and operative treatment of intracavitary liposarcoma of the right ventricle. J Thorac Cardiovasc Surg 81:137, 1981.
53. Poole GV Jr, Meredith JW, Breyer RH, et al: Surgical implications in malignant cardiac disease. Ann Thorac Surg 36:484, 1983.
54. Longino LA, Meeker IA Jr: Primary cardiac tumors in infancy. J Pediatr 43:724, 1953.
55. Scannell JG, Grillo HC: Primary tumors of the heart: A surgical problem. J Thorac Surg 35:23, 1958.
56. Schmaltz AA, Apitz J: Primary heart tumors in infancy and childhood: Report of four cases and review of literature. Cardiology 67:12, 1981.
57. Gabelman C, Al-Sadir J, Lamberti J, et al: Surgical treatment of recurrent primary malignant tumor of the left atrium. J Thorac Cardiovasc Surg 77:914, 1979.
58. Cooley DA, Reardon MJ, Frazier OH, et al: Human cardiac explantation and autotransplantation: Application in a patient with a large cardiac pheochromocytoma. Tex Heart Inst J 12:171, 1985.
59. Jamieson SW, Gaudiani VA, Reitz BA, et al: Operative treatment of an unresectable tumor of the left ventricle. J Thorac Cardiovasc Surg 81:797, 1981.
60. Armitage JM, Kormos RL, Griffith BP, et al: Heart transplantation in patients with malignant disease. J Heart Transplant 9:627, 1990.
61. Aravot DJ, Banner NR, Madden S, et al: Primary cardiac tumors–Is there a place for cardiac transplantation? Eur J Cardiothorac Surg 3:521, 1989.
62. Lockwood WB, Broghamer WL Jr: The changing prevalence of secondary cardiac neoplasms as related to cancer therapy. Cancer 45:2659, 1980.
63. Klatt EC, Heitz DR: Cardiac metastases. Cancer 65:1456, 1990.
64. Roberts WC, Glancy DL, DeVita VT Jr: Heart in malignant lymphoma (Hodgkin's disease, lymphosarcoma, reticulum cell sarcoma and mycosis fungoides): A study of 196 autopsy cases. Am J Cardiol 22:85, 1968.
65. McDonnell PJ, Mann RB, Bulkley BH: Involvement of the heart by malignant lymphoma: A clinicopathologic study. Cancer 49:944, 1982.
66. Kaul S, Fishbein MC, Seigel RJ: Cardiac manifestations of acquired immune deficiency syndrome: A 1991 update. Am Heart J 122:535, 1991.
67. Malaret GE, Aliaga P: Metastatic disease to the heart. Cancer 22:457, 1968.
68. Redwine DB: Complete heart block caused by secondary tumors of the heart: Case report and review of literature. Tex Med 70:59, 1974.
69. Smith LH: Secondary tumors of the heart. Rev Surg 33:223, 1976.
70. Bailey CP, Schechter DC, Folk FS: Extending operability in lung cancer involving the heart and great vessels. Ann Thorac Surg 11:140, 1971.
71. Glazer M, Kioschos JM, Kroetz FW, et al: Simulation of right atrial myxoma by metastatic leiomyosarcoma. Cancer 27:238, 1971.
72. Gordon R, Kimbiris D, Segal BL: Obstruction of the right ventricular outflow tract due to metastatic hypernephroma. Vasc Surg 7:213, 1973.
73. Hammond GL, Strong WW, Cohen LS, et al: Chondrosarcoma simulating malignant atrial myxoma. J Thorac Cardiovasc Surg 72:575, 1976.
74. Orsmond GS, Knight L, Dehner LP, et al: Alveolar rhabdomyosarcoma involving the heart: An echocardiographic, angiographic and pathologic study. Circulation 54:837, 1976.
75. Keir P, Keen G: Secondary leiomyosarcoma of the right ventricle: A surgical report. Br Heart J 40:328, 1978.
76. Ritcher N, Yon JL Jr: Squamous cell carcinoma of the cervix metastatic to the heart. Gynecol Oncol 7:394, 1979.

77. Magovern GJ, Yusuf MF, Liebler GA, et al: The surgical resection and chemotherapy of metastatic osteogenic sarcoma of the right ventricle. Ann Thorac Surg 29:76, 1980.

78. Martin JL, Boak JG: Cardiac metastasis from uterine leiomyosarcoma. J Am Coll Cardiol 2:383, 1983.

79. Utley JR, Mobin-Uddin K, Segnitz RH, et al: Acute obstruction of tricuspid valve by Wilms' tumor. J Thorac Cardiovasc Surg 66:626, 1973.

80. Murphy DA, Rabinovitch H, Chevalier L, et al: Wilms' tumor in right atrium. Am J Dis Child 126:210, 1973.

81. Aytac A, Tuncali T, Tinaztepe K, et al: Metastatic Wilms' tumor in the right atrium propagated through the inferior vena cava. Vasc Surg 10:268, 1976.

82. Vaughan ED Jr, Crosby IK, Tegtmeyer CJ: Nephroblastoma with right atrial extension: Preoperative diagnosis and management. J Urol 117:530, 1977.

83. Lam CR, Webb D, Green E: Primary liver tumor presenting as right atrial tumor: A case report. Surgery 59:872, 1966.

84. Ehrich DA, Widmann JJ, Berger RL, et al: Intracavitary cardiac extension of hepatoma. Ann Thorac Surg 19:206, 1975.

85. Boland TW, Winga ER, Kalfayan B: Chondrosarcoma: A case report with left atrial involvement and systemic embolization. J Thorac Cardiovasc Surg 74:268, 1977.

86. Gardner MAH, Bett JHN, Stafford EG, et al: Pulmonary metastatic chondrosarcoma with intracardiac extension. Ann Thorac Surg 27:238, 1979.

87. Rote AR, Flint LD, Ellis FH Jr: Intracaval recurrence of pheochromocytoma extending into right atrium: Surgical management using extracorporeal circulation. N Engl J Med 296:1269, 1977.

88. Ciafone RA, Galle JS, Chawla SK: Carcinoma of the lung invading the left atrium. Conn Med 44:773, 1980.

89. Kaku K, Kawashima Y, Kitamura S, et al: Resection of leiomyosarcoma originating in internal iliac vein and extending into heart via inferior vena cava. Surgery 89:604, 1981.

90. Marshall FF: Surgery of renal cell carcinoma with inferior vena cava involvement. Semin Urol 7:186, 1989.

91. Stewart JR, Carey JA, McDougal WS, et al: Cavoatrial tumor thrombectomy using cardiopulmonary bypass without circulatory arrest. Ann Thorac Surg 51:717, 1991.

92. Klein EA, Kaye MC, Novick AC: Management of renal cell carcinoma with vena caval thrombi via cardiopulmonary bypass and deep hypothermic circulatory arrest. Urol Clin North Am 18:445, 1991.

93. Barone GW, Kahn MB, Cook JM, et al: Recurrent intracaval renal cell carcinoma: The role of intravascular ultrasonography. J Vasc Surg 13:506, 1991.

94. Choh JH, Gurney R, Shenoy SS, et al: Renal-cell carcinoma: Removal of intracardiac extension with aid of cardiopulmonary bypass. NY State J Med 81:929, 1981.

95. Thompson WR, Newman K, Seibel N, et al: A strategy for resection of Wilms' tumor with vena cava or atrial extension. J Pediatr Surg 27:912, 1992.

96. Hancock EW: Neoplastic pericardial disease. Cardiol Clin 8:673, 1990.

97. Olopade OI, Ultmann JE: Malignant effusions. CA Cancer Clin J 41:166, 1991.

98. Fraser RS, Viloria JB, Wang N-S: Cardiac tamponade as a presentation of extracardiac malignancy. Cancer 45:1697, 1980.

99. Haagensen CD, Feind CR, Herter FP, et al: The Lymphatics in Cancer. Philadelphia, WB Saunders, 1972.

100. Caro DM, Berjon A, Teijeira J, Duran CG: Étude anatomique des lymphatiques cardiaques: Leur participation pathogénique dans les épanchements péricardiques. Ann Chir Thorac Cardiovasc 11:373–376, 1972.

101. Miller AJ, Jain S, Leven B: Radiographic visualization of the lymphatic drainage of heart muscle and pericardial sac in the dog. Chest 59:271, 1971.

102. Hanfling SM: Metastatic cancer to the heart: Review of the literature and report of 127 cases. Circulation 22:474, 1960.

103. Nelson BE, Rose PG: Malignant pericardial effusion from squamous cell cancer of the cervix. J Surg Oncol 52:203, 1993.

104. Abraham KP, Reddy V, Gattuso P: Neoplasms metastatic to the heart: Review of 3314 consecutive autopsies. Am J Cardiovasc Pathol 3:195, 1990.

105. Wiener HG, Kristensen IB, Haubek A, et al: The diagnostic value of pericardial cytology: An analysis of 95 cases. Acta Cytol 35:149, 1991.

106. Roberts WC, Spray RL: Pericardial heart disease: A study of its causes, consequences and morphologic features. Cardiovasc Clin 7:11, 1976.

107. Kline IK: Cardiac lymphatic involvement by metastatic tumor. Cancer 29:799, 1972.

108. Onuigbo WIB: The spread of lung cancer to the heart, pericardium, and great vessels. Jpn Heart J 15:234, 1974.

109. Abubakar S, Malik I, Ali SM, Khan A: Management of malignant pericardial effusion with tetracycline induced pericardiodesis. JAMA 266:119, 1991.

110. Theologides A: Neoplastic cardiac tamponade. Semin Oncol 5:181, 1978.

111. Thurber DL, Edwards JE, Anchor RWP: Secondary malignant tumors of the pericardium. Circulation 26:228, 1972.

112. Fincher RME: Case report: Malignant pericardial effusion as the initial manifestation of malignancy. Am J Med Sci 305:106, 1993.

113. Little AG, Kremser PC, Wade JL, et al: Operation for diagnosis and treatment of pericardial effusions. Surgery 96:738, 1984.

114. Appelqvist P, Maamies T, Grohn P: Emergency pericardiotomy as primary diagnostic and therapeutic procedure in malignant pericardial tamponade: Report of three cases and review of the literature. J Surg Oncol 21:18, 1982.

115. Lopez JM, Delgado JI, Tovar E, Gonzalez AG: Massive pericardial effusion produced by extracardiac malignant neoplasms. Arch Intern Med 143:1815, 1983.

116. Krisanda TJ: Atrial fibrillation with cardiac tamponade as the initial manifestation of malignant pericarditis. Am J Emerg Med 8:531, 1990.

117. Glazer GM, Gross BH, Orringer MB, et al: Computed tomography of pericardial masses: Further observation and comparison with echocardiography. J Comput Assist Tomogr 8:895, 1984.

118. Johnson FE, Wolverson MK, Sundaram M, Heiberg E: Unsuspected malignant pericardial effusion causing cardiac tamponade: Rapid diagnosis by computed tomography. Chest 82:501, 1982.

119. Coplan NL, Kennish AJ, Burgess NL, et al: Pericardial mesothelioma masquerading as a benign pericardial effusion. J Am Coll Cardiol 4:1307, 1984.

120. Hayward R, Treasure T, Swanton H, Emanuel R: Drainage of neoplastic pericardial effusions. Lancet 1:108, 1983.

121. Davis S, Rambotti P, Grignani F: Intrapericardial tetracycline sclerosis in the treatment of malignant pericardial effusion: An analysis of thirty-three cases. J Clin Oncol 2:631, 1984.

122. Wong B, Murphy J, Chang CJ, et al: The risk of pericardiocentesis. Am J Cardiol 44:1110, 1979.

123. Gatenby RA, Hertz WH, Kessler HB: Percutaneous catheter drainage for malignant pericardial effusion. J Vasc Interv Radiol 2:151, 1991.

124. Alcan KE, Zabetakis PM, Marino ND, et al: Management of acute cardiac tamponade by subxyphoid pericardiotomy. JAMA 247:1143, 1982.

125. Hankins JR, Satterfield JR, Aisner J, et al: Pericardial window for malignant pericardial effusion. Ann Thorac Surg 30:465, 1980.

126. Millaire A, Wurtz A, deGroote P, et al: Malignant pericardial effusions: Usefulness of pericardioscopy. Am Heart J 124:1030, 1992.

127. Cham WC, Freiman AH, Carstens HB, Chu FCJ: Radiation therapy of cardiac and pericardial metastases. Radiology 114:701, 1975.

128. Smith FE, Lane M, Hudgins PT: Conservative management of malignant pericardial effusions. Cancer 33:47, 1974.

129. Nanjo R: Intracavitary injection of OK-432 for malignant pericardial effusion: A case report. Radiat Med 8:155, 1990.

130. Celermajer DS, Boyer MH, Bailey BP, et al: Pericardiocentesis for symptomatic malignant pericardial effusion: A study of 36 patients. Med J Aust 154:19, 1991.

131. Grau JJ, Estapé J, Palombo H: Intracavitary oxytetracycline in malignant pericardial tamponade. Oncology 49:489, 1992.

132. Cormican MC, Nyman CR: Intrapericardial bleomycin for the management of cardiac tamponade secondary to malignant pericardial effusion. Br Heart J 63:61, 1990.

133. Chan A, Rischin D, Clarke CP, et al: Subxyphoid partial pericardiectomy with or without sclerosant instillation in the treatment of symptomatic pericardial effusions in patients with malignancy. Cancer 68:1021, 1991.

134. Martini N, Freiman AH, Watson RC, et al: Intrapericardial instillation of radioactive chromic phosphate in malignant pericardial effusion. Am J Roentgenol 128:639, 1977.

135. Lokich JJ: The management of malignant pericardial effusions. JAMA 224:1401, 1973.

136. Terry LN Jr, Klingerman MM: Pericardial and myocardial involvement by lymphomas and leukemias: The role of radiotherapy. Cancer 25:1003, 1090.

137. Rinkevich D, Borovik R, Bendett M, et al: Malignant pericardial tamponade. Med Pediatr Oncol 18:287, 1990.

138. Posner MR, Cohen GI, Skarin AT: Pericardial disease in patients with cancer: The differentiation of malignant from idiopathic and radiation induced pericarditis. Am J Med 71:407, 1981.

139. Kiser JC: Discussion of paper by Hankins JR, et al: Pericardial window for malignant pericardial effusion. Ann Thorac Surg 30:469, 1980.

140. Keane D, Jackson G: Managing recurrent malignant pericardial effusions: Percutaneous balloon pericardiotomy may have a role. Br Med J 305:729, 1992.

141. Palacios IF, Tuzcu EM, Ziskind AA, et al: Percutaneous balloon pericardial window for patients with malignant pericardial effusions and tamponade. Cathet Cardiovasc Diagn 22:224, 1991.

142. Caccavale RJ, Sisler GE, Newman J, Lewis RH: Pericardial disease. In Kaiser LR, Daniel TM (eds): Thoracoscopic Surgery. Boston, Little, Brown and Co, 1993, pp 177–187.

143. Ruckdeschel JC, Chang P, Martin RG, et al: Radiation-related pericardial effusion in patients with Hodgkin's disease. Medicine 54:245, 1975.

144. Martin RG, Ruckdeschel JC, Chang P, et al: Radiation-related pericarditis. Am J Cardiol 35:216, 1975.

145. Byhardt R, Brace K, Ruckdeschel JC, et al: Dose and treatment factors in radiation-related pericardial effusion associated with the mantle technique for Hodgkin's disease. Cancer 35:795, 1975.

Part IV

MALIGNANCIES OF THE CHEST WALL AND PLEURA

31 OVERVIEW OF MALIGNANCIES OF THE CHEST WALL AND PLEURA

Thomas H. Weisenburger

CHEST WALL TUMORS

Chest wall tumors constitute fewer than 1% of all tumors and, when present, are malignant approximately 60% of the time. Of those that are malignant, a little more than half are primary tumors of the chest wall; the remainder are metastatic. (See Tables 32–1 to 32–3 for frequency of various primary and metastatic tumors to the chest wall.)

The initial evaluation after the discovery of a chest wall tumor consists of a thorough physical examination to locate the tumor, which may indicate its histology (e.g., chondrosarcomas tend to recur along the costochondral junctions[1]), and routine laboratory tests to determine any signs of systemic involvement, which may indicate metastatic disease. Useful radiographic studies are posteroanterior and lateral chest views, and computed tomography and magnetic resonance imaging, which can be most useful in determining what anatomic structures are involved and whether lung metastases are present. A bone scan should be performed not only to determine whether there is periosteal or rib involvement at the site but also to screen for the presence of metastatic disease. Further work-up, including pulmonary function tests, should be performed selectively, depending on the extent of resection involved and the findings on the physical examination and radiographs.

As pointed out in Chapter 32, it is no longer necessary or mandatory to perform an excisional biopsy on chest wall tumors. Tissue may be obtained by needle aspiration, with or without core biopsy, to establish the diagnosis. If insufficient material for permanent sections and immunohistochemical and electron microscopic studies is obtained with needle biopsy, an incisional biopsy using a transverse incision is recommended. After the histologic type of chest wall tumor is established, a therapeutic plan is developed that must consider the use of adjuvant therapies, depending on the microscopic diagnosis.

Chondrosarcomas generally are treated with surgery alone. Low-grade tumors that can be completely excised with negative margins are associated with an excellent prognosis. Higher grade tumors and larger tumors are more difficult to control, and combination therapy using radiation and surgery must be investi-gated to evaluate the efficacy of these more difficult lesions.

Approximately 6.5% of Ewing's tumors will be primary rib lesions,[2] and half of the affected patients will present with metastatic disease.[3] Multimodality therapy has become the standard, with the best results obtained in patients who have had complete resection followed by chemotherapy or radiotherapy.

Osteogenic sarcoma of the chest wall is an infrequent sign of presentation for osteogenic sarcoma. These lesions are generally resected, with postoperative adjuvant chemotherapy considered in those patients without metastatic disease.[4]

Plasmacytoma of the chest wall usually is a manifestation of systemic multiple myeloma and should be managed with chemotherapy. Radiation therapy should be considered if it is apparently a solitary plasma cell tumor.

Surgery alone for soft tissue sarcomas of the chest wall is associated with a high incidence of local recurrence.[5] Therefore, adjuvant therapy in the form of radiotherapy and chemotherapy has been evaluated. Because of the usefulness of adjuvant radiotherapy in soft tissue sarcomas at other sites,[6] it is reasonable to consider preoperative or postoperative radiotherapy in this situation. Whether chemotherapy should be used in this specific subgroup of chest wall soft tissue sarcomas has not as yet been answered. Although the major study on this point indicated increased disease-free survival, there was no difference in overall 3-year survival.[7]

Special consideration should be given to peripheral neuronepitheliomas and rhabdomyosarcomas, which, after a generous biopsy, should be treated with combined radiotherapy and chemotherapy. Surgery should be considered to remove gross residual disease after radiotherapy and chemotherapy if it is possible to ensure negative margins.

Desmoid tumors or low-grade fibrosarcomas of the chest wall are best treated with wide excision, with overall survival approaching 95% at 10 years.[8]

Pass provides an excellent discussion in Chapter 32 of the surgical approach, with an emphasis on the principle of obtaining negative surgical margins and a description of new techniques available to reconstruct the soft tissues and bony structures of the chest wall.

TUMORS OF THE PLEURA

Mesotheliomas of the pleura can be benign or malignant and, if malignant, either localized or diffuse. Usually, localized malignant mesotheliomas can be managed reasonably well with local resection. The major challenge to the physician managing these tumors is diffuse malignant mesothelioma, a rare and usually fatal tumor. Most but not all of these tumors are related to asbestos exposure.[9]

Mesotheliomas are either the epithelial type which is more likely to produce fluid and have a longer course, or the mesenchymal type, which is more likely to be dry and infiltrative and is associated with shorter survival.[10] The histologic diagnosis may be elusive, since reactive mesothelial cells may resemble malignant mesothelial cells. Pleural biopsy is frequently required.

Sugarbaker notes that an aggressive surgical approach is generally limited to Stage I tumors, defined as disease localized to the parietal and visceral pleura without lymph node involvement. Surgical treatment with pleural pneumonectomy has a high mortality rate and yields relatively low survival rate. Because of this, adjuvant treatment is desirable to treat any microscopic disease left behind. Sugarbaker reported a 17% overall survival rate (50% in patients with epithelial type) with a trimodality program of extrapleural pneumonectomy plus four to six cycles of chemotherapy followed by 55 Gy radiotherapy to the hemithorax.[11] Several other series with extrapleural pneumonectomy are presented in Table 33–1.

Unfortunately, chemotherapy for malignant mesothelioma, with single or combination agents, has not been impressive (see Tables 33–2 to 33–4). Intracavitary instillation of cisplatin has been reported but appears to be less effective than in peritoneal mesothelioma.[12]

There is little experience with combined chemotherapy and radiotherapy, although a small series using intermittent doxorubicin and radiotherapy appeared to indicate increased survival.[13] A randomized intergroup study comparing radiotherapy with or without doxorubicin is under way.

Because of the infrequency of this tumor, the difficulty in management, and the lack of randomized studies, firm conclusions as to treatment are difficult to draw. Combined modality therapy using surgery, radiation, and chemotherapy must be evaluated to determine the optimal management of this difficult clinical problem. Referral of these patients to centers that specialize in the treatment of malignant mesothelioma will facilitate the search for more active protocols.

Moores and Ruckdeschel present an excellent discussion of the anatomy and physiology of the pleural space and the path of physiology of fluid formation. After the discovery of a pleural effusion and its confirmation on radiographs, thoracentesis should be performed. Approximately 50% of malignant pleural effusions are diagnosed on the first thoracentesis. The figure increases to 70% by the third tap. Thoracoscopy with direct biopsy of the pleura is positive in 97% of the patients with malignant pleural effusions.[14] Moores and Ruckdeschel recommend thoracoscopy with biopsy if the diagnosis is not established after the second thoracentesis.

They point out that treatment in the vast majority of patients is palliative, and they emphasize that rapid diagnosis and treatment are important in the successful management of patients with malignant pleural effusions (see Fig. 34–1).

The treatment will depend on the histology of the malignancy. If the pleura is the initial site of metastasis from chemotherapy-sensitive tumors, effusions are usually treated with systemic agents, with resolution in most instances. If, however, the patient is refractory to this treatment and for most other solid tumors, tube thoracostomy and pleurodesis are indicated. Talc, now available asbestos free and sterile, appears to be more effective than tetracycline or bleomycin.[15, 16]

REFERENCES

1. Marcove RC, Huvos AG: Cartilaginous tumors of the ribs. Cancer 27:794–801, 1971.
2. Thomas PR, Foulkes MA, Gilula LA, et al: Primary Ewing's sarcoma of the ribs. Cancer 51:1021–1027, 1983.
3. Hayes FA, Thompson EI, Houstu HO, et al: The response of Ewing's sarcoma to sequential cyclophosphamide and Adriamycin induction therapy. J Clin Oncol 1:45–51, 1983.
4. Link MD, Gorin AM, Miser AW, et al: The effect of adjuvant chemotherapy on relapse-free survival in patients with osteosarcoma of the extremity. N Engl J Med 314:1600–1606, 1986.
5. Romsdahl MM, Lindberg RR, Martin RG, et al: Patterns of failure after treatment of soft tissue sarcomas. Cancer Treat Symp 2:251–258, 1983.
6. Lindberg RD, Martin RG, Romsdahl MM, et al: Conservative surgery and postoperative radiotherapy in 300 patients with soft tissue sarcomas. Cancer 47:2391–2397, 1981.
7. Glenn J, Kinsella T, Glatstein E, et al: A randomized prospective trial of adjuvant chemotherapy in adults with soft tissue sarcomas of the head and neck, breast, and trunk. Cancer 55:1206–1214, 1985.
8. Brodsky JT, Gordon MS, Hajdu SI, et al: Desmoid tumors of the chest wall. J Thorac Cardiovasc Surg 104:900–903, 1992.
9. Wagner JC, Sleggs CA, Marchand P: Diffuse pleural mesothelioma and asbestos exposure in the Northwestern Cape Province. Br J Ind Med 17:260–270, 1960.
10. Elmes PC, Simpson MJC: The clinical aspects of mesothelioma. Q J Med 45:427–429, 1976.
11. Sugarbaker DJ, Strauss GM, Lynch TJ, et al: Node status has prognostic significance in the multi-modality therapy of diffuse, malignant mesothelioma. J Clin Oncol 11:1172–1178, 1993.
12. Markman M, Cleary S, Pfeifle CL, et al: Cisplatin administered by the intracavitary route as treatment for malignant mesothelioma. Cancer 58:18–21, 1986.
13. Sinoff C, Falkson G, Sandison AG, et al: Combined doxorubicin and radiation therapy in malignant pleural mesothelioma. Cancer Treat Rep 66:1605–1607, 1982.
14. Boutin C, Viallat JR, Cargnino P, et al: Thoracoscopy in malignant pleural effusions. Am Rev Respir Dis 124:588, 1981.
15. Fentimen IS, Rubens RD, Hayward JL: A comparison of intracavitary talc and tetracycline for the control of pleural effusions secondary to breast cancer. Eur J Cancer Clin Oncol 22:1079, 1986.
16. Hamed H, Fentimen IS, Chaudary MA, et al: Comparison of intracavitary bleomycin and talc for control of pleural effusion secondary to carcinoma of the breast. Br J Surg 76:1266, 1989.

32 PRIMARY AND METASTATIC CHEST WALL TUMORS

Harvey I. Pass

Chest wall tumors can originate in any of the histologic elements of the thorax, including muscle, nerve, bone, cartilaginous elements, and soft tissue. Moreover, the presence of a neoplasm of the external thorax could be a metastatic lesion from a previously treated or occult primary tumor. Until recently, it has been difficult to report on a large series of patients in a prospective manner to assess the adequacy of current surgical techniques and the influence of adjunctive therapy on survival owing to the paucity and inhomogeneity of the histologic types of tumors reported.

This chapter emphasizes malignant chest wall lesions, both primary and metastatic. The role of surgery in the diagnosis and management is described, and the importance of uniform treatment of defined histologic categories of chest wall neoplasms is emphasized. Many aspects of treatment, ranging from diagnosis to the use of adjunctive therapies, continue to cause controversies that can be settled only by carefully performed multi-institutional, prospective, randomized trials. It is hoped that the recognition of the limits of past reports will stimulate these types of trials.

HISTORICAL ASPECTS

Paget[1] is credited with reporting in 1896 the first accounts of chest wall neoplasms, of which 24 were malignant. The first report of the use of surgery to treat such tumors was made in 1898 by Parham[2], who is generally given credit, along with Rudolf Matas, for performing the first successful resections. These earliest resections were made possible by the advent of positive-pressure ventilation. From the early 1900s to the middle of the twentieth century, there were scattered reports of resections and literature reviews that involved local resectional therapy. In 1921, Hedgeblom[3] described 313 cases of patients with chest wall tumors, of which 74% were malignant. In 1951, O'Neal and Ackerman[4] reported 96 cases of patients with cartilaginous tumors of the ribs and sternum, of which two-thirds were malignant. In 1953, Hochberg[5] described 205 cases, of which 50% were malignant.

These reports were important in that they paralleled a period of increased patient survival with larger resections due to the use of improved anesthetic techniques; better understanding of pleural physiology, including the use of closed water seal drainage; and the advent of antibiotics. The reports also served as the foundations for classifying chest wall tumors by histology and location.

The modern era of treatment of malignant chest wall neoplasms began in the 1960s with the reporting of treatment of histologically uniform tumors. This allowed greater understanding of the biologic variability of cell types, specifically regarding the tendency to either recur locally or metastasize. With a greater understanding of the natural history, newly developed chemotherapeutic regimens were added and radiotherapy techniques were refined, so this method could be used as a primary or adjunctive treatment. Also, musculocutaneous flap procedures as well as innovative uses for newly developed prosthetic materials were developed to aid in the reconstruction of the chest wall.

INCIDENCE AND HISTOLOGIC TYPES

The incidence of chest wall neoplasms has been estimated to be less than 1% of all tumors,[6] and the majority of the tumors originate in cartilage or bone. A 71-year series from the Mayo Clinic reported 6221 patients with primary bony tumors, of which only 263 (4.2%) originated in the chest wall.[7] During a similar period, 120 cartilaginous neoplasms of the chest wall were recorded, of which 96 (80%) were malignant.

Many studies have reported that metastatic (solitary) lesions occur with about the same frequency as primary tumors. This finding was reported by Ochsner and associates[8] in 1966; in their series of 134 chest wall neoplasms, 50 were metastatic and 36 were primary malignant chest wall lesions. This proportion differs from that reported by Blades and Paul[9] (9% metastatic), as well as from the findings of a number of current reviews (Table 32–1). When multiple sites of involvement are noted, metastatic malignancy should be considered. The most likely tumors causing solitary metastatic lesions of the bony thorax are genitourinary, thyroid, colonic, and sarcomatous primaries.[10] Renal cell and thyroid malignancies have a high propensity for sternal metastases, occasionally appearing as pulsatile masses.[11]

TABLE 32–1. Incidence of Primary Versus Metastatic Tumors Found at Chest Wall Resection

STUDY	YEAR	NO. OF PRIMARY TUMORS	NO. OF METASTATIC TUMORS	TOTAL
McCormack et al[55]	1981	60	32	92
Rami-Porta et al[76]	1985	15	36	51
Perry[45]	1985	17	7	24
Pairolero and Arnold[64]	1985	50	32	82
Total (%)		57	43	

TABLE 32–2. Chest Wall Tumors: Benign Versus Malignant

STUDY	YEAR	NO. OF BENIGN TUMORS	NO. OF MALIGNANT TUMORS	TOTAL
Threlkel and Adkins[78]	1971	22	23	45
Teitlebaum[38]	1972	29	32	61
Graeber[77]	1982	51	59	110
Sabanathan et al[12]	1985	26	27	53
Rami-Porta et al[76]	1985	12	15	27
McAfee et al[7]	1985	24	96	120
Pairolero and Arnold[64]	1985	18	26	44
King et al[81]	1986	19	71	90
Ala-Kulju et al[82]	1988	24	10	34
Ryan et al[83]	1989	5	88	93

A review of the literature confirms that 60% of chest wall tumors prove to be malignant (Table 32–2). Tissue of origin of the malignancy is overwhelmingly bone or cartilage, with rib primaries more common than sternum primaries (Table 32–3). Soft tissue sarcomas are the third most common cause of chest wall malignancies.

SYMPTOMS AND PHYSICAL FINDINGS

Depending on the tumor stage at presentation, patients will present with variable symptoms referable to a chest wall neoplasm. Approximately 20% of patients with chest wall neoplasms are asymptomatic.[12] The presence of a mass possibly associated with localized or referred pain will be the most common presenting complaint. Eighty per cent of the patients will have an enlarging mass, of which 50% to 60% are painful. A history of chest trauma is occasionally encountered, and although certain histologic types of chest wall tumors have a higher incidence in certain age groups, chest wall tumors can occur in patients of all ages.

Examination of the patient should concentrate on evaluation of tumor location and size and possible invasion of contiguous structures. Malignant chest wall tumors are usually fixed to the bony thorax, and their size may vary. Consistency may vary with his-

tologic type, with bony tumors feeling harder than soft tissue tumors.

Location of the lesion may give a clue to the histologic type of tumor; the majority of tumors of cartilaginous origin occur along the costochondral junctions.[13] Tumors located away from the costal cartilages on the chest wall are of bony or soft tissue origin.

In examining the patient, one should keep in mind the location of the tumor in relation to major neurovascular components and contiguous structures. Lesions high in the axilla may require further work-up to rule out the necessity of forequarter amputation. Posterior lesions may require neurosurgical guidance if examination reveals the tumor to be close to the thoracic spine. Inferior lesions could require partial resection of the diaphragm.

RADIOGRAPHIC ASSESSMENT

Radiographic assessment of the chest wall mass provides the most information regarding the origin of the mass (bone, cartilage, or soft tissue) as well as the planning of subsequent surgical or nonsurgical therapy. The standard posteroanterior and lateral chest radiographs can be used to define in a nonspecific

TABLE 32–3. Primary Malignant Chest Wall Tumors

STUDY	CHONDROSARCOMA	FIBROSARCOMA	OSTEOSARCOMA	MULTIPLE MYELOMA	EWING'S SARCOMA	OTHER TUMOR	TOTAL
McAfee et al[7]	96	0	0	0	0	0	96
Sabanathan et al[12]	13	0	0	8	6	0	27
Teitlebaum et al[38]	10	0	3	10	2	7	32
Perry et al[45]	0	0	3	0	3	22	28
Pairolero and Arnold[64]	7	9	3	2	2	27	50
McCormack et al[55]	13	10	17	1	4	15	59
Rami-Porta et al[76]	1	0	0	1	4	0	6
Graeber[77]	10	19	4	8	6	12	59
Threlkel and Adkins[78]	3	7	2	3	2	6	23
Watkins and Gerard[79]	7	9	0	1	1	18	36
Golladay et al[80]	0	1	0	0	1	6	8
King et al[81]	17	0	3	2	4	45	71
Ala-Kulju et al[82]	4	1	1	1	1	3	10
Ryan et al[83]	3	3	4	0	6	16	32
Burt et al[25]	88	0	38	0	0	0	126

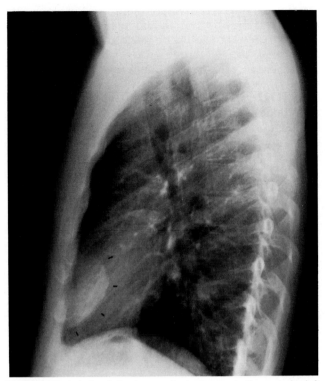

FIGURE 32–1. Lateral chest x-ray study demonstrating anterior left-sided chest wall mass (*small arrows*).

manner the location of the mass (Fig. 32–1). Rib destruction, either as the primary site of origin of the tumor or due to invasion, may be present (Fig. 32–2). Careful scrutiny of the lung fields should be performed to rule out intraparenchymal lesions. The presence of a pleural effusion should be noted; further work-up of an effusion is needed to rule out malignant cells resulting from transthoracic invasion or discontinuous pleural disease.

Computed tomography (CT) is the most valuable tool in the evaluation of a chest wall tumor.[14] The 1-cm axial cuts provide the best way to define the limits of the lesion in both a superoinferior plane and the depth of the tumor. By carefully noting the superior and inferior extents of the lesion and the relation to the intercostal spaces, the surgeon will know which interspace can be safely entered for intrapleural assessment of disease without violating the tumor. CT can be used to define, albeit incompletely, the relation between the mass and contiguous structures such as the scapula, root of the neck, diaphragm, lung, and axillary contents. Examination of the lung windows will uncover any synchronous metastatic disease, which would dictate the use of a median sternotomy if it is technically feasible[15] (Figs. 32–3 and 32–4). The mediastinal and bone windows provide the best information regarding the dimensions of the lesion, i.e., the depth as well as the consistency of the tumor. Inhomogeneity within the tumor may indicate the presence of focal necrosis.

The relation of the mass to the chest wall musculature can also be well defined by CT scanning. Depending on the location of the mass as pictured on CT, surgical flaps can be planned that will leave sufficient tumor-free margins of musculature while sparing sufficient muscle to be rotated for chest wall reconstruction. Assessment of the pleura can also be performed by CT scanning to try to rule out discontinuous pleural disease and pleural fluid. Finally, if the patient is not a surgical candidate but satisfies a protocol situation that dictates innovative preoperative therapy before resection, CT serves as the best predictor of measurable disease, allowing more objective conclusions to be made with regard to responses to treatment.

Magnetic resonance imaging (MRI) has become increasingly popular to supplement or replace CT of the chest wall lesion. The ability to image in the transverse, sagittal, and coronal planes as well as the use of different MRI sequences has added to definition of

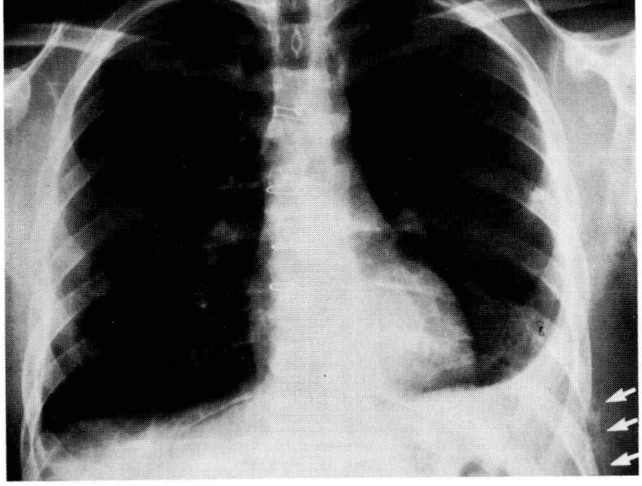

FIGURE 32–2. PA chest x-ray study demonstrating destruction of left eighth rib by metastatic osteogenic sarcoma (*arrows*).

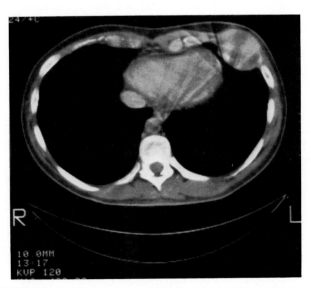

FIGURE 32–3. CT scan demonstrates the chest wall tumor seen in Figure 32–1.

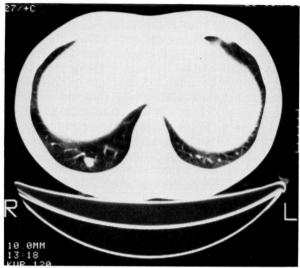

FIGURE 32–4. Synchronous lung metastasis in patient with chest wall tumor demonstrated by CT in Figure 32–3. Simultaneous median sternotomy and chest wall resection were performed in this patient (see Fig. 32–12).

the precise anatomic situation of the tumor before treatment. Although not subjected to head-to-head comparison, it is generally believed that MRI allows superior anatomic definition, qualification of disease extent, and definition of bone involvement compared with CT.

Angiography can be used selectively in the work-up of the patient with a chest wall neoplasm[16] (Fig. 32–5). When the lesion is close to or in the axilla, angiography may define invasion or abutment of the axillary artery and help determine whether the patient will require concomitant forequarter resection. If a muscle flap is to be used that has already been in an irradiated field, selective angiography can define the integrity of the appropriate vascular pedicle.

Bone scanning should be performed in all cases of chest wall, rib, or sternal neoplasms. Periosteal involvement in proximity to the tumor, as well as other sites of peripheral involvement with metastatic disease, can be defined. The absence of rib involvement on a bone scan in the region of the chest wall mass should not lead one to compromise the resection by trying to avoid rib resection and thus violate the tumor pseudocapsule.

Pulmonary function testing can be used selectively in patients undergoing chest wall resection. If invasion of the lung is suspected on the basis of CT findings and major pulmonary resection is being contemplated, pulmonary function and arterial blood gases with the patient inspiring room air should be determined.

Further work-up is dictated by history and physical examination to locate the primary tumor if the chest wall lesion is believed to be a metastasis. Primary renal and lung lesions are most highly suspect and can be studied accordingly.

DIAGNOSIS

Most surgeons stress that all chest wall tumors should be considered malignant until proved to be otherwise and that wide excision should be carried out.[5, 8, 9, 12] Others have placed size restrictions (i.e., 4 cm) on malignancy potential, stating that smaller lesions should, if possible, be totally excised without preliminary biopsy. Newer developments in the diagnosis and treatment of chest wall neoplasms, however, have forced a reappraisal of this approach in that neoplasms incompletely cured by single modality ther-

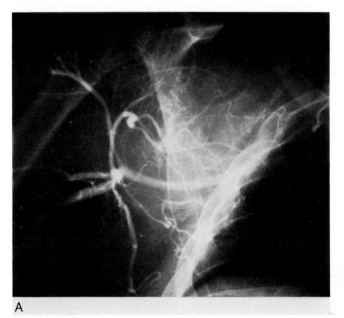

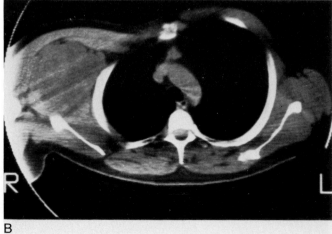

FIGURE 32–5. Axillary artery displacement by a large right axillary tumor (*A*). CT scan in the same patient (*B*). This patient required chest wall resection and forequarter.

apy are now responding to combination chemotherapy, radiation, and surgery, and the temporal order of therapies for histologic type of tumor has yet to be defined.[17] Moreover, pathologists are able to give more accurate diagnoses as to the origin of the neoplasm through the use of monoclonal antibodies and other immunohistochemical techniques, along with electron microscopy.[18] Finally, local recurrence due to initial "nonexcisional" biopsy techniques has not been proved to occur, nor does a reasonable delay in waiting for the preoperative diagnosis appear to affect survival.

A generous specimen of the tumor that is free from necrosis should be obtained as an initial step.[19] Needle aspiration cytology with or without core-cutting biopsy has been shown to be effective in making a diagnosis. Core-cutting biopsy has a higher accuracy (96%) than fine-needle aspiration (64%). Such core biopsies not only have been successful in making the diagnosis but also frequently provide sufficient tissue for grading.[20] Excisional biopsy is appropriate for lesions less than 2 cm or those that appear to be benign by roentgenographic examination.

If no diagnosis can be made by needle or core-cutting biopsy in a large lesions, an incisional biopsy should be performed. The biopsy should be made by a transverse incision (Fig. 32–6), which can easily be excised when skin flaps are begun at the later definitive procedure. The biopsy should not cause extensive contamination of the surrounding skin and fascial planes by hematoma formation and should not require the insertion of a drain. Sufficient material must be collected for permanent histopathology, immunohistochemical verification, and electron microscopy. Treatment options can then be guided, especially in the pediatric age group, by the definitive cell type of the tumor, and the appropriate adjuvant therapy can be considered.

THERAPY

Once the histologic type of chest wall tumor has been determined, an appropriate therapeutic plan must be formulated that takes into account the usefulness of adjuvant therapy. The majority of chest wall tumors will need surgical therapy as first-line treatment; however, a subset of tumors has emerged that may dictate the preoperative or postoperative use of adjuvant chemotherapy, radiation, or both (Fig. 32–7). A discussion, therefore, of the pathophysiology, methods of spread, and past as well as current therapies for the major chest wall tumors is in order, with the recognition that the literature is deficient in large-scale, prospective studies for individual tumor types.

Chondrosarcoma

Chondrosarcoma is the most common of the chest wall neoplasms, representing 20% of all bony neoplasms. Chondrosarcomas are usually solitary, primarily affecting the top four ribs. They can involve the sternum and are usually seen in individuals older than 40 years. They are usually found arising anteriorly from either the costochondral or sternochondral junction (66%), with 25% arising posteriorly from the rib head.[7]

Most patients will have a long duration of symptoms, finally presenting with a painful, firm mass. Symptoms of invasion (hemoptysis, spinal cord compression, Horner's syndrome) or metastases may occur initially.

The presumptive diagnosis of chondrosarcoma can be made on roentgenographic examination, on which a lobulated mass is seen arising in the medullary portion of the rib or sternum.[21] Cortical bone is typically destroyed, and the margins of the tumor are poorly

FIGURE 32–6. Transversely placed previous biopsy of chest wall sarcoma. Transverse orientation lends itself to easier excision in raising the skin flaps at time of definitive resection.

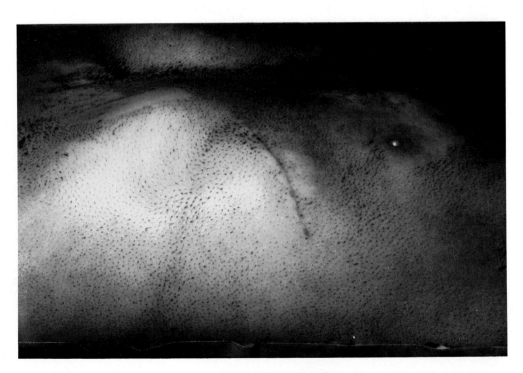

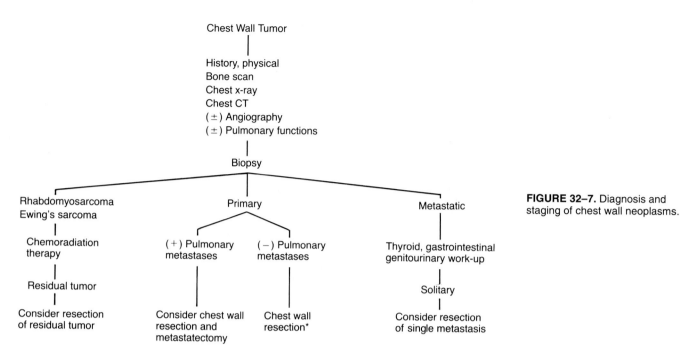

Chest Wall Tumor
|
History, physical
Bone scan
Chest x-ray
Chest CT
($\pm$) Angiography
($\pm$) Pulmonary functions
|
Biopsy

Rhabdomyosarcoma
Ewing's sarcoma
|
Chemoradiation
therapy
|
Residual tumor
|
Consider resection
of residual tumor

Primary

(+) Pulmonary
metastases
|
Consider chest wall
resection and
metastatectomy

(−) Pulmonary
metastases
|
Chest wall
resection*

Metastatic
|
Thyroid, gastrointestinal
genitourinary work-up
|
Solitary
|
Consider resection
of single metastasis

FIGURE 32–7. Diagnosis and staging of chest wall neoplasms.

*If chest wall lesion is too large to ensure negative margins, consider primary radiation therapy or preoperative best-choice chemotherapy with tumor resection after objective response.

defined. A mottled type of calcification is usually present.

Cartilaginous tumors such as chondrosarcoma are difficult to grade histologically. In the past, grading systems have been based on the degree of cellularity and pleomorphism (Fig. 32–8). Recently, newer cytologic, histochemical, and biochemical analyses have been used in grading.[22] Cytologic analysis of the nuclear abnormalities and histologic evaluation of the bone-tumor interface will best predict local aggressiveness. DNA content of tumor as well as flow cytometry studies may grade chondrosarcoma more precisely. At present, the grading classification correlates with clinical behavior of the tumor, with high-grade (Grade III) tumors having a stronger propensity for metastatic potential (75%) than low-grade (15%) or moderate-grade (40%) tumors.[23]

The natural history of chest wall chondrosarcoma usually consists of slow growth and local recurrence. More than half of the tumors that are excised incompletely or without adequate margins recur, either locally or with metastasis. Metastasis occurs mainly in lymph nodes and lung; other sites of metastatic disease include bone, liver, pleura, and subcutaneous tissue.[24]

In a review from the Mayo Clinic,[7] the estimated 10-year survival rate for 72 patients with chest wall chondrosarcoma was 53.4%, and the 5-year survival rate of 88 patients treated at Memorial Sloan-Kettering Cancer Hospital (MSK) was 64%.[25] Patients with a wide resection had a 96% 10-year survival rate compared with 65% for local excision and 14% for palliative excision.[7] Survival in the Mayo Clinic experience

was influenced by tumor size, grade, and location (sternal primaries faring better than rib tumors). No patient with Grade III tumor survived longer than 2 years. In the MSK series, survival was favorably influenced by age of less than 50 years, absence of synchronous metastases, and complete rather than incomplete resection. There was a 28% chance of local recurrence, and those patients had a greater chance of developing metastases than the group without local recurrence. Grade of the lesion did not influence survival in the MSK series.[25]

Chondrosarcomas are extremely radioresistant and chemoresistant, and controlled trials evaluating che-

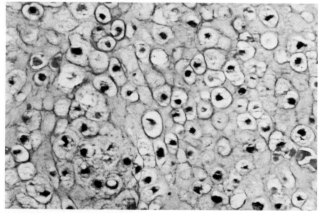

FIGURE 32–8. Chondrosarcoma, histologic view ($\times$15), well differentiated, with chondroid lacunar formation.

moradiation for these tumors are few. For high-grade unresectable chondrosarcomas, high-dose (50 to 55 Gy) radiotherapy may be warranted.[26] Local control may require as much as 75 Gy. There is some suggestion that a combination of radiotherapy and surgery may have a high potential for improving local control rates for chondrosarcomas of the axilla, mandible, and skull.[27] Further controlled investigations must be performed to evaluate the efficacy of this treatment for chest wall lesions.

Ewing's Sarcoma

Ewing's sarcoma accounts for 10% to 15% of bone tumors in children and adolescents and is distinguished from other bony tumors by its relative radiation sensitivity. In the largest series, the median patient age was 16 years. Fifteen per cent of Ewing's sarcomas involve the chest wall, and approximately 6.5% are primary rib lesions.[28] Ewing's sarcoma is unique histologically, consisting of broad sheets of small polyhedral cells with pale cytoplasms, small hyperchromatic nuclei, well-defined borders, and a complete absence of intracellular material (Fig. 32–9). Ewing's sarcoma is periodic acid–Schiff (PAS) positive, but differentiating it from the other round cell tumors of childhood necessitates a comprehensive approach combining light microscopy, special stains, and electron microscopy.[29] The tumor is markedly vascular and has widespread necrosis.

A painful mass with a large soft tissue component is the most common presentation, along with pleural effusion. Systemic symptoms include fatigue, weight loss, and intermittent fever. The most consistent radiographic finding is evidence of destruction of bone lysis. Occasionally, there is a diffuse expanded bone lesion with little periosteal reaction and irregular absorption of the medullary area. Widening and sclerosis of the cortex with multiple layers of new bone formation produce the characteristic onion peel appearance. It is not uncommon for more than one rib to be involved.

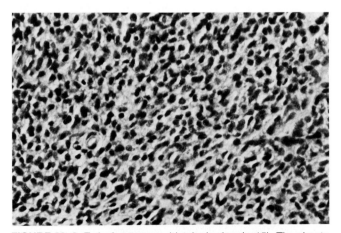

FIGURE 32–9. Ewing's sarcoma, histologic view (×15). The sheets of uniform, round, closely packed cells with minimal cytoplasm are typical of the tumor.

As many as 50% of patients present with metastatic disease, usually via hematogenous spread to lung and central nervous system. Lymph node involvement may also occur.[30]

There is no uniform staging system for Ewing's sarcoma, and most studies classify patients in Groups I through IV, depending on the presence or absence of gross residual disease or metastases. In a patient with the diagnosis of Ewing's sarcoma of rib, bone marrow aspirates, bone scanning, CT scan of the chest, radiography of the primary lesion, and cardiac evaluation should be performed (in anticipation of adriamycin therapy).[31]

Despite the response of this tumor to radiation therapy, the prognosis for patients before the advent of chemotherapy was poor, with 5-year survival rates of 5% to 15%. Surgery has been recognized as integral in the treatment of patients with the disease; the impression is verified in retrospective studies by the Mayo Clinic[32] in which the 10-year survival rate was 30% for patients with surgery versus 8% for patients without surgery. Currently, surgery is recommended as primary therapy if the lesion is expendable bone, such as the ribs. However, tumors more than 10 cm in diameter and tumors with significant soft tissue extension have a worse prognosis than smaller tumors. Therefore, multimodality therapy has become the rule for the treatment of Ewing's sarcoma.

The Intergroup Ewing's Sarcoma Study reported 21 patients with localized disease of the rib.[28] The patients were treated with surgical excision or biopsy followed by local radiotherapy and randomization to chemotherapy. The radiotherapy consisted of treatment of the entire rib with a 5-cm margin to a disc of 55 Gy over 5.5 weeks, followed by an optional boost of 20 Gy over the subsequent week. Chemotherapy usually consisted of multidrug treatment with vincristine, cytoxan, dactinomycin, and adriamycin. Complications of therapy included myelosuppression, skin reactions, and cardiomyopathy, with approximately 50% of patients having serious to life-threatening toxicities. Local control was excellent (95%), and disease-free survival at 3 years approached 50%. The best survival occurred in patients who had complete surgical excision followed by chemotherapy or radiotherapy.

A modification of this protocol is being used at the National Cancer Institute (NCI), where patients with localized Ewing's sarcoma of rib are treated with chemotherapy and localized radiotherapy, followed by wide excision of residual tumor. After surgery, total body irradiation and additional chemotherapy are given, followed by bone marrow reinfusion using cryopreserved autologous bone marrow.

The MSK group recently published their results with 62 patients with primary Ewing's sarcoma of the chest wall.[33] The majority (73%) received chemotherapy with local therapy, either irradiation or resection. Despite having local disease only at presentation, 71% developed metastases, and the overall survival was a median of 57 months (48% survived 5 and 10 years).

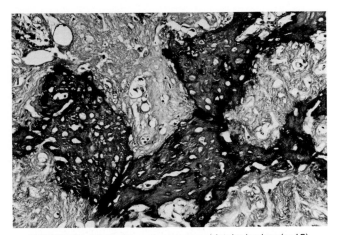

FIGURE 32–10. Osteogenic sarcoma, histologic view (×15).

Only the development of metastases at any time during the course of the disease was correlated with a poor outcome.

Osteogenic Sarcoma

Osteogenic sarcoma usually appears in the extremity[34]; therefore, innovative treatment with adjuvant therapy of truncal osteogenic sarcoma is largely anecdotal (Fig. 32–10). The tumor chiefly occurs during childhood and adolescence and is associated with a painful, firm soft tissue mass fixed to the underlying bone. Osteogenic sarcoma has one of the more characteristic radiographic appearances, with a starburst pattern due to intramedullary radiodensity and radiolucency (of nonossified tumor) with cortical destruction, periosteal elevation, and extraosseous extension.[35]

Vascular invasion leads to pulmonary metastases early in the course. Therefore, in recent years there has been interest in adjuvant therapy of osteosarcomas with preoperative or postoperative chemotherapy (Fig. 32–11). The Mayo Clinic series did not find a significant difference in the disease-free survival between patients given chemotherapy with surgery and those undergoing surgery alone.[36] Other investigators, however, are reporting 90% disease-free survival with preoperative use of multidrug chemotherapy (vincristine, high-dose methotrexate, doxorubicin [Adriamycin], bleomycin, dactinomycin, and cytoxan).[37] There has been a corresponding decrease in the number of local recurrences, at least in the amputation series of osteosarcomas, with the institution of multimodality therapy.

A proportion of chest wall osteosarcomas develop after radiotherapy to the chest wall—as many as 30% in the MSK series.[25] Resection of these as well as de novo chest wall sarcomas is the standard of treatment. There are no data with regard to the use of the above regimens for these truncal osteosarcomas, and overall survival is poor, with a 15% 5-year survival rate. Median survival is approximately 1 year. Synchronous pulmonary metastases portends an even poorer survival (median, 5-month survival). Such data mitigate strongly for further trials of adjuvant therapy for chest wall osteosarcomas.

Plasmacytoma

Solitary plasmacytoma constitutes 15% to 30% of all chest wall tumors, most often presenting in middle-aged to older individuals (median age, approximately 60 years) as a well-defined, punched-out lytic lesion in the rib.[38] The bone lesions of plasmacytoma are similar in appearance, distribution, and multiplicity to those of multiple myeloma. Plasmacytoma, a systemic disease characterized by fever, weakness, and abnormal serum protein, usually occurs in patients younger than those with multiple myeloma and is associated with longer survival. Presentation can occur usually as chest wall pain, with or without an associated mass. The majority arise in the rib or clavicle.

Diagnosis of solitary plasmacytoma is confirmed by biopsy of a lytic lesion composed of plasma cells and marrow aspiration containing less than 5% plasma cells.[39] Plasmacytoma is very responsive to alkylating agents (melphalan) and prednisone combinations.[40] Some institutions are investigating the addition of vincristine, cytoxan, and carmustine.[41] Radiotherapy also gives effective palliation (8 to 20 Gy), with small

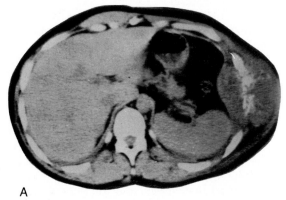

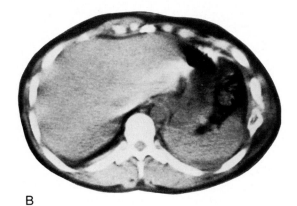

FIGURE 32–11. CT scan of metastatic osteogenic sarcoma, left chest. Note the starburst appearance (*A*). After preoperative treatment with ifosfamide chemotherapy, there is marked decrease in the size of the tumor (*B*), allowing a margin-free chest wall resection.

doses used for the ribs.[39] Unfortunately, the majority of patients with solitary plasmacytoma will subsequently develop multiple myeloma. The only role for surgery in plasmacytoma is in diagnosis of the condition. Overall 5-year survival rates range from 37% to 45%, with a median survival of 56 months.[12]

Soft Tissue Sarcomas

Sarcomas are a group of rare malignant tumors with similar morphologic and histologic characteristics as well as natural history. A sarcoma is virtually always surrounded by a pseudocapsule that is invaded by malignant tissue and can spread along muscle bundles, blood vessels, nerves, and fascial planes. Local recurrence can occur despite supposedly adequate surgical resection, and sarcomas share the tendency to manifest pulmonary metastases early in the clinical course (within the first 2 years).[42] Soft tissue sarcomas represent approximately 20% of malignant lesions affecting the chest wall. Soft tissue sarcomas are graded on a scale of from I to III, with Grade III tumors having the most aggressive local biology as well as the greatest propensity for metastases. The degree of necrosis in the surgical specimen is the best histopathologic parameter for predicting time to recurrence and overall survival.[39] The most common histologic types of soft tissue sarcomas are fibrosarcoma, leiomyosarcoma, liposarcoma, synovial sarcoma, neurofibrosarcoma, and malignant fibrous histiocytoma.

Surgery alone for the sarcomas just listed has been associated with a high incidence of local recurrence (10%).[43] Thus, recent investigations have evaluated the impact of adjuvant radiotherapy, chemotherapy, or both on local recurrence rates, distant treatment failure, and survival. Present studies have not determined the efficacy, with regard to local failure or survival, of preoperative or postoperative radiotherapy for chest wall lesions. At the NCI, radiotherapy is administered after surgery to all truncal sarcomas, with or without chemotherapy.[44]

At the NCI, 28 patients had chest wall resection for high-grade primary, metastatic, or recurrent sarcoma.[45] All deaths were related to sarcoma recurrence, usually to the lungs. The overall actuarial survival rate was 85% at 1 year, 65% at 3 years, and 59% at more than 5 years. This compares favorably with a series from MSK[46] in which 90 patients with resected high-grade soft tissue sarcomas had a 5-year survival rate of 49%. The local recurrence in the MSK series was 27% compared with 16% in the NCI series. Development of metastases correlated with decreased survival in both series; however, in the NCI group, synchronous pulmonary metastases at the time of chest wall resection were a poor prognostic indicator. Moreover, the inability to obtain tumor-free margins at the time of resection correlated with decreased survival time.

Special Consideration in Soft Tissue Sarcomas

For the pediatric and adolescent age groups, special consideration must be given regarding treatment of specific histologic soft tissue sarcomas, namely, peripheral neuroepithelioma and rhabdomyosarcoma. Neuroepithelioma commonly occurs on the chest wall and has features similar to those of Ewing's sarcoma, yet there usually is evidence of neural differentiation.[47] Tests for immunocytochemical markers (neuron-specific enolase) are positive,[48] and on electron microscopy, unequivocal dense-core granules or neurites are seen.[49]

Patients with chest wall rhabdomyosarcoma (representing approximately 7% to 9% of all patients with rhabdomyosarcoma[50]) are considered a poor risk for surgery alone. During the past decade, the results of treatment have improved remarkably with the use of combined modality therapy consisting of local radiotherapy and chemotherapy.[51] The most effective chemotherapeutic agents have been Adriamycin, cytoxan, dactinomycin (Actinomycin D), and vincristine. Patients with localized tumors are reported to have an 80% complete response rate.[52] Considering the effectiveness of this therapy, the role of surgery in chest wall rhabdomyosarcoma should be limited to generous biopsy by incision of the tumor at a site free of necrosis to obtain the diagnosis and to remove gross residual disease after radiotherapy and chemotherapy. The operation to remove the gross residual disease must be planned to ensure negative margins. Depending on the situation (protocol or nonprotocol), decisions regarding the need and type of postresectional therapy can be based on histologic examination of the specimen, with quantification of preoperative therapy–induced tumor necrosis.

Low-Grade Chest Wall Sarcomas: Desmoid tumors

Desmoid tumors are low-grade fibrosarcomas known for their local recurrence propensity. They have well-differentiated fibroblasts and fibrocytes with an abundant intercellular matrix. The absence of necrosis and mitoses classifies them as Grade I sarcomas. Wide local resection frequently involves full-thickness chest wall resection and reconstruction. The overall survival rate approaches 95% at 10 years, and the disease-free survival rate at 10 years is 71%. The local recurrence rate at 5 years is 30%, and older patients, at least in one series, appear to have lower recurrence rates than individuals less than 30 years of age.[53]

CHEST WALL RESECTION: SURGICAL TECHNIQUE

Chest wall resection and reconstruction can be performed with low mortality and morbidity, even with wide removal of the bony thorax. Mortality ranges from 1% to 4.5% regardless of cell type,[54, 55] and the most common complications include pulmonary insufficiency, infection, hemorrhage, and flap loss.

Position

Positioning of the patient for a chest wall resection depends on the location of the chest wall mass. For anterior lesions, the patient may be in the supine position, with slight lateral elevation to assist in thoracotomy. The majority of lesions of the chest wall are most easily resected with the patient in the decubitus position as for a posterolateral thoracotomy. The position of the patient also depends on the extent of the metastatic work-up, in that if bilateral or contralateral synchronous pulmonary metastatic disease is present and is considered to be resectable, the initial approach may be median sternotomy with metastatectomy. With a sternotomy, the extent of the chest wall involvement can be easily assessed, and the limits of the resection can be easily defined. Standard sternotomy closure after resection and reconstruction of the chest wall mass can be performed in the usual fashion, and this approach is well tolerated by the patient.

Anesthesia

Standard inhalational and narcotic techniques can be used for the patient undergoing chest wall resection. Patients previously treated with Adriamycin may require judicious monitoring of fluids by central venous pressure monitoring or use of a Swan-Ganz catheter. If the patient has been previously treated with bleomycin, low inspired oxygen fractions should be used. Selective ventilation using a double-lumen endotracheal tube has proved extremely useful, especially to define any adhesions between the chest wall mass and the lung and to aid in their resection in continuity with the neoplasm. Use of a double-lumen system should always be monitored via an indwelling arterial line for pressure and blood gas monitoring. At the conclusion of the operation, if further respiratory support is needed, the double-lumen tube should be replaced by an endotracheal tube of appropriate size.

The Procedure

The skin incision must be planned so that if the patient has had a previous incisional biopsy, the surgeon can excise en bloc the old biopsy scar as well as any scars from drain placement. Without violating the pseudocapsule of the tumor, a superior skin flap is raised to an intercostal space clearly above the superior margin of the neoplasm. The superior musculature (latissimus, pectoralis, and serratus) is then divided down to that intercostal space. An exploratory thoracotomy is performed through the intercostal space after deflation of the lung if a double-lumen endotracheal tube has been used. This thoracotomy incision will be used to determine the presence or absence of discontinuous malignant pleural disease, the invasiveness and exact location of the chest wall mass in relation to the ribs and sternum, and the presence or absence of pleural fluid, all of which may influence the extent of the operation. The presence or absence of adhesions to the lung can also be assessed

by this initial thoracotomy, as well as the relation of the tumor to the ribs that will serve as the superior, medial, and lateral margins. Adhesions between the lung and the chest wall should not be violated; they can easily be divided after complete or three-fourth mobilization of the chest wall mass.

After the chest has been assessed and the rib above which the intercostal incision was made is judged to be completely clear of tumor, this intercostal incision can be extended anteriorly and posteriorly to such an extent that division of the rib would start a resection line that is at least 3 in from the edge of the tumor in all directions. Instead of cutting the rib once anteriorly, we prefer to excise 1-cm sections of rib anteriorly and posteriorly by scoring the rib with electrocautery and excising the segment with guillotine bone cutters. The intercostal bundle is then encircled with a right-angle clamp and divided between ties of nonabsorbable suture. The anterior ribs are similarly divided into a sequential fashion down to the anterior and inferior edge of the skin flap. Any musculature overlying the ribs can be divided with electrocautery, with care taken to maintain adequate margins from the pseudocapsule. The posterior rib division is performed in a similar fashion.

A lower skin and subcutaneous flap is then created, with care taken to avoid the muscle and fascia overlying the tumor. An inferior thoracotomy incision can then be made, and again the relation of the tumor to the pericardium, diaphragm, and lung is assessed. Contiguous involved structures should be widely excised (i.e., leaving grossly negative margins). Rib resection then proceeds anteriorly and posteriorly, with a small segment of each rib excised. All of these rib segments can be processed as the bony margin of the resection. After all of the intercostal bundles are secured and the rib segments have been excised down to the inferior thoracotomy, the portion of the chest wall should be completely free except for any attachments to the lung or diaphragm. With the TA-90 or TA-55 4.8 stapling device, the lung can be divided under direct vision so the resection will include any adhesions. The diaphragm can be excised wide of the adhesions to the tumor and usually reapproximated using mattress sutures.

The extent of the chest wall resection with regard to the amount of muscle overlying the mass that should be excised must be guided by the principle of producing negative margins rather than conserving tissue for reconstruction. Overlying serratus or latissimus muscle should not be violated, especially if the tumor is a soft tissue sarcoma. Violation of the pseudocapsule with these sarcomas by stripping off the fascia and muscle, possibly to conserve the tissue for wound closure, will only lead to a positive margin with a significant chance for tumor recurrence.[56] The principle of "never seeing the tumor" during the resection necessitates this approach. In cases of metastatic tumor to rib or a primary rib tumor, there may not be a significant soft tissue component, and more overlying muscle may be preserved. Preoperative bone scanning and CT may provide more insight as to the presence or absence of a soft tissue component of this bony tumor and help guide the resection.

When a rib is clearly involved by tumor, it should be completely excised with its cartilaginous articulation. It is impossible to predict marrow extension of tumor involvement. Uninvolved ribs or articular cartilage above and below the tumor mass may be partially excised; however, the extent of excision should leave no doubt in the operating room about the presence of negative margins.

Involvement of Contiguous Structures

High lesions in the axilla may require concomitant forequarter amputation and chest wall resection. Roth and associates[57] described a useful technique for this procedure that involves removal of the arm, shoulder girdle, and chest wall from the angle of the ribs to the middle of the sternum. Involvement of the subscapular muscle or the scapula itself can be addressed by removing the scapula partially or in toto, with resuturing of the uninvolved musculature to the residual chest wall.[58]

CHEST WALL RECONSTRUCTION

When a patient requires chest wall resection for a malignant chest wall tumor, careful preoperative planning is crucial, not only as described to ensure a negative margin but also to produce a physiologically and cosmetically acceptable result at the conclusion of the procedure. Operations must be individualized with regard to bony and soft tissue coverage. The ideal approach involves a plastic surgery–thoracic surgery team that handles the resection and reconstruction problems in a consistent way.

There are many ways to deal with chest wall reconstruction considering the options that have been available since the first description of the use of Marlex for chest wall replacement and the first use of myocutaneous flaps. This section describes what we consider to be the most important considerations in how to "close the wound" after major chest wall resection.

Influence of Preoperative Treatment, Specifically Radiotherapy

Patients with radioresponsive tumors (Ewing's sarcoma, rhabdomyosarcoma) who receive localized preoperative radiotherapy between 50 and 65 Gy may show early erythematous and edematous skin changes, which can progress to fibrosis, contracture, indolent ulceration, and infection.[59] During chest wall resection after a good tumor response to radiotherapy without removal of all bony or soft tissue components within the radiation ports, some tissue may be left in which the vascularity has been compromised by irradiation. The irradiation may also have a stabilizing fibrotic effect on the chest wall, especially if the resulting rib deficit is less than three ribs, possibly ensuring stability of the chest wall without bony reconstruc-

tion.[60] Most surgeons have been reticent to reconstruct the bony thorax with a component of synthetic material after significant local high-dose irradiation, especially if the wound is contaminated. In this situation, muscle transposition provides adequate soft tissue coverage and chest stabilization.

Influence of the Magnitude of Surgery, Location, and Preoperative Pulmonary Physiology Regarding "Bony" Reconstruction

The magnitude of surgery with regard to the extent of rib resection should influence the surgeon's judgment about the need for reconstruction. Since 1977, the approach at the NCI has been that no patient with three or fewer resected ribs has had bony reconstruction, regardless of location. When a minor portion of the chest wall is sacrificed with a forequarter resection, reconstruction usually is not required; however, if the forequarter resection is performed because of invasion by a chest wall tumor that involves a larger portion of the chest wall, reconstruction may be necessary. With resection involving four or more ribs, along with significant muscle and integumentary removal to ensure negative margins, reconstruction can be considered necessary (1) to obtain sufficient chest wall fixation in a vulnerable area for vital respiratory effort, (2) to achieve additional chest wall fixation for more adequate respiratory function, (3) to provide additional support for the heart or lung, (4) to reduce paradox, or (5) to secure optimal chest function in a vigorous patient with a long life expectancy.[61]

Anterior or inferior defects of more than three ribs usually need repair with autogenous or prosthetic material.[54] When the resection lies posterior or superior under the scapula and the large muscles of the back, reconstruction usually is not needed. Defects that include the manubrium, upper sternum, and sternoclavicular junction cause a significant paradox; reconstruction should be performed not only to avoid paradox but also to protect the underlying viscera and great vessels.

Methods of Bony Reconstruction

When bony reconstruction of the chest wall is considered essential, the surgeon has a variety of materials from which to choose. For lesions involving the manubrium and sternum, autogenous rib grafts from the opposite chest have been used,[62] although the long-term fate of these rib grafts is unknown. More recently, synthetic material has been preferred.

The ability of Marlex mesh to stabilize the bony chest wall and to prevent paradox over the long term has been debated in the literature. Crucial to the use of any synthetic material is that it be placed under tension when sewn into place to the ribs of the chest wall defect. Prolene sutures are placed through muscle and fascia and around or through the ribs and cartilage to secure the mesh (Fig. 32–12). When placement is completed, the Marlex should be stretched "tight as a drum." With its initially high tensile strength, it may ensure a stable thoracic wall early; however, many observers remark on the loss of support with time. The Marlex usually is incorporated in the chest wall by infiltration of its interstices with fibrous tissue.

Another polypropylene mesh, Prolene, also has been used for chest wall reconstruction. Prolene differs from Marlex in that the former is a double-stitch knit, whereas Marlex is only a single-stitch knit.[63] Prolene is rigid in all directions, whereas Marlex is rigid in only one direction.

The 2-mm-thick Gore-Tex Soft Tissue Patch has also been used because it is impervious to flow of both air and water across the chest wall.[54] This feature would be ideal for a large defect with concomitant pneumonectomy.

A rigid chest wall replacement covering all dimensions of the defect is accomplished with the use of the "Marlex sandwich," as developed by McCormack and associates.[55] Two pieces of Marlex mesh slightly larger than the skeletal defect are cut. As the methyl methacrylate begins to set, it is spread over one layer of the mesh to a size smaller than the defect. Steel mesh is added to prevent fragmentation, followed by another Marlex layer. The prosthesis is then molded to the shape of the defect and sutured to the edges. Muscle and skin closures are then performed. Claims have been made that when a rigid chest wall is reconstructed with the Marlex sandwich, respirator time is decreased due to reduced paradox.

At the NCI, a modification of this technique is performed in which the Marlex is first sutured drum tight to the edges of the defect, and the lung is deflated (Fig. 32–13). The methyl methacrylate is then spread on the Marlex, and steel mesh is placed on the still hardening and warming methyl methacrylate. A final layer of Marlex mesh is placed over the steel mesh. In our experience, no immediate problems have been associated with this in situ technique as long as the methyl methacrylate is allowed to set before inflating the lung or closing the wound.

Occasionally, reversible metabolic acidosis occurs due to anion release when methyl methacrylate is used. Seroma formation requiring long-term closed drainage has been associated with the Marlex sandwich technique. The objection to the use of the Marlex sandwich is that it is a large foreign body that, if infected, would have to be completely removed; another technique of reconstruction would then have to be used.[64] Similarly, delay in postoperative chemotherapy may result if persistent seroma formation occurs. Finally, the long-term inertness of the sandwich in the face of postoperative adjuvant therapy, specifically radiotherapy, has not been sufficiently tested. We removed a methacrylate sandwich 1 year after implantation because of infection secondary to skin and subcutaneous necrosis after postoperative radiotherapy.

Muscle Flaps and Transpositions

With a soft tissue sarcoma that has been previously sampled, a situation in which all drain and biopsy skin sites must be removed without violating the pseudocapsule, it is necessary to accomplish full-thickness removal of skin, subcutaneous tissue, muscle, and bony chest wall. In general, if primary closure cannot be performed, muscle transposition best accomplishes soft tissue reconstruction. For defects of three ribs or less in an area that would not produce much paradox, simple subcutaneous and skin closure may be acceptable, yet the majority of resections will require some sort of tissue transposition.

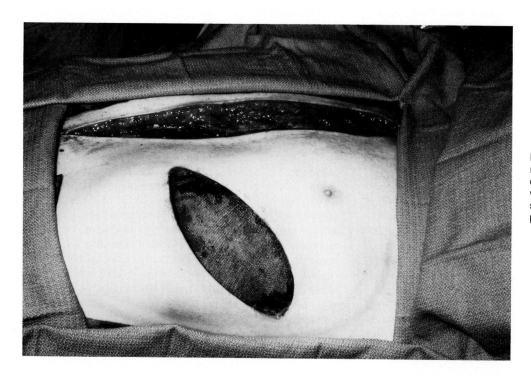

FIGURE 32–12. Marlex reconstruction of an anteriolateral chest wall resection combined with simultaneous median sternotomy for synchronous pulmonary metastatic disease.

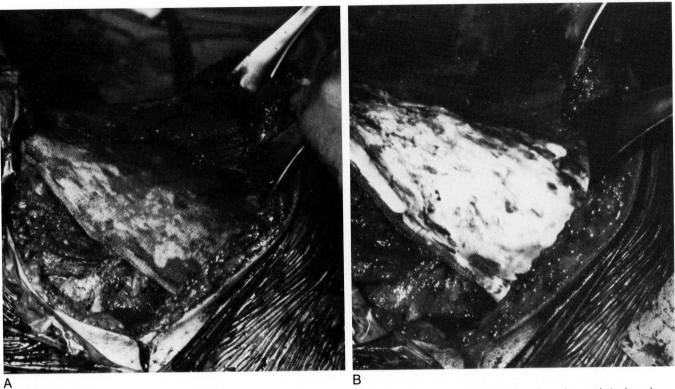

A B

FIGURE 32–13. Chest wall resection. Marlex has been sewn drum tight to the edges of the wound (*A*). Methyl methacrylate and steel mesh are then applied to the Marlex base to form a rigid chest wall replacement (*B*).

In 1950, Campbell[65] first reported the use of a latissimus dorsi muscle flap, which he transferred on its thoracodorsal blood supply with a fascia lata graft beneath a split-thickness skin graft over its surface for reconstruction of a full-thickness defect of the chest wall. In 1968, Hueston and McConchie[66] used a pectoralis major myocutaneous flap to close a manubrial defect. In 1978, Arnold and Pairolero[62] first described the closure of a chest wall defect with a rotated pectoralis muscle flap; flail chest was prevented by autogenous rib grafts.

Myocutaneous flaps differ from other skin flaps in that the muscle underlying the skin is included in the myocutaneous flap and the entire unit is rotated on a single pedicle. This will usually provide safe wound coverage and add a minimal to moderate amount to chest stability. The most commonly used muscle flaps are pectoralis major, latissimus dorsi, and transverse rectus abdominal muscle (TRAM) flaps. Size and location of the chest wall defect and preservation of blood supply to the desired flap dictate the appropriate reconstruction. Larson and associates[67] believe that the presence of a flap's nutritional vessels in a previously irradiated field does not compromise flap viability. When there is any question of nutrient vessel patency, the appropriate preoperative angiographic assessment should be performed.

Defects of the lower neck and upper third of the sternum are best covered by the pectoralis major myocutaneous flap, whereas wounds of the anterior chest wall requiring removal of three or more ribs and the resection of less than 3 cm of skin call for latissimus dorsi flaps. The TRAM flap can be reserved for larger defects that preserve at least one internal mammary vessel and can easily cover an entire hemithorax.[68]

Pectoralis Flaps. The blood supply to the pectoralis major muscle is the pectoral branch of the thoracoacromial artery, which enters the muscle just lateral to the midclavicular line. After complete mobilization along with the neurovascular bundle, the muscle can be rotated and advanced across the midline. Further coverage can be accomplished by mobilization of the opposite pectoralis major muscle. Functional disability is minimal. If desired, the pectoralis can be segmentally split according to three segmental branches.[69] The pectoralis can be taken as a muscle flap or as a myocutaneous unit because of the multiple perforators entering the skin through the muscle. Transection of the lateral tendinous insertion of the muscle provides greater mobility.[62]

Latissimus Dorsi Flaps. As with the pectoralis muscle, the latissimus dorsi muscle can be elevated with or without the overlying skin. The thoracodorsal artery, a terminal branch of the subscapularis artery, is the major blood supply. It enters the undersurface of the muscle about 10 cm from its insertion. A fairly extensive collateral plexus in the area of the serratus anterior muscle will occasionally supply the muscle if the thoracodorsal artery has been previously divided.

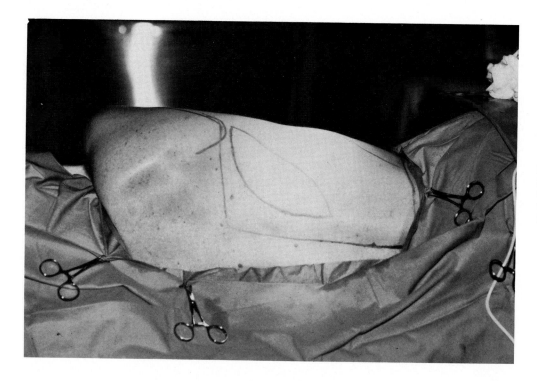

FIGURE 32–14. Outline of tip of scapula, latissimus muscle, and skin island prior to mobilization of right-sided latissimus dorsi myocutaneous flap.

The muscle is dissected from the tip of the scapula, separating it from the serratus anterior. A 10- × 16-cm island of the skin can be taken safely[70] (Figs. 32–14 to 32–17). Because of its long pedicle, a latissimus dorsi flap can be used to cover any area of the chest wall and can be rotated medially as a turnover flap across the midline to fill opposite posterior wall defects. The muscle then gets its blood supply from mul-

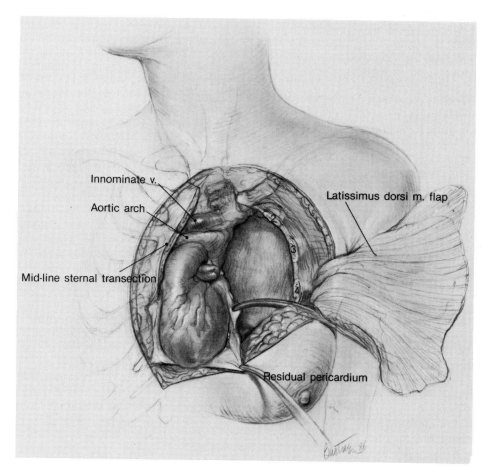

FIGURE 32–15. Chest wall resection, illustrating removal of the second, third, and fourth ribs and a portion of the sternum. A latissimus dorsi flap has been mobilized to cover the defect. Note that a partial pericardiectomy was necessary to ensure negative margins in this case.

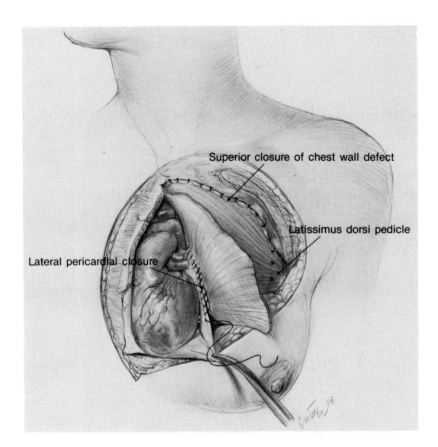

FIGURE 32–16. The muscle flap has been sutured to the edges of the wound—to the remaining intercostal muscle, rib, or presternal fascia—to close the defect. In this case, the edges of the pericardium have been sewn to the inferior surface of the flap, both to support the heart and to prevent herniation.

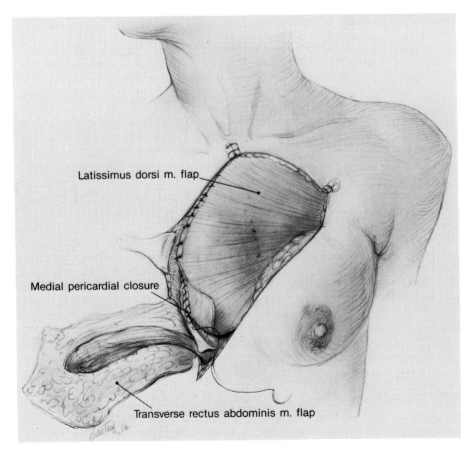

FIGURE 32–17. Completed coverage of the chest wall defect with the latissimus flap. Skin coverage could be obtained by means of transplanted skin island on the flap via skin grafting or by the use of a second myocutaneous flap, such as transverse rectus abdominis muscle (TRAM) flap, which is depicted.

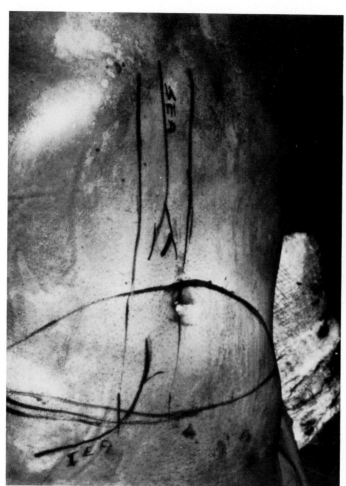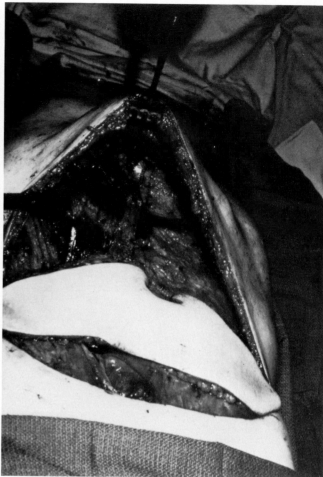

FIGURE 32–18. Procedural outlines for right-sided TRAM flap. SEA = superior epigastric artery. IEA = inferior epigastric artery. This TRAM flap is used for reconstruction of a left-sided chest wall resection (*A*). Flap mobilization completed for TRAM flap: retractor is under the right rectus muscle: rake retractor elevates the superior flap under which the elliptical myocutaneous skin flap will be directed to the left chest (*B*).

tiple branches of the intercostal and upper lumbar arteries.[71]

TRAM Flaps. The TRAM flap, described by Robbins[72] in 1979 for breast reconstruction, is extraordinarily useful in the construction of full-thickness chest wall defects. The vascular supply to the muscle and skin is bipedicular, with both the superior and inferior epigastric arteries coursing on the posterior surface of the muscle. Usually the flap is based superiorly on the ipsilateral or contralateral internal mammary artery and will reach to the most anterior chest or inferior portion of the axilla (Figs. 32–18 and 32–19). If a cuff of fascia is retained, the abdominal wall can be closed without herniation.

Other Pedicle Flaps. For lower chest wall and upper abdominal defects, the external oblique muscle can be used.[73] Serratus anterior muscle has been used on occasion for anterior defects. Fasciocutaneous flaps are based on the premise that skin flaps from muscles can be extended beyond distal muscle borders by preserving vascular connections that extend to adjacent myocutaneous territories in the muscle fascia and in

the overlying subcutaneous tissue.[74] In the thorax, this approach can be used to carry either abdominal or presternal skin on a pectoralis major muscle flap. Rectus abdominis fascia and epigastric skin carried on pectoralis major fasciocutaneous flaps substantially lengthen the flaps. Vertical abdominal fasciocutaneous flaps based on the superior epigastric artery have also been described.

Free Flaps. With the advent of microsurgical techniques, free flaps consisting of tensor fascia lata muscle with fascia lata and overlying skin can be based on the lateral femoral circumflex vessels.[60] These vessels are anastomosed to the transverse cervical or thoracoacromial vessels. Fascia lata muscle is sutured to the periosteal margin of rib and sternum and may contribute to chest wall stabilization as well as coverage. Boyd and associates[60] at New York University reported a 96% success rate.

Omentum. When muscle flaps are not available or large enough, omentum based on the right or left gastroepiploic vessels can be transposed over bone grafts or mesh.[75] Omentum will not provide chest wall

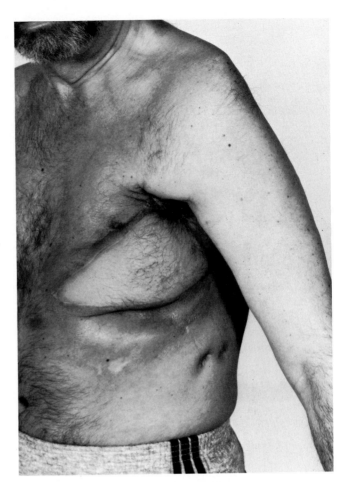

FIGURE 32–19. TRAM flap depicted 6 months after surgery.

stability, and complications are more common than with muscle flaps, requiring repeated débridements and skin grafting.

SELECTED REFERENCES

Burt M, Fulton M, Wessner-Dunlap S, et al: Primary bony and cartilaginous sarcomas of chest wall: Results of therapy. Ann Thorac Surg 54:226–232, 1992.
This is a complete review of the 40-year experience with chest wall osteosarcomas and chondrosarcomas managed at the Memorial Sloan-Kettering Cancer Center. The overall 5-year survival rate was 64% for the 88 patients with chondrosarcoma and 15% for those with osteosarcoma. Prognostic indicators are well detailed and include synchronous metastases or development of metastases at any time during the patient's course.

Burt M, Karpeh M, Ukoha O, et al: Medical tumors of the chest wall. J Thorac Cardiovasc Surg 105:89–96, 1993.
A complete 40-year experience with the more unusual tumors of the chest wall is discussed, including 24 patients with plasmacytoma and 62 patients with Ewing's sarcoma. This unique series comments on the role of adjuvant systemic as well as local radiotherapy in addition to surgery in the management of these patients.

Perry RR, Roth JA, Pass HI: Survival after surgical resection for high-grade chest wall sarcomas. Ann Thorac Surg 49:363–369, 1990.
In this summary of the mangement of truncal sarcomas involving the chest wall, primary, recurrent, and metastatic tumor management is considered, and prognostic factors are detailed. The 59% 5-year survival, 0% surgical mortality, and 16% local recurrence rates compare favorably with those of other studies in the literature.

Seyfer AE, Graeber GM: Chest-wall reconstruction. Surg Clin North Am 69:899–1122, 1989.
This is a monograph that summarizes virtually all aspects of management of the patient with the chest wall lesion. The preoperative work-up, radiographic evaluation, and specific techniques for reconstruction are adequately covered. It does not, however, give all inclusive data on the individual benign and chest wall masses.

Seyfer AE, Graeber GM, Wind G: Atlas of Chest Wall Reconstruction. Rockville, Maryland, Aspen Publishers, Inc, 1986.
This definitive text is beautifully illustrated to demonstrate the anatomy and physiology necessary to be known to manage patients with a chest wall problem. Superbly geared toward the practicing thoracic and plastic surgeon, the book emphasizes a team approach for management.

REFERENCES

1. Paget S: The Surgery of the Chest. Bristol, Wright, 1896, p 479.
2. Parham FW: Thoracic wall resection for tumors growing from the bony wall of the chest. Trans South Surg Gyn Assoc 11:233, 1899.
3. Hedgeblom C: Tumors of the bony chest wall. Arch Surg 3:56–85, 1921.
4. O'Neal LW, Ackerman LV: Cartilaginous tumors of ribs and sternum. J Thorac Surg 21:71–108, 1951.
5. Hochberg LA: Primary tumors of the rib. Arch Surg 67:566–594, 1953.
6. Adkins P: Chest wall tumors. *In* Shields T (ed): General Thoracic Surgery. Philadelphia, Lea & Febiger, 1972.
7. McAfee MK, Pairolero PC, Bergstrahl EJ, et al: Chondrosarcoma of the chest wall: Factors affecting survival. Ann Thorac Surg 40:535–540, 1985.

8. Ochsner A, Lucus GL, McFarland GB: Tumors of the thoracic skeleton. J Thorac Cardiovasc Surg 52:311–321, 1966.
9. Blades B, Paul JS: Chest wall tumors. Ann Surg 131:976–984, 1950.
10. Stelzer P, Gay WA: Tumors of the chest wall. Surg Clin North Am 60:779–786, 1980.
11. Crile G: Pulsating tumors of the sternum. Ann Surg 103:199–209, 1936.
12. Sabanathan S, Salama FD, Morgan WE, et al: Primary chest wall tumors. Ann Thorac Surg 39:4–15, 1985.
13. Marcove R, Huvos A: Cartilaginous tumors of the ribs. Cancer 27:794–801, 1971.
14. Leitman BS: The use of computed tomography in evaluating chest wall pathology. J Comput Tomogr 7:399–408, 1983.
15. Pass HI, Dwyer A, Makuch R, et al: Detection of pulmonary metastases in patients with osteogenic and soft-tissue sarcomas: The superiority of CT scans compared with conventional linear tomograms using dynamic analysis. J Clin Oncol 3:1262–1265, 1985.
16. Martini N, Huvos A, Smith J, et al: Primary malignant tumors of the sternum. Surg Gynecol Obstet 138:391–395, 1974.
17. Kumar AM, Green A, Smith JW, et al: Combined therapy for malignant tumor of the chest wall in children. J Pediatr Surg 12:991–999, 1977.
18. Linnoila RI, Tsokos M, Triche TJ, et al: Evidence for neural origin and periodic-Schiff-positive variants of the malignant small cell tumor of thoracopulmonary region. Lab Invest 48:514, 1983.
19. Benfield JR: Primary chest wall tumors. Ann Thorac Surg 39:1, 1985.
20. Barth RJ, Merino MJ, Solomon D, et al: A prospective study of the value of core needle biopsy and fine needle aspiration in the diagnosis of soft tissue masses. Surgery 112:536–543, 1992.
21. Wilner D: Radiology of Bone Tumors and Allied Disorders. Philadelphia, WB Saunders, 1982.
22. Sanerkin NG: The diagnosis and grading of chondrosarcoma of bone: A combined cytologic and histologic approach. Cancer 45:582–594, 1980.
23. Pritchard DJ, Lurke RJ, Taylor WF, et al: Chondrosarcoma: A clinicopathologic statistical analysis. Cancer 45:149–157, 1980.
24. Marcove RC: Chondrosarcoma: Diagnosis and treatment. Orthop Clin North Am 8:811–820, 1977.
25. Burt M, Fulton M, Wessner-Dunlap W, et al: Primary bony and cartilaginous sarcomas of chest wall: Results of therapy. Ann Thorac Surg 54:226–232, 1992.
26. Harwood AG, Kragbich JI, Fornasier VL: Radiotherapy of chondrosarcoma of bone. Cancer 45:2769–2777, 1980.
27. Arlen M, Tollefson HR, Huvos AG, et al: Chondrosarcoma of the head and neck. Am J Surg 120:456–460, 1970.
28. Thomas PR, Foulkes MA, Gilula LA, et al: Primary Ewing's sarcoma of the ribs. Cancer 51:1021–1027, 1983.
29. Triche TJ, Askin LB: Neuroblastoma and the differential diagnosis of small, round blue-cell tumors. Hum Pathol 44:569–595, 1983.
30. Hayes FA, Thompson EI, Hutsu HO, et al: The response of Ewing's sarcoma to sequential cyclophosphamide and induction therapy. J Clin Oncol 1:45–51, 1983.
31. Pizzo PA, Miser JS, Cassady JR, et al: Solid tumors of childhood. In DeVita VT Jr, Hellman S, Rosenberg SA (eds): Cancer: Principles and Practice of Oncology. Philadelphia, JB Lippincott, 1985.
32. Pritchard DJ, Dahlin D, Dauphine R, et al: Ewing's sarcoma. J Bone Joint Surg 57:10–16, 1975.
33. Burt M, Karpeh M, Ukoha O, et al: Medical tumors of the chest wall. J Thorac Cardiovasc Surg 105:89–96, 1993.
34. Friedman MA, Carter SK: The therapy of osteogenic sarcoma. J Surg Oncol 4:482–510, 1972.
35. Enneking WF: Musculoskeletal Tumor Society, Vol. 2. New York, Churchill-Livingstone, 1976.
36. Taylor WF, Ivins JC, Dahlin DC, et al: Trends and variability in survival from osteosarcoma. Mayo Clin Proc 53:695–700, 1978.
37. Rosen G, Caparros B, Huvos AC, et al: Preoperative chemotherapy for osteogenic sarcoma: Selection of postoperative adjuvant chemotherapy based upon the response of the primary tumor to preoperative chemotherapy. Cancer 49:1221–1230, 1982.
38. Teitlebaum S: Twenty-year experience with intrinsic tumor of the bony thorax at a large institution. J Thorac Cardiovasc Surg 63:776–782, 1972.
39. Crowin J, Lundberg RD: Solitary plasmacytoma of bone vs extramedullary plasmacytoma and their relation to multiple myeloma. Cancer 43:1007–1013, 1979.
40. McElwain TJ, Poules RL: High dose intravenous melphalan for plasma-cell leukemia and myeloma. Lancet 2:822–824, 1983.
41. Alexanian R, Dreuer R: Chemotherapy for multiple myeloma. Cancer 53:583, 1984.
42. Potter DA, Glenn J, Kinsella T, et al: Patterns of recurrence in patients with high grade soft tissue sarcomas. J Clin Oncol 3:353–356, 1985.
43. Romsdahl MM, Lundberg RR, Martin RG, et al: Patterns of failure after treatment of soft tissue sarcomas. Cancer Treat Symp 2:251–258, 1983.
44. Glenn J, Kinsella T, Glatstein E, et al: A randomized prospective trial of adjuvant chemotherapy in adults with soft tissue sarcomas of the head and neck, breast, and trunk. Cancer 55:1206–1214, 1985.
45. Perry RR, Venzon D, Roth JA, Pass HI: Survival after surgical resection for high-grade chest wall sarcomas. Ann Thorac Surg 49:363–369, 1990.
46. Gordon MS, Hajdu SI, Bains MS, Burt ME: Soft tissue sarcomas of the chest wall. J Thorac Cardiovasc Surg 101:843–854, 1991.
47. Schmidt D, MacKay B, Ayala AG: Ewing's sarcoma with neuroblastoma-like features. Ultrastruct Pathol 3:143–151, 1982.
48. Tsokos M, Linnoila RI, Triche TJ, et al: Neuron-specific enolase as an aid to the diagnosis of primitive small round cell tumor of neural origin. Lab Invest 48:874, 1983.
49. Marangos PJ: Isolation and characterization of the nervous system specific protein 14–3–2 from rat brain. J Biol Chem 250:1884–1891, 1975.
50. Raney RB, Rajab AH, Ruymann FB, et al: Soft tissue sarcoma of the trunk in childhood. Cancer 49:2612–2616, 1982.
51. Raney RB, Gehan EA, Maurer HM, et al: Evaluation of intensified chemotherapy in children with advanced rhabdomyosarcoma. Cancer Clin Trials 2:19–28, 1979.
52. Maurer HM, Foulkes M, Gehan EA, et al: Intergroup rhabdomyosarcoma study (IRS): II. Preliminary report. Proc Am Soc Clin Oncol 2:70, 1983.
53. Brodsky JT, Gordon MS, Hajdu SI, Burt M: Desmoid tumors of the chest wall. J Thorac Cardiovasc Surg 104:900–903, 1992.
54. Pairolero PC, Arnold PG: Chest wall tumors. J Thorac Cardiovasc Surg 90:367–372, 1985.
55. McCormack P, Bains M, Beattie EJ, et al: New trends in skeletal reconstruction after resection of chest wall tumors. Ann Thorac Surg 31:45–52, 1981.
56. Canton J, McNeer GD, Chu FC, et al: The problem of local recurrence after treatment of soft tissue sarcoma. Ann Surg 168:47–53, 1968.
57. Roth JA, Sugarbaker P, Baker A: Forequarter amputation and chest wall resection. Ann Thorac Surg 37:423–427, 1984.
58. Sugarbaker P: Scapulectomy. In Sugarbaker P (ed): Atlas of Surgery for Soft Tissue Sarcomas. Philadelphia, JB Lippincott, 1985.
59. Pantoja E, Frede T, Kanchala S: Complications of postoperative radiation in breast cancer. Breast 4:4, 1978.
60. Boyd AD, Shaw WW, McCarthy JG, et al: Immediate reconstruction of full thickness chest wall defects. Ann Thorac Surg 32:337–346, 1981.
61. Martini N, Starzynski TE, Beattie EJ: Problems in chest wall resection. Surg Clin North Am 49:313–322, 1969.
62. Arnold PG, Pairolero PC: Use of pectoralis major muscle flap to repair defects of the anterior chest wall. Plast Reconst Surg 63:205–213, 1979.
63. Arnold PG, Pairolero PC: Chest wall reconstruction. Ann Surg 199:725–732, 1984.
64. Pairolero PC, Arnold PG: Chest wall reconstruction. Ann Thorac Surg 32:325–326, 1981.
65. Campbell DA: Reconstruction of the anterior thoracic wall. J Thorac Surg 19:456–461, 1950.
66. Hueston JT, McConchie IH: Compound pectoral flap. Aust N Z J Surg 38:61–63, 1969.
67. Larson DC, McMurtrey MJ, Howe HJ, et al: Major chest wall reconstruction after chest wall irradiation. Cancer 49:1286–1293, 1982.

68. Larson DI, McMurtrey MJ: Musculocutaneous flap reconstruction of chest wall defects: An experience with 50 patients. Plast Reconst Surg 73:734–740, 1984.

69. Tobin GR, Mavroudis C, Howe WR, et al: Reconstruction of complex thoracic defects with myocutaneous and muscle flaps. J Thorac Cardiovasc Surg 85:219–228, 1983.

70. Dingman R, Argenta IC: Reconstruction of the chest wall. Ann Thorac Surg 32:203–208, 1981.

71. Bostwick J, Scheflan M, Nahai F, et al: The "reverse" latissimus dorsi muscle and musculocutaneous flap: Anatomical and clinical considerations. Plast Reconst Surg 65:395–399, 1980.

72. Robbins TH: The rectus abdominis myocutaneous flap for breast reconstruction. Aust N Z J Surg 49:527–530, 1979.

73. Hodgkinson DJ, Arnold PG: Chest wall reconstruction using the external oblique muscle. Br J Plast Surg 33:216–220, 1980.

74. Maruyama Y, Ohnishi K, Chung CC: Vertical abdominal fasciocutaneous flaps in the reconstruction of chest wall defects. Br J Plast Surg 38:230–233, 1985.

75. Arnold PG, Witzke DJ, Irons GB, et al: Use of omental transposition flaps for soft tissue reconstruction. Ann Plast Surg 11:508–512, 1983.

76. Rami-Porta R, Bravo-Bravo JL, Aroca-Gonzalez MJ, et al: Tumors and pseudotumors of the chest wall. Scand J Thorac Cardiovasc Surg 19:97–103, 1995.

77. Graeber GM: Initial and long-term results in the management of primary chest wall neoplasms. Ann Thorac Surg 34:664–673, 1982.

78. Threlkel JB, Adkins RB: Primary chest wall tumors. Ann Thorac Surg 11:450–459, 1971.

79. Watkins E, Gerard FP: Malignant tumors involving the chest wall. J Thorac Cardiovasc Surg 39:117–129, 1960.

80. Golladay ES, Hale JA, Mollitt DL, et al: Chest wall masses in children. South Med J 78:191–195, 1985.

81. King RM, Pairolero PC, Trastek VF, et al: Primary chest wall tumors: Factors affecting survival. Ann Thorac Surg 41:597–601, 1986.

82. Ala-Kulju K, Ketonen P, Järvinen A, et al: Primary tumors of the ribs. Scand J Thorac Cardiovasc Surg 22:97–100, 1988.

83. Ryan MB, McMurtrey MJ, Roth JA: Current management of chest-wall tumors. Surg Clin North Am 69:1061–1080, 1989.

33 MULTIMODALITY THERAPY OF MALIGNANT MESOTHELIOMA

David J. Sugarbaker, Michael T. Jaklitsch, Alexander D. Soutter, Joseph Aisner, and Karen Antman

THE ROLE OF SURGERY IN THE TREATMENT OF MALIGNANT MESOTHELIOMA

Malignant pleural mesothelioma has two gross pathologic presentations. There is the rare presentation of a locally confined, aggressively invasive malignant mesothelioma. Surgery alone in the treatment of localized malignant pleural mesothelioma has been limited to the tumor that could be completely removed with wide local excision. The vastly more common form of gross pathologic presentations is a diffuse malignant mesothelioma that extends into every fissure and pleural reflection, trapping the lung and invading surrounding structures. The role of surgery in the treatment of diffuse malignant mesothelioma has traditionally been limited to pleural biopsy to establish a histologic diagnosis and pleurodesis for palliation.

Despite the dismal survival statistics, mesothelioma is recognized to be a locally aggressive tumor that metastasizes late in the normal clinical course. Most patients die as the result of the primary lesion invading local organs (heart, liver, esophagus, tracheobronchial tree) and not of distant metastasis. Improved local control of this tumor should lead to marked palliation and may produce improved long-term survival.

Efforts to improve local control have stimulated several multimodality protocols that are in use in institutions with a large referral base for these patients. The technique of extrapleural pneumonectomy, herein described, is most appropriate when combined with additional oncologic therapies in a multimodality protocol.

Several investigators have tried pleurectomy without pneumonectomy, followed by adjuvant chemotherapy or radiotherapy, as an alternate surgical approach for diffuse malignant pleural mesothelioma.[1–3] This approach seems to offer good local control and significant palliation. We have used this approach for the dyspneic patient who is not a candidate for our trimodality extrapleural pneumonectomy protocol. However, it still remains unclear whether this less radical alternative approach can produce a comparable rate of 5-year survivals.

An aggressive trimodality protocol combining extrapleural pneumonectomy with sequential postoperative chemotherapy (doxorubicin, 60 mg/m²; cyclophosphamide, 600 mg/M²; and cisplatin, 70 mg/M² for four to six cycles) and 55 Gy of adjuvant radiotherapy to the postoperative hemithorax, has been used at the Brigham & Women's Hospital in Boston since 1985.[4] This operative approach differs from other descriptions in the literature.[5–7] This chapter provides a detailed description of the current operative technique of extrapleural pneumonectomy for diffuse malignant mesothelioma in use at Brigham & Women's Hospital.

THERAPEUTIC APPROACH

Preoperative Evaluation

The first challenge facing the thoracic surgeon who is evaluating a patient suspected of having diffuse malignant mesothelioma is to establish clearly a histologic diagnosis. Reactive mesothelial cells can be difficult to distinguish from cancerous mesothelioma cells in pleural fluid cytology samples, unless the pathologist reading the specimen has considerable experience. Frequently, a pleural biopsy is required by the least invasive method, yet with sufficient material to establish clearly a histologic diagnosis as well as the cell type. Video-assisted thoracoscopy has been extremely effective in accomplishing this goal.

Radiographic imaging studies are obtained to determine the extent of intrathoracic and extrathoracic disease. Magnetic resonance imaging (MRI) of the chest has recently been shown to be an important adjunct to computed tomography (CT).[8] Sagittal MRI views are especially useful in detecting tumor invasion of the paravertebral sulcus or mediastinum, particularly the vena cava, aorta, trachea or esophagus. Involvement of any of these anatomic structures (Butchart Stage II, Table 33–1)[5, 9] or evidence of transdiaphragmatic extension (Butchart Stage III) has not been associated with any long-term survivors. Based on this data, surgical resection is indicated only for patients with Butchart Stage I disease. In cases in which there

538

is equivocal radiographic evidence of abdominal extension, laparoscopy or limited laparotomy is planned to examine the liver for signs of invasion. This approach has proved very effective in reducing the incidence of exploratory thoracotomy without resection.

All potentially resectable patients must undergo a thorough preoperative team evaluation by a thoracic surgeon, a medical oncologist, and a radiotherapist. Each prospective surgical candidate is then subjected to routine pulmonary function testing with dynamic spirometry, functional oximetry, and arterial blood gas measurement. Any patient with an initial forced expiratory volume in one second (FEV_1) of less than 2 liters, or with a predicted postoperative FEV_1 of less than 1.2 liters, undergoes quantitative ventilation-perfusion scanning as an estimate of postoperative lung function.

Echocardiography is useful for a number of reasons. Direct mediastinal invasion frequently is detected by this technique. As a preoperative gauge of ventricular function, it is a useful predictor of perioperative morbidity and mortality. It also serves as a standard against which any subsequent doxorubicin-induced cardiac toxicity can be measured. Echocardiography is repeated halfway through the postoperative chemotherapeutic regimen to detect any deterioration in cardiac function. All patients with a predicted postoperative FEV_1 of less than 1 liter, an ejection fraction of less than 45% on echocardiogram, a room-air arterial carbon dioxide tension greater than 44 mm Hg, or oxygen tension less than 65 mm Hg are palliated without extrapleural pneumonectomy.

Those patients who are found suitable for surgery are administered prophylactic antibiotics, have pneumatic stockings (Kendall Healthcare Products Co., Mansfield, MA) put on, and have arterial and central venous lines placed. A thoracic epidural catheter is placed for intraoperative and postoperative anesthesia. After induction of general anesthesia, the patient is intubated with a Robertshaw double-lumen endotracheal tube and a nasogastric tube. The nasogastric tube is used to facilitate dissection around the esophagus intraoperatively.

The patient is positioned in the left lateral decubitus position for the right pleuropneumonectomy, which is detailed in the following sections; the modifications necessary for resection of left-sided lesions are covered briefly after that description.

Operative Technique

When radiographic studies cannot exclude transdiaphragmatic extension, the initial step in the procedure must be laparoscopy, or limited laparotomy via a subcostal incision, to inspect the liver for signs of invasion. Biopsy-proven abdominal disease precludes any attempt at thoracic resection.

When there is no evidence of peritoneal disease, an extended right thoracotomy is performed. An incision is made along the bed of the sixth rib, from the costochondral junction to a point 2 cm lateral to the costovertebral junction (Fig. 33–1).[10] The sixth rib is stripped of its periosteum and completely resected to provide wide exposure and easy access to the extrapleural plane of dissection.

The periosteum is incised, and dissection is directed toward the apex of the lung, freeing the parietal pleura from the chest musculature both sharply and bluntly. This technique requires meticulous attention to hemostasis, which is best achieved by the liberal use of electrocautery. Newly dissected regions are then packed with Mikulicz pads to maintain hemostasis throughout the pleuropneumonectomy.

The dissection is first completed anteriorly, from the apex to the diaphragm, to provide adequate exposure for the posterior dissection that follows. Two chest retractors are then placed anteriorly and posteriorly to ensure a controlled approach to the brachial triangle and posterior mediastinal structures. As dissection

TABLE 33–1. Butchart Staging System for Malignant Pleural Mesothelioma

STAGE	CHARACTERISTIC
I	Within the capsule of the parietal pleura: ipsilateral pleura, lung, pericardium, diaphragm
II	Invading chest wall or mediastinum: esophagus, heart, opposite pleura + Lymph nodes within the chest
III	Through diaphragm to peritoneum. Opposite pleura + Lymph nodes outside the chest
IV	Distant blood-borne metastases

Adapted from Butchart EG, Ashcroft T, Barnsley WC, Holden MP: Pleuropneumonectomy in the management of diffuse malignant mesothelioma of the pleura. Experience with 29 patients. Thorax 31:15–24, 1976; and Antman K, Pass HI, Recht A: Benign and malignant mesothelioma. *In* DeVita VT Jr, Hellman S, Rosenberg SA (eds): Cancer: Principles and Practice of Oncology. 3rd Ed. Philadelphia, J.B. Lippincott, 1989, pp 1399–1414.

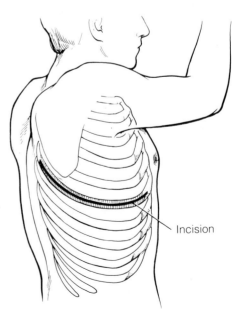

FIGURE 33–1. The extended right thoracotomy incision. (From Sugarbaker DJ, Mentzer SJ, Strauss G: Extrapleural pneumonectomy in the treatment of malignant pleural mesothelioma. Ann Thorac Surg 54:941–946, 1992.)

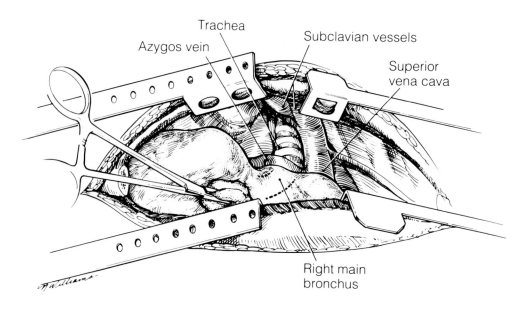

FIGURE 33–2. The right mainstem bronchus identified. (From Sugarbaker DJ, Mentzer SJ, Strauss G: Extrapleural pneumonectomy in the treatment of malignant pleural mesothelioma. Ann Thorac Surg 54:941–946, 1992.)

continues up to the cupola, particular care is taken to remain in the plane between the pleurae and the subclavian vessels. In a similar fashion, the internal mammary artery and vein are carefully identified and preserved; avulsion of these vessels from the subclavian artery or superior vena cava can be avoided if the dissection stays close to the parietal pleura, within the extrapleural fat.

The posterior mediastinal structures are approached from the apex. The extrapleural dissection proceeds inferiorly until the right upper lobe and main stem bronchus are clearly identified (Fig. 33–

2).[10] The azygous vein and superior vena cava are then freed of the investing parietal pleurae, and the dissection is carried circumferentially around the margins of the diaphragm to the anterior border of the pericardium. Every effort is made to preserve the continuity of the pleural envelope, and this necessitates resection of the diaphragm with the pleura (Fig. 33–3).[10] The peritoneum is freed from the undersurface of the diaphragm using a sponge stick (Fig. 33–4).[10] The diaphragm is then divided anteriorly as far as the pericardium. The inferolateral border of the pericardium must be entered in order to define adequately

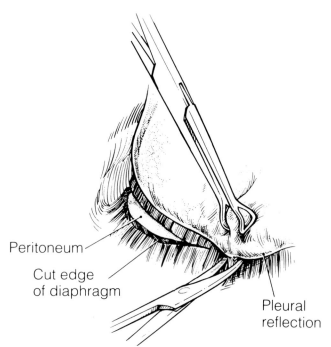

FIGURE 33–3. Dissection of the pleural envelope off the diaphragm. (From Sugarbaker DJ, Mentzer SJ, Strauss G: Extrapleural pneumonectomy in the treatment of malignant pleural mesothelioma. Ann Thorac Surg 54:941–946, 1992.)

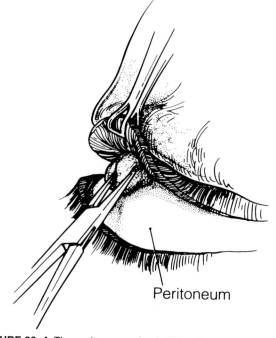

FIGURE 33–4. The peritoneum wiped off the diaphragm with a sponge. (From Sugarbaker DJ, Mentzer SJ, Strauss G: Extrapleural pneumonectomy in the treatment of malignant pleural mesothelioma. Ann Thorac Surg 54:941–946, 1992.)

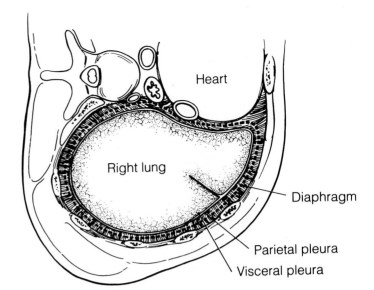

FIGURE 33–5. Diaphragm and pleural envelope divided lateral to inferior cava and esophagus. (From Sugarbaker DJ, Mentzer SJ, Strauss G: Extrapleural pneumonectomy in the treatment of malignant pleural mesothelioma. Ann Thorac Surg 54:941–946, 1992.)

the walls of the inferior vena cava and protect this structure from injury. The pleural envelope and diaphragm are divided posteriorly along the caval and esophageal hiatuses to complete the incision (Fig. 33–5).[10] Special care is taken to preserve the integrity of the pleural envelope.

The pericardium is then incised anteromedially to the phrenic nerve (Fig. 33–6).[10] Dissection is carried posteriorly along the pericardium, and the phrenic nerve is sacrificed. The main pulmonary artery is dissected away from the superior vena cava and superior pulmonary veins, and it is divided between two lines of vascular staples (Fig. 33–7).[10] The superior and inferior pulmonary veins are transected in a similar fashion. The pericardial resection is completed by dividing the pericardium posterior to the hilum. Retrac-

tion of the specimen anteriorly improves exposure posterior to the pericardium and lateral to the esophagus. This maneuver also facilitates a subcarinal lymph node dissection, which is performed at this time. The main bronchus is dissected to the carina and is transected at that level with a bronchial stapler (Fig. 33–8).[10] The specimen is removed en bloc and submitted for frozen-section analysis of resection margins. Any unresectable regions of gross disease are outlined with radio-opaque clips to guide subsequent radiotherapy or are treated intraoperatively with the application of radioactive seeds. Sheets of Surgicel (Johnson & Johnson, Arlington, TX) are placed over the denuded chest wall and are covered with dry packs; several minutes of tamponade are usually sufficient to ensure adequate hemostasis.

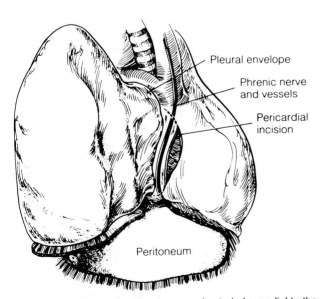

FIGURE 33–6. The pericardium is opened anteriorly, medial to the phrenic nerve and hilar vessels. (From Sugarbaker DJ, Mentzer SJ, Strauss G: Extrapleural pneumonectomy in the treatment of malignant pleural mesothelioma. Ann Thorac Surg 54:941–946, 1992.)

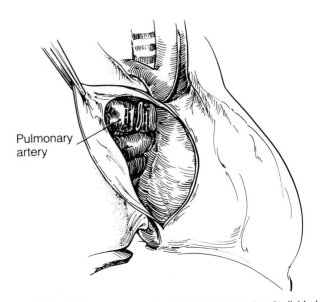

FIGURE 33–7. The intrapericardial right pulmonary artery is divided by two staple lines. (From Sugarbaker DJ, Mentzer SJ, Strauss G: Extrapleural pneumonectomy in the treatment of malignant pleural mesothelioma. Ann Thorac Surg 54:941–946, 1992.)

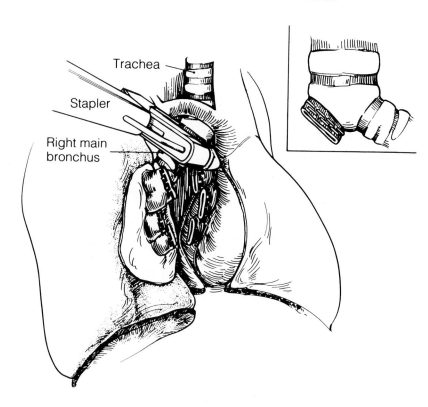

FIGURE 33–8. The main bronchus is dissected to the carina and stapled. (From Sugarbaker DJ, Mentzer SJ, Strauss G: Extrapleural pneumonectomy in the treatment of malignant pleural mesothelioma. Ann Thorac Surg 54:941–946, 1992.)

A flap of pericardial fat is wrapped around the bronchial stump. To prevent cardiac herniation, the remaining pericardium is repaired using a prosthetic patch and running 0 monofilament suture; fenestrations in the patch prevent tamponade (Fig. 33–9).[10]

Attention is then turned to the diaphragmatic defect. If the peritoneum remains intact, the peritoneum may be merely reinforced with multiple reefing stitches of 0 Vicryl (Fig. 33–10)[10] anchored in the chest wall. If the peritoneum has been excised, the diaphragmatic defect is repaired with an impermeable prosthetic patch sewn in place with running 0 monofilament suture (Fig. 33–11).[10] This watertight technique prevents rapid peritoneal fluid leakage into the thorax, where it can result in mediastinal shift or cardiac tamponade in the early postoperative period. An advantage of routine diaphragmatic reconstruction with prosthetic mesh is that it prevents the displacement of abdominal contents into the hemithorax after surgery. Upward displacement of the liver and bowel may limit the dose of adjuvant radiotherapy that can be delivered to the diseased hemithorax. The dose of radiotherapy to the posterior costophrenic sulcus may be particularly compromised should displacement occur.

The chest is closed in multiple layers to ensure an airtight seal, and a red rubber catheter is left in the lateral margin of the wound. This catheter is used to remove air (750 ml in women, 1000 ml in men) in the operating room before the patient is extubated. A postoperative chest roentgenogram is obtained to detect any mediastinal shift. Air is then injected or aspirated to balance the mediastinum, and the catheter is removed in the recovery room. In the event of imperfect hemostasis, a standard chest tube is inserted and placed to drainage on water seal without suction overnight. It can usually be removed on the first postoperative day. Blood loss for right pleuropneumonectomy is typically 750 ml.

Left Pleuropneumonectomy

The anatomy of the left hemithorax requires several modifications in technique. Because placement of a

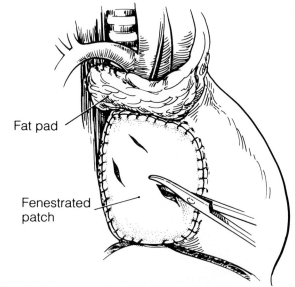

FIGURE 33–9. A pericardial fat pad has been sewn to cover the bronchial stump; the pericardium is closed with a patch, and fenestrations are made in the patch. (From Sugarbaker DJ, Mentzer SJ, Strauss G: Extrapleural pneumonectomy in the treatment of malignant pleural mesothelioma. Ann Thorac Surg 54:941–946, 1992.)

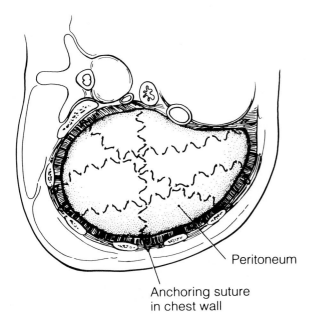

FIGURE 33–10. Reconstruction of the diaphragm, using multiple sutures of O Vicryl in reefing fashion, is carried out; the sutures are anchored to the chest wall. (From Sugarbaker DJ, Mentzer SJ, Strauss G: Extrapleural pneumonectomy in the treatment of malignant pleural mesothelioma. Ann Thorac Surg 54:941–946, 1992.)

Peritoneum

Anchoring suture in chest wall

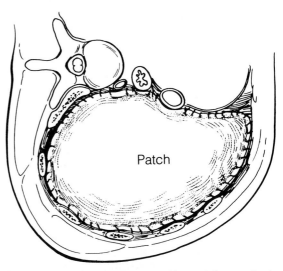

FIGURE 33–11. A prosthetic impermeable patch is sewn in place at the point where the peritoneum has been removed. (From Sugarbaker DJ, Mentzer SJ, Strauss G: Extrapleural pneumonectomy in the treatment of malignant pleural mesothelioma. Ann Thorac Surg 54:941–946, 1992.)

Patch

right double-lumen endotracheal tube can be difficult, an endobronchial blocker is often necessary for control of the left mainstem bronchus. The patient is placed in the right lateral decubitus position.

Left pleuropneumonectomy initially proceeds as on the right. Dissection of the left pleural envelope is technically easier than resection of right-sided disease, because of the absence of the caval and esophageal hiatuses. However, particular care must be taken during dissection posteromedially. In this region, it is critically important to remain in the preaortic plane; entrance into a retroaortic plane can result in avulsion of intercostal arteries from the aorta and attendant hemorrhage that is difficult to control. Tumor extension must be carefully assessed at this point because involvement of the aorta may preclude resection.

After dissection of the pleural envelope from the chest wall, the diaphragm is incised radially along the left side, with special care taken to protect the aorta during dissection of the hiatus. The left main pulmonary artery is identified as it courses out of the pericardium and into the left hemithorax (Fig. 33–12).[10] Unlike the technique on the right, the artery is divided at the extrapericardial, extrapleural point with a double vascular staple line. The pericardium is then entered inferiorly, the phrenic nerve is sacrificed, the pulmonary veins are divided within it, and the pericardial resection is completed posteriorly. The left mainstem bronchus is divided near the carina, and the resulting short bronchial stump is covered with a pericardial fat pad.

The pericardial defect is not routinely reconstructed on the left because there is no risk of cardiac herniation. The diaphragm is reconstructed and the chest is

closed as on the right. Because of the smaller size of the left hemithorax, less air is removed (500 ml in women, 750 ml in men) through the red rubber catheter at the end of the procedure. Blood loss for left pleuropneumonectomy is usually less than on the right, approximately 500 ml.

Postoperative Management

Postoperatively, patients are monitored in a thoracic unit with arterial lines, central venous lines, continuous oximetry, and telemetry. Epidural catheters are

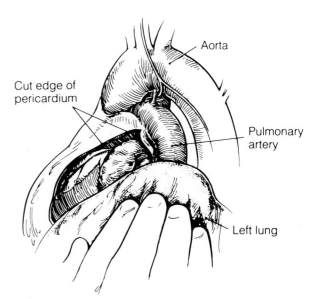

Aorta

Cut edge of pericardium

Pulmonary artery

Left lung

FIGURE 33–12. The extrapericardial and extrapleural pulmonary arteries are ready to be dissected. (From Sugarbaker DJ, Mentzer SJ, Strauss G: Extrapleural pneumonectomy in the treatment of malignant pleural mesothelioma. Ann Thorac Surg 54:941–946, 1992.)

TABLE 33–2. Select Series of Extrapleural Pneumonectomy in the Treatment of Pleural Mesothelioma

AUTHOR	YEAR	NUMBER OF PATIENTS	ADJUVANT THERAPY	2-YEAR SURVIVAL (%)	5-YEAR SURVIVAL (%)	OPERATIVE MORTALITY (%)
Worn	1974[11]	62	None	37	10	Not Stated
Butchart	1976[5]	29	None	10	4	31
Rusch	1991[12]	20	None	33	NA§	15
Sugarbaker	1993[4]	52	†EP + CAP 4 to 6 cycles then 55 Gy radiotherapy	17 (overall) 50 (epithelial) 8 (other types)	4 45* 0	6
Allen	1994[13]	40	EP + CAP†	23	10	8
		56	Pleur + CAP‡	9	5	5

*Five-year survival is for patients with epithelial histology and no positive mediastinal nodes at resection.
†EP + CAP = Extrapleural pneumonectomy followed by cyclophosphamide, adriamycin, and cisplatin (CAP).
‡Pleur + CAP = Pleurectomy followed by CAP.
§NA = Data not available.

used for 3 to 5 days after surgery to minimize atelectasis. Individual nursing care, including chest physiotherapy, is performed with the wound side down for 2 days. Pneumatic stockings should be worn for several days to protect against deep vein thrombosis.

The immediate postoperative course following extrapleural pneumonectomy is frequently complicated by fluid retention and capillary leak of the remaining lung. For this reason, patients should be restricted to one liter per 24 hours for 3 days postoperatively. Should desaturation occur, diuresis, chest physiotherapy, or bronchoscopy can be used.

Chest films are evaluated immediately after surgery and daily for mediastinal shift, which could produce tamponade or in-flow obstruction. Aggressive diagnosis and treatment of contralateral infiltrates is necessary for these patients.

Removal of nasogastric tubing is based on clinical signs and can be performed on Day one postoperatively. It is a significant clinical decision because aspiration can be fatal in these patients whose pulmonary capacity has been reduced.

Although it is a rare complication, cardiac herniation should be considered should there develop sudden hemodynamic collapse after repositioning the patient either supinely or in the right lateral decubitus position. In the face of cardiac arrest, no matter what the cause, open cardiac massage must be performed because closed compressions will not work owing to the absence of the resected lung. The heart is not compressed between the sternum and vertebral column, but instead is displaced into the vacant hemithorax with closed compressions. Thus, closed cardiac compressions worsen the hemo-dynamic compromise of cardiac herniation. Care of these patients requires rapid recognition of the complication, immediate thoracotomy, and return of the heart into the pericardial sac. This measure alone will dramatically reverse the hemodynamic compromise.

Hemodynamic compromise of a more insidious nature may be due to cardiac tamponade. The pericardial patch is fenestrated to prevent this complication, but if these fenestrations are not adequate in size or are occluded with clot, tamponade may still develop.

The most common complication of this operation is

postoperative arrhythmias. Thirty-seven percent of the patients treated with extrapleural pneumonectomy at the Brigham & Women's Hospital experienced supraventricular dysrhythmia with a peak incidence between 2 and 6 postoperative days. The vast majority of these patients respond to digitalization, and few require cardioversion. Continuous telemetry is recommended for at least 6 days after this operation.

Results

Several authors have explored the impact of extrapleural pneumonectomy used as a single modality in the treatment of diffuse malignant pleural mesothelioma (Table 33–2).[5, 11, 12]

In 1974, Worn reported his experience with 62 extrapleural pneumonectomies without adjuvant therapy and 186 patients treated with palliative operations. Many current items of interest are lacking in this report, including the histologic subtypes, pathologic stage, and operative mortality rate. However, his results are the best of any series of single modality therapy with a 37% 2-year survival and a 10% 5-year survival.[11]

Butchart and colleagues reported results of extrapleural pneumonectomy in 29 patients in 1976.[5] This has become one of the most quoted papers on the subject. Advocates of extrapleural pneumonectomy point out the 2 long-term survivors without disease, while opponents of the procedure quote the high 31% operative mortality rate in this series. The authors carefully analyzed the histology of the tumors removed and found a significantly higher survival rate in the patient group with epithelial histology. Furthermore, they established a clinicopathologic staging system of diffuse malignant pleural mesothelioma, and found survival was better in Butchart Stage I patients (tumor confined to the homolateral pleura, lung, and pericardium without invasion of the chest wall, mediastinum, or mediastinal lymph nodes).

Rusch and associates reported a prospective but nonrandomized trial for the Lung Cancer Study Group.[12] From 1985 to 1988, 63 patients who were not acceptable candidates for extrapleural pneumonectomy were treated according to the preference of their physicians: 26 patients had a parietal pleurectomy with a variety of adjuvant therapies, whereas 37 patients had no surgical therapy. It is unclear what therapy, if any, this latter group received. Twenty patients were treated with extrapleural pneumonectomy without adjuvant therapy unless they developed recurrent disease. In this series, extrapleural pneumonectomy had an associated 15% operative mortality rate. The patients treated with extrapleural pneumonectomy had a palliative benefit manifested by a significantly increased disease-free time for the first 14 postoperative months, compared with the other two groups, but there was no difference in overall survival. Furthermore, the pneumonectomy group had marked improvement in local control of the tumor.

Allen, Faber, and Warren have updated the ongoing series of patients treated at the Rush–Presbyterian–St. Luke's Medical Center of Chicago.[13] Since 1958, they have treated 40 patients with extrapleural pneumonectomy and 56 patients with pleurectomy. Seventy-three per cent of both of these groups have also received adjuvant chemotherapy. A variety of agents have been used without a specific protocol, although their recent experience has been with cyclophosphamide, doxorubicin, and cis-platinum (CAP). Radiotherapy has also been used but is generally reserved for local recurrence. Using modern intraoperative monitoring and intensive care, they report similar operative mortality rates for the two procedures: 7.5% for extrapleural pneumonectomy and 5.4% for pleurectomy. The extrapleural pneumonectomy patients had a 2-year survival of 22.5% and a 5-year survival of 10%, whereas the pleurectomy patients had a 2-year survival of 8.9% and a 5-year survival of 5.4%. This trend did not reach statistical significance in their series.

The Memorial Sloan-Kettering Cancer Center of New York (MSKCC) has also developed an extensive experience with pleurectomy in the surgical treatment of this disease.[1, 14, 15] In 1993, Rusch reported the most recent update of their ongoing studies.[3] Pleurectomy is possible only in a free pleural space, where the lung is not heavily encased in a thick, noncompliant rind of tumor. It entails the complete removal of all gross tumor and usually the pericardium and diaphragm, while leaving the lung in place. The initial experience at MSKCC combined pleurectomy with either external beam radiation or intracavitary brachytherapy. From 1976 to 1988, 105 patients were treated in this manner with an operative mortality of 1.5%, which is less than the best reports of extrapleural pneumonectomy.[14] Although the overall median survival was 12.6 months, patients with the epithelial histology had a median survival time of 22.5 months. Since 1988, MSKCC has initiated a new trial combining pleurectomy with intrapleural cisplatin, 75 mg/m², and mitomycin, 8 mg/M².[3] Systemic chemotherapy consisting of two cycles of cisplatin, 50 mg/m²/week, and mitomycin, 8 mg/M², is then given beginning 1 month postoperatively. As of the last report, 23 patients had been treated with this protocol and were followed beyond the immedi-

ate postoperative period. After a median follow-up of 11 months, 12 were free of disease, two were alive with disease, and six had died of disease. Most recurrences had been local. It is hoped that further follow-up from this study will establish whether long-term disease-free survival can be anticipated with this treatment option.

Our experience has been with the use of extrapleural pneumonectomy as cytoreductive surgery, combined with aggressive systemic chemotherapy followed in turn by external radiation to the diseased hemithorax. This approach has several advantages to previously reported protocols. We believe pneumonectomy provides greater palliation for those patients who are not cured by removing the shunt of nonoxygenated blood through the diseased lung when disease recurs after pleurectomy or approaches end-stage without previous surgical therapy. This elimination of the shunt fraction of blood prevents the debilitating dyspnea and orthopnea that marks the terminal stages of advanced disease in the chest. Also, the radiation dose that can be delivered to the hemithorax is greatly increased without the native lung. In the MSKCC experience with pleurectomy and radiotherapy, there was a significant incidence of radiation pneumonitis and pericarditis.[3] Finally, the combination of extrapleural pneumonectomy combined with adjuvant chemotherapy and radiotherapy seems to offer the best chance for cure in carefully selected patients, even though the majority will experience a relapse and die of the disease.

From 1980 to 1992, 52 selected patients at the Brigham & Women's Hospital have received a trimodality protocol, which has included extrapleural pneumonectomy, adjuvant chemotherapy (cyclophosphamide, 600 mg/m²; doxorubicin, 60 mg/m²; and cisplatin, 70 mg/m² for four to six cycles, to a cumulative doxorubicin dose of 450 mg/m²), and 55-Gy adjuvant radiotherapy. The median age was 53 years (ranging from 33 to 69 years). The 30-day mortality rate in this group was 5.8%, with a 17% morbidity rate.[4]

Median survival for patients with diffuse malignant mesothelioma without trimodality therapy ranges between 4 to 12 months.[9, 11–13, 16–18] Median survival of the overall Brigham & Women's Hospital series was 16 months. Patients with the epithelial histologic variant had improved median survival of 24 months. Furthermore, the subgroup of 25 patients with the epithelial cell type and no mediastinal nodal metastases at resection did well, with a 5-year survival of 45%.[4]

Multivariate analysis of this series revealed that cell type and mediastinal node status had prognostic significance in diffuse malignant mesothelioma. Epithelial cell type and no nodal metastases are separate predictors of long-term survival. Separate analysis is not available between sarcomatous cell type and mixed sarcomatous-epithelial cell type. Based on this data, a pathologic modified Butchart staging system has been proposed (Table 33–3).[4]

Patient selection for extrapleural pneumonectomy is critical for both those who are deemed appropriate and those who are not. Operative mortality for this procedure has been higher than that for intrapleural pneumonectomy in several reports.[5, 12, 19] Furthermore, the adjuvant chemotherapy and radiotherapy bring an additional risk for morbidity and mortality. Counterbalancing these disadvantages are the dismal survival statistics of diffuse malignant mesothelioma, as well as the significant morbidity of the disease.[20]

The palliation given to these patients with surgical interventions, through either pleurectomy or pneumonectomy, is dramatic and difficult to capture by examining just the survival statistics. The natural course of this disease is frequently a rapid and dramatic decline with progressive dyspnea, orthopnea, cachexia, and chest wall pain that is poorly controlled with narcotics. Fever associated with a large tumor burden adds to the cachexia, as does the protein loss of repetitive thoracentesis to improve lung function. Pleurodesis is frequently unsuccessful or only partially successful. By eliminating the shunt fraction of the diseased lung, pneumonectomy can paradoxically produce greater pulmonary palliation than pleurectomy alone once disease has progressed to end-stage, provided there is not disease in the contralateral hemithorax.

At present, the groups that are reporting improved outcomes with extrapleural pneumonectomy are using the operation in conjunction with other adjuvant therapies to increase local control.[21–23] Standardized treatment of large patient groups with the same stage of disease is still required for adequate analysis of treatment options. All reports to date have had a mixed population in regard to several prognostic factors, and many of the groups have been treated with a mixture of protocols.

The combination of multiple modalities seems to offer the best treatment for these unfortunate patients. New protocols should be aimed at treatment combinations designed to give maximal local control. One possibility would be to combine concomitant adjuvant chemotherapy and radiotherapy after extrapleural pneumonectomy. The role of extrapleural pneumonectomy in the treatment of mesothelioma is a matter of controversy.

CHEMOTHERAPY OF MALIGNANT MESOTHELIOMA

Malignant mesothelioma was rarely reported before 1960, when Wagner and colleagues[24] established the association between malignant mesothelioma and asbestos exposure. A similar association was described in the United States by Selikoff and associates in 1964.[25] Since then, malignant mesothelioma, which remains a relatively rare tumor, has been reported more frequently.[26, 27] This is due, in part, to the increased use of asbestos products during and following the Second World War. Therapeutic approaches for mesothelioma, however, have been very slow to develop. Between 1960 and 1980, the chemotherapy experience with single agent or combination regimens derived

TABLE 33–3. A Proposed Staging System for Mesothelioma Patients Based on the Survival Rate of 52 Patients*

STAGE	CHARACTERISTIC
I	Disease confined to within capsule of the parietal pleura: ipsilateral pleura, lung, pericardium, diaphragm* or chest wall disease limited to previous biopsy sites
II	All of Stage I with positive intrathoracic (N1 or N2) lymph nodes
III	Local extension of disease into: chest wall or mediastinum; heart, or through diaphragm, peritoneum; with or without extrathoracic or contralateral (N3) lymph node involvement
IV	Distant metastatic disease

*Butchart Stages II and III[5] are combined into Stage III. Stage I represents resectable patients with negative nodes. Stage III patients are resectable but have positive nodal status.

Adapted from Antman K, Pass HI, Recht A: Benign and malignant mesothelioma. In DeVita VT Jr, Hellman S, Rosenberg SA (eds): Cancer: Principles and Practice of Oncology. 3rd Ed. Philadelphia, J.B. Lippincott, 1989, pp 1399–1414; and Sugarbaker DJ, Mentzer SJ, Strauss G: Extrapleural pneumonectomy in the treatment of pleural mesothelioma. Ann Thorac Surg 54:941–946, 1992.

mostly from relatively few and small, single institution series or as part of broad Phase II studies, or as part of sarcoma studies. Despite this experience, difficulty in defining reliable response rates to chemotherapy (either single agent or combination) resulted from a number of factors. First, because of a lack of defined criteria for diagnosis, many pathologists were reluctant to diagnose mesothelioma definitively except at autopsy. Except for the less common mixed fibrosarcomatous and epithelial form, mesothelioma often remained a diagnosis of exclusion. This diagnostic reluctance made it difficult to gather sufficient numbers of patients for disease-focused treatment protocols.

Another factor that confounded data from past trials derives from the fact that most mesotheliomas are not strictly measurable on chest x-ray studies. Pleural thickening or a chest wall mass, required for reliable response assessment, is frequently obscured by an effusion, the volume of which is notoriously unreliable in determining responsiveness to therapy. Thus past trials may have been biased by either including patients with metastatic disease or overinterpreting subjective criteria. The wide availability of (CT) scanning, which reliably assesses extent of disease[28]; the increased incidence of the disease[26, 27]; and the development of multi-institutional cooperative group trials have recently allowed a more systematic approach to mesothelioma.

Another potential problem with some of the earlier data is seen in some of the reported small studies with positive results. Slightly larger series with lower or negative response rates may never have been published, thus sometimes producing an erroneous view of an agent's activity. A good example of small favorable report bias is seen in the early report of responsiveness to 5-fluorouracil (5-FU) in two of three patients.[29] No large study of this agent in mesothelioma was published until a full decade later.[30] However, the activity of 5-FU is still not established, because the larger study employed approximately half of the dose rate of the earlier, smaller study. Other confounding problems in the evaluation of chemotherapy in mesothelioma include the extent of prior treatment and performance status, which are seldom reported. The discrepancy in response rates seen in sequential trials may result from differences in these parameters because these are among the most important prognostic factors in human cancers.

Today, there are better established criteria for histologic and immunocytochemical diagnosis of mesothelioma.[31] Also, most Phase II chemotherapy trials now focus on mesothelioma specifically and require good performance status and no prior chemotherapy. Nevertheless, the response rates for many of the standard chemotherapeutic agents have not yet been definitively established. For example, the reported response rate of mesothelioma to doxorubicin varies from 0% to 40% in various series (Table 33–4).[29, 30, 32–42] Generally, the higher response rates were observed at larger institutions or cancer centers. However, patients referred to these institutions are usually younger and have better performance status and less advanced disease. Intensive supportive care is available at these institutions as well, allowing higher dose treatment.

SINGLE AGENT ACTIVITY

The reported activities of the single agents remain somewhat difficult to interpret because of the above-mentioned limitations and are considered as compilations of the various published reports listed in Table 33–4.[29, 30, 32–127] Based on these compilations, which ignore dosing and scheduling features of the agents, doxorubicin and cyclophosphamide appear to possess modest activity against mesothelioma. Methotrexate with rescue, 5-azacytidine, and 5-FU also appear to have modest activity as single agents (Table 33–4). Because only the recent trials have specifically focused on mesothelioma, response frequencies are stated only when the number of evaluable cases exceeds 10. Cisplatin as a single agent appears to possess a marginal level of activity in mesothelioma, with 12 of a total of 67 patients (18%) responding in several Phase II studies (Table 33–4). One trial by Planting and colleagues[80] suggests that the dose and schedule may be important. Because the response frequency overall has been disappointing, further studies of single agents in previously untreated patients is needed in order to identify active agents for combination chemotherapy and combined modality studies.

COMBINATION CHEMOTHERAPY

Combinations of chemotherapy have also been tested in patients with mesothelioma in small series or as part of broad Phase II studies. Therefore, past information regarding the role of various combinations is also subject to the same errors and biases as the single agent data. The majority of such combinations were based on doxorubicin, cyclophosphamide, or cisplatin, and are presented as a compilation of the trials according to the inclusion of anthracyclines in Table 33–5* or exclusive of anthracyclines in Table 33–6.† As in the Table 33–4, the response frequencies are listed only for those combinations for which the accumulated experience exceeds 10 patients. Although some single institutions reported response rates of 30% to 40% for doxorubicin- or cisplatin-containing regimens in small series containing 10 to 20 patients, cooperative group trials for the same combinations reported much lower response rates.[37, 42, 78, 143] One should note that the overall 20% response rate for doxorubicin-containing regimens shown in Table 33–5 and the 19% response rate for the non–anthracycline-containing combinations listed in Table 33–6 do not appear strikingly different from the 18% response rate for doxorubicin used as a single agent (see Table 33–4). These compilations, however, do not take into account any dose or schedule dependency of either the single agents or their combinations. Because dose intensity is often compromised for combinations, higher doses of doxorubicin could be equivalent to lower doses as part of combinations. Further studies of dose dependency and drug resistance thus may be of some value in the treatment of this tumor.

The usual approach of combining active agents also has not proved particularly valuable in the treatment of mesothelioma. For example, an intergroup study combined doxorubicin and cyclophosphamide with or without dacarbazine (DTIC) and reported response rates of 7% for both arms of the randomized trial.[143] The results of this study may be somewhat difficult to interpret and lower than expected because this study was composed of patients with advanced disease at the same time that another study of ipsilateral radiotherapy plus or minus doxorubicin was composed of patients with earlier stage (Stage I or II) mesothelioma. Thus, the patients with better prognostic factors were treated with the second protocol. Not surprisingly, we have observed that early peritoneal mesotheliomas seem to respond to chemotherapy more frequently than advanced peritoneal mesotheliomas[159]; thus, some of the discrepancies in the response rate may have resulted from a selection bias of patients with more extensive disease.

Although the reported activity of cisplatin as a single agent is unimpressive, more recent series using cisplatin combinations have suggested a possible role for these protocols in the treatment of mesothelioma. Cisplatin is known to be synergistic with other agents using in vitro experimental systems, and synergy has been suggested clinically in testicular cancer and in small cell lung cancer. Doxorubicin, 50 mg/m², and cisplatin, 50 mg/m², resulted in four responses among six patients with mesothelioma.[135] Responses continued between 5 and 17 months. Several additional trials of the combination of doxorubicin and cisplatin

---

*See references 29, 32, 33, 35, 38, 39, 52, 57, 95, 105, and 128–147.
†See references 32, 33, 36, 41, 52, 57, 64, 91, 95, 104, 129, 136, and 148–158.

TABLE 33–4. Single Agent Response Rates in Malignant Mesothelioma

AGENT	NUMBER EVALUABLE	NUMBER RESPONDING	% RESPONDING	REFERENCES
Anthracyclines				
Doxorubicin	164	29	18	29, 30, 32–42
Detorubicin	21	9	43	43
Pirarubicin	100	12	12	44–47
Epirubicin	69	8	12	48, 49
Mitoxantrone	46	1	2	50
Aclacinomycin-A	10	1	10	51
Actinomycin D	3	0		52, 53
Alkylating Agents				
Cyclophosphamide	14	4	28	29, 54–57
Ifosfamide	84	6	7	58–60
Mechlorethamine	6	2		61–66
Thiotepa	7	1		34, 54, 64, 66, 67
Melphalan	3	2		33, 67
Procarbazine	6	2		32, 68
Mitomycin-C	19	4	21	69
Dacarbazine (DTIC)	4	1		29, 70, 71
Cisplatin	56	8	14	32, 72–79
Cisplatin (weekly)	11	4	36	80
Carboplatin	97	11 (2 CR)	11	81–86
Iproplatin (JM9)	7	0		85, 86
Dibromodulcitol	5	0		87, 88
Antimetabolites				
5-Fluorouracil	28	4	14	29, 30, 89, 90
Methotrexate, high dose	9	4		91
Methotrexate, standard	1	0		92
Baker's antifol	3	0		93
Dideazafolic acid (CB3717)	18	1	6	86, 94
Dichloromethotrexate	1	0		95
5-Azacytidine	7	0	7	96, 97
Dihydro 5 azacytadine	55	4 (1 CR)		98, 99
Bleomycin	6	1		38, 95
6 Diazo-5-oxo-L-norleucine	7	0		51
Ara C, high dose	1	1		100
Nitrosoureas				
PCNU	34	0	0	101
BCNU	2	0		92, 102
Methyl CCNU	3	0		103–105
ACNU	2	0		106
Streptozotocin	1	0		32
Vincas and Related Compounds				
Vincristine	23	0		107
Vindesine	37	1	3	108, 109
Etoposide (VP16)	51	3	6	110–113
Miscellaneous				
M AMSA	19	1	5	114
AZQ	20	0	0	115
Maytansine	5	0		88, 95
Methyl-G	2	1		95
Glucosamine	2	0		29, 64
Hydroxyurea	2	0		33, 52
DDMP	2	0		116
Bruceantin	1	0		117
Cycloleucine	7	2		38
Biologic Response Modifiers				
BCG (after surgery)	30	NE	NE	118
RNA (intrapleural)	10	8		119
interferon				
alpha	25(1 CR)	3	12	120
beta	14	0		121
gamma (intrapleural)	99	24(7 CR)	24	122–125
IL2 (intrapleural)	24	10	42	123, 126, 127

CR = Complete response; NE = Not evaluable; ACNU = Nimustine; AZQ = Aziridinyl benzoquinone; BCG = Bacillus Calmette-Guérin vaccine; BCNU = Carmustine; DDMP = Metoprine; IL2 = Interleukin-2; MAMSA = Amsacrine; Met-CCNU = Semustine; PCNU = 1(2-chloroethyl)-3-(2,6-dioxo-3-piperidyl)-1-nitrosourea.

TABLE 33–5. Combinations Containing Anthracyclines

COMBINATION	NUMBER EVALUABLE	NUMBER RESPONDING	RESPONSE RATE (%)	REFERENCES
Dox + VCR	6	0		35
Dox + DTIC	8	4		39, 128
Dox + 5-AZA	36	8	27	95, 129
Dox + ACTD	3	0		130
Dox + ICRF	1	1		131
Dox + IFOS	47	12	26	132–134
Dox + DDP	59	16	27	135–139
Dox + DDP + VDS	9	0		140
Dox + DDP + BLEO + MMC + IP HD	25	11 (1CR)	44	141
Dox + DDP + CYC	23	6	26	142
Dox + CYC	6	1		32, 52
Dox + CYC + VCR	15	5	33	29, 35
Dox + CYC ± DTIC	81	6	7	143
Dox + CYC + DTIC + VCR	30	8	21	57, 104, 144
Dox + CYC + DTIC + VCR + ACTD	5	1		33
Dox + CYC + MTX + VCR + VP16	12	2	17	145
Dox + DTIC + VCR	4	0		104
Dox + High dose MTX, VCR	5	3		52
Dox + Various other agents	66	7	11	38, 39
TOTAL DOX COMBINATIONS	441	91	44	
Other Anthracyclines				
Pirarubicin + DDP	39	6	15	46, 139
Epirubicin + IFOS	17	1	6	146
Rubidizone + DTIC	23	0	0	147

ACT D = Actinomycin D; 5-AZA = 5-azacytidine; BLEO = bleomycin; DDP = cisplatin; CYC = cyclophosphamide; DTIC = dacarbazine; Dox = doxorubicin; VP16 = etoposide; IFOS = ifosfamide; ICRF = Imperial Cancer Research Fund drug; IP HD = intrapleural hyaluronidase; MTX = methotrexate; MMC = Mitomycin-C; VCR = vincristine; VDS = vindesine.

have been completed and the composite response is only 27%, however.[136–139] A combination of cisplatin and Mitomycin-C, at doses of 50 and 10 mg/m², respectively, resulted in four objective responses in 12 patients.[153] This regimen design was rationally based on in vitro sensitivity to these two agents, using hu-

man malignant mesothelioma xenografts that were serially transplanted in nude mice and tested against a series of single agents. The cisplatin analogues carboplatin and iproplatin were tested in these cell lines as well and exhibited some activity that did not correlate totally with sensitivity to cisplatin.[153] The Cancer and

TABLE 33–6. Combination Chemotherapy Regimens Without Anthracyclines

DRUG COMBINATION	NUMBER EVALUABLE	NUMBER OF RESPONDERS	RESPONSE RATE (%)	REFERENCES
CYC + VCR	1	0		52
CYC + VCR + ACTD	4	0		104
CYC + VCR + ACTD + DTIC	14	1	7	57
CYC + VCR + 5FU	2	0		64, 148
CYC + VBL + 5FU	9	2		129
CYC + VCR + 5FU + MTX	7	4		33, 36, 41, 148
DDP + CYC + MTX	9	1		95
DDP + 5FU	12	0		95, 150
DDP + VP16	26	3	12	151
DDP + VBL + BLEO	1	0		152
DDP + MMC	51	13	25	136, 153, 154
DDP + high dose MTX	6	4		91
DDP + dihydro-5-azacytidine	30	4	13	155
CBP + MMC	5	1		134
VDS + MMC	12	0	0	156
VCR + high-dose MTX	9	6		157
5FU + MeCCNU	2	0		52, 95
5FU + VBL + BCNU + MTX	1	0		158
VBL + BLEO	2	0		32, 52
Total	194	38	20	

ACTD = Actinomycin D; BLEO = bleomycin; CBP = carboplatin; BCNU = carmustine; DDP = cisplatin; CYC = cyclophosphamide; DTIC = dacarbazine; VP16 = etoposide; 5FU = 5-fluorouracil; MTX = methotrexate; MMC = Mitomycin-C; MeCCNU = semustine; VBL = vinblastine; VCR = vincristine; VDS = vindesine.

TABLE 33–7. Combined Modality Therapies

THERAPY	NUMBER IN STUDY	NUMBER RESPONSES	PER CENT RESPONSE	MDS MONTHS	REFERENCE
PLX + (DDP + MMC)*	12	NA	NA	NA	173
EPX + CYC + DOX + DDP + RT	44	NA	NA	21	176
PLX or EPX + (DDP + MMC)*	14	NA	NA	<18	177
PLX or EPX + PRPHYN + light	NA	NA	NA	NA	178
PLX or EPX + DOX + VDS + CYC + RT	57	NA	NA	NA	179
DOX + RT	14	3	21	NA	95
DOX + RT	10	1	10	NA	180
DDP + TAM + IFNα	25	3	12	8.3	181

*Chemotherapy intraoperative and postoperative
DDP = Cisplatin; CYC = cyclophosphamide; EPX = extrapleural pneumonectomy; IFNα = interferon; MMC = Mitomycin-C; PLX = pleurectomy; PRPHYN = protoporphyrin; RT = radiotherapy; TAM = tamoxifen; VDS = vindesine; NA = data not available.

Leukemia Group B (CALGB) subsequently reported the results of a study in which patients with measurable mesothelioma received either cisplatin and Mitomycin-C or cisplatin and doxorubicin.[136] The objective response rates (13%) were similar for the two combinations in patients with measurable disease, but there were more regressions with mitomycin plus cisplatin if patients with evaluable nonmeasurable disease were included in the response rate (28% versus 13%).

INTRACAVITARY DELIVERY OF CHEMOTHERAPY

Because mesothelioma begins and spreads superficially within the pleural and peritoneal cavities, intracavitary instillation of chemotherapy or radioisotopes could potentially treat the early regional disease in the chest when a cavity still exists. The proclivity of peritoneal mesothelioma to remain localized even when advanced has also fostered the use of intraperitoneal chemotherapy. Early anecdotal reports of prolonged survival with certain radioisotopes[160, 161] also stimulated interest in this approach. Delivery of high intracavitary concentrations of chemotherapeutic agents could capitalize on a steep dose-response curve and enhance local control. The major theoretic obstacle to intracavitary chemotherapy is the shallow depth of drug penetration. Debulking or peeling of the tumor with repetitive chemotherapy exposure may avoid this theoretical limitation. In addition, if substantial intravenous drug levels result from peritoneal absorption, such as occurs with cisplatin, then the combination of free surface diffusion and intracapillary drug exposure may be potentially more efficacious than the intravenous therapy alone.

Cisplatin is the most extensively studied agent for intracavitary use.[158–164] The pharmacokinetic parameters show that the exposure (concentration X time) is 30-fold greater, and the peak levels 20 to 200 times greater with intracavitary than intravenous cisplatin.[162, 164] Although intracavitary cisplatin appears to have considerable efficacy in peritoneal mesothelioma, it appears less promising in pleural disease.[164] Other agents have also been tested for intracavitary

administration including doxorubicin, cytosine arabinoside, Mitomycin-C, and interferon.[165–172]

COMBINED MODALITY THERAPY

One logical outcome of testing individual therapeutic maneuvers would be to combine them in order to improve the therapeutic margin. Thus surgery, chemotherapy, radiosensitizers, and radiotherapy might be used in sequence or together to reduce tumor burden and destroy residual or microscopic tumor. The experience with combined modalities is relatively limited and is listed in Table 33–7.[95, 173, 176, 177, 179–181]

Surgical Adjuvant Therapy

Although many investigators are exploring surgical methods of tumor debulking (decortication) or complete resection (extrapleural pneumonectomy), by the time most patients present with pleural mesothelioma, surgical resection is rarely feasible. Even in those cases in which surgical resections are attempted, including radical extrapleural pneumonectomy, a high rate of local and systemic recurrences lead to ultimate treatment failure. Local recurrences with tumor growth into and through surgical scars are seen frequently. Thus, recent studies of the management of pleural mesothelioma have emphasized the need for adjuvant intraoperative or postoperative therapies. Rusch and colleagues at the Memorial Sloan-Kettering Cancer Center have instilled cisplatin and Mitomycin-C into the pleural space following pleurectomy and decortication.[173] The pharmacokinetic assessment of this approach suggests a high intracavitary concentration of drug with adequate systemic levels as well. They have also added postoperative systemic cisplatin and mitomycin chemotherapy.[174] Sugarbaker and colleagues have tested combined modality therapy using extrapleural pneumonectomy followed by cisplatin, doxorubicin, and cyclophosphamide chemotherapy and external beam irradiation.[175] In a group of 44 patients who were able to tolerate aggressive treatment from 1980 to 1991, all of whom were either Stage I or Stage II, the combined modality program resulted in a 45% 2-year survival among the 34 patients with negative mediastinal lymph nodes.[176] Epithelial cell type was also a favorable prognostic factor in this report. Combined modality studies with adjuvant chemotherapy are also receiving attention by other investigators.[177] Further study is needed to assess whether surgery plus adjuvant therapies can improve survival or whether the favorable results represent a selection bias.

Another approach to adjuvant therapy has been to administer a photoactivated dye such as protoporphyrin and to activate the dye within the hemithorax after a debulking surgical procedure such as a modified extrapleural pneumonectomy or pleural decortication. The initial Phase I dosimetry studies have been conducted at the National Cancer Institute by Pass and colleagues,[178] and further Phase II testing is awaited. Such trials will, however, also be subject to the same concern about selection bias as other surgical based trials.

Combined Chemotherapy and Radiotherapy

Because most patients are not good candidates for surgical resections, another approach that could be considered is the use of chemotherapy with radiotherapy. There is, however, only very limited experience with this approach, and there has been little reported on testing radiosensitizers or radioprotective agents. Doxorubicin plus radiotherapy has been studied in two small trials.[97, 180] A small group of patients in the large series reported from South Africa treated with doxorubicin and radiation of 10 Gy every 6 weeks for four courses appeared to show prolonged survival, with a median survival time of 22.6 months.[180] At present, a randomized intergroup (ECOG, RTOG, SECSG, and SWOG) study is testing the role of radiotherapy with and without the subsequent administration of doxorubicin.

Another approach to combined modality therapy has been to combine biologic agents, chemotherapy resistance modulators, and chemotherapeutic agents.[181] Whether this approach will prove useful remains to be confirmed.

Although the role of combined modality therapies can not easily be distinguished from the contribution of its component therapies, at least one nonrandomized study from Hamburg has suggested a prolongation of life expectancy with multimodal treatment compared with best supportive care.[179] Aggressive treatment included surgery with either pleurectomy and decortication or extrapleural pneumonectomy. Chemotherapy included doxorubicin, vindesine, and cyclophosphamide. Patients in the aggressive treatment group who were in partial or complete remission without progression at the completion of their chemotherapy underwent 45 to 60 Gy of irradiation. The median survival time in the treated patients was 13 months compared with 7 months for those receiving best supportive care. However, the patients in the aggressively treated group had better prognostic fac-

tors such that the outcome may be an artifact of this imbalance of the prognostic factors.

FUTURE DIRECTIONS

Because mesothelioma remains a rare and usually fatal tumor, accrual of patients unto organized clinical trials must remain a high priority. Although several single agents and some combination regimens show some modest antitumor activity, none are so beneficial in overall outcome as to suggest a standard therapeutic approach. New treatment protocols for mesothelioma are thus needed, including new drug discovery (Phase II) studies, combinations of active single agents, and the development of rational combined modality programs. Although any approach that produces a significant percentage of disease-free survival would obviate the need for randomization, several approaches such as the surgical adjuvant programs have been shown to be feasible, and their general applicability may need more formalized study. The comparative assessment of chemotherapeutic regimens, and different surgical approaches will, however, require intergroup cooperative randomized trials. Until highly active and effective therapeutic regimens are identified, referral of patients with malignant mesothelioma to centers that specialize in the treatment of this disease will aid in the identification of such active therapies.

SELECTED REFERENCES

Sugarbaker DJ, Strauss GM, Lynch TJ, et al: Node status has prognostic significance in the multimodality therapy of diffuse, malignant mesothelioma. J Clin Oncol 11:1172–1178, 1993.
Multimodality therapy including extrapleural pneumonectomy had acceptable rates of morbidity and mortality for 52 selected patients. Multivariate analysis showed histologic subtype and mediastinal node status were independent predictors of long-term survival. A modification of the Butchart staging system was suggested. Prolonged survival occurred in patients with the epithelial histologic variant and negative mediastinal lymph nodes.

Rusch VW: Pleurectomy/decortication and adjuvant therapy for malignant mesothelioma. Chest 103(suppl):382S–384S, 1993.
A comparison of the recent literature advocating extrapleural pneumonectomy with the literature advocating pleurectomy and decortication followed by adjuvant therapy. The operative technique of pleurectomy is briefly described, along with its advantages and disadvantages. The operative mortality rate for this operation may be as low as 1.8%.

Lewis RJ: Malignant pleural mesothelioma: A nonsurgical problem. In Kittle CF (ed): Current Controversies in Thoracic Surgery. Philadelphia, W.B. Saunders, 1986, pp 61–84.
This is the opposing opinion that surgery has no role in the management of malignant pleural mesothelioma. It includes a review and criticism of several reports of successful application of extrapleural pneumonectomy to the treatment of mesothelioma. It raises several points to consider when selecting patients for possible operative therapy.

Patz EF Jr, Shaffer K, Piwnica-Worms DR, et al: Malignant pleural mesothelioma: Value of CT and MR imaging in predicting resectability. AJR Am J Roentgenol 159:961–966, 1992.
CT and MRI findings in 41 consecutive patients referred for extrapleural pneumonectomy were examined before surgery. Of 34 patients sent to thoracotomy after CT and MRI evaluation, 24 had tumors that were resectable. The sensitivity was high (>92%), but

specificity was low (25% to 50%). MRI was slightly better than CT in predicting resectability of tumors involving the diaphragm and chest wall, whereas CT was slightly better in predicting resectability of tumors involving the mediastinum.

REFERENCES

1. Hilaris BS, Nori D, Kwong E, et al: Pleurectomy and intraoperative brachytherapy and postoperative radiation in the treatment of malignant pleural mesothelioma. Int J Radiat Oncol Biol Phys 10:325–331, 1984.
2. Rusch VW, Niedzwiecki D, Tao Y, et al: Intrapleural cisplatin and mitomycin for malignant mesothelioma following pleurectomy: Pharmacokinetic studies. J Clin Oncol 10:1001–1006, 1992.
3. Rusch VW: Pleurectomy/decortication and adjuvant therapy for malignant mesothelioma. Chest 103(Suppl):382S–384S, 1993.
4. Sugarbaker DJ, Strauss GM, Lynch TJ, et al: Node status has prognostic significance in the multimodality therapy of diffuse, malignant mesothelioma. J Clin Oncol 11:1172–1178, 1993.
5. Butchart EG, Ashcroft T, Barnsley WC, Holden MP: Pleuropneumonectomy in the management of diffuse malignant mesothelioma of the pleura. Experience with 29 patients. Thorax 31:15–24, 1976.
6. Faber LP: Malignant pleural mesothelioma: Operative treatment by extrapleural pneumonectomy. In Kittle CF (ed): Current Controversies in Thoracic Surgery. Philadelphia, W.B. Saunders, 1986, pp 80–84.
7. DaValle MJ, Faber LP, Kittle CF, Jensik RJ: Extrapleural pneumonectomy for diffuse, malignant mesothelioma. Ann Thorac Surg 42:612–618, 1986.
8. Patz EF Jr, Shaffer K, Piwnica-Worms DR, et al: Malignant pleural mesothelioma: Value of CT and MR imaging in predicting resectability. AJR Am J Roentgenol 159:961–966, 1992.
9. Antman K, Pass HI, Recht A: Benign and malignant mesothelioma. In DeVita VT Jr, Hellman S, Rosenberg SA (eds): Cancer: Principles and Practice of Oncology. 3rd Ed. Philadelphia, J.B. Lippincott, 1989, pp 1399–1414.
10. Sugarbaker DJ, Mentzer SJ, Strauss G: Extrapleural pneumonectomy in the treatment of malignant pleural mesothelioma. Ann Thorac Surg 54:941–946, 1992.
11. Worn H: Moglichkeiten und Ergebnisse der chirurgischen Behandlung des malignen Pleuramesothelioma. Thoraxchir Vask Chir 22:391–393, 1974.
12. Rusch VW, Piantadosi S, Holmes EC: The role of extrapleural pneumonectomy in malignant pleural mesothelioma. A Lung Cancer Study Group Trial. J Thorac Cardiovasc Surg 102:1–9, 1991.
13. Allen KB, Faber LP, Warren WH: Malignant pleural mesothelioma: Extrapleural pneumonectomy and pleurectomy. Chest Surg Clin North Am 4:113–126, 1994.
14. McCormack PM, Nagasaki F, Hilaris BS, Martini N: Surgical treatment of pleural mesothelioma. J Thorac Cardiovasc Surg 84:834–842, 1982.
15. Martini N, McCormack PM, Bains MS, et al: Pleural mesothelioma. Ann Thorac Surg 43:113–120, 1987.
16. Chahinian AP, Pajak TF, Holland JF, et al: Diffuse malignant mesothelioma: Prospective evaluation of 69 patients. Ann Intern Med 96(6 Pt 1):746–755, 1982.
17. Law MR, Hodson ME, Turner-Warwick M: Malignant mesothelioma of the pleura: Clinical aspects and symptomatic treatment. Eur J Respir Dis 65:162–168, 1984.
18. Law MR, Gregor A, Hodson ME, et al: Malignant mesothelioma of the pleura: A study of 52 treated and 64 untreated patients. Thorax 39:255–259, 1984.
19. Sugarbaker DJ, Body SC: Technique of pleural pneumonectomy in diffuse mesothelioma. In Shields TW (ed): General Thoracic Surgery. 4th Ed. Malvern, Pennsylvania, Lea & Febiger, 1994; 749–756.
20. Lewis RJ: Malignant pleural mesothelioma: A nonsurgical problem. In Kittle CF (ed): Current Controversies in Thoracic Surgery. Philadelphia, W.B. Saunders, 1986, pp 61–84.
21. Bamler KJ, Maassen W: The percentage of benign and malignant pleura tumors among the patients of a clinic of lung surgery with special consideration of the malignant pleuramesothelioma and its radical treatment, including results of a diaphragm substitution of preserved dura mater [Ger]. (Author's translation.) Thoraxchir Vask Chir 22:386–391, 1974.
22. DeLaria GA, Jensik R, Faber LP, Kittle CF: Surgical management of malignant mesothelioma. Ann Thorac Surg 26:375–382, 1978.
23. Sugarbaker DJ, Heher EC, Lee TH, et al: Extrapleural pneumonectomy, chemotherapy, and radiotherapy in the treatment of diffuse malignant pleural mesothelioma. J Thorac Cardiovasc Surg 102:10–14, 1991.
24. Wagner JC, Sleggs EA, Marchand P: Diffuse pleural mesothelioma and asbestos exposure in the North Western Cape Province. Br J Industr Med 17:260–271, 1960.
25. Selikoff IJ, Churg J, Hammond EC: Asbestos exposure and neoplasia. J Am Med Assoc 188:142, 1964.
26. Driscoll TR, Bakar GJ, Daniels S, et al: Clinical aspects of malignant mesothelioma in Australia. Aust NZ J Med 23:19–25, 1993.
27. Connelly RR, Spirtas R, Myers MH, et al: Demographic patterns for mesothelioma in the United States. J Natl Cancer Inst 78:1053, 1987.
28. Mirvis S, Dutcher JP, Haney PJ, et al: CT of malignant pleural mesothelioma. Am J Roentgenol 140:665, 1983.
29. Gerner RE, Moore GE: Chemotherapy of malignant mesothelioma. Oncology 30:152–155, 1974.
30. Harvey VJ, Slevin ML, Ponder BA, et al: Chemotherapy of diffuse malignant mesothelioma: Phase II trials of single agent 5-fluorouracil and adriamycin. Cancer 54:961–964, 1984.
31. Corson J: Pathology of malignant mesothelioma. In Antman K, Aisner J (eds): Asbestos Related Malignancy. Orlando, Florida, Grune and Stratton, 1987, pp 179–200.
32. Aisner J, Van Echo DA, Wiernik PH: Unpublished data.
33. Yap BS, Benjamin RS, Burgess MA, et al: The value of Adriamycin in the treatment of diffuse malignant pleural mesothelioma. Cancer 42:1692–1696, 1978.
34. Bonadonna G, Ueretta G, Tancini G, et al: Adriamycin (NSC 123127) studies at the Instituto Nazionale Tumori, Milan. Cancer Chemother Rep III 6:231–245, 1975.
35. Gottlieb JA, Baker LH, O'Bryan RM, et al: Adriamycin (NSC 123127) used alone and in combination for soft tissue and bony sarcomas. Cancer Chemother Rep 6:271–282, 1975.
36. Kucuksu N, Thomas W, Ezdinli E: Chemotherapy of malignant diffuse mesothelioma. Cancer 37:1265–1274, 1976.
37. Lerner H, Amato D, Shiraki M, et al: A prospective study of Adriamycin programs in malignant mesothelioma. Proc Am Soc Clin Oncol 2:230, 1983.
38. Lerner H, Schoenfeld D, Martin A, et al: Malignant mesothelioma: The Eastern Cooperative Oncology Group (ECOG) experience. Cancer 52:1981–1985, 1983.
39. Mischler NE, Chuprevich T, Johnson RO, et al: Malignant mesothelioma presenting in the pleura and peritoneum. J Surg Oncol 11:185–191, 1979.
40. O'Bryan RM, Luce JK, Talley RW, et al: Phase II evaluation of Adriamycin in human neoplasia. Cancer 32:1–8, 1973.
41. Stock RJ, Fu YS, Carter JR: Malignant peritoneal mesothelioma following radiotherapy for seminoma of the testis. Cancer 44:914–919, 1979.
42. Van Dyk JJ, Van Der Merwe AM, Falkson HC, et al: Adriamycin in the treatment of cancer. S Afr Med J 50:61–66, 1976.
43. Colbert N, Izrael V, Vannetzel JM, et al: A prospective study of detorubicin in malignant mesothelioma. Proc Am Soc Clin Oncol 4:127, 1985.
44. Kaukel E, Koschel G, Gatzemeyer U, Salewski E: A phase II study of pirarubicin in malignant pleural mesothelioma. Cancer 66:651–654, 1990.
45. Sridhar KS, Doria R, Hussein AM, et al: Activity and toxicity of 4'-0-tetrahydropyranyladriamycin (pirarubicin) in malignant mesothelioma. Proc Am Soc Clin Oncol 11:A1225, 1992.
46. Koschel G, Calavrezos A, Kaukel E, et al: Phase III randomized comparison of pirarubicin vs. pirarubicin and cisplatin for treatment of pleural mesotheliomas. Proc Eur Congress Contra Oncol 6, 1991.
47. Ruffie P, Salomon C, Herait P, et al: Phase II study of THP-

Adriamycin (THP-A) in malignant pleural mesothelioma (MPM). 1st International Mesothelioma Conference. Paris, France, 1991, p 40.

48. Magri MD, Veronesi A, Foladore S, et al: Epirubicin in the treatment of malignant mesothelioma: A Phase II cooperative study. The North-Eastern Italian Oncology Group—Mesothelioma Committee. Tumori 77:49–51, 1991.

49. Mattson K, Giaccone G, Kirkpatrick A, et al: Epirubicin in malignant mesothelioma: A phase II study of the E.O.R.T.C. lung cancer cooperative group. J Clin Oncol 10:824–828, 1992.

50. van Breukelen FJ, Mattson K, Giaccone G, et al: Mitoxantrone in malignant pleural mesothelioma: A study by the EORTC Lung Cancer Cooperative Group. Eur J Cancer 27:1627–1629, 1991.

51. Earhart RH, Amato DJ, Chang AY, et al: Phase II trial of 6-diazo-5-oxo-L-norleucine versus aclacinomycin-A in advanced sarcomas and mesotheliomas. Invest New Drugs 8:113–119, 1990.

52. Antman K, Blum R, Greenberger J, et al: Multimodality therapy for mesothelioma based on a study of natural history. Am J Med 68:356–362, 1980.

53. Oels HC, Harrison EG, Carr DT, et al: Diffuse malignant mesothelioma of the pleura: A review of 37 cases. Chest 60:564–570, 1971.

54. Butt WO: Mesothelioma of the pleura. J Can Assoc Radiol 13:40–49, 1962.

55. DiPietro S, Gennari L: Successful cyclophosphamide treatment in a case of diffuse pleural mesothelioma. Tumori 49:69–73, 1963.

56. Hitchcock HT: Mesothelioma of the pleura. Ir J Med Sci 3:453–456, 1970.

57. Legha SS, Muggia FM: Therapeutic approaches in malignant mesothelioma. Cancer Treat Rev 4:13–23, 1977.

58. Falkson G, Hunt M, Borden EC, et al: An extended phase II trial of ifosfamide plus mesna in malignant mesothelioma. Invest New Drugs 10:337–343, 1992.

59. Zidar BL, Metch B, Balcerzak SP, et al: A phase II evaluation of ifosfamide and mesna in unresectable diffuse malignant mesothelioma: A South West Oncology Group study. Cancer 70:2547–2551, 1991.

60. Krarup-Hansen A, Martensson G, Hansen HH: Phase II trial of high-dose ifosfamide (IFS) + mesna in malignant mesothelioma. Ann Oncol 1(suppl):57, 1990.

61. Cafrey PR, Lucido JL: The clinical and pathologic aspects of pleural mesotheliomas. Surgery 49:690–695, 1961.

62. Champion P: Two cases of malignant mesothelioma after exposure to asbestos. Am Rev Respir Dis 103:821–826, 1971.

63. Gray FW, Tom BCK: Diffuse pleural mesothelioma: A survival of one year following nitrogen mustard therapy. J Thorac Cardiovasc Surg 44:73–77, 1962.

64. Jara F, Takita H, Rao UN: Malignant mesothelioma: Clinicopathologic observation. NY State J Med 77:1885–1888, 1977.

65. Jones DEC, Silver D: Peritoneal mesotheliomas. Surgery 86:556–560, 1979.

66. Kaplan WD, Zimmerman RE, Bloomer WD, Knapp RC: Therapeutic intraperitoneal 32P: A clinical assessment of the dynamics of distribution. Radiology 138:683–688, 1981.

67. McGowan L, Bunnag B, Arias LF: Mesothelioma of the abdomen in women; monitoring of therapy by peritoneal fluid study. Gynecol Oncol 3:10–14, 1975.

68. Falkson G, DeVilliers PC, Falkson HC: N-isopropyl-alpha-(2methylhydrazino)-p-toluamide hydrochloride (NSC-77213) for the treatment of cancer patients. Cancer Chemother Rep 46:7–16, 1965.

69. Bajorin D, Kelsen D, Mintzer DM: Phase II trial of mitomycin in malignant mesothelioma. Cancer Treat Rep 71:857–858, 1987.

70. Gottlieb JA, Benjamin RS, Baker LH, et al: Role of DTIC (NSC 45388) in the chemotherapy of sarcomas. Cancer Treat Rep 60:199–203, 1976.

71. Gottlieb JA, Serpick AA: Clinical evaluation of 5-(3,3-dimethyl-1-triazeno) imidazole-4-carboxamide in malignant melanoma and other neoplasms: Comparison of twice-weekly and daily administration schedules. Oncology 25:225–233, 1971.

72. Dabouis G, LeMevel B, Corroller J: Treatment of diffuse pleural malignant mesothelioma by cis-dichloro diammine platinum in nine patients. Cancer Chemother Pharmacol 5:209–210, 1981.

73. Dabouis G, Delajartre MB, LeMevel BP: Treatment of diffuse pleural malignant mesothelioma by cis-diaminedichloroplatinum: Preliminary results in eleven patients. Med Oncol Soc, Nice, France 52:98, 1979.

74. Glatstein E, Fuks Z, Bagshaw M: Diaphragmatic treatment in ovarian carcinoma: A new radiotherapeutic technique. Int J Radiat Oncol Biol Phys 2:357–362, 1977.

75. Hayes DM, Cvitkovic E, Golbey RB, et al: High dose cisplatinum diaminedichloride. Cancer 39:1372–1381, 1977.

76. Mintzer D, Kelson D, Frimmer D, et al: Phase II trial of high dose cisplatin in patients with malignant mesothelioma. Proc Am Soc Clin Oncol 3:258, 1984.

77. Rossoff AH, Slayton RE, Perlia CP: Preliminary clinical experience with cisdiammine dichloroplatinum (II) (NSC 119875 CACO). Cancer 30:1451–1456, 1972.

78. Samson MK, Baker LH, Benjamin RS, et al: Cis dichlorodiammine-platinum (II) in advanced soft tissue and bony sarcomas: A South West Oncology Group Study. Cancer Treat Rep 63:11–12, 1979.

79. Rebattu P, Riou R, Pacheco Y, et al: Phase II study of very high dose cisplatin in the treatment of malignant mesothelioma. 1st International Mesothelioma Conference. Paris, France, 36, 1991.

80. Planting A, Goey H, Verweij J: Phase II study of six weekly courses of high dose cisplatin in mesothelioma. Proc Am Assoc Cancer Res 32:194, 1991 (abstract 1158).

81. Raghavan D, Gianoutsos P, Bishop J, et al: Phase II trial of carboplatin in the management of malignant mesothelioma. J Clin Oncol 8(1):151–154, 1990.

82. Vogelzang NJ, Goutsou M, Corson JM, et al: Carboplatin in malignant mesothelioma: A phase II study of the Cancer and Leukemia Group B. Cancer Chemother Pharmacol 27(3):239–242, 1990.

83. Mbidde EK, Harland SJ, Calvert AH, Smith IE: Phase II trial of carboplatin (JM8) in treatment of patients with malignant mesothelioma. Cancer Chemother Pharmacol 18:284–285, 1986.

84. Mbidde EK, Smith IE, Harland S: Phase II trial of carboplatin (JM8) in the treatment of patients with mesothelioma (M). Br J Cancer 54:215, 1986.

85. Cantwell BMJ, Harris AL, Ghani S: Phase II studies of a novel antifolate CB3717, and the platinum analogues JM8 and JM9, in mesothelioma of pleura and peritoneum. Br J Cancer 54:216, 1986.

86. Cantwell BMJ, Franks CR, Harris AL: A phase II study of the platinum analogues JM8 and JM9. Cancer Chemother Pharmacol 18:286–288, 1986.

87. Andrews N, Weiss A, Ansfield F, et al: Phase I study of dibromodulcitol (NSC 104800). Cancer Chemother Rep 1971; 55:61–65.

88. Borden E, Ash A, Rosenbau C, et al: Phase II evaluation of dibromodulcitol, ICRF 159, and maytansine in sarcomas and mesotheliomas. Proc AACR/ASCO 21:479, 1980.

89. Ratzer ER, Pool JL, Melamed MR: Pleural mesotheliomas: Clinical experience with thirty-seven patients. Am J Roentgenol 99:863–880, 1967.

90. Riddell RJ: Three cases of mesothelioma. Med J Aust 2:554–559, 1966.

91. Djerassi I, Kim JS, Kassarov L, et al: Response of mesothelioma to large doses of methotrexate with rescue (HDMTXCF) used alone or with cis platinum. Proc Am Soc Clin Oncol 4:191, 1985.

92. Kovarik JL: Primary pleural mesothelioma. Cancer 38:1816–1825, 1976.

93. Thigpen JT, O'Bryan RM, Benjamin RS, et al: Phase II trial of Baker's antifol in metastatic sarcoma. Cancer Treat Rep 61:1485–1487, 1977.

94. Cantwell MJ, Earnshaw M, Harris AL: Phase II study of a novel antifolate, N10-Propargyl-5,8 dideazafolic acid (CB3717), in malignant mesothelioma. Cancer Treat Rep 70(10):1335–1336, 1986.

95. Chahinian AP, Pajak T, Holland J, et al: Diffuse malignant mesothelioma: Prospective evaluation of 69 patients. Ann Intern Med 96:746, 1982.

96. Vogler WR, Arkun S, Velez-Garcia E: Phase I study of twice-weekly azacytidine. Cancer Chemother Rep 58:895–899, 1974.

97. Vogler WR, Miller DS, Keller JW: 5-Azacytidine: A new drug for the treatment of myeloblastic leukemia. Blood 48:331–337, 1976.

98. Harmon D, Vogelzang N, Roboz J, et al: Dihydro-t-azacytidine (DHAC) in malignant mesothelioma (Meso) using serum hyaluronic acid (SHA) as a tumor marker: A phase II trial of the CALGB. (Abstract 1248.) Proc Am Soc Clin Oncol 10:351, 1991.

99. Dhingra HM, Murphy WK, Winn RJ, et al: Phase II trial of 5, 6-dihydro-5-azacytidine in pleural malignant mesothelioma. Invest New Drugs 9:69–72, 1991.

100. Kirshner J, Delosantos R, Ziegler P, et al: Phase I/II study of high dose ara-C in solid tumors. (Abstract.) Am Soc Clin Oncol 3:44, 1984.

101. Wasser L, Hunt M, Lerner H, et al: Phase II trial of PCNU in malignant mesothelioma: An ECOG trial. Proc Am Soc Clin Oncol 8:A1238, 1989.

102. Iriarte PV, Hananian J, Cortner JA: Central nervous system leukemia and solid tumors of childhood: Treatment with 1,3 bis-(2-chloroethyl)-1-nitrosourea (BCNU). Cancer 19:1187–1194, 1966.

103. Chang P, Levine MA, Wiernik PH, et al: A phase II study of intravenously administered methyl CCNU in the treatment of advanced sarcomas. Cancer 37:615–619, 1976.

104. Creagen ET, Hahn RG, Ahmann DL, et al: A comparative clinical trial evaluating the combination of adriamycin, DTIC and vincristine, the combination of actinomycin D, cyclophosphamide and vincristine, and a single agent, methylCCNU, in advanced sarcomas. Cancer Treat Rep 60:1385–1387, 1976.

105. Spremulli E, Wampler G, Regelson E, et al: Chemotherapy of malignant mesothelioma. Cancer 40:2038–2045, 1977.

106. Saijo N, Nishiwaki Y, Kawase 1, et al: Effect of ACNU on primary lung cancer, mesothelioma and metastatic pulmonary tumors. Cancer Treat Rep 62:139–141, 1978.

107. Martensson G, Sorenson S: A phase II study of vincristine in malignant mesothelioma—a negative report. Cancer Chemother Pharmacol 24:133–134, 1989.

108. Boutin C, Irisson M, Guerin J, et al: Phase II trial of vindesine on malignant pleural mesothelioma. Cancer Treat Rep 71:205–206, 1987.

109. Kelsen D, Gralla R, Chang E: Vindesine in the treatment of malignant mesothelioma: A phase II study. Cancer Treat Rep 67:821–822, 1983.

110. Falkson G, Falkson H: Clinical trial of the oral form 4'-dimethyl epipodophyllotoxin-β-D ethylidene glucoside (NSC 141540) and VP-16-213. Proc Am Assoc Cancer Res 1:160, 1978.

111. Nissen NI, Larsen V, Pederson H, et al: Phase I clinical trial of a new antitumor agent, 4'dimethylepipodophyllotoxin-9-(4,6-O-ethylidene-beta-D-glucopyranoside) (NSC 141540). Cancer Chemother Rep 56:769–777, 1972.

112. Nissen NI, Dombernowsky P, Hansen HH, et al: Phase I clinical trial of an oral solution of VP16-213. Cancer Treat Rep 60:943–945, 1976.

113. Smit EF, Berendsen HH, Postmus PE: Etoposide and mesothelioma [letter]. J Clin Oncol 8:1281, 1990.

114. Falkson G, Vorobiof DA, Lerner JH: A phase II study of M-AMSA in patients with malignant mesothelioma with cyclophosphamide, Adriamycin and vincristine. Cancer Chemother Pharmacol 4:135, 1980.

115. Eagan R, Frytak S, Richardson R, et al: Phase II trial of diaziquone in malignant mesothelioma. Cancer Treat Rep 70:429, 1986.

116. Price LA, Hill BT, Goldie JH: DDMP and selective folinic acid protection in the treatment of malignant disease: A further report. Clin Oncol 3:281–286, 1977.

117. Garnick MB, Blum RH, Canellos GP, et al: Phase I trial of Brucceantin. Cancer Treat Rep 63:1929–1932, 1979.

118. Webster I, Cochrane JWC, Burkhardt KR: Immunotherapy with BCG vaccine in 30 cases of mesothelioma. S Afr Med J 81:277–278, 1982.

119. Esposito S: RNA therapy for pleural mesothelioma. Lancet II:1203–1204, 1969.

120. Christmas TI, Manning LS, Gerlepp MJ, et al: Effect of interferon-alpha 2 on malignant mesothelioma. J Interferon Res 13:9–12, 1993.

121. Von Hoff DD, Metch B, Lucas JG, et al: Phase II evaluation of recombinant interferon-beta (IFN-beta ser) in patients with diffuse mesothelioma: A Southwest Oncology Group study. J Interferon Res 10(5):531–534, 1990.

122. Brandely M, Sousell Sante R. A Phase II multicentre study of recombinant interferon (R-IFNγ) in malignant mesothelioma. 1st International Mesothelioma Conference. Paris, France, 5, 1991 (abstract).

123. Boutin C, Viallat JR, Astoul P: Treatment of mesothelioma with interferon gamma and interleukin 2. Rev Pneumol Clin 46:211–215, 1990.

124. Boutin C: Treatment of malignant mesothelioma using intrapleural gamma interferon. Bull Acad Natl Med 174:421–426, 1990 (discussion 427).

125. Boutin C, Viallat JR, Zandwijk NV, et al: Activity of intrapleural recombinant gamma-interferon in malignant mesothelioma. Cancer 67:2033–2037, 1991.

126. Stoter G, Goey SH, Slingerland R, et al: Intrapleural interleukin-2 (IL-2) in malignant pleural mesothelioma: A phase I-II study. Proc Am Assoc Cancer Res 31:A1630, 1990.

127. Robinson BWS, Bowman RV, Christmas TI, et al: Clinical experience using immunotherapy (IL-2/LAK cells or interferon alpha 2a) in malignant mesothelioma. 1st International Mesothelioma Conference. Paris, France, 38, 1991.

128. Gottlieb J, Baker L, Quagliana J, et al: Chemotherapy of sarcomas with a combination of Adriamycin and dimethyl triazeno imidazole carboxamide. Cancer 30:1632–1638, 1972.

129. Chahinian AP, Holland JF: Treatment of diffuse malignant mesothelioma: A review. Mt Sinai J Med 45:54–67, 1978.

130. Brenner DE, Chang P, Wiernik PH: Adriamycin and actinomycin-D therapy for advanced sarcomas. Cancer Treat Rep 65:231–236, 1981.

131. Chlebowski R, Pugh R, McCracken J, et al: A phase I–II trial of combination therapy with adriamycin and ICRF. Proc Am Assoc Cancer Res 20, 1979.

132. Carmichael J, Cantwell BM, Harris AL: A phase II trial of ifosfamide/mesna with doxorubicin for malignant mesothelioma. Eur J Cancer Clin Oncol 25(5):911–912, 1989.

133. Alberts AS, Falkson G, van ZL: Ifosfamide and mesna with doxorubicin have activity in malignant mesothelioma [letter; comment]. Eur J Cancer 26(9):1002, 1990.

134. Van Meerbeek J, Dirix L, Prove A, et al: A phase II trial of ifosfamide/mesna and doxorubicin with growth factor support in mesothelioma. Proc Am Soc Clin Oncol 12:A1371, 1993.

135. Zidar B, Pugh R, Schiffer L, et al: Treatment of six cases of mesothelioma with doxorubicin and cis-platinum. Cancer 52:1788–1791, 1983.

136. Chahinian AP, Antman K, Goutsou M, et al: Randomized phase II trial of cisplatin with mitomycin or doxorubicin for malignant mesothelioma. J Clin Oncol 11(8):1559–1565, 1993.

137. Ardizzoni A, Rosso R, Salvati F, et al: Activity of doxorubicin and cisplatin combination chemotherapy in patients with diffuse malignant pleural mesothelioma. An Italian Lung Cancer Task Force Phase II study. Cancer 67(12):2984–2987, 1991.

138. Niki Y, Nakayama S, Soga T, et al: [A case of remission induced in diffuse pleural malignant mesothelioma by the treatment with cisplatin and doxorubicin]. Gan To Kagaku Ryoho 16(11):3635–3638, 1989.

139. Niki Y, Soga T, Nishimura A, et al: [A diffuse, pleural, malignant mesothelioma kept in long remission by chemotherapy combining pirarubicin and cisplatin.] Gan No Rinsho 36:2463–2467, 1990.

140. Nakano T, Maeda MMJ, Iwahashi N, et al: Combination chemotherapy of cisplatin, doxorubicin and vindesine in malignant pleural mesothelioma. 1st International Mesothelioma Conference. Paris, France, 32, 1991.

141. Breau JL, Boaziz C, Morere JJF, et al: Combination chemotherapy with cisplatinum, adriamycin, bleomycin and mitomycin C, plus systemic and intrapleural hyaluronidase in 25 consecutive cases of Stages II, III pleural mesothelioma. 1st International Mesothelioma Conference. Paris, France, 5, 1991.

142. Shin DM, Fossella FV, Putnam JB, et al: Phase II study of combination chemotherapy with cytoxan (C), Adriamycin (A), and cisplatin (P) for unresectable or metastatic malignant pleural mesothelioma (MPM). Proc Am Soc Clin Oncol 12:A1362, 1993.

143. Samson MK, Wasser LP, Borden EC, et al: Randomized comparison of cyclophosphamide, imidazole carboxamide, and Adriamycin versus cyclophosphamide and adriamycin in patients with advanced stage malignant mesothelioma: A sarcoma intergroup study. J Clin Oncol 5:86–91, 1987.

144. Gottlieb JA, Bodey GP, Sinkovics JG, et al: An effective new four-drug combination regimen (CY-VA-DIC) for metastatic sarcomas. Proc AACR/ASCO 15:162, 1974.

145. Jett JR, Eagan RT: Chemotherapy for malignant mesothelioma: CAMEO. Am J Clin Oncol 5:429–431, 1982.

146. Magri MD, Foladore S, Veronesi A, et al: Treatment of malignant mesothelioma with epirubicin and ifosfamide: A phase II cooperative study. Ann Oncol 3:237–238, 1992.

147. Zidar BL, Benjamin RS, Frank J, et al: Combination chemotherapy for advanced sarcomas of bone and mesothelioma utilizing rubidazone and DTIC: A South West Oncology Group Study. Am J Clin Oncol 6(1):71–74, 1983.

148. Tucker WG, Talley RW, Brownlee RW, et al: Preliminary trials with combination therapy of cyclophosphamide, vincristine and 5-fluorouracil. Cancer Chemother Rep 52:593–596, 1968.

149. Gerner RE, Moore GE: Multiple drug therapy for malignant solid tumors in adults. Cancer Chemother Rep 57:237–239, 1973.

150. Ellerby RA, Ansfield FJ, Davis HL: Preliminary report on phase I clinical experience with combined cis-diaminedichloride platinum and 5FU. Recent Results Cancer Res 48:153–159, 1974.

151. Eisenhauer EA, Evans WK, Murray N, et al: A Phase II study of VP-16 and cisplatin in patients with unresectable malignant mesothelioma. An NCI Canada clinical trials group study. Invest New Drugs 6:327–329, 1988.

152. Samson MK, Baker LH, Devos JM, et al: Phase I clinical trial of combined therapy with vinblastine, bleomycin and cis-dichloro-diammine-platinum. Cancer treat Rep 60:91, 1976.

153. Chahinian AP, Norton L, Holland JF, et al: Experimental and clinical activity of Mitomycin C and cis-diamminedichloroplatinum in malignant mesothelioma. Cancer 44:1688–1692, 1984.

154. Thomas CR Jr, Leslie WT, Purl S, Bonomi P: Phase II study of carboplatin (CBDCA) or cisplatin (CDDP) and mitomycin c (MC) in patients (PTS) with pleural mesothelioma. Proc Am Soc Clin Oncol 10:A1060, 1991.

155. Samuels BL, Herndon J, Vogelzang NJ, et al: Dihydro-5-azacytidine (DHAC) and cisplatin (DDP) in mesothelioma (CALGB 9031). Proc Am Soc Clin Oncol 13:A 1994.

156. Gridelli C, Pepe R, Airoma G, et al: Mitomycin c and vindesine: An ineffective combination chemotherapy in the treatment of malignant pleural mesothelioma. Tumori 78:380–382, 1992.

157. Dimitrov NV, Egner J, Balcueva E, et al: High-dose methotrexate with citrovorum factor and vincristine in the treatment of malignant mesothelioma. Cancer 50:1245–1247, 1982.

158. Omura GA, Roberts GA: Combination therapy of solid tumors using 1,3-bis(2-chlorethyl)-1-nitrosourea (BCNU), vincristine, methotrexate and 5-fluorouracil. Cancer 31:1374–1381, 1973.

159. Antman K, Osteen R, Klegar K, et al: Early peritoneal mesothelioma: A treatable malignancy. Lancet 2:977–981, 1985.

160. Richert R, Sherman CD: Prolonged survival in diffuse pleural mesothelioma treated with Au[198] Cancer 12:799–805, 1959.

161. Rogoff EE, Hilaris BS, Hulvos AG: Long-term survival in patients with malignant peritoneal mesothelioma treated with irradiation. Cancer 35:656–664, 1973.

162. Casper ES, Kelsen DP, Alcock NW, Lewis JL: IP cisplatin in patients with malignant ascites: Pharmacokinetic evaluation and comparison with the IV route. Cancer Treat Rep 67:235–238, 1985.

163. Howell SB, Pfeifle CL, Wung WE, et al: Intraperitoneal cisplatin with systemic thiosulfate protection. Ann Intern Med 97:845–851, 1982.

164. Markman M, Cleary S, Pfeifle C, Howell SB: Cisplatin administered by the intracavitary route as treatment for malignant mesothelioma. Cancer 58:18–21, 1986.

165. Markman M, Howell SB, Lucas WE, et al: Combination intraperitoneal chemotherapy with cisplatin, cytarabine, and doxorubicin for refractory ovarian cancer and other malignancies principally confined to the peritoneal cavity. J Clin Oncol 2:1321–1326, 1984.

166. Markman M, Kelsen D: Efficacy of cisplatin-based intraperitoneal chemotherapy as treatment of malignant peritoneal mesothelioma. J Cancer Res Clin Oncol 118:547–550, 1992.

167. Lederman GS, Recht A, Herman T, et al: Long-term survival in peritoneal mesothelioma. The role of radiotherapy and combined modality treatment. Cancer 59:1882–1886, 1987.

168. Vlasveld LT, Gallee MP, Rodenhuis S, Taal BG: Intraperitoneal chemotherapy for malignant peritoneal mesothelioma. Eur J Cancer 27(6):732–734, 1991.

169. Tattersall M, Newlands E, Woods R: Intracavitary doxorubicin in malignant effusions. Lancet 1:390, 1979.

170. Langer C, O'Dwyer P, Nash S, et al: Intraperitoneal (IP) cisplatin (CDDP) and etoposide (VP16) in malignant peritoneal mesothelioma: Favorable outcome with combined modality therapy. Proc Am Soc Clin Oncol 12:A1365, 1993.

171. Rosso R, Rimoldi R, Salvati F, et al: Intrapleural natural beta interferon in the treatment of malignant pleural effusions. Oncology 45:253–256, 1988.

172. Stathopoulis GP, Baxevanis CN, Dedoussis GV, et al: Intracavitary infusion of interferon-alpha in nonresponsive malignancies to chemotherapy. Proc Am Assoc Cancer Res 34:A1306, 1993.

173. Rusch VW, Niedzwiecki D, Tao Y, et al: Intrapleural cisplatin and mitomycin for malignant mesothelioma following pleurectomy: Pharmacokinetic studies. J Clin Oncol 10:1001–1006, 1992.

174. Rusch VW: Pleurectomy/decortication and adjuvant therapy for malignant mesothelioma. Chest 103(suppl):382S–384S, 1993.

175. Sugarbaker DJ, Lee TH, Coupe G, et al: Extrapleural pneumonectomy, chemotherapy and radiotherapy in the treatment of diffuse malignant pleural mesothelioma. J Thorac Cardiovasc Surg 102:10–15, 1991.

176. Sugarbaker DJ, Strauss G, Lynch T, et al: Trimodality therapy of malignant mesothelioma (MPM). Proc Am Soc Clin Oncol 11:A1209, 1992.

177. Netaji B, Adelstein DJ, Rice TW, et al: Aggressive combined modality treatment for malignant mesothelioma. Proc Am Soc Clin Oncol 11:A1217, 1992.

178. Pass H, Tochner Z, DeLaney T, et al: Intraoperative photodynamic therapy after resection of pleural malignancies. Proc Third Biennial Mtg International Photodynamic Assoc. July 17–21, 1990, Buffalo, New York, p 26.

179. Calavrezos A, Koschel G, Husselmann H, et al: Malignant mesothelioma of the pleura. Klin Wochenschr 66:607–635, 1988.

180. Sinoff C, Falkson G, Sandison AG, et al: Combined doxorubicin and radiation therapy in malignant pleural mesothelioma. Cancer Treat Rep 66:1605–1607, 1982.

181. Pogrebniak H, Kranda K, Steinberg S, et al: Cisplatin, interferon-alpha, and tamoxifen (CIT) for malignant pleural mesothelioma. Proc Am Soc Clin Oncol 12:A1363, 1993.

34 PLEURAL EFFUSIONS IN PATIENTS WITH MALIGNANCY

Darroch W.O. Moores and John C. Ruckdeschel

Pleural effusion is a common occurrence in patients with malignancy. In fact, pleural effusion is often the first manifestation of disease. Although the length of a patient's life is more often determined by the progress of the systemic cancer, the quality of life can be improved significantly by accurate diagnosis and successful management of the effusion.

NORMAL ANATOMY AND PHYSIOLOGY OF THE PLEURAL SPACE

The normal pleural space measures approximately 10 to 20 μ in width, and the areas of the pleural surfaces are each approximately 2000 cm^2 in a 70-kg human.[1] The volume of pleural fluid in the normal space is 0.1–0.2 ml/kg of body weight.[2] Normal pleural fluid is a clear, colorless fluid with a protein concentration of less than 1.5 gm/dl.[1-3] The visceral and parietal pleural surfaces consist of a single layer of pleomorphic mesothelial cells containing microvilli. Within this single layer there is basement membrane, collagen, elastic tissue, blood vessels, and lymphatics. The density of microvilli is higher on the visceral than on the parietal mesothelial surface.[4]

The blood supply of the visceral pleura is derived from the bronchial arteries that drain into the pulmonary venous system.[2, 5, 6] The parietal pleura is supplied by the systemic circulation through arteries that supply the chest wall, diaphragm, and mediastinal pleura.[7]

Lymphatic drainage of the pleural space begins with openings between the mesothelial cells called stomata. Stomata, found only on the parietal pleura, are the usual exit point for pleural fluid, protein, and cells that are removed from the pleural space.[2, 8] There is controversy regarding the extent of the stomata on the parietal surface. They are located mainly in the mediastinal pleura caudally and on the intercostal and diaphragmatic pleural surfaces.[8] The stomata connect via lymphatic lacunae with lymphatic channels that run along the intercostal space and drain into the mediastinum.[7] Pulmonary lymphatics consist of a superficial plexus situated below the visceral pleura and a deep plexus located around blood vessels and bronchioles.[9] The subpleural lymphatic plexus is denser over the lower lobes than upper lobes. Pulmonary

lymphatic flow is toward the hilum. A disturbance in lymphatic drainage of the pleural space is a major contributor to the development of pleural effusion. In the normal state, the volume of fluid and concentration of protein in the pleural space is balanced. Changes in microvascular pressure or permeability disturb this equilibrium, leading to the accumulation of fluid and a change in protein concentration.

Pleural fluid is essentially interstitial liquid of the parietal pleura.[2] The parietal pleura is supplied by the systemic circulation. The pressure in the pleural space is subatmospheric and probably is less than the pressure in the interstitium of the subpleural space. The parietal pleura contributes the protein and fluid; the contribution from the visceral pleura is probably minimal in the normal person. Lymphatic drainage capacity of the pleural space appears to have a large reserve so that when abnormal amounts of pleural fluid accumulate, as in disease, it usually represents a combination of increased formation of liquid and impaired lymphatic drainage (Table 34–1).

PATHOPHYSIOLOGY OF PLEURAL FLUID FORMATION

It was previously thought that the pulmonary artery supplied the visceral pleura, that protein-free liquid was absorbed across the visceral pleura, and that there was a high rate of pleural fluid and protein turnover. New information requires rethinking of these concepts.[2, 10]

Based on work in sheep, it appears that there is a low rate of pleural liquid formation within the pleural space, in the order of 0.01 ml/(kg × hr) or approximately 7 ml/day in a 30-kg sheep.[2] This information is in contradistinction to the previously held concept of high fluid turnover within the pleural space. It is believed that pleural catheter irritation and inflammation were responsible for previous reports of high fluid turnover.[11] It is believed that pleural fluid is formed and removed slowly from the pleural space and has a lower protein concentration than lung and systemic lymph.[7] The parietal pleura is responsible for most of the protein-fluid exchange within the pleural space. A low-protein filtrate from the systemic circu-

TABLE 34–1. Causes of Pleural Effusion*

REFERENCE	(69)	(70)	(71)	(72)	(21)	(73)	(74)	TOTAL
Patients	271	436	274	133	73	182	300	1669
Malignancy	95	229	169	64	34	50	117	758 (45%)
Congestive heart failure	46	44	42	18	6	43	5	204 (12%)
Infectious								372 (22%)
Tuberculous	56	24	16	1	6	17	53	173 (10%)
Bacterial	45	7	26	5	3	26	38	150 (9%)
Viral	7	5			1	7	1	21 (1%)
Fungal	2	2		1		1		6 (<1%)
Empyema		10	1		8			19 (1%)
Parasitic			2					2 (<1%)
Indeterminant		75		25	7	3	62	172 (10%)
Pulmonary embolus or infarct	11	13		3	2	8	2	39 (3%)
Cirrhosis		9	8	1		5	3	28 (2%)
Collagen disease	5	4	1	5	3	2	2	22 (1%)
Other†	4	14	8	10	3	20	17	76 (5%)

*The causes of pleural effusions as reported in seven large and frequently cited studies are listed in this table and are summated in the last column.

†Includes causes of pleural effusion, each less than 1%: nephrosis, trauma, pneumothorax, postoperative, subdiaphragmatic abcess, hypoproteinemia, pulmonary fibrosis, pancreatitis, pseudocyst, Dressler's syndrome, hepatitis, uremia, Meig's syndrome, asbestosis, and chylothorax.

References cited in this table are from Hausheer FH and Yarbro JW.[14]

(From Hausheer FH, Yarbro JW: Diagnosis and treatment of malignant pleural effusion. Semin Oncol 12:54, 1985; with permission.)

lation enters via the parietal pleura and exits via the parietal pleural stomata.

There are six mechanisms responsible for the accumulation of an abnormal amount of pleural fluid[7]:

1. Increase in hydrostatic pressure in the microvascular circulation, as occurs in patients with congestive heart failure.

2. Decreased oncotic pressure in the microvascular circulation, occurring in patients with low serum albumin.

3. Decrease in pressure in the pleural space, as occurs in patients with atelectasis.

4. Increased permeability of the microvascular circulation occurring with inflammatory processes, both benign and malignant, occurring within the pleural space.

5. Impaired lymphatic drainage from the pleural space, which can occur in patients with pneumonia or malignant obstruction of the lymphatic spaces within the lung. Increased fluid formation in malignancy may occur from altered microvascular permeability, but large effusions result only with involvement of the lymphatic system by the malignancy.

6. Movement of fluid from the peritoneal space. Patients with ascites can develop pleural effusion due to passage of fluid through either diaphragmatic lymphatics or diaphragmatic anatomic defects.

Lymphatic obstruction, a predominant mechanism of pleural fluid formation in malignancy, can occur with blockage of the lymphatic system from any point from the stomata of the parietal pleura to the mediastinal lymph nodes.[12] Tumor invasion of the pleura either seeds the mesothelial surface or invades the subserosal layer. With seeding of the mesothelial surface, there is an exfoliation of tumor cells into the pleural fluid. If there is submesothelial involvement, a paucity of malignant cells are found in the fluid. The types of cancer usually associated with malignant effusion are shown in Table 34–2.

CLINICAL MANIFESTATIONS

Virtually all patients with malignant pleural effusion are symptomatic. Shortness of breath, cough, chest pain, and a sense of fullness within the chest are common presenting complaints. Physical findings include decreased breath sounds, increased dullness to percussion, decreased tactile fremitus, and decreased diaphragmatic excursion. Contralateral tracheal deviation is found in association with large effusions.

Pleural effusion is often the initial manifestation of patients with malignancy. Chernow and Sahn reported that of 96 patients with malignant effusion, 44 (46%) had no prior history of cancer.[13]

DIAGNOSIS

Chest x-ray study is the most useful screening tool used in determining the presence, distribution, and significance of pleural effusion. Following radiographic confirmation of pleural effusion, needle thoracentesis should be performed.

The conventional diagnostic tests applied to pleural fluid are cell count with differential; cytologic examination; direct smear and cultures for bacteria, fungi, and acid-fast bacilli; protein and lactate dehydrogenase (LDH) determination; glucose; and pH. For patients with known or suspected malignancy, cytology, protein and LDH is all that is required. Table 34–3 outlines the fluid characteristics in patients with malignant and paramalignant pleural effusion.

The diagnosis of malignant pleural effusion depends on finding malignant cells in the pleural fluid or pleural tissue. Cytologic examination of pleural fluid should be performed at the time of first thoracentesis. Approximately half of malignant pleural effusions are diagnosed on the basis of the first cytologic analysis. Second and third thoracenteses increase the incidence of positive findings to about

TABLE 34–2. Malignant Neoplasms Associated with Pleural Effusion*

REFERENCE	(69)	(75)	(71)	(70)	(37)	(74)	TOTAL
Patients	95	96	141	229	133	117	811
Malignancy							
Lung	42	32	47	95	32	34	282 (35%)
Breast	24	20	42	53	35	12	186 (23%)
Lymphoma/leukemia	11			28	33	7	79 (10%)
Adenocarcinoma, unknown primary	17		12	19	6	41	96 (12%)
Reproductive tract		11	12	12	13	4	52 (6%)
Gastrointestinal tract		14	11	9	1	3	38 (5%)
Genitourinary tract		4	10	4	2		20 (3%)
Primary unknown		13	2		2	5	22 (3%)
Other†	1	2	5	9	9	11	37 (5%)

*The table presents data fro six large and representative studies that report the type of cancer associated with malignant pleural effusions. The total of these series and the percentage for each malignancy is shown in the last column.

†Includes causes of 1% or less of malignant pleural effusion: endocrine, thoracic carcinoma, cutaneous, head and neck, mesothelioma, extremity, bone, and myeloma.

References cited in this table are from Hausheer FH and Yarbro JW.[14]

(From Hausheer FH, Yarbro JW: Diagnosis and treatment of malignant pleural effusion. Semin Oncol 12:54, 1985; with permission.)

65% and 70%, respectively.[14] Closed pleural biopsy has a diagnostic yield of approximately 50%. Cytologic examination of pleural fluid and closed pleural biopsy are complementary; however, closed pleural biopsy adds little to cytology alone in diagnosing malignancy.[7] Thoracoscopy with direct pleural biopsy has a diagnostic yield of approximately 97% in patients with malignant effusion.[15] Patients with suspected malignant effusion who are without diagnosis following two-needle thoracenteses should be referred to thoracic surgery for thoracoscopy. A small number of patients who have pleural effusion associated with malignancy do not have malignant cells demonstrated in the pleural fluid or from pleural tissue at biopsy. These effusions are related to the underlying cancer but are not due to direct pleural involvement; they are called paramalignant effusions. These effusions may be due to the direct local effect of the tumor causing lymphatic obstruction or to bronchial obstruction, leading to pneumonitis or atelectasis.

Malignancy accounts for approximately 50% of all new pleural effusions in the adult. Congestive heart failure, however, is probably the single most common cause of pleural effusion overall. Malignant pleural effusion may be serous, serosanguineous, or grossly bloody. Red cell counts most commonly range from 30,000 to 50,000/μl. When red cell counts are higher than 100,000/μl in the absence of trauma, malignancy is the most likely diagnosis. The majority of non–red blood cells are lymphocytes, macrophages, and mesothelial cells, with lymphocytes representing more than 50% of the cell population half of the time.[16]

Pleural fluid associated with malignancy is usually exudative, with protein concentration from 1.5 to 8.0 gm/dl, and a pleural fluid to serum LDH ratio greater than 0.6.[7] The specific gravity of the fluid is frequently, but not always, more than 1.016.[14] The glucose level is variable but may fall to less than 60 mg/dl[12] if the effusion has been present for a long period of time. Low pH–low glucose malignant pleural effusion is usually associated with a large tumor burden and fibrosis of the pleura.[17]

Approximately two-thirds of all malignant effusions are accounted for by lung cancer, breast cancer, and lymphoma.[14] Carcinoma from any organ can metastasize to the pleura;[12] however, lung cancer is the tumor to most commonly result in malignant and paramalignant effusion. Adenocarcinoma of the lung is the most common cell type to involve the pleura owing to its usually peripheral location and propensity for contiguous spread. In approximately 15% of patients with malignant pleural effusion, the primary lesion is unknown.[14]

An assortment of techniques and laboratory tests have been used to increase the diagnostic yield of pleural fluid examination and closed pleural biopsy. The application of the immunoperoxidase staining technique to needle biopsy specimens of the pleura may be helpful in distinguishing reactive mesothelial cells from malignant cells.[18] Placing pleural fluid in a specially prepared tissue culture medium may allow easier identification of malignant cells based on the ability of the tissue culture medium to transform mesothelial cells into fibroblasts. Against a background of fibroblasts, clumps of adenocarcinoma cells are more easily identified.[19] Cytogenetic analysis of pleural fluid used in conjunction with standard cytologic techniques may increase the yield over standard cytologic analysis from 50% to 81%.[20] Cytogenetic analysis of a pleural effusion is expensive and not readily available in all laboratories. It may be of value in equivocal cases if other means of diagnosis have provided negative results. Pleural fluid carcinoembryonic antigen has not been found to be of diagnostic value in malignant effusion.[21] Elevated levels of hyaluronic acid in pleural fluid are supportive but not diagnostic for the diagnosis of mesothelioma. Electron microscopic examination of pleural fluids seems to offer little over standard cytologic evaluation in the majority of patients.[22]

To date, some of the new techniques have improved diagnostic yield of pleural fluid, especially in equivocal cases, but in general they are either too slow, too expensive, or nonspecific. Although it is academically

TABLE 34–3. Characteristics of Malignant and Paramalignant Pleural Effusions

APPEARANCE	CLASSIFICATION	PROTEIN	LDH	RED BLOOD CELLS	WHITE BLOOD CELLS	DIFFERENTIAL	GLUCOSE	pH	AMYLASE
Malignant Serous, sanguineous, bloody, milky	Exudate or transudate (5–10%)	4 gm/dl; range 1.5–8.0 gm/dl	300 u/L; can be >1000 U/liter; exudate by LDH only suggests malignancy	Few to 1 million/ μl; >100,000, cancer likely	2500–4000/μl; rarely >10,000/ μl	>50% lymphocytes in 50% of patients; 5% with eosinophilia; polymorphonuclear cells <25% of cells	<60% mg/dl or pleural fluid to serum ratio <0.5 (30%)	<7.30 (30%)	↑ <10%
Paramalignant Serous, sanguineous, bloody, milky, turbid, purulent	Exudate or transudate	Variable; pleural fluid to serum ratio >0.5 or <0.5	Pleural fluid to serum ratio >0.6 or <0.6	Usually <10,000/ μl	Low counts; except parapneumonic effusions or pulmonary embolism	Lymphocyte most common cell; may be poly- morphonuclear predom- inant (parapneumonic)	>60 mg/dl except in empyema	>7.30 except in empyema	Less than serum

LDH = lactate dehydrogenase.
From Sahn SA: Malignant pleural effusions. Semin Respir Med 9:43–53, 1987. Reprinted with permission from Seminars in Respiratory Medicine, 9, 43–53, 1987, Thieme Medical Publishers, Inc.

interesting to explore methods of improving yield of malignancy on pleural fluid analysis, standard cytologic analysis and thoracoscopy with direct biopsy are the gold standard diagnostic tools.

MANAGEMENT OF MALIGNANT PLEURAL EFFUSION

When treating patients with malignant pleural effusion, it is important to keep the patient and disease in proper perspective. The vast majority of these patients are not curable, and treatment is aimed toward the most effective type of palliation. If the malignancy is likely to be highly sensitive to systemic chemotherapy, such therapy should be given as in patients with lymphoma or small cell lung cancer. When the tumor is unlikely to be responsive to systemic therapy, as in patients with non–small cell lung cancer or pancreatic cancer, tube thoracostomy drainage with subsequent chemical pleurodesis is the treatment of choice. Repeat thoracenteses are not useful in controlling effusion, and the control rate for tube thoracostomy alone is low.[14]

We believe that rapid diagnosis and therapy is important in the successful management of patients with malignant pleural effusions. The algorithm in Figure 34–1 serves as our framework for prompt diagnosis and management of patients with malignant effusion.

Malignant pleural effusion is a local problem in a patient with systemic disease. Many patients have systemic as well as local therapy; management of the effusion itself is usually achieved by local means. Local therapy includes intrapleural chemical therapy, pleuroperitoneal shunts, thoracoscopy with pleurodesis, or open thoracotomy with pleurectomy.

Intrapleural Chemical Therapy

A wide array of agents has been used over the past for intrapleural therapy of malignant pleural effusion. Austin and Flye reviewed much of the published literature on management of malignant pleural effusion and assembled the aggregate response rate of various treatment modalities (Table 34–4).[23] These agents may be introduced into the pleural space through conventional chest tube catheters or through soft small-bore catheters placed in the outpatient setting.[24, 25] Sonography can assist in locating the fluid collection.[25]

AGENTS WITH CYTOREDUCTIVE ACTIVITY

Cytoreductive agents are thought to resolve the pleural effusion by directly reducing the tumor burden. Initially it was thought that this was the mode of action of intrapleurally placed radioactive isotopes and nitrogen mustard when used for malignant pleural effusion. Autopsy data, however, showed that

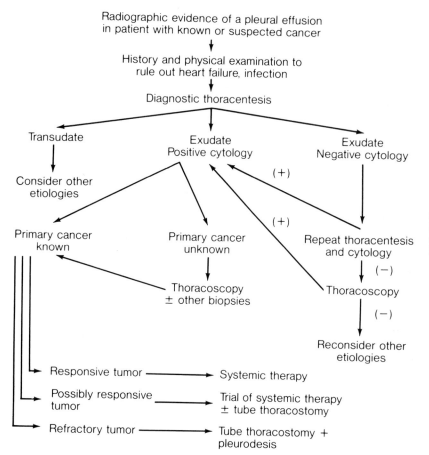

FIGURE 34–1. Approach to diagnosis and therapy of malignant pleural effusion. (From Ruckdeschel JC: Management of malignant pleural effusion: An overview. Semin Oncol 15[Suppl 3]:24–28, 1988. Reprinted with permission.)

TABLE 34–4. Effectiveness of Techniques to Control Malignant Pleural Effusion Due to Various Primary Tumors

TECHNIQUE	OBJECTIVE RESPONSE RATE (ORR)*						RANGE OF ORR AMONG STUDIES REVIEWED (%)‡
	Lung	Breast	Lymphoma	Ovary	Other	Overall	
Intrapleural techniques or agents							
Radioisotopes	54% (102/190)	57% (234/413)	50% (22/44)	59% (32/54)	48% (85/177)	55% (536/980)	25% to 100%
Nitrogen Mustard	66% (35/53)	48% (100/208)	37% (7/19)	73% (8/11)	46% (11/24)	52% (177/338)	28% to 87%
Talc							
General anesthetic	93% (42/45)	96% (26/27)	100% (1/1)	100% (1/1)	87% (27/31)	92% (97/105)	76% to 100%
Suspension	86% (12/14)	96% (27/28)	100% (3/3)	88% (7/8)	67% (4/6)	90% (53/59)	83% to 93%
Quinacrine	83% (30/36)	80% (37/46)	78% (7/9)	50% (3/6)	77% (17/22)	80% (102/128)	57% to 100%
Tetracycline	100% (7/7)	86% (6/7)	—	0% (0/1)	100% (4/4)	87% (27/31)	83% to 100%
Thiotepa	0% (0/1)	52% (11/21)	—	100% (2/2)	0% (0/2)	46% (18/39)	30% to 63%
5-Fluorouracil	—	—	—	—	—	66%§ (23/35)	—
Bleomycin	100% (3/3)	100% (8/8)	50% (2/4)	100% (3/3)	100% (1/1)	90% (17/19)	—‖
Chest tube alone	100% (1/1)	53% (17/32)	—	—	14% (1/7)	55% (38/69)	0% to 100%
Pleurectomy	100% (41/41)	100% (33/33)	100% (1/1)	100% (1/1)	100% (30/30)	99% (145/147)	95% to 100%

*Objective response rate was calculated as the number of objective responses divided by number of evaluable patients. An objective response was defined as no requirement for thoracentesis for at least 1 month following the procedure. An evaluable patient was defined as one who survived at least 1 month following the procedure.
‡The studies reviewed in compilation of these data are listed in the source of the original table.
§Only one study using this agent was found, and the data were not broken down according to primary malignancy.
‖Only one study using this agent was reviewed.
Modified from Austin EH, Flye MW: The treatment of recurrent malignant pleural effusion. Ann Thorac Surg 28:190–203, 1979. Modified with permission from the Society of Thoracic Surgeons (The Annals of Thoracic Surgery, 1979, 28, 190–203).

they actually produce a dense pleurodesis, like the agents discussed later. Cisplatin has been used, both alone and in combination with cytosine arabinoside, for intraperitoneal and intrapleural chemotherapy of a variety of solid tumors.[26–29] Subsequent examination of the thorax of treated patients at surgery suggests that these drugs produce true cytoreduction rather than sclerosis.[30] This suggestion is supported by the finding that complete removal of pleural fluid is not necessary in order to achieve control of the pleural effusion when treated with cisplatin and cytosine arabinoside.[31] Rusch and associates at Memorial Sloan-Kettering Hospital have performed pharmacokinetic studies in patients given intrapleural mitomycin and cisplatin for mesothelioma.[32, 33] Their studies show that intrapleural chemotherapy has a distinct local pharmacologic advantage and also produces significant and sustained drug plasma levels.[32]

AGENTS THAT PRODUCE CHEMICAL PLEURODESIS

The list of chemicals that produce pleurodesis is long, but the selection is made easy by practical considerations of availability, cost, patient acceptance, and comfort. All of these drugs act nonspecifically, producing adhesions between the visceral and parietal pleura and obliterating the pleural space.[34, 35] The degree to which each agent achieves this goal depends on the ability of (1) the lung to fully expand and provide complete contact between the pleural surfaces and (2) the agent to induce a chemical pleuritis. The following agents fit into this category.

Radioactive Isotopes. These were first tried during the 1940s after attempts to control malignant pleural effusions proved unsuccessful. The isotopes used include ^{198}Au and Cr^{34}PO$_4$ (which is less expensive and less hazardous). The response rate for radioisotopes is in the range of 55% to 60%. Side effects are primarily nausea (25% of patients) and vomiting (5% of patients). Their short half-lives (2.7 days for ^{198}Au and 14.3 days for Cr^{34}PO$_4$) limit their availability. Their use is also hindered by the need to protect hospital personnel from radiation.

Nitrogen Mustard. This agent has been used intrapleurally since 1949. When administered in doses of 0.4 mg/kg up to 20 mg, it can be very effective, with success rates reported as high as 87% with long-term follow-up.[36] The drawbacks of nitrogen mustard are its side effects: pain, nausea, vomiting, and occasional bone marrow suppression.[37, 38] Because equal success can be achieved with less toxic drugs, nitrogen mustard is rarely used today.

Bleomycin. Unlike nitrogen mustard, bleomycin

appears to have little local or systemic toxicity and is well tolerated even by neutropenic patients. Response rates of 60% to 85% have been reported with doses of 15 to 240 mg.[39, 40] A recently completed prospective randomized trial comparing tetracycline with bleomycin (60 units) showed bleomycin to be significantly superior to tetracycline (1 gm) in controlling malignant pleural effusions at 30 and 90 days following intrapleural injection.[41]

Quinacrine. This agent is effective in producing pleurodesis and controlling effusions in at least 70% of patients.[42] A trial comparing tetracycline with quinacrine, however, suggests that tetracycline is equally effective but is associated with less fever and pleuritic pain.[43] Owing to its toxicity, quinacrine is no longer used.

Talc. Talc is the oldest, cheapest, and perhaps most effective agent for pleurodesis.[44–49] Use of talc results in control of the effusion in approximately 90% of patients.[46–48] It produces a severe pleuritis, resulting in dense pleural adhesions. Talc can be sterilized by dry heat oven, gas,[45] or gamma irradiation.

Talc may be administered at the bedside by slurry[45] but is best insufflated at thoracoscopy or scattered across the pleural surfaces at thoracotomy. Bedside instillation of a talc suspension via thoracostomy tube is reported to be effective in the management of malignant pleural effusion (MPE) without the extreme pleural pain that accompanies poudrage application. Chambers initially reported successful pleurodesis in 17 of 20 patients with MPE using a suspension of talc in 1% procaine.[50] More recently, Webb and colleagues treated 34 patients with 5 gm of iodized talc mixed with lidocaine.[47] Of the 28 patients with MPE, 100% achieved control of effusion; two of the treated patients had previously failed tetracycline pleurodesis.

Two small randomized studies have suggested that talc is more effective than bleomycin or tetracycline for control of MPE. Fentiman and associates randomly assigned 33 evaluable breast cancer patients to receive talc (n = 12) via thoracoscopic insufflation, or tetracycline, 500 mg, via chest tube (n = 21).[51] Successful sclerosis was achieved in 92% of the talc-treated patients versus 48% of those treated with tetracycline. In addition, 11 tetracycline failures were subsequently salvaged by talc. Hamed compared intracavitary bleomycin (n = 15) with talc insufflation (n = 10) in 25 evaluable breast cancer patients.[52] With a mean follow-up of 9 months, they reported 100% control with talc versus 66% control after bleomycin. One-half of bleomycin failures were successfully salvaged with talc. Of note, pleuritic pain was not observed in the talc group. In both of these studies, talc was administered by insufflation under general anesthesia, any reaccumulation of effusion was called a treatment failure, and the patient population under study consisted of only breast cancer patients.

The short-term morbidity with intrapleural talc appears to be minimal.[47] Pain is thought not to be as great in patients with cancer compared with those being treated for recurrent pneumothorax.[47] Most reports have advocated the use of general anesthesia for talc insufflation, but all the above-referenced reports of bedside instillation of a talc suspension have given only local anesthesia with no reports of severe or unmanageable pain. Other adverse reactions reported after the instillation of talc include a report of adult respiratory distress syndrome (ARDS) in three patients after intrapleural instillation of 10 gm of talc[53] and acute respiratory failure with diffuse bilateral interstitial infiltrates a few hours after the administration of 2 gm of talc in another report.[54] Adler and Sayek also describe two steroid-dependent patients with transient hypotension following instillation of talc by poudrage; symptoms rapidly resolved with intravenous fluids and intravenous steroids.[45] In the Fentiman study, two patients in the talc group had an unexplained asystolic arrest while under general anesthesia while being turned after the poudrage procedure.[51] The other risks associated with talc include the concern about asbestos contamination; at present, all medical-grade talc is certified to be asbestos free. Dissemination of talc to other organs has not been described.

There has been a resurgence in the use of talc owing to recent availability of talc in a sterile preparation. Talc is packaged by the Axion Corp of France (Axion Corp., Avenue Du Vent Des Dames—Z.1 Les Paluds, 13685 Aubagne, France) in a sterile aerosol form. It is distributed in the USA by the Bryan Corporation (Bryan Corp., 4 Plympton Street, Woburn, MA 01801, Tel: 617/935-0000). Concerns about its carcinogenic potential[55, 56] are probably not valid now that asbestos-free preparations are available[57] and certainly do not apply in patients with malignant effusions.

Tetracycline. Tetracycline was the most popular agent for achieving pleurodesis until it was withdrawn from the market by the manufacturer.[58] It was cheap, easily available, and easily administered at the bedside via a chest tube. Its disadvantages were that it frequently produced severe pleuritic pain that was difficult to control even with good premedication,[59] and had a failure rate of approximately 25–50%.[41]

Use of doxycycline, a tetracycline derivative, has been reported for control of malignant pleural effusions, with success rates equivalent to that reported for tetracycline.[60, 61]

REFRACTORY MALIGNANT PLEURAL EFFUSION

If tube thoracoscopy and chemical pleurodesis fail to control malignant pleural effusion, a second attempt at tube thoracoscopy with drainage and sclerosing agent is indicated. Patients who fail subsequent attempts at chemical pleurodesis are difficult to manage. Young patients with good performance status, particularly those with trapped lungs that do not fully re-expand following fluid evacuation, may be good candidates for placement of a pleuroperitoneal shunt (Fig. 34–2).[62–65] Pleuroperitoneal shunts require significant patient participation, and therefore, the patients must be in generally good physical condition, alert, intelligent, and motivated. We do not advocate using these shunts as a first-line treatment for malignant pleural effusion but have found them to be successful in the appropriate patient with refractory effusion.

Robinson and his colleagues from Toronto report the use of a percutaneous Tenckhoff catheter for the management of malignant pleural effusion in nine patients.[66] Four of their nine patients had undergone previously unsuccessful chemical pleurodesis. The Tenckhoff catheters were placed under local anesthesia and left as external drainage tubes. The catheters were opened, and the pleural effusion was allowed to drain whenever the patient became symptomatic. The author reported success in all nine patients treated in this manner. This is a limited report, but this technique may well be a viable therapeutic option in patients with refractory effusion. The disadvantage of an indwelling catheter is the discomfort of the drain; however, the Tenckhoff catheter is small and, according to the authors, was well tolerated in all nine patients.

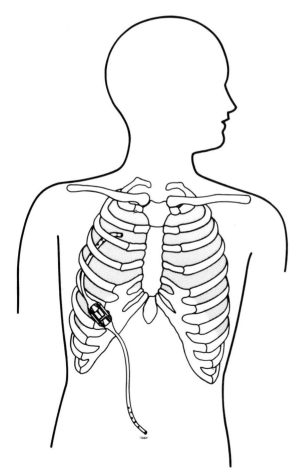

FIGURE 34–2. Denver pleuroperitoneal shunt in place.

THORACOSCOPY IN THE MANAGEMENT OF MALIGNANT PLEURAL EFFUSION

Thoracoscopy has been used for the diagnosis and management of malignant pleural effusion with excellent results for many years. It can be performed under local or general anesthesia.[46–49] Diagnostic and therapeutic thoracoscopy with talc insufflation does not require sophisticated equipment. The mediastinoscope, which is available in all thoracic operating rooms, serves well as a thoracoscope for this purpose. Single-lung anesthesia using a double-lumen endotracheal tube facilitates access to the thorax. With the lung collapsed and with the patient under general anesthesia, the thoracic contents can be readily examined, loculations broken down, biopsies taken, and chemical pleurodesis carried out. We prefer talc insufflation as the agent of choice for pleurodesis in this setting. Other thoracoscopic options used to create pleural adhesions, apart from agents used for chemical pleurodesis, include direct argon beam coagulation or Yag laser fulguration of the parietal pleura.

SURGERY

A final option in the management of malignant pleural effusions is thoracotomy with mechanical pleurodesis by pleurectomy. Understandably, this procedure is associated with a prohibitive morbidity and mortality rate, even in experienced hands (10% perioperative death rate, 23% complication rate according to Martini and colleagues[67]) because of the generally poor performance status of these patients. Although the operation is successful in controlling the effusion in 85% to 100% of patients, it has largely been abandoned for safer, less invasive alternatives. Pleurectomy as treatment of malignant pleural disease should be reserved for patients who are found to have unsuspected malignant pleuritis at time of thoracotomy.

CLINICAL TRIALS IN MALIGNANT PLEURAL EFFUSION

Much has been published about the management of malignant pleural effusions, but there have been few well-designed prospective trials evaluating the optimal treatment of this common and disabling problem. This is partly because of the special problems patients with malignant pleural effusions pose for the design of clinical trials.

Patients with malignant pleural effusions have a limited life expectancy even if they have a good performance status at the time of entry into the study. About half of the patients die within 3 months of entry into the study. Thus, large numbers of patients must be entered into a study in order to have statistically adequate numbers of patients available for the analysis of response rates. Many of these patients require ongoing radiotherapy or systemic treatment for disease at extrathoracic sites. Withholding or failing to modify medically indicated treatment in order to evaluate pleurodesis as the sole variable would be unwise and unethical. Patients with malignant pleural effusion often have underlying pulmonary parenchymal disease, bulky pleural disease, or some degree of a so-called trapped lung; these conditions make it difficult to interpret the patient's radiologic response after pleurodesis. Ideally, such patients should be excluded from a clinical trial. In contradistinction to clinical trials of other diseases, studies of malignant pleural effusions have no standard way to measure response. The most objective definition of recurrence is, we feel, the one reported by us: no radiographic evidence of any pleural fluid reaccumulation.[41] Other authors attempt to quantitate the amount of pleural fluid seen on chest radiograph as a partial or a complete response;[61] others simply record whether or not patients redeveloped symptoms. Unfortunately, the issue of how best to define response remains unsettled. Finally, because the management of malignant pleural effusion is primarily palliative, clinical trials should include a careful examination of the toxicity, the cost of treatment, and the need for retreatment in patients who have recurrent disease.

GUIDELINES FOR THE DESIGN OF PROTOCOLS

Experience gained from a recent multi-institutional prospective clinical trial has helped in the ongoing development and refinement of guidelines for the design of protocols for the treatment of malignant pleural effusion.[41, 68] These guidelines apply to protocols in which either sclerosing or cytotoxic intrapleural therapy is evaluated. Also, they aim not only to answer questions specific to each study but to provide consistency in comparing the results of different clinical studies. These guidelines include the following eligibility criteria and treatment modalities.

Eligibility Criteria

1. Histologic or cytologic proof of malignancy involving the pleura should be required.

2. Re-expansion of the lung must be demonstrated on chest x-ray study after insertion of a chest tube to drain the effusion. Such a demonstration obviates entering study patients whose effusions cannot be controlled by pleurodesis because they have a so-called trapped lung and a fixed pleural space.

3. For agents being administered at the bedside through a chest tube, patients should not have undergone a previous pleurodesis. This issue is less important if an agent is being administered by thoracoscopy, during which pleural adhesions can be lysed and good intrapleural dispersion of the agents ensured.

4. Patients should have a good performance status (0 to 2 in the Southwest Oncology Group or Eastern Cooperative Oncology Group scale) at the time of entry into the study. Otherwise they may not survive

long enough for the results of their treatment to be evaluated.

5. Patients should be entered into the study only if their effusion is refractory to standard treatment. For instance, pleural effusions present at the initial diagnosis of a lymphoma are very likely to resolve after chemotherapy or radiotherapy without further intervention. Patients with pleural effusions secondary to solid tumors that are highly responsive to chemotherapy, such as germ cell tumors, breast cancer, or ovarian cancer, should be entered on a protocol only if the effusion has failed to respond to chemotherapy.

Treatment Modalities

1. The timing of pleurodesis after insertion of a chest tube is controversial. At a minimum, the chest x-ray study should demonstrate complete evacuation of the pleural space. Waiting more than 3 or 4 days may allow loculation of the pleural space and prevent adequate dispersion of the sclerosing agent. Whatever timing for pleurodesis is selected must be carefully specified in the treatment section of the protocol.

2. Guidelines for the administration of intrapleural therapy must be specified. These guidelines include dilution of the agent, method and length of time of intrapleural instillation, and management of the chest tube after both instillation and drainage of the agent.

3. The length of time a chest tube is left in place after pleurodesis is also controversial. Common practice is to remove the chest tube when the drainage is less than 150 ml/24 hours. Presumably, this method promotes pleurodesis by ensuring maximal contact between the pleural surfaces after scleroses.

4. Protocols evaluating cytotoxic rather than sclerosing agents should mandate instillation of the intrapleural agent immediately after the re-expansion of the lung and removal of the chest tube immediately after completing intrapleural treatment. This approach decreases the chance that the effect of cytotoxic therapy is masked or altered by pleural adhesions.

5. The success of an agent for pleurodesis should be judged by the recurrence or absence of an effusion on serial chest x-ray studies. The noting of symptoms is an inaccurate way to assess response in these patients, who usually have multiple reasons to be dyspneic. Survival is also not an appropriate endpoint in studies of agents for pleurodesis. Control of a malignant pleural effusion can affect the quality of life or the need for hospitalization, but it usually does not significantly influence survival.

6. Simple, reproducible criteria for radiographic response should be used. The assessment of response on chest x-ray study is often complicated by the presence of underlying pulmonary parenchymal disease, pleural thickening, or pleural masses. This makes it difficult to classify patients as having a complete response, partial response, or stable disease, as would be done in most cancer trials. The simplest, most reproducible criterion is to determine whether the patient has or has not reaccumulated any fluid. The

chest x-ray study taken immediately after removal of the chest tube should serve as a baseline reference.

7. The length and timing of follow-up by chest x-ray study must be specified. In general, a follow-up period of 3 months with monthly chest x-ray studies is adequate. Beyond that, patient attrition due to death from underlying disease precludes the assessment of response in a significant number of patients.

8. Because intrapleural therapy primarily affects the patient's quality of life, data collection should include a careful assessment of toxicity and pain associated with treatment.

Prospective clinical trials for malignant pleural effusions will be a major contribution to the management of this common and morbid problem. However, trial design needs to be far more stringent than it has been in the past.

SUMMARY

The proper management of a pleural effusion in a patient with malignancy is based on an understanding of the normal anatomy and physiology of the pleural space and the ways in which they are altered by disease. The major challenge in diagnosing and treating a cancer patient who develops a pleural effusion is to accurately and quickly determine the etiology of the effusion and to choose a treatment best suited to the individual patient. Careful selection of the treatment of pleural effusions should result in relief of symptoms in the vast majority of patients with little accompanying morbidity. Delay in diagnosis and management should be avoided to prevent loss of valuable time in this group of terminally ill patients.

ANNOTATED REFERENCES

Hausheer FH, Yarbro JW: Diagnosis and treatment of malignant pleural effusion. Semin Oncol 12:54, 1985.
This is an excellent review article of the diagnosis and treatment of malignant pleural effusion. The authors have conducted an extensive review of the literature and treatment options.
Sahn SA: State of the art. The pleura. Am Rev Respir Dis 138:184, 1988.
This report by Sahn is the best review of pleural effusion currently in print. It is highly recommended to all readers.
Staub NC, Wiener-Kronish JP, Albertine KH: Transport through the pleura. Physiology of normal liquid and solute exchange in the pleural space. In Chretien J, Bignon J, Hirsch A (eds): The Pleura in Health and Disease. New York, Marcel Dekker, 1985, pp 169–193.
This is an excellent review article of the modern concepts of normal pleural physiology and solute exchange in the pleural space. The article outlines our current concepts and knowledge and puts to rest some of the previous misunderstanding on the topic.

REFERENCES

1. Agostoni E, D'Angelo E: Thickness and pressure of the pleural liquid at various heights and with various hydrothoraces. Respir Physiol 6:330, 1969.
2. Staub NC, Wiener-Kronish JP, Albertine KH: Transport through the pleura. Physiology of normal liquid and solute exchange in the pleural space. In Chretien J, Bignon J, Hirsch A (eds): The Pleura in Health and Disease. New York, Marcel Dekker, 1985, pp 169–193.
3. Agostoni E: Mechanics of the pleural space. Physiol Rev 52:57, 1972.
4. Wang NS: The regional difference of pleural mesothelial cells in rabbits. Am Rev Respir Dis 110:623, 1974.
5. McLaughlin RF: Bronchial artery distribution in various mammals and in humans. Am Rev Respir Dis 128S:S57, 1983.
6. McLaughlin RF, Tyler WS, Canada RO: Subgross pulmonary anatomy of the rabbit, rat, and guinea pig, with additional notes on the human lung. Am Rev Respir Dis 94:380, 1966.
7. Sahn SA: State of the art. The pleura. Am Rev Respir Dis 138:184, 1988.
8. Wang, NS: The preformed stomas connecting the pleural cavity and the lymphatics in the parietal pleura. Am Rev Respir Dis 111:12, 1975.
9. Nagaishi C: Functional anatomy and histology of the lung. Baltimore, University Park Press, 1972, 107–179.
10. Wiener-Kronish JP, Albertine KH, Licko V, et al: Protein egress and entry rates in pleural fluid and plasma in sheep. Appl Physiol 56:459–463, 1984.
11. Wiener-Kronish JP, Albertine KH, Roos PJ, et al: Pleural fluid dynamics in sheep are altered by a pleural catheter. Fed Proc 41:1127, 1982.
12. Sahn SA: Malignant pleural effusions. Semin Respir Med 9:43, 1987.
13. Chernow B, Sahn SA: Carcinomatous involvement of the pleura: An analysis of 96 patients. Am J Med 63:695, 1977.
14. Hausheer FH, Yarbro JW: Diagnosis and treatment of malignant pleural effusion. Semin Oncol 12:54, 1985.
15. Boutin C, Viallat JR, Cargnino P, et al: Thoracoscopy in malignant pleural effusions. Am Rev Respir Dis 124:588, 1981.
16. Yam LT: Diagnostic significance of lymphocytes in pleural effusions. Ann Intern Med 66(Pt 2):972, 1967.
17. Sahn SA, Good JT, Jr: Pleural fluid pH in malignant effusions. Diagnostic, prognostic, and therapeutic implications. Ann Intern Med 108:345, 1988.
18. Herbert A, Gallagher PJ: Interpretation of pleural biopsy specimens and aspirates with the immunoperoxidase technique. Thorax 37:822, 1982.
19. Monif GRG, Stewart BN, Block AJ: Living cytology. A new diagnostic technique for malignant pleural effusions. Chest 69:626, 1976.
20. Dewald GW, Hicks GA, Dines DE, et al: Cytogenetic diagnosis of malignant pleural effusions. Mayo Clin Proc 57:488, 1982.
21. McKenna JM, Chandrasekhar AJ, Henkin RE: Diagnostic value of carcinoembryonic antigen in exudative pleural effusions. Chest 78:587, 1980.
22. Gondos B, McIntosh KM, Renston RH, et al: Application of electron microscopy in the definitive diagnosis of effusions. Acta Cytol 22:297, 1978.
23. Austin EH, Flye MW: The treatment of recurrent malignant pleural effusion. Ann Thorac Surg 28:190, 1979.
24. Walsh FW, Alberts WM, Solomon DA, et al: Malignant pleural effusions: Pleurodesis using a small-bore percutaneous catheter. South Med J 82:963, 1989.
25. Morrison MC, Mueller PR, Lee MJ, et al: Sclerotherapy of malignant pleural effusion through sonographically placed small-bore catheters. AJR 158:41, 1992.
26. Bergerat J-P, Drewinko B, Corry P, et al: Synergistic lethal effect of cis-dichlorodiammineplatinum and 1-beta-D-arabinofuranosylcytosine. Cancer Res 41:25, 1981.
27. Kern DH: In vitro pharmacokinetic studies of cytosine arabinoside (ARA-C; Cytostar-U); synergy of anti-tumor activity with cis-platinum (abstract). Proceedings, International Conference on Advances in Regional Cancer Therapy, Giessen, West Germany, August 1985.
28. Markman M, Howell SB, Green MR: Combination intracavitary chemotherapy for malignant pleural disease. Cancer Drug Deliv 1:333, 1984.
29. Rusch VW, Figlin R, Godwin D, et al: Intrapleural cisplatin and cytarabine in the management of malignant pleural effusions: A Lung Cancer Study Group Trial. J Clin Oncol 9:313, 1991.

30. Markman M: Melphalan and cytarabine administered intraperitoneally as single agents and combination intraperitoneal chemotherapy with cisplatin and cytarabine. Semin Oncol 12(3) Suppl 4:33, 1985.
31. Markman M, Cleary S, King ME, et al: Cisplatin and cytarabine administered intrapleurally as treatment of malignant pleural effusions. Med Pediatr Oncol 13:191, 1985.
32. Rusch VW, Niedzwiecki D, Tao Y, et al: Intrapleural cisplatin and mitomycin for malignant mesothelioma following pleurectomy: Pharmacokinetic studies. J Clin Oncol 10(6): 1001, 1992.
33. Rusch V, Kelsen D, Saltz L, et al: A phase II trial of intrapleural and systemic chemotherapy after pleurectomy/decortication for malignant pleural mesothelioma (MPM). Proc Am Soc Clin Oncol (ASCO) #1211, 1992.
34. Frankel A, Krasna I, Baronofsky ID: An experimental study of pleural symphysis. J Thorac Cardiovasc Surg 42:43, 1961.
35. Sahn SA, Good JT, Potts DE: The pH of sclerosing agents: A determinant of pleural symphysis. Chest 76:198, 1979.
36. Kinsey DL, Carter D, Klassen KP: Simplified management of malignant pleural effusion. Arch Surg 89:389, 1964.
37. Anderson CB, Philpott GW, Ferguson TB: The treatment of malignant pleural effusions. Cancer 33:916, 1974.
38. Greenwald DW, Phillips C, Bennett JM: Management of malignant pleural effusion. J Surg Oncol 10:361, 1978.
39. Paladine W, Cunningham TJ, Sponzo R, et al: Intracavitary bleomycin in the management of malignant effusions. Cancer 38:1903, 1976.
40. Bitran JD, Brown C, Desser RK, et al: Intracavitary bleomycin for the control of malignant effusions. J Surg Oncol 16:273, 1981.
41. Ruckdeschel JC, Moores D, Yee JY, et al: Intrapleural therapy for malignant pleural effusions: A randomized comparison of bleomycin and tetracycline. Chest 100:1528, 1991.
42. Taylor SA, Hooton NS, MacArthur AM: Quinacrine in the management of malignant pleural effusion. Br J Surg 64:52, 1977.
43. Bayly TC, Kisner DL, Sybert A, et al: Tetracycline and quinacrine in the control of malignant pleural effusions. Cancer 41:1188, 1978.
44. Shedbalkar AR, Head JM, Head LR, et al: Evaluation of talc pleural symphysis in management of malignant pleural effusion. J Thorac Cardiovasc Surg 61:492, 1971.
45. Adler RH, Sayek I: Treatment of malignant pleural effusion: A method using tube thoracostomy and talc. Ann Thorac Surg 22:8, 1976.
46. Pearson FG, MacGregor DC: Talc poudrage for malignant pleural effusion. J Thorac Cardiovasc Surg 51:732, 1966.
47. Webb WR, Ozmen V, Moulder PV, et al: Iodized talc pleurodesis for the treatment of pleural effusions. J Thorac Cardiovasc Surg 103:881, 1992.
48. Daniel TM, Tribble CG, Rodgers BM: Thoracoscopy and talc poudrage for pneumothoraces and effusions. Ann Thorac Surg 50:186, 1990.
49. Hartman DL, Gaither JM, Kesler KA, et al: Comparison of insufflated talc under thoracoscopic guidance with standard tetracycline and bleomycin pleurodesis for control of malignant pleural effusions. J Thorac Cardiovasc Surg 105:743, 1993.
50. Chambers JS: Palliative treatment of neoplastic pleural effusion with intercostal intubation and talc instillation. West J Surg Obstet Gynecol 66:26, 1958.
51. Fentiman IS, Rubens RD, Hayward JL: A comparison of intracavitary talc and tetracycline for the control of pleural effusions secondary to breast cancer. Eur J Cancer Clin Oncol 22(9):1079, 1986.
52. Hamed H, Fentiman IS, Chaudary MA, et al: Comparison of intracavitary bleomycin and talc for control of pleural effusions secondary to carcinoma of the breast. Br J Surg 76:1266, 1989.
53. Rinaldo JE, Owens GR, Rogers RM: Adult respiratory distress syndrome following intrapleural instillation of talc. J Thorac Cardiovasc Surg 85:523, 1983.
54. Bouchama A, Chastre J, Gaudichet A, et al: Acute pneumonitis with bilateral pleural effusion after talc pleurodesis. Chest 85:795, 1984.
55. Henderson WJ, Joslin CAF, Turnbull AC, et al: Talc and carcinoma of the ovary and cervix. J Obstet Gynecol Br Commonwealth 78:266, 1971.
56. Longo DL, Young RC: Cosmetic talc and ovarian cancer. Lancet 2:349, 1979.
57. Chappell AG, Johnson A, Charles J, et al: (Research Committee of the British Thoracic Association and the Medical Research Council Pneumoconiosis Unit): A survey of the long-term effects of talc kaolin pleurodesis. Br J Dis Chest 73:285, 1979.
58. Heffner JE, Unruh LC: Tetracycline pleurodesis: Adios, farewell, adieu. Chest 101:5, 1992.
59. Bezanilla AR: Treatment for malignant pleural effusions. (Letter to the editor.) Chest 70:408, 1976.
60. Gericke KR: Doxycycline as a sclerosing agent. Ann Pharmacother 26:648, 1992.
61. Robinson LA, Fleming WH, Galbraith TA: Intrapleural doxycycline control of malignant pleural effusions. Ann Thorac Surg 55:1115, 1993.
62. Weese JL, Schouten JT: Pleural peritoneal shunts for the treatment of malignant pleural effusions. Surg Gynecol Obstet 154:391, 1982.
63. Little AG, Kadowaki MH, Ferguson MK, et al: Pleuro-peritoneal shunting: Alternative therapy for pleural effusions. Ann Surg 208:443, 1988.
64. Reich H, Beattie EJ, Harvey JC: Pleuroperitoneal shunt for malignant pleural effusions: A one-year experience. Semin Surg Oncol 9:160, 1993.
65. Tsang V, Fernando HC, Goldstraw P: Pleuroperitoneal shunt for recurrent malignant pleural effusions. Thorax 45:369, 1990.
66. Robinson RD, Fullerton DA, Albert JD, et al: Use of pleural Tenckhoff catheter to palliate malignant pleural effusion. Ann Thorac Surg 57:286, 1994.
67. Martini N, Bains MS, Beattie EJ Jr: Indications for pleurectomy in malignant effusion. Cancer 35:734, 1975.
68. Moores DW, Rusch VW: Malignant pleural effusions. In Rusch VW, Ginsberg RJ, Holmes EC (eds): A Thoracic Surgical Handbook for Clinical Trials. New York Memorial Sloan-Kettering Cancer Center, 1993, pp 39–41.
69. Salyer WR, Eggleston JC, Erozan YS: Efficacy of pleural needle biopsy and pleural fluid cytopathology in the diagnosis of malignant neoplasm involving the pleura. Chest 67:536, 1975.
70. Leuallen EC, Carr DT: Pleural effusion—a statistical study of 436 patients. N Engl J Med 252:79, 1955.
71. Tinney WS, Olsen AM: The significance of fluid in the pleural space: A study of 274 cases. J Thorac Surg 14:248, 1946.
72. Storey DD, Dines DE, Coles DT: Pleural effusion: A diagnostic dilemma. JAMA 236:2183, 1976.
73. Light RW, Macgregor MI, Luchsinger PC, et al: Pleural effusions: The diagnostic separation of transudates and exudates. Ann Intern Med 77:507, 1972.
74. Hirsch A, Ruffie P, Nebut M, et al: Pleural effusion: Laboratory tests in 300 cases. Thorax 34:106, 1979.
75. Chernow B, Sahn SA: Carcinomatous involvement of the pleura: An analysis of 96 patients. Am J Med 63:695, 1977.

Part V

PULMONARY METASTASES

35 RESECTION OF PULMONARY METASTASES

Louis A. Lanza and Joe B. Putnam Jr.

Patients with malignant solid tumors often present with metastases at some time during the course of their disease. The majority of such patients have multiple sites of metastases not amenable to resection. Despite its limitations, chemotherapy remains the preferred method of treatment for these patients, although long-term survival remains elusive. The best treatment for isolated pulmonary metastases is unknown. As predicted by autopsy studies, approximately one-third of patients will die with pulmonary metastases and a portion of these patients will have metastases isolated to the lungs.

Although numerous clinical studies support resection, no controlled study exists comparing surgical resection of isolated pulmonary metastases from selected solid tumors with other available treatment options. Many authors report a 5-year survival rate of 25% to 40% following resection of isolated pulmonary metastases. Because of the survival advantage identified following complete resection, pulmonary metastasectomy continues to be advocated for such treatment of isolated pulmonary metastases from a variety of solid tumors.

HISTORICAL PERSPECTIVE

Pulmonary resection for chest wall sarcoma or incidental to chest wall resection was reported in the early 1880s by Weinlechner and Kronlein.[1, 2] Resection of a pulmonary metastasis as a separate procedure was described in 1930 by Torek.[3] Barney and Churchill[4] noted long-term survival in a patient following resection of a pulmonary metastasis from hypernephroma. Local control of the primary tumor was also achieved, and the patient survived 23 years and died from unrelated causes. Alexander and Haight[5] summarized the first large series of 25 patients following metastasectomy in 1947 that included one patient who underwent a lobectomy for a sarcomatous metastasis. Ehrenhaft[6] reported on 37 patients with pulmonary metastasectomy (1946 through 1957) for lesions of various histologic types. Three of 28 patients with primary carcinoma and one of nine patients with sarcomatous histology remained alive at 5 years. Most resections were offered to patients with a single metastasis following a long disease-free interval. Multi-

ple pulmonary metastases from osteochondroma of the tibia were resected in 1953 by Mannix, with the patient surviving for more than 2 years.[1] Martini and associates[7] in 1971 reported a series of patients with metastatic osteosarcoma treated with aggressive pulmonary metastasectomy and multiple procedures. Twenty-two patients underwent a total of 59 thoracotomies and 152 total metastases were removed, with 53 of 59 thoracotomies being performed for multiple rather than single metastases. The survival rate at 3 years was 45%. Following this report, a more aggressive approach to pulmonary metastasectomy for sarcomatous disease was more widely adopted. In the past 20 years, resection of solitary and multiple pulmonary metastases from numerous primary neoplasms has been performed, resulting in long-term survival in up to 40% of patients so treated.[8]

PATHOLOGY

Pulmonary metastases may develop by hematogenous, lymphatic, or aerogenous routes, or by direct invasion. Biology of the primary tumor or of the population of cells prone to metastases as well as host resistance determines mechanisms of spread, location(s) of metastases, and growth. Tumor cells that reach the blood stream frequently are filtered by the liver or the lung. Cells may preferentially adhere to the underlying capillary endothelium. Tumor cells may travel by lymphatics and occupy a discrete position within the lung or may diffusely involve the entire lung, as is seen with lymphangitic spread of breast carcinoma or other metastatic adenocarcinomas. Direct invasion of other structures may occur as the metastasis grows. Aerogenous spread of tumor from one site within the bronchus to another site rarely occurs.

DIAGNOSIS

Few patients (<5%) with pulmonary metastases present with symptoms. Hemoptysis, dyspnea, cough, pain, or pneumothorax rarely occurs from pulmonary metastases. Most metastatic lesions appear in a peripheral location, although they may occur in any lo-

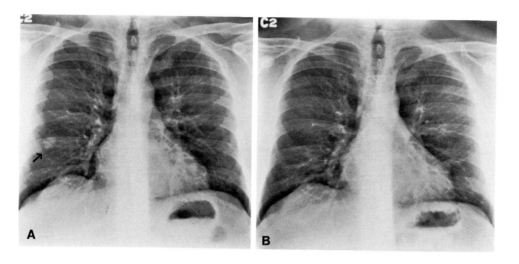

FIGURE 35–1. A 28-year-old man with myxoid liposarcoma of the right gluteal region underwent tumor resection surgery with wide local excision nine months previously. A right lung nodule was identified on chest x-ray study *(A)* and confirmed as a solitary nodule on computed tomography of the chest. At median sternotomy, three nodules were found—one on the right and two occult metastases on the left. A complete resection was performed *(B)*.

cation within the lung. Diagnosis is routinely made on follow-up chest roentgenograms after primary tumor resection. Pulmonary osteoarthropathy has been reported.[9] The majority of symptomatic patients do not have resectable disease at presentation.

The standard chest roentgenogram remains the most cost-effective tool for screening for pulmonary metastases (Fig. 35–1). Duda and colleagues examined 130 patients with soft tissue and bone sarcomas. Sixty-six patients had no evidence of pulmonary metastases on chest x-ray study and subsequently had linear tomography or computed tomography (CT) of the chest.

Only one patient of 53 with a normal chest x-ray study and no local recurrence had an abnormal tomogram. Two patients of 13 with locally recurrent sarcoma and a normal chest x-ray study had an abnormal tomogram. The authors concluded that a screening chest x-ray study in the absence of local recurrence would be most cost effective; however, tomograms should be performed for evaluation of the extent of disease (e.g., pulmonary metastases) in patients with locally recurrent sarcomas.[10]

CT of the chest (Fig. 35–2) can detect smaller pulmonary nodules at an earlier time than can a chest x-

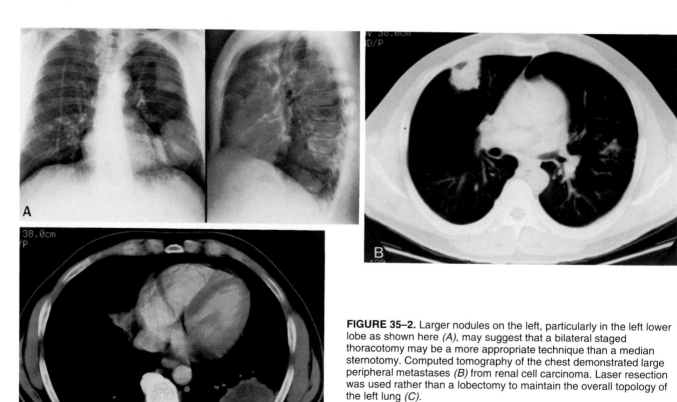

FIGURE 35–2. Larger nodules on the left, particularly in the left lower lobe as shown here *(A)*, may suggest that a bilateral staged thoracotomy may be a more appropriate technique than a median sternotomy. Computed tomography of the chest demonstrated large peripheral metastases *(B)* from renal cell carcinoma. Laser resection was used rather than a lobectomy to maintain the overall topology of the left lung *(C)*.

ray study or linear tomography; however, its cost effectiveness in screening is low. No data suggest that earlier detection with CT yields improved survival. Theoretically earlier detection and treatment of metastases could improve survival; however, in one study that detected occult metastases during median sternotomy with bilateral lung exploration, survival was not improved over that in patients who had a single thoracotomy, even though a significant percentage of patients would be expected to have occult metastases.[11]

The cost of CT scanning and radiation exposure may exceed many times that of a chest x-ray study.[12] Screening with conventional chest x-ray study, with chest CT used selectively for evaluation of chest x-ray study abnormalities or for potential pulmonary metastases in patients with recurrent primary tumor, may prove a more efficient approach for detecting pulmonary metastases in patients at risk. Patients without evidence of metastases on chest x-ray study rarely have metastases demonstrated by tomography. Lien and colleagues,[13] however, showed that approximately half of the patients with nonseminomatous testicular tumors have negative chest x-ray studies but abnormalities identified on CT scans. Chang and associates[14] prospectively evaluated the role of CT in the detection of pulmonary metastases. In 25 patients with a known history of malignancy, CT detected 69 nodules, of which only 31 proved to be malignant at thoracotomy. Linear tomography detected 38 nodules, of which 25 were malignant, while chest x-ray study detected 21 nodules, of which 19 proved malignant. Overall, CT detected 58% of the total number of metastatic nodules; linear tomography, 47%; and chest x-ray study, 36%. Only six of the 31 additional nodules detected by CT scan (compared with tomography) proved to be metastases. Pass and colleagues[15] prospectively evaluated CT scanning in the detection of pulmonary metastases in patients with osteogenic and soft tissue sarcoma. Compared with linear tomography, CT detected more pulmonary metastases at an earlier time (56 by CT versus 7 by full lung tomography, p = .001) and of a smaller size (7.6 mm by CT versus 13.2 mm by full lung tomography, p < .05). They recommended that surgical decisions for resection of pulmonary metastases be based on CT rather than full lung tomography findings.

In patients with a known malignancy who present with multiple pulmonary nodules, the probability of metastatic disease approaches 100%. However, the etiology of single nodules may be determined only with excision, particularly when the nodule is small. Benign granulomatous disease may mimic metastases. Johnson and coworkers[16] reported only a 33% true positive yield in patients with known malignancies undergoing pulmonary resection of nodules that were less than 0.5 cm in diameter. Tumors were benign or surgically removed in 33% of children with known malignant disease who developed new pulmonary nodules. Cahan and associates[17] reported on 54 patients with colon cancer who developed solitary pulmonary nodules on follow-up. Of the 54 patients treated with pulmonary resection, 25 were found to have metastatic lesions whereas 29 were found to have primary lung carcinomas. Clinical Stage I or II primary lung carcinoma may be indistinguishable from a solitary metastasis, particularly if the primary tumor is squamous cell carcinoma or adenocarcinoma. Similar findings have been described in patients with breast carcinoma and new pulmonary nodules.[18] Recently, positron-emission tomography (PET) has shown promise of distinguishing benign from malignant pulmonary nodules based on patterns of 2-[F-18]-fluoro-2-deoxy-D-glucose uptake in preliminary reports.[19] However, at present, patients who have known malignancies and indeterminate pulmonary nodules should be offered pulmonary resection for both diagnoses and potential treatment.

TREATMENT OF PULMONARY METASTASES

At present, treatment options are limited for patients with metastatic solid tumors. Curative treatment remains elusive, and few effective agents exist for the majority of patients with metastatic solid tumors. In patients with additional disseminated extrathoracic disease, resection is of no value. However, in patients with isolated pulmonary metastases, resection may offer a viable treatment option with potential for long-term survival with little treatment-related risk.

Chemotherapy

Salvage chemotherapy with surgical resection may be effective in prolonging survival in patients who develop pulmonary metastases from osteogenic sarcoma, as suggested by Marina and coworkers[20] and Pastorino and associates[21]; however, Bacci and colleagues[22] and others have not seen a benefit. Bacci[22] examined patients with osteogenic sarcoma of the extremity who presented with pulmonary metastases. Chemotherapy (doxorubicin [Adriamycin], methotrexate, cisplatin) followed by surgery failed to provide disease-free or overall survival equivalent to that for patients without metastases at presentation. Postoperative chemotherapy (ifosfamide, VP-16) was also given. Seventy-three per cent of patients with metastases at presentation experienced a recurrence within 3.5 years compared with 27% of patients without metastases at presentation. Glasser and colleagues[23] showed that histologic response to chemotherapy (per cent necrosis) was the only independent predictor of enhanced survival in a study of 279 patients with Stage II osteogenic sarcoma.

In 50 patients with metastatic breast cancer whose first metastases were found in the lungs, Schlappack and associates[24] reported a median survival time of only 11.5 months for single pulmonary metastases and 10.5 months in those patients with more than one metastases.

Completeness of resection after chemotherapy remains crucial and may have a significant impact on subsequent survival. Kim and Louie[25] treated patients with metastatic renal cell carcinoma with interleukin-2 prior to surgical resection of residual tumor. Nine of 11 patients are alive and have no evidence of disease at a median follow-up of 21 months. Lanza and associates[26] examined the response of soft tissue sarcoma metastases that were treated with chemotherapy prior to surgery. Patients were graded as having complete, partial, or no response or progression resulting from the chemotherapy. Survival could not be predicted on the basis of the patient's response to chemotherapy alone.

Radiation Therapy

The role of radiation therapy in the treatment of pulmonary metastasis remains limited. Baeza and coworkers[27] reported on 62 patients who were treated with whole lung irradiation for pulmonary metastases from a variety of histologies. The incidence of radiation pneumonitis was 23% in those receiving 15 Gy or more. In three patients, it was fatal. With the exception of patients with Wilms' tumor, only three patients were alive at 24 months. In patients with resected osteogenic sarcoma, prophylactic whole lung irradiation reduces the incidence of pulmonary metastases, as does adjuvant chemotherapy.[28] At present, radiation therapy is most widely used for palliation of symptoms in patients with advanced unresectable disease.

Immunotherapy

Immunotherapy for the treatment of solid tumor remains experimental.

Surgery

Resection for metastases regardless of site presumes a favorable biology producing only isolated single-organ metastases. Existing clinical data support the concept that in a subset of patients with isolated metastases, visible disease comprises the only metastases, whose resection proves curative. In a larger proportion of patients, recurrence occurs, which is likely due to subclinical disease present at the time of metastasectomy. At present, our knowledge does not allow accurate differentiation between these subgroups. Future research may identify biologic prognostic factors or metastatic determinants predictive of disseminated or limited metastatic disease. In addition, advances in treatment strategies may improve the efficacy of treatment modalities. Until then, patient selection for pulmonary metastasectomy should remain liberal in otherwise viable patients without significant alternative treatment options.

A substantial number of patients at multiple institutions have been reported who have undergone pulmonary metastasectomy with favorable long-term results. Appelquist and associates[29] reported a 10% seven-year survival rate in 42 patients who had isolated pulmonary metastases from tumors of varied histologic type. McCormack and Martini[30] described the experience at Memorial Sloan-Kettering Cancer Center with 663 pulmonary metastasectomies performed on 448 patients with either metastatic sarcoma or carcinoma over a 17-year period. The operative mortality rate was 1.0%. Two hundred and forty-six patients had carcinomatous histologic type, whereas 202 patients had sarcomatous histologic type. The overall 5-year survival rate for patients with completely resected carcinoma histologic type was 25%, whereas the 5-year survival rate of patients with sarcomatous histologic type was 18% to 29%, depending on the specific histologic type. Mountain and coworkers[31] reported on 556 patients treated with pulmonary metastasectomy at M.D. Anderson Cancer Center over a 20-year period. The operative mortality rate was again low (1.5%). The overall 5-year survival rate following thoracotomy was 35%, with survival varying by histologic type. Wilkins and colleagues[32] reported on 163 pulmonary resections performed on 142 patients with a variety of histologies at the Massachusetts General Hospital with a mortality rate of 1.2%. The cumulative 5-year survival rate for patients who underwent resection was 30%. They advocated a continued aggressive surgical approach for the treatment of isolated pulmonary metastases. Wright and associates[33] reported on 153 thoracotomies performed on 142 patients over a 22-year period for the removal of pulmonary metastases at the University of Iowa. The operative mortality rate was 0.7%. The actuarial 5-year survival rate for patients with metastatic carcinoma was 24% and for sarcoma, 29%. The histology did not appear to influence survival significantly. Morrow and associates[34] described 207 thoracotomies performed on 167 patients for metastasectomy at the University of Minnesota. The operative mortality rate was 0.6%. The cumulative survival rate at 5 years was 29% and, at 10 years, it was 20% for a variety of histologies. The most favorable outcome was found in patients with testicular and renal cell carcinomas, whereas the least favorable results were found in patients with melanomas and colon and uterine carcinomas. Marks and associates,[35] Valente and colleagues,[36] van Dongen and coworkers,[37] Van de Wal and associates,[38] Vogt-Moyhopf and coworkers,[39] Eckersberger and colleagues,[40] McCormack,[41] and Stewart and associates[42] have reported similar experiences with large groups of patients undergoing pulmonary metastasectomies for a variety of tumor histologies.

SELECTION CRITERIA FOR RESECTION OF PULMONARY METASTASES

Selection criteria for patients undergoing pulmonary metastasectomy were described in 1958 by Ehrenhaft and Lawrence and have not changed significantly since that time.[6] Potential candidates for pulmonary resection should meet these criteria:

1. Pulmonary nodules consistent with metastases,
2. Control of primary tumor,

addition, concomitant cardiovascular disease should be appropriately investigated prior to surgery. Strict adherence to these guidelines ensures safe resection with minimal morbidity and mortality.

SURGICAL TECHNIQUES AND INCISIONS

Various surgical approaches and resection techniques have been described for the resection of pulmonary metastases. These include median sternotomy (Fig. 35–3), posterolateral thoracotomy, transsternal bilateral thoracotomies, and video-assisted thoracic surgery (VATS). The optimal approach depends on the individual patient, tumor histology, the location of the nodules requiring resection, the number of lesions, and laterality of the disease (Table 35–1). In some cases, the patient's functional status may also influence the surgical approach.

Johnston[48a] reported his experience with 53 median sternotomies in 46 patients undergoing pulmonary metastasectomy. Forty of the 46 patients had either metastatic osteosarcoma or soft tissue sarcoma. Fifty-three per cent more tumor nodules were found on median sternotomy than on full lung tomograms. Sixty-one per cent of patients thought to have unilateral disease by tomography were found to have bilateral disease on exploration. In a subsequent study, Roth and colleagues[11] retrospectively compared median sternotomy to thoracotomy in 65 patients with soft tissue sarcomas treated at the National Cancer Institute with pulmonary metastasectomy. The complication rate did not differ between the two groups. Forty-five per cent of patients with unilateral metastases on preoperative CT scan were found to have bilateral metastases at exploration. Actuarial post-thoracotomy survival did not differ between the two

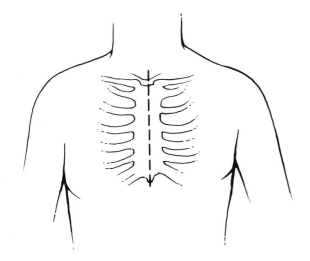

FIGURE 35–3. A median sternotomy incision provides access to both the right and the left thoraces. Resection of nodules in the posteromedial aspect of the left hilum is difficult to perform without displacing the heart.

3. All nodules potentially resectable with planned surgical procedures,

4. Adequate postoperative pulmonary reserve anticipated, and

5. No extrathoracic metastases.

In addition to these anatomic criteria, however, standard functional criteria for pulmonary resection should be observed to allow for safe resection. Although the majority of patients who undergo pulmonary metastasectomy are subject to single or multiple wedge resections, occasionally anatomic pulmonary resection is required to remove all metastatic disease. A residual postoperative FEV_1 of 30% predicted should be ensured, taking into account the number of metastases resected and technique of resections. In

TABLE 35–1. Comparison of Surgical Incisions for Resection of Metastases

MEDIAN STERNOTOMY

For:	Bilateral thoracic explorations with one incision
	Less patient discomfort
Against:	Metastases near the hilum difficult to resect
	Difficult exposure of the left lower lobe in patients with obesity, cardiomegaly, or an elevated left hemidiaphragm

POSTEROLATERAL THORACOTOMY

For:	Common approach to the hemithorax
	Excellent exposure to all components and areas of the hemithorax
Against:	More patient discomfort
	Muscles may be divided (except for muscle sparing technique)
	Only one hemithorax may be explored at one operation; a second operation is needed for bilateral metastases

THORACOSCOPIC OR VIDEO-ASSISTED THORACIC SURGERY FOR RESECTION

For:	Excellent visualization
	Minimal morbidity and discomfort
	Excellent exposure for visceral pleural metastases
Against:	Unable to fully evaluate metastases in the lung parenchyma
	Unable to completely palpate lung
	Learning curve
	Length of procedure
	Operating room costs may be higher with multiple resections

groups. It seems likely that sternotomy represents the preferred approach to pulmonary metastasectomy in patients with osteogenic and soft tissue sarcomas because it is associated with low operative risk and reduced postoperative discomfort, and allows for single-staged exploration and resection of disease in both hemithoraces.

Recent reports[43] have advocated thoracoscopic resection of pulmonary metastases (Fig. 35–4). Twenty-one thoracoscopic resections using varied techniques were described in 15 patients with minimal morbidity and no deaths. The mean postoperative hospital stay was 3.3 days. Although it is possible that thoracoscopic resection may result in decreased postoperative stay, based on data presented earlier, it is unlikely that thoracoscopic resection results in complete metastasectomy, especially in patients with sarcomatous histologies. Additional follow-up will be needed before thoracoscopic metastasectomy replaces open resection.

In patients with single or unilateral metastases from nonsarcomatous histologies, little data exist supporting one approach over the other. Patients with single nodules and a history of carcinoma may have new primary lung cancers, and although median sternotomy has been advocated as the preferred approach for pulmonary resections of all types,[44] posterolateral thoracotomy remains the preferred approach for unilateral anatomic pulmonary resections.

Extent and Technique of Resection

Most metastatic nodules in the lung appear in subpleural locations and can be easily removed by wedge excision. This accomplishes the goals of total tumor excision with maximal preservation of lung parenchyma. Occasional patients display metastases in locations that require larger pulmonary resections, such as lobectomy or pneumonectomy. Putnam and associ-

ates[45] described treatment of pulmonary metastases by pneumonectomy or en bloc resection with chest wall or other thoracic structures such as the diaphragm, pericardium, and superior vena cava in a small group of patients, with good results. Nineteen patients underwent pneumonectomy, and another 19 patients underwent other extended pulmonary resections. The 5-year actuarial survival rate was 25%. The mortality rate was 5%, and these deaths occurred in patients undergoing pneumonectomy following prior wedge resections. Wright and coworkers[33] reported on 153 thoracotomies performed on 142 patients at the University of Iowa over a 20-year period for a variety of histologic types of tumor. Eight patients underwent pneumonectomy, 42 patients underwent lobectomy, 13 patients underwent segmentectomy, and 50 patients underwent wedge resections. There was no statistical difference in the actuarial 5-year survival rates according to the type of resection performed. McGovern and associates[46] reported results of completion pneumonectomy performed at the Mayo Clinic. One hundred and thirteen patients underwent the procedure over a 27-year period, of whom 20 patients had pulmonary metastasis as the operative indication. In the subgroup of 20 patients undergoing completion pneumonectomy for metastatic disease, no postoperative deaths occurred and only one patient experienced postoperative complications. Interestingly, the 5-year actuarial survival rate in the 20 patients undergoing completion pneumonectomy for pulmonary metastases was 40.8%, which was significantly higher than that of patients undergoing completion pneumonectomy for either lung cancer (26.4%) or benign lung disease (27.2%).

In patients undergoing wedge metastasectomy, the decision regarding the adequacy of margin of resection often must be made by the surgeon alone. Distortion of lung parenchyma following wedge resection may simulate close or positive resection margins after

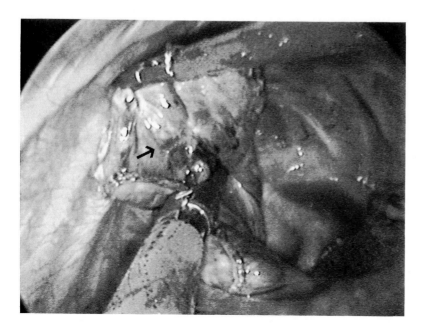

FIGURE 35–4. Video-assisted thoracic surgery (VATS) techniques may be considered as a surgical treatment option in carefully selected patients. The metastasis is shown. Disadvantages of this technique include the inability of the surgeon to palpate the lung parenchyma.

histologic fixation and processing. Ballantine and co-workers[47] have called into question the adequacy of wedge resection for pulmonary metastases. Eighteen children underwent wedge resection of pulmonary metastases over a 10-year period for a variety of child-hood cancers. Approximately 50% of patients experienced local recurrences in the lungs near the sites of resection. Based on the data presented, it is difficult to determine whether recurrence in the lung represented progression of disease or inadequate resection.

At present, most surgeons perform pulmonary wedge resections with the aid of surgical staplers. Staplers expedite nonanatomic pulmonary resection and provide good protection against prolonged air leaks. Depending on anatomic determinants, either the GIA or TA stapler may be used. Most patients are ventilated using a double-lumen endotracheal tube to facilitate selective pulmonary deflation, which allows careful pulmonary palpation. Other techniques of pulmonary resection may be used, however. Cooper and colleagues[48] described precision cautery excision of pulmonary lesions. Seventeen patients underwent cautery excision of pulmonary lesions, seven of which were metastatic tumors. Postoperative complications, including prolonged air leaks, were minimal. The authors concluded that precision cautery excision of pulmonary lesions allows limited excision of deep-seated nodules with maximal conservation of lung tissue. More recently, neodymium-yttrium-aluminum-garnet laser has been advocated as a useful tool in pulmonary metastasectomy. Branscheid and associates,[49] Miyamoto and coworkers,[50] and Kodama and colleagues[51] have described facile resection of multiple metastases with minimal morbidity. Either contact or noncontact techniques have been described. The technique does not appear to differ significantly from precision cautery excision, except that light energy is employed instead of electrical energy. Its increased cost may not warrant widespread application.

A median sternotomy is recommended for initial exploration and resection of unilateral or bilateral nodules in patients with pulmonary metastases from osteogenic or soft tissue sarcomas and should be considered the procedure of choice in patients with suspected bilateral metastases from any primary neoplasm. A thorough exploration for unilateral or bilateral nodules as well as resection of these nodules may be accomplished through a median sternotomy incision. Prior to surgery, the patient is examined thoroughly to determine the extent of metastases and whether or not an operation can be safely performed (Table 35–2). The chest roentgenograms and chest CT scans are reviewed and displayed prominently in the operating room. After intubation with a single-lumen endotracheal tube, bronchoscopy is performed to evaluate the tracheobronchial tree. A double-lumen endotracheal tube is placed. Sequential deflation of each lung aids in exposure and palpation of the pulmonary nodules.

All nodules are resected with a margin of normal

tissue. Nodules should not be shelled out because viable tumor cells remain on the periphery of the resected area. Often the decision of adequacy of margin is the surgeon's alone because lung parenchyma may become distorted around the nodule after resection, giving the illusion of a positive or close margin. Mediastinal lymph node metastases rarely result from pulmonary metastases (see the articles by Putnam and colleagues[52] and Udelsman and coworkers[53]). Laser-assisted pulmonary resection using the neodymium-yttrium-aluminum-garnet laser may provide a better means of resecting pulmonary metastases than surgery with the surgical stapler as recommended by Kodama and colleagues,[51] Branscheid and coworkers,[49] Miyamoto and associates,[50] and Landreneau and colleagues.[54] Disadvantages of laser resection may include longer operating time and potential for prolonged postoperative air leaks; however, use of the laser may enhance preservation of lung parenchyma with less distortion (see Fig. 35–6). Bovie electrocautery may also spare the lung parenchyma by removing the metastases with minimal distortion of the remaining lung. Air leaks can be sealed with fibrin glue.

Median Sternotomy

The patient is positioned supine with the entire anterior thorax exposed from the neck to the umbilicus and laterally to each anterior axillary line. The sternum is divided. The pulmonary ligament is divided on each side to mobilize the lung completely. The lungs are sequentially deflated and palpated. Metastases are identified and resected, and then the deflated lung is reinflated. The deflated right lung may be brought completely into the field, attached by only the hilar structures. Exposure of the left lower lobe may be more difficult than exposure of the other lobes because of the overlying heart. With appropriate gentle traction on the pericardium, the left lower lobe can be exposed readily and brought into the operative field. Various techniques (e.g., surgical packs behind the hilum of the deflated lung to elevate the parenchyma to better visualize the lung) or technical aids (e.g., an internal mammary artery retractor to expose basilar tumors or posterior hilar left lower lobe masses) may be employed.

Posterolateral Thoracotomy

The posterolateral thoracotomy is a familiar and standard approach to pulmonary resection for carcinoma of the lung, although Urschel and Razzuk[44] have advocated median sternotomy for resection of lung carcinoma. Posterolateral thoracotomy may provide better exposure for metastases located posteriorly near the hilum on the left side. The surgeon is limited to one hemithorax. Rarely would bilateral thoracotomies be performed at the same operation.

TABLE 35–2. Algorithm for Management of Suspected Pulmonary Metastases

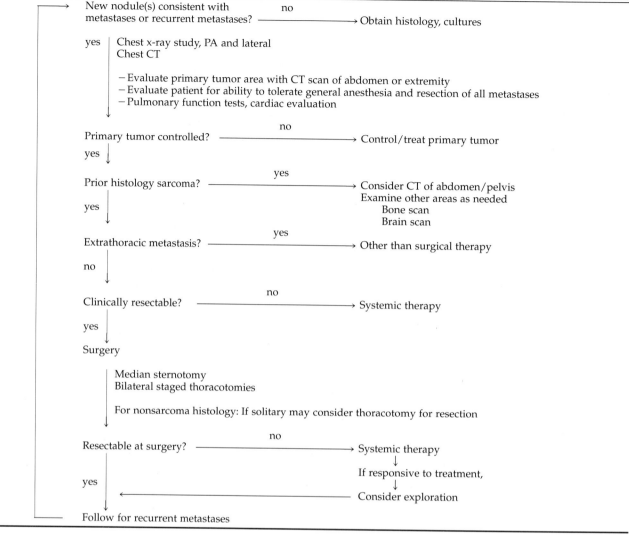

CT = computed tomography.

Video-Assisted Thoracic Surgery

VATS using high-resolution video imaging may be helpful for diagnosis, staging, and resection of metastases, as suggested by Kodama and colleagues[51] and Miller and associates[55]; however, its usefulness is limited because metastases can best be identified on the surface of the lung. Metastases within the lung parenchyma may be undetectable with this technique. Landreneau and associates[56] have described minimal morbidity and no mortality in 61 patients who underwent 85 thoracoscopic pulmonary resections. Lesions were small (<3 cm) and were located in the outer third of the lung parenchyma. Metastases in 18 patients were resected via thoracoscopy in this series. VATS was the only procedure performed in these patients. At present, this approach can be advocated only for diagnosis or staging of the extent of metastases (Fig. 35–4). Complications of VATS may include failure to resect all metastases, leaving positive margins, or pleural seeding with extraction of the metastasis.

Extended Resection of Pulmonary Metastases

Pneumonectomy or other extended resection of pulmonary metastases may be performed safely in selected patients, with some patients achieving long-term disease-free survival. Less than 3% of all patients undergoing resection of pulmonary metastases require such an extended resection. Putnam and associates[45] performed pneumonectomy or en bloc resection of pulmonary metastases with the chest wall or other thoracic structures such as the diaphragm, pericardium, or superior vena cava in a small percentage of patients, with good results. Nineteen patients had a pneumonectomy, and another 19 patients had other types of extended resection. The 5-year actuarial survival rate was 25%. The mortality rate was 5%, and the deaths occurred in those patients having pneumonectomy, often after undergoing multiple prior wedge resections for metastases.

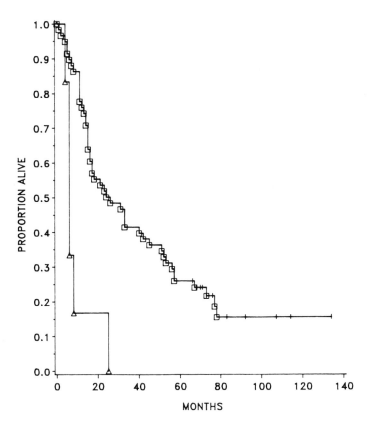

FIGURE 35–5. Overall survival following thoracotomy for resectable (□) and unresectable (Δ) metastases from adult soft tissue sarcomas. The median survival times were 25 months and 6 months, respectively (p = .0002, n = 69; eleven patients were unresectable).

PROGNOSIS AND SURVIVAL ANALYSIS

An evaluation of results of resection for pulmonary metastasectomy is difficult because numerous primary histologies are often combined. Although the identification of trends is helpful, a critical analysis of results and factors that influence survival depends on single primary histology (e.g., breast, colon, melanoma) or similar histology (e.g., soft tissue sarcomas) and sufficient numbers of patients. Prognostic indicators have been reviewed to assess their influence singularly and in combination on postresection survival in patients with pulmonary metastases and to assist clinically in better selecting appropriate patients for resection of pulmonary metastases. Age, gender, histology, grade, and location of the primary tumor, stage of primary tumor, disease-free survival time, number of nodules on preoperative radiologic studies, unilateral or bilateral metastases, tumor doubling time (TDT), and synchronous or metachronous metastases may be evaluated preoperatively. Postoperatively, resectability, technique of resection, nodal spread, number of metastases and location, re-resection post-thoracotomy disease-free survival, and overall survival may be examined.

Survival Analysis

Prognostic Variables

Initial pulmonary metastasectomies were performed on patients with single metastases and long disease-free intervals. Presumably, this reflected a favorable

tumor biology, and patients not meeting these criteria were excluded from thoracotomy. As experience with resection of pulmonary metastases grew, it became clear that patients not meeting these criteria could potentially benefit from pulmonary metastasectomy. Investigators have searched for clinical criteria that may predict a more favorable outcome. However, most reports were difficult to interpret because mixed histologies were analyzed together. More recently, investigators have attempted to report on homogeneous histologic groups in an attempt to determine prognostic factors to guide selection of patients for pulmonary metastasectomy. These prognostic factors include clinical, biologic, and molecular criteria that describe the biologic interaction between the metastases and the patient and the association of these metastases with prolonged survival. These prognostic indicators may be used to identify those patients who are most likely to benefit after resection of pulmonary metastases. To date, no single factor or group of factors has been found reliable enough to warrant exclusion of patients without other curative treatment options from resection.

Resectability

Resectability appears to be the most constant single variable reflecting prolonged post-thoracotomy survival (Fig. 35–5). Resectability is applicable to all histologic types. In all solid tumor histologies investigated to date, inability to perform complete resection at the time of thoracotomy predicts a shortened and often limited survival after thoracotomy. Despite the use of other modalities to treat residual disease, patients with disease not completely resectable survive for shorter intervals compared with patients undergoing complete resection.

Age, Gender, Location, and Stage of Primary Tumor

Age and gender do not usually influence post-thoracotomy survival and, generally, should not be considered as prognostic factors. In addition, postresection survival is not usually influenced by the specific anatomic location of the primary tumor. Postresection survival in patients with more advanced stage primary neoplasms does not usually differ from patients with earlier stage disease. Still, initial or primary stage may suggest the biologic aggressiveness of the tumor. Schlappack and colleagues[24] found that a negative nodal status predicted improved postresection survival for patients with breast cancer. McCormack and associates[57] found better post-thoracotomy survival in patients with Dukes' Stage A colorectal carcinoma (5-year survival rate, 37.5%) compared with Dukes' Stage C patients (5-year survival, 15%), although this was not confirmed by the recent study by McAfee and coworkers.[58] Gorenstein and associates[59] found that patients with earlier stage primary melanoma had a longer duration of survival following resection of pulmonary metastases than did patients with more advanced stage primary melanoma.

Disease-Free Interval

Disease-free interval is determined from the time of control of the primary tumor, usually by resection, to the time metastases are detected. The interval may be determined by the biologic aggressiveness of the tumor, but other unknown host and tumor factors may also play a role. In patients with osteogenic sarcoma,[60] soft tissue sarcoma,[61] colorectal carcinoma,[62] renal cell carcinoma,[63] and breast carcinoma,[64] a disease-free interval of more than 12 months is associated with prolonged post-thoracotomy survival.

Number of Nodules on Preoperative Studies

The number of nodules on preoperative studies has not been examined for all histologies to date. In patients with osteogenic sarcomas, improved post-thoracotomy survival was found in patients with three or less nodules on linear tomography.[65] In patients with soft tissue sarcomas, four or less nodules predicted improved outcome (Fig. 35–6).[52] Other studies have described similar findings for these same histologies.[66, 67]

Number of Metastases Resected

In general, patients with fewer metastases found and resected at thoracotomy experience a longer post-thoracotomy survival than do patients with numerous metastases. In patients with osteogenic sarcoma, pa-

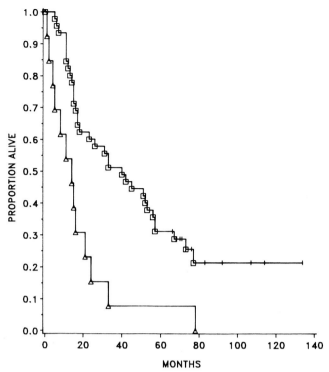

FIGURE 35–6. Patients with three or fewer nodules identified on preoperative computed tomogram of the chest (□) had a better survival (40 months median survival rate) than patients with four or more nodules (Δ). (Fourteen months median survival, p = .0006.)

tients with four or less nodules resected at thoracotomy experience longer survival.[65] In patients with soft tissue sarcomas, less than 16 resected nodules predicted a more favorable outcome.[52] In patients with Ewing's sarcoma, less than four nodules also predicted a more favorable survival following complete resection.[68] Patients with colorectal metastases and a single nodule experienced prolonged survival compared with others.[58] However, in patients with breast carcinoma,[64] renal cell carcinomas[69] and melanomas,[59] the survival was not influenced by the number of nodules resected.

Unilateral or Bilateral Metastases

Initial pulmonary metastasectomies were performed on patients with single unilateral metastases. Subsequent data have shown that survival is not affected by bilaterality.

Tumor Doubling Time

The use of TDT to select patients for pulmonary metastasectomy was first described by Joseph,[70] based on observation by Collins.[71] Its prognostic significance has been analyzed for a variety of histologies (Fig. 35–7). Previously, doubling times were calculated by plotting the diameter of the largest nodule on semilogarithm paper using measurements made at least 14 days apart. A mathematical formula may more accurately determine the TDT by minimizing graphical error:

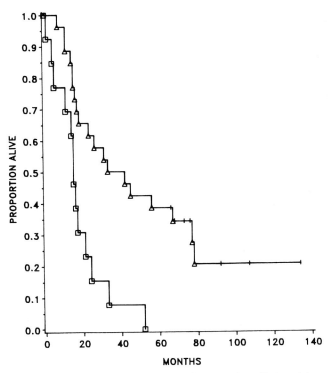

FIGURE 35–7. Tumor doubling times of greater than 40 days (□) were compared with those with doubling rates of less than 40 days (△). (The median survival was 37 months and 15 months, respectively; p = .002.)

$$\text{TDT} = \text{T}\left(\ln\frac{2}{3} \times \ln\frac{\text{M2}}{\text{M1}}\right)$$

where T = time interval between measurements, M1 = measurement 1, and M2 = measurement 2. Simplified, it becomes:

$$\text{TDT} = 0.231\,\text{T} - \ln\left(\frac{\text{M2}}{\text{M1}}\right)$$

The use of this formula assumes an exponential growth curve throughout the clinical life of the metastases. In biologic systems, gompertzian growth curves may more accurately describe patterns of growth.

In patients with pulmonary osteogenic sarcoma, no correlation could be found between TDT and post-thoracotomy survival.[65] In some reports[52] but not others,[67] a TDT of greater than 20 days predicted a more favorable post-thoracotomy survival in patients with soft tissue sarcomas.

Response to Chemotherapy

Intuitively, one would predict that patients with pulmonary metastases showing a favorable response to chemotherapy would experience a prolonged post-thoracotomy survival. In patients with metastatic soft tissue sarcomas, Lanza and coworkers[26] found no correlation between response to preoperative chemotherapy and post-thoracotomy survival. Twenty-six patients were treated with intensive preoperative

chemotherapy prior to pulmonary metastasectomy. Two patients were found to have benign disease at thoracotomy. Of the remaining 24 patients, five achieved a complete radiographic response, but all had recurrence in the lungs and were referred for resection. Seven patients achieved a partial response and had residual disease resected. Twelve patients experienced either no response or disease progression during chemotherapy and were referred for surgery. The post-thoracotomy disease-free interval and overall survival did not differ significantly between the three groups (Fig. 35–8). Additional data are needed to determine the optimal use of chemotherapy in patients undergoing pulmonary metastasectomy.

RESULTS OF RESECTION OF PULMONARY METASTASES

Until recently, most reports describing pulmonary metastasectomy analyzed results for a variety of histologies combined. Owing to this factor, analysis of outcome was difficult, because natural history and survival following resection may vary widely with histologic type. Critical analysis of results and evaluation of factors that may influence survival depend on careful evaluation of patients with homogeneous histologies.

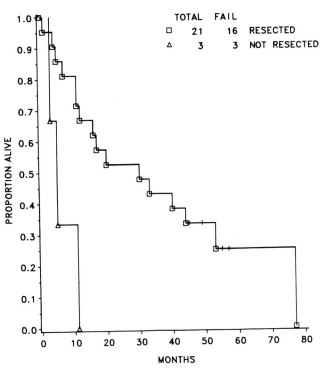

FIGURE 35–8. Survival after thoracotomy for patients with resectable lesions (□) treated with salvage chemotherapy (30 months median survival) was better than that for patients with unresectable lesions (△). (Six months median survival, p = .0053). Even when treated with chemotherapy, unresectable patients had poor survival rates.

Sarcomas

Sarcomas preferentially metastasize to the lungs. These metastases commonly are isolated and resectable and do not consistently represent diffuse systemic or untreatable spread of the primary sarcoma. Surgery alone cannot control micrometastases; however, selected patients with isolated pulmonary metastases have prolonged survival after resection of their metastases. These patients may represent a unique population with a particular tumor biology. After complete resection of pulmonary metastases (including multiple and bilateral metastases), long-term survival (>5 years) may be expected in approximately one-third of patients.

Osteogenic Sarcoma

The major site of metastases in patients with osteogenic sarcoma is the lungs. Prior to the development of effective chemotherapeutic agents, over 90% of patients with this disease died of pulmonary metastases. In 1971, Martini and associates[7] reported a series of 22 patients treated with aggressive pulmonary resection. Prior to this time, patients with osteosarcoma metastatic to the lungs had been offered pulmonary metastasectomy on a selected basis, mostly only to those patients with a limited number of nodules who had a long disease-free interval. In 1965, a policy of aggressive metastasectomy was initiated at Memorial Sloan-Kettering Cancer Center. Twenty-two patients underwent a total of 59 thoracotomies, during which 152 total metastatic nodules were resected. The 3-year absolute survival rate was 45%. Marcove and associates[72] updated the Memorial Sloan-Kettering Cancer Center experience with metastatic osteosarcoma in 1975. The 5-year survival rate of 22 patients undergoing aggressive pulmonary metastasectomy was compared with that of a control cohort of 145 patients who were treated without thoracotomy. The 5-year survival rate of the patients treated with aggressive metastasectomy was 31%, whereas that of patients treated without thoracotomy was only 2%.

The development of effective chemotherapeutic regimens improved the outlook of patients with metastatic osteogenic sarcoma. Giritsky and coworkers[73] reported improved survival in patients who were treated with chemotherapy combined with aggressive resection and irradiation. Twelve patients received intensive chemotherapy following amputation, followed by a total of 19 thoracotomies for the group for pulmonary metastasectomy. Seventeen of the 19 patients were disease free at thoracotomy. The 3-year survival rate for the group was 57.8%, which compared favorably with historical controls. More recently, Skinner and colleagues[74] reported similar improved outcomes in patients treated with aggressive chemotherapy combined with pulmonary metastasectomy. Two hundred and forty-seven patients with Stage I osteogenic sarcoma were treated at the University of California at Los Angeles (UCLA) between 1971 and 1991 using four sequential treatment strategies. Group I was treated with surgery alone, whereas groups II through IV received various combinations of chemotherapeutic agents. Group I experienced a 92% incidence of pulmonary metastases, of which only 17% underwent resection. The 5-year survival rate for this group of patients was zero. The incidence of lung metastases in the most recent group dropped to 31%, and most patients (82%) underwent resection of metastases. The 5-year actuarial survival rate in this group was 41%.

Carter and associates,[75] Snyder and colleagues,[76] and Belli and coworkers[77] have described similar favorable survival times with the use of chemotherapy and aggressive pulmonary resection. Putnam and associates[65] reported on a group of 80 patients with osteogenic sarcoma treated with aggressive pulmonary metastasectomy over an 8-year period at the National Cancer Institute and used multivariate analysis to determine prognostic factors. Forty-three of the 80 patients developed pulmonary metastases as the initial site of failure, and 39 underwent one or more thoracotomies for resection. The actuarial 5-year survival rate of the 43 patients was 40%. By regression analysis, prognostic factors that influenced survival included the number of nodules on preoperative tomograms, the disease-free interval, resectability, and the number of metastases resected at thoracotomy. The single most useful predictor of a favorable postthoracotomy survival was the presence of three or fewer nodules on preoperative linear tomography.

Long-term follow-up has been reported in patients who appear to be cured following aggressive pulmonary metastasectomy. Beattie and colleagues[78] reported a 67% 19-year survival rate in patients surviving 10 years or more despite multiple resections and as many as nine thoracotomies. However, a significant proportion of 10-year survivors was noted to develop secondary malignancies during the second decade of follow-up.

Soft Tissue Sarcoma

The majority of patients with soft tissue sarcomas who fail treatment have recurrences in the lungs. Potter and colleagues[79] described patterns of recurrence in a large group of patients with soft tissue sarcomas treated at the National Cancer Institute over a 7-year period. Of 563 total patients, 307 were treated for cure with surgery alone or in combination with chemotherapy and radiation therapy. One hundred and seven patients developed recurrent disease with a median disease-free interval of 18 months. Isolated pulmonary metastases were the most common pattern of recurrence (52%), followed by isolated local recurrence (20%). Patients not rendered surgically disease free following the first recurrence had a median survival of only 7.4 months, whereas 45% of patients rendered surgically disease free at first recurrence were disease free at a median follow-up of 28 months. A similar experience was reported by Huth and Elber.[80] They treated 255 patients with combined modality therapy. Eighty-five of 255 patients suffered recurrences, of which 43 were confined to the lungs.

Putnam and associates[52] described predictors of improved postoperative survival in patients undergoing resection of pulmonary metastases from soft tissue sarcomas. The most significant predictors of survival were a TDT of more than 20 days, four or less nodules on preoperative linear tomography, and a disease-free interval of more than 12 months. Combining the three prognostic factors improved the predictive accuracy above that found using the factors individually. Roth and colleagues[61] further analyzed prognostic factors in patients with soft tissue and osteogenic sarcomas to determine the general applicability of factors between the two histologic groups. The number of metastases on preoperative tomography was found to be the best predictor of survival for both patients with soft tissue sarcomas and those with osteogenic sarcomas, whereas other factors could not be generalized for the two groups.

Casson and associates[81] examined predictors of 5-year survival in a group of 58 patients undergoing pulmonary metastasectomy for soft tissue sarcomas. Fifteen patients (25%) survived 5 years. Independent prognostic indicators associated with improved survival included a TDT of more than 40 days, unilateral disease on preoperative studies, three or less nodules on chest CT scan, two or fewer resected nodules, and histology of malignant fibrous histiocytoma (Fig. 35–9).

Ewing's Sarcoma

Ewing's sarcoma is the second most common childhood bone tumor, exceeded in frequency only by osteogenic sarcoma. The lung is the most common site of metastatic disease at presentation and is also the most common site of initial relapse. Lanza and coworkers[68] reported results in 19 patients who underwent thoracotomy for suspected pulmonary metastases from Ewing's sarcoma over a 20-year period. Three patients (16%) were found to have benign nodules and 10 patients (53%) were rendered disease free; however, six patients (32%) were found to have unresectable disease at thoracotomy. The actuarial 5-year survival rate for the 10 patients rendered disease free was 15%, and their median post-thoracotomy survival was 28 months. In contrast, the median post-thoracotomy survival of the six patients not rendered disease free was only 12 months, and no patient was alive 22 months following thoracotomy (p2 = 0.004). Patients undergoing resection of fewer than four malignant nodules survived longer than those undergoing resection of four or more nodules.

Breast Carcinomas

Systemic chemotherapy has been shown to prolong survival of patients with breast cancer when used as adjuvant treatment following complete resection of primary tumor. The survival of patients with documented metastatic disease still remains limited. Most

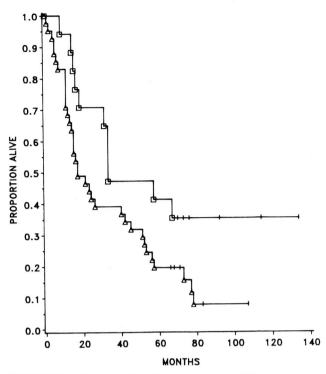

FIGURE 35–9. Patients with histology of malignant fibrous histiocytoma (□) had a longer survival (33 months median survival) than all other histologic types combined (△). (Seventeen months' survival, p = .04.)

patients with breast cancer develop visceral or bone metastases in unresectable sites, but the lung is the site of first recurrence in approximately 12%. Schlappack and associates[24] described the survival of 50 breast cancer patients whose first recurrence was in the lungs and who were treated with chemotherapy or hormonal therapy. Only three patients were referred for pulmonary resection from the group. Eleven patients achieved a complete clinical response, three of which were surgical. The median survival of the group from the time of detection of pulmonary metastases was only 13 months. Patients with solitary metastases had a median survival of 11.5 months compared with 10.5 months for patients with multiple metastases. Patients with a disease-free interval of more than 18 months had a median survival of 15 months compared with 8 months for those patients with a disease-free interval of less than 18 months. Patients who were estrogen-receptor positive survived longer (median 21 months) than those who were estrogen-receptor negative (median 4.5 months).

In contrast, Lanza and colleagues[64] described significant long-term survival in 44 patients who underwent surgical resection of isolated pulmonary metastases from carcinoma of the breast from 1981 through 1991. The 44 women underwent a total of 47 thoracotomies with no operative mortality and only three minor postoperative complications (3 of 47, 6.4%). The median post-thoracotomy survival was 47 ± 5.5 months and the actuarial 5-year survival rate was 49.5% (Fig. 35–10). Patients with a disease-free interval of more than 12 months had a median survival of

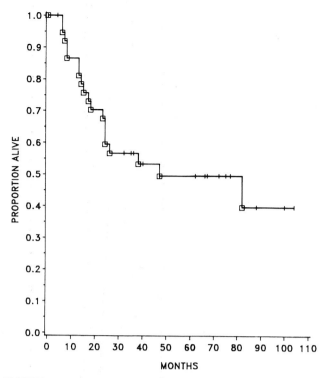

FIGURE 35–10. Overall actuarial survival for patients with breast carcinoma following surgical resection of pulmonary metastases. (Forty-seven months median survival; 37 patients; 18 deaths.)

82 ± 6 months and an actuarial 5-year survival rate of 57%, whereas patients with disease-free intervals of less than 12 months had a median survival of only 15 ± 3.6 months and 0% 5-year survival rate (see Fig. 35–4). Patients who were estrogen-receptor positive tended to have a longer post-thoracotomy survival time, but the differences did not reach statistical significance (p = .098). Other analyzed variables, including the number of metastases resected and axillary nodal status, did not predict outcome. The authors concluded that pulmonary metastasectomy could be performed safely in patients with breast cancer with isolated pulmonary metastases and could result in significant long-term survival. Staren and associates[82] compared the outcome of 33 patients with metastatic breast cancer isolated to the lung treated primarily with pulmonary metastasectomy with that of 30 patients treated primarily with chemohormonal therapy. The mean survival in the surgical group was significantly longer than that in the medical group, even when only those patients with single pulmonary metastases were compared (58 months versus 34 months). Similarly, the overall 5-year survival rate was significantly better in the surgical group (36%) than in the medical group (11%). They concluded that surgical resection should be strongly considered for patients with isolated pulmonary metastases from carcinoma of the breast.

Colorectal Carcinomas

The survival of patients with metastatic colorectal cancers remains limited, and nonsurgical complete re-

sponses using available chemotherapeutic agents remain elusive. Although the majority of patients will fail with liver metastases or with disseminated disease, a proportion will develop only isolated pulmonary metastases. The optimal treatment for these patients remains unknown.

Mansel and coworkers[83] described the experience at the Mayo Clinic with pulmonary metastasectomy for patients with colorectal cancer. Sixty-six patients underwent pulmonary resection over a 10-year period. The median post-thoracotomy survival was 3.5 years, and the cumulative survival rate at 5 years was 38%. Patients with solitary metastases survived longer than those with multiple metastases. This experience has been recently updated by McAfee and associates,[58] who reported on 139 patients who underwent pulmonary metastasectomy for colorectal cancer with an operative mortality of 1.5% at the same institution. The overall 5-year actuarial survival rate was 30.5%. Patients with low (<4 mg/ml) levels of preoperative carcinoembryonic antigen and a single metastasis survived longer than others.

Goya and colleagues[84] reported 10-year results following resection of pulmonary metastases from colorectal primaries. Sixty-two patients underwent thoracotomy, with cumulative 5- and 10-year survival rates of 42% and 22%, respectively. Four of 13 patients who survived 5 years died of metastases during later follow-up. Patients with solitary metastases smaller than 3 cm in diameter had more favorable survival times.

Although resection of hepatic metastases is the accepted treatment for patients with isolated resectable liver metastases, little data exist comparing results of this procedure with those for resection of metastases present in other sites. Sauter and coworkers[85] compared the survival of 31 patients undergoing hepatic resection for metastatic colorectal cancer with that of 18 patients undergoing resection of isolated pulmonary metastases. The 5-year actuarial survival rate was 47% for patients undergoing pulmonary resection and 19% for patients undergoing hepatic resection. Patients with single pulmonary metastases experienced the longest post-thoracotomy survival.

It has been postulated that differing patterns of venous drainage for colon and rectal cancer may determine patterns of tumor recurrence and therefore survival following pulmonary metastasectomy. Scheele and associates[86] compared the post-thoracotomy survival of 25 patients with primary tumor in the portal drainage bed with that of 19 patients with primaries in the middle and lower rectum (systemic drainage bed). Although patients with colon primaries tended to experience a longer post-thoracotomy survival when compared with patients with rectal primaries, the differences in survival were not statistically significant. They concluded that the site of the primary tumor cannot accurately predict survival following complete resection of pulmonary metastases from colorectal carcinomas.

Recurrence in the lung may occur following pulmonary metastasectomy for colorectal cancer. Mori and coworkers[87] reported on 35 patients undergoing pulmonary metastasectomy with a 38% 5-year survival rate. Seven of the 35 patients underwent two or more resections for pulmonary recurrences, with four of seven patients remaining disease free for a mean of 33.5 months (range 5 to 58 months) following thoracotomy. Repeat pulmonary metastasectomy may further extend survival in selected patients with isolated pulmonary metastases from colorectal primaries.

Renal Cell Carcinomas

Barney and Churchill[4] first reported long-term survival following pulmonary metastasectomy for renal cell carcinoma. Since that initial report, various authors have described their own experiences. Katzenstein and coworkers[88] reported on 44 patients with pulmonary metastases from renal cell carcinomas who were treated with pulmonary resection. The authors concluded that resection of the primary tumor was warranted if the metastases were unilateral. Mayo and colleagues[89] reported a 42% five-year survival rate and a 25% 10-year survival rate. Dernevick and associates[90] reported a 21% 5-year survival rate in 33 patients who were treated with pulmonary metastasectomy for renal cell carcinoma. Patients with a disease-free interval of less than 1 year had a shortened post-thoracotomy survival. Pogrebniak and coworkers[91] more recently reported the experience from the National Cancer Institute on 23 patients over a 6-year period who underwent metastasectomy for pulmonary metastases from renal cell carcinoma. Eighteen patients also received interleukin-2–based immunotherapy prior to resection. Mean survival following resection was 43 months and did not correlate with the number of tomographic nodules, the number of nodules resected, or the preoperative disease-free interval. Patients who were disease free at thoracotomy survived significantly longer than patients who were not rendered disease free, with two of 15 patients whose disease was completely resected reported alive without disease more than 45 months following thoracotomy.

Testicular Neoplasms

Testicular cancer is a potentially curable neoplasm that has become a model for curable neoplasms using combined modality treatment. Cytoreductive surgery has been used effectively in patients with testicular neoplasms who do not achieve a complete response following chemotherapy. Accurate serum markers have predicted viable tumor burden and facilitated therapeutic decision making. Because metastatic lesions that do not completely respond to chemotherapy may be of a benign histologic type (mature teratoma), resection also provides diagnostic information that is important in treatment planning.

Stahel and coworkers[92] reported results on 15 patients with nonseminomatous testicular cancer who underwent surgical resection of residual disease following chemotherapy. Nine patients had disease in the lungs or the mediastinum. The presence of ne-

crotic tumor, mature teratoma, or immature or mature teratomas with only foci of malignancy predicted a favorable outcome. Whillis and associates[93] reported on 72 patients treated for metastatic nonseminomatous testicular cancer over an 11-year period. Thirty-seven patients did not achieve a complete response to chemotherapy. Sixteen of these patients had normal tumor markers and had residual disease resected surgically, nine of whom remain disease free (56%), including two patients who were found to have malignant teratoma in the resected specimen.

Gynecologic Neoplasms

A small proportion of patients with primary gynecologic neoplasms develop isolated pulmonary metastases. Fuller and colleagues[94] reported on 15 patients treated with pulmonary metastasectomy over a 39-year period at the Massachusetts General Hospital. The histologies varied, with two patients having ovarian primaries, six patients having cervical primaries, three patients having endometrial primaries, two patients having uterine sarcomas, and two patients having choriocarcinomas. The 5-year actuarial survival rate was 36%. A prolonged disease-free interval and a solitary pulmonary lesion of less than 4 cm predicted a better post-thoracotomy survival. Levenbach and coworkers[95] reported results in 45 patients with primary uterine sarcomas treated with pulmonary metastasectomy over a 29-year period at Memorial Sloan-Kettering Cancer Center. Seventy-one per cent had unilateral metastases, 51% had single metastases, and 70% had nodules larger than 2 cm. Complete resection of metastatic disease was achieved in only 64% of patients. The actuarial 5-year post-thoracotomy survival rate was 54%, and the 10-year survival rate was 35%. Unilaterality predicted improved post-thoracotomy survival. Smaller numbers of patients with primary cervical cancer[96] or gestational choriocarcinomas,[97, 98] who were treated in part with pulmonary metastasectomy, have also been described.

Head and Neck Neoplasms

Patients with primary tumors of the head and neck have an increased risk for developing other primaries of the aerodigestive tract. Differentiation between primary and secondary pulmonary neoplasms can be difficult in this population. Rendina and colleagues[99] reported on 11 patients with primary laryngeal tumors who developed pulmonary lesions. Three patients (27%) were found to have primary lung cancer at thoracotomy. Six patients were treated with metastasectomy, four of whom remain disease free after a mean of 46 months (range 40 to 55 months) following thoracotomy. Two patients were not resected, and both were dead of disease at 12 months. Mazer and associates[100] reported their experience with 44 patients treated at M.D. Anderson Cancer Center. The cumulative 5-year survival rate following pulmonary resection was 43%. Patients with primary laryngeal tumors experienced the best post-thoracotomy survival. Locoregional recurrence, the stage of the primary neoplasm, and the presence of multiple metastases did not predict a shortened survival. Unfavorable prognostic factors were the presence of nodal metastases at the primary site, the presence of mediastinal lymph node metastases, and the presence of an oral cavity primary. Finley and associates[101] reviewed the experience with 58 patients who had primary squamous cell cancer of the head and neck and pulmonary metastases treated with metastasectomy at Roswell Park Cancer Institute. Twenty-four of the 58 patients underwent thoracotomy for resection of metastases. Four were found to have primary tumor of the lung. Of the remaining 20 patients, 18 (90%) were rendered disease free at thoracotomy and experienced a 29% actuarial five-year survival. The preoperative disease-free interval predicted post-thoracotomy survival while the number of resected metastases was not predictive.

Melanoma

Failure patterns of patients with malignant melanoma remain unpredictable, and the majority of patients develop disseminated disease. Effective systemic therapy for these patients remains elusive. Patients with limited resectable systemic disease likely benefit from resection.[102]

Mathiesen and coworkers[103] examined the results in 33 patients undergoing pulmonary resection for suspected metastatic melanoma over a 21-year period. Eleven patients (33%) were found to have benign disease at thoracotomy, and 10 patients could not be rendered disease free. Twelve patients underwent complete resection of metastatic melanoma, with a median post-thoracotomy survival of 12 months (range 3 to 35 months). There were no 5-year survivals. Based on this experience, the authors concluded that the major role for surgery in these patients was diagnostic. Pogrebniak and associates[104] examined the National Cancer Institute experience over a 16-year period. Forty-nine patients underwent thoracotomy for presumed metastatic melanoma. Sixteen patients (32%) were found to have benign disease at thoracotomy. The median survival of patients with malignant disease was 13 months, and two patients who underwent resection of a single nodule remained disease free at 88 and 120 months, respectively, post-thoracotomy. The duration of post-thoracotomy survival did not correlate with the depth of the primary tumor, lymph node status, disease-free interval, or number of nodules on preoperative tomograms.

Wong and colleagues[105] examined the experience at UCLA with 47 patients over a 15-year period. The median survival of the 47 patients was 19 months, and the actuarial 5-year survival rate was 25%. Thirty-eight patients who were rendered disease free at thoracotomy had improved survival (median, 24 months; 5-year survival rate, 31%) when compared with patients not rendered disease free (median, 6 months; 5 years, 0%). The use of adjuvant therapy or the disease-free interval did not appear to influence the length of post-thoracotomy survival.

Gorenstein and coworkers[59] examined the experience at M.D. Anderson Cancer Center. Fifty-six patients underwent 65 pulmonary resections for metastatic melanoma over an 8-year period. In one-half of the patients undergoing resection, the lungs were the initial site of failure. Fifty-four of 56 patients (96%) were rendered disease free at thoracotomy, and there were no operative deaths. The median post-thoracotomy survival was 18 months, and the actuarial 5-year survival rate was 25% (Fig. 35–11). Patients who initially had pulmonary metastases had a median survival of 30 months, compared with 17 months for patients with initial locoregional failure (Fig. 35–12).

Harpole and associates[106] have examined the extensive experience with malignant melanoma at Duke University Medical Center. Over a 20-year period, 7564 patients were treated, of whom 945 patients (12%) developed pulmonary metastases. Resection of pulmonary disease predicted improved survival. Patients with a single pulmonary nodule survived longer following resection than did patients with a single nodule treated without surgery.

Childhood Tumors

Osteogenic Sarcomas

The majority of patients treated for osteogenic sarcoma are children or young adults. The results of surgical resection of osteogenic sarcoma are discussed in a previous section (see section on Osteogenic Sarcoma).

Wilms' Tumor

Recent advances in the treatment of children with Wilms' tumor have improved the outcome in this disease. Pulmonary metastases may be safely resected in children with isolated lesions, but a recent report by Green and colleagues[107] failed to show a survival advantage for children treated with pulmonary resection compared with those treated with chemotherapy and whole lung irradiation.

Hepatoblastoma

The outlook for children who develop recurrent disease from hepatoblastoma remains poor. Feusner and associates[108] examined the role of resection of isolated pulmonary metastases in children with initial Stage I hepatoblastoma. Ten of 33 children developed recurrent disease; in six of the children, the recurrence was isolated to the lungs. Three of the six patients remain disease free 64 to 104 months following pulmonary metastasectomy. Similar favorable results were reported by Black and colleagues.[109]

RECURRENT PULMONARY METASTASES

The lungs remain the most common site of failure following pulmonary metastasectomy in patients with

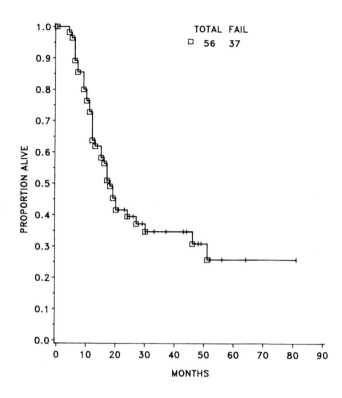

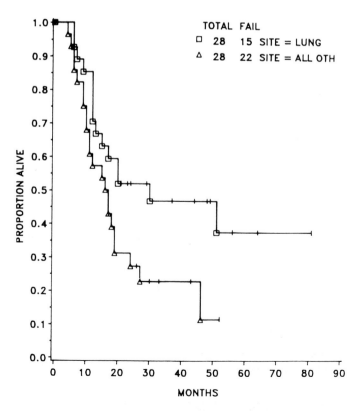

FIGURE 35–11. Overall actuarial survival for patients with melanoma following surgical resection of pulmonary metastases. (Eighteen months median survival.)

FIGURE 35–12. Survival for patients with melanoma following surgical resection of pulmonary metastases. (□ = Initial recurrence in the lungs; Δ = initial recurrence outside the lungs [p = .037; logrank].)

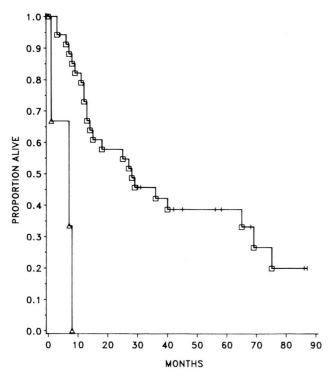

FIGURE 35–13. Survival of patients following thoracotomy and resection of recurrent pulmonary metastases from soft tissue sarcomas. Patients with resectable recurrent metastases (□) had a longer survival (28 months median) after resection than unresectable patients (Δ). (Seven months median survival, p = .0001). Survival in patients with resectable lesions was similar to that in patients with initial (nonrecurrent) metastases.

sarcomatous metastases. Rizzoni and associates[110] examined the results of repeat pulmonary metastasectomy in patients with soft tissue sarcoma. Twenty-nine patients underwent two or more resections (a total of 40 resections) over a 7-year period, with no operative deaths and three complications (7.5%). Complete resectability and a disease-free interval of more than 6 months predicted improved survival. In addition, the TDT of the first recurrence and the pres-

ence of three or fewer lung nodules on linear tomography prior to first resection predicted the length of survival following subsequent resections. The post-thoracotomy actuarial survival rates for patients undergoing one, two, three, or more resections did not differ significantly (see Fig. 35–6). Pogrebniak and colleagues[69] updated this experience. The actuarial median survival following repeat metastasectomy was 25 months in patients rendered disease free at

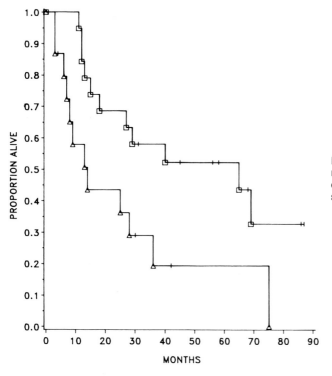

FIGURE 35–14. Survival following resection of a solitary recurrent metastasis (□) (65 months median survival) was better than for resection of two or more recurrent metastases (Δ). (Fourteen months median survival, p = .01.)

repeat metastasectomy. Casson and coworkers[111] confirmed these findings in a separate group of patients with adult soft tissue sarcoma treated at M.D. Anderson Cancer Center. Twenty-nine patients underwent resection of recurrent pulmonary metastases. The median survival of patients rendered disease free at second resection was 28 months (Fig. 35–13). Patients undergoing resection of a single recurrent pulmonary metastasis had a median post-thoracotomy survival of 65 months, whereas patients who had two or more nodules resected had a median survival only 14 months following the second resection (Fig. 35–14).

CONCLUSIONS

Surgical resection of isolated pulmonary metastases can be performed safely in patients from a spectrum of histologic tumor types. Uncontrolled data suggest that a subset of patients obtain long-term survival following complete resection of metastatic disease confined to the lungs. For the majority of malignant solid tumor histologic types, long-term survival has remained elusive with non-surgical treatment modalities. To date, no randomized study has provided definitive data comparing resection of isolated pulmonary metastases with other forms of therapy. In addition, clinical prognostic variables have not proved accurate enough to allow exclusion of otherwise viable patients from pulmonary metastasectomy. As such, resection of pulmonary metastases remains a viable option for the treatment of patients with isolated pulmonary metastases.

SELECTED REFERENCES

Martini N, Huvos A, Mike G, et al: Multiple pulmonary resections in the treatment of osteogenic sarcoma. Ann Thorac Surg 12:271–280, 1971.
    One of the first studies to suggest that pulmonary metastases could be resected on multiple occasions with associated survival.
Putnam JB, Roth JA, Wesley MN, et al: Analysis of prognostic factors in patients undergoing resection of pulmonary metastases from soft tissue sarcomas. J Thorac Cardiovasc Surg 87:260–267, 1984.
    An accurate and rapid method to identify preoperatively those patients who will maximally benefit from resection of pulmonary metastases.
Roth JA, Putnam JB, Wesley MN, Rosenberg SA: Differing determinants of prognostic factors in patients undergoing resection of pulmonary metastases from soft tissue sarcomas. J Thorac Cardiovasc Surg 87:260–267, 1983.
    This paper shows that the prognostic factors vary among patients with pulmonary metastases.

REFERENCES

1. Meade RH: A History of Thoracic Surgery. 1st Ed. Springfield, Illinois, Charles C Thomas, 1961, pp 194–197.
2. Kronlein RU: Ueber Lungenchirirugie. Berlin Klin Wochenschr 9:129–132, 1884.
3. Torek F: Removal of metastatic carcinoma of the lung and mediastinum: Suggestions as to technic. Arch Surg 21:1416–1421, 1930.
4. Barney JD, Churchill EJ: Adenocarcinoma of the kidney with metastasis to the lung cured by nephrectomy and lobectomy. J Urol 42:269–276, 1939.
5. Alexander J, Haight C: Pulmonary resection for solitary metastatic sarcoma and carcinoma. Surg Gynecol Obstet 85:129–146, 1947.
6. Ehrenhaft JL, Lawrence MS, Sevsindy DM: Pulmonary resections for metastatic lesions. Arch Surg 77:606, 1958.
7. Martini N, Huvos A, Mike G, et al: Multiple pulmonary resections in the treatment of osteogenic sarcoma. Ann Thorac Surg 12:271–280, 1971.
8. Putnam JB Jr, Roth JA: Prognostic indicators in patients with pulmonary metastases. Semin Surg Oncol 6:291–296, 1990.
9. Goldstraw P, Walbaum PR: Hypertrophic pulmonary osteoarthropathy and its occurrence with pulmonary metastases from renal carcinoma. Thorax 31:205, 1976.
10. Duda RB, Beatty JD, Kokal WA, et al: Radiographic evaluation for pulmonary metastases in sarcoma patients. J Surg Oncol 38:271–274, 1988.
11. Roth JA, Pass HI, Wesley MN, et al: Comparison of median sternotomy and thoracotomy for resection of pulmonary metastases in patients with adult soft-tissue sarcomas. Ann Thorac Surg 42:134–138, 1986.
12. DiMarco AF, Briones B: Is CT performed too often? (Editorial.) Chest 103:985, 1993.
13. Lien HH, Lindskold L, Fossa SD, Aass N: Computed tomography and conventional radiography in intrathoracic metastases from non-seminomatous testicular tumor. Acta Radiol 29:547–549, 1988.
14. Chang AE, Schaner EG, Conkle DM, et al: Evaluation of computed tomography in the detection of pulmonary metastases: A prospective study. Cancer 43:913–916, 1979.
15. Pass HI, Dwyer A, Makuch R, Roth JA: Detection of pulmonary metastases in patients with osteogenic and soft-tissue sarcomas: The superiority of CT scans compared with conventional linear tomograms using dynamic analysis. J Clin Oncol 3:1261–1265, 1985.
16. Johnson H Jr, Fantone J, Flye MW: Histological evaluation of the nodules resected in the treatment of pulmonary metastatic disease. J Surg Oncol 21:1–4, 1982.
17. Cahan WG, Castro EB, Hajdu SI: The significance of a solitary lung shadow in patients with colon carcinoma. Cancer 33:414–421, 1974.
18. Cahan WG, Castro EB: Significance of a solitary lung shadow in patients with breast cancer. Ann Surg 181:131–143, 1975.
19. Gupta NC, Frank AR, Dewan NA, et al: Solitary pulmonary nodules: Detection of malignancy with PET with 2-[F-18]-fluoro-2-deoxy-D-glucose. Radiology 184:441, 1992.
20. Marina NM, Pratt CB, Rao BN, et al: Improved prognosis of children with osteosarcoma metastatic to the lung(s) at the time of diagnosis. Cancer 70:2722–2727, 1992.
21. Pastorino U, Gasparini M, Valente M, et al: Primary childhood osteosarcoma: The role of salvage surgery. Ann Oncol 3(Suppl 2):S43–S46, 1992.
22. Bacci G, Picci P, Briccoli A, et al: Osteosarcoma of the extremity metastatic at presentation: Results achieved in 26 patients treated with combined therapy (primary chemotherapy followed by simultaneous resection of the primary and metastatic lesions). Tumori 78:200–206, 1992.
23. Glasser DB, Lane JM, Huvos AG, et al: Survival, prognosis, and therapeutic response in osteogenic sarcoma. The Memorial Hospital experience. Cancer 69:698–708, 1992.
24. Schlappack OK, Baur M, Steger G, et al: The clinical course of lung metastases from breast cancer. Klin Wochenschr 66:790–795, 1988.
25. Kim B, Louie AC: Surgical resection following interleukin 2 therapy for metastatic renal cell carcinoma prolongs remission. Arch Surg 127:1343–1349, 1992.
26. Lanza LA, Putnam JB Jr, Benjamin RS, Roth JA: Response to chemotherapy does not predict survival after resection of sarcomatous pulmonary metastases. Ann Thorac Surg 51:219–224, 1991.
27. Baeza MR, Barkley HT, Fernandez CH: Total lung irradiation in the treatment of pulmonary metastases. Radiology 116:151, 1975.
28. Burgers JM, van Glabbeke M, Busson A, et al: Osteosarcoma of the limbs. Report of the EORTC-SIOP 03 trial 20781 investi-

gating the value of adjuvant treatment with chemotherapy and/or prophylactic lung irradiation. Cancer 61:1024–1031, 1988.

29. Appelqvist P, Koikkalainen K, Tala P, Kuisman A: Surgical treatment of pulmonary metastases. Int Surg 64:13–16, 1979.

30. McCormack PM, Martini N: The changing role of surgery for pulmonary metastases. Ann Thorac Surg 28:139–145, 1979.

31. Mountain CF, McMurtrey MJ, Hermes KE: Surgery for pulmonary metastasis: A 20-year experience. Ann Thorac Surg 38:323–330, 1984.

32. Wilkins EW Jr, Head JM, Burke JF: Pulmonary resection for metastatic neoplasms in the lung. Experience of the Massachusetts General Hospital. Am J Surg 135:480, 1978.

33. Wright JO III, Brandt B III, Ehrenhaft JL: Results of pulmonary resection for metastatic lesions. J Thorac Cardiovasc Surg 83:94–99, 1982.

34. Morrow CE, Vassilopoulos PP, Grage TB: Surgical resection for metastatic neoplasms of the lung: Experience at the University of Minnesota Hospitals. Cancer 45:2981–2985, 1980.

35. Marks P, Ferag MA, Ashraf H: Rationale for the surgical treatment of pulmonary metastases. Thorax 36:679, 1981.

36. Valente M, Pastorino U, Gandi C, et al: Secondary lung cancer resection with curative intent: Causes of success and failure and prognostic factors. Tumori 68:337, 1986.

37. van Dongen JA, Hart AA, Jonk A, et al: Resection of pulmonary metastases—results, prognostic factors, reappraisal of selection criteria. Thorac Cardiovasc Surg 34:140–142, 1986.

38. Van de Wal H, Verhagen A, Lecluyse A, et al: Surgery of pulmonary metastases. J Thorac Cardiovasc Surg 34:153–156, 1986.

39. Vogt-Moykopf I, Meyer G, Merkle NM, et al: Late results of surgical treatment of pulmonary metastases. Thorac Cardiovasc Surg 34:143–148, 1986.

40. Eckersberger F, Moritz E, Wolner E: Results and prognostic factors after resection of pulmonary metastases. Eur J Cardiothorac Surg 2:433–437, 1988.

41. McCormack P: Surgical resection of pulmonary metastases. Semin Surg Oncol 6:297–302, 1990.

42. Stewart JR, Carey JA, Merrill WH, et al: Twenty years' experience with pulmonary metastasectomy. Am Surg 58:100–103, 1992.

43. Dowling RD, Wachs ME, Ferson PF, Landreneau RJ: Thoracoscopic neodymium:yttrium aluminum garnet laser resection of a pulmonary metastasis. Cancer 70:1873–1875, 1992.

44. Urschel HC Jr, Razzuk MA: Median sternotomy as a standard approach for pulmonary resection. Ann Thorac Surg 41:130–134, 1986.

45. Putnam JB, Suell D, Roth JA: Extended resection of pulmonary metastases: Is the risk justified? Ann Thorac Surg 55:1440–1446, 1992.

46. McGovern EM, Trastek VF, Pairolero PC, Payne WS: Completion pneumonectomy: Indications, complications, and results. Ann Thorac Surg 46:141–146, 1988.

47. Ballantine TVN, Wiseman NE, Filler RM: Assessment of pulmonary wedge resection for the treatment of lung metastases. J Pediatr Surg 5:671–676, 1975.

48. Cooper JD, Perelman M, Todd TRJ, et al: Precision cautery excision of pulmonary lesions. J Pediatr Surg 41:51, 1986.

48a. Johnston MR: Median sternotomy for resection of pulmonary metastases. J Thorac Cardiovasc Surg 85:516, 1983.

49. Branscheid D, Krysa S, Wollkopf G, et al: Does ND-YAG laser extend the indications for resection of pulmonary metastases? Eur J Cardiothorac Surg 6:590–596, 1992.

50. Miyamoto H, Masaoka T, Hayakawa K, Hata E: Application of the Nd-YAG laser for surgical resection of pulmonary metastases. Kyobu Geka 45:56–59, 1992.

51. Kodama K, Doi O, Higashiyama M, et al: Surgical management of lung metastases. Usefulness of resection with the neodymium:yttrium-aluminum-garnet laser with median sternotomy. J Thorac Cardiovasc Surg 101:901–908, 1991.

52. Putnam JB Jr, Roth JA, Wesley MN, et al: Analysis of prognostic factors in patients undergoing resection of pulmonary metastases from soft tissue sarcomas. J Thorac Cardiovasc Surg 87:260–267, 1984.

53. Udelsman R, Roth JA, Lees D, et al: Endobronchial metastases from soft tissue sarcoma. J Surg Oncol 32:145–149, 1986.

54. Landreneau RJ, Herlan DB, Johnson JA, et al: Thorascopic neodymium:yttrium-aluminum-garnet laser-assisted pulmonary resection. Ann Thorac Surg 52:1176–1178, 1991.

55. Miller DL, Allen MS, Trastek VF, et al: Videothoracoscopic wedge excision of the lung. Ann Thorac Surg 54:410–413, 1992.

56. Landreneau RJ, Hazelrigg SR, Ferson PF, et al: Thoracoscopic resection of 85 pulmonary lesions. Ann Thorac Surg 54:415–419, 1992.

57. McCormack PM, Attiyeh FF: Resected pulmonary metastases from colorectal cancer. Dis Colon Rectum 22:553–556, 1979.

58. McAfee MK, Allen MS, Trastek VF, et al: Colorectal lung metastases: Results of surgical excision. Ann Thorac Surg 53:780–785, 1992.

59. Gorenstein LA, Putnam JB, Natarajan G, et al: Improved survival after resection of pulmonary metastases from malignant melanoma. Ann Thorac Surg 52:204–210, 1991.

60. Pastorino U, Valente M, Gasparini M, et al: Lung resection as salvage treatment for metastatic osteosarcoma. Tumori 74:201–206, 1988.

61. Roth JA, Putnam JB, Wesley MN, Rosenberg SA: Differing determinants of prognosis following resection of pulonary metastases from osteogenic and soft tissue sarcoma patients. Cancer 55:1361–1366, 1985.

62. Brister SJ, de Varennes B, Gordon PH, et al: Contemporary operative management of pulmonary metastases of colorectal origin. Dis Colon Rectum 31:786–792, 1988.

63. Jett JR, Hollinger CG, Zinsmeister AR, Pairolero PC: Pulmonary resection of metastatic renal cell carcinoma. Chest 84:442–445, 1983.

64. Lanza LA, Natarajan G, Roth JA, Putnam JB Jr: Long term survival following resection of pulmonary metastases from carcinoma of the breast. Ann Thorac Surg 54:244–248, 1992.

65. Putnam JB Jr, Roth JA, Wesley MN, et al: Survival following aggressive resection of pulmonary metastases from osteogenic sarcoma: Analysis of prognostic factors. Ann Thorac Surg 38:516–523, 1983.

66. Meyer WH, Schell MJ, Kumar AP, et al: Thoracotomy for pulmonary metastatic osteosarcoma. An analysis of prognostic indicators of survival. Cancer 59:374–379, 1987.

67. Jablons D, Steinberg SM, Roth J, et al: Metastasectomy for soft tissue sarcoma. Further evidence for efficacy and prognostic indicators. J Thorac Cardiovasc Surg 97:695–705, 1989.

68. Lanza LA, Miser JS, Pass HI, Roth JA: The role of resection in the treatment of pulmonary metastases from Ewing's sarcoma. J Thorac Cardiovasc Surg 94:181–187, 1987.

69. Pogrebniak HW, Roth JA, Steinberg SM, et al: Reoperative pulmonary resection in patients with metastatic soft tissue sarcoma. Ann Thorac Surg 52:197–203, 1991.

70. Joseph WL, Morton DL, Adkins PC: Prognostic significance of tumor doubling time in evaluating operability in pulmonary metastatic disease. J Thorac Cardiovasc Surg 61:23–32, 1971.

71. Collins VP, Loeffler RK, Tivey H: Observations on growth rates of human tumors. Am J Roentgenol 76:988–1000, 1956.

72. Marcove RC, Martini N, Rosen G: The treatment of pulmonary metastases in osteogenic sarcoma. Clin Orthop 111:65, 1975.

73. Giritsky AS, Etcubanas E, Mark JBD: Pulmonary resection in children with metastatic osteogenic sarcoma. J Thorac Cardiovasc Surg 75:354–362, 1978.

74. Skinner KA, Eilber FR, Holmes EC, et al: Surgical treatment and chemotherapy for pulmonary metastases from osteosarcoma. Arch Surg 127:1065–1070, 1992.

75. Carter SR, Grimer RJ, Sneath RS, Matthews HR: Results of thoracotomy in osteogenic sarcoma with pulmonary metastases. Thorax 46:727–731, 1991.

76. Snyder CL, Saltzman DA, Ferrell KL, et al: A new approach to the resection of pulmonary osteosarcoma metastases. Results of aggressive metastasectomy. Clin Orthop 247:253–253, 1991.

77. Belli L, Scholl S, Livartowski A, et al: Resection of pulmonary metastases in osteosarcoma. A retrospective analysis of 44 patients. Cancer 63:2546–2550, 1989.

78. Beattie EJ, Harvey JC, Marcove R, Martini N: Results of multiple pulmonary resections for metastatic osteogenic sarcoma after two decades. J Surg Oncol 46:154–155, 1991.

79. Potter DA, Glenn J, Kinsella T, et al: Patterns of recurrence in patients with high-grade soft-tissue sarcomas. J Clin Oncol 3:353–366, 1985.

80. Huth JF, Elber FR: Patterns of metastatic spread following resection of extremity soft-tissue sarcomas and strategies for treatment. Semin Surg Oncol 4:20, 1988.

81. Casson AG, Putnam JB, Natarajan G, et al: Five-year survival after pulmonary metastasectomy for adult soft tissue sarcoma. Cancer 69:662–668, 1992.

82. Staren ED, Salerno C, Rongione A, et al: Pulmonary resection for metastatic breast cancer. Arch Surg 127:1282–1284, 1992.

83. Mansel JK, Zinsmeister AR, Pairolero PC, Jett JR: Pulmonary resection of metastatic colorectal adenocarcinoma. A ten year experience. Chest 89:109–112, 1986.

84. Goya T, Miyazawa N, Kondo H, et al: Surgical resection of pulmonary metastases from colorectal cancer: 10-year follow-up. Cancer 64:1418–1421, 1989.

85. Sauter ER, Bolton JS, Willis GW, et al: Improved survival after pulmonary resection of metastatic colorectal carcinoma. J Surg Oncol 43:135–138, 1990.

86. Scheele J, Altendorf Hofmann A, Stangl R, Gall FP: Pulmonary resection for metastatic colon and upper rectum cancer. Is it useful? Dis Colon Rectum 33:745–752, 1990.

87. Mori M, Tomoda H, Ishida T, et al: Surgical resection of pulmonary metastases from colorectal adenocarcinoma. Special reference to repeated pulmonary resections. Arch Surg 126:1297–1301, 1991.

88. Katzenstein AL, Purvis RJ, Gmelich J, Askin F: Pulmonary resection for metastatic renal adenocarcinoma. Cancer 41:712–723, 1978.

89. Mayo P, Saha SP, McElvein RB: Long term survival after resection of multiple pulmonary metastases from adenocarcinoma of the kidney. South Med J 74:161, 1981.

90. Dernevik L, Berggren H, Larsson S, Roberts D: Surgical removal of pulmonary metastases from renal cell carcinoma. Scand J Urol Nephrol 19:133–137, 1985.

91. Pogrebniak HW, Haas G, Linehan WM, et al: Renal cell carcinoma: Resection of solitary and multiple metastases. Ann Thorac Surg 54:33–38, 1992.

92. Stahel RA, Van Hochstetter AR, Largiado R, et al: Surgical resection of residual tumor after chemotherapy in non-seminomatous testicular cancer. Eur J Cancer Clin Oncol 18:1259, 1982.

93. Whillis D, Coleman RE, Cornbleet MA, Blah: Failure of salvage treatment in metastatic testicular teratoma. Clin Oncol 3:141, 1991.

94. Fuller AF Jr, Scannell JG, Wilkins EW Jr: Pulmonary resection for metastases from gynecologic cancers: Massachusetts General Hospital experience, 1943–1982. Gynecol Oncol 22:174–180, 1985.

95. Levenback C, Rubin SC, McCormack PM, et al: Resection of pulmonary metastases from uterine sarcomas. Gynecol Oncol 45:202–205, 1992.

96. Seki M, Nakagawa K, Tsuchiya S, et al: Surgical treatment of pulmonary metastases from uterine cervical cancer. Operation method by lung tumor size. J Thorac Cardiovasc Surg 104:876–881, 1992.

97. Saitok K, Harada K, Nakayama H, et al: Role of thoracotomy in pulmonary metastases from gestational choriocarcinoma. J Thorac Cardiovasc Surg 85:815–820, 1983.

98. Sink JD, Hammond CB, Young WG Jr: Pulmonary resection in the management of metastases from gestational choriocarcinoma. J Thorac Cardiovasc Surg 81:830–834, 1981.

99. Rendina EA, de Vincentiis M, Primerano G, et al: Pulmonary resection for metastatic laryngeal carcinoma. J Thorac Cardiovasc Surg 92:114–117, 1986.

100. Mazer TM, Robbins KT, McMurtrey MJ, Byers RM: Resection of pulmonary metastases from squamous carcinoma of the head and neck. Am J Surg 156:238–242, 1988.

101. van Overhagen H, Lameris JS, Berger MY, et al: Improved assessment of supraclavicular and abdominal metastases in oesophageal and gastro-oesophageal junction carcinoma with the combination of ultrasound and computed tomography. Br J Radiol 66:203–208, 1993.

102. Fern LG, Gutterman J, Burgess MA, et al: The natural history of resectable metastatic melanoma (Stage IV A melanoma). Cancer 50:1656, 1982.

103. Mathisen DJ, Flye MW, Peabody J: The role of thoracotomy in the management of pulmonary metastases from malignant melanoma. Ann Thorac Surg 27:295–299, 1979.

104. Pogrebniak HW, Stovroff M, Roth JA, Pass HI: Resection of pulmonary metastases from malignant melanoma: Results of a 16-year experience. Ann Thorac Surg 46:20–23, 1988.

105. Wong JH, Euhus DM, Morton DL: Surgical resection for metastatic melanoma to the lung. Arch Surg 123:1091–1095, 1988.

106. Harpole DH Jr, Johnson CM, Wolfe WG, et al: Analysis of 945 cases of pulmonary metastatic melanoma. J Thorac Cardiovasc Surg 103:743–748, 1992.

107. Green DM, Breslow NE, Ii Y, et al: The role of surgical excision in the management of relapsed Wilms' tumor patients with pulmonary metastases: A report from the National Wilms' Tumor Study. J Pediatr Surg 26:728–733, 1991.

108. Feusner JH, Krailo MD, Haas JE, et al: Treatment of pulmonary metastases of initial Stage 1 hepatoblastoma in childhood. J Pediatr Surg 26:778, 1991.

109. Black CT, Luck SR, Musemeche CA, et al: Aggressive excision of pulmonary metastases is warranted in the management of childhood hepatic tumor. J Pediatr Surg 26:1082, 1991.

110. Rizzoni WE, Pass HI, Wesley MN, et al: Resection of recurrent pulmonary metastases in patients with soft-tissue sarcomas. Arch Surg 121:1248–1252, 1986.

111. Casson AG, Putnam JB, Natarajan G, et al: Efficacy of pulmonary metastasectomy for recurrent soft tissue sarcoma. J Surg Oncol 47:1–4, 1991.

Index

Note: Page numbers in *italics* refer to illustrations; page numbers followed by (t) refer to tables.

ISBN 0-7216-4769-3

90038

9 780721 647692